ORTHODONTICS
Current Principles and Techniques

THOMAS M. GRABER, D.D.S., M.S.D., Ph.D., Odont. Dr., D.S.C.

Director, G.V. Black Institute for Continuing Education and Kenilworth Dental Research Foundation;
Former Professor and Chairman, Section of Orthodontics, University of Chicago, Chicago, Illinois;
Editor-in-Chief, *American Journal of Orthodontics and Dentofacial Orthopedics;*
Visiting Professor, Department of Orthodontics, University of Michigan, Ann Arbor;
Recipient, Albert H. Ketcham Award; Private Practice, Evanston, Illinois

ROBERT L. VANARSDALL, Jr., D.D.S.

Professor and Chairman, Department of Orthodontics,
School of Dental Medicine, University of Pennsylvania;
Staff, Children's Hospital of Philadelphia; Albert Einstein Medical Center, and the Medical College of
    Pennsylvania;
Co-editor, *Journal of Adult Orthodontics and Orthognathic Surgery;*
Private Practice, Philadelphia, Pennsylvania

SECOND EDITION

with 2744 illustrations

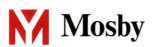 **Mosby**

St. Louis Baltimore Boston Chicago London Madrid Philadelphia Sydney Toronto

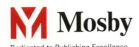

Mosby

Dedicated to Publishing Excellence

Publisher: George Stamathis
Editor: Linda L. Duncan
Developmental Editor: Jo Salway
Project Manager: Patricia Tannian
Production Editor: Barbara Jeanne Wilson
Senior Designer: Gail Morey Hudson
Manufacturing Supervisor: Karen Lewis

SECOND EDITION

Printed in the United States of America
Composition by Graphic World, Inc.
Printing/binding by Walsworth Publishing Co.

Mosby–Year Book, Inc.,
11830 Westline Industrial Drive,
St. Louis, Missouri 63146

Library of Congress Cataloging in Publication Data

Orthodontics : current principles and techniques / [edited by] Thomas M. Graber, Robert L. Vanarsdall.—2nd ed.
  p. cm.
 "Fourth version"—Pref.
 First two editions published by W.B. Saunders; subsequent editions renumbered by Mosby.
 Includes bibliographical references and index.
 ISBN 0-8016-6590-6
 1. Orthodontics. I. Graber, T. M. (Thomas M.), 1917-
II. Vanarsdall, Robert L.
 [DNLM: 1. Orthodontics. WU 400 0776 1994]
RK521.G673 1994
617.6′43—dc20
DNLM/DLC   93-42589
for Library of Congress   CIP

94 95 96 97 98 / 9 8 7 6 5 4 3 2 1

ORTHODONTICS

Current Principles and Techniques

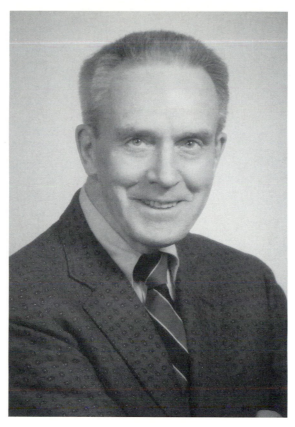

Dr. Brainerd F. Swain

The authors who have contributed to this book are sharing knowledge that they have accumulated from many years of study, research, and practice. These practitioners differ in background and technique, but they have a common commitment in seeking to improve orthodontic treatment. One who has served as an inspiration to us all by personal example of a lifetime dedicated to the highest standards of orthodontics is Dr. Brainerd F. Swain. Always in search of new information and eager to share it, Dr. Swain has remained both student and teacher throughout his professional life; a legacy of his lifetime achievements has been set down in the previous editions of this text, which he coauthored.

Dr. Swain is revered as the great gentleman of our specialty. His participation, along with his gracious manner and ethical values, elevates the quality of every meeting he attends. His wonderful personality and willingness to do more than his share benefit his patients and friends, as well as assorted organizations, societies, and universities. It was a proud moment for orthodontics when Dr. Swain received the Ketcham Award. His professional accomplishments and creative contributions are astonishing in number, but the chief reason for the enormous respect and love we have for Barney is his unique, warm, and honorable character.

We take special pride in dedicating this book to you, Barney.
We thank you for your cherished friendship and for your passion for orthodontics!

The Authors

CONTRIBUTORS

James L. Ackerman, D.D.S.

Clinical Professor, Department of Periodontology,
School of Dentistry, Temple University,
Philadelphia, Pennsylvania

Charles J. Burstone, D.D.S., M.S.

Professor, Department of Pediatric Dentistry
and Orthodontics,
School of Dental Medicine,
The University of Connecticut Health Center,
Farmington, Connecticut

Jack G. Dale, B.A., D.D.S., Postdoctoral Fellowship in Orthodontics (Harvard)

Associate Professor, Faculty of Dentistry,
University of Toronto;
President and Co-Founder, Harvard Society
for the Advancement of Orthodontics;
Co-Chairman of the Board, The Charles H.
Tweed International Foundation for
Orthodontic Research;
Past President, American Board of Orthodontics;
Private Practice, Toronto, Ontario, Canada

Thomas M. Graber, D.M.D., M.S.D., Ph.D., Odont. Dr., D.S.C.

Director, G.V. Black Institute for Continuing
Education and Kenilworth Dental Research Foundation;
Former Professor and Chairman, Section of Orthodontics,
University of Chicago, Chicago, Illinois;
Editor-in-Chief, *American Journal of Orthodontics
and Dentofacial Orthopedics;*
Visiting Professor, Department of Orthodontics,
University of Michigan, Ann Arbor;
Recipient, Albert H. Ketcham Award;
Private Practice, Evanston, Illinois;

Donald R. Joondeph, D.D.S., M.S.

Associate Professor and former Chairman,
Department of Orthodontics,
University of Washington,
Seattle, Washington

Herbert A. Klontz, D.D.S.

Associate Professor,
Department of Orthodontics,
University of Oklahoma,
Oklahoma City, Oklahoma

James A. McNamara, Jr., D.D.S., Ph.D.

Professor of Dentistry,
Department of Orthodontics and Pediatric Dentistry,
School of Dentistry;
Professor of Anatomy and Cell Biology,
School of Medicine;
Research Scientist, Center for Human Growth
and Development,
University of Michigan,
Ann Arbor, Michigan

David R. Musich, D.D.S., M.S.

Clinical Professor,
Department of Orthodontics,
University of Pennsylvania,
Philadelphia, Pennsylvania

William R. Profitt, D.D.S., Ph.D.

Kenan Professor and Chairman,
Department of Orthodontics,
School of Dentistry,
University of North Carolina,
Chapel Hill, North Carolina

Kaare Reitan, D.D.S., M.S.D., Ph.D.

Formerly, Research Fellow,
Institute of Experimental Research;
Lecturer in Applied Histology,
Department of Graduate Orthodontics,
University of Oslo, Oslo, Norway;
Recipient, Albert H. Ketcham Award

Richard A. Riedel, D.D.S., M.S.D.

Professor Emeritus,
Department of Orthodontics,
School of Dentistry,
University of Washington,
Seattle, Washington;
Recipient, Albert H. Ketcham Award

W. Eugene Roberts, D.D.S., Ph.D.

Professor and Chairman,
Department of Orthodontics,
Indiana University,
Indianapolis, Indiana

Ronald H. Roth, D.D.S., M.S.

Clinical Professor of Orthodontics,
Department of Growth and Development,
Division of Orthodontics,
University of California, San Francisco,
San Francisco, California;
Clinical Professor of Orthodontics,
Department of Orthodontics,
University of Detroit/Mercy,
Detroit, Michigan

Per Rygh, D.D.S., Ph.D.

Professor and Chairman,
Department of Orthodontics and Facial
Orthopedics,
University of Bergen,
Bergen, Norway

Paul W. Stöckli, Dr. Med. Dent., M.S.

Professor and Chairman,
Department of Dentofacial Orthopedics
and Pedodontics,
Dental School,
University of Zürich,
Zürich, Switzerland

Ullrich M. Teuscher, PD Dr. Med.

Senior Lecturer,
Department of Dentofacial Orthopedics
and Pedodontics,
Dental School,
University of Zürich,
Zürich, Switzerland

James L. Vaden, D.D.S., M.S.

Associate Professor,
Department of Orthodontics,
University of Tennessee,
Memphis, Tennessee;
Adjunct Professor, University of Michigan;
Private Practice,
Cookeville, Tennessee

Robert L. Vanarsdall, Jr., D.D.S.

Professor and Chairman,
Department of Orthodontics,
School of Dental Medicine,
University of Pennsylvania;
Staff, Children's Hospital of Philadelphia,
Albert Einstein Medical Center, and the Medical College of
Pennsylvania;
Co-editor, *Journal of Adult Orthodontics and
Orthognathnic Surgery;*
Private Practice, Philadelphia, Pennsylvania

Richard P. Walker, D.D.S., M.S.C.

Associate in Dentistry,
Department of Orthodontics,
Faculty of Dentistry,
University of Toronto, Ontario, Canada;
Private Practice, Toronto, Ontario, Canada

Bjorn U. Zachrisson, D.D.S., M.S.D., Ph.D.

Professor II,
Department of Orthodontics,
Faculty of Dentistry,
University of Oslo,
Oslo, Norway

PREFACE

This is actually the fourth version of our graduate text. Starting in 1969 the first two texts were published by W.B. Saunders. The next version by Graber and Swain was published by Mosby–Year Book. The new team of Graber and Vanarsdall has intensively analyzed the biological and technical developments in orthodontics and associated fields and has incorporated many of them with the time-tested concepts and methodologies of our previous volumes.

The success of the earlier versions has been beyond expectations, and we have built on this success, using questionnaires to orthodontists, teachers, and clinicians. No book can completely cover all aspects of a discipline, but with the feedback we have received and with the efforts of our outstanding contributors, we feel that we have achieved an excellent overview.

Of the 16 chapters, three are by new authors on new subjects: bone physiology and metabolism, by Roberts; computers in orthodontics, by Walker; and early treatment, by McNamara. The Tweed-Merrifield edgewise chapter is written by three new authors: Vaden, Dale, and Klontz.

Other chapters have been revised to incorporate advances in *materia technica* and treatment. The increased emphasis on periodontal considerations is evident in the special Vanarsdall chapter and the chapter on adult orthodontics by Vanarsdall and Musich. Orthodontic aspects of orthognathic surgery is state of the art.

The result is a compendium of orthodontic knowledge and clinical techniques that is unique and practical.

CHAPTER ONE

Diagnosis and Treatment Planning in Orthodontics, by William R. Proffit and James L. Ackerman, is an in-depth analysis of the multifaceted aspects of diagnosis and treatment implications. Whereas there is more than one mechanical *road to Rome,* the critical basis of all therapeutic measures is a proper synthesis of information gleaned from essential diagnostic criteria.

CHAPTER TWO

Biomechanical Principles and Reactions, by the world's leading authorities Kaare Reitan and Per Rygh, has been updated by continuing research and remains the most complete and current contribution on tissue changes in any orthodontic textbook. Recent litigious experience by orthodontists emphasizes the need for more attention to both favorable and unfavorable tissue reactions from more efficient appliances. The latest electron microscope research has po-

tent clinical implications on the amount, type, duration, and direction of force, which is even more important with the increasing numbers of adult orthodontic patients.

CHAPTER THREE

Bone Physiology, Metabolism, and Biomechanics in Orthodontic Practice, by W. Eugene Roberts, is at the cutting edge of orthodontic research. Together with the Reitan-Rygh chapter on tissue change, it provides the most current and comprehensive information available for student, researcher, and clinician. Expediting treatment objectives by manipulation of biochemical factors of the dentoalveolar environment is now a reality—the result of outstanding research by Dr. Roberts and his colleagues.

CHAPTER FOUR

Application of Bioengineering to Clinical Orthodontics, by Charles Burstone, remains the preeminent source of information on biomechanics and physical science principles. Carefully coordinated with all the other chapters, this chapter is the culmination of the rapid advances in *materia technica* in the past 10 years. Like the previous three chapters, Chapter Four is the common denominator for all subsequent sections of the book.

CHAPTER FIVE

Computer Applications in Orthodontics, by Richard Walker—a developer, innovator, and leader in computer science—augments the traditional diagnostic criteria, enhancing their three-dimensionality and interrelationships. This chapter provides guidance to students, researchers, and clinicians for use of an essential diagnostic tool.

CHAPTER SIX

Interceptive Guidance of Occlusion with Emphasis on Diagnosis, by Jack Dale, completes the diagnosis and treatment section, melding developmental diagnostic and biomechanical principles to provide a rationale for interceptive procedures, where there are arch deficiency considerations. The best possible biologic guidance and the adjustive phenomena for the growing child are elucidated by outstanding and profuse illustrations. This chapter is the bridge to Section II and to its first chapter on functional appliance therapy.

CHAPTER SEVEN

Functional Appliances, by Thomas M. Graber, ties in with the philosophy propounded by Teuscher and Stöckli in Chapter Eight as well as that of McNamara in Chapter Nine on mixed dentition. Functional orthopedic principles are delineated historically, as well as developmentally. A new section on the use of rare earth magnets enhances dentofacial orthopedic potential. The pitfalls of this approach, functional orthopedics, are described for an increasingly used and abused technique.

CHAPTER EIGHT

Combined Activator Headgear Orthopedics, by Ullrich M. Teuscher and Paul Stöckli, is a logical continuation of the previous chapter. Principles and causal therapy in Class II malocclusion are applied via fixed and functional adjuncts. The clinical implications and applications are significant.

CHAPTER NINE

Mixed Dentition Treatment, by James McNamara, Jr., is a new and needed discussion of the expanding role of transitional dentition therapy in modern orthodontic practice. Beautifully organized and presented with multiple, magnificent drawings by Bill Brudon, this chapter is even more meaningful to the teacher and clinician alike.

CHAPTER TEN

Bonding in Orthodontics, by Bjorn U. Zachrisson (another world-class leader), has been extensively updated to reflect the latest advances in a rapidly advancing field. It remains the ultimate source for state-of-the-art information and application of bonding techniques.

CHAPTER ELEVEN

The Tweed-Merrifield Edgewise Appliance, by Jim Vaden, Jack Dale, and Herbert Klontz, is a new chapter by three outstanding and experienced clinicians. The principles and techniques that have withstood the test of time, that have been exhaustively tested, with thousands of patients, and that have been modified by the latest and best armamentaria are magnificently illustrated and make this chapter the most current and complete presentation on this appliance technique that exists today. Knowledge acquired from Chapter Eleven serves as the basis for all subsequent chapters.

CHAPTER TWELVE

Treatment Mechanics for the Straight Wire Appliance, by Ronald H. Roth, continues the development of this widely used appliance by its most eminent and experienced teacher. The chapter is the result of years of experience, clinical research, and appliance modification by the author.

CHAPTER THIRTEEN

Periodontal/Orthodontic Interrelationships, by Robert L. Vanarsdall, is unique in the literature. Double specialty training and experience by the author provide unparalleled exposition of the subject in an area becoming more subject to litigious actions.

CHAPTER FOURTEEN

Adult Orthodontics: Diagnosis and Treatment, by Robert L. Vanarsdall and David R. Musich, is a classic example of the best possible teamwork on this important and expanding part of orthodontic practice by eminent teachers, authors, and clinicians. The special diagnostic and therapeutic demands are described in a comprehensive manner.

CHAPTER FIFTEEN

Orthodontic Aspects of Orthognathic Surgery, by David Musich, highlights the teamwork necessary in correcting skeletal malocclusions. This chapter, by one of the country's leading and experienced clinicians and teachers, is a frank presentation of the potential therapeutic goals, together with a discussion of problems that may occur along the way.

CHAPTER SIXTEEN

Retention and Relapse, by Donald R. Joondeph and Richard A. Riedel, discusses one of the most important aspects of orthodontic treatment, regardless of the means of achieving the results. Despite the rapid development of therapeutic armamentaria, the major challenge of retaining the greatest amount of correction remains. Detailed guidance on this subject is given, optimizing the results attained with the greatest possible stability.

The editors and authors sincerely hope that this combined effort will help students and practitioners alike to serve their patients better. Gratitude is expressed to all who made this prodigious effort possible.

Editors

Thomas M. Graber
Robert L. Vanarsdall

CONTENTS

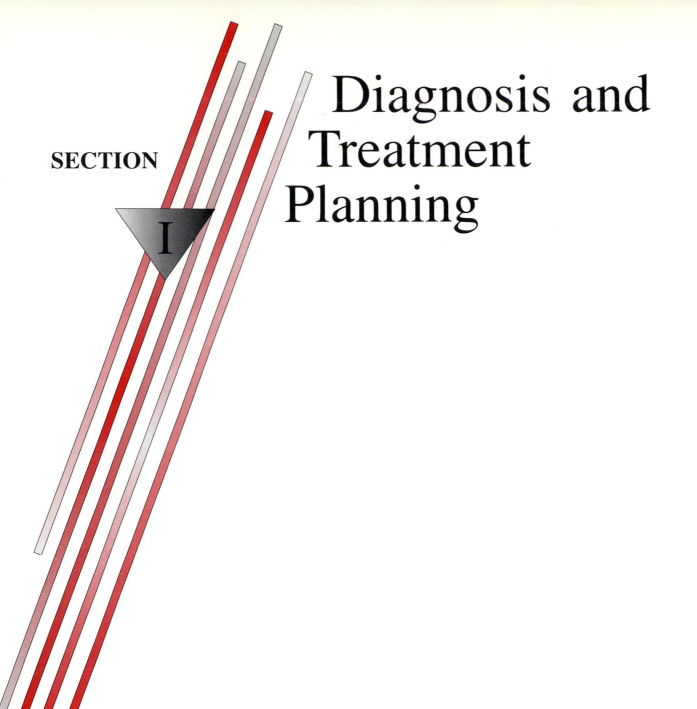

SECTION

I

Diagnosis and Treatment Planning

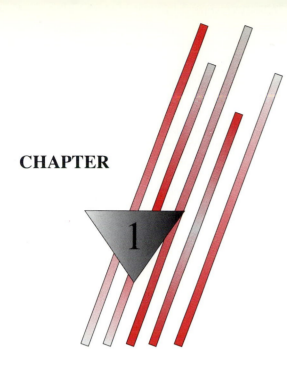

CHAPTER

1

Diagnosis and Treatment Planning in Orthodontics

WILLIAM R. PROFFIT
JAMES L. ACKERMAN

"Diagnosis in orthodontics requires the synthesis of manifold factors into a discrete list of problems each defined so clearly that the treatment alternatives become evident."

THE DIAGNOSTIC AND TREATMENT PLANNING PROCESS IN ORTHODONTICS

In a general sense the goal of orthodontic treatment is to improve the patient's life adjustment by enhancing dental and jaw function and dentofacial esthetics. From this perspective the role of orthodontics is analogous to several other medical specialties, such as orthopedics and plastic surgery, in which the patient's problems often are not due to disease but rather result from distortions of development. As the paradigm of health care has evolved from a disease-oriented focus to a wellness model,[94] orthodontics now is viewed more clearly as a health service related to establishing and maintaining physical and emotional fitness. Malocclusion of the teeth is not a disease; it is a disability with potential impact on physical and mental health, and appropriate treatment is important for the patient's well-being.

More specifically, the goal of orthodontics is to obtain optimal proximal and occlusal contact of the teeth (occlusion) within the framework of normal function and physiologic adaptation, acceptable dentofacial esthetics and self-image, and reasonable stability. Because of the enormous variation in dental and facial relationships and the large number of available treatment options, the decision-making process in orthodontics can be challenging, even to the experienced orthodontist. It usually is disconcerting to the neophyte to learn that often more than one treatment plan will successfully resolve an orthodontic problem. It is perhaps even more unsettling to realize that there may not necessarily be a single, best treatment strategy for a specific problem. The fact that equally tenable treatment alternatives may exist does not mean that the treatment planning process can be taken lightly—just the reverse is true. After the patient's problems have been identified and placed in priority order (which constitutes diagnosis), the treatment plan must consist of a series of logical steps that will produce maximum benefit to the patient.

Orthodontic diagnosis has changed somewhat in the last several years. Diagnosis now includes a greater emphasis on the functional and psychosocial ramifications of dentofacial deformity. At the same time a more dramatic change has occurred in treatment planning, which has become a more interactive process between the patient and/or parents and the orthodontist. This shift has taken place because of a change in the ethical view of the doctor-patient relationship. Previously, the orthodontist decided on the most ideal treatment plan for the patient, and the patient (or parent) either accepted or rejected the plan, with little room for considering alternatives. Today the orthodontist is expected to outline the patient's problems, use input from the patient to establish priorities in dealing with the problems, present reasonable treatment alternatives, and explain the risk-benefit considerations of each alternative, including the option of no treatment. Then the patient, considering the orthodontist's recommendations, elects the plan that best suits his or her needs. The decision-making paradigm has shifted from the doctor as the decision maker toward the patient as the co-decision maker.

The orthodontist's dilemma now is how to adhere to the obligation set forth in the American Association of Orthodontists Code of Ethics to "perform the highest quality orthodontic services within his/her power to perform," while at the same time respecting the patients' right to decide the treatment best suited to their needs. Conflict may arise concerning what the patient wants and what the doctor thinks the patient ought to have. As part of self-determination, individuals should be responsible for determining what is or what is not done. The American Dental Association (ADA) Principles of Ethics has been modified recently to state, "The dentist's primary professional obligation shall be service to the public. The competent and timely delivery of quality care within the bounds of the clinical circumstances presented by the patient, with due consideration being given to the needs and desires of the patient, shall be the important aspect of that obligation." This contrasts with the earlier ADA Code of Ethics, which stated, "The dentist's primary duty of serving the public is discharged by giving the highest type of service of which he is capable. . . ." The major issue is whether the doctor or the patient decides if treatment will be done and what the nature of that treatment will be.

This conflict is between paternalism and autonomy. Paternalism describes actions taken by one person in the presumed best interest of another person, without that person's consent. Autonomy demands that the individual consent to any action taken on his or her behalf and reflects a belief in the merit of individual self-determination. The natural tendency is toward paternalism in the doctor-patient relationship, which comes into focus with respect to the information that is provided to the patient. The doctor who fails to disclose certain facts to the patient is acting paternalistically because the patient cannot choose rationally if he or she is not fully informed.

Patient autonomy has become more than a moral doctrine. It is now a legal requirement and is the philosophical and ethical basis for the doctrine of informed consent. At the end of this chapter we discuss in some detail informed consent in orthodontics and its role in minimizing allegations of negligence on the part of the orthodontist. To obtain informed consent, the proper presentation of a treatment plan is a necessary part of risk management in orthodontic practice.

ORTHODONTIC PROBLEMS AND TREATMENT POSSIBILITIES

In diagnosis and treatment planning, the orthodontist must:

1. Recognize the various characteristics of malocclusion and dentofacial deformity
2. Define the nature of the problem, including the etiology if this is possible
3. Design a treatment strategy based on the specific needs and desires of the individual

The goal of the diagnostic process is to produce a comprehensive but concise list of the patient's problems and to synthesize the various treatment possibilities into a rational

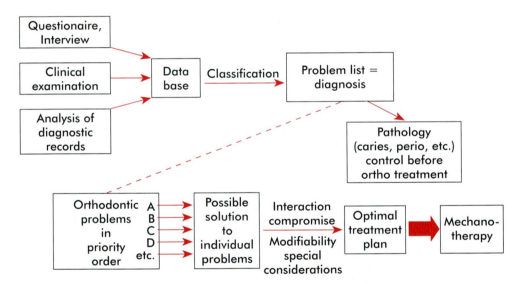

Fig. 1-1 This flow chart illustrates the sequence of problem-oriented diagnosis and treatment planning. Diagnosis requires the acquisition of adequate data, organized into a data base with three components, from which a problem list is abstracted. The problem list is the diagnosis.

Treatment planning begins with the separation of pathologic and structural (developmental) problems. Pathologic problems (periodontal disease, for example) must be treated first and brought under control before treatment of structural problems can proceed. The first step in the plan for orthodontic treatment is to put the structural problems in priority order. Then the possible solutions to these problems are considered as if each problem were the only one the patient had, and the interactions among the possible solutions and cost-risk/benefit ratios are considered in synthesizing the possibilities into a plan designed to maximize benefit to the patient.

This method of separating the problems, while considering possible solutions and then synthesizing the possibilities, merely formalizes the thought processes used by many experienced orthodontists. The advantages of this method are that the patient's problems are considered broadly and that the plan is developed in a way that is quite compatible with obtaining informed consent to treatment.

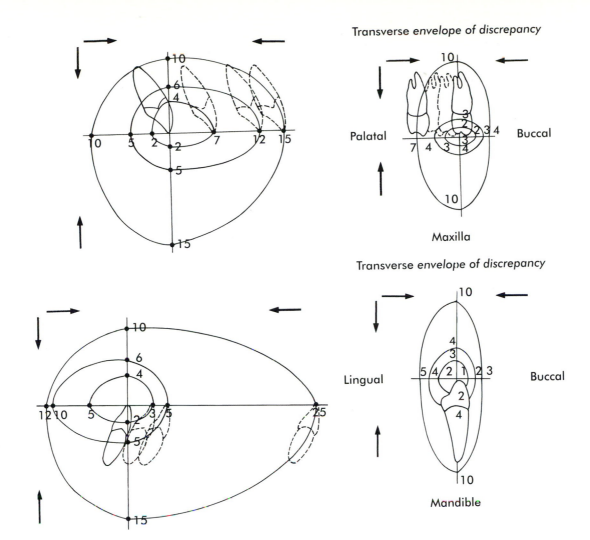

Fig. 1-2 The *envelope of discrepancy* for the maxillary and mandibular arches in three planes of space. The ideal position of the upper and lower incisor in the anteroposterior and vertical planes is shown in the center of the incisor diagrams. The millimeters of change to retract a protruding incisor, to move forward an incisor that is posteriorly positioned, or to extrude or intrude an incisor that is not correctly positioned vertically are shown along the horizontal and vertical axes respectively. The limits of orthodontic tooth movement alone are represented by the inner envelope; possible changes in incisor position from combined orthopedic and orthodontic treatment in growing individuals are shown by the middle envelope; and the limits of change with combined orthodontic and surgical treatment are shown by the outer envelope.

For example, the inner envelope for the upper arch suggests that maxillary incisors can be brought back a maximum of 7 mm by orthodontic tooth movement alone to correct protrusion but can be moved forward only 2 mm. The limit for retraction is established by the lingual cortical plate and is observed in the short term; the limit for forward movement is established by the lip and is observed in long-term stability or relapse. Upper incisors can be extruded 4 mm and depressed 2 mm, with the limits being observed in long-term stability rather than as limits on initial tooth movement.

Observe that the envelopes of discrepancy for the transverse dimension in the premolar areas are much smaller than incisors in the A-P plane of space. The transverse dimension can be critical to long-term stability, periodontal health, and frontal dentofacial esthetics (see Chapter 13).

The orthodontic and surgical envelopes can be viewed separately for the upper and lower arches, but the growth modification envelope is the same for both: 5 mm of growth modification in the A-P plane of space to correct Class II malocclusion is the maximum that should be anticipated, whether occlusion is achieved by acceleration of mandibular growth or restriction of maxillary growth. The outer envelope suggests that 10 mm is the limit for surgical maxillary advancement and intrusion although the maxilla can be retracted or brought downward a maximum of 15 mm; the mandible can be surgically set back 25 mm but can be advanced only 12.

These numbers, of course, are guidelines and may underestimate or overestimate the possibilities for any given patient; however, they serve to place the potential of the three major treatment modalities in perspective.

plan that maximizes benefit to the patient. The problem list should lead logically to the treatment plan. Fundamental to this process is an adequate collection of relevant information: the data base. The data base is organized into three major categories of descriptive elements: general evaluative, functional, and structural. Then a problem list is derived from the data base and set in order of priority according to the individual patient's needs and desires. Treatment possibilities are examined and formulated into the optimal approach for this particular patient; then the treatment plan is presented so that informed consent can be obtained. This separation-synthesis approach is outlined in Fig. 1-1. It is the basis of organization for the diagnostic and treatment planning approach we recommend and for the remainder of this chapter.

Although the specific type of treatment should not be considered until complete diagnostic information has been evaluated, it is helpful in the beginning to consider how orthodontic treatment can be accomplished. The four basic treatment modalities that the orthodontist can use (either separately or in combination) are:

1. Repositioning the teeth through orthodontic tooth movement (The biology of tooth movement is described in Chapters 2 and 3.)
2. Redirection of facial growth through functional alteration or the use of strong modifying forces (This concept is explained in greater detail in Chapter 7.)
3. Dentofacial orthopedics in which dentofacial growth is altered through the use of strong modifying forces (Chapters 7 and 8 describe orthodontic appliances that are commonly used in conjunction with orthopedic forces.)
4. Surgical-orthodontic treatment (Chapter 15) (The recent text by Proffit and White[118] offers a thorough discussion of the surgical correction of dentofacial deformity.)

The treatment modality (or combination of modalities) that is best for an individual patient is determined by the nature and severity of the orthodontic problem. This can be visualized by considering an *envelope of discrepancy* based on the degree of disparity in occlusal relationships (Fig. 1-2). For any characteristic of malocclusion there are three ranges of correction: (1) a range of correction that can be accomplished by orthodontic tooth movement alone; (2) a larger range of correction that can be achieved by tooth movement plus functional or orthopedic treatment; and (3) a still larger range of correction that requires surgery as part of the treatment plan. This *envelope of discrepancy* is not symmetric. In general the greater discrepancy can be corrected better by orthodontic and orthodontic-functional treatment in the sagittal (A-P) than in the vertical or transverse planes of space. The orthodontist has greater latitude for correcting maxillary protrusion than mandibular protrusion because of the anatomic and physiologic constraints that are present. The oral cavity can be thought of as a closed container. Orthodontics alone rearranges the contents of the container; orthopedic-functional treatment and sur-

gical treatment change the container's shape. Timing of treatment also is a factor. The orthodontic range is about the same in children as it is in adults. The same can be said of the possible amount of surgical correction; however, the orthopedic-functional range diminishes steadily as a child matures, and it disappears after the adolescent growth spurt.

NORMAL OCCLUSION VS MALOCCLUSION
Characteristics of Ideal Occlusion

What we call ideal occlusion today was described as early as the eighteenth century by the famous anatomist John Hunter. Carabelli (in the midnineteenth century) was probably the first to describe abnormal relationships of the upper and lower dental arches in a systematic way. The terms *edge-to-edge bite* and *overbite* are derived from Carabelli's system of classification. The term *orthodontics* was coined by Lefoulon of France at approximately the same time as interest in correcting malocclusion became widespread.[160] Even though several treatises on orthodontics had already been written by the beginning of the twentieth century (most notably, the treatise by Kingsley[72]) these authors had no acceptable method for describing irregularities and abnormal relationships of the teeth and jaws.

The ideal arrangement of the teeth can be defined clearly and described geometrically. Angle's *line of occlusion* (Fig. 1-3) continues to serve this purpose well. It shows that the

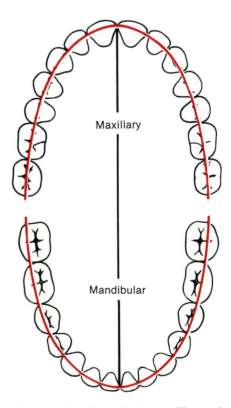

Fig. 1-3 The line of occlusion for the maxillary and mandibular arches passes through the central fossae and along the cingulae of maxillary teeth, and through the buccal cusps and incisal edges of mandibular teeth.

buccal cusps and incisal edges of the mandibular teeth should be concordant with the central fossae and cingulae of the maxillary teeth when the teeth are normally occluded.[9] The line of occlusion is a smooth, continuous, symmetric curve. From the first molar forward, it is best described as a catenary curve (the curve formed when a chain or rope is hung by both ends). Brader[16] demonstrated that the total arch form is better fitted by a *tri-focal ellipse:* a curve that is mathematically complex but easily constructed geometrically. The preformed arch wires now offered to orthodontists either follow the catenary form or, alternatively, follow an adaptation of the Brader arch form.

Each tooth's position spatially within the arch can be described in relation to the line of occlusion. Angle termed the tooth movements necessary to bring a tooth to the line of occlusion first, second, and third order, according to the type of movement required. A horizontal change relative to the line of occlusion represents a first order movement, a vertical change represents a second order movement, and a torsional change (with the line of occlusion serving as the axis) represents a third order movement.

The original definitions have been changed somewhat as more positioning has been built into orthodontic brackets. It has become accepted to refer to first order positioning as *in-out,* second order positioning as *tip* or *angulation,* and third order positioning as *torque* or *inclination.* In addition, *offset* and *cusp height positioning* now are recognized as being important. These terms can be defined as follows:

1. *In-out.* Faciolingual relationships of the tooth crowns to the line of occlusion (Thus the labial surface of the crown can be facially or lingually placed.)

2. *Tip.* Relative mesial or distal angulation of the crown and the root along the line of occlusion (e.g., mesial crown tip, same as distal root tip; distal crown tip, same as mesial root tip)

3. *Torque.* Relative crown and root inclination perpendicular to the line of occlusion (e.g., lingual crown torque, same as labial or buccal root torque; labial or buccal crown torque, same as lingual root torque)

4. *Offset.* Rotations, described by the position of mesial and distal proximal tooth contacts in relation to the line of occlusion (e.g., mesiolingual rotation, same as distofacial rotation; mesiofacial rotation, same as distolingual rotation)

5. *Cusp height positioning.* Described on the basis of the position of the occlusal surfaces incisogingivally in relation to the occlusal plane (The possibilities are infra-occlusion and supra-occlusion, which serve to establish cusp heights in excursive functions, and not so much to describe the relationships in static occlusion.)

Since each of these parameters of tooth position is related to the imaginary ideal, it is necessary to define what the ideal positions are. To do this, it is helpful to use the technique of orthogonal projection, which enables the three-dimensional dentition to be graphically represented as three separate two-dimensional views that allow plane geometric description. When orthogonal projection is applied to the skull and dentition, the planes of projection are the occlusal, sagittal, and transverse (coronal) (Fig. 1-4).

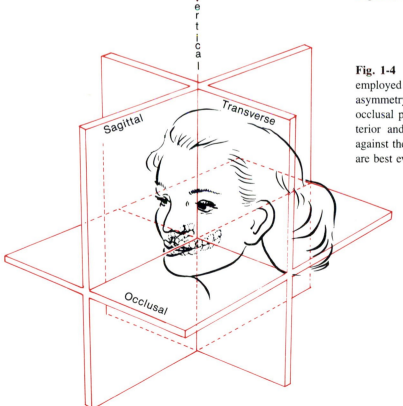

Fig. 1-4 Perspective view of the planes of reference normally employed for orthodontic examination. The alignment of teeth and asymmetry of dental arches are best seen in projection against the occlusal plane; profile and facial esthetics along with anteroposterior and vertical relationships are best studied in projection against the sagittal plane; and transverse dentofacial relationships are best evaluated in projection against the transverse plane.

Andrews[8] described six keys to normal occlusion: (1) molar relationship; (2) crown angulation (tip); (3) crown inclination (torque); (4) absence of rotations; (5) tight contacts; and (6) a flat occlusal plane or slight curve of Spee. These characteristics can be visualized in orthogonal projection, viewing the dentition from the occlusal, sagittal, and transverse projections.

Occlusal Projection

In the occlusal view the important relationships can be enumerated as follows:

1. Tight proximal tooth contacts, with no interdental spacing
2. No rotations (except for the maxillary molars)
3. Marginal ridges that are level

In this view the 10 degree distolingual offset of the maxillary first and second molars can be visualized (Fig. 1-5). This rotation is important in establishing the correct anteroposterior position of the buccal cusps of the maxillary molars in relation to their respective mandibular landmarks.

Sagittal Projection

In the sagittal view the important considerations are:

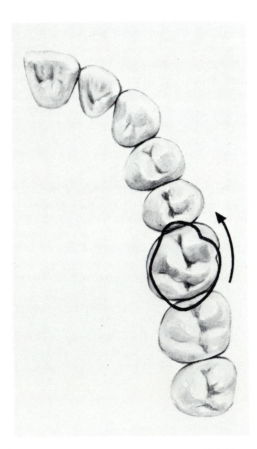

Fig. 1-5   Rotated teeth occupy more space within the arch, affecting occlusal relationships. Correction of mesiolingual rotation of the upper first molars is particularly important in establishing correct occlusion. (From Andrews LF: *Am J Orthod* 62:296, 1972.)

1. *Molar relationship.* The distal surface of the distobuccal cusp of the maxillary first permanent molar should make contact and occlude with the mesial surface of the mesiobuccal cusp of the lower second molar. The mesiobuccal cusp of the maxillary first permanent molar should fall within the groove between the mesial and middle cusps of the lower first permanent molar[147] (Fig. 1-6).

2. *Posterior crown angulation.* In the sagittal projection the facial surfaces of the crowns of all the posterior teeth distal to and including the canines can be visualized. The gingival portion of the long axis of each crown should be distal to the incisal portion. The amount of angulation of the posterior teeth can be described by relating the long axis of each tooth crown to a true vertical line constructed perpendicular to the occlusal plane (Fig. 1-7).

3. *Incisor crown inclination (torque).* In this projection the incisors (centrals and laterals) are seen in labiolingual view, showing their inclination or torque. Upper and lower incisor inclination should be sufficient to resist overeruption of the incisors, and to allow proper distal positioning of the contact points of the upper teeth in their relations to the lower teeth, permitting proper occlusion.

   The inclination of the incisor teeth when projected in the sagittal plane can be described by relating a line tangent to the facial contour of the tooth crown to a true vertical line constructed perpendicular to the occlusal plane (Fig. 1-8).

4. *Occlusal plane.* The plane of occlusion should vary from generally flat to a slight curve of Spee (Fig. 1-9).

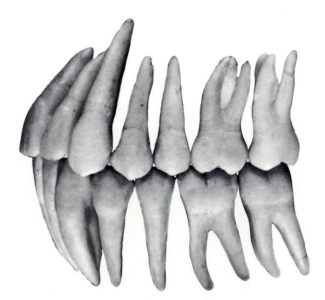

Fig. 1-6   The *ideal* occlusion (buccal view). (From Kraus BS, Jordan RE, Abrams L: *Dental anatomy and occlusion: a study of the masticatory system*, Baltimore, 1969, Williams & Wilkins.)

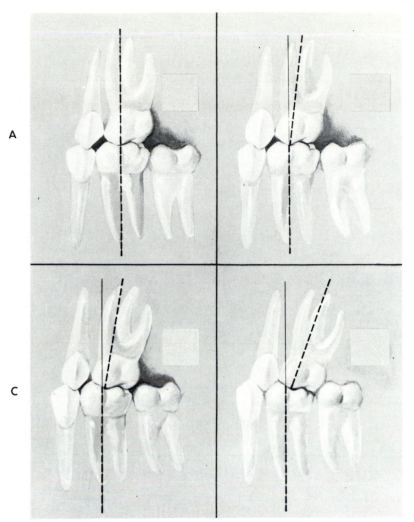

A

B

C

D

Fig. 1-7   The posterior crown angulation (tip) is measured by the inclination of the long axis of the crown to a line perpendicular to the occlusal plane. Note that distal inclination of the upper molar, *B* to *D*, brings the distobuccal cusp down into contact with the lower molar. Even if the mesiobuccal cusp of the upper molar articulates in the mesial groove of the lower molar, proper occlusion will not result if the upper molar is too vertically upright. (From Andrews LF: *Am J Orthod* 62:296, 1972.)

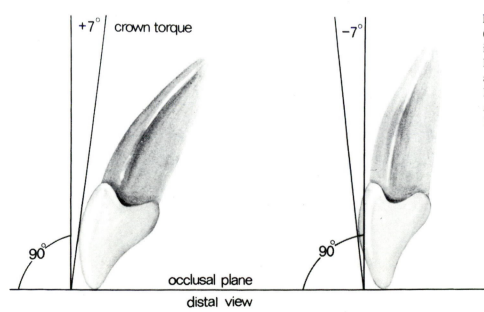

Fig. 1-8   Crown inclination or torque (e.g., of the upper left central incisor) is determined by the angle between a line perpendicular to the occlusal plane and one tangent to the middle of the labial or buccal clinical crown. (From Andrews LF: *Am J Orthod* 62:296, 1972.)

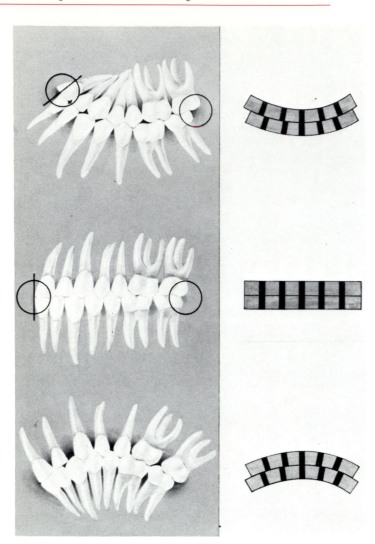

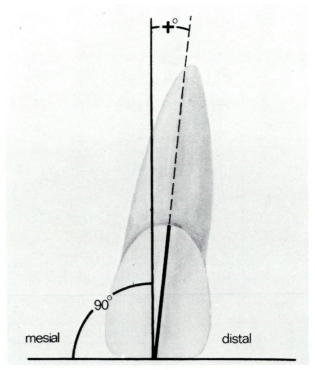

Fig. 1-9   If the curve of Spee is not relatively flat, teeth in one arch will be crowded, while those in the other will tend to be spaced. It should be kept in mind, however, that this does not mean the arch should be perfectly flat. It is an error in orthodontic treatment to extrude maxillary second molars in order to totally flatten the posterior end of the dental arch. (From Andrews LF: *Am J Orthod* 62:296, 1972.)

Fig. 1-10   Incisor crown angulation (tip) is measured by the inclination of the long axis of the crown to a line perpendicular to the occlusal plane. The incisal edge normally is parallel to the occlusal plane when incisor crown angulation is correct. (From Andrews LF: *Am J Orthod* 62:296, 1972.)

Transverse Projection

In the transverse projection the labial surfaces of the crown of the incisor teeth (centrals and laterals) can be visualized, as can the facial surfaces of all the posterior teeth, including the canines:

1. *Incisor crown tip (angulation).* The gingival portion of the long axis of each crown should be distal to the incisal portion (Fig. 1-10).
2. *Posterior crown inclination (canines through molars).* Crown inclination refers to the buccolingual inclination of the long axis of the crown, not to the long axis of the entire tooth.
   a. *Maxillary.* A lingual crown inclination should exist. It is constant and similar from the canines through the second premolars and slightly more pronounced in the molars.
   b. *Mandibular.* The lingual crown inclination of the lower posterior teeth progressively increases from the canines through the second molars (Fig. 1-11).

The posterior view of the dentition (transverse projection) shows that the maxillary roots converge and the mandibular roots diverge (Fig. 1-12). The salient point is that the long axes of the maxillary and mandibular first molars form a straight line; thinking teleologically, this configuration is to best resist the forces of occlusion. Whatever the reason, it causes the maxillary bony base (basal bone, facial base) to represent a smaller area (in the occlusal view) than the mandibular bony base. The smaller maxillary base can be observed particularly well in the relationship of the maxillary and mandibular edentulous ridges when a full denture setup is being done.

Finally, it is clear now that the relationship of the mandibular condyles to the glenoid fossae must be considered in determining occlusal relationships. A gross discrepancy

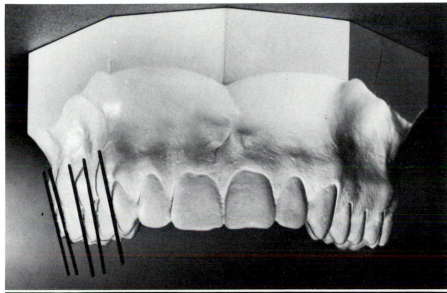

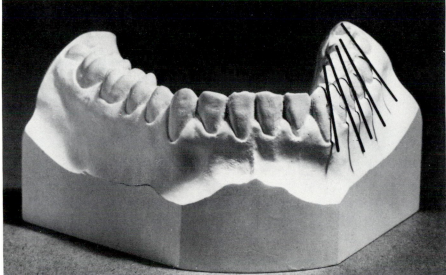

Fig. 1-11 Lingual crown inclination is present for the maxillary and mandibular posterior teeth (including canines). (From Andrews LF: *Am J Orthod* 62:296, 1972.)

Fig. 1-12 The occlusion (lingual view). In this orientation the relationships of the supporting cusps and their fossae can be observed. The normal first molar occlusion should have the mesiolingual cusp of the maxillary first molar resting in the central fossa of the mandibular first molar. (Modified from Kraus BS, Jordan RE, Abrams L: *Dental anatomy and occlusion: a study of the masticatory system,* Baltimore, 1969, Williams & Wilkins.)

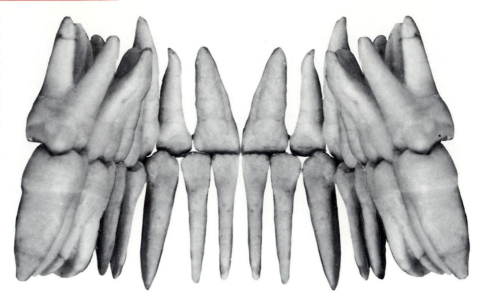

between maximum intercuspation and the position of the mandible when it is seated by muscular guidance can be termed *deflective malocclusion.*[162] For any concept of ideal occlusion to be biologically sound, it must ultimately consider function.

Distinguishing Normal Occlusion from Malocclusion

Fundamental to orthodontic diagnosis is understanding the concept of *normal occlusion.* Traditionally, any deviation from *ideal occlusion* has represented what Guilford[53] termed malocclusion. Of course, ideal occlusion rarely exists in nature, and so perhaps it is better to call this concept the *imaginary ideal* (see Fig. 1-6). Unfortunately, there is no clearcut or acceptable definition of *normal occlusion;* thus much of our diagnosis in orthodontics is based on this highly arbitrary concept of the ideal.

Severe malocclusion is often accompanied by disproportions of the face and jaws. When this occurs, the problems are commonly referred to as dentofacial deformities; however, malocclusion should not be thought of as a pathologic condition but merely as human morphologic variation. (Exceptions occur in genetic disorders of the face and jaws, such as craniofacial dysostosis or cleft lip and/or palate, when growth is distorted in the aftermath of trauma, and in other special circumstances.)

Part of the dilemma in differentiating normal occlusion from malocclusion stems from our inability to measure or quantify the functional characteristics of occlusion. One of the first and still one of the few biometric studies of occlusion was Hellman's.[56] However, his was a rather static approach to occlusion. He believed that in the maximum intercuspal position, specific landmarks in the opposing dental arches should contact. As long as the orthodontist's view of occlusion remains largely in this realm of static descriptive morphology, a problem lies in being able to define the

individual norm. Of course, the *individual norm* is difficult to define because function and physiologic adaptation must be considered when deciding whether a given individual's occlusion is normal. By default, clinical orthodontics has accepted a therapeutic goal that Fischer[44] called the *achieveable optimum.* In this approach the orthodontist attempts to achieve ideal occlusion for each patient, knowing that the true norm for a particular individual can only be ascertained after treatment and retention have been completed.

In summary, the current view is that a malocclusion exists when a misarrangement of the teeth creates a problem for the individual, whether functionally or psychosocially. Admittedly, this definition is, in part, a cultural one—the same arrangement of teeth could be a functional or psychosocial problem in one setting and not in another. A patient should have reasonable alignment and occlusion of the teeth (the severity of any malocclusion is determined at least in part by the reaction of the patient and others), and should have normal jaw function (i.e., no significant handicap) in any of the oral activities (chewing, swallowing, speaking). Because neither the reactions nor the impact on function can be predicted confidently from the morphology (at least with present knowledge) it is difficult to draw a line based on morphology alone that differentiates normal occlusion from malocclusion. Efforts to develop an *index of malocclusion* to determine priority for treatment run into problems at precisely this point.[101]

EPIDEMIOLOGIC STUDIES OF MALOCCLUSION

As a background for orthodontic diagnosis and treatment planning, it is necessary to understand something of the *prevalence* of problems relating to occlusal disharmony, the actual *need* for treatment of these problems, the *demand* for this treatment on the part of patients, and the *effectiveness* of various treatment procedures. Progress has been made toward all these goals, but the amount of epidemiologic information about malocclusion still is insufficient, and few studies have been made since the 1970s. At least some data are now available for all the points emphasized, and these will be discussed in turn. Some orthodontic information was obtained during the large-scale survey by the United States Public Health Service (USPHS) of the health of the US population in 1991 through 1992 (N-HANES III), and this should be available in 1994.

The incidence of malocclusion varies widely in different countries of the world. In primitive and isolated societies there is less variation in occlusal patterns than in more heterogeneous populations.[37] Dental crowding and malalignment are rare in nearly all primitive populations. Among Australian aborigines, for example, ideal occlusion frequently is observed. This variation between primitive and modern groups has been attributed to the effect of natural selection, inbreeding versus outbreeding, and environmental factors. None of the explanations at present seems entirely satisfactory, and therefore we must consider that we simply do not know why an increase in malocclusion accompanies

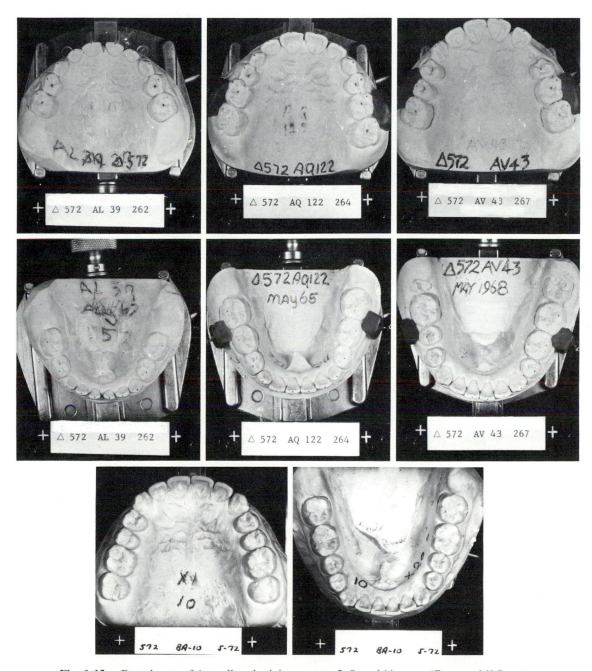

Fig. 1-13 Dental casts of Australian aborigines at ages 5, 8, and 11 years. (Courtesy MJ Barrett, University of Adelaide.)

Continued.

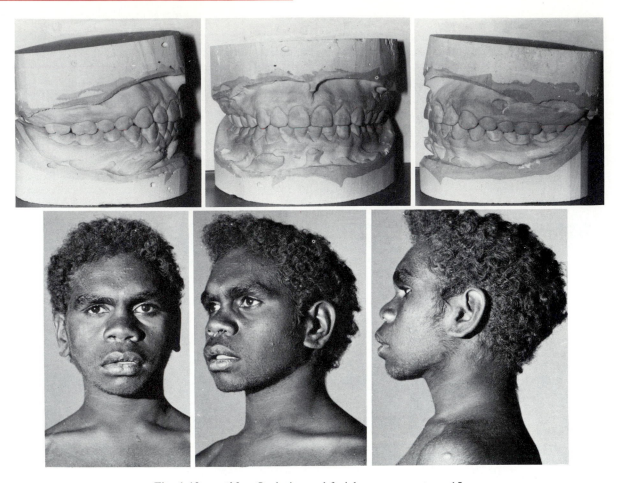

Fig. 1-13, cont'd   Occlusion and facial appearance at age 15.

development of a society.[28] Sometimes the stable occlusal pattern in a primitive group is not the imaginary ideal occlusion. In certain Melanesian islanders, the usual condition is what we would call a skeletal Class III malocclusion, with good dental alignment. Thus incisal guidance, cusp protection, and the like, which are useful therapeutic concepts, are apparently not selective in an evolutionary context. Raymond Begg[11] theorized that the increased attrition of teeth caused by primitive diets prevents the development of crowding and justified frequent extraction of premolars as compensation for the lack of wear in modern populations; however, this explanation is not supported by current data.[29] Teenage Australian aborigines whose modern diet has prevented significant attrition still do not develop crowding of incisors (Fig. 1-13).

The reported rate of malocclusion is higher in developed countries than it is in primitive countries and appears to be slightly higher in the United States than anywhere else. Until the 1970s, widely varying estimates for malocclusion in the United States were produced by a series of small-scale epidemiologic studies. In 1970 the USPHS published two important studies of dental relationships, the first provides data for children ages 6 to 11 years[66] and the second provides

data for youths 12 to 17.[65] Data from these studies are presented in Table 1-1. In both studies a sample of nearly 8000 individuals was chosen to represent the approximately 25 million Americans between 6 years and 17 years, excluding only Indians on reservations.

Based on these figures it appears that 75% of American children and youths have some degree of occlusal disharmony, which therefore must be considered typical rather than atypical. In the USPHS study the Treatment Priority Index (TPI)[49] was used to indicate degree of disharmony. This index is calculated from a detailed evaluation of the occlusal relationships of the teeth. Fig. 1-14 displays the percentages of children with given TPI scores: the higher the score, the greater the disharmony.

Although orthodontists may differ with both the TPI method and the suggested interpretation of scores, this index gives a known starting point for assessing malocclusion. When this approach is used, 37% of American children are judged, by a score of 4 or more, to have definite malocclusions (which does not mean that every person with a score of 4 needs treatment, nor does it mean that many of those with scores of 2 or 3 would not benefit from treatment). Of all children, 40% have some malalignment of teeth; 17%

TABLE 1-1

Number and Percent of Children and Youths in the United States with High Priority for Orthodontic Treatment, by Specified Malocclusion Findings and Race

Finding and race	Number (thousands)		Percent of those measured	
	Age 6 to 11*	12 to 17†	6 to 11	12 to 17
Tissue impingement				
Total‡	711	201	4.0	0.9
White	697	192	4.6	1.0
Black	31	9	1.2	0.3
Posterior crossbite 4 teeth or more to lingual				
Total‡	261	334	1.1	1.5
White	224	268	1.1	1.4
Black	55	54	1.7	1.8
Posterior crossbite 4 teeth or more to buccal				
Total‡	24	22	0.1	0.1
White	20	19	0.1	0.1
Black	—	3	—	0.1
Tooth displacement scores 7 or more				
Total‡	665	7368	2.8	32.5
White	571	6544	2.8	33.5
Black	52	776	1.6	25.7
TPI scores 7 to 9 (severe handicap with treatment highly recommended)				
Total‡	1525	2896	8.6	13.0
White	1299	2492	8.6	13.0
Black	218	365	8.6	12.2
10 or more (severe handicap with treatment mandatory)				
Total‡	975	3564	5.5	16.0
White	771	3106	5.1	16.2
Black	211	454	8.3	15.2
Overbite 6 mm or more				
Total‡	1169	2281	6.6	10.3
White	1147	2230	7.6	11.7
Black	20	42	0.8	1.4
Open bite 2 mm or more				
Total‡	443	509	2.5	2.3
White	211	229	1.4	1.2
Black	244	300	9.6	10.1
Upper overjet 7 mm or more				
Total‡	1672	1783	9.4	8.0
White	1471	1611	9.7	8.4
Black	201	165	7.9	5.5
Lower overjet 1 mm or more				
Total‡	142	201	0.8	0.9
White	121	153	0.8	0.8
Black	15	36	0.6	1.2

*From Kelly JE, Sanchez M, Van Kirk LE: DHEW Publication no. (HRA) 74-1612, 1973.
†From Kelly J, Harvey C: DHEW Publication no. (HRA) 77-1644, 1977.
‡Includes data from "other races," which are not shown separately.

have significant protrusion of maxillary incisors, and 20% a Class II molar relationship; less than 1% have lower overjet, although 5% have a Class III molar relationship; and 4% have an anterior open bite. The incidence varies according to social, sexual, and regional groupings. For example, open bite is 4 times more common in blacks than in whites and slightly more common in girls than in boys. Findings for 6 to 11 and 12 to 17 years are similar but with some interesting changes: the incidence of crowding increases, while open bite decreases. The American data are more complete than those available for other countries; however, the same general picture emerges: in developed nations

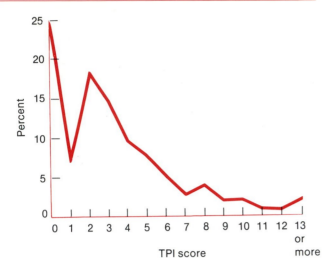

Fig. 1-14 Percent of children with specified TPI scores. Interpretation of these scores (as suggested by Grainger) is as follows: *0*, virtually classic normal occlusion; *1* to *3*, minor manifestations of occlusal disharmony; *4* to *6*, definite malocclusion; *7* to *9*, severe handicap, treatment highly desirable; *10* or greater, severe handicap, treatment mandatory. (From Kelly JE, Sanchez M, Van Kirk LE: DHEW Publication no. [HRA] 74-1612, 1973.)

a surprisingly high percentage of the population has dental disharmony and malocclusion, despite racial and ethnic differences.

NEED FOR TREATMENT

A major difficulty in assessing the need for orthodontic treatment is that one person's acceptable condition may be another's problem: anatomically similar malocclusions may cause difficulty for one person but not for another. Malocclusion creates problems in three major circumstances: (1) when it causes or predisposes to disease; (2) when it leads to disturbances in jaw function (temporomandibular dysfunction [TMD] and related conditions) or affects other oral functions (e.g., mastication, speech); and (3) when its effect on facial esthetics causes psychosocial problems. To evaluate the need for orthodontic treatment, it is necessary that all these aspects be considered.

Malocclusion and Oral Disease

Although it seems intuitively obvious that malocclusion should contribute to periodontal disease and caries by making it harder to care for the teeth, modern studies indicate that this effect is small. An individual's willingness and motivation determine oral hygiene much more than how well the teeth are aligned. Individuals with malocclusion are not more prone to tooth decay,[57] and only a tenuous link exists between the presence or absence of malocclusion and the development of periodontal problems in later life.[112] It was thought at one time that trauma from occlusion played

a significant role in the pathogenesis of periodontal problems; however, recent research has led to a much decreased emphasis on occlusal trauma as a primary causal factor in periodontal disease.[78] If plaque is controlled, so is periodontal disease; if not, periodontal problems will ensue. The patient's occlusal status seems to make little if any difference in whether periodontal problems develop, although it can affect the progress once disease is present.

Another indication that there is little need for orthodontic treatment to prevent the development of periodontal disease comes from two studies of the long-term effects of orthodontic treatment. The studies, carried out under contract from the National Institute of Dental Research in the late 1970s, one at the University of Rochester[111] and the other at the University of Illinois,[127] involved more than 100 patients who were carefully examined 10 to 20 years after the completion of their orthodontic treatment. When these patients were compared with untreated individuals in the same age group, there was no evidence that their periodontal status was better (or worse). Since their functional occlusions were improved as a result of the previous treatment, a beneficial effect on periodontal health would have been expected if the occlusion had played a major role.

On the other hand, some periodontists have pointed to a disproportionate number of patients seeking care for periodontal problems who previously had undergone orthodontic treatment, and suggested that the orthodontic treatment may have had long-term detrimental periodontal effects, perhaps because of inflammation that was created during the orthodontic treatment. This also is not the case. There is no evidence that orthodontic treatment leads to periodontal problems. It seems to be true that periodontists are more likely to see patients who have had orthodontic treatment previously—not because they are more likely to develop periodontal problems but because they represent a group of patients who seek dental care.

Malocclusion and Functional Problems

It is certain that malocclusion can lead to functional problems; however, the relationship between morphologic deviations from the ideal and impaired function has not been studied adequately. This is particularly true for masticatory activity and chewing efficiency. It is obvious that if only a few teeth meet, the patient may have difficulty masticating; however, we know little or nothing about the compromises and adaptations that malocclusion may require, except for extreme cases in which nutritional inadequacy becomes obvious. Patients with severe malocclusion often complain about difficulty in eating. Many patients report that they have learned to avoid certain foods that they cannot manage. The same patients usually indicate that they can eat better after treatment and often consider ease in masticating as a major benefit of orthodontic treatment. The orthodontist's problem is the lack of an instrument for measuring masticatory activity. When a child walks, an observer can note whether the gait is even or whether the child stumbles. What

TABLE 1-2
Speech Difficulties Related to Dental Problems

Speech sound	Type	Dental problems
/s/, /z/	Sibilant	*Lisp* related to large gap between incisors or missing incisors, open bite
/t/, /d/	Linguoalveolar stop	*Difficulty in production* related to irregular incisors (especially lingual position of maxillary incisors or supernumerary teeth); tongue-tie
/f/, /v/	Labiodental fricative	*Distortion* related to excessive protrusion of mandible
th, sh, ch (voiced or voiceless)	Linguodental fricative	*Distortion* related to severe open bite, missing incisors
/l/	Linguoalveolar continuant	*Distortion* related to tongue-tie

From Bell WH, Proffit WR, White RP: *Surgical correction of dentofacial deformities,* Philadelphia, 1980, WB Saunders, p. 113.

is the equivalent for chewing? Clinically applicable tests are urgently needed in this area.

A link between malocclusion and speech problems also is obvious in some patients. In the presence of severe malocclusion, it can be difficult or impossible to produce certain sounds, and effective speech therapy may require orthodontic treatment first. The assessment is complicated because neuromuscular problems that cause speech problems also can be causative agents for malocclusion. It can be difficult to know whether the malocclusion is contributing to the speech problem or vice-versa. In this area the situation is somewhat clearer. The relationships between certain dental and speech sounds are illustrated in Table 1-2.

The functional problem of most concern to orthodontists and the one whose relation to malocclusion is least well established is a difficulty in jaw function manifested as pain in and around the temporomandibular joint. TMD may be attributed to pathologic changes in the TM joint, but more often it is due to muscle fatigue, spasm, and resulting pain. The presence of malocclusion is not highly correlated with the presence of TMD.[36,127] Even though some correlations are statistically significant, the highest correlation coefficients typically are between 0.3 and 0.4, which means that there is only a 10% to 15% chance of predicting TMD from the occlusion or vice-versa. Patients with pain in the muscles almost always have a history of clenching and grinding their teeth, presumably in response to stress. Perhaps the conclusion is that some types of malocclusion make it easier for a patient to hurt himself with parafunctional activity.

Some clinicians feel that even minor imperfections in the occlusion can serve as a trigger for bruxism, which, if true, would indicate a real need for perfecting the occlusion in everyone. Scientific evidence on this point is lacking; however, it seems unlikely because the number of people with moderate degrees of malocclusion far exceeds the number of TMD patients. However, if a patient responds to stress by increased oral muscle activity, improper occlusal relationships may make the problem harder to control. Therefore malocclusion coupled with pain and spasm in the muscles of mastication may indicate a need for orthodontic treatment

(or other occlusal therapy). Obviously, if the problem is some sort of pathologic condition within the joint itself, occlusal therapy of any type, including orthodontics, would not be a total answer to the problem.

The role of orthodontic treatment as a cause of TMD also has been controversial. The weak link between occlusion and TM joint function suggests that orthodontics probably would have little effect, as suggested by a number of recent studies.[35,58,126] Despite concerns expressed by some dentists that premolar extraction or interarch elastics could trigger TMD, it is not likely to occur.[74,121]

Esthetic and Psychosocial Considerations

Concern about the appearance of the teeth and face is widely acknowledged to be a major motivating factor for orthodontic treatment.[20,70,135] Obvious malocclusion can be a major social handicap. Individuals who have a dentofacial deformity may encounter social responses that can severely affect their life adaptation. Perceived dentofacial esthetics and social aspects may be more influential in the decision to seek orthodontic treatment than the clinical status, because an unattractive appearance often evokes an unfavorable social response and negative stereotyping.[25,67]

Psychic distress caused by facial disfigurement is not in direct proportion to its anatomic severity. A grossly disfigured person, being able to predict a consistently negative response, develops techniques for coping. An individual with an apparently less severe problem, such as a receding chin or irregular upper incisors, is sometimes ridiculed or ignored. These unpredictable responses produce anxiety and can have strong deleterious effects.[86] On the other hand, good dental appearance is desired by essentially all persons and is highly correlated with successful and prestigious occupations.[146]

In 1976 the United States Department of Defense requested that the National Research Council (operating arm of the National Academy of Sciences) conduct a study of severely handicapping orthodontic conditions and provide guidelines that might be used to select personnel or dependents most in need of orthodontic treatment. The resulting report[101] specifically recognized the role of all the afore-mentioned factors in determining the need for orthodontic treatment, and it emphasized the psychologic component. The recommendations suggested that orthodontic handicap could be functional or psychosocial and that both factors should be taken into account when determining the need for treatment. The best available evidence is that approximately 5% of U.S. children and youths have severely handicapping malocclusion. In these patients both functional and psychosocial aspects are present. Although the NRC committee's recommendations focused on this most severely affected subset of all persons with malocclusion, its approach provides an excellent perspective on the need for orthodontic treatment and the factors that must be considered during evaluation. Since esthetic concerns can affect the way an individual lives, the esthetic component of malocclusion cannot be minimized.

DEMAND FOR TREATMENT AND ITS EFFECTIVENESS

Just as not all patients with dental problems seek dental care, so, too, not all patients with malocclusion (even the most severe) seek orthodontic treatment. If need for treatment is defined as malocclusion of a certain degree of anatomic severity, need and demand may be quite different. Patients often respond more to what they perceive than to what dentists recommend. If the estimate of need takes into account the psychosocial impact of malocclusion (or the lack of it), demand and need move closer together. Unfortunately, data are not available to allow a comparison of the number of people who think they need treatment with the number of people who have varying degrees of malocclusion. The USPHS data from the 1970s[65,66] suggest that (as might be expected) the perceived need varies with social and cultural conditions. Children who are being raised in urban areas are more often thought (by their parents and peers) to need treatment than are those who live in rural areas, even though the prevalence of occlusal disharmony is similar in both areas. In typical middle-class suburbs about 35% of children are thought by parents and peers to need orthodontic treatment. Facial appearance is a major factor in this determination of need (and therefore subsequent demand) for treatment.

Family income also is strongly related to demand. The higher the family income, the greater the demand for orthodontic treatment is likely to be. Higher income groups can more easily afford orthodontics, and higher socioeconomic groups place greater value on facial appearance. The effect of financial considerations on demand is revealed most clearly by the response to third party payment plans. When third party copayment is available, the number of individuals seeking treatment rises considerably.[46] The growth of third party payment plans has contributed significantly to the increase in delivery of orthodontic treatment, and as these plans become more widely available, it is likely that demand

for treatment will more closely approach the 35% level that is thought by the public to need treatment.[88]

The effectiveness of orthodontic treatment has received remarkably little study. This area now is becoming the subject of investigation, stimulated by two factors from opposite points on the professional compass. Those who support orthodontic treatment financially through the various third party plans want proof that their funding is producing results. At the same time the professionals are bombarded by an increasing number of new technical approaches, and they are inclined to compare the effectiveness of radically different treatment approaches, as for instance the use of functional appliances versus traditional fixed appliance therapy for Class II malocclusion.

Data from two early studies on the effectiveness of interceptive mixed dentition orthodontic treatment illustrate the value of this type of information. Both the Burlington, Ontario, study in the 1950s,[113] which is better known for its long-term growth records, and a 1970s study at the University of Pennsylvania[5] suggest that only about 15% of children thought by their parents to need orthodontic treatment (95% of whom did need treatment in the opinion of the orthodontist who examined them) were judged to have benefited from preventive and interceptive treatment alone. In other words, data now are available to show that if orthodontic treatment is begun in the mixed dentition, even for what appears to be relatively minor problems, further treatment usually will be needed as the child matures. Preventive and interceptive treatment has been emphasized in the teaching of children's dentistry for the past three decades, and most dentists believe that such treatment is more effective than it actually turns out to be.

A major reason for orthodontic treatment is the correction of malaligned anterior teeth, and although ideal alignment typically exists at the end of active treatment, it is known now that this often is not maintained long-term. With or without orthodontic treatment, some degree of crowding of the lower incisors is found in the majority of adults. To provide more space for alignment, extraction was introduced into modern orthodontics, primarily to reduce the chance of relapse after crowded teeth were aligned. Although nonextraction treatment seems to be somewhat more prone to posttreatment relapse,[47] return of crowding is distressingly frequent, even with extraction treatment.[80,81,93] It is important to judge the effectiveness of orthodontic treatment in terms of benefits larger than long-term maintenance of perfect alignment.

Recently the National Institute of Dental Research has funded studies on the effectiveness of orthodontic treatment, with a special focus on the alternative approaches to Class II malocclusion. Preliminary results from a randomized clinical trial of early (preadolescent) versus late (adolescent) treatment of Class II patients indicate that significant growth modification can be obtained; however, it is not yet clear whether these changes will be maintained through the second phase of comprehensive treatment that all these patients will receive.[152] In a comparison of orthodontic camouflage versus surgical-orthodontic correction in nongrowing patients, both types of treatment corrected the buccal occlusion; however, 95% of the surgical-orthodontic patients and only 74% of the orthodontics-only patients had acceptable overjet at the conclusion of treatment.[116] It appears that in adolescents, successful orthodontic treatment is unlikely if the overjet is greater than 10 mm; beyond that, especially if other signs of skeletal dysplasia are present, surgery is needed for successful treatment.[117]

Although the data for treatment effectiveness still are quite limited, it is comforting to orthodontists to know that when patients who have undergone orthodontic treatment are surveyed, the majority believe that they benefited from the treatment and are pleased with the results—an indication that the social-behavioral component of need is being addressed reasonably well.[106]

ETIOLOGY OF ORTHODONTIC PROBLEMS

It is commonly accepted that the etiology of any problem should be contained in the diagnosis. In the early part of this century, medical success in dealing with bacterial and viral diseases for which a single major cause could be identified, led to great emphasis on identifying causative agents. Unfortunately, a single clearly identifiable agent is not always apparent, and it is recognized now that multifactorial causes must be considered in even apparently straightforward bacterial illnesses. For instance, whether you catch the flu depends not only on whether you were exposed to the virus but also on the circumstances under which the exposure occurred and your level of resistance at that time. Malocclusion is a developmental problem, not a pathologic one, and although we can say that both hereditary and environmental factors are important influences on development, often we are not able to ascertain which malocclusions are determined largely on a genetic basis, which result largely from environmental factors, and which are a combination of hereditary and environmental factors (Fig. 1-15).

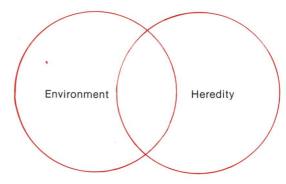

Fig. 1-15   Malocclusion may be caused by heredity, environment, or a combination of the two. The relative importance of environment vs. heredity has been controversial since the days of Angle. There is now little question that both are important; probably, hereditary influences are more prominent in skeletal proportions and environmental influences are more important in determining dental relationships.

At the two extremes it is sometimes easy to place the patient in one of these two categories. A chronic thumbsucker with an anterior open bite, for example, can most likely be labeled as having a problem stemming from local causes (Fig. 1-16). A patient who has a normal dentition except for one or more congenitally missing teeth can probably be classified as having a problem of genetic origin. However, the majority of patients whom the orthodontist treats are not easily placed in one of these categories.

Genetic Syndromes

A relatively small number of orthodontic patients are affected by known genetic syndromes that affect the oral structures. Tables 1-3 to 1-6 give a partial listing of these syndromes and their oral manifestations. By far, the most common orthodontic problem that may be part of a genetic syndrome is cleft lip and palate; however, there are many causes for facial clefting conditions and not all of the causes can be traced to genetics.[64]

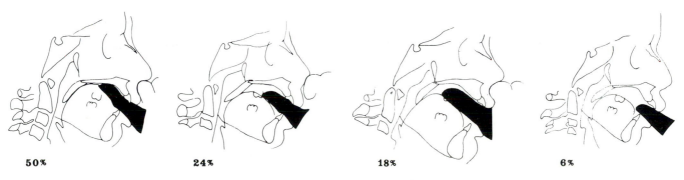

50%   **24%**   **18%**   **6%**

Fig. 1-16   Four individual acts of thumbsucking (tracings of cineradiographs). Each presents a variable pattern in thumb posture. The type and extent of open bite associated with thumbsucking varies with the thumb posture. (From Subtelny JD: *Angle Orthod* 43:347, 1973.)

TABLE 1-3

Malformation Syndromes Associated with Mandibular Deficiency

Condition	Striking features	Etiology
Robin complex	Micrognathia, cleft palate, and glossoptosis; occurs as isolated malformation complex or as part of broader pattern of abnormalities; of the many syndromes with the Robin complex as one component, Stickler syndrome is most common	Etiologically heterogeneous; Stickler syndrome is autosomal dominant
Treacher Collins syndrome	Symmetrically hypoplastic low-set ears; down slanting palpebral fissures; micrognathia; sometimes cleft palate	Autosomal dominant
Nager acrofacial dysostosis	Symmetrically hypoplastic ears; down slanting palpebral fissures; micrognathia; cleft palate; in some cases, preaxial upper limb deficiency	Autosomal recessive
Wildervanck-Smith syndrome	Symmetrically hypoplastic ears; down slanting palpebral fissures; micrognathia; cleft lip and palate in some cases; limb reduction defects of upper and lower limbs	Unknown; all cases to date sporadic
Hemifacial microsomia (Goldenhar syndrome)	Unilateral or bilateral asymmetrically hypoplastic ears and mandibular ramus; ear tags and/or pits, micrognathia; variably cleft lip or palate; epibulbar dermoids; vertebral anomalies; cardiac defects; renal anomalies; other abnormalities	Most cases sporadic; few familial instances in which pedigrees are compatible with autosomal dominant or autosomal recessive inheritance
Möbius syndrome	Bilateral sixth and seventh nerve palsy and (variably) other cranial nerve involvement; high broad nasal bridge; epicanthic folds; micrognathia; talipes equinovarus; limb reduction defects; mental deficiency	Unknown; almost all cases sporadic; rare familial instances
Hallermann-Streiff syndrome	Dyscephaly; hypotrichosis; congenital cataracts; beaked nose; micrognathia; anteriorly placed mandibular condyles; natal teeth; oligodontia; short stature	Unknown; all cases to date sporadic

From Cohen M: In Bell WH, Proffit WR, White RP: *Surgical correction of dentofacial deformities*, Philadelphia, 1980, WB Saunders, p.23.

The greatest value of knowing that a patient has a particular syndrome is that it allows much better prediction of future development in this individual who will not grow in the normal pattern.[48] Sometimes, recognizing a syndrome is made more difficult by incomplete expression of the gene or genes involved (called partial penetrance). If a genetic syndrome is suspected, the orthodontist should have the patient evaluated through a clinic that specializes in such matters. Most university medical centers now have craniofacial teams. A listing of recognized groups can be obtained from the American Cleft Palate Association (Salk Hall, University of Pittsburgh, Pittsburgh, Pa, 15261). Dental crown and root morphologic traits sometimes serve as genetic markers in these situations.[3] A patient who has anomalous teeth should be examined carefully for ear, hand, or other deformities that may indicate a genetic syndrome.

Genetic Influences

It is widely acknowledged that most malocclusions have a genetic component; however, it is extremely difficult to quantify how much of a given problem is genetic and how much is due to prenatal or postnatal environmental factors. Although genealogies and pedigrees are helpful in recording the patient's family history, they are not revealing in regard to exact patterns of dentofacial inheritance. Because of the polygenic inheritance of craniofacial and dental characteristics or traits, it is unlikely that simple methods will reveal the genetic component of most malocclusions. However, certain malocclusions show a familial tendency, such as some Class III malocclusions and some open bite problems (Fig. 1-17). Continued mandibular growth and the development of true prognathism are found more often when there is a familial incidence of such a condition. Studies of

TABLE 1-4

Malformation Syndromes Associated with Mandibular Prognathism

Condition	Striking features	Etiology
Basal cell nevus syndrome (Gorlin syndrome)	Macrocephaly; frontal and biparietal bossing; dystopia canthorum or ocular hypertelorism; mild mandibular prognathism; jaw cysts; multiple basal cell carcinomas; bifid ribs; spina bifida occulta; short fourth metacarpals	Autosomal dominant
Klinefelter syndrome	Skeletal disproportion; small testes; increased urinary gonadotrophins; gynecomastia and mental deficiency in some cases; mandibular prognathism occasionally (somewhat dependent upon increased number of X chromosomes); overall condition becomes more severe as number of X chromosomes increases	Commonly XXY karyotype, but XXXY and XXXXY also occur
Marfan syndrome	Marfanoid habitus; dolichostenomelia; arachnodactyly; ectopia lentis; fusiform and dissecting aneurysms of aorta; mandibular prognathism	Autosomal dominant
Osteogenesis imperfecta	Fragile bones; blue sclerae; deafness; loose ligaments; dentinogenesis imperfecta-like tooth condition; mandibular prognathism	Autosomal dominant (common type); etiologically heterogeneous
Waardenburg syndrome	White forelock; dystopia canthorum; heterochromia irides, synophrys, mild hypoplasia of alar cartilages; mild mandibular prognathism; sensorineural deafness	Autosomal dominant (common type); etiologically heterogeneous, with three other types known

From Cohen M: In Bell WH, Proffit WR, White RP: *Surgical correction of dentofacial deformities*, Philadelphia, 1980, WB Saunders, p. 23

TABLE 1-5

Malformation Syndromes Associated with Problems of Facial Height

Condition	Striking features	Etiology
Amelogenesis imperfecta	Discolored teeth; hypomaturation, hypoplasia, or hypocalcification of enamel; anterior open bite	Etiologically heterogeneous; several modes of inheritance depending upon type of enamel defect and family history
Beckwith-Wiedemann syndrome	Macroglossia; anterior open bite; mandibular prognathism; earlobe grooves; depressions on posterior rim of ear; omphalocele or umbilical hernia; neonatal hypoglycemia; visceromegaly; postsomatic gigantism; other abnormalities	Unknown; most cases sporadic; few familial instances

From Cohen M: In Bell WH, Proffit WR, White RP: *Surgical correction of dentofacial deformities*, Philadelphia, 1980, WB Saunders, p. 37.

twins[82,84] and of triplets[73] have shown a high concordance of dentofacial traits in monozygotic individuals, which suggests a large heritable component in the etiology of malocclusion. From an examination of longitudinal data from the Bolton-Brush growth study, Harris and Johnson[54] concluded that the heritability of skeletal characteristics was high, but that of dental characteristics was low. To the extent that facial proportions and jaw relationships determine the characteristics of a malocclusion, an hereditary component is likely to be present; however, dental variation seems to be determined more often by the environment.

TABLE 1-6

Malformation Syndromes Associated with Facial Asymmetry

Condition	Striking features	Etiology
Hemifacial microsomia (Goldenhar syndrome)	Unilateral or bilateral asymmetrically hypoplastic ears and mandibular ramus; ear tags and/or pits; micrognathia; variably cleft lip and/or palate; epibulbar dermoids; vertebral anomalies; cardiac defects; renal anomalies; other abnormalities	Most cases sporadic; few familial instances in which pedigrees are compatible with autosomal dominant and autosomal recessive transmission
Hemihypertrophy	Hemihypertrophy involving head, limbs, and body; expression variable; hypertrophy involves both bone and soft tissue; tongue, mandible, and teeth may be unilaterally enlarged; occasionally associated with Wilms' tumor, adrenocortical carcinoma, or hepatoblastoma; may be associated with a variety of other anomalies	Unknown; sporadic occurrence
Neurofibromatosis	Café-au-lait spots, neurofibromas, other hamartomas and neoplasms; skeletal defects; endocrine disturbances; some patients have macrocephaly, craniofacial asymmetry, mandibular asymmetry, or hypertrophy of facial soft tissue	Autosomal dominant
Romberg syndrome	Hemiatrophy involving muscle, bone, and cartilage (progressive); involves lip and tongue; left-side predilection; epilepsy in some cases; migraine in some cases; small percentage have body involvement	Unknown

From Cohen M: In Bell WH, Proffit WR, White RP: *Surgical correction of dentofacial deformities,* Philadelphia, 1980, WB Saunders, p. 38.

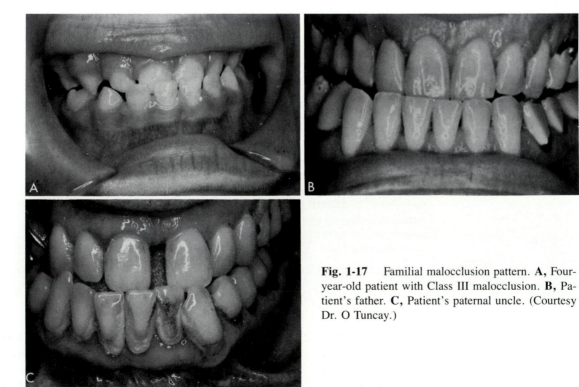

Fig. 1-17   Familial malocclusion pattern. **A,** Four-year-old patient with Class III malocclusion. **B,** Patient's father. **C,** Patient's paternal uncle. (Courtesy Dr. O Tuncay.)

Intrauterine and Neonatal Environment

Although it is not uncommon for parents to believe that a child with a genetic syndrome is suffering from the effects of a birth injury, dentofacial problems related to either birth trauma or the intrauterine environment are relatively unusual. One unusual but striking condition that is related to the intrauterine environment (Fig. 1-18) is intrauterine molding, in which the pressure during fetal growth distorts the developing face. The most frequent problem of this type is the Pierre Robin anomaly (Fig. 1-19).

Postnatal Environment

The role of the postnatal environment in the etiology of malocclusion continues to be vigorously debated. The environment in this sense refers to all the nongenetic influences that may be brought to bear on the developing individual and refers particularly to the effects of muscle function and neuromuscular adaptation. Alteration of the growth pattern is the mechanism by which the environment can produce occlusal disharmony. Since genetic influences also affect growth, it may be difficult to judge whether it is heredity or environment that is the cause of growth problems. If both heredity and environment are involved, it may be difficult to decide which part of the problem is genetic and which is environmental. Nevertheless, the distinction is important because the orthodontist's concept of the relative importance of environment versus heredity can directly influence the approach to orthodontic treatment.

Implicit in Edward Angle's ideal of 32 natural teeth in perfect occlusion is his belief that perfect occlusion is possible for every individual, and that when malocclusion exists, it is because environmental influences have prevented the ideal potential from being realized. The use of various exercises and physical therapy in an orthodontic practice, which found its greatest exponent in Alfred P. Rogers,[125] is based on a belief in the importance of environmental influences to the exclusion of genetic factors. Conversely, the reintroduction of extraction treatment into orthodontic therapy in the 1930s and 1940s was accompanied by an emphasis on the probability of a hereditary discrepancy between tooth mass and jaw size. The extraction philosophy was accompanied for a time by an almost total rejection of environmental factors as causal agents.

The orthodontist who believes that growth problems leading to skeletal malocclusion are largely if not entirely genetic has little hope of altering growth patterns and tends to focus treatment on adapting the dentition to a skeletal pattern that cannot be controlled. The orthodontist who believes that the same growth problems are environmentally determined becomes an activist in attempting to alter the environment and expects therapeutic success as a result. With the reintroduction of functional appliances into American orthodontics came, not surprisingly, an increase in the presumed importance of environmental factors as causes.

The scientific background for more emphasis on environmental causes of malocclusion rests primarily on findings with experimental animals.[55,90,92,110] Under certain experimental conditions growth can be modified quite extensively,

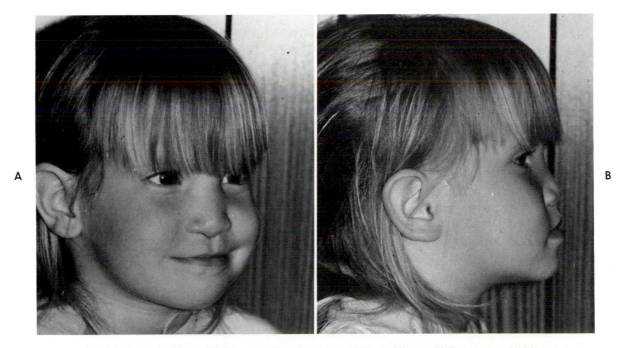

Fig. 1-18   **A,** Midface deficiency attributed to intrauterine molding at birth; one arm had been compressed across the middle of the face. **B,** At age 3 the depression of the midface is less obvious but can still be observed. (From Bell WH, Proffit WR, White RP: *Surgical correction of dentofacial deformities,* Philadelphia, 1980, WB Saunders.)

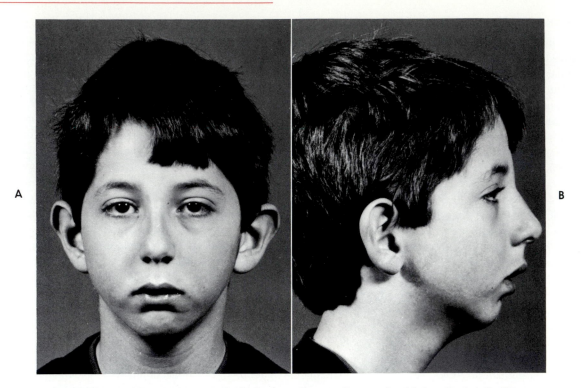

Fig. 1-19   Facial appearance at age 9 of a boy who was diagnosed at birth as having the Pierre Robin syndrome; extreme mandibular deficiency can be traced to mechanical pressure that restricts its intrauterine growth. Some individuals with this syndrome eventually have enough catch-up growth to produce an almost normal mandible, but not all are so fortunate. Although this boy has had considerable postnatal growth of the mandible, severe mandibular deficiency persists. (From Proffit WR, White RP: *Surgial-orthodontic treatment,* St Louis, 1991, Mosby.)

and in some circumstances growth can be stimulated. Some results with functional appliances in human patients support the interpretations of the animal work as directly applicable to humans. Other functional appliance experiences are less encouraging.[40,107,108] Considering the amount of time this question has been under study, a surprisingly small amount of good data exist to support the hypothesis that growth can be modified in a major way.

If unfavorable environmental factors might cause malocclusion, what functional influences should be suspected and how would they operate? Studies of form-function relationships in recent years have clarified this complex and frequently confusing area, particularly with regard to influences on tooth position. Now it is clear, for instance, that the duration rather than the magnitude of soft tissue pressure against the teeth is more important. Even light pressures, if maintained for a period of hours, have the potential to move teeth. On the other hand, heavier pressures like those exerted during swallowing and speaking, and the very heavy pressures exerted during chewing, have little effect on tooth position because of their short duration.[114] The work of Davidovitch et al[31] with cats indicates that about 4 hours of pressure is necessary to induce changes in cyclic AMP in the periodontal ligament. Cyclic AMP represents the *second*

messenger system through which cell-mediated responses occur. This duration of pressure to produce a response corresponds well to clinical experience with patients, which indicates that hours of pressure are needed to produce orthodontic tooth movement. Thus pressures by the tongue during swallowing, once widely suspected of being the cause of anterior open bite, are too short in duration to be effective. For the same reason it is doubtful that the way one speaks influences the position of the teeth (despite the suspicions of French writers years ago who thought that the protruding teeth of the English were caused by their peculiar /th/ sound). On the other hand, sucking habits that persist for many hours per day or pressures by the soft tissues as they rest passively against the teeth for many hours per day have the potential to affect tooth position. A search for environmental causes of malocclusion, therefore, should focus on three areas: (1) habits of long duration—primarily sucking habits; (2) influences on posture of the head, mandible, and tongue because posture determines resting soft tissue pressures; and (3) influences on tooth eruption.

It is widely believed that thumbsucking can cause both protrusion of the maxillary incisor teeth and an anterior open bite. The USPHS epidemiologic surveys[65,66] revealed a statistically significant association between reported thumbsucking and both of these orthodontic problems. Interestingly, the number of children of all ages who have an open bite is fewer than the number who suck their thumbs. Nearly all children who have an open bite suck their thumbs; however, the reverse is not true. The duration of sucking (number of hours per day), not its intensity, probably determines whether an open bite results.

Posture of the head, mandible, and tongue determines the pattern of resting pressures on the teeth and has the potential to affect tooth position. Head posture also correlates with facial proportions and the facial growth pattern: a head-forward, chin-extended posture is associated with a long face, whereas a military-appearing, head-back, chin-down posture is associated with a short face.[141] Scientific history is replete with errors caused by confusing correlation with cause and effect. The variations in posture may not cause the facial proportions. Both posture and facial proportions probably are related to unknown additional factors.

In recent years several clinicians have revived the idea that the long-face, skeletal-open bite pattern of facial development is caused by mouth breathing. Since a change from nasal to oral respiration is associated with postural changes[157] and since a variety of malocclusions can be produced in primates by obstructing the nares,[55] this suggestion seems plausible. Linder-Aronson[77] showed that in Swedish children referred for tonsillectomy and adenoidectomy, there is a statistically significant increase in face height compared to untreated controls. This difference diminishes after removal of the tonsils and adenoids.[68] On the other hand, although the differences pointed out by Linder-Aronson are undoubtedly real, they are small and do not account for the severe long-face patterns that are difficult orthodontic problems. English workers in the 1950s reported that children attending upper respiratory infection clinics appeared to have the same incidence and variety of malocclusions as other children.[76] This suggests that for most patients, mouth breathing may not be a potent influence on facial growth. At the present state of knowledge, nasopharyngeal surgery for orthodontic purposes should be recommended with great caution.

Influences on eruption of the teeth also may contribute to development of malocclusion. A force generated within the periodontal ligament initially elevates the teeth into occlusion then causes them to erupt further as jaw growth continues and facial height increases. The mechanism by which this eruption force is generated has never been clarified, although its location within the PDL now is known.[144] If teeth fail to erupt properly, one possible cause is an interference from soft tissue pressures or from a mechanical obstruction at eruption. Another possibility involves some problem with the eruption mechanism itself. Until recently this possibility was largely overlooked; however, it is now clear that a few patients with posterior open bite have an abnormal periodontal ligament and a failure of the normal eruption mechanism (Fig. 1-20).[119]

Finally, a factor that can cause malocclusion is trauma. Trauma to the teeth may lead to ankylosis and subsequent failure of eruption. Trauma to the mandible may result in fracture at the neck of the mandibular condyle, that is followed by displacement of the condyle and resorption of the condylar fragment. Trauma to the mandible occurs more frequently than once was thought, often with such minimal pain and discomfort to the child that the diagnosis is not made at the time of injury. After fracture of the condyles at an early age there is an excellent chance of regeneration and continued normal development; however, 10% to 15% of children have varying degrees of growth arrest after early fracture and a few may show excessive growth.[83] In a survey of patients referred to the University of North Carolina for surgical-orthodontic evaluation,[120] it was found that approximately 5% of severe mandibular deficiency problems requiring surgical correction appeared to be related to early fracture of the condyles (Fig. 1-21). In many of these patients the diagnosis had been missed initially. Whether prompt and appropriate management of condylar fractures would have decreased the incidence of future growth prob-

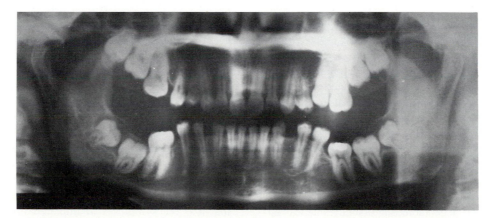

Fig. 1-20 Typical signs of primary failure of eruption: posterior teeth are differentially affected, and the affected teeth have not erupted, even though overlying bone has been resorbed.

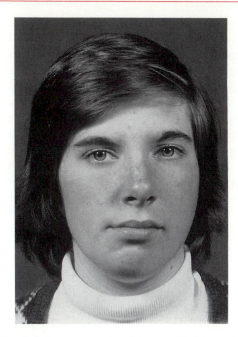

Fig. 1-21   Facial asymmetry in a 15-year-old girl that developed following a fall at age 8. In retrospect a fracture of the right condylar process at that time led to diminished growth on the affected side and an asymmetry of both the mandible and the maxilla. The secondary maxillary deformity, with lateral canting of the occlusal plane and the mouth opening, occurs because vertical development of both jaws is inhibited when the mandible cannot grow vertically the normal amount.

lems is unknown; however, the possibility that a unilateral growth disturbance leading to asymmetry or mandibular deficiency could be caused by an old mandibular fracture and must be kept in mind.

ORTHODONTIC DIAGNOSIS

Meaning of the Term Diagnosis in Orthodontics

The concept of diagnosis in orthodontics has been interpreted in several ways, and thus the term *diagnosis* has been used by different authors to mean different things. In the words of Strang[149]:

"There is nothing complicated about making a diagnosis in orthodontia, for the moment one has detected a deviation from normal occlusion and so determines that there is malocclusion, the diagnosis is complete."

Those who subscribe to this limited definition of diagnosis prefer to call the complex reasoning needed to determine the treatment strategy simply *case analysis*. This process could be called the traditional approach, since it was made popular by Angle. In Angle's view normal occlusion, favorable function, and acceptable dentofacial esthetics represented an identity. It was not possible to have one without the others. Normal occlusion was the central theme that

brought about perfect harmony and balance in function and esthetics. This view included favorable physiologic adaptation because normal occlusion was thought to stimulate alveolar bone formation and, in turn, periodontal health and tooth stability. Clinical experience has shown that these concepts, however attractive, are incorrect.

Early critics of the traditional diagnostic approach (e.g., Case; Hellman; Simon) maintained that proper diagnosis required a deeper understanding of the orthodontic problem. The concepts of dental and skeletal components of malocclusion can be credited to these men. They challenged Angle's idea of the constancy of position of the maxillary first molars, and suggested that it is an insufficient diagnosis to say, for example, "Class II, division 1 malocclusion." Rather, it is necessary to ascertain whether the maxillary teeth are positioned too far anteriorly or the mandibular teeth too far posteriorly, the maxilla is prognathic or the mandible retrognathic, or any combination of these factors. This approach to diagnosis can be called the rational approach. Perhaps it achieved its fullest expression with Sassouni,[131] who suggested that there are 128 different types of Class II, division 1 malocclusions.

A third view of diagnosis, which Moorrees and Gron termed *overall diagnosis*,[98] takes into consideration not only the dental, skeletal, and muscular factors considered by Hellman, Simon, and others, but also the somatic and emotional development of the individual and a host of personal and societal factors. In this chapter the overall approach to diagnosis is recommended. In our view, the goal of the diagnostic process in orthodontics is to produce a list of *all* the patient's problems and to state them clearly and concisely.

Orthodontic Diagnosis Compared with Medical Diagnosis

Although in orthodontics the term *diagnosis* is used in contexts similar to its use elsewhere in medicine and dentistry, there is a subtle but important difference in meaning. In medical diagnosis one attempts to understand the nature of a disease process through observation, interpretation, and labeling or symbolization. A disease results from a host-disorder interaction and is manifested as a deviation from normal. Disease manifestations are objective signs that can be seen or measured by the physician, and subjective symptoms that can be reported by the patient. Underlying a patient's signs and symptoms are physiologic or pathologic processes that are triggered by etiologic or causative factors.

Malocclusion is the result of a developmental process, not pathology, and the objective signs typically measured by the orthodontist are morphologic characteristics rather than the physiologic measurements of function (temperature, fluid compositions, etc.) used by the physician treating an illness. Nevertheless, the orthodontist needs to keep in mind that it is the symptoms of impaired function and/or psychosocial acceptance that has led the patient to seek treatment, not the morphologic signs per se.

The Diagnostic Process in Orthodontics

For nongrowing patients, the variables that should be evaluated and correlated in orthodontic diagnosis are those represented in Table 1-7. Although this table is a theoretical construct, most of the situations listed in the table not only are possible, but also occur frequently. The table merely describes groupings of signs and symptoms; it does not imply causality. Occlusal disharmony does not necessarily determine poor function, just as good occlusion does not always result in good physiologic adaptation. The same is true of facial imbalance and psychosocial difficulties. An apparently minor esthetic disproportion may have major consequences for the patient, or alternatively, a major facial imbalance may have little impact.

The table, however, is not sufficient for diagnosis. In the typology, the variables are treated as if they were discrete, discontinuous traits, such as eye color or blood group antigens; however, occlusion, dentofacial esthetics and self-image, and function-physiologic adaptation really are continuous variables (like height and weight). For this reason there are a large number of combinations or permutations rather than just the 16 shown in the typology.

In addition, the orthodontist most often treats young, growing patients. Thus it is necessary to forecast changes in occlusion, esthetics, and function attributed to growth and to forecast the likely impact of these changes. Other interesting challenges arise in evaluating a child patient: e.g., the orthodontist must consider the face and dentition in five dimensions—three of space and two of time. In terms of time the dentofacial complex may be viewed from the standpoint of evolution (e.g., phylogenetic and ontogenetic time) or from the standpoint of the development of the individual (chronologic time).

Perhaps an even more difficult condition of orthodontic diagnosis is that some of our standards in orthodontics are culturally imposed. Peck and Peck[109] have shown that the esthetic standards of the public do not always correlate with the accepted esthetics for orthodontists. The choice of treatment in orthodontics depends to some extent on social, ethical, and economic factors regarding the patient, the patient's family, and the society in which they live. When the clinician is forced to make esthetic and ethical judgments about a fundamentally biologic problem, art (not science) is being invoked, and the final decision should represent wisdom and not necessarily truth in a scientific sense.[1]

The more systematically an orthodontist approaches the collection of adequate diagnostic data and the more thoroughly those data are interpreted in terms of expected treatment responses, the better will be the probability of successful treatment.

Problem-Oriented Diagnosis and Treatment Planning

An approach to decision making in orthodontics that simplifies this complex but often diverse cognitive process is a modification of Weed's[158] problem-oriented approach to medical records (see Fig. 1-1). In this approach the goal of the diagnostic process is to produce a list of the individual patient's problems, taking into account both subjective and objective findings.

For the clinician to separate the various elements of the orthodontic problem into a rational diagnosis, it is fundamental that an adequate data base be established. Usually, too little time is devoted to this aspect of orthodontics. When work is begun from such a data base, orthodontic diagnosis becomes the process of synthesizing the manifold factors

TABLE 1-7

General Indications for Orthodontic Treatment

Signs	With dysfunction With psychosocial implications	With dysfunction Without psychosocial implications	Without dysfunction With psychosocial implications	Without dysfunction Without psychosocial implications
	← Symptoms →			
Major malocclusion Major facial imbalance	Treatment needed	Treatment needed	Treatment needed	Treatment desirable
Major malocclusion Minor facial imbalance	Treatment needed	Treatment needed	Treatment needed	Treatment desirable
Minor malocclusion Major facial imbalance	Treatment mandatory	Treatment desirable	Ortho elective May require surgery	Treatment effective
Minor malocclusion Minor facial imbalance	Treatment mandatory	Treatment desirable	Treatment elective	No treatment

of a complex situation into a discrete list of problems, each of which suggests a tentative solution. Proper diagnosis in clinical orthodontics is equivalent to a good hypothesis in basic research. A well-stated hypothesis is a question so well phrased that an answer is inherent in the question. A well-conceived diagnosis automatically suggests appropriate treatment plans.

THE DATA BASE FOR ORTHODONTIC DIAGNOSIS: GENERAL CONSIDERATIONS

One of the major appeals of the Angle classification for the orthodontist has been that it represents a shorthand or abbreviated description of a complex problem. Angle's genius in this regard is undisputed. Nevertheless, other descriptors of orthodontic problems are equally as powerful as Angle's morphologic description and conjure for the orthodontist a picture of the type of problem under discussion. For instance, both *amelogenesis imperfecta* and *airway obstruction* suggest that the patient has some type of skeletal open bite malocclusion. Amelogenesis imperfecta is a general evaluative characteristic derived from the dental history of the patient and confirmed by clinical examination; airway obstruction is a functional characteristic noted clinically. Another general evaluative characteristic, McGregor's Index Degree 4 (definitely shocking and repelling to others; evokes violent reaction of horror, repulsion, and pity)[87] obviously describes a patient with a craniofacial anomaly.

The goal in orthodontic diagnosis and the goal of the classification process that in orthodontics is used to organize the diagnostic data base is to fully describe the patient's problems with the best possible economy of words, using as few descriptors as possible to portray a clear picture of situation. A systematic description in orthodontics requires that three major categories be considered for each patient: general evaluative, functional, and structural. Within each category are five descriptors and a number of collateral descriptive characteristics. The 15 descriptive elements are:

General evaluative
   Psychosocial (self-image, self-esteem, reaction of others)
   Medical-dental history
   Genetic history
   Social-behavioral history
   Physical and growth-maturation status
Functional
   Condylar position/pathologic occlusion/TMD symptoms
   Habits
   Tongue and lip posture/airway
   Speech
   Eating/masticatory efficiency
Structural
   Alignment/symmetry within dental arches
   Facial esthetics/profile

Transverse dental/jaw relationships (posterior crossbite)
Sagittal (A-P) dental/jaw relationships (Angle Class)
Vertical dental/jaw relationships (deep/open bite)

Thus, to fully describe an orthodontic condition requires consideration of three major areas, each with five or fewer descriptive elements. The general evaluative elements are derived mostly from the patient's history. The functional elements are elucidated mostly from clinical examination of the patient, and the structural elements are defined in greatest detail by an analysis of the patient's diagnostic records. This organizational approach serves as the format for collecting and organizing the orthodontic data base, and provides the foundation for a problem-oriented treatment planning scheme as outlined in Fig. 1-1. Much of the emphasis will be on the data base; of necessity, a major focus also will be on the use of structural analysis in establishing problem lists. The final section of the chapter illustrates the integration of problems, goals, and practical considerations into a treatment plan that can be presented to the patient for informed consent.

INTERVIEW DATA: GENERAL EVALUATION
Initial Patient Contact

Data collection for the orthodontist begins with the first encounter with the patient and/or parent. This first contact is usually by telephone, and certain demographic information should be recorded then. The patient's age, the source of referral, the family's dentist, and (by inference) the orthodontist's other patients who live in that particular neighborhood are all clues to what this family's orthodontic awareness may be. The ease or difficulty with which the receptionist can schedule the first appointment may also indicate the type of demands this family may make in the future and the amount of cooperation that may be forthcoming during treatment.

When the patient arrives for the first appointment, the *chief orthodontic concern* can be revealing. "What aspect of Jane's orthodontic problem concerns you most?" will elicit a variety of answers. These can range from "The space between her front teeth" to "None, it was our dentist's idea that we come for an evaluation." Whether the parents' orientation is primarily cosmetic or whether their greatest concern is with function and oral health will usually be revealed in this interview.

Medical-Dental History

In obtaining the medical history a few major questions must always be asked (Fig. 1-22). Since many patients and parents do not realize the relationship that overall health has to dentofacial development, persistence in the pursuit of answers to these questions is important.

The patient is asked when he or she last saw a physician, and why. Next, the patient is asked whether he or she has ever been hospitalized. If the hospitalization was for tonsillectomy and adenoidectomy, the orthodontist now has a clue that the patient may have had earlier difficulties with breathing and tongue posture—factors that are associated with vertical problems such as open bites. Sometimes the patient's admission to the hospital may have been the result of a traumatic experience, such as a car accident, and it is important to find out whether the patient's teeth or jaws were affected. What the examiner is searching for is whether the patient has had any serious health problems.

Next, the question should be asked: Is the patient taking any medication? A parent who is reluctant to tell the orthodontist or the assistant that a child is epileptic will nevertheless usually be open about reporting that the patient takes Dilantin or other anticonvulsant drugs. It is important to know that anticonvulsant drugs are in use if a seizure or other medical emergency occurs. These drugs also can influence orthodontic tooth movement if gingival hyperplasia occurs. Chronic steroid medication reduces resistance to infection and may lead to problems in tolerating orthodontic appliances. The reasons for medication should be followed up with the patient's physician.

Other important areas to explore are: allergies, especially latex sensitivity or nickel sensitivity (latex gloves and elastics, and wires and brackets containing nickel will be encountered during orthodontic treatment); history of blood transfusions (greatly increased chance of hepatitis or AIDS virus exposure); and heart problems, such as mitral valve prolapse or rheumatic fever (antibiotic prophylaxis is required for invasive procedures such as banding). Other questions and the potential importance of the answers for orthodontic treatment are shown in the annotations to Fig. 1-22.

The dental health status of the parents, particularly regarding loss of teeth, sometimes indicates the patient's potential susceptibility to periodontal disease. Questions regarding the family's dental history often reveal the parent's oral health awareness. Another question should be asked specifically: Has the patient ever had a traumatic accident involving the teeth? Orthodontic treatment can exacerbate periapical symptoms in teeth that are already marginal because of trauma. Usually the tooth movement alone is blamed if problems arise.

Genetic History

A genetic history can begin with an inquiry as to whether any siblings have required orthodontic treatment and a discussion about the nature of their problems. Inquiries should also be made as to whether either or both of the parents received orthodontic treatment. If the answer is *yes*, the orthodontist will need to know the reasons for their treatment. It is not unusual today to have a parent respond that a close relative had a significant malocclusion that required surgery. When examining the child, the orthodontist should be alert to facial characteristics that might be associated with a craniofacial syndrome (see Tables 1-3 through 1-6).

Social-Behavioral History

Part of the evaluation of a patient should also focus on the social and behavioral history. This information is more difficult to obtain, since parents are often reluctant to speak about a child's emotional problems. A question about progress in school can be helpful in this regard. If the orthodontist suspects that there might be an emotional problem because of findings, such as a prolonged thumbsucking habit, poor progress in school, sleepwalking in a young child, or enuresis in an older child, it is often easiest to ask whether the child or the family is receiving counseling. If any major problems exist, it is usually at this point that a mother will tell of a divorce, a husband's death or illness, or another major problem in the home.

Questions about school progress may reveal that the child has a learning disability. If this is the case the orthodontist should modify somewhat the approach to the child. Since learning-disabled patients may have a short attention span,

---

Fig. 1-22 (see pp. 30-31)   A form for obtaining the medical/dental history for a child or adolescent seeking orthodontic treatment. A similar but modified form is needed for older patients. The annotations below indicate the orthodontic relevance of selected items, with the numbers keyed to the form:

3. *This helps establish the possibility of previous trauma and injury to the face (condylar fracture) or teeth.*
4. *If trauma occurs during treatment, the DPT status is important, and oral soft tissue lacerations are more likely if orthodontic appliances are in place.*
8b,c,d,f. *These patients need antibiotic coverage during orthodontic banding and debanding procedures (but not for routine appliance adjustments).*
8g,h,i,j,k. *With modern infection control procedures, these patients can be treated, but the treatment may need to be modified to limit its scope or invasiveness.*
8n. *Diabetic patients who slip out of control can experience rapid periodontal degeneration during orthodontic treatment.*
9-12. *These questions help establish growth status.*
16. *The parent and patient's concerns must be considered carefully when the treatment objectives are established.*
19a. *It is better radiation hygiene to obtain recent radiographs from referring practitioners, rather than retaking them.*
19g. *Bleeding on probing is the major clinical sign of active periodontal disease, which must be controlled before orthodontic treatment begins.*
19i. *Careful pretreatment investigation of any tendency toward temporomandibular dysfuncton is necessary.*
19j. *There is a familial tendency toward some facial patterns (especially mandibular prognathism, and to a lesser extent long face problems). Congenitally missing teeth also have a documented genetic component.*
19k. *Dental trauma increases the chance of endodontic complications during orthodontic treatment.*
(Adapted from Proffit WR: *Contemporary orthodontics*, St Louis, 1993, Mosby.)

MEDICAL HISTORY
(Child/Adolescent)

PATIENT NAME: _____   DATE: _____

BIRTH DATE: _____

Name of your child's Physician: _____   Office Phone: _____

Address of your child's Physician: _____   Date of last exam: _____

1. Is your child in good health: .... Yes No Don't Know

2. Does your child have a health problem? .... Yes No Don't Know
   If yes, explain: _____

3. Has your child ever been hospitalized, had general anesthesia or emergency
   room visits: .... Yes No Don't Know
   If yes, explain: _____

4. Are your child's immunizations up to date: .... Yes No Don't Know

5. Allergies (please list): _____

6. Past medications taken by child: _____

7. Daily medications child is now taking: _____

8. Has your child ever had or been treated by a physician for:

Check

Yes	No	?	
			a. Problems at birth
			b. Heart murmur
			c. Heart disease
			d. Rheumatic fever
			e. Anemia
			f. Sickle cell anemia
			g. Bleeding/hemophilia
			h. Blood transfusion
			i. Hepatitis
			j. AIDS or HIV+
			k. Tuberculosis
			l. Liver disease
			m. Kidney disease

Check

Yes	No	?	
			n. Diabetes
			o. Arthritis
			p. Cancer
			q. Cerebral palsy
			r. Seizures
			s. Asthma
			t. Cleft lip/palate
			u. Speech or hearing problems
			v. Eye problems/contact lenses
			w. Skin problems
			x. Tonsil/adenoid problems
			y. Sleep problems
			z. Emotional/behavior problems

Fig. 1-22 See legend on p. 29.

9. Has your child had any recent rapid growth? _____ If so, how much? _____

10. Parents: (Father) Ht: _____ Wt: _____ (Mother) Ht: _____ Wt: _____

11. Older brothers and sisters: (1) Ht: _____ Wt: _____ (2) Ht: _____ Wt: _____ (3) Ht: _____ Wt: _____

12. Females: Has menstruation begun? _____ If yes, when: _____ Pregnant: _____

13. If yes to any above, please explain this or any other problem: _____

14. Child's grade in school: _____ Child's school: _____

15. Do you consider your child to be (check one): Advanced in learning ☐ Progressing normally ☐
    Slow learner ☐

DENTAL HISTORY

16. What is your main concern about your child's dental condition:_____

17. Has your child been to a dentist before? No Yes If yes, date of last visit:_____

18. Regular dentist's name: _____

19. Check

Yes	No	?	
			a. Has your child ever had dental x-rays? Date of last x-rays: _____
			b. Will your child be uncooperative? Is yes, explain: _____
			c. Has your child experienced any complications following dental treatment? If yes, explain____
			d. Has your child had cavities and/or toothaches?
			e. Are your child's teeth sensitive to temperature or food?
			f. Did you or your child ever get instructions in brushing?
			g. Do your child's gums bleed when brushed?
			h. Does your child use fluoride products: rinses, drops, tabs?
			i. Has your child had any clicking or pain in the jaw joints? If yes, explain: _____
			j. Has your child inherited any family facial or dental characteristics? If yes, explain:_____
			k. Has your child ever injured his or her teeth?
			l. Has your child ever injured his or her jaws or face?
			m. Did your child use a pacifier?
			n. Did your child suck a finger or thumb?

20. Does your child have any other dental problems we should know about? ____ Please explain: _____

21. Whom may we thank for referring you to our office? _____

22. PERSON COMPLETING THIS FORM: Signature _____

    Relationship to patient: _____

Fig. 1-22, cont'd See legend on p. 29.

it is unwise to offer them information that is too detailed or to give them too much information during the consultation. It is also not a good idea to introduce alternatives about which they must make decisions, since decision-making can often frustrate and produce anxiety for the learning-disabled person. In designing a treatment strategy for the learning-disabled patient, it may be preferable, whenever possible, to reduce the patient's responsibility in carrying out the treatment. For example, if a crossbite requires correction, it would be better to use a fixed rather than a removable appliance.

After hearing about a learning disability the interviewer must judge whether the patient would respond well to the additional attention that he or she would receive during orthodontics or whether treatment would represent one more insult (the proverbial last straw). Many children and almost all adolescents have some kind of minor or major emotional problem. Adults, whom the children see often and with whom they relate well, can have a positive influence on them during orthodontic treatment. The orthodontist often inadvertently serves in this role, and the astute clinician who realizes that treatment should be of the whole child can put forth a concerted effort when a problem is known to exist.

It is important to realize that the patient's behavior at home and in school may be different than it is in the orthodontist's office; however, the clinician does not truly know the patient without having a broad overview of behavior. Therefore an attempt should be made to elicit the child's feelings of self-worth. If a facial protrusion is the problem, how does it affect the child's self-evaluation? These are not questions that can be asked of the average youngster or parent, so the orthodontist must listen with a third ear. Do the other children at school call the child a funny name that relates to the appearance? Does the family inadvertently focus on one or more of the child's facial features? A child with an orthodontic problem, who has an accurate self-image and diminished self-esteem because of it, is likely to be a cooperative and appreciative patient. Frequently, the emotional outlook of this kind of patient will be improved after the appliances are placed. Sometimes teasing from peers stops as soon as they see the appliances in place.

Finally, it is wise to ask such patients, no matter what their age, how they think they will react to having orthodontic treatment and whether they think they will be cooperative patients. Children are very candid. They will usually say what they fear and what they dislike if they are approached in a nonthreatening fashion. Under almost any circumstances it is counterproductive to perform orthodontics for an antagonistic patient regardless of how severe the malocclusion may be. It is a good idea before beginning a course of treatment to wait until an uncooperative child sees the light or until the parents convince the child of the merit of orthodontics.

Although the social-behavioral history is important when a child patient is being evaluated, it is even more important

for an adult. The answer to two questions must be carefully sought from adults: "Why are you seeking orthodontic treatment now?" (as opposed to last year or next year) and "What do you expect from orthodontic treatment?" An adult patient who seeks treatment as an attempt to deal with social problems and who expects a change in life status as a result will be a much greater treatment (and posttreatment) problem than will the patient who is well adjusted socially and who now can afford the correction of an orthodontic problem (for example, dental protrusion) that has been a long-time annoyance. A surprising number of adults bring a hidden agenda to the orthodontist, and time spent exploring their motivations and expectations can be time well spent. The patient who has a minor deformity (e.g., crowded incisors) and a major complaint related to it ("I can't find a decent job because my teeth are so ugly") can be a definite problem during and after treatment if the dissatisfaction persists, as it almost always does.

Physical Growth Status

In the overall evaluation of a patient, it is important to judge general physical development in relation to the amount of growth that has occurred and the potential for future growth that remains. The beginning student in orthodontics usually must be convinced that the emphasis in orthodontic education on craniofacial growth and development is merited. Any experienced orthodontist knows that the best results are achieved in good growers (Figs. 1-23 and 1-24) and that the poorest clinical results occur in the poor growers (Fig. 1-25). By good grower the clinician means an amount, rate, direction, and pattern of growth that facilitates treatment. The degree to which orthodontic treatment affects growth is still debatable; however, the great extent to which craniofacial growth affects treatment is undisputed. Therefore the modifiability of a problem and the treatment prognosis are strongly influenced by growth. The acceleration of facial growth at puberty is mild compared to that occurring in the extremities of the body; however, it is significant, nevertheless, and the most favorable time to attack many orthodontic problems with skeletal manifestations is during this period of growth acceleration. Thus predicting the nature and timing of the onset of pubertal growth is important in planning orthodontic therapy.

One method of evaluating the growth status of a child is to plot the child's height and weight on standard growth charts. This method is particularly valuable in longitudinal studies of children, because the height-weight data indicate a channel of growth in which a particular child is likely to remain. A rise in the body height increment is a reasonably good indication that the acceleration in facial growth at puberty is beginning.

Another physical characteristic that should be noted is the general body build of the child; which is most frequently described in terms of Sheldon's somatotypes,[136] using the terms ectomorphic, mesomorphic, and endomorphic to describe tall and thin, average, or short and fat children, re-

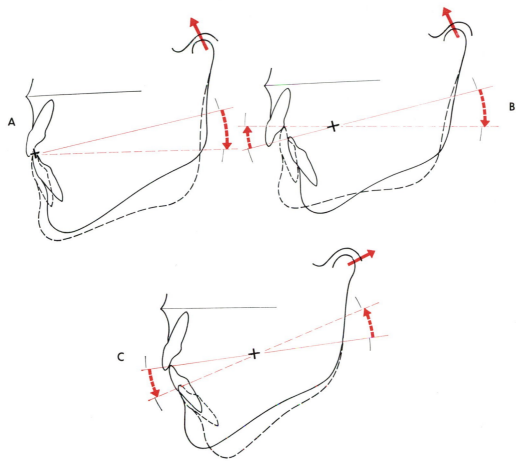

Fig. 1-23   Three types of rotation of the mandible during growth. **A,** Forward rotation, with the center at the mesial edges of the lower incisors. **B,** Forward rotation, with the center at the premolars. **C,** Backward rotation, with the center at the occluding third molars. The forward-rotating patterns are favorable for Class II treatment (provided the tendency toward deepening of the bite can be controlled) but not for Class III. Backward rotation increases the chance of open bite and makes open bite more difficult to correct. (From Björk A, Skieller V: *Am J Orthod* 62:339, 1972.)

spectively. This description has certain implications regarding somatic growth and development. Ectomorphic children tend to grow more slowly and to reach the pubertal growth spurt later than do mesomorphic or endomorphic children.[151] Thus certain types of therapy might be deferred for ectomorphic patients beyond the time at which they would be instituted in children with a different body build. Not all tissues of the body grow at the same rate, of course. The well-known growth curves originally presented by Scammon[133] demonstrate the different pattern of growth for nervous tissues, lymphatic tissue, the genital organs, and the general body. Craniofacial growth is affected by the differential between neural growth and the general bodily curve. An intermediate position between these differing curves best represents the growth of the face and jaws, as shown in Fig. 1-26. Maxillary growth precedes mandibular growth somewhat.

As Fig. 1-26 indicates, the acceleration of general body

growth that occurs at puberty is directly and causally related to sexual maturation and the onset of rapid sexual development. The relation of various markers of sexual maturation to the somatic growth spurt is indicated in Figs. 1-27 and 1-28. Perhaps the most straightforward indicator of sexual maturation is the beginning of menstruation in females; however, if a female has achieved menarche, the greatest part of her skeletal growth has already occurred. Thus menarche can be used only retrospectively as an indicator that the peak of the pubertal growth spurt has passed. The earlier, more subtle signs of sexual maturation in males and females must be used to obtain insight into the stages of sexual development and degrees of progress into the adolescent growth spurt.

Just as a patient's dental age can be established by comparing the eruption pattern and amount of root development of permanent teeth with those expected at a given age, skeletal age can be established by comparing ossification

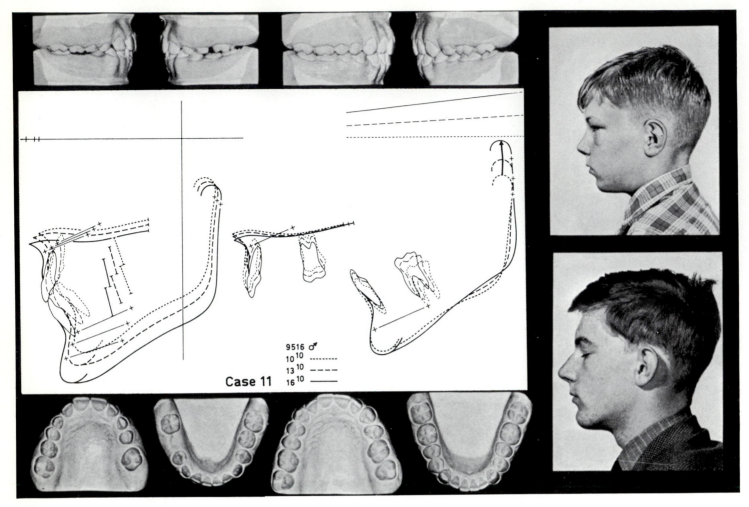

Fig. 1-24 Favorable forward-rotating mandibular growth pattern. (From Björk A, Skieller V: *Am J Orthod* 62:339, 1972.)

patterns of various skeletal elements. Dental development correlates with other aspects of general body development, but the correlation is relatively poor. Dental age is not a good indicator of the timing of skeletal growth and the adolescent growth spurt. Skeletal age, on the other hand, correlates reasonably well with the physical growth status and, accordingly, has been used in orthodontic diagnosis for this purpose. Usually, the ossification stage of the hand and wrist bones is employed. It is easy to obtain a wrist film with the standard cephalometric x-ray unit or even with a dental x-ray machine. Skeletal age is established from the film using the standards of Greulich and Pyle.[51] Unfortunately, the relationship between physical growth and skeletal maturity is least reliable in children who are most deviant from the general population: in the children with severe malocclusion in whom information about growth status is most needed.

Specific indicators of the pubertal growth spurt have been sought on wrist films (Fig. 1-29). The beginning of ossi-

fication of the adductor sesamoid and the appearance of the hook of the hamate serve to some extent as indicators of the onset of puberty.[50] Unfortunately, establishing the timing of puberty from wrist films is only marginally better than guessing, and this method should be used only in conjunction with the other indicators of overall bodily growth, with a full understanding that errors can occur when wrist films are used alone.[60]

In the general evaluation it is important not to overlook the child's neuromuscular status and level of physiologic, as opposed to anatomic, maturation. An evaluation of these factors can begin with observing the child's general muscular coordination. Serious problems will be revealed immediately in difficulties with gait and posture. Many factors that in the past were grouped under the general heading of habits may instead be either necessary physiologic adaptations (e.g., mouth breathing in a child who has nasal obstruction) or behavior that was appropriate at an earlier age but now represents some developmental immaturity (e.g.,

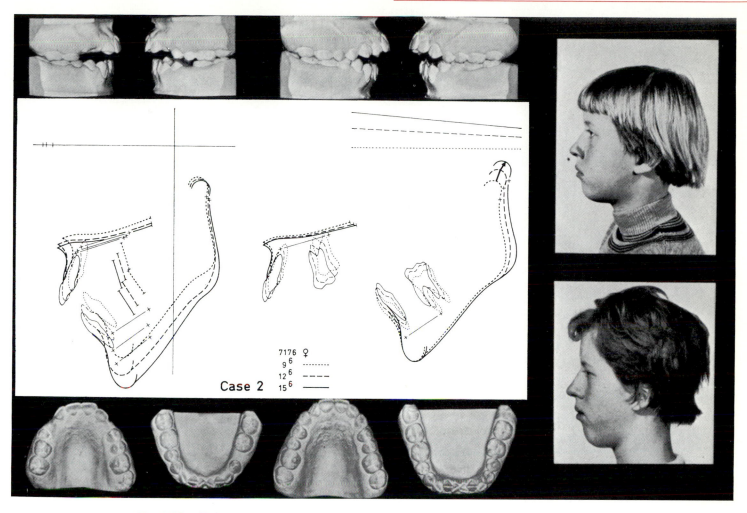

Fig. 1-25 Unfavorable backward-rotating mandibular growth pattern. (From Björk A, Skieller V: *Am J Orthod* 62:339, 1972.)

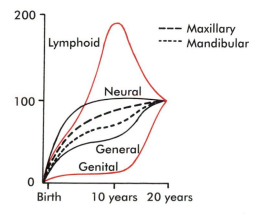

Fig. 1-26 Growth curves for various tissue systems (modified from Scammon). The curves for growth of the jaws are intermediate between the neural and general body growth curves; however, the maxilla is slightly closer to the neural curve and therefore slightly accelerated relative to the mandible.

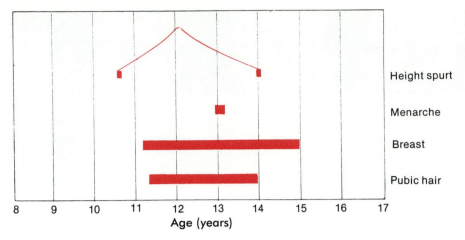

Fig. 1-27   Sequence of events of puberty in girls at various ages. The peak of the height curve represents the peak velocity of the spurt. The bars represent the beginning and the completion of the events of puberty. Although the adolescent growth spurt for girls typically begins at 10.5 years and ends at 14 years of age, it can start as early as 9.5 years and end as late as 15 years. Similarly, menarche can come at any time between the ages of 10 and 16.5 and tends to be a late event of puberty. Some girls begin to show breast development as early as 8 years and have completed it by age 13; others may not begin breast development until 13 years and complete it at age 18. Pubic hair first appears after the beginning of breast development in two thirds of all girls. (From Tanner JM: *Sci Am* 229:34, 1973. *All rights reserved.*)

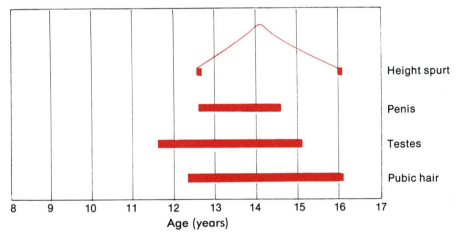

Fig. 1-28   Sequence of events of puberty in boys. The adolescent growth spurt of boys can begin as early as 10.5 years or as late as 16 years and can end anywhere from 13.5 years to age 17.5. Elongation of the penis can begin from age 10.5 years to age 14.5 and can end from 12.5 years to 16.5. Growth of the testes can begin as early as 9.5 years or as late as age 13.5 and can end at any time between the ages of 13.5 and 17. (From Tanner JM: *Sci Am* 229:34, 1973. *All rights reserved.*)

tongue thrusting in many young patients). Thumbsucking, finger sucking, lip biting, and nail biting are examples of common childhood habits that affect the developing dentition. The specific oral behaviors affecting the teeth will be discussed more thoroughly in the section on oral examination; however, it should be remembered that these factors relate to the overall stage of physiologic maturation just as

the amount of future craniofacial growth relates to general bodily development.

In this section we have tried to point out the vast amount of information that can be learned about a patient before an oral examination is performed or a set of orthodontic records is obtained and analyzed. The orthodontist who does not take advantage of this information in formulating a diagnosis

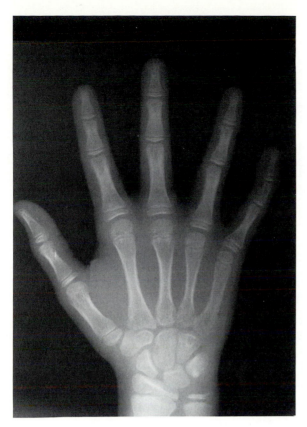

Fig. 1-29 A hand-wrist radiograph is used to obtain the skeletal age of a boy undergoing growth modification treatment for Class II malocclusion. The skeletal age is established by comparing the pattern of ossification with a standard atlas of the hand and wrist[88]; specific indicators of the adolescent growth spurt also can be evaluated.[89] One method that is quite successful for clinical use is to evaluate the status of several anatomical landmarks, such as the distal and middle epiphyseal plates of the fifth phalanx (little finger) and the epiphyseal plates of the radius and ulna, to gain a sense of where the patient is along the statural growth curve and then to use the presence or absence of the sesamoids and the hook of the hamate as additional indicators of the adolescent growth spurt.

and plan of treatment is potentially penalizing himself or herself as well as the patient. The technique of effective history taking is asking the right questions and listening to what the patient or parent says and discerning the meaning of the replies.

CLINICAL EXAMINATION DATA: ORAL HEALTH, FUNCTION, DENTOFACIAL PROPORTIONS/ESTHETICS

A careful clinical examination is an essential part of orthodontic diagnosis. It should include three major areas: (1) health of the intraoral soft and hard tissues; (2) function of the oral structures (this includes an evaluation of condylar position and TMD signs/symptoms, and of tooth wear and/

or gingival recession related to the occlusion [which Amsterdam[7] called evidence of *pathologic occlusion*]; habits; airway and tongue/lip posture; eating and masticatory efficiency; and speech); and (3) dentofacial proportions and facial esthetics. The examination has two goals: to provide diagnostic data, and to determine what diagnostic records are needed.

Health of Teeth and Intraoral Soft Tissues

The initial examination of any patient should include a careful analysis of the health and function of the hard and soft tissues. The availability of rapidly processed panoramic dental radiographs has changed routine clinical examination. A better clinical evaluation can be done with a panoramic radiograph at hand. Questions about whether teeth are missing or unerupted can be answered immediately, bony defects can be observed, a good view of the mandibular condyles usually is available, and supplementary radiographs can be ordered as needed. We assume in this discussion that a panoramic radiograph is available at the time of the clinical examination, and we recommend that this radiograph be taken at the patient's initial appointment, not deferred until other diagnostic records are collected.

As part of visual and tactile examination of the dentition, it is important to count the teeth. A quick check should be made for mobility of the primary or permanent teeth. In the mixed dentition one should palpate for unerupted maxillary canines, since it often is not possible from the radiographs to ascertain whether these teeth are erupting labially or palatally. It should be possible to palpate a labially positioned canine. Ankylosed primary teeth usually appear submerged (Fig. 1-30). Tapping these with the handle of a dental instrument usually produces a somewhat higher *ring* than that from a normal tooth. Any other abnormalities of the hard tissues should be noted, such as enamel defects and internal or external resorption.

From the panoramic radiograph, numerous aspects of the dentition can be assessed: teeth that are present yet unerupted, teeth that are impacted, supernumerary teeth, unusual crown forms or other abnormalities, and any congenitally missing teeth (Fig. 1-31). Furthermore, the panoramic film will reveal any periapical pathosis or periodontal breakdown. The caries incidence should be judged from the oral examination. Although gross caries can be detected on the panoramic film, if there is evidence of active caries or previous caries activity, bitewing film should supplement the panoramic survey in the complete examination (see Table 1-8 for the current USPHS recommendations for dental radiographic examination for pathology).

From the panoramic radiograph also, an assessment can be made of the amount of calcification of unerupted teeth and, by means of root calcification norms, the dental age of a patient can be established[92] (Fig. 1-32). In addition, the amount of root calcification can be used for predicting the timing of tooth emergence.[52] It is also a good idea to establish the dental age based on eruptive norms, and for

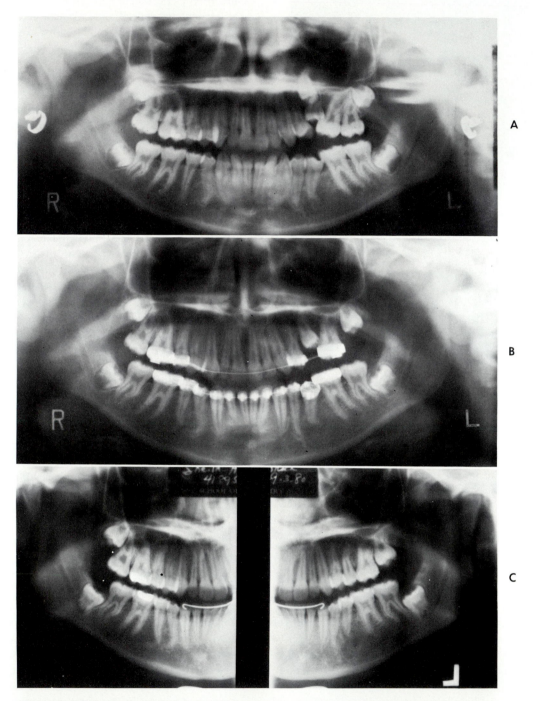

Fig. 1-30 Failure of eruption of the maxillary second premolar because of mechanical obstruction. **A,** Age 13. The left maxillary deciduous second molar is ankylosed and submerging, with obstruction and displacement of the permanent successor. **B,** After the ankylosed deciduous molar and the permanent second molar has been extracted, there is spontaneous eruption of the premolar toward the space produced by distal movement of the first molar. **C,** Final position of the second premolar in functioning occlusion, after completion of orthodontic treatment. (From Proffit WR et al: *Am J Orthod* 80:181, 1981.)

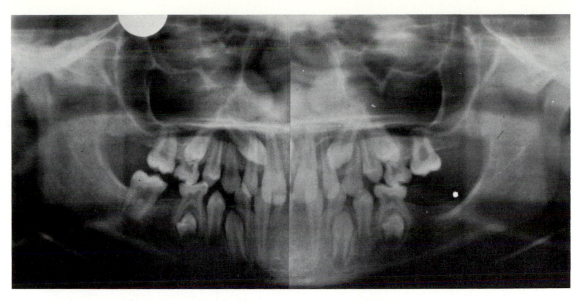

Fig. 1-31 Multiple congenital absence of teeth and poorly erupting and impacted permanent teeth. It is not unusual to find these two conditions occurring together.

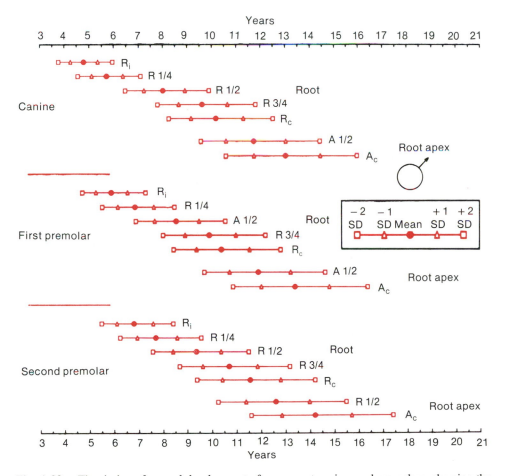

Fig. 1-32 The timing of normal development of permanent canines and premolars, showing the times at which root formation begins; the root is ¼, ½, ¾ and totally completed, the apex is ½ closed, and the apex is totally closed. Two standard deviations in either direction are indicated. This chart is particularly useful in comparing the development of one tooth in a child's mouth (for example, a suspiciously slow second premolar) to the other teeth. (From Moorrees CFA et al: *Angle Orthod* 33:44, 1963.)

TABLE 1-8

Orthodontic Radiographic Examination Developmental Status, Dental Pathology*

No clinical caries, history of fluoridation	Panoramic only
Clinical caries and/or restorations present	Panoramic plus posterior bitewings
Deep clinical caries	Panoramic, posterior bitewings, periapicals of affected teeth
Periodontal involvement	Panoramic, posterior bitewings, periapicals of affected teeth

*Recommendations from US Department of Human Services: *The selection of patients for x-ray examination: dental radiographic examination,* Pub No FDA 88-8273, Rockville, Md, 1987, US Food and Drug Administration.

this purpose the standards of Hurme[61] can be used (Fig. 1-33).

Supplemental periapical radiographs may be needed in some children with no evidence of pathology if there is reason to suspect abnormalities of unerupted teeth or if the incisor roots cannot be seen clearly on the panoramic film. These should be obtained only if needed and not taken routinely.

Examination of the soft tissues should begin with the buccal and labial mucosa, taking special note of the frenal attachments. Is there a heavy frenum in the area of a maxillary midline diastema? Surgical removal of the attachment before orthodontic tooth movement is contraindicated in most instances; however, surgical removal of excess tissue

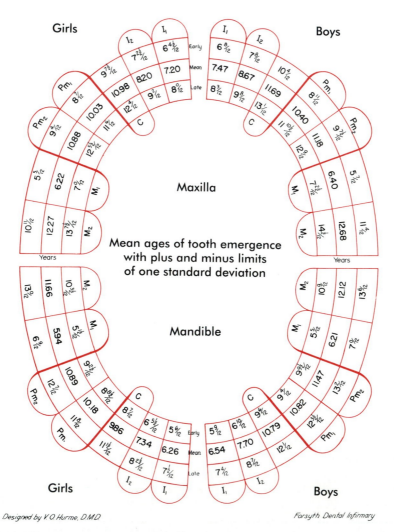

Fig. 1-33 This chart, developed by Hurme, shows the time of emergence of the permanent teeth for boys and girls. The maxillary teeth are shown in the upper half of the chart and the mandibular teeth are below; girls are on the left, and boys are on the right. The mean age for appearance of each tooth is shown in the middle row, with one standard deviation above and below the mean indicated. Note that girls have earlier eruption on the average and that there is considerable normal variation. Clinically, it is more significant if one tooth deviates from the pattern for the rest of the teeth for a particular patient rather than all the teeth being advanced or delayed. (From Hurme VO: *J Dent Child* 16:11, 1949.)

may be required after the space has been closed if the initial diastema was greater than 3 mm.[34] Is there gingival clefting or recession in the lower incisor region near a high frenum? Such an attachment often causes periodontal problems and may require early intervention.

After examination of the mucosa the health of the gingiva should be addressed. Gingivitis is common in children; however, severe periodontal problems are uncommon, even in the presence of severe malocclusion. The discovery of bone loss in a child should lead to the suspicion of an underlying systemic illness (e.g., diabetes, blood dyscrasia) or hormonal imbalance. Occasionally, juvenile periodontitis, with rapid bone loss around first molars and central incisors, will be observed. Orthodontic treatment to close the space where first molars have been lost may be needed in such children; and once the periodontal problem has been brought under control, this treatment can be carried out without recurrence of the periodontitis, even if it was severe enough to lead to loss of multiple teeth initially.[89]

Two other periodontal problems often are observed in patients who are candidates for orthodontic treatment: (1) clefts of the gingiva around severely retrusive or badly rotated mandibular incisors; and (2) gingival hyperplasia and fibrosis in children receiving anticonvulsive medication such as phenytoin (Dilantin). Gingival clefts usually reflect a lack of attached gingiva and may occur in any area of the mouth, although they are most common in the mandibular anterior region. Periodontal surgery to provide a wider zone of attached gingiva, usually accomplished by a free gingival graft, is the usual treatment for patients with gingival clefts. Patients taking Dilantin or equivalent drugs may need gingivectomy or gingivoplasty while under orthodontic treatment. If there are concerns about the periodontal condition, the periodontist should be consulted early, before the orthodontic treatment plan is formulated. It is much easier to prevent periodontal complications from orthodontic treatment than to correct them once they have occurred (Fig. 1-34). In adult orthodontic patients a periodontal consultation and preliminary periodontic treatment should be routine.

When the incisors are protrusive, the alveolar bone will be thin, with an occasional dehiscence (vertical splitting) or with fenestrations (round holes) in the bone wall. Such defects can be detected with a periodontal probe. Expansion of the dental arch has reached its biologic limit when these defects begin to appear, and further expansion of the arch during orthodontic treatment is contraindicated.

As a final step in the soft tissue examination, the tautness or flaccidity of the lips and cheeks should be noted. Since resting pressures are an important determinant of stable tooth positions, they can provide valuable insight into the possibilities for arch expansion or, conversely, the need for extraction to deal with crowding.

Functional Evaluation

Condylar position, TMD signs/symptoms. In orthodontics the analysis of jaw function and functional occlusion now receives much greater emphasis. Many clinicians have strong opinions about what constitutes proper jaw function and how to analyze this diagnostically. Unfortunately, these opinions are widely divergent. The same diagnostic information often is said to be vital or unimportant depending upon how the clinician intends to use it for treatment planning. It is fair to say that scientific evidence for many current views is lacking. In this section we attempt to provide a conservative view of an evolving situation, emphasizing established findings and attempting to place controversial aspects in perspective.

The first step in functional analysis is to examine the patient's maximum jaw opening. For adults, the maximum opening should be 45 mm or more; for children it is proportionally smaller. In neither children nor adults should the mandible deviate laterally upon opening.

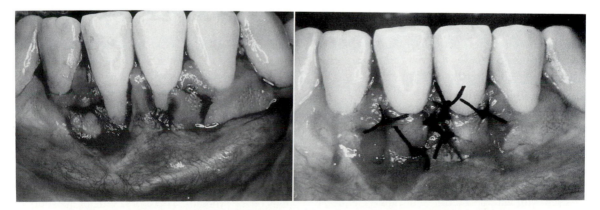

Fig. 1-34 When lower incisors are advanced orthodontically or when a lower border osteotomy to reposition the chin is planned, an adequate gingival attachment is necessary to prevent gingival recession from occurring later. It is much easier to prevent this complication by placing a gingival graft early than to attempt to correct stripping of the tissue later with laterally repositioned flaps, as shown here or in similar periodontal surgery techniques. (Courtesy John Moriarty.)

In children, either limitation of opening or lateral deviation usually is the result of previous injury to one or both condyles. Fracture of the condyles at an early age is more common than once thought, but in the majority of patients an early subcondylar fracture results in no permanent deformity. If scarring in the TM joint area occurs, however, so that translation of the mandible is impeded, there will be an interference with normal growth. This situation is best described as a *functional ankylosis* and its recognition is clinically quite important because the prognosis for orthodontic treatment based on growth modification is poor. If a child can open only on a hinge movement, the resulting limitation of maximum opening may be the first sign of a potentially serious difficulty.

In adults, limitation of opening can be produced by a number of factors, and the most common factor is muscle spasm. When limitation of opening is present or when facial pain is noted, palpation to detect sore spots of not only the joint but also the muscles of the head and neck is important. TM joint crepitus or clicking should be noted—the possible significance is discussed in the ensuing paragraphs.

A second important step in analysis of jaw function is to establish the path of closure of the mandible and to determine whether the maximum intercuspal position (centric or habitual occlusion) corresponds to the retruded position (centric relation). The proper registration of centric relation is extremely controversial. Placing the mandible in its most posterosuperior position by heavy pressure on the jaw, as was commonly recommended a decade ago, is not physiologic. Treating patients to this position may create functional problems rather than solve them. Almost all patients have a small (1 to 2 mm) forward shift from the posterior position to centric occlusion, and careful studies by Stockli[148] and others have shown that even if orthodontic treatment is done to eliminate this discrepancy, it will reappear. Arthrographic and magnetic resonance imaging (MRI) studies of the TM joint show that in some patients the articular disk can be displaced[24,104]; if this has occurred, it is easy to understand how the mandible could be forced too far posteriorly. It is an error, therefore, to assume automatically that the most posterosuperior position into which the mandible can be manipulated is the true centric relation.

Disk displacements and internal derangements of the TM joint are quite rare in children, so the establishment of a discrepancy between centric relation and centric occlusion (CR-CO) is much less problematic in younger patients. However, CR-CO discrepancies are often found in children, and it is important that these be noted clinically. Shifts of the mandible to an acquired centric occlusion (which can be considered deflective malocclusions) are particularly likely in children with anteroposterior and transverse problems. Unilateral crossbites are usually the result of a lateral shift of the mandible in response to narrow width of the maxillary arch. Obviously it is important to distinguish this condition from a true skeletal asymmetry. In children with either a Class II or a Class III malocclusion there can be a tendency to posture the jaw forward into an acquired occlusion, which makes the Class III situation look worse and the Class II situation look better. The mandibular deficient patient who postures the mandible forward, concealing the severity of the skeletal problem, can be a real embarrassment if treatment is planned without recognition of the true extent of the discrepancy.

The situation for postpubertal adolescents and adults is more complex, especially if there are TMD symptoms. Some patients tolerate degrees of occlusal disharmony that would evoke severe symptoms in others. Bruxing or clenching habits are an essential component of TMD symptomatology. In the absence of internal joint problems or other pathologic conditions, symptoms are almost never produced by normal function but instead relate to the extent of parafunctional activity and the amount of muscle spasm that results.

When the true centric relation for an older patient is difficult to ascertain because of the presence of muscle spasm, it may be necessary to use an interocclusal splint to disclude the teeth before making the determination. Such a splint also often improves TMD symptoms. The use of thin plastic strips (leaf gauges) to disclude anterior teeth as a routine method for establishing centric relation results in a more upward and forward position of the condyle than is achieved by pressure on the chin. As a general rule, in patients with TMD the mandibular musculature will tend to seat the condyles upward and forward when a disclusion splint is placed.

A more extreme approach to allowing the muscles to determine condylar position is the use of electrical stimulation to obtain centric relation.[63] Centric relation determined in this way routinely is anterior to the centric relation produced by the disclusion approach and often is several millimeters forward from the most retruded position to which the mandible can be pushed. Since surface electrodes are used in the *myocentric* technique and since this results in greater stimulation of superficial than deep muscles, the validity of the electrical stimulation approach remains questionable.

The final step in analysis of jaw function is to examine functional excursions. If TMD symptoms are present, accurate analysis may require mounting diagnostic casts on an adjustable articulator. Determining the centric relation position is the critical step, and articulator mountings are no better than the centric relation recording on which they are based.

It is important for the orthodontist to realize that jaw function problems are not always related to the occlusion. Especially in older patients, internal pathology of the joint may be the problem. Therefore, a major question for clinical examination is whether any special diagnostic procedures should be carried out. If internal derangements are suspected, special radiographic or MRI studies of the joint may be indicated (see below).

Habits. The role of habits as causal factors for malocclusion probably has been overstated in the past (see the section on etiology, above). Nevertheless, habits can be important, especially in patients who have anterior open bite and incisor protrusion. Part of the clinical examination should involve a careful examination of the patient for habits that might be causal agents. The prime suspects are thumb-sucking or other sucking habits, lip biting, nail biting, or related biting habits (unilateral posterior open bite has been traced on occasion to the habit of biting the cap to a ballpoint pen for most of the school day). Tongue thrust swallow is always present when there is an open bite. In itself, this is of little significance; however, it may reflect an altered tongue posture that is important. In the past, musical instruments have been indicted as the cause of various malocclusions. Current evidence suggests that unless the patient plays the instrument for far more hours per day than any but the most dedicated musician would devote, there will be little or no impact on the dentition[71]—which does not

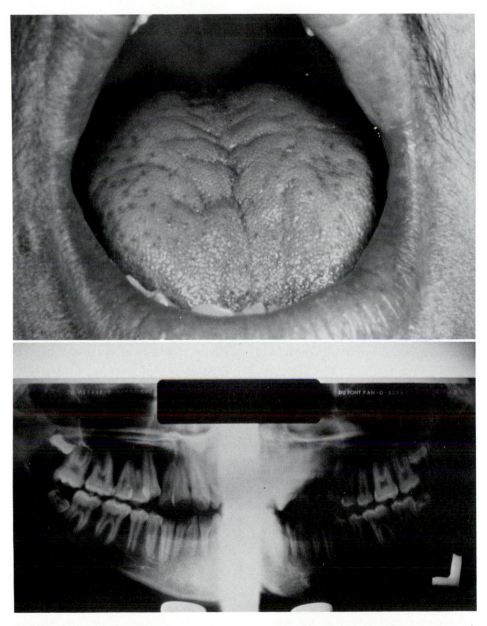

Fig. 1-35   Clinical and radiographic views of a 15-year-old patient with a large tongue and a history of long-term medication for hypothyroidism. Infraeruption of all mandibular teeth suggests that the tongue lies passively over the teeth at rest. Note the short distance from the root apices to the lower border of the mandible. Infraeruption allows the mandible to rotate upward and forward in occlusion; thereby, the Class III malocclusion is accentuated. True macroglossia is difficult to distinguish clinically from a normal but large tongue. Both the history and the interference with normal eruption suggest that this is true macroglossia. (From Bell WH, Proffit WR, White RP: *Surgical correction of dentofacial deformities*, Philadelphia, 1980, WB Saunders.)

mean that there can be no effect in a patient who may practice for many hours per day.

Tongue and lip posture/airway. Two aspects of the tongue deserve attention: (1) resting posture and size; and (2) function. Although the size of the tongue is difficult to assess, its general dimensions can be evaluated visually. If the tongue covers or overlaps the posterior mandibular teeth when it is maximally protruded, or if the patient can touch the tip of the nose or chin with the tongue, the tongue is probably large.

The orthodontist can most accurately assess the resting posture of the tongue by observing its position when the teeth are just slightly parted. Resting tongue posture also can be evaluated from a cephalometric radiograph taken with the patient at rest just after swallowing. True macroglossia is rare, and what appears clinically to be a large tongue usually is the result of a forward tongue posture. On the other hand, if a forward tongue posture cannot be changed, which may be difficult to accomplish because it is part of the patient's overall physiologic adaptation, retraction of protruding teeth may be difficult. A low, forward tongue position is associated with a broad shallow mandibular dental arch and a V-shaped maxillary arch (Fig. 1-35). Tongue posture usually depends on anatomic relationships in the pharynx, but occasionally it is dictated by a tight lingual frenum. To evaluate the lingual frenum the orthodontist should ask the patient to raise the tongue to the roof of the mouth while the mouth is open. If the patient cannot do this, the lingual frenum may be too tight and a simple surgical procedure to release it may be helpful.

Tongue position often is an adaptation to the position of the jaws or teeth; if this is the case, orthodontic treatment itself will correct the apparently faulty position. The most effective treatment for tongue thrust swallow is to correct the open bite malocclusion. Some patients, of course, do have motor or sensory deficiencies that affect oral function. If this is suspected, both motor ability and sensory ability should be tested. Gymnastic techniques such as tongue curling, moving the tongue in a four leaf clover pattern, and touching the tip of the protruded tongue laterally and vertically indicate the status of motor control. Whether the patient can recognize plastic forms introduced into the oral cavity will provide information about sensory abilities. This testing of oral stereognosis has not yet been standardized for routine clinical use; however, it is potentially useful when neurologic problems are suspected. On the other hand, some tests recommended by orthodontic clinicians in the past (e.g., the measurement of maximum lip force)[62] add little or nothing to the diagnostic evaluation because the results correlate poorly with either the anatomic situation or the response to treatment.

Airway obstruction can be a causal agent for malocclusion (see etiology section above), but the degree and duration of obstruction that are needed to affect dentofacial relationships are now known, and this whole area can be extremely difficult to evaluate on clinical examination. The orthodontist needs to know if the patient is enough of a mouth breather to cause problems during orthodontic treatment. The difficulty is that many patients who clinically look as if they are mouth breathers (the *adenoid facies* of many anecdotal reports) prove on laboratory evaluation to be breathing normally through the nose. A child (but not necessarily an adult) who snores may have a significant airway problem and may well be mostly a mouth breather during the day. Laboratory tests that evaluate nasal-oral breathing ratios are becoming available (and are much preferred over measurements of nasal resistance, which can be misleading). Referral of some patients for more detailed airway evaluation is recommended.

Speech. Speech evaluation properly belongs in the hands of trained speech specialists, but an orthodontist should be able to detect errors in speech and recognize those that may be related to malocclusion. Lisping, the most common speech articulation error, may be caused in part by irregularities of the anterior teeth. There is no evidence, however, that lisping can cause dental problems. Other fricative (f, v) and alveolar stop (t, d, n) consonants also may be affected by malaligned teeth (see Table 1-2). Correcting the malocclusion is unlikely to remedy even these related speech errors without associated speech therapy. Of course, orthodontic treatment will, have no effect on other common speech errors of children, such as substituting one sound for another.

Speech problems are particularly severe in persons with a history of cleft palate. Cleft defects occur over a spectrum from most anterior (notching of the vermillion border of the lip) to most posterior (affecting only the soft palate). A patient with a bifid uvula is better described as having a cleft of the soft palate; this is significant for speech function because the central muscular mass of the uvula, required for its elevation and function, is missing. In patients with these problems, speech difficulties may appear during adolescence because the normal loss of adenoid tissue at that age unmasks the functional problem for which the lymphoid tissue previously compensated. In submucous clefts, palpation of the posterior edge of the hard palate usually reveals a slight notching. A patient with suspected abnormalities of the soft palate and/or cleft palate speech with obvious cleft deformity should be referred to a university cleft palate center for further evaluation.

It also should be kept in mind that orthodontic appliances can affect speech. Bonded palatal expanders, for instance, pose difficult adaptation problems for many patients. A child who has speech problems should have orthodontic therapy that does not make normal speech more difficult. Consultation with the patient's speech therapist before beginning treatment for a child who has speech problems can be helpful.

Eating/masticatory efficiency. Orthodontists traditionally have paid little attention to mastication, apparently on the theory that, with the modern soft diet, masticatory effectiveness is almost irrelevant. Many orthodontic patients recognize that they have difficulty when eating (about 25% of those attending a dentofacial deformity clinic report problems of this type). Clarification can be gained by asking whether there are certain foods that the patient does not eat because he or she knows they are difficult to manage. Often pizza is on the list because it requires normal incisor function to bite through the toppings and crust in a socially acceptable manner. Unfortunately, there are no good tests of masticatory function at present, and it is difficult to quantify the degree of handicap the patient has. If masticatory function is impaired, however, it is reasonable to expect that orthodontic treatment can improve it.

Visual Examination of Dentofacial Proportions and Facial Esthetics

The orthodontist can make some diagnostic determinations from the examining room doorway regarding the patient's face, posture, and expression. It can often be determined from the patient's facial proportions whether the orthodontic problem will be largely a dental one or will relate to difficult skeletal or facial problems.

In assessing the face in its broadest context, the clinician should try to rule out any genetic defects or partial expression of genetic defects. The space separating the eyes can often give a clue to this kind of problem. In a number of genetic defects affecting the face and teeth, one finds hypertelorism. Malformation of the ears may be associated with one of the branchial arch syndromes, which can affect the mandibular condyle.[48] Although the orthodontist in pri-

vate practice rarely treats patients with malformations other than cleft lip and/or palate, it is important to consider the possibility of other syndromes. Some malocclusions represent microforms of recognized syndromes. A patient with a severe maxillary deficiency at age 13 years, for instance, may be a mild Crouzon syndrome patient (Fig. 1-36). Frequently this knowledge does not markedly affect the treatment plan; however, it often influences the therapeutic modifiability and thereby the treatment goals. Sometimes a surgical approach to treatment will be selected based on the recognition that the orthodontist is dealing with the result of a process other than normal variation.

For clinical examination of facial proportions and facial esthetics it is better to have the patient standing in a relaxed manner or seated in a straight chair rather than reclining in a dental chair; the upright position allows the head to assume its natural position (which is determined physiologically, not anatomically). A person looking at a distant object assumes a head position that will keep the visual axis level. This position is characteristic for the individual and is the way the head is normally oriented. Clinical examination, photographs, and cephalometric radiographs all should be taken in natural head position.

Before the advent of cephalometric radiography, orthodontists often used anthropometric measurements (external measurements made directly on the patient) to help establish facial proportions. Milo Hellman, who was well known both as an influential orthodontist and a prominent physical anthropologist (and who is now known to young orthodontists

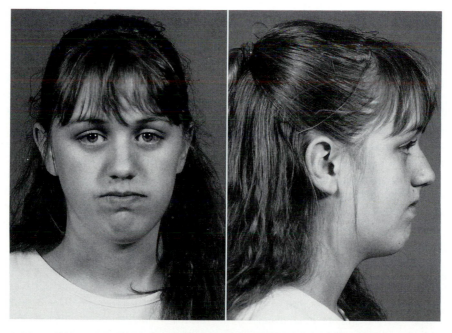

Fig. 1-36 Midface deficiency coupled with moderate hypertelorism may indicate a mild Crouzon syndrome. Syndrome identification is important when possible because it greatly improves the clinician's ability to predict the pattern of subsequent growth and development. It is quite unlikely that this patient will have excessive mandibular growth; however, the maxillary deficiency will persist and may worsen.

TABLE 1-9

Facial Anthropometric Measurements (Young Adults)

Parameter	Male	Female
1. Zygomatic width (zy-zy) (mm)	137 (4.3)	130 (5.3)
2. Gonial width (go-go)	97 (5.8)	91 (5.9)
3. Intercanthal distance	33 (2.7)	32 (2.4)
4. Pupil-midfacial distance	33 (2.0)	31 (1.8)
5. Nasal base width	35 (2.6)	31 (1.9)
6. Mouth width	53 (3.3)	50 (3.2)
7. Face height (N-gn)	121 (6.8)	112 (5.2)
8. Lower face height (subnasale-gn)	72 (6.0)	66 (4.5)
9. Upper lip vermilion	8.9 (1.5)	8.4 (1.3)
10. Lower lip vermilion	10.4 (1.9)	9.7 (1.6)
11. Nasolabial angle (degrees)	99 (8.0)	99 (8.7)
12. Nasofrontal angle (degrees)	131 (8.1)	134 (1.8)

Data from Farkas LG: *Anthropometry of the head and face in medicine,*
New York, 1981, Elsevier Science.
Standard deviation is in parenthesis.

TABLE 1-10

Facial Indices (Young Adults)

Index	Measurements	Male	Female
Facial	n-gn/zy-zy	88.5 (5.1)	86.2 (4.6)
Mandible-face width	go-go/zy-zy	70.8 (3.8)	70.1 (4.2)
Upper face	n-sto-/zy-zy	54.0 (3.1)	52.4 (3.1)
Mand. width—face height	go-go/n-gn	80.3 (6.8)	81.7 (6.0)
Mandibular	sto-gn/go-go	51.8 (6.2)	49.8 (4.8)
Mouth-face width	ch-ch × 100/zy-zy	38.9 (2.5)	38.4 (2.5)
Lower face—face height	sn-gn/n-gn	59.2 (2.7)	58.6 (2.9)
Mandible-face height	sto-gn/n-gn	41.2 (2.3)	40.4 (2.1)
Mandible-upper face height	sto-ng/n-sto	67.7 (5.3)	66.5 (4.5)
Mandible-lower face height	sto-ng/sn-gn	69.6 (2.7)	69.1 (2.8)
Chin-face height	sl-gn × 100/sn-gn	25.0 (2.4)	25.4 (1.9)

From Farkas LG, Munro JR: *Anthropometric facial proportions in medicine,* Springfield, Ill, 1987, Charles C Thomas.
Standard deviation is in parenthesis.

for the research prize in his name), determined both normal facial proportions and growth changes during development in this way. Although this approach was largely replaced by cephalometric analysis, it still can be quite useful. Clinical anthropometry has undergone a revival recently because of current data provided by Farkas,[38] whose studies of Canadians of northern European origin provided the data for Tables 1-9 and 1-10. The proportional relationships (e.g., the relationship between height and width of the face) are more important than the absolute values. The orthodontist must be careful to avoid treatment that would alter the ratios in the wrong direction: treatment with Class II elastics that could rotate the mandible downward in a patient whose face is already too long for its width.

Frontal view. Full face examination traditionally receives less emphasis in orthodontics than in profile evaluation, but it is nevertheless an important part of the clinical examination. Lateral cephalometric radiographs will be obtained routinely; however, unless there are special indications, posteroanterior (PA) cephalometric radiographs may be omitted. Therefore the full face clinical examination assumes even greater importance. Normal facial proportions for an individual in natural head position facing the examiner are shown in Fig. 1-37, and the ratios shown in Table 1-10 are important.

Facial asymmetries are a major focus of the full-face examination. A mild asymmetry may be of greater concern to the patient than a mild profile disproportion, since patients usually view themselves and others face-to-face, not in profile. In patients with questionable ocular or orbital asymmetry or deformity, interpupillary and intercanthal distances should be checked against standards (Table 1-9). Neurocranial growth is virtually complete by 6 years of age, so adult standards apply to essentially all patients in the orthodontic age group. With ocular hypertelorism the interpupillary distance is increased. With telecanthism, distortion

of the bridge of the nose increases the intercanthal distance. The distinction can be important in evaluating genetic syndromes.

Symmetry in the middle and lower thirds of the face is particularly concerned with the relative positions of the nose and chin. Since either or both of these structures can be deviated, careful analysis is indicated. For some patients cosmetic nasal surgery after orthodontics may be required to correct a nasal deformity. In evaluating asymmetry in the lower third of the face, it is important to record the relationship of the dental midlines; however, the important factor in this examination is not the relation of the dental midlines to each other (the dental casts will record that) but rather the relation of the maxillary dental midline to the skeletal midline, and the mandibular dental midline to both the chin and the midline of the face.

A second important consideration in the full face clinical examination is the vertical relation of the dentition to the lips. At rest, the lips should be in contact or nearly so. Up to 4 mm of lip separation at rest is within normal limits, particularly for younger children.[156] Lip incompetence is defined as inability to seal the lips without excessive strain; however, this should not be taken to mean that the lips should always be in contact when the patient is at rest. Patients with lip strain often manifest hyperactivity of the mentalis muscle, which clinically appears as a kind of peach pitting of the soft tissue chin.

When soft tissue and hard tissue vertical relationships are correct, the incisal edges of maxillary teeth are exposed at rest, and only a small amount of gingiva is exposed on full smile. Excessive vertical development of the maxilla often

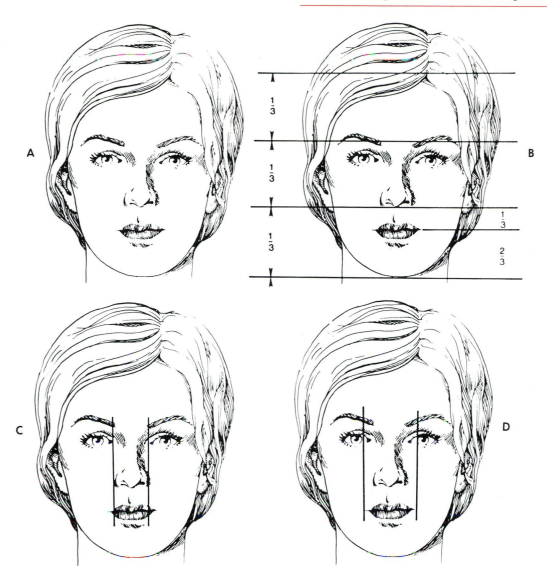

Fig. 1-37 Normal facial proportions. **A,** Natural head position, while facing the examiner. **B,** Thirds of the face are roughly equal in vertical dimension. **C,** Intercanthal distance is about equal to the alar-nasal base width. **D,** The mouth is as wide as the distance from the right to the left medial limbus. (From Bell WH, Proffit WR, White RP: *Surgical correction of dentofacial deformities,* Philadelphia, 1980, WB Saunders.)

occurs along with lip incompetence. However, some patients have a short upper lip, and it is important to distinguish excessive exposure of the teeth caused by overeruption of incisors from that caused by underdevelopment of the upper lip.

Profile view. On clinical examination of the profile the relative positions of the forehead, nose, lips, and chin should be evaluated. Lip contour is usually described as convex, straight, or concave, and this judgment is made relative to the nose and chin. A large nose and a well-developed chin can easily mask a protrusive dentition. Similarly the opposite situation, a small nose and a receding chin, can make a face appear more convex.

The orthodontist should realize that the chin is a relatively recent evolutionary addition. DuBrul and Sicher[32] suggest that the human chin replaced the simian shelf of lower primates as the bracing for the anterior part of the mandible. The human neonate does not have a prominent chin, and a salient feature of craniofacial growth and development is the growth of the chin. The growth of the nose, particularly during puberty, is also a dramatic aspect of human craniofacial growth and development. Unfortunately, the ultimate size of the nose or chin in a young child can not be predicted; however, an examination of the child's parents and older siblings may reveal some hint regarding final dimensions of these structures. The nasolabial and nasofrontal angles can also be useful in deciding how the nose relates to the upper and lower face.

The clinical examination of facial proportions must be recognized as a vital step in the overall diagnostic procedure. Decisions involving extraction vs. nonextraction treatment, the degree of retraction for protruding incisors, and whether orthodontics alone will be sufficient or whether surgery is needed depend heavily on this information.

Diagnostic Records Needed

Diagnostic records for orthodontic purposes may be divided into three major categories: (1) dental casts and occlusal records, (2) photographic records, and (3) radiographic records.

Dental casts and occlusal records. Dental casts for orthodontic purposes differ from those taken for many other dental purposes in two ways: (1) the impressions are extended maximally to allow as much as possible of the alveolar process and teeth to be displayed, and (2) the casts are trimmed with a symmetric base to allow better visualization of asymmetries in arch form and tooth position. Casts should be trimmed to centric (habitual) occlusion unless a gross discrepancy is evident; if one exists, a centric relation record should be made, at least statically (i.e., nonarticulated casts trimmed to represent the retruded position, which is acceptable for preadolescent children) or via an articulator mounting with a record of functional excursions (sometimes indicated for older patients).

Photographic records. For ideal photographic representation of the face, at least six different views are recommended (Fig. 1-38). The patient assumes a natural head position, and frontal and lateral facial photographs are taken showing (1) the teeth in maximum intercuspal position with the lips closed, even if this strains the patient and (2) the mandible in rest position with the lips in repose. A three-quarters view, smiling photograph frequently reveals what the patient looks like to others. The smiling view will reveal a short upper lip, if it is present, and will demonstrate how much gingiva the patient shows when smiling. A silhouette photograph with the teeth in intercuspal position and the lips closed is a dramatic way of representing the soft tissue profile. These facial photographs are intended to capture the aspects of facial esthetics already reviewed during the patient's clinical examination. A minimum set of three facial views consists of a full face view, with lips relaxed; a full face, smiling view; and a lateral view, with lips relaxed. We recommend a standard set of four views, including lateral, frontal, and three-quarter views (see Fig. 1-39). These should be supplemented with additional views in patients with severe facial distortions, especially if skeletal asymmetry is present.

The intra-oral photographic series consists of five views: right and left lateral, anterior, and upper and lower occlusal (Fig. 1-39). The occlusal photographs should be taken using a front surface mirror to allow a direct view. Mirrors can be used for the lateral views to obtain a more direct view of the buccal occlusion. Since occlusal relationships are captured more accurately on casts, mirror views of the lateral occlusion are not usually necessary. The major purpose of the intraoral photographs is to enable the orthodontist to review again the hard and soft tissue findings when all the diagnostic data are being analyzed. It is surprising how often a finding is discovered on the photographs that was overlooked at the time of the oral examination. Another purpose of the intraoral photographs is to record hard and soft tissue conditions as they existed before treatment. Photographs that show white spot lesions of the enamel, hypoplastic areas and gingival clefts are essential to document that such preexisting conditions were not caused by any subsequent orthodontic treatment. Since it is impossible to anticipate which patients will need defensive documentation, it is important to do it routinely.

Radiographic records. As noted above, we advocate having a panoramic radiograph available when the patient is initially examined clinically. Current US guidelines for additional radiographs in screening for dental pathology are shown in Table 1-8.

Periapical radiographs. For most orthodontic patients the additional information gained from routine periapical films is not justified by the increased radiation exposure. If there is any suspicion of root resorption in the anterior area, periapical films of the maxillary and mandibular incisors may be needed. Any areas of special interest noted on the panoramic film should also be viewed in greater detail on a periapical film.

The adult orthodontic patient with periodontal disease is now the prime candidate for a full intraoral series and a panoramic radiograph. If periodontal disease is suspected, periapical radiographs of suspicious areas are required.

Cephalometric radiographs. A lateral cephalometric radiograph is needed routinely. Lateral cephalometric films have two purposes: (1) they reveal details of skeletal and dental relationships that cannot be observed in other ways, and (2) they allow a precise evaluation of treatment response. In many instances an adequate orthodontic diagnosis can be made without a cephalometric radiograph; however, it is practically impossible to assess accurately a patient's response to treatment without being able to compare cephalometric films before and after treatment. For this reason, even in patients whose dental and skeletal relationships seem perfectly straightforward (e.g., Class I crowding problems), a lateral cephalometric film is needed. It is a serious error to treat skeletal malocclusions without a cephalometric evaluation.

The diagnostic value of lateral cephalometric films can be improved by taking the films with the patient in natural head position rather than orienting the head to an anatomic plane as was done in the original cephalometric techniques. Cephalometric head holders fix the patient's head at three points: the external auditory canals bilaterally and the bridge of the nose or forehead. It is possible to obtain a natural head position cephalometric film, controlling both the

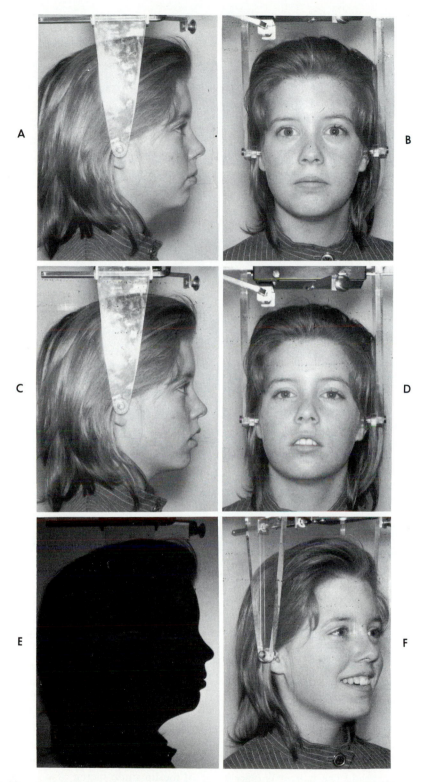

Fig. 1-38   An ideal set of facial photographs for orthodontic records of a typical patient consists of six photographs taken in natural head position. **A** and **B,** Maximum intercuspal position, lips sealed. **C** and **D,** Rest position. **E,** Silhouette, intercuspal position. **F,** Three-quarters view, smiling.

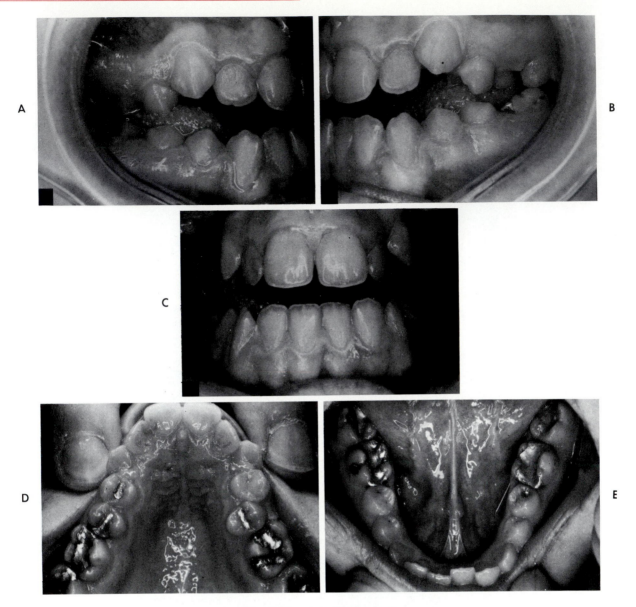

Fig. 1-39 **A** to **E**, Intra-oral.

source to subject and the subject to film distances, without using a head holder at all.[27] Such films are made by having the patient orient the midline of the face (midsagittal plane) to the midsagittal plane of the head holder, without actually attaching the head holder. For occasional patients with gross deformities this may be the only feasible approach because the ears are malpositioned.

In most patients the major difference between a natural head position film and an anatomically positioned one is in the vertical orientation of the head. The patient is placed lightly into the ear rods, gently manipulated into a relaxed position while looking either into his own eyes in a mirror a few feet away or out a window at a distant horizon, and then fixed in the cephalostat.

It also is of diagnostic importance when the cephalometric film is made to have the patient's lips relaxed rather than pulled into a strained closure. This is particularly true when vertical repositioning of the teeth, whether by orthodontic intrusion or extrusion or by surgical repositioning of segment, is contemplated. A number of the published soft tissue cephalometric analyses have been derived from cephalograms with the subject's lips in closed position even if strained. These analyses neglect the vertical component and may present a distorted view of the A-P lip position because of the lip strain factor.

The teeth should be held lightly together in centric (habitual) occlusion when the cephalogram is obtained. If a severe CR-CO discrepancy exists, obtaining a second film with the mandible retruded may be helpful; but it must be recognized that getting the patient into a true centric relation

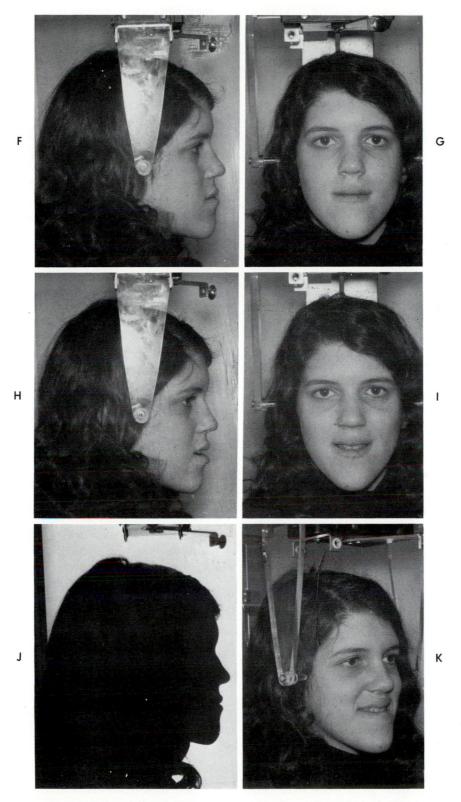

Fig. 1-39, cont'd   F to **K,** Facial views of a complex and severe malocclusion.

position, however it is defined, can be extremely difficult while in the cephalometric head holder. For this reason the centric relation film is of less diagnostic value than might be thought initially, and taking two lateral head films is rarely indicated.

A posteroanterior cephalometric film should be taken if an asymmetry is noted in the clinical examination or if skeletal transverse problems exist (e.g., a transverse maxillary deficiency that may require maxillary expansion). P-A films, with the face to the cassette, are preferred over A-P films because facial magnification is less. As with the full intraoral series, the additional diagnostic information available from PA films justifies taking them only in special circumstances.

TM joint images. Imaging of the temporomandibular joint may be indicated in patients who have TMD symptoms, but this is not indicated routinely in orthodontic patients.

Possible TM joint images fall into five categories: (1) standard radiographic views, especially the transcranial, obtained by using special positioning devices; (2) laminographic radiographs of the joint, which can be obtained with or without the patient positioned in a cephalostat; (3) TM joint arthrography; (4) computed tomographic (CT) scans; and (5) MRI scans.

Transcranial and similar views of the TM joint, though widely used through the 1970s, are not longer considered adequate for diagnosis of TM joint pathology. Laminographic or MRI views (see below) have largely replaced this radiographic technique.

Cephalometric laminagraphy, particularly from a series of cuts at various depths across the condyle, can be quite valuable in revealing irregularities in the condylar outline related to trauma or disease. When needed, such films can be obtained by using medical equipment found in the radiology department of most hospitals. This method has been advocated as a way to visualize whether the condyles are correctly positioned in the articular fossae, and thereby to check on whether proper centric relation has been achieved, and some clinicians have suggested taking two lateral cephalograms, with a cut through the condyle on each side. Unfortunately, the condyle anatomically is a cylinder at least 1 cm in transverse width positioned at approximately a 30 degree angle to the midsagittal plane. Thus the depth of the laminagraphic cut influences the resulting picture. For this reason information on condylar position from single laminagraphic films is of limited diagnostic value.

Arthrography of the TM joint, using injection of a radiopaque material into the upper or lower joint spaces, first demonstrated anterior displacement of the disk and the relationship of disk displacement to clicking noises within the joint. At this point, however, much of the information initially obtained from arthrography can be obtained from clinical examination. Arthrography as a routine diagnostic procedure is contraindicated because there is some risk with the arthrographic injections and treatment planning rarely depends on the radiographic demonstration of disk displacement.

If hard tissue pathology is suspected in or around the TM joint (arthritic degeneration, for instance), the preferred imaging approach at present is CT. This technique provides the equivalent of multiple laminographic cuts with less radiation and greater flexibility.

When the orthodontist infers from clinical examination that there is an internal derangement of the TM joint or other soft tissue pathology in or around the joint, MRI is now the preferred imaging technique. Unlike arthrography, it is noninvasive, and it also has the advantage of not involving ionizing radiation. The imaging of soft tissues often is superior to that which is obtained from CT; however, the hard tissue contours are less accurately depicted.

In our view, images of the TM joint should be ordered only if there is a specific reason for doing so. The primary indication would be the suspicion, based on clinical examination, that internal joint pathology is present. For adult patients with TMD, orthodontic treatment aimed at establishing a new occlusal relationship closer to the correct centric relation position should be undertaken only after careful consideration of the etiology of the TMD symptoms.

COMPLETING THE DATA BASE: EVALUATION OF DIAGNOSTIC RECORDS
Modern Approach to Classification

In orthodontics, classification of a case traditionally has meant using the Angle classification scheme of the early 1900s. Edward Angle contributed the concept that if the mesiobuccal cusp of the maxillary first molar rests in the buccal groove of the mandibular first molar and if the rest of the teeth in the arch are aligned, then ideal occlusion will result. Angle described three basic types of malocclusion, all of which represented deviations in an anteroposterior dimension. Lischer[79] later termed Angle's Class I occlusion *neutro-occlusion,* his Class II relationship *disto-occlusion,* and his Class III relationship *mesio-occlusion.*

The Angle classification was readily accepted by the dental profession, since it brought order out of what previously had been confusion regarding dental relationships. Almost immediately, however, deficiencies were recognized in the Angle system. Two severe critics were Van Loon[155] and Case,[22] who pointed out that Angle's method disregarded (in treatment planning as well as in classification) the relationship of the teeth to the face (i.e., the profile). Another criticism by Case as well as others was that, although malocclusion was a three-dimensional problem, in the Angle system only AP deviations (sagittal plane) were taken into consideration. To quote Case:

For the very advantage of perfect harmony and unanimity in our literature and teaching, the author would gladly have adopted the Angle classification, were it not for the fact that as it now stands it cannot be made to express a large number of very important characters of malocclusion which should be full recognized and systematically included. . . . Furthermore, the Angle classification does not recognize those wide differences in the character of certain malocclusions which have the same distomesial occlusion of the buccal teeth.

In 1912, in a report to the British Society for the Study of Orthodontics, Norman Bennett[12] suggested that malocclusion be classified with regard to deviations in the transverse dimension, the sagittal dimension, and vertical dimension. This recommendation, rejected at the time, was later realized in the work of Simon[138] and the development of his system of gnathostatics. Simon related the teeth to the rest of the face and cranium in all three dimensions of space. His approach, although somewhat complex, clearly represented an advance. If it had not been for the introduction of radiographic cephalometrics in the 1930s and 1940s, gnathostatics probably would have made a greater impact on present-day orthodontics. With the advent of the lateral cephalogram, many of the relationships that could be determined from gnathostatic casts were more easily observable on the cephalometric head film.

Another early criticism of the Angle system was that it merely described the relationship of the teeth and did not include a diagnosis. Simon, Hellman,[56] Lundstrom,[85] and Horowitz and Hixon[59] recognized the need to differentiate between dentoalveolar and skeletal discrepancies and to evaluate their relative contributions toward the creation of a malocclusion. These authors suggested that a classification should include this type of diagnosis and should point logically to a treatment plan.

The difficulty becomes apparent when it is recognized that malocclusions having the same Angle classification may, indeed, be only analogous (having only the same occlusal relationships) and not homologous (having all characteristics in common). Despite the informal additions to Angle's system that most orthodontists use, there is a tendency to treat malocclusions of the same classification in a similar manner. Homologous malocclusions require similar treatment plans whereas analogous malocclusions may require different treatment approaches. Some poor responses to treatment are undoubtedly related to this fault in diagnosis. Fig. 1-40 illustrates two nearly identical Angle Class II, division 1, malocclusions in children of the same age. There are differences in skeletal proportions and in the relationships of the teeth to their respective jaws, and both affect the profile. Although individual orthodontists may differ concerning treatment plans, the two cases should not be treated exactly the same. These are analogous malocclusions.

Since Angle and his followers did not recognize any need for the extraction of teeth, the Angle system does not take into account the possibility of arch perimeter problems. The reintroduction of extraction into orthodontic therapy has made it necessary for orthodontists to add arch perimeter analysis as an additional step in classification.

A final, but not inconsequential, difficulty with Angle's classification procedure is that it does not indicate the complexity and severity of the problem.

The Angle system has remained the accepted method of classifying malocclusions for nearly a century because of its simplicity and because many of the malocclusions referred to orthodontists include an AP problem. (In surveys of large population groups AP problems are less common.) For many years orthodontists have extended the Angle classification in a nonstandard and nonsystematic way. To quote Simon, "If one asks an experienced orthodontist: How do you treat Class I (Angle)? he usually replies with the question: Which kind of malocclusion do you really mean?"

To overcome these difficulties, and to provide a systematic way to evaluate the orthodontic diagnostic records, we recommend a classification scheme for malocclusions in which five characteristics and their interrelationships are assessed. Our representation of malocclusion, using a modified Venn diagram, is shown in Fig. 1-41. Common to all dentitions is the degree of alignment and symmetry within the dental arches. We represent this in the diagram as the universe, the frame of reference within which all patients and malocclusions exist. Many but not all malocclusions affect facial esthetics, particularly when the incisors protrude, and this is represented as a major set within the universe. Lateral (transverse), anteroposterior (sagittal) and vertical deviations from ideal, and their interrelationships, are represented by three interlocking subsets within the esthetics set.

The diagram is another way of representing the fact that alignment of the teeth relative to Angle's line of occlusion is common to all patients, who may also have esthetic problems and improper occlusal relationships in all three planes of space. If the teeth are perfectly aligned in both arches, ideal occlusion will occur when the mesiolingual cusps of the maxillary first molars rest in the central fossae of the mandibular first molars, provided the curves of Spee are harmonious and there is no tooth size discrepancy. This, of course, is the traditional Angle concept. Esthetic ideals vary because of racial, ethnic, and cultural differences, and the patient must be viewed relative to an appropriate reference group. Patients with occlusal deviations are likely to have more than one plane of space affected, as for example the Class II division 1 patient who usually also has a deep bite anteriorly.

Experience has confirmed that describing a malocclusion in terms of the five major characteristics provides an economical and efficient way to detect all important points, without overlooking important aspects. Perhaps more importantly, it provides a systematic way to examine the diagnostic records while keeping all aspects of the patient's dentofacial condition in perspective.

Steps in Reviewing the Diagnostic Records

Step 1 is to analyze the alignment and symmetry of the teeth in the dental arches (interproximal and contact relationships). This is done by examining the dental casts, looking down on the occlusal surfaces of the teeth (casts not in occlusion). Alignment is the key word of Step 1; among the possibilities are ideal, crowded (arch length deficiency), spaced, and mutilated. To ascertain which teeth are present or absent, it is obviously important to count them. Irregu-

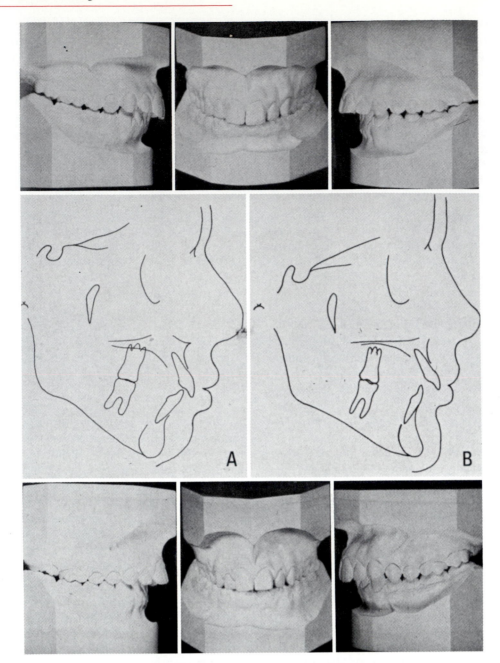

Fig. 1-40   Clinical records of apparently similar malocclusions. Despite the almost identical dental casts, the malocclusions are analogous but are not homologous because of the differences in skeletal patterns. Different treatments will be required. (From Ackerman JL, Proffit WR: *Am J Orthod* 56:443, 1969.)

larities of individual teeth are described if desired by the method of Lischer: the use of the suffix version to describe the direction of individual tooth malalignments (e.g., labioversion; linguoversion). It is important also to evaluate the symmetry of each dental arch, looking at both arch form and the position of the teeth within the arch. Many (but not all) Angle Class I malocclusions have no other problems and can be described solely in terms of intra-arch alignment and symmetry.

Step 2 is to review the findings from the clinical exam-

ination of the face and to confirm these from the photographs. Of particular interest and relevance is the protrusion (or retrusion) of the incisors. It is important to keep in mind that crowding and protrusion are different aspects of the same thing: the degree of crowding depends on whether the incisors are protrusive or retrusive, as well as on how much space exists within the arch.

Step 3 is to place the dental casts in occlusion and note the buccolingual relationships of the posterior teeth and the lateral (transverse) relationships of the jaws. A judgment is

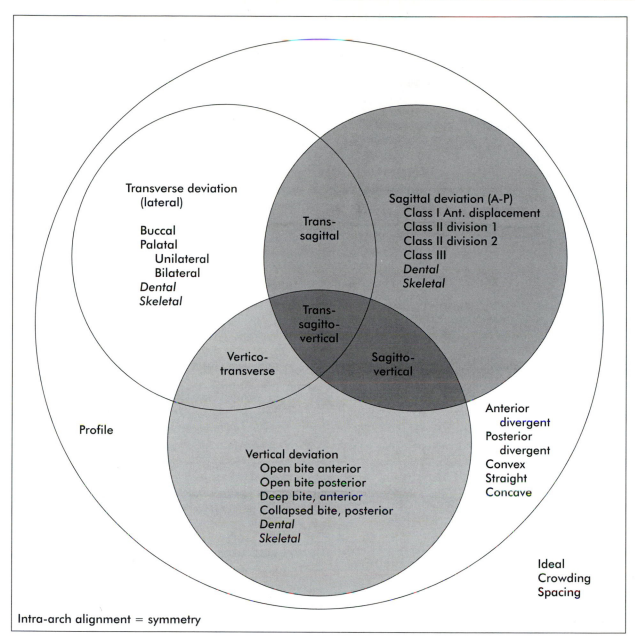

Fig. 1-41   A Venn diagram can be used to represent the five major characteristics of malocclusion and their interaction. The sequential description of the major characteristics is the key to the Ackerman-Proffit classification system; however, the interaction of the tooth and jaw relationships with dental alignment and facial appearance must be kept in mind.

also made to determine whether a transverse problem—typically, posterior crossbite—is basically dentoalveolar, skeletal, or a combination of the two. A continuous range of problems exist: those that are entirely skeletal to those that are entirely dental, with components of both in most instances. Because skeletal width dimensions can be seen on the dental casts, a PA cephalometric radiograph is not necessary unless skeletal asymmetry is suspected; however, if a PA ceph is available, it also is evaluated at this stage. If a bilateral palatal crossbite is entirely due to constriction of the maxilla, it is labeled as a skeletal problem. A similar

crossbite caused by constriction of the maxillary dental arch alone, with normal width of the base of the palatal vault, would be dentoalveolar in nature. As a general rule, maxillary or mandibular is used to indicate where the problem is located. *Maxillary palatal crossbite* implies a narrow maxillary arch; *mandibular buccal crossbite,* describing the same dental relationship, indicates excess mandibular width as the cause.

Step 4 is to evaluate the face and dental arches in the AP dimension (sagittal plane), using both the dental casts in occlusion and the lateral cephalometric radiograph. In this dimension the orthodontist uses the Angle classification and merely supplements it by stating whether a deviation is skeletal, dentoalveolar, or both. The skeletal possibilities are normal, maxillary excess, mandibular deficiency, maxillary deficiency, mandibular excess, and combinations of these.

Step 5 is to evaluate the face and dentition from the standpoint of the vertical dimension, again using both the articulated dental casts and the lateral cephalometric film. Bite depth is used to describe the occlusal relationship. The possibilities are anterior open bite, anterior deep bite, posterior open bite, and posterior collapsed bite. Again, the orthodontist must determine whether the problem is skeletal, dentoalveolar, or a combination of both. Most of the published cephalometric analyses are weak in this area. Appropriate measurements for evaluation of vertical relationships are discussed in the section on vertical analysis.

At each step, as any problem is noted, it should be judged as mild, moderate, or severe in terms of its deviation from the ideal. Of course, it is possible to use linear and angular measurements to supplement other descriptors, but measurements are most useful when considered as evidence by which severity is judged, not as evaluations in their own right.

This method automatically produces a list of the patient's orthodontic problems, in the sequence of the five steps. If there is no problem in a given area, then there is nothing to list. Thus the review of the diagnostic records for a patient might produce a problem list such as the following:

Alignment/Symmetry	Mild mandibular, moderate maxillary crowding
Esthetics	Convex profile, mild bimaxillary dentoalveolar protrusion
Transverse	[no problem]
Sagittal	½ cusp Class II dental, skeletal Class I
Vertical	Deep bite, dental, extrusion of lower incisors

In the following sections of the chapter, we present information in considerable detail about how to judge deviations from the ideal at each of these steps. The clinician's judgment must be based on evidence and must be done carefully; however the evaluation is not complete until measurements from casts and radiographs have been reduced to a series of statements in the problem list like those above. It is easy for the novice to bog down in the details of the diagnostic workup and lose sight of the ultimate goal, which is the problem list.

EVALUATION OF STRUCTURAL PROBLEMS
Intra-arch Alignment, Symmetry, and Arch Form

In the clinical evaluation certain judgments are made, such as crowding, spacing, and rotations. When this particular dimension is considered in greater detail, the occlusal view of the orthodontic casts is used. It is surprisingly easy to overlook missing teeth, and for this reason the teeth that are present should be noted in the record. The symmetry of the Palmer notation for teeth (1 to 8 in each quadrant) has advantages for orthodontics because it emphasizes the analogy of corresponding teeth. Unfortunately, this system is poorly compatible with computer records. The Fédération Dentaire Internationale (FDI) tooth code[39] is a much better choice for orthodontists who are moving to computer record systems than is the military (1 to 32) system, which often is employed in restorative dentistry.

The congenital absence of a tooth cannot be established accurately unless one knows the dental age of the individual and the approximate timing of the onset of calcification of the crowns under normal circumstances. For example, if a mandibular second premolar does not appear to be forming on the panoramic radiograph of a 6-year-old child, the tooth may be congenitally absent if the dental age of this child is 6 or 7 years. However, if the child's dental age is approximately 4, it may simply be that the developing bud of the premolar has not yet begun to calcify.

For a patient whose dental age is lagging considerably behind the chronologic age, the orthodontist frequently would prefer to wait until the late stages of the transitional dentition before applying active mechanotherapy. However, if the skeletal age is advanced and there is a skeletal problem, it may be necessary to start treatment based more on the timing of skeletal growth than on the dental age.

When crowding is present, an analysis of the space available for the teeth of both the maxillary and the mandibular arches is needed. The underlying principle of this analysis is that only a certain amount of arch perimeter is available, whatever the mesiodistal dimensions of the teeth may be. Lundström,[85] and later Tweed,[154] pointed out that the orthodontist is limited by the apical base or basal bone to the degree to which the line of occlusion can be changed.

Although several methods have been suggested for establishing the apical base (one of which is viewing the cast by x-ray projection, a suggestion originated by Downs and followed up by Brodie[19]), it is difficult to establish the normal relationship between the dental arch and the apical base. The present position of the teeth seems to be the best single guide to stable future position, as indicated by the usual stability of intermolar and intercanine width dimension.

There are exceptions to this stability of arch dimension, as was shown by Sillman,[137] Baume,[10] and Moorrees[99] in their classic studies of the developing dentition. In most individuals an increase in width of the first permanent molar by 2 mm to as much to 5 mm occurs after these teeth erupt. Intercanine width, particularly in the mandible, changes least and can be thought of as a *constant* after these teeth erupt. Premolar width does not seem to be so tightly controlled.

Particularly in planning treatment for patients in the mixed dentition stage, it is desirable to do a space analysis, calculating the arch perimeter available for alignment of teeth (space available) and comparing this dimension to the total mesiodistal diameter of the permanent teeth (space required). This diagnostic step was originally proposed by Nance.[105]

When doing a space analysis procedure, the first step is to establish the amount of space required. This is the sum of the mesiodistal diameters of the teeth measured with either a bow divider or a sharpened Boley gauge. Both prediction tables and measuring the teeth on the bitewing radiograph have been advocated to obtain the size of unerupted teeth, and both are reasonably successful techniques. The best combination of precision and ease of measurement (for appropriate populations of northern European origin) currently is obtained with the Tanaka-Johnston method,[150] which uses the width of the lower incisors to predict the size of both the lower and upper canines and premolars. This method has good accuracy, and requires neither radiographs nor reference tables (when the method is memorized), which make it convenient (Table 1-11). For a patient from a different racial background, measurements of unerupted teeth on radiographs, using a control for radiographic magnification, is recommended.

The method of establishing the amount of space available, which is the arch perimeter, is a bit more difficult. A number of methods have been suggested. The important point to remember is that we do not understand the factors responsible for determining dental arch form, and therefore it is not possible to establish the dental arch form for a specific individual. We know that there may be an inherent morphogenetic pattern for the dental arch that the orthodontist should maintain during treatment. If the dental arch is somewhat V-shaped, it behooves the orthodontist not to change this into a U-shaped configuration. To do so would merely invite collapse. Because the mandibular arch clinically appears to be less adaptable to arch form changes, the mandibular arch perimeter is usually the more critical to determine.

One method that has been used traditionally to measure the arch perimeter is a brass wire contoured over the buccal cusps and incisal tips of the lower teeth from molar to molar and then straightened out. As Currier[30] pointed out, however, arch length and the geometric form of the arch are affected by whether the orthodontist uses the buccal cusp tips, the central fossa line, or the arch described by the lingual cusps of the teeth. The wire should be contoured along the line of occlusion: the central fossa line of the

upper and the buccal cusp line of the lower. The brass wire method requires considerable judgment regarding proper arch form. Another suggestion is to use a bow divider to measure segments along the arch at the alveolar crest and add the segments (Fig. 1-42). Musich and Ackerman[102] suggest using a hanging chain, which automatically establishes a catenary curve, as a rapid and reliable method for establishing mandibular arch perimeter (Fig. 1-43).

Another aspect that must be considered in this analysis is the curve of Spee. If this curve is basically flat (as can be determined merely by placing the occlusal surfaces of the teeth over the flat base of the other cast), then there is no influence on the space analysis. If however, there is a deep curve that the orthodontist plans to flatten, additional arch perimeter will be required to accomplish this (Fig. 1-44). Slightly less than 1 mm of additional arch perimeter is needed for each millimeter of leveling of the curve of Spee, if the arch is leveled through the second molars.[45] A deep curve is frequently accompanied by mesially tipped mandibular posterior teeth.

Since one of the major treatment planning decisions in orthodontics is whether it is necessary to extract teeth, space analysis is a critical determination. If there is less space available than required, the orthodontist must decide whether it will be necessary to extract teeth to produce the space required, whether the dental arch can be slightly expanded in the premolar region to gain additional space, or whether some reduction of tooth size can be accomplished by stripping enamel from the interproximal surfaces of teeth. Many other factors are related to this decision, such as the inclination of the incisor teeth. The decision cannot be based simply on the analysis of arch form, symmetry, and tooth alignment.

Two other important factors must be considered at this stage of analysis. One is the relative tooth size between the

TABLE 1-11

Tanaka and Johnston Prediction Values

One half of the mesiodistal width of the four lower incisors	+ 10.5 m =	Estimated width of mandibular canine and premolars in one quadrant
	+ 11.0 mm =	Estimated width of maxillary canine and premolars in one quadrant

From Tanaka MM, Johnston LE: *J Am Dent Assoc* 88:798, 1974.

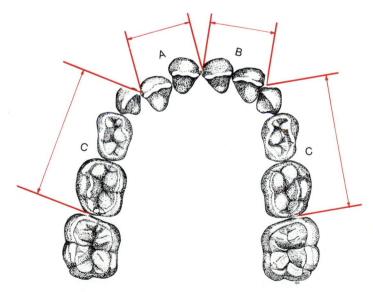

Fig. 1-42 Arch perimeter measurement by segments.

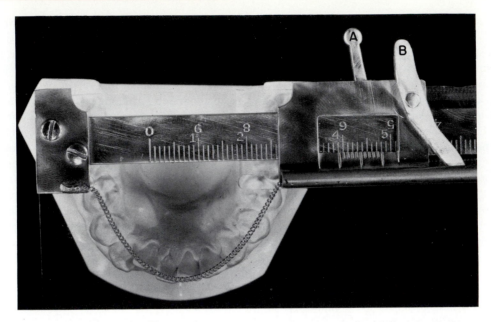

Fig. 1-43 The *hanging chain* method of estimating arch perimeter. The chain naturally forms a catenary curve, eliminating judgment of arch form. (From Musich DR, Ackerman JL: *Am J Orthod* 63:366, 1973.)

TABLE 1-12

Expected Tooth Size Relationships*

Maxillary anteriors	Mandibular anteriors	Maxillary anteriors	Mandibular anteriors	Maxillary anteriors	Mandibular anteriors
40.0	30.9	45.5	35.1	50.5	39.0
40.5	31.3	46.0	35.5	51.0	39.4
41.0	31.7	46.5	35.9	51.5	39.8
41.5	32.0	47.0	36.3	52.0	40.1
42.0	32.4	47.5	36.7	52.5	40.5
42.5	32.8	48.0	37.1	53.0	40.9
43.0	33.2	48.5	37.4	53.5	41.3
43.5	33.6	49.0	37.8	54.0	41.7
44.0	34.0	49.5	38.2	54.5	42.1
44.5	34.4	50.0	38.6	55.0	42.5
45.0	34.7				

Modified from Bolton WA: *Am J Orthod* 48:504, 1962.

*Differences of more than 2 mm from these relationships indicate the probability of a tooth-size discrepancy.

mandibular and maxillary teeth, particularly in the anterior region. Are the sizes of these teeth in harmony, and under ideal circumstance would these teeth fit together properly? The tooth size analysis suggested by Bolton[15] is a useful index for this particular judgment (Table 1-12). To a certain extent, tooth size ratios depend on the amount of overbite and overjet; a final decision cannot be made about a tooth-size discrepancy until all the tentative treatment plans from the problem list are synthesized. Stripping the teeth to reduce their width or to increase mesiodistal width with composite buildups[41] are possibilities for correcting tooth-size discrepancy. The correct procedure depends on the magnitude of the discrepancy. Another possibility, of course, is asymmetric extraction.

A diagnostic setup, made by cutting the teeth off the base and resetting them in wax,[69] is needed to confirm the indication for stripping or for asymmetric extraction in cases of tooth-size discrepancy (Fig. 1-44). If a satisfactory arrangement of teeth cannot be achieved in a setup, it is certainly unrealistic to think that it can be done in the mouth. Stripping incisors purely for increased stability is usually done after treatment rather than before and is preferred when tooth size discrepancy is proved.

Several other details should be noted from the casts, such

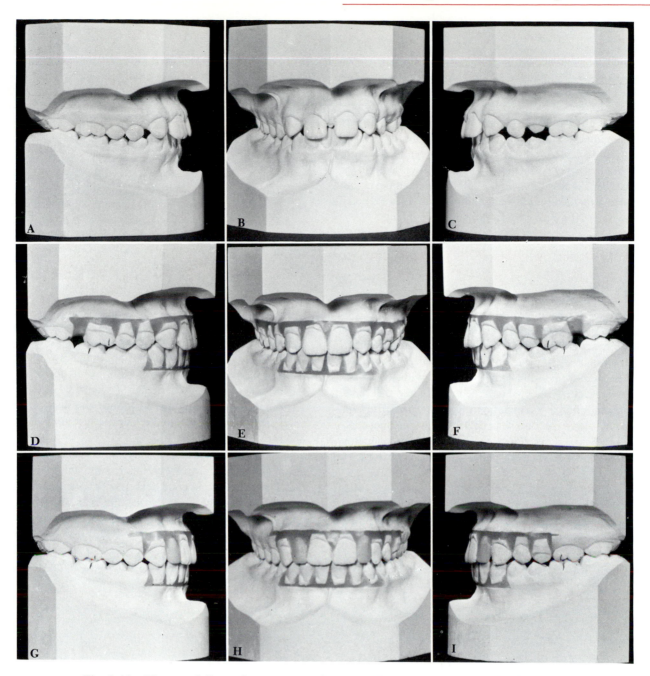

Fig. 1-44   The use of diagnostic set-ups to evaluate possible treatment outcomes. **A** to **C**, Casts of the malocclusion. **D** to **F**, Possible occlusion with closure of the lateral incisor space, bringing the posterior teeth into a Class II relationship. **G** to **I**, Possible occlusion with prosthetic replacement of the missing laterals.

as the marginal ridge heights in the premolar and molar region. In general, the marginal ridges should be the same height so that contact areas of the teeth are optimal and the architecture of the interproximal alveolar bone can follow the cementoenamel junctions of the teeth. A large discrepancy vertically between marginal ridges usually indicates poor axial inclination of the teeth. This may cause greater susceptibility to vertical bony defects. Also teeth in this condition are targets for food impaction.

If the maxillary first molars are rotated mesially, this may indicate that these teeth have slipped anteriorly, rotating around the large palatal root. Because of the rhomboidal shape of the maxillary first molar, this mesially rotated position also takes up additional arch perimeter (see Fig. 1-5). If the maxillary molars can be rotated to their correct positions,[147] additional space can be gained and also the AP positions of the upper buccal cusps can be corrected. Rotation alone frequently will correct an end-on molar relationship.

During the clinical examination note the midline of the dentition in relation to the midline of the face. The skeletal midline is indicated by the midpalatal raphe and by the incisive papillae on the maxillary cast. If there are discrepancies, the true midline should be indicated on the lower cast. It is important to differentiate intra-arch midline shifts caused by displaced incisors from serious symmetry problems. Often simply correcting the alignment will correct the midline. This is less likely to be true if a skeletal deviation, as revealed by facial midlines that do not coincide, is noted or if there is an asymmetry in the buccal segments.

Facial Esthetics: Analysis of Photographs and Soft Tissue Profile

The ideal photographic representation of the face has been discussed in connection with diagnostic records, and the evaluation of facial balance was discussed in the section on clinical examination. The patient's facial balance can be further evaluated by means of standardized facial photography and soft tissue cephalometrics. Even with a good soft tissue image, however, it should be remembered that three-dimensional clinical examination provides a better evaluation of soft tissue contours than does two-dimensional cephalometric analysis. Notes from the clinical examination should be available when the photographs and cephalometric film are being evaluated.

Evaluation of the facial profile can be done best when two aspects are considered separately in the beginning. First, the anterior or posterior *divergence* of the total facial profile should be examined (Fig. 1-45). This can be done best by examining the inclination of a line dropped from soft tissue nasion to soft tissue pogonion as it relates to the true hor-

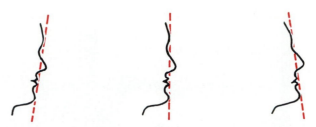

Fig. 1-45 Divergence of the face (a term coined by Milo Hellman) is defined as anterior or posterior inclination of the lower face relative to the forehead. Divergence of a straight profile line does not indicate facial or dental disproportions. To some extent this characteristic is a racial and an ethnic one. Posterior divergence is most likely to be found in Caucasians of northern European descent; an anteriorly divergent profile is common in both blacks and Orientals. (Redrawn from Proffit WR: *Contemporary orthodontics,* St Louis, 1993, Mosby.)

izontal plane (the patient's visual axis). The intersection of these planes defines the facial angle. In an orthognathic (straight) face the facial angle is approximately 90 degrees. If the mandible is positioned posteriorly, as indicated by a facial angle significantly less than 90°, the face is *posteriorly divergent*. If the mandible is positioned anteriorly, the facial angle is greater than 90° and the descriptive term *anteriorly divergent* would apply.

It should be noted that reasonable degrees of both posterior and anterior divergence are compatible with good facial proportions and good dental occlusion. Obviously this would be true only when the maxilla is in an intermediate position between the divergent mandible and upper facial structures. There are significant racial differences in facial divergence. Northern Europeans tend to be posteriorly divergent, whereas Orientals and American Indians often are

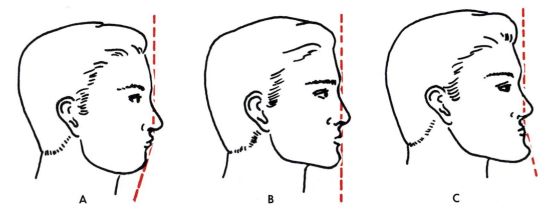

Fig. 1-46 Profile convexity or concavity, with a bend in the profile line, results from a disproportion of the jaws but does not in itself indicate which jaw is at fault. **A,** Convex profile indicates a Class II malocclusion, usually from a mandible that is positioned too far posteriorly. **B,** Illustration of a normal profile. **C,** A concave profile indicates a Class III malocclusion, which may be due to a maxilla that is too far back or a mandible that is too far forward. (Redrawn from Proffit WR: *Contemporary orthodontics,* St Louis, 1993, Mosby.)

anteriorly divergent. How harmoniously the jaws are related is reflected in the curvature of a line from soft tissue nasion to the upper lip and then to soft tissue pogonion (Fig. 1-46). If this line is relatively straight, as it might be even in the presence of anterior or posterior divergence, better facial proportions are present than if there is significant convexity (indicating a probable Class II relationship) or concavity (indicating a Class III relationship).

A second aspect of the profile that must be considered is the prominence of the lips, which is related in part to the position of the incisors and the amount of support provided by the dentition. The relative prominence of the chin also is a factor, since prominence of the lips is visually evaluated relative to the chin.

Both facial photographs and the lateral cephalogram can be helpful in assessing the chin-lip relationship. Photographs and clinical examination show whether the soft tissue chin is recessive, adequate, or prominent. On the cephalogram a line perpendicular to the mandibular plane drawn from the lower border of the mandible to point B reveals the *actual* bony chin (Fig. 1-47). A line drawn vertically from nasion through point B will indicate the amount of bony chin anterior to this line, which can be thought of as the *effective* chin. Holdaway originated the concept, later incorporated into the Steiner cephalometric analysis,[145] that the amount of effective chin should equal the distance that the lower incisors are in front of the line B. This *Holdaway ratio* can help establish lower incisor position when the orthodontist is considering altering the AP position of the incisors, keeping in mind that moving the incisors in itself

changes the amount of effective chin. The Holdaway ratio also is useful when the chin is to be repositioned surgically. In recent years this ratio has been adjusted to allow greater prominence of the incisor and thus more relative protrusion of the lips. The present general guideline is that the incisor should be approximately 2 mm and no more than 4 mm further in front of the N-B line than pogonion (i.e., ideal values would be 3:1, 4:2, 5:3, 6:4; acceptable would be 5:1, 6:2, etc.).

A number of lines across the soft tissue profile have been advocated as helpful in assessing facial balance and soft tissue proportions. Of these perhaps the most useful is the line from the most anterior point on the chin across the anterior point of the upper lip and extending across the nose. The outline of the nose anterior to this line and the curve of the upper lip posterior to it should form a reasonably symmetric S curve (Fig. 1-48). The upper sulcus, which is the deepest point of the soft curvature beneath the nose, should fall 5 ± 2 mm behind this line in typical white patients. Because this line, like all of the profile indicators, is influenced considerably by racial characteristics and lip thickness, it must be used cautiously as a general guideline.

When assessing facial contours and the profile, the orthodontist must keep in mind that the face tends to become more orthognathic with growth. Young children normally have relatively receding chins and convex profiles. As

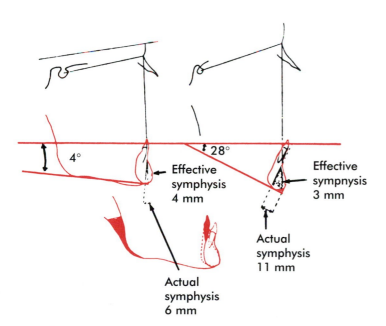

Fig. 1-47 The actual chin (the bony anterior buttress of the mandible) is not affected by the position of the mandible; however, the effective or visual chin is influenced. A steeper mandibular plane means a less effective chin. (Modified from Schudy FF: *Angle Orthod* 33:69, 1963.)

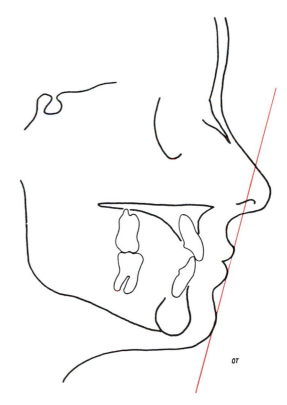

Fig. 1-48 The chin-lip line gives an indication of nose size relative to existing lip position. (From Bell WH, Proffit WR, White RP: *Surgical correction of dentofacial deformities*, Philadelphia, 1980, WB Saunders.)

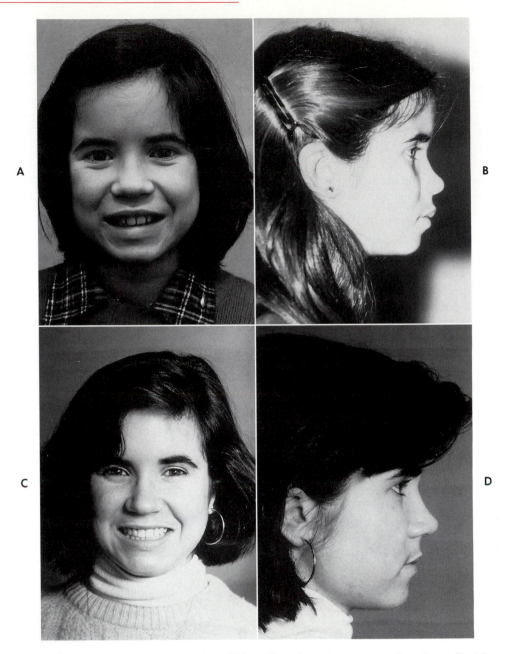

Fig. 1-49 **A** and **B,** Before correction of bimaxillary dentoalveolar protrusion. **C** and **D,** After correction of bimaxillary dentoalveolar protrusion. The incisors were retracted after extraction of first premolars.

growth continues, the hard and soft tissue chin becomes more prominent, as does the nose. General proportions tend to be maintained, however. Children who already have favorable Holdaway ratios are likely to become adults with prominent chins whereas those who are severely deficient at an early age are likely to stay that way. The earthy aphorism of Cecil Steiner—"them that has, gets"—is still a good rule of thumb. Valuable information as to the probable type of facial growth also can be obtained by examining the parents and older siblings of the parent.

Occasionally young patients are brought for orthodontic evaluation who have perfectly normal dental occlusion yet extreme facial convexity. Case called this condition bimaxillary protrusion, and modern orthodontists use this term; however, the condition is really bimaxillary dentoalveolar protrusion: protrusion of the alveolar processes relative to the basal bone of the maxilla and mandible. The terminology leads to occasional confusion with the physical anthropologists' bimaxillary protrusion, which is protrusion of both jaws relative to the cranium. In this kind of dental protrusion

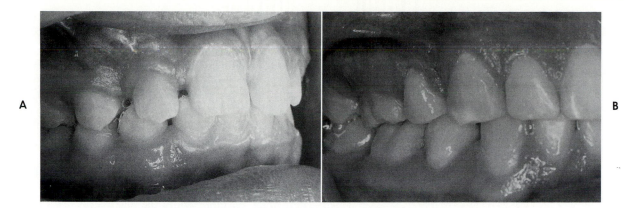

Fig. 1-50 Occlusal relationships. **A,** Before correction of the bimaxillary protrusion of the patient in Fig. 1-49. **B,** After the correction of bimaxillary protrusion of the same patient.

problem, the orthodontist must decide what the patient's face will look like after full growth has occurred. Some patients with bimaxillary dentoalveolar protrusion benefit from having four premolars extracted and fixed appliance orthodontic therapy instituted (Figs. 1-49 and 1-50). The desired amount of retraction of the incisor teeth requires careful consideration. If patients with protrusion have too much incisor retraction, their faces look prematurely aged. Facial esthetic norms vary especially in different ethnic and racial groups.[6,159] Esthetic values definitely come into play in making the decision about how much the incisors should be retracted, and some convexity of the profile is acceptable in screen and public personality figures. The "straight face" standards invoked by some orthodontists in the past require modification to match esthetic standards of the public today.

Transverse Relationships

Problems in the transverse plane of space are seen primarily as posterior crossbites, which may be due to displacement of the teeth relative to their supporting bone (dental crossbite), or to a narrow maxilla or wide mandible (skeletal crossbite). The objective in analyzing the diagnostic records is to accurately describe the occlusion and distinguish between skeletal and dental contributions to this aspect of the malocclusion.

Posterior crossbite is described relative to the normal position of the upper molars (Fig. 1-51). Thus a bilateral maxillary lingual (or palatal) crossbite means that the upper molars are lingual to their normal position on both sides. A unilateral mandibular buccal crossbite would mean that the mandibular molars are buccally positioned on one side. The terminology specifies which teeth (maxillary or mandibular) are displaced from their normal positions.

It is important to specify, in the sense of the location of the anatomic abnormality, why the crossbite exists: whether it is skeletal, dental, or some combination of the two. Because skeletal width dimensions can be seen on the dental

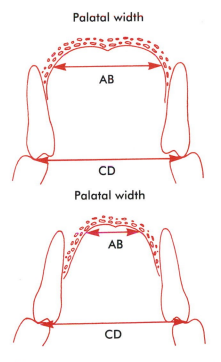

Fig. 1-51 Maxillary posterior crossbite can be purely dental or purely skeletal, or it can have elements of both. A purely dental crossbite implies normal width of the palate (distance *AB*), with the teeth tilted toward the midline so that the intermolar distance (distance *CD*) is small and a crossbite exists. For these patients, dimensions *AB* and *CD* are approximately equal. A purely skeletal crossbite implies that the palatal width is inadequate: both distance *AB* and *CD* are smaller than normal; however, *CD* is considerably larger than *AB*. When *CD* is much larger than *AB*—the teeth tilt outward more than the normal amount—partial dental compensation for the skeletal deficiency has developed.

TABLE 1-13
Arch Width Measurements (Young Adults)

Tooth	Maxillary (mm)		Mandibular (mm)	
	Male	Female	Male	Female
Canines	32*	31	25	23
First premolar	37	35	33	31
Second premolar	41	40	38	36
First molar	47	45	43	42
Second molar	52	49	49	47

*All distances are measured between the centroids of the teeth; standard deviation is approximately 2 mm for all measurements.
Data from Moyers RE, van der Linden FPGM, Riolo ML: *Standards of human occlusal development*, Ann Arbor, 1976, University of Michigan.

casts, this can be deduced from the casts, without having to make measurements on a P-A cephalometric film (which is a major reason why the P-A film is not required routinely). If the base of the palatal vault is wide but the dentoalveolar processes lean inward, the crossbite is dental in the sense that it is caused by distortion of the dental arch. If the palatal vault is narrow and the maxillary teeth lean outward but nevertheless are in crossbite, the problem is skeletal in the sense that it results from the narrow width of the maxilla. Just as there are dental compensations for skeletal deformity in the A-P and vertical planes of space, the teeth can compensate for transverse skeletal problems. It is not unusual to see a constricted maxilla with the maxillary teeth tipped outward in partial compensation.

Transverse displacement of the lower molars relative to the mandible is rare, so measuring the width of the mandibular arch can indicate whether the maxilla or mandible is at fault in a posterior crossbite. If there is a crossbite and measurements across the arch show that the mandible is wide while the maxillary arch is normal, a skeletal mandibular discrepancy probably is present.

Tabulated data for normal molar and canine widths are shown in Table 1-13.

Anteroposterior (Sagittal) Relationships

Skeletal vs. Dental Components of A-P Problems

Skeletal and dental aspects of Angle classification. The Angle classification has been used in orthodontics for nearly a century. Because it refers primarily to the characteristics of the AP or sagittal plane of space, characteristics of malocclusion in this plane are rarely overlooked. However, the Angle classification does not distinguish skeletal and dental components, and it is important to make this decision when patients with malocclusion are being evaluated (even in those with less severe problems).

Although Angle's classification is done entirely from dental relationships, a link to skeletal jaw relationships is implied. Angle observed that the maxillary first molar is found

under the lateral buttress of the zygomatic arch, which he termed the *key ridge* of the maxilla. He considered this relationship to be biologically invariant and made it the basis for his classification. Accordingly, he considered *disto-occlusion* an acceptable synonym for his Class II, since this implied a distal position of the mandible. Similarly, Class III was referred to as *mesio-occlusion,* relating to a mesial position of the mandible. A faulty position of the maxillary dentition or maxilla was not allowed.

McNamara[91] showed that about two thirds of a typical group of Class II malocclusions are due to mandibular retrusion (the rest are due primarily to excessive vertical, not horizontal, development of the maxilla, as described in the section on vertical problems below). A broader view makes it apparent that there are more possibilities for deviations in the AP plane of space than Angle envisioned, or at least than he had included in his classification system. Angle's classes are used now to describe four different thought related perspectives: molar relationship, type of malocclusion, skeletal jaw relationship, and direction of growth. Any time the Angle classes are employed, it is important to specify which is meant.

Cast vs. cephalometric analysis of relationships. For an appropriate evaluation of the A-P plane of space, six essential relationships must be established: maxilla to cranium, mandible to cranium, maxilla to mandible, maxillary teeth to maxilla, mandibular teeth to mandible, and maxillary teeth to mandibular teeth. Only the last relationship can be evaluated from dental casts alone. The dental casts are used primarily to confirm relationships noted clinically. One of the major advantages of dental casts, aside from their being a permanent record, is that they allow the occlusion to be visualized from the lingual aspect. Thus the relationships of supporting cusps and fossae can be assessed only on dental casts. The other A-P relationships may be deduced from clinical examination and from photographs; however, a lateral cephalogram is necessary for accuracy and detail, and is used routinely for this purpose.

Cephalometric analysis is almost always carried out on a tracing of the radiograph that emphasizes the relationship of selected points, not the radiograph itself. Tracings have two advantages: they reduce the amount of information on the film to a manageable level, and they can be superimposed to show changes caused by growth and/or treatment. The landmarks used in tracings can be represented as coordinate points on an (x,y) graph, and the digital coordinates can readily be placed into computer memory. There is an increasing trend toward use of computers in cephalometric analysis (Chapter 5). An adequate digital model is required, which means that at least 50 and preferably 100 or more points should be digitized (Fig. 1-52). Excellent software programs are available to calculate angles and distances, and to superimpose digitized tracings.

The underlying principle of cephalometric analysis, however, is not different when computers are used. In diagnosis, the patient's facial and dental proportions are compared to

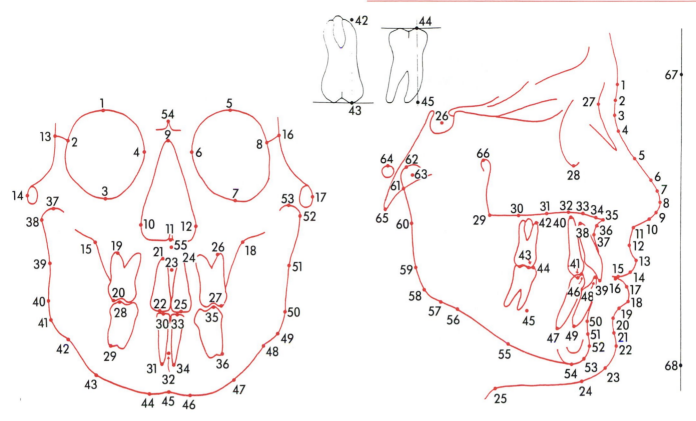

Fig. 1-52   The standard digitization models for P-A and lateral cephalometric radiographs used in a current cephalometric analysis and prediction program (Dentofacial planner, DFP). Like other modern programs, DFP allows customization of the digitization model, with up to 180 points available.

a reference group, so that differences between the patient and normal values can be highlighted. Cephalometric analysis was developed initially by selecting measurements that were most useful in differentiating patients with the various Angle classifications. The objective was to produce a reasonably finite number of measurements that would serve as guides in evaluating particular relationships. The original analysis, Down's, had five skeletal and five dental criteria, each meant to evaluate a particular relationship.

To a surprising extent, even when computers are used, much cephalometric analysis remains cast in this pattern. At present there are many named cephalometric analyses, each based on choosing one or two specific measurements from the multitude that might be used to evaluate a single relationship. In truth, there is not and will not be any single analysis that is ideal for every patient, simply because certain measurements will be useful in providing information about certain patients but not useful for others. For some individuals an accurate evaluation of dental and skeletal relationships can be achieved without making any measurements at all on the cephalometric film. For others a detailed cephalometric workup using measurements included in a broad data base of cephalometric norms will be required. The goal of cephalometric analysis must be evaluation of the under-

lying relationships, not the recording of any particular set of measurements. The measurements themselves are always a means to this end. Making decisions based solely on a given set of measurements, without thinking about the underlying relationships, has been correctly condemned by perceptive orthodontists as playing the numbers game, and unfortunately computers can be used only to make the numbers game easier and more attractive.

The concept of evaluating the underlying relationships can be grasped most readily by thinking in terms of dentofacial units, as illustrated in the block diagrams shown in Fig. 1-53. The goal is to describe the relationships in a meaningful way. At a minimum, that requires using cephalometric measurements as data, and reducing it to words and qualifying adjectives. SNA = 82 degrees and SNB = 76 degrees is not a diagnosis. Moderate skeletal mandibular deficiency is (but that judgment should not be made from a single angular measurement like SNB).

Normal dental and facial proportions can be represented in two ways: as tabulated measurements, or as a normal tracing produced by averaging the coordinates for the reference sample. Therefore comparison of a patient to a reference sample can be done in two ways: by comparing selected measurements for the patient to the same mea-

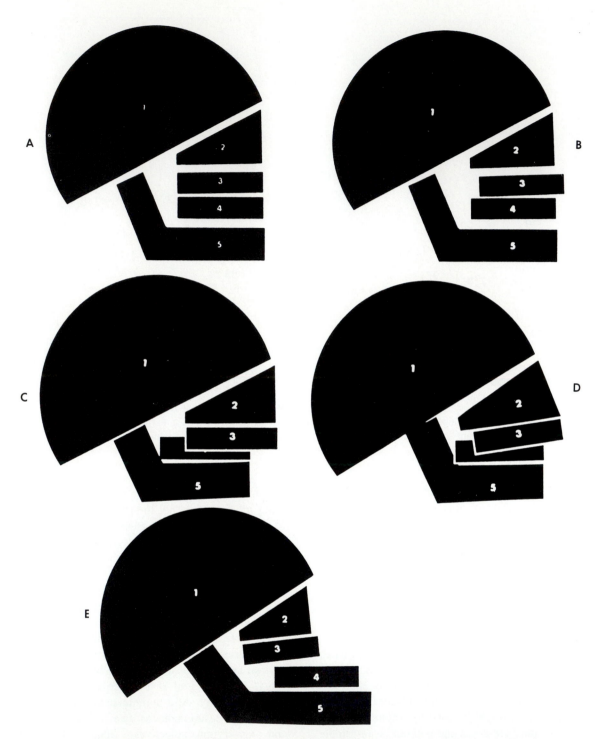

Fig. 1-53 Dentofacial relationships: *1,* Upper face and cranium; *2,* nasomaxillary complex; *3,* maxillary dentition; *4,* mandibular dentition; *5,* mandible. **A,** Normal (orthognathic) skeletal and dental relationships. **B,** Malocclusion caused solely by maxillary dental protrusion. **C,** Mandibular skeletal retrusion plus deep bite, with mandibular overclosure. **D,** Maxillary skeletal protrusion and skeletal open bite tendency resulting from an upwardly inclined palatal plane. This type of skeletal sagittovertical interaction occurs frequently in Class II open bite problems. **E,** Combination of maxillary skeletal retrusion and mandibular skeletal protrusion. The maxillary teeth are shifted forward on their base, whereas the mandibular teeth are shifted backward. Thus there is a partial dental compensation for the skeletal jaw discrepancy. (From Bell WH, Proffit WR, White RP: *Surgical correction of dentofacial deformities,* Philadelphia, 1980, WB Saunders.)

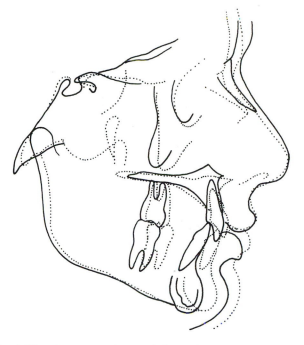

Fig. 1-54 One approach to cephalometric analysis is to visually compare the patient's tracing to a normal reference tracing. The Bolton standards, derived from the Bolton growth study, are often used for this purpose. Note the differences between the tracing of this patient *(solid lines)* and the Bolton standard *(dashed lines)*. From visual inspection alone and without the necessity for measurements, it is apparent that the patient (whose other diagnostic records are shown in Figs. 1-67 to 1-69) has an anterior cranial base that is tilted up anteriorly, a maxilla that is in good position but with the upper incisor tipped lingually, and skeletal mandibular deficiency. The mandible is rotated down slightly anteriorly, and its effective length is lessened by the posterior positioning of the temporomandibular joint. (See Fig. 1-67 to compare with a more conventional cephalometric analysis.)

surements on the reference sample, which is the typical cephalometric analysis approach; or by superimposing the normal tracing on the patient's tracing and visually comparing the two (Fig. 1-54). The latter method is called *template analysis.* This approach is just as valid as the comparison of measurements. The measurements look more scientific but have the disadvantage that only a few measurements are made in the typical analysis, and those may not be the correct ones for a given patient. In the discussion below we refer to classic cephalometric measurements, but we recommend use of the template method, especially as an initial step in determining how the patient differs from the norm. Experienced orthodontists often hold up the cephalometric radiograph and look at it—which is a type of template analysis, as the clinician compares this film to what he knows the normal facial proportions to be.

Before cephalometric radiographs were available, orthodontists were able to deduce skeletal relationships with rea-

sonable accuracy from analysis of the soft tissue profile. Some clinicians recently have advocated analyzing a video image of the patient's profile instead of a cephalometric radiograph, on the basis that the same information is available without the necessity of radiation, and that predictions of growth and treatment outcomes are more useful when the video image is used. It should be kept in mind that the high correlations between hard and soft tissue contours are not perfect—which means that carrying out treatment without serial cephalometric films carries with it a risk of serious error. In our view, video images are quite acceptable to supplement cephalometric radiographs (Fig. 1-55) but the images are not acceptable as replacements.

Relation of Maxilla to Cranium

When dentofacial proportions and relationships are evaluated in a patient with malocclusion, the orthodontist must be aware that the cranium may not be perfectly normal. Especially in patients with more severe problems, cephalometric measurements relating the maxilla to the cranial base may appear abnormal because of deviations in the cranial base. The problem of establishing a reference point is greatest in patients who have the most severe dentofacial deformity. It is particularly easy to see in these individuals that no point within the facial skeleton is likely to be unaffected by the deformity.

Because deviations and compensations in the cranium and cranial base can be present even in patients with relatively modest malocclusion, it is best to use an external reference that does not relate to the skeleton at all: the patient's visual axis. This is the position assumed by an individual looking at an object on the far horizon; the head is oriented level, physiologically rather than anatomically. This position is reproducible for any individual. The same effect as looking at the distant horizon (though with greater variability) can be obtained by having the patient look straight into a mirror.

This position, with the visual axis level, is the *natural head position.* We have already described its use in clinical evaluation and photographic recording, and we strongly recommend its use in cephalometric radiography. The original cephalometric technique called for using the external auditory meatus and the anterior inferior rim of the orbit as reference points to orient the patient's head, placing the Frankfort plane level. The Frankfort plane was selected originally by anatomists as the best approximation to natural head positioning if physiologic positioning were no longer possible (in studies of skulls from burial mounds, for instance). More accurate diagnostic data can be obtained from cephalometric films with the patient in natural head position, using techniques described originally by Moorrees and Kean.[99] For most patients and for routine purposes it is better to use a conventional head holder but to establish a vertical head position by having the patient look into the distance instead of leveling the Frankfort plane. Only if one or both of the patient's ears are displaced is it necessary to dispense completely with the head positioning device.

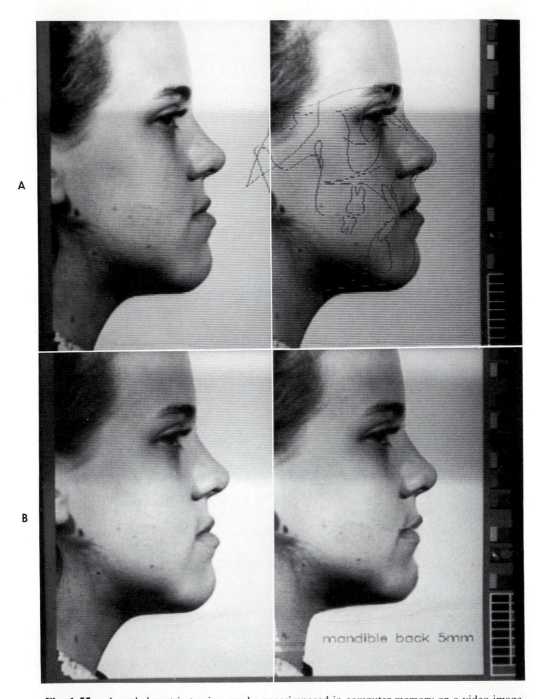

Fig. 1-55 A cephalometric tracing can be superimposed in computer memory on a video image of the patient, so that soft tissue characteristics can be visualized more clearly. When treatment is planned, the superimposed image has the advantage in that manipulation of hard tissue structures can be linked to changes in the soft tissue profile, which can help both the doctor and the patient understand more clearly the esthetic implications of alternative treatment approaches. **A,** A simultaneous view (split screen) of the patient's initial facial appearance with and without the superimposed cephalometric tracing. **B,** Split screen comparison of the initial image, and the prediction of a 5 mm mandibular setback. (Courtesy Dr. David Sarver.)

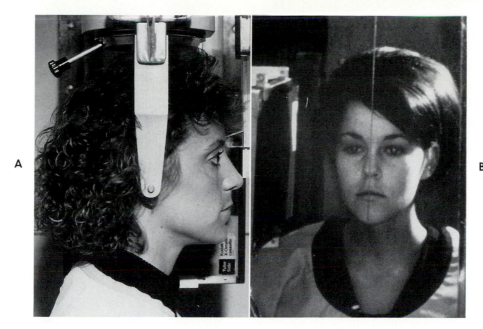

Fig. 1-56 Taking cephalometric radiographs in natural head position provides superior diagnostic information, even though the reproducibility of head position is not quite as good as it is with standard head positioning. The simplest technique for NHP is to use the standard cephalostat (unless it is obvious that the ears are on different levels [which is rare but not impossible]). **A,** Instead of placing the Frankfort plane in a level position, let the patient level his or her head and look into his or her eyes in a mirror; then place the nasal bar to maintain the patient's position while radiograph is obtained. **B,** If the ear rods cannot be used because of an asymmetric ear, the chain in the midline is employed to orient the patient's head to the midsagittal plane. A mirror may need to be added to the wall of the cephalometric area to change to NHP from the standard technique.

On a film taken with the patient assuming the natural head position, the lower border is parallel with the patient's visual axis (if the cassette was level) and a line paralleling the vertical edges of the film represents the *true vertical*. One simple but effective method of analysis is to evaluate the relative position of the anterior maxilla to the anterior extent of the cranial base (nasion). These should fall approximately on the same true vertical line. If angular measurements are to be used, the first step in analyzing maxilla-cranium relationships is to check the inclination of the cranial base (the S-N line) against the *true horizontal,* which is parallel with the visual axis. If the inclination differs from the norm of 6°, a correction must be made in the SNA reading so the anteroposterior position of the anterior maxilla can be evaluated. For example, SNA may be 75° in a patient who has a 15° angle between the SN and true horizontal planes. If a 9° correction is made in SNA, the corrected value becomes 84° and it is this corrected value that should be compared to the norms. This indicates slight protrusion of the maxilla rather than the retrusion suggested by the original 75° (Fig. 1-56).

The best cephalometric indicator of the posterior border of the maxilla is the pterygomaxillary fissure (Ptm). Both the anterior nasal spine (ANS) and point A (at the base of the alveolar ridge) can be used as anterior limits. Table 1-14 summarizes useful measurements relating these points to the cranium.

Relation of Mandible to Cranium

The position of the anterior portion of the mandible relative to the cranium is affected by not only the size (length) of the mandible itself but also the position of the TM joint. This in turn is influenced by the angle of cranial flexure at sella turcica, often referred to as the saddle angle. A sharp cranial flexure puts the TM joint relatively forward, whereas a more obtuse flexure places the point of articulation more posteriorly (Fig. 1-57). Depending on the location of the mandibular fossa, a mandible of normal size might therefore be either deficient or excessive in its anterior projection. This can be evaluated indirectly from the cranial flexure itself, defined as N-S-Ar, or more directly by applying standards relating the condyle position to sella or to the pterygomaxillary fissure.

Relative to a true vertical line, the mandible should be 2 to 3 mm behind the maxilla. Provided a correction for any cranial base inclination is made, the angle SNB can be used to indicate the position of the anterior mandible relative to the cranium. Although the angle ANB serves as an indicator

TABLE 1-14

Normal Cranial Base and Maxillary Relationships

Relationships	Cephalometric values		
	Males		Females
CRANIAL BASE RELATIONSHIPS			
SN-Ba (saddle length)		130° ± 6°	
S-N length	83 ± 4 mm		77 ± 4 mm
S-Ba length	50 ± 4 mm		46 ± 4 mm
Ba-N length	120 ± 4 mm		112 ± 5 mm
SN-FH		5° ± 6°	
MAXILLA TO CRANIUM			
Horizontal (anteroposterior)			
SNA		82° ± 4°	
SN-ANS		87° ± 4°	
FH-NA		85° ± 4°	
SN-PM vert (Eth-Ptm)		106° ± 6°	
Ba-PNS	52 ± 4 mm		50 ± 4 mm
Ba-ANS	113 ± 5 mm		106 ± 5 mm
Vertical			
Na-ANS	60 ± 4 mm		56 ± 3 mm
Orb-Pal pl	27 ± 3 mm		25 ± 2 mm
Eth-PNS	55 ± 4 mm		50 ± 3 mm
INTERNAL MAXILLARY MEASUREMENTS			
PNS-ANS	62 ± 4 mm		57 ± 4 mm
Ptm-ANS	65 ± 3 mm		61 ± 4 mm
PM vert-A (perpendicular)	59 ± 3 mm		57 ± 4 mm

From Bell WH, Proffit WR, White RP: *Surgical correction of dentofacial deformities*, Philadelphia, 1980, WB Saunders, p. 142.

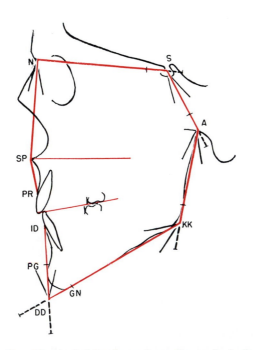

Fig. 1-57 Björk's facial polygon is another method of graphically illustrating the interaction among the proportional skeletal contributions to the dentofacial complex. A change in the cranial flexure angle at sella, for instance, will affect both face height and the prominence of the mandible.

of the difference in position between the maxilla and mandible, it can be misleading if the face has significant divergence or if there are vertical disproportions. What really counts is the millimeter difference in anteroposterior position between the two jaws. This can be measured directly as the millimetric A-B difference projected to the true horizontal line.

The effective length of the mandible is that which is projected horizontally (Fig. 1-58). Vertical-horizontal interactions in establishing mandibular position are important. Data for mandibular positions are displayed in Table 1-15.

Relation of Maxillary Teeth to Maxilla

In establishing the position of the teeth to their own supporting bone, it is important to evaluate both the inclination and the position of the tooth crowns. In the Steiner analysis the inclination of the upper incisor to the N-A line and the distance (in millimeters) of the tip of the incisor from this line are measured. These values give an excellent estimate of incisor position, provided facial divergence is not too great. Since inexperienced tracers frequently show point A forward of its anatomic location, incisor protrusion may be understated. The inclination of the upper incisor to the true horizontal line can be used to check on the Steiner figures.

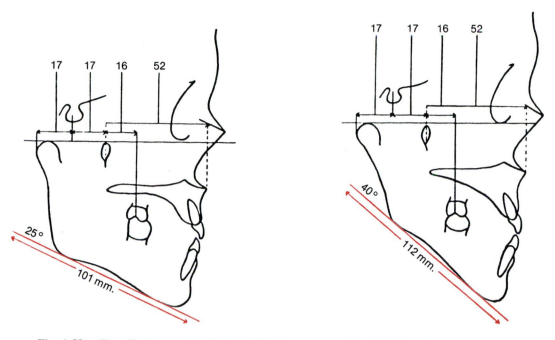

Fig. 1-58   The effective length of the mandible in anteroposterior dysplasia is that which projects horizontally. The Wylie analysis, one of the original cephalometric methods, takes this into account. (From Wylie WL: *Angle Orthod* 17:97, 1947.)

TABLE 1-15
Normal Mandibular Relationships

Relationship	Cephalometric values		
	Males		Females
MANDIBLE TO CRANIUM			
SNB		79° ± 3°	
SN-Pog		79° ± 3°	
NPog-FH (facial pl)		85° ± 5°	
	83° ± 4°		86° ± 3°
FH-NB		82° ± 3°	
NPog-Mand pl		68° ± 3°	
Ba-Gn	128 mm ± 5		120 mm ± 6
INTERNAL MANDIBULAR MEASUREMENTS			
Condyle-B	117 ± 5 mm		102 ± 6 mm
Co-Pog	131 ± 6 mm		121 ± 4 mm
Co-Gn (ramal length)	66 ± 4 mm		60 ± 3 mm
Go-B	81 ± 4 mm		76 ± 4 mm
Go-Gn (body length)	86 ± 4 mm		81 ± 4 mm
Ramal thickness at midpoint	40 ± 3 mm		36 ± 3 mm
Co-Mand pl perp	58 ± 5 mm		55 ± 3 mm
MANDIBLE TO MAXILLA			
ANB		3° ± 2°	
Pal pl-NB		85° ± 3°	
Pal pl-BPog		86° ± 3°	
Pal pl-Mand pl		82° ± 4°	
Condyle-PNS	48 ± 3 mm		45 ± 3 mm

From Bell WH, Proffit WR, White RP: *Surgical correction of dentofacial deformities,* Philadelphia, 1980, WB Saunders, p. 143.

Relation to Mandibular Teeth and Chin to Mandible

The relation of the lower incisors to the N-B line, in both inclination and position, can be used in the same way as for the maxilla. Chin position is indicated by the N-B to Pog distance. Chin position is related to incisor position by the Holdaway ratio: lower incisors should be forward of the N-B line by at least as much as the chin point is, and a 2 mm greater incisor protrusion probably is ideal for best esthetics in most Caucasians. The ideal protrusion is larger in blacks and Orientals.

When facial divergence is considerable, the Steiner figures accept some compensatory displacement of the mandibular teeth relative to the mandible as normal or desirable. Standards relating incisor position to the A-Pog line produce even greater compensation of tooth position if there is a significant discrepancy in jaw position. The A-Pog reference line should be used with an understanding of the compromised tooth position it may dictate in patients with skeletal discrepancies. The initial cephalometric analysis should not be one predicated on an assumption that correction of jaw relationships by orthopedic, functional, or surgical treatment is impossible and that treatment must be accomplished by tooth movement alone.

Cephalometric norms for tooth-jaw relationships are shown in Table 1-16.

Vertical Relationships

The lateral cephalometric film, facial photographs, and dental casts are needed for analysis of vertical relationship. Originally the focus of cephalometric analysis was on the

TABLE 1-16
Normal Dentoskeletal Relationships

Relationship	Cephalometric values		
	Males		**Females**
MAXILLARY TEETH TO OTHER STRUCTURES			
1-NA		22° ± 6°	
1-NA		4 ± 3 mm	
Max arch length (mesial 6-labial 1)	27 ± 2 mm		25 ± 2 mm
ANS-1	33 ± 3 mm		30 ± 3 mm
Pal pl-1	33 ± 3 mm		30 ± 3 mm
Pal pl-6	28 ± 3 mm		25 ± 2 mm
1-SN		104° ± 6°	
1-FH		109° ± 7°	
1-Pal pl		112° ± 6°	
Pal pl-Func occ pl		7° ± 3°	
MANDIBULAR TEETH TO OTHER STRUCTURES			
1-APog	3 ± 3 mm		1 ± 3 mm
1-NB	6 ± 3 mm		3 ± 3 mm
1-SN		52° ± 8°	
1-FH		56° ± 8°	
1-Pal pl		59° ± 7°	
1-Mand pl		95° ± 7°	
1-APog		24° ± 5°	
1-NB		25° ± 6°	
Go-LIE (lower incisor incisal edge)	88 ± 5 mm		80 ± 5 mm
Mand arch length	27 ± 2 mm		25 ± 2 mm
6-Mand pl	33 ± 3 mm		33 ± 3 mm
1-Mand pl	49 ± 3 mm		42 ± 3 mm
Infradentale-Me	38 ± 3 mm		31 ± 3 mm
CHIN PROMINENCE			
Pog-NB		2 ± 2 mm	
MAXILLARY TO MANDIBULAR TEETH			
1-1		129° ± 10°	
1-Func occ pl		61° ± 7°	
1-Func occ pl		67° ± 7°	

From Bell WH, Proffit WR, White RP: *Surgical correction of dentofacial deformities*, Philadelphia, 1980, WB Saunders, p. 146.

A-P plane of space, primarily because the first workers attempted to relate cephalometric findings to the Angle classification. Although much work in recent years has been devoted to vertical relationships, the usual cephalometric analysis presented as a diagnostic package for clinicians remains incomplete in this area.

As with the A-P plane of space, it is important to distinguish skeletal and dental effects when the vertical plane is analyzed. Since bite depth is determined by the contact relationships of the teeth, there is an inherent contradiction in the terms *skeletal open bite* and *skeletal deep bite*. Based on the work of Sassouni,[130] however, these terms have come to be defined as indicating skeletal proportions that cause a built-in tendency toward deep bite or open bite relationships (Fig. 1-59). As the jaw rotates downward, there is an increasing tendency toward an open bite relation anteriorly; as it rotates upward, there is an increasing tendency toward deep bite. The relation of the vertical position of the mandible to the anterior position must also be noted at this point. A downward rotation of the mandible is a backward rotation, leading to a relatively weaker and more distally positioned chin. Similarly, as the vertical dimension decreases, the mandible rotates upward and forward and the chin becomes more prominent.

Skeletal Vertical Relationships

The first step in assessing the vertical relationships of the maxilla and mandible to the cranium is to measure anterior face height. This is more important proportionally than absolutely: the lower face (lips to chin) should be 55% of the total nasion-pogonion distance (Table 1-17 and Fig. 1-60). To assess the skeletal situation, the orthodontist must also evaluate posterior vertical dimensions. However, direct measurement of the posterior vertical is difficult. Both the relative angulation and the position of the maxilla and mandible are significant. Posterior vertical distances in relation to anterior measurements establish the angulation. Thus if angulation plus anterior vertical is measured, posterior vertical can be evaluated indirectly.

Wylie and Johnson[164] proposed an analysis of vertical dysplasia not long after Wylie had published his method for analyzing anteroposterior dysplasia,[163] but the measurements were not especially successful in defining the vertical relationships. Since the height of faces varies considerably, proportionate rather than absolute standards are required. The Coben analysis[26] (Fig. 1-61), in which linear measurements expressed as percentages and proportions are emphasized, can be useful in evaluating vertical dysplasias. Moorrees and Lebret[100] proposed a system in which a reg-

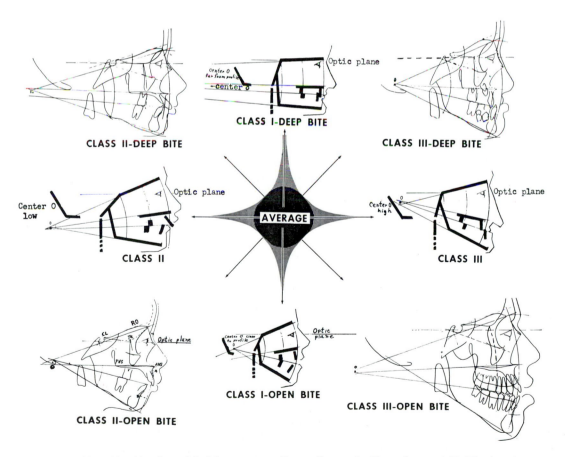

Fig. 1-59 Classification of facial types according to Sassouni. (From Sassouni V: *The face in five dimensions,* ed 2, Morgantown, 1962, West Virginia University Press.)

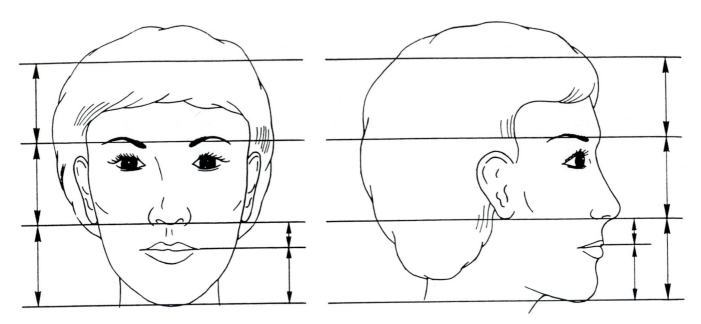

Fig. 1-60 Horizontal lines are used to establish the vertical proportions of the face. The ideal face has classically been considered to divide into approximately equal thirds, as illustrated here. Within the lower face, the mouth should be one third of the way from the base of the nose to the chin. Farkas' data (see Tables 1-9 and 1-10) indicate that the normal lower face may be slightly longer than this one; however, the classic proportions still are a good starting point for clinical examination. Gross deviations from these proportions are abnormal. (From Proffit WR, White RP: *Surgical-orthodontic treatment,* St Louis, 1991, Mosby.)

TABLE 1-17
Normal Vertical Dentofacial Relationships

Relationship	Cephalometric values	
	Males	**Females**
SN-Pal pl	7° ± 3°	
SN-Func occ pl	14° ± 4°	
SN-GoGn	32° ± 5°	
SN-Ramal pl	89° ± 4°	
FH-Func occ pl	11° ± 3°	
FH-Ramal pl	85° ± 4°	
Pal pl-NA	88° ± 4°	
Ramal pl-Mand pl	123° ± 5°	
Me-ANS	80 ± 6 mm	70 ± 5 mm
Me-Pal pl perp	76 ± 6 mm	67 ± 4 mm
Me-N	137 ± 8 mm	123 ± 5 mm
S-PNS	56 ± 4 mm	51 ± 3 mm
S-ANS	100 ± 5 mm	93 ± 6 mm
S-Gn	144 ± 7 mm	131 ± 5 mm
S-Go	88 ± 6 mm	80 ± 5 mm

From Bell WH, Proffit WR, White RP: *Surgical correction of dentofacial deformities,* Philadelphia, 1980, WB Saunders, p. 149.

ularly spaced grid, whose spacing is determined by the size of the individual patient's cranial base, is projected over the facial area. Deviations from normal proportionality are then expressed graphically by distortions of the grid as it fits over the patient's actual cephalometric landmarks (Fig. 1-62). The Moorrees mesh, as it is called, by its absence of numbers forces its user to focus on the relationships themselves. Its greatest virtue, the graphic presentation, has also been its greatest disadvantage since the flexibility of the approach and the lack of standards are conducive to some artistic license.

Another method for evaluating vertical proportions relies on the convergence (or parallelism) of the mandibular plane, occlusal plane, and palatal plane, as suggested by Sassouni.[132] If these planes rapidly converge and meet at a point close behind the face, posterior vertical dimensions are relatively smaller than anterior vertical ones. This produces a skeletal tendency toward anterior open bite, which is now routinely called *skeletal open bite.* It also implies a short ramus and an obtuse gonial angle, although these features do not necessarily have to be present. The open bite tendency is accentuated if the palatal plane is tipped up anteriorly and down posteriorly, a condition seen often enough to demonstrate that the skeletal problems leading to open bite are not exclusively in mandibular positioning. Palatal, occlusal, and mandibular planes running almost parallel, on

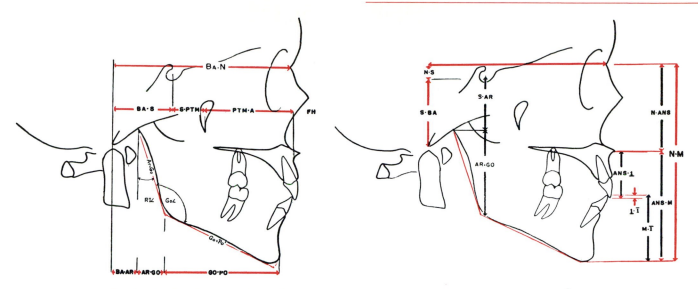

Fig. 1-61 The Coben analysis, which emphasizes proportional relationships of measured distances rather than angular relationships. (From Coben SE: *Am J Orthod* 41:407, 1955.)

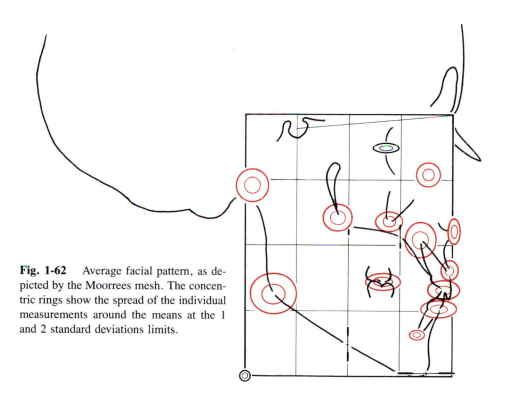

Fig. 1-62 Average facial pattern, as depicted by the Moorrees mesh. The concentric rings show the spread of the individual measurements around the means at the 1 and 2 standard deviations limits.

the other hand, lead to a skeletal predilection toward anterior deep bite. Individuals with this condition tend to have a longer ramus and a less obtuse gonial angle.

Normative data for percentage of upper to lower face height in children[103] and adults[134] have been published. When these standards were applied to a clinically determined group of long face children and adults, Fields et al.[42] found that nearly half were misclassified. The study showed that no single cephalometric variable reliably separates nor-

mal from vertically abnormal patients. Statistical evaluation of their data indicated that efficient and accurate classification required use of at least three of the many significantly different cephalometric values between the two groups. For example, the combination of anterior total face height, and S-N-mandibular plane angle provides accurate classification. This result reinforces the comment just made: To evaluate vertical proportions, it is necessary to have information about both anterior and posterior vertical dimensions; however, posterior vertical can be evaluated indirectly from angular data if the anterior vertical dimension is known.

AP/Vertical Interaction

When either plane of space is being considered, the interaction between sagittal and vertical factors must be kept constantly in mind. This interaction is perhaps nowhere better seen than in the person who has a short mandibular ramus, steep and convergent mandibular plane angle, and Class II malocclusion including elements of true as well as relative mandibular deficiency. Antegonial notching of the mandible often is present in these individuals. This condition now is frequently called the long face syndrome, a term that appropriately emphasizes the primarily vertical nature of the problem. Orthodontic management can be extremely difficult, and surgical treatment involving vertical repositioning of the maxilla often is the only way to achieve a satisfactory result.

The interaction between skeletal, sagittal, and vertical relationships extends also into an interaction between facial components and the structure of the cranial base. Bjork's facial polygons[128] emphasize the interaction between facial and cranial base factors (see Fig. 1-57) and demonstrate how variations in a cranial base relationship (i.e., the cranial base flexure angle) can require compensatory changes in facial relationships (i.e., the mandibular plane angle or anterior vertical dimensions).

Recognition of Dental Vertical Problems

Dental vertical relationships can be divided into four major categories: anterior open bite, anterior deep bite, posterior open bite, and posterior collapsed bite with overclosure. Since the same occlusal relations can result from skeletal jaw proportions or from infraeruption or supraeruption of teeth, the descriptive terminology should be as precise as possible in indicating whether jaw or tooth positions are basically at fault in producing a vertical problem.

A deep bite anteriorly could be caused by supraeruption of upper and/or lower incisors or infraeruption of posterior teeth. Similarly, an anterior open bite could be caused by infraeruption of incisors in either arch or supraeruption of the posterior teeth. A posterior open bite could be caused by lack of eruption of posterior teeth in one part of the arch or on one side. However, if the posterior teeth failed to erupt bilaterally, the jaw would rotate upward and forward and, instead of a posterior open bite, the situation might be described as posterior bite collapse. The true posterior open bite for such a patient would be revealed when proper anterior vertical dimension was reestablished. One might think that this could be done simply by having the patient assume the physiologic rest position, as is done with edentulous patients who require fabrication of dentures; but the rest position of the mandible when natural teeth are present is influenced by the position of the teeth, so if only some posterior teeth have been lost, rest position may not adequately reveal the extent of infraeruption. Early loss of max-

illary and mandibular first molars is a common cause of this type of bite collapse. With second molars replacing first molars, even if these have achieved normal vertical development, the patient will tend to be rotated closed even in the postural position of the mandible. (In mild skeletal open bite problems, the orthodontist can take advantage of this effect, reducing excess face height by extracting first molars and slipping the second molars anteriorly.)

To evaluate whether infraeruption or supraeruption is present, the orthodontist must use linear measurements from the base of the alveolar process. Cephalometric standards containing this information are available in the data from the Michigan growth study. Tabulated data for adults are provided in Table 1-17. Age values for males and females are contained in the *Atlas of Craniofacial Growth* by Riolo et al.[124] When these data are used, the amount of eruption anteriorly or posteriorly can be established. For example, supraeruption of mandibular incisors often contributes to the anterior deep bite that accompanies most Class II malocclusions. To evaluate whether this is the case, one can measure the distance from the incisal edge vertically to the lower border of the mandible and compare this with the cephalometric standards for that patient's age and sex. If the distance is increased, supraeruption of the incisors has occurred. If a deep bite exists but the lower incisors have not supraerupted, another cause for the deep bite must be sought. Similar measurements can be made posteriorly, from the palatal plane to the cusp tip of the upper first molar and from the lower border of the mandible to the cusp tip of the lower first molar.

In judging the amount of eruption the orthodontist must take the overall proportions into account, since deviations in eruption often accompany skeletal vertical dysplasias. Supraeruption of maxillary posterior teeth typically accompanies a skeletal open bite pattern. The relation of the upper molar roots to the height of the palatal vault, which is easily observed cephalometrically, can aid a quick evaluation. The root apices of the upper molar in an adult should be 2 to 3 mm below the height of the palatal vault. Distances in excess of this probably represent some supraeruption of the upper molar, whereas roots that are above the height of the palatal vault probably represent a deficiency in vertical development. More precise information can be obtained from the linear measurements.

Skeletal components of vertical dysplasia are revealed in rotation of the mandible—upward and forward in skeletal deep bite and downward and backward in skeletal open bite. The amount of rotation of the jaw interacts strongly with posterior eruption—which will be deficient in skeletal deep bite and excessive in skeletal open bite. Dental compensation for the skeletal jaw relationships can occur in the amount of eruption of the anterior teeth. For instance, in a patient with a skeletal deep bite pattern, a deep bite still would not be present if there were less than normal eruption of anterior teeth. Similarly, in a skeletal open bite pattern, an actual open bite might not exist if there were excessive eruption of upper and lower incisors so that the teeth fitted together despite the jaw rotation.

Understanding that a skeletal open bite may or may not be accompanied by an open bite relationship of the anterior teeth can be extremely difficult for the neophyte. However, the distinction is critical. For example, it is quite conceivable that a patient could present with a Class II deep bite dental relationship despite the presence of a skeletal open bite pattern. In this instance the cause of the Class II relationship would be the downward and backward rotation of the mandible while the deep bite was due to excessive eruption of the incisors. Obviously the treatment for such a Class II deep bite problem would differ from that for a Class II deep bite relationship in an individual who had a skeletal deep bite problem.

Problems Related to Failure of Eruption

One possible cause of open bite is failure of eruption of teeth. This can be due to either interference with normal eruption (by far the more common cause) or abnormalities in the periodontal ligament that affect the eruption mechanism.

Ankylosis of a primary or permanent tooth is defined as fusion of cementum directly to alveolar bone. When this occurs, even in a small area, further eruption of the tooth is impossible. If ankylosis occurs in a growing child, continued vertical development of other teeth leaves the ankylosed tooth behind so it appears submerged. An ankylosed primary tooth will impede eruption of the underlying permanent tooth and sometimes can lead to gross displacement of the permanent tooth bud. When normal eruption has been interfered with by such a mechanical obstruction, removal of the obstruction usually is followed by renewed eruption

of the impacted tooth. Even if the tooth whose eruption has been blocked does not erupt on its own into a normal position, it usually can be brought to that position by orthodontic tooth movement (see Fig. 1-30).

In the well-defined syndrome of cleidocranial dysplasia, generalized failure of eruption of succedaneous teeth occurs. Primary teeth, by contrast, erupt normally. The first permanent molars also erupt, befitting their status as an extension of the primary dental lamina. The problem is the lack of normal resorption of bone overlying the permanent teeth; thus eruption is impossible. If the overlying bone, and with it the obstruction, is removed, eruption of permanent teeth will occur.[140] Patients in whom eruption is being blocked mechanically, whether by an ankylosed primary tooth or by failure of bone resorption, can be recognized by lack of resorption over the crowns and a downward lengthening of the roots.

In the condition called primary failure of eruption,[119] abnormalities of the periodontal ligament cause eruption failure. The condition dramatically illustrates that eruptive movements of a tooth do not cause the resorption of alveolar bone that is a necessary part of eruption. In situations in which the eruption mechanism cannot express itself (Figs. 1-20 and 1-63), resorption of overlying bone creates large cystic-appearing areas around the unerupted teeth, but eruption does not occur. Primary failure of eruption differentially affects the posterior teeth. It appears that all teeth distal to the first affected tooth also are affected. In other words, if the first molars are affected, the second and third molars will be affected also but the premolars will be normal; however, if the premolars are affected, all molars will be affected also. The abnormal periodontal ligament does not respond to orthodontic tooth movement, even though the unerupted

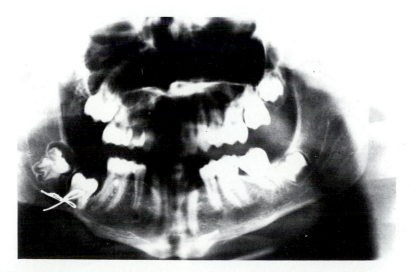

Fig. 1-63   Effect of wire ligature on eruption of the second molar for a patient in whom the ligature inadvertently trapped this tooth when a mandibular fracture was wired. Note that the ligature has mechanically prevented eruption, but bone over the unerupted molar has resorbed. Compare to the situation in Fig. 1-23. Note also that the mandibular left canine is unerupted. This tooth was in the line of a second fracture and is now ankylosed as a result of the trauma.

teeth are not ankylosed, as can be demonstrated by their normal mobility when they are surgically exposed. The affected teeth do become ankylosed when orthodontic forces are applied. Since this makes orthodontic treatment impossible, it is fortunate that the condition is rare; still, most practicing orthodontists encounter a few such patients during their career.

Radiographic Evaluation of Airway Status

With the recent emphasis on nasal obstruction as a potential contributor to the development of malocclusion, especially vertical dysplasia of the long face type, the use of lateral or PA cephalometric films to evaluate airway status has been suggested.[122] The shadow of the adenoids is clearly revealed on most lateral cephalometric films, and it seems reasonable to assume that measuring the distance between the adenoid mass and the surface of the soft palate (Fig. 1-64) would give an assessment of the posterior nasal airway. It must be remembered, however, that the two-dimensional cephalometric radiograph is an imperfect representation of the complex three-dimensional structure of the airway. Laboratory tests show that some patients with little or no apparent space for a posterior nasal airway on a cephalometric film do in fact have an adequate airway.[43] This can occur because of airflow on each side of the midline adenoid mass. A more important cephalometric relationship than the apparent width of the posterior airway is the position of the adenoid mass relative to the posterior nasal choanae (posterior wall of the maxilla). If the adenoid mass covers the posterior choanae, nasal obstruction is likely, but laboratory tests are required to confirm the radiographic finding.

Evaluating airway obstruction from P-A cephalometric films is even more subjective than doing this from lateral films. The tortuous nature of the nasal airway can be seen clearly on consecutively deeper tomographic films.[95] In a single film, the overlap makes it impossible to determine the point of minimum diameter, and thereby the limiting factor in nasal airflow.

A radiographic search for airway obstruction in deep nasal and pharyngeal structures may be somewhat misguided in any event, based on laboratory findings indicating that the opening of the nostril, which forms the liminal valve of the nasorespiratory system, often is the point of maximum resistance to airflow.[142] Dilating the nares with a piece of tubing typically decreases nasal resistance. This observation helps explain the otherwise puzzling finding that surgical procedures which move the maxilla upward, thereby reducing the volume of the nasal chamber, usually decrease resistance to nasal airflow rather than increase it.[153] One response to the maxillary surgery is widening of the alar base and flaring of the nostrils.

STEPS IN PLANNING TREATMENT

The last step in diagnosis is to generate a list of discrete and carefully designed problems. If the data base has been developed as suggested, it is in fact a list of problems under the following major headings:

- General and overall health problems (including self-image)
- Oral health and functional problems (including habits)
- Structural problems

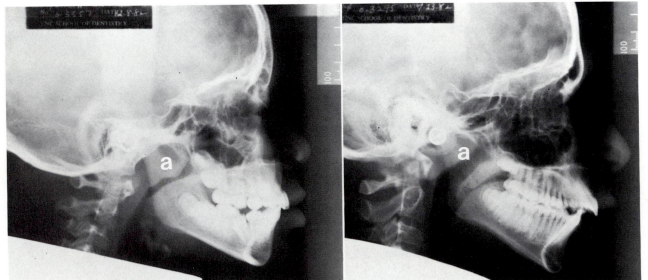

A   B

Fig. 1-64 **A,** Relatively large adenoids. **B,** Relatively small adenoids. The two-dimensional width of the airway between the adenoid mass *(a)* and the soft palate is not a good indicator of the three-dimensional volume of the actual airway.

TABLE 1-18

Possible Solutions to Some Typical Dentofacial Deformity Problems*

Problem	Possible solution
Protruding lips due to incisor protrusion	Premolar extraction, orthodontic retraction of incisors Premolar extraction, surgical retraction of incisor dentoalveolar segment Camouflage: genioplasty Incisor extraction, prosthodontic replacement

Skeletal mandibular deficiency (anteroposterior)	Differential mandibular growth
	   Headgear
	   Functional appliance
	Surgical mandibular advancement
	Camouflage: orthodontic or surgical retraction of maxillary incisors
	Camouflage: genioplasty

Excess anterior vertical dimension	Orthodontic treatment during growth: prevent molar eruption Rotate mandible closed surgically Surgical maxillary posterior intrusion Total maxillary intrusion Reduction genioplasty

*The proper choice depends on the *total* problem list for the individual patient. There is a best way for each patient, but it is not the same for all patients.

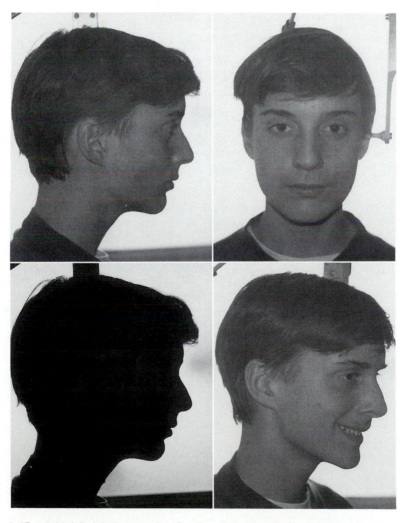

Fig. 1-65 Initial facial photographs of patient T.T. Mandibular deficiency is apparent.

- The subheadings under structural problems are the five characteristics of malocclusion: problems of
  - Alignment/symmetry within the dental arch
  - Profile and dentofacial esthetics
  - Transverse dental and skeletal relationships
  - Sagittal dental and skeletal relationships
  - Vertical dental and skeletal relationships

The diagnostic evaluation and development of a problem list for a typical orthodontic patient are illustrated in Figs. 1-65 to 1-67 and Table 1-18.

Treatment planning then is carried out in a series of steps:

1. *Separate pathologic from structural problems.* Differentiate the problems that will be handled with orthodontic treatment from those that will require other types of treatment
2. *Place the structural problems in priority order.* The most important problem comes first
3. *Consider the possible solutions to each problem.* Take them one at a time, with the most important first
4. *Review the interactions among the possible solutions.* Note that some possible solutions solve more than one problem, while others might solve one problem but make another worse
5. *Synthesize the possible solutions into a final plan.* Consider the interactions and practical considerations of cost and risk vs benefit, in order to maximize benefit to the patient

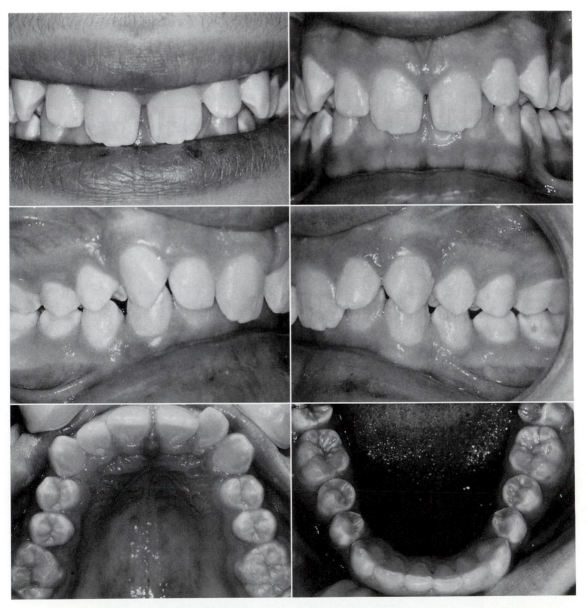

Fig. 1-66   Initial intra-oral photographs of patient T.T. Note the Class II, division 2, dental pattern but with normal exposure of the upper incisors beneath the lip.

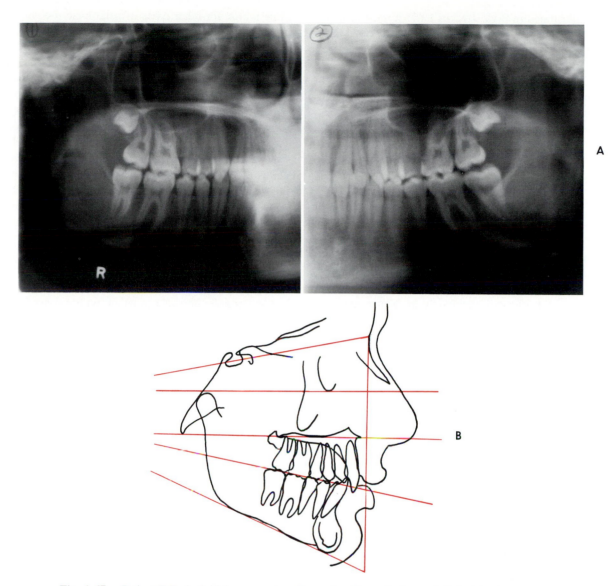

Fig. 1-67 Patient T.T. **A,** Initial panoramic radiograph, with no findings of clinical importance. **B,** Initial cephalometric tracing. For this patient, the relationship of the horizontal reference lines shows reasonably good vertical proportions, with the maxilla tipped slightly down posteriorly. The relationship of the maxilla and mandible to the N-perpendicular line suggests that the maxilla is slightly posteriorly to the normal position, and the mandible is more so. The mandibular plane to SN is 36°, SNA angle is 73°, and SNB is 69°; however, in this patient, these numbers are misleading and must be corrected if they are to be used at all. The problem is that the anterior cranial base is 11° to the Frankfort plane and the true horizontal (i.e., the SN line is tipped up anteriorly) (see Fig. 1-54 to note the same information in a template superimposition), which means that a 5° correction is needed (in measurements to SN). Even so, with the anterior position of nasion relative to the jaws, the ANB angle underestimates the severity of the skeletal Class II relationship. The A-B difference of 12 mm parallel to the true vertical line gives a clearer picture of the severity of the skeletal Class II. Because of the position of nasion and the resulting posterior inclination of the NA and NB lines, the Steiner figures for the relationship of the incisors to the NA and NB lines (maxillary incisor to NA, 6°, 4 mm; mandibular incisor to NB, 25°, 5 mm) are also somewhat misleading. Any particular set of cephalometric measurements must be made with an understanding of how they should be interpreted for a particular patient.

These sequential steps are discussed in detail below, and are illustrated in the development of a treatment plan for the patient illustrated in Figs. 1-65 to 1-67. It must be kept in mind that diagnosis (the formulation of the problem list) is a scientific and objective procedure. Its objective can be considered scientific truth. In contrast, the goal of treatment planning is wisdom, and subjective judgment must be used in developing the best plan for a specific patient. Judgment is first introduced at the point when the problems are prioritized. Inevitably, the same problem list prioritized differently will result in different treatment plans.

Pathologic vs Structural Problems

Priority for treatment has two aspects. First, pathologic problems must be brought under control; then attention can be turned to the structural problems of malocclusion and dentofacial deformity. This does not mean that the pathologic problems are necessarily more important, but rather that they are more time urgent. Thus the first step in planning treatment is to consider any pathologic problems, and arrange for proper treatment. The orthodontist does not have to treat periodontal breakdown discovered during the orthodontic diagnostic evaluation, but he or she is responsible for bringing it to the patient's attention and arranging a proper referral. Orthodontic treatment cannot begin until periodontal problems have been brought under control. The same is true for other types of pathologic problems.

Prioritizing the Problem List

Prioritizing the structural problem list is done to concentrate attention on what is most important for a particular patient. Edward Angle thought that there was a single ideal state for everyone, in which the best possible occlusion, facial esthetics, function, and stability coexisted. Unfortunately, that is not correct. The best occlusion may not be compatible with the best esthetics, or the best esthetics may not be compatible with the best function and stability. The patient's perception of his or her condition is important in setting these priorities. It is always difficult for clinicians to avoid imposing their own beliefs at this stage, and it is not totally inappropriate to do so; however, ignoring the patient's chief concern can lead to serious errors in planning treatment and potential litigious consequence.

For example, consider a patient with a Class II, division 1, malocclusion with mandibular deficiency and a weak chin. If the clinician concentrates on the occlusion and ignores the patient's concerns about the deficient chin, and formulates a treatment plan built around correcting the malocclusion by retracting the maxillary incisors, it is unlikely that the patient will be happy with the treatment result. The plan did not deal with the patient's major problem and was therefore inappropriate.

The prioritized problem list for the patient is shown in Figs. 1-65 to 1-67 (also see box below).

Possible Solutions to Problems

The next step is to review possible solutions to the individual problems, starting with the most severe and ending with the least severe. These tentative plans or solutions should be in broad terms, not yet to the stage of specific mechanotherapy.

There are two major advantages to this individual problem-individual plan approach before a final synthesis into a

---

 PROBLEM LIST, T.T.

FROM INTERVIEW:
None

FROM CLINICAL EXAMINATION:

Tissue health
- Wear facets on teeth
- Hypertrophied maxillary labial frenum

Jaw function
- Parafunction: probable nocturnal bruxism

Facial proportions
- Mandibular deficiency

FROM DIAGNOSTIC RECORDS:

Dental alignment/symmetry
- Crowded maxillary incisors, II/2 pattern
- Maxillary midline diastema
- Tooth size discrepancy, narrow maxillary lateral incisors

Profile/esthetics
- Mandibular deficiency

Transverse relationships
- Unilateral maxillary buccal crossbite tendency, left, dental

Sagittal (A-P) relationships
- Skeletal Class II, mandibular deficiency

Vertical relationships
- Anterior deep bite, skeletal and dental, with palatal impingement

---

 PRIORITIZED PROBLEM LIST, T.T.

A. PATHOLOGIC PROBLEMS
1. Wear facets on mandibular incisors (nocturnal bruxing?)
2. Hypertrophied maxillary labial frenum

B. STRUCTURAL PROBLEMS
1. Skeletal Class II, division 2, mandibular deficiency
2. Anterior deep bite, skeletal and dental
3. Unilateral buccal crossbite tendency, dental
4. Maxillary midline diastema
5. Tooth size discrepancy, small maxillary lateral incisors

unified plan takes place. The first is that there is less chance of rejecting a treatment possibility too soon or never thinking of it at all. The second, which is even more important, is that this approach allows the orthodontist to keep the patient's various problems in perspective and in priority order. The reason for listing the problems in priority order is to maintain a focus on what is most important for a particular individual. With a compulsion for ideal occlusion, orthodontists sometimes overlook the patient's chief concern. We must satisfy not only ourselves but the patient as well.

A possible solution is merely a general strategy for correcting the individual problems (e.g., tooth extractions, orthopedics, surgical orthodontics, functional orthodontics, control of tooth eruption). The treatment strategy is then translated into biomechanical terms and a specific mechanotherapy prescribed.

Treatment Possibilities

Before considering specific possibilities in detail, it is helpful to review the possibilities for orthodontic treatment more generally. These are outlined in Table 1-18. The specific possibilities for any patient will be combinations of these general possibilities, and key questions for planning treatment usually revolve around how to correct intra-arch crowding and malalignment (expansion or extraction?) and how to correct occlusal malrelationships (growth modification, orthodontic camouflage, or surgery?).

Crowding and Malalignment: To Extract or Not to Extract?

To satisfy the criteria *acceptable esthetics and reasonable stability*, the orthodontist frequently must consider extracting teeth. In 1921 Case observed the following:[22]

> *No matter how irregular the teeth, however bunched, malaligned, or malposed, they can always be placed in their respective places in the arch and in normal occlusion; therefore, so far as the relations of the teeth to others are concerned, no dental malposition should be taken as a basis for extraction. The only excuse for the extraction of saveable teeth must be that it is inexpedient or impossible to correct their positions that way without producing facial protrusion.*

The only thing that we would currently add to Case's dictum is that, in some cases, aligning malposed teeth without extraction might markedly affect the stability of the result. If we accept esthetics and stability as the valid criteria for extraction in orthodontics, how well can we determine in a child what the face will look like in adulthood and what the new functional environment will be after treatment?

Part of the answer was pointed out by Tweed in 1945.[154] He found that a group of patients whom he had treated without extractions showed a great tendency toward dental collapse. Since these dentitions had been expanded during treatment, he correctly reasoned that in these cases there was a greater tendency toward contraction of the arches than toward slight growth (expansion). When he removed teeth in these patients and closed spaces, stability was improved (but current data show that extraction is by no means a guarantee of long-term stability).[80,81] After retreatment with extraction, according to Tweed, these patients' profiles also were much improved as excessive protrusion was corrected.

It is important to note that Tweed's seminal cases had been treated initially without extraction, and were retreated with extraction. The orthodontist cannot always make the extraction decision on a priority basis. It is not always possible to predict what the profile will look like if teeth are not extracted. In many cases in which teeth have been extracted the profile appears less pleasing after treatment. In some mixed dentition cases in which serial extractions have been performed, it appears later that sufficient space has developed for all the permanent teeth.

Margolis[86] popularized the view that the most effective extraction strategy to relieve crowding is to extract the premolar teeth closest to the site of the crowding. Since most patients have incisor crowding, this would dictate extracting first premolars in most cases. Unfortunately, this rule has led to overretraction of anterior teeth in many cases. Carey[21] and Williams[161] showed evidence years ago for the benefit of extracting second premolars or even first molars to alleviate crowding but at the same time to reduce the degree of retraction of the anterior teeth. More recently, extraction of second molars has been advocated for the same reason.[13] In theory this provides some additional space and assumes that eventually the third molars will erupt into the second molar position. Although second molar extraction is an alternative in some cases, there is no documentation that second molar extraction offers greater stability than nonextraction treatment with later third molar extraction.[143]

Recent advocates of nonextraction treatment have suggested that expanding the arches early, in the mixed dentition, would overcome some of the esthetic and stability problems experienced during the post-Angle and pre-Tweed era. There are simply no long-term data available now to support this contention—which does not mean that it is wrong, only that it is unproven.

In orthodontics we have tended to be extreme in our views regarding extractions. In Angle's era it was considered a sin to extract in any case; later, at the height of Tweed and Begg's influence, nearly all irregularities became extraction cases; recently, the pendulum has again swung strongly toward nonextraction treatment. For years orthodontists considered that there were only a few borderline cases in which a decision to extract or not to extract was somewhat difficult. It is rather unsettling that borderline category probably encompasses more cases than we ever suspected. The ultimate facial appearance is affected by the growth of several structures (soft tissue, nose, chin), which at this time we cannot govern or predict. Stability of the dentition depends on factors that we know little about and over which we have little control. If we do not know the cause of a malocclusion, unless we remove the causal factors by chance, there is no reason to expect physiologic recovery. It may be necessary to observe the patient's response to the initial stages of treatment before making the final decision regarding whether extraction is required.

Skeletal Discrepancies: Growth Modification vs Camouflage vs Surgery

There are only three possibilities for treatment of a malocclusion caused by skeletal discrepancy: growth modification so that growth corrects the problem; orthodontic camouflage: moving teeth so the occlusion is corrected although the skeletal discrepancy remains; or surgical repositioning of the jaws. Each of the possibilities can be the appropriate choice in the right circumstance. Growth modification, if possible, provides the ideal result. Orthodontic camouflage represents a compromise. It can be quite acceptable and is the best choice in moderate discrepancies but is less acceptable in more severe problems. Surgery is reserved for the more severe problems but should not be overlooked.

Growth modification. The orthodontic pioneers took it for granted that their treatment could modify jaw proportions. They felt that environmental influences were the main cause of malocclusion. For example, allowing a child to sleep on his stomach so there was pressure on the chin that retarded mandibular growth, was considered a major cause of Class II problems. Angle assumed that Class II elastics significantly changed jaw growth, and attributed much of the occlusal correction to this. He abandoned his earlier use of headgear, not because it was ineffective, but because he thought it unnecessary when intraoral elastics could produce the same result.

Early cephalometric studies showed that the effects of the fixed orthodontic appliances of that era were almost totally caused by tooth movement, with little skeletal change. Accordingly, efforts at growth modification were largely abandoned in the United States in midcentury. In Europe, attempts at growth modification continued, using functional appliances that postured the mandible forward to stimulate the growth of deficient mandibles.

Headgear to influence maxillary growth was reintroduced in the United States in the late 1950s and was widely accepted by American orthodontists; however, functional appliances were used rarely until the 1970s. At present, opinions still differ regarding the effectiveness of growth modification, but the possibility is accepted by most clinicians. To briefly summarize an involved and important subject, a reasonable, current view follows:

1. Growth modification is possible, in patients who are growing actively—meaning that growth modification treatment must be carried out during the mixed dentition for many patients. By the time the premolars erupt, it is too late for most girls and many boys.
2. The amount of skeletal change that can be produced is significant but limited. More than 5 to 6 mm of differential growth between the maxilla and mandible is unlikely.

3. The skeletal effects of headgear and functional appliances are remarkably similar, despite their focus on the maxilla in the first instance and the mandible in the latter.
4. Restraint of excessive mandibular growth is extremely difficult to achieve, which means that a relatively high proportion of patients with mandibular prognathism will require surgery.
5. Because growth modification treatment changes the expression of growth but has little or no effect on the underlying growth pattern, treatment must continue, at least at a reduced level, until growth is essentially complete after adolescence.

For a more complete review of this subject, see Chapters 7, 8, 9, as well as 14 which is in *Contemporary Orthodontics*.[115]

Camouflage. If extractions are used to provide space, it is possible to correct molar and incisor relationships despite an underlying skeletal Class II or Class III jaw relationship. This method was developed as extractions were reintroduced into orthodontics in the 1930s and 1940s, and was most widely employed at the peak of orthodontic pessimism about growth modification.

The term camouflage implies that repositioning the teeth will not have a detrimental effect on facial esthetics. A considerable amount of retraction of protruding upper incisors in skeletal Class II patients can be carried out before prominence of the nose and too obtuse a nasolabial angle become an esthetic problem. Recent work suggests that in adolescents (who are the major candidates for camouflage, being too old at that point for effective growth modification), camouflage is unlikely to be successful if overjet is greater than 10 mm, especially if the mandible is short, lower incisors are already protrusive relative to the mandible, or face height is increased.[117]

Camouflage is less successful in Class III problems. Although the lower incisors can be retracted and the upper incisors protracted to correct reverse overjet (crossbite), the effect is to make the chin even more prominent. For this reason, camouflage is limited to mild Class III problems.

The AP movement of incisors to correct overjet does not improve excessive vertical exposure of incisors, and often makes this problem worse because intra-arch elastics have an extrusive component. Camouflage, therefore, is not indicated as an approach to long face problems.

Surgery. From the time of Angle, it was recognized that the only solution to mandibular prognathism in many instances was surgery to shorten the mandible. Until the 1960s, orthognathic surgery was almost entirely limited to this procedure. Since then, the technical problems have been overcome, and it is now possible to reposition both jaws in all three planes of space. Surgical intervention should be limited to the most severe problems, but when camouflage would not be satisfactory, it is the alternative of choice. For further information on surgical treatment possibilities and the interaction between orthodontist and surgeon, see Chapter 15 and *Surgical-Orthodontic Treatment*.[118]

Synthesizing Possible Solutions into a Final Treatment Plan

With the list of treatment possibilities complete, the treatment plan can be completed. The objective, of course, is to come up with the plan that is best for that individual patient, and the steps in planning treatment are designed to produce that outcome.

Three things must be considered: interactions among the treatment possibilities, cost and risk vs benefit, and *practical considerations* such as the patient's willingness and ability to cooperate with various types of treatment. Prediction of treatment results can be an important tool in choosing among treatment alternatives (Table 1-19).

Interactions Among Treatment Possibilities

When problems and their possible solutions are listed in priority order, it becomes apparent what possibilities would solve more than one problem, while some other solutions.

TABLE 1-19

Prioritized Problem List and Synthesis of Treatment Possibilities into a Final Plan

Patient: T. T.
Chronological age: 13 yr 5 mo
Dental age: Commensurate with chronologic age
Skeletal age: 12 yr 6 mo
Behavioral characteristics: Well adjusted psycholosocially
Growth forecast: Potential for favorable mandibular growth
Anticipated cooperation: Hopefully good

Prioritized problem list	Treatment possibilities	Unified treatment plan
A. Pathologic problems		
Problem 1: Wear facets on mandibular incisors caused by nocturnal bruxing.	Use niteguard as retainer post active treatment.	
Problem 2: Hypertrophied maxillary labial frenum.	Consider frenectomy if necessary.	
B. Structural problems		Level and align maxillary and mandibular teeth, flaring maxillary incisors, closing maxillary midline diastema, creating curve of Spee in the maxillary arch and reducing curve of Spee in mandibular arch to open the bite. Consider frenectomy before active treatment complete.
Problem 1: Class II, division 2, skeletal and dental.	Convert to Class II, division 1; restrain maxillary growth and use forward growth of mandible. Reevaluate, depending on facial growth pattern and patient compliance, for possible mandibular advancement surgery.	Use extraoral traction to restrain maxillary growth and use intermaxillary elastics as needed to correct sagittal problem. Reevaluate if necessary for possible mandibular advancement surgery.
Problem 2: Anterior deep bite with palatal impingement of mandibular incisors, dental, and skeletal.	Open bite through differential eruption of posterior teeth; anterior intrusion unnecessary if growth occurs and undesirable for preparation for surgery.	Post treatment consider bonding of maxillary lateral incisors if necessary. Use niteguard as maxillary retainer and use fixed retention in mandibular anterior region.
Problem 3: Maxillary buccal crossbite tendency left side, skeletal, and dental.	Constrict maxillary left buccal segment and expand mandibular left buccal segment; arch wires should be adequate, unilateral crosselastics undesirable.	
Problem 4: Maxillary midline diastema.	Condense space.	
Problem 5: Anterior tooth size discrepancy caused by narrow maxillary lateral incisors.	Consider bonding of maxillary lateral incisors post treatment if spacing has occurred.	

Rentention requirements: Indefinite retention may be required.
Overall prognosis: Guarded depending on patient compliance and facial growth pattern.

are incompatible because solving one problem would make another worse.

An important interaction is the relationship between vertical and horizontal changes in the position of the mandible. For instance, in the case of a patient with overjet and a deep bite, attempts to open the bite with conventional orthodontic mechanics could make the overjet worse (in the absence of growth) because the mandible would rotate downward and backward if posterior teeth were extruded. In an older patient, this interaction might dictate use of intrusive mechanics. Considerations of this type become second nature to the experienced clinician, but the process of listing the possibilities and then thinking about their interactions can be a great help in dealing with complex cases and multiple problems.

Prediction of Outcomes as a Treatment Planning Tool

Interactions among treatment possibilities are easiest to see when the probable outcomes are predicted. Prediction now takes three forms: setups of the teeth so the clinician can view the way they would fit if rearranged in a certain way (with or without extraction, for instance, or if the jaws were moved surgically to a different position); cephalometric prediction of changes caused by growth or treatment; and profile prediction, based on computer manipulation of video images of the patient's profile.

Orthodontic tooth prediction on dental casts. If the teeth are to be reset on casts to determine the potential result of orthodontic tooth movement, it is better not to move the last molars from their original positions even if these teeth will be moved during treatment (Fig. 1-68). Leaving this last tooth in place has two advantages: (1) the vertical dimension is maintained and (2) the tooth serves as a reference point for the initial position of the teeth and jaws. When the other teeth are removed, cuts should be made up beneath but not through the contact points. Then the individual teeth can be broken apart so their widths are not reduced.

Special attention should be paid to considerations as the teeth are reset:

1. The amount of space required to level the arches. Leveling out the curve of Spee always requires more space (Fig. 1-69). Without extraction, the incisors will be thrown forward as the arch is leveled; with extraction, some extraction space will be closed as the arch is leveled out. A guide for planning purposes is that approximately 0.75 mm of additional arch length is required for each millimeter of vertical leveling if the total arch including the second molars is levelled; 0.25 mm is needed for each millimeter if the second molars are not leveled.[45]

2. The relative amount of any extraction space to be closed by retracting the anterior teeth versus mesial movement of posterior teeth. This is affected by both

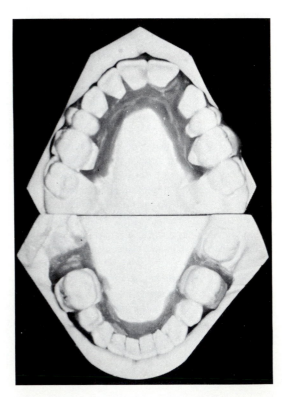

Fig. 1-68 Diagnostic setup for evaluating possible posttreatment tooth positioning in a patient with crowding, a missing maxillary lateral incisor, and incisor protrusion. Note that first premolars have been removed. Leaving the last molars on the cast allows evaluation of the posterior anchorage requirements; it is apparent that no forward movement of the upper molars could be tolerated in this patient, while the lower molars should come forward during closure of the lower extraction spaces.

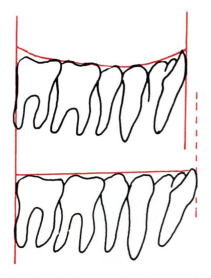

Fig. 1-69 Leveling the lower arch when there is an excessive curve of Spee inevitably increases arch length, which leads to incisor protrusion, unless the arch is expanded laterally or the molars are moved distally (which is difficult). The effect on arch length is nonlinear—relatively more arch expansion is needed to level a deep curve of Spee rather than a shallow one.

the type of mechanotherapy and by which teeth were extracted. Extractions at the posterior part of the arch produce much less potential for incisor retraction than do extractions that are more anterior. Extraction of the second molar provides only 1 to 2 mm additional space for decrowding of the arch, and it leaves little possibility for incisor retraction. Moving the extraction site more anteriorly leaves greater possibilities for incisor retraction, as opposed to mesial movement of posterior teeth. When the extraction is within the dental arch (so there are anterior and posterior anchorage units), the orthodontic mechanotherapy also can be varied to maximize or minimize incisor retraction as desired, within the limits established by which teeth were extracted. When first premolars are selected for extraction, the space closure can be managed with a maximum 3:1 differential in either direction. It is important that the cast setup be realistic in showing tooth movement possibilities. An overly optimistic prediction is not helpful in producing a rational treatment plan.

When orthodontic tooth movement will be done in preparation for surgical repositioning of the jaws, the repositioned teeth on the cast represent a dental prediction for the first phase of treatment (there should also be a corresponding cephalometric prediction). These casts are moved to a new occlusal relationship on an articulator for a prediction of the occlusion after the surgical treatment. When the first phase of treatment has been completed, new records must be taken; and these records, of actual relationships at the conclusion of presurgical orthodontic treatment, are used in the final planning for the second (surgical) phase of correction.

Cephalometric visualized treatment objectives. One method of representing the treatment goals two-dimensionally (sagittally and vertically) is by outlining the proposed skeletal and dental changes on the cephalometric tracing. This approach produces a blueprint or architectural plan, which then is carried out through the appropriate mechanotherapy. This is particularly effective in planning treatment for nongrowing patients (adults) and for planning surgical treatment.[139] (See Chapter 14.)

It is somewhat more difficult to accomplish this for the growing patient because of the limitations in our ability to forecast growth, which does not, however, diminish the importance of attempting to adopt this kind of thinking in treatment planning. The concepts of Bjork and Skieller[14] related to forward and backward rotating growth patterns have markedly improved our previous understanding of facial growth patterns. It is no longer acceptable to rely on the constancy of growth pattern concepts of Broadbent[17] and Brodie,[18] since it is now clear that increments of facial growth are not uniform in either direction or rate. Even the paths of eruption of the teeth are quite variable and difficult to predict.

Methods for growth prediction continue to improve, but since the current approaches are based on relatively small samples and use average growth increments, accuracy in the more deviant cases is lacking. Templates are as effective as current computer methods, since both use the method of adding average growth increments to the present relationships. A different approach to growth forecasting, perhaps using innovative mathematical approaches but probably requiring more complete data sets, will be necessary to make growth prediction precise enough to be of real clinical value.

Video image predictions of profile changes. In the absence of growth, prediction can be quite accurate. Prediction of treatment changes in the absence of growth is especially useful when surgical treatment is being considered for an adult, and computer manipulation of digitized tracings has the advantage of making it quick and easy to do multiple predictions. (See Chapter 5.) The recent introduction of video images of the patient's profile superimposed in computer memory on the tracing makes it possible to make hard tissue changes and visualize the probable soft tissue effects (but the accuracy is limited to the quality of the algorithms linking hard tissue change to soft tissue change, and these are somewhat questionable). Nevertheless, both the clinician and the patient can more readily grasp the esthetic impact of the proposed treatment when video images are available,[129] and this method of prediction is likely to be even more useful in the future as both hardware and software are improved.

Cost and Risk vs Benefit

This evaluation is a way of expressing what Moorrees and Gron[98] called *therapeutic modifiability*. The greater the effort is to achieve a small change, the less is the therapeutic modifiability, and vice versa. In a sense, the orthodontist's goal is economy of effort and resources, so that the benefit to the patient is maximized while the risk and cost are minimized. The desired economy is obtained when the cost-risk vs benefit ratio, and the therapeutic modifiability, are high.

The risk of any treatment procedure and its cost (considered broadly, not just in money but also in cooperation, discomfort, aggravation, and time) must be compared to its benefit to the patient. For example, the risk and cost of surgery to correct a jaw discrepancy would be higher than the risk and cost of inter-arch elastics to correct the incisor relationship, or the risk and cost of extraction treatment to correct incisor crowding would be greater than that of nonextraction treatment (in terms of the treatment difficulty and cooperation required, even if the fee was the same). But if the simpler and less risky procedures would provide little real benefit to the patient, while the more involved procedures would be of considerable benefit, the analysis might still favor surgery or extraction. The question "Is it worth it?" is an important one. It must be answered from the patient's perspective, and must be discussed during the case presentation designed to obtain informed consent.

In considering therapeutic modifiability, the orthodontist should regard two points in time: (1) when active treatment will be completed; and (2) when the patient will no longer be wearing orthodontic appliances, either active or passive. If teeth are moved to unstable positions, there is every likelihood that relapse will occur, unless permanent retention is employed—and if this is planned, its cost in patient cooperation should be considered.

Integrally involved with the concept of modifiability is the assessment of possible contraindications to treatment. The risks increase as treatment goals are pushed to the limits of what is possible. For example, an overly zealous treatment plan for alignment by expansion can result in well-aligned tooth crowns but with severe root resorption, devitalization or fenestration of the labial cortical plate of bone (Figs. 1-70 to 1-72).

Practical Considerations

For many patients, there are pertinent special considerations to be taken into account. In planning treatment for maximum benefit to the patient, it is equally important not to introduce these considerations too soon, so that treatment possibilities are ignored, and not to overlook them altogether. For example, in a periodontally involved adult, it may be important to minimize treatment time to help maintain periodontal control. (See Chapter 13.) If the growth pattern is uncertain, it may be important to keep treatment options open. If the appearance of the appliance is important to the patient, it may be important to use lingual brackets, even if this makes treatment more difficult, expensive, and time consuming. These considerations can be addressed rationally only when the treatment possibilities and the other factors influencing the final treatment plan are known.

Testing Treatment Response

No treatment plan should be considered final, because midcourse corrections can be made at any time depending on treatment response, patient cooperation, growth, or any

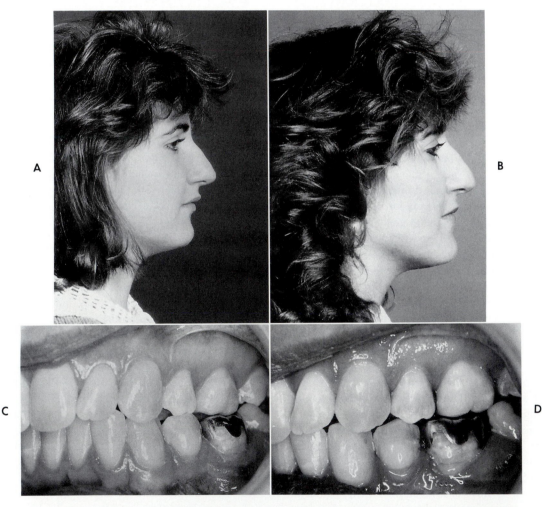

Fig. 1-70 Patient N.A. **A,** Profile and, **B,** occlusal relationships after initial orthodontic treatment. **C,** Profile and, **D,** occlusal relationships after retreatment with surgical mandibular advancement. The initial treatment was attempted orthodontic camouflage of skeletal mandibular deficiency. The patient was not happy with the esthetics; a Class II molar relationship and an excess overjet persisted long-term.

unforeseen events. A number of orthodontic diagnostic systems have been devised that project a rigid treatment plan from limited cephalometric and dental cast measurements. By offering a format for establishing and analyzing the data base, we have not meant to imply that a treatment plan which will require no changes can be generated for all patients. Rigid systems or definitive treatment plans succeed for the majority of patients but fail for others. The difficulty is that of the weather forecasts of years past, which said flatly: rain or clear, with no allowance for uncertainty.

There are several sources of uncertainty in orthodontic treatment plans. A major difficulty is that the cause of a malocclusion is rarely known; as long as this is the case, there must be some uncertainty in the treatment plan for correction of the problem. An orthodontic treatment plan is quite likely to be the same whether the malocclusion is caused by genetic influences on jaw morphology or by neuromuscular influences on tooth position, but the treatment response may not be the same at all. Also the mechanotherapy required to achieve the goals of orthodontic treatment in adults may be considered against a background of unchanging jaw relationships, whereas in growing children it must be considered against the changes that will occur because of growth as well as those that will occur because

of treatment. Growth prediction introduces another uncertainty into the diagnostic procedure.

One way to deal with diagnostic uncertainty is to use the treatment response as another diagnostic criterion.[4] With this procedure an initial diagnosis is made, in the face of some uncertainty, as to the nature of the problem. An initial stage of specifically directed treatment is based on this diagnosis, and the treatment response is used to confirm or reject the original diagnosis. For example, an anterior open bite may be diagnosed as caused by thumbsucking, and treatment to correct the sucking habit may be started. If the open bite is eliminated without further treatment, the diagnosis is supported. If the open bite persists, the diagnosis will have to be modified, perhaps to include excessive posterior vertical development. If the patient responds well to a functional appliance that controls posterior eruption, this diagnosis is confirmed. If not, other factors will have to be considered. This approach is called *therapeutic diagnosis*.

In fact, all interceptive procedures in orthodontics are exercises in therapeutic diagnosis. For example, if a problem of maxillary incisor protrusion and open bite is resolved with the use of such devices as thumb-guard appliances and lip bumpers, then the indictment of a habit as the cause is confirmed. If the malocclusion persists, a new hypothesis

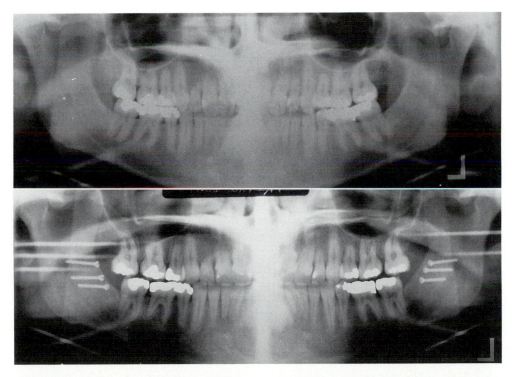

Fig. 1-71 Patient N.A. Panoramic radiographs before and after surgical-orthodontic retreatment. Note the severe resorption of the maxillary incisors (especially on the right side) that occurred during the initial orthodontic treatment. Resorption is particularly likely to occur during attempts to camouflage skeletal Class II or Class III problems, apparently because this tends to throw the maxillary incisor roots against the lingual cortical plate. No further resorption occurred during the retreatment because care was taken to avoid contact of the roots with the cortical plate.

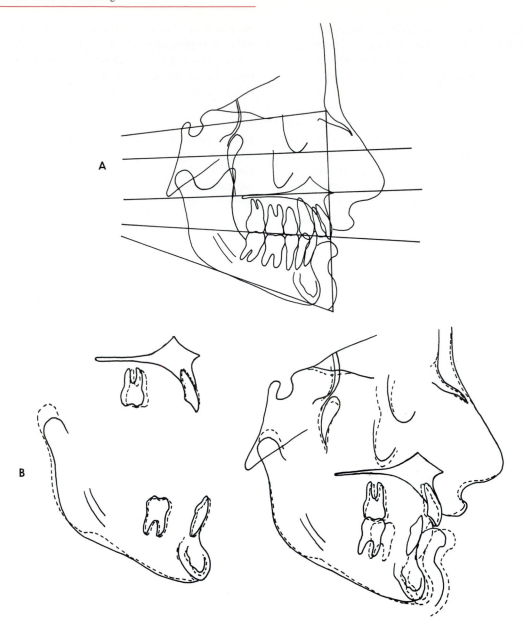

Fig. 1-72   Patient N.A. **A,** Cephalometric tracing at age 20 (5 years after initial orthodontic treatment was completed). **B,** Cephalometric superimposition showing the change produced by surgical retreatment with mandibular advancement. Rotating the mandible at surgery so the chin moves both downward and forward improves face height and enhances stability.

or diagnosis must be formulated and a new treatment plan must be established.

The use of therapeutic diagnosis implies that the cause of the problem is not known. For this reason a concerted effort has been made in medicine to move beyond therapeutic diagnosis. As we learn more about the etiology of malocclusion, we should also strive to perfect our diagnostic abilities in orthodontics. On the other hand, it is important to recognize that a diagnosis that does not include the cause

of the problem, as many orthodontic diagnoses do not, is incomplete and leaves room for error.

Therapeutic diagnosis is not a substitute for established diagnostic procedures; nor should it become a cover for fuzzy thinking in diagnosis. However, when uncertainty exists despite a careful diagnostic evaluation, it is dangerous to formulate a rigid treatment plan. Systematic evaluation of the initial response to orthodontic treatment can help a great deal in making difficult diagnostic and treatment planning decisions, especially concerning the basic question of extraction or nonextraction. Borderline cases, in which the treatment response should be considered before the orthodontist decides to extract, are more common than many diagnostic systems indicate. It is strength, not weakne. recognize true uncertainty.

If doubt exists about a borderline case, evaluation of response to treatment can begin with the first phase of treatment. While applying separators in a crowded case, the orthodontist can determine whether all the contacts are tight. Do the separators stay in with minimal effect, or do they fall out a few days later because of space between the teeth? How sore do the teeth become from the separators? When the posterior bands are fit, how difficult is it to seat them? When the orthodontist is working in the patient's mouth, how tight is the labial and buccal musculature? Does the tongue protrude over the teeth? Do the preformed bands demonstrate significant tooth-size discrepancies between the right and left sides? During the seating of bands, how hard can the patient bite?

At the next visit the patient's oral hygiene can be checked, and the orthodontist can also observe whether the patient deformed the archwires and whether the patient has a grinding or a clenching habit. All these factors are likely to influence the course of treatment.

From this frame of reference, much of orthodontic treatment is based on a type of therapeutic diagnosis. If a child is treated successfully (occlusally and facially) without extractions and remains stable, we assume that a correct decision was made and that some of the causes of the problem were also eliminated. If, on the other hand, nonextraction treatment proceeds with difficulty, adversely affecting facial esthetics or indicating the prospect of an unstable denture, we can then presume that extraction might alleviate the problem. When extraction cases are selected on this basis, the results are more consistently successful. It is not surprising that in these cases the residual extraction spaces close rapidly after treatment and facial esthetics improve.

It is impractical to perform a therapeutic diagnosis for every orthodontic patient. Many cases need a decision to extract from the start (e.g., a bimaxillary dentoalveolar protrusion with crowding). If therapeutic diagnosis were carried to an extreme, the increase in treatment time in many cases would make the approach unrealistic. The final decision in a therapeutic diagnosis should be made within the first 6 months of treatment. The increase in treatment time is minimal if an extraction decision is made after the first few months, since the first phases of treating extraction and nonextraction cases involve the same basic elements of alignment and leveling.

The importance of assessing the patient's cooperation with regard to wearing appliances and to practicing oral hygiene, should not be minimized. Since our treatment planning in orthodontics always calls for some type of therapy that requires the patient's diligence in wearing appliances, this factor can be tested only by instituting treatment. If oral hygiene is poor, the hazard of decalcification becomes great. It is sometimes comforting to be able to attenuate the treatment goals and reduce treatment time.

PRESENTING THE PLAN TO THE PATIENT: INFORMED CONSENT

Informed consent is a social policy based on ethical guidelines and supported by legal precedents. In order for consent to be legally valid, it must be obtained voluntarily from a mentally competent person of legal age. The landmark decisions regarding what constitutes informed consent are based on the patient's right to autonomy.

The positive value of informed consent is that it enhances the doctor/patient relationship through better communication. As Chiccone[23] suggested, we recommend that the following points be discussed with the patient:

1. Diagnosis, presented in language the patient can understand
2. Comprehensive treatment plan, explaining what procedures are recommended and how they will be performed
3. Overview of reasonable alternative treatments that are available, whether or not you perform them
4. Probable sequelae of electing nontreatment
5. Potential risks, consequences and likelihood of secondary treatment (It is the complication not discussed with the patient that triggers a liability claim. Some states have adopted legislation that defines by percent occurrence the need to discuss a potential risk; for example, in Montana a 0.5% to 3% risk need not be disclosed to the patient.)
6. Predicted outcome of treatment, including how the patient will benefit and the probability of success (Keep in mind that reality should always supersede optimism.)

Chiccone goes on to say that there are three caveats to be heeded in implementing the doctrine of informed consent:

1. The greater the potential injury, even if the risk is minimal, the greater the obligation to inform the patient (So if the orthodontist is recommending orthognathic surgery, the risk of death from general anesthesia should be discussed even though it is extremely small.)
2. The greater the chance of a risk occurring even if the injury would be minimal, the greater the obligation to inform the patient (So the orthodontist should point out that minimal, almost undetectable, root resorption occurs in nearly all teeth in nearly all patients who undergo tooth movement.)
3. The more elective the proposed treatment, the more invasive the bodily intrusion will be considered in the event of an injury (So surgery for minor esthetic reasons should be discussed carefully.)

Although originally the doctrine of informed consent was grounded in assault and battery theory, this has largely been replaced by the negligence theory. According to Kukafka,[75] the elements of an informed consent cause of action in negligence are:

1. A patient-doctor relationship existed
2. The provider had a duty to disclose relevant information
3. The provider failed to provide this information and failure cannot be excused
4. If the provider had furnished the patient with the undisclosed information, the patient would not have consented to treatment
5. The plaintiff's injury and damages claimed were a reasonably foreseeable consequence of the inadequate information: proximate cause

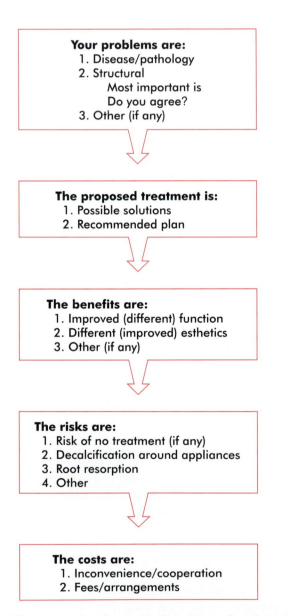

Fig. 1-73 A flow chart for consultation with a patient that ends with informed consent.

There are two standards for an orthodontist's duty to disclose information under the informed consent doctrine. The first of these is known as the *professional standard*. This standard is merely that the orthodontist proceeds as any competent orthodontist would do under a similar circumstance. The other standard, which has now replaced the professional standard in most states, is the *reasonable person standard*. The courts have decided that the standard for disclosure should not rest in the practitioner community but should be based on the standard that doctors are required to disclose information based on a reasonable patient's judgment as to whether disclosure would aid his or her consent decision. With this standard, the decision-making power is assigned to the patient only to the extent to which the doctor feels a reasonable patient would require this information in order to make an informed decision. In short the doctor is not required to give a mini-course in orthodontics. If the issues are complex, they should be put into simple language so the patient can understand them. The key is presenting the information so that the patient has autonomy in deciding what treatment he or she will receive.[2]

The problem-oriented approach to orthodontic diagnosis and treatment planning recommended in this chapter facilitates obtaining true informed consent. Note that the diagnostic information is obtained and can be presented to the patient in exactly the format Chiccone recommends. We suggest that the consultation appointment follow the outline shown in Fig. 1-73.

In this chapter we have outlined the general principles of diagnosis and treatment planning in orthodontics. The separation-synthesis approach to the decision-making process reduces complex problems to simple terms. Since variation is the theme in orthodontics, this method allows the flexibility of individualizing treatment for any patient, whether the problem is common or uncommon, mild or severe. On the one hand we offer a format that is useful in assessing orthodontic problems; on the other hand we emphasize that there are no rigid procedures required in every case. There is no more creative aspect of orthodontics than treatment planning. Each patient's problems, if viewed with an open mind and freshness of view, can offer a stimulating challenge to even an experienced clinician. We hope that we have captured some of the excitement and satisfaction that can be derived from approaching this subject from this perspective.

REFERENCES

1. Ackerman JL: Orthodontics: art, science, or trans-science? *Angle Orthod* 44:243, 1974.
2. Ackerman JL: Ethics and risk management in orthodontics, *Proc Harvard Soc Advance Orthod,* 1992.
3. Ackerman JL, Ackerman AL, Ackerman AB: Taurodont, pyramidal and fused molar roots associated with other anomalies in a kindred, *Am J Phys Anthropol* 38:681, 1973.
4. Ackerman JL, Proffit WR: Treatment response as an aid in diagnosis and treatment planning, *Am J Orthod* 57:490, 1970.
5. Ackerman JL, Proffit WR: Preventive and interceptive orthodontics: a strong theory proves weak in practice, *Angle Orthod* 50-75, 1980.

6. Altemus LA: Cephalofacial relationships, *Angle Orthod* 38:275, 1968.

7. Amsterdam M: Periodontal prosthesis, twenty-five years in retrospect, *Alpha Omegan* 67:8, 1972.

8. Andrews LF: The six keys to normal occlusion, *Am J Orthod* 62:296, 1972.

9. Angle EH: *Treatment of malocclusion of the teeth and fractures of the maxillae,* ed 6, Philadelphia, 1900, SS White Dental Manufacturing.

10. Baume LJ: Physiological tooth migration and its significance for the development of occlusion, *J Dent Res* 29:123, 331, 338, 440, 1950.

11. Begg PR, Kesling PC: *Begg orthodontic theory and technique,* ed 3, Philadelphia, 1977, WB Saunders.

12. Bennett NG: Report of the committee on orthodontic classification, *Oral Health* 2:321, 1912.

13. Bishara SE, Burkey PS: Second molar extractions: a review, *Am J Orthod Dentofac Orthop* 89:415, 1986.

14. Bjork A, Skieller V: Facial development and tooth eruption: an implant study at the age of puberty, *Am J Orthod* 62:339, 1972.

15. Bolton WA: The clinical application of a tooth-size analysis, *Am J Orthod* 48:504, 1962.

16. Brader AC: Dental arch form related with intraoral forces: PR = C, *Am J Orthod* 61:541, 1972.

17. Broadbent BH: The face of the normal child, *Angle Orthod* 7:183, 1937.

18. Brodie AG: On the growth pattern of the human head: from the third month to the eighth year of life, *Am J Anat* 68:209, 1941.

19. Brodie AG: The apical base: zone of interaction between the intestinal and skeletal systems, *Angle Orthod* 36:136, 1966.

20. Brown DF, Spencer AJ, Tolliday PD: Social and psychological factors associated with adolescents' self-acceptance of occlusal conditions, *Comm Dent Oral Epidemiol* 15:70-73, 1987.

21. Carey CW: Light force technique combining the sliding section and laminated arches, *Am J Orthod* 52:85, 1966.

22. Case CS: *A practical treatise on the technics and principles of dental orthopedia and prosthetic correction of cleft palate,* Chicago, 1921, CS Case.

23. Chiccone MU: *Informed consent: in perspective, Dental Rx* 3(2): Newark, 1990 (Publication of Mid-Atlantic Medical Insurance).

24. Christiansen EL, Thompson JR: *Temporomandibular joint imaging,* St Louis, 1990, Mosby.

25. Clifford MM: Physical attractiveness and academic performance, *Child Study* 5:201-209, 1975.

26. Coben SE: Basion horizontal coordinate tracing film, *J Clin Orthod* 13:598, 1979.

27. Cooke MS: Five-year reproducibility of natural head posture: a longitudinal study, *Am J Orthod Dentofac Orthop* 97:487, 1990.

28. Corrucini RS: An epidemiologic transition in dental occlusion in world populations, *Am J Orthod* 86:419, 1984.

29. Corrucini RS: Australian aboriginal tooth succession, interproximal attrition and Begg's theory, *Am J Orthod Dentofac Orthop* 97:347-357, 1990.

30. Currier JH: A computerized geometric analysis of human dental arch form, *Am J Orthod* 56:164, 1969.

31. Davidovitch Z, Montgomery PC, Yost RW, Shanfeld JL: Immuno-histochemical localization of cyclic nucleotides in the periodontium: mechanically stressed cells in vivo, *Anat Rec* 192:351, 1978.

32. DeBrul EL, Sicher H: *The adaptative chin,* Springfield, Ill, 1954, Charles C Thomas.

33. DeFriese GH, editor: *Planning for dental care on a statewide basis,* Chapel Hill, North Carolina, 1981, Dental Foundation of North Carolina.

34. Edwards JG: The diastema, the frenum, the frenectomy: a clinical study, *Am J Orthod* 71:489, 1977.

35. Egermark I, Thilander B: Craniomandibular disorders with special reference to orthodontic treatment: an evaluation from childhood to adulthood, *Am J Orthod Dentofac Orthop* 101:28, 1992.

36. Egermark–Ericsson I, Carlsson GE, Magnusson T: A long-term epidemiologic study of the relationship between occlusal factors and mandibular dysfunction in children and adolescents, *J Dent Res* 66:67, 1987.

37. El Mangoury NH, Mostafa YA: Epidemiologic panorama of malocclusion, *Angle Orthod* 60:207, 1990.

38. Farkas LG, Munro IR: *Anthropometric facial proportions in medicine,* Springfield, Ill, 1987, Charles C Thomas.

39. Fédération Dentaire Internationale: 58th Annual Session (S. Keiser-Nielson, Chairman), Bucharest, 1971.

40. Fields HW: *Treatment of skeletal problems in preadolescent children.* In Proffit WR: *Contemporary orthodontics,* ed 2, St Louis, 1993, Mosby.

41. Fields HW Jr: Orthodontic-restorative treatment for relative mandibular anterior excess tooth-size problems, *Am J Orthod* 79:176, 1981.

42. Fields HW, Proffit WR, Nixon WL et al: Facial pattern differences in long-faced children and adults, *Am J Orthod* 85:217, 1984.

43. Fields HW, Warren DW, Black K, Phillips C: Relationship between vertical dentofacial morphology and respiration in adolescents, *Am J Orthod Dentofac Orthop* 99:147, 1991.

44. Fischer B: *Clinical orthodontics,* Philadelphia, 1957, WB Saunders.

45. Germane N, Staggers JA, Rubenstein L, Revere JT: Arch length considerations due to the curve of Spee: a mathematical model, *Am J Orthod Dentofac Orthop* 102:251, 1992.

46. Glasser MA, Hoffman WS: *Demand for care: the effects of prepayment on the utilization of dental services.* In Bawden JW, DeFriese GH, editors: *Planning for dental care on a statewide basis,* Chapel Hill, North Carolina, 1981, Dental Foundation of North Carolina.

47. Glenn G, Sinclair PM, Alexander RC: Non-extraction orthodontic therapy: posttreatment dental and skeletal stability, *Am J Orthod Dentofac Orthop* 91:321, 1987.

48. Gorlin RJ, Pindborg JJ, Cohen MM: *Syndromes of the head and neck,* ed 2, New York, 1990, McGraw-Hill.

49. Grainger RM: *Orthodontic treatment priority index,* Series 2, no. 25, Washington, DC, 1965, National Center for Health Statistics.

50. Grave KC, Brown T: Skeletal ossification and the adolescent growth spurt, *Am J Orthod* 69:611, 1976.

51. Greulich WW, Pyle SL: *Radiographic atlas of skeletal development of the hand and wrist,* ed 2, Stanford, Calif, 1959, Stanford University Press.

52. Gron AM: Prediction of tooth emergence, *J Dent Res* 41:573, 1962.

53. Guilford SH: *Orthodontia or malposition of human teeth, prevention and remedy,* Philadelphia, 1889, Spangler.

54. Harris EF, Johnson MG: Heritability of craniometric and occlusal variables: a longitudinal sib analysis, *Am J Orthod Dentofac Orthop* 99:258, 1992.

55. Harvold EP, Tomer BS, Vargervik K et al: Primate experiments on oral respiration, *Am J Orthod* 79:359, 1981.

56. Hellman M: Variations in occlusion, *Dent Cosmos* 63:608, 1921.

57. Helm S, Peterson PE: Causal relationship between malocclusion and caries, *Acta Odontol Scand* 47:217, 1989.

58. Hirata RH, Heft MW, Hernandez B, King GJ: Longitudinal study of signs of temporomandibular disorders (TMD) in orthodontically treated and nontreated groups, *Am J Orthod Dentofac Orthop* 101:35, 1992.

59. Horowitz SL, Hixon EH: *The nature of orthodontic diagnosis,* St Louis, 1966, Mosby.

60. Houston WJB, Miller JC, Tanner JM: Prediction of the timing of the adolescent growth spurt from ossification events in hand-wrist films, *Br J Orthod* 6:145, 1979.

61. Hurme VO: Ranges of normalcy in the eruption of permanent teeth, *J Dent Child* 16:11, 1949.

62. Ingervall B, Janson T: The value of clinical lip strength measurements, *Am J Orthod* 80:495, 1981.

63. Jankelson B: Electronic control of muscle contractions—a new era in occlusion and prosthodontics, *Sci Educ Bull Coll Dent* 2:29, 1969.

64. Johnston MC, Bronsky PT: Abnormal craniofacial development: an overview, *J Craniofac Genet Dev Biol.*

65. Kelly J, Harvey C: *An assessment of the teeth of youths 12-17 years,* DHEW Publication no. (HRA) 77-1644, Washington, DC, 1977, National Center for Health Statistics, USPHS.

66. Kelly JE, Sanchez M, Van Kirk LE: *An assessment of the occlusion of teeth of children,* DHEW Publication no. (HRA) 74-1612, Washington, DC, 1973, National Center for Health Statistics, USPHS.

67. Kenealy P, Frude N, Shaw W: An evaluation of the psychological and social effects of malocclusion: some implications for dental policy making, *Soc Sci Med* 28:583, 1989.

68. Kerr WJ, McWilliam JS, Linder-Aronson S: Mandibular form and position related to changed mode of breathing—a five-year longitudinal study, *Angle Orthod* 59:91, 1989.

69. Kesling HD: Predetermined pattern as a diagnostic aid, *Am J Orthod* 33:42, 1947.

70. Kilpelainen PVJ, Phillips C, Tulloch JFC: Anterior tooth position and motivation for early treatment, *Angle Orthod* 63:171, 1993.

71. Kindisbacher I, Hirschl U, Ingervall B, Geering A: Little influence on tooth position from playing a musical instrument, *Angle Orthod* 60:223, 1990.

72. Kingsley NW: *Treatise on oral deformities as a branch of mechanical surgery,* New York, 1880, Appleton.

73. Kraus BS, Wise WJ, Frei RH: Heredity and the craniofacial complex, *Am J Orthod* 45:172, 1959.

74. Kremenak CR, Kinser DD, Harman HA et al: Orthodontic risk factors for temporomandibular disorders (TMD), I: Premolar extractions, *Am J Orthod Dentofac Orthop* 101:13, 1992.

75. Kukafka AL: Informed consent in law and medicine: autonomy vs paternalism, *J Law Ethics in Dent* 2:132-142, 1989.

76. Leech HL: A clinical analysis of orofacial morphology and behaviour of 500 patients attending an upper respiratory research clinic, *Dent Pract* 9:57, 1958.

77. Linder-Aronson S: Adenoids, their effect on mode of breathing and nasal airflow and their relationship to characteristics of the facial skeleton and the dentition, *Acta Otolaryngol Suppl* 265:1, 1970.

78. Lindhe J: Trauma from occlusion, *Dtsch Zahnaerztl Z* 35:680, 1980.

79. Lischer BE: *Principles and methods of orthodontia,* Philadelphia, 1912, Lea & Febiger.

80. Little RM, Riedel RA, Engst ED: Serial extraction of first premolars-postretention evaluation of stability and relapse, *Angle Orthod* 60:225, 1990.

81. Little RM, Wallen TR, Riedel RA: Stability and relapse of mandibular alignment: first premolar extraction cases treated by traditional edgewise orthodontics, *Am J Orthod* 80:349, 1981.

82. Lobb WK: Craniofacial morphology and occlusal variation in monozygous and dizygous twins, *Angle Orthod* 57:291, 1987.

83. Lund K: Mandibular growth and remodelling processes after condylar fractures, *Acta Odontal Scand 33 Suppl* 64:1, 1974.

84. Lundström A: Nature vs nurture in dentofacial variation, *Eur J Orthod* 6:77-91, 1984.

85. Lundström AF: Malocclusion of the teeth regarded as a problem in connection with the apical base, *Sven Tandlak Tidskr* 16:147, 1923.

85a. Lundstrom F, Lundström A: Natural head position as a basis for cephalometric analysis, *Am J Orthod Dentofac Orthop* 101:244, 1992.

86. Margolis H: Personal communication, 1984.

87. McGregor FC: Social and psychological implications of dentofacial disfigurement, *Angle Orthod* 40:231, 1969.

88. McLain JB, Proffit WR: The prevalence of malocclusion and its relation to need and demand for orthodontic treatment, *J Dent Educ* 49:386, 1985.

89. McLain JB, Proffit WR, Davenport RH: Adjunctive orthodontic therapy in treatment of juvenile periodontitis, *Am J Orthod* 83:290, 1983.

90. McNamara JA: Functional determinants of craniofacial size and shape, *Eur J Orthod* 2:131, 1980.

91. McNamara JA: Components of Class II malocclusion in children 8-10 years of age, *Angle Orthod* 51:177, 1981.

92. McNamara JA, Carlson DS: Quantitative analysis of temporomandibular joint adaptations to protrusive function, *Am J Orthod* 76:593, 1979.

93. McReynolds DC, Little RM: Mandibular second premolar extraction-postretention evaluation of stability and relapse, *Angle Orthod* 61:133, 1991.

94. Mohs E: General theory of paradigms on health, *Scand J Soc Med Supp* 46:14-24, 1991.

95. Montgomery WM, Vig PS, Staab EV, Matteson SR: Computed tomography: a three-dimensional study of the nasal airway, *Am J Orthod* 76:363, 1979.

96. Moorrees CFA: *The dentition of the growing child,* Boston, 1959, Harvard University Press.

97. Moorrees CFA, Fanning EA, Gron AM: The consideration of dental development in serial extraction, *Angle Orthod* 33:44, 1963.

98. Moorrees CFA, Gron AM: Principles of orthodontic diagnosis, *Angle Orthod* 36:258, 1966.

99. Moorrees CFA, Kean MR: Natural head position: a basic consideration for analysis of cephalometric radiographs, *Am J Phys Anthropol* 16:213, 1958.

100. Moorrees CFA, Lebret L: The mesh diagram and cephalometrics, *Angle Orthod* 32:214, 1962.

101. Morris AL et al: *Seriously handicapping orthodontic conditions,* Washington, 1977, National Academy of Sciences.

102. Musich DR, Ackerman JL: The catenometer: a reliable device for estimating dental arch perimeter, *Am J Orthod* 63:366, 1973.

103. Nahoum HI: Vertical proportions and the palatal plane in anterior open-bite, *Am J Orthod* 59:273, 1971.

104. Nance EP, Powers TA: Imaging of the temporomandibular joint, *Radiol Clin North Am* 28:1019, 1990.

105. Nance HN: The limitations of orthodontic treatment. I and II, *Am J Orthod* 33:177, 253, 1947.

106. Ostler S, Kiyak HA: Treatment expectations vs outcomes in orthognathic surgery patients, *Int J Adult Orthod Orthognath Surg* 6:247, 1991.

107. Pancherz H, Fackel U: The skeletofacial growth pattern pre- and post-dentofacial orthopedics: a long-term study of Class II malocclusions treated with the Herbst appliance, *Eur J Orthod* 12:209-218, 1990.

108. Pancherz H, Malmgren O, Haag U et al: Class II correction in Herbst and Bass therapy, *Eur J Orthod* 11:17, 1989.

109. Peck H, Peck S: A concept of facial esthetics, *Angle Orthod* 40:284, 1970.

110. Petrovic A, Stutzmann J, Oudet C: Condylectomy and mandibular growth in young rats: a quantitative study, *Proc Finn Dent Soc* 77:139, 1981.

111. Polson AM: *Long-term effect of orthodontic treatment on the periodontium.* In McNamara JA, Ribbens KA, editors: *Malocclusion and the periodontium,* Ann Arbor, 1987, University of Michigan Press, pp. 89-100.

112. Polson AM, Heil LC: Occlusion and periodontal disease, *Dent Clin North Am* 24:783, 1980.

113. Popovich F, Thompson GW: *Evaluation of P and I orthodontic treatment between 3 and 18 years of age.* In Cook JT, editor: *Transactions of the Third International Orthodontic Congress,* London, 1975, Staples Press.

114. Proffit WR: Equilibrium theory revisited: factors influencing position of the teeth, *Angle Orthod* 48:175, 1978.

115. Proffit WR: *Contemporary orthodontics,* ed 2, St Louis, 1993, Mosby.

116. Proffit WR, Phillips C, Douvartzidis N: The effects and efficacy of orthodontic vs surgical-orthodontic treatment of Class II malocclusion in non-growing patients, *Am J Orthod Dentofac Orthop* 101:556, 1992.

117. Proffit WR, Philips C, Tulloch JFC, Medland PH: Orthognathic vs orthodontic correction of skeletal Class II malocclusion in adolescents: effects and indications, *Int J Adult Orthod Orthognath Surg* (in press).

118. Proffit WR, White RP Jr: *Surgical-orthodontic treatment,* St Louis, 1992, Mosby.
119. Proffit WR, Vig KWL: Primary failure of eruption: a possible cause of posterior open bite, *Am J Orthod* 80:173, 1981.
120. Proffit WR, Vig KWL, Turvey TA: Early fracture of the mandibular condyles: frequently an unsuspected cause of growth disturbances, *Am J Orthod* 78:1, 1980.
121. Rendell JK, Norton LA, Gay T: Orthodontic treatment and temporomandibular joint disorders, *Am J Orthod Dentofac Orthop* 101:84, 1992.
122. Ricketts RM: Respiratory obstruction syndrome, *Am J Orthod* 54:495, 1968.
123. Riolo ML, Brandt D, TenHoeve TR: Association between occlusal characteristics and signs and symptoms of TMJ dysfunction in children and young adults, *Am J Orthod* 92:467, 1987.
124. Riolo ML, Moyers RE, McNamara JA Jr, Hunter WS: *An atlas of craniofacial growth.* Monograph 2, Craniofacial Growth Series, Ann Arbor, 1974, Center for Human Growth and Development, University of Michigan.
125. Rogers AP: A restatement of the myofunctional concept in orthodontics, *Am J Orthod* 36:845, 1950.
126. Sadowsky C: The risk of orthodontic treatment for producing temporomandibular disorders: a literature overview, *Am J Orthod Dentofac Orthop* 101:79, 1992.
127. Sadowsky C, BeGole EA: Long-term effects of orthodontic treatment on periodontal health, *Am J Orthod* 80:156, 1981.
128. Salzmann JA: *Practice of orthodontics,* Philadelphia, 1966, WB Saunders.
129. Sarver DM, Johnston MW, Matukas VJ: Video imaging for planning and counselling for orthognathic surgery, *J Oral Maxillofac Surg* 46:939, 1988.
130. Sassouni V: *The face in five dimensions,* ed 2, Morgantown, West Virginia, 1962, West Virginia University Press.
131. Sassouni V: The Class II syndrome: differential diagnosis and treatment, *Angle Orthod* 40:334, 1970.
132. Sassouni V, Forrest EJ: *Orthodontics in dental practice,* St Louis, 1971, Mosby.
133. Scammon RE: *The measurement of the body in childhood.* In Harris JA, editor: *The measurement of man,* Minneapolis, 1930, University of Minnesota Press.
134. Scheideman GB, Bell WH, Legan HL et al: Cephalometric analysis of dentofacial normals, *Am J Orthod* 78:404, 1980.
135. Shaw WC, Humphreys S: Influence of children's dentofacial appearance on teacher expectations, *Community Dent Oral Epidemiol* 10:313-319, 1982.
136. Sheldon WH: *The varieties of human physique,* New York, 1940, Harper.
137. Sillman JH: Dimensional changes of the dental arches: longitudinal studies from birth to 25 years, *Am J Orthod* 50:824, 1964.
138. Simon P: *Fundamental principles of a systematic diagnosis of dental anomalies,* Boston, 1926, Stratford (Translated by BE Lischer).
139. Sinclair PM, Thomas PM, Proffit WR: *Combined surgical and orthodontic treatment.* In Proffit WR: *Contemporary orthodontics,* ed 2, St Louis, 1993, Mosby.
140. Smylski PT, Woodside DG, Harnett BE: Surgical and orthodontic treatment of cleidocranial dysostosis, *Int J Oral Surg* 3:380, 1974.
141. Solow B, Siersbaek-Nielsen S: Cervical and craniocervical posture as predictors of craniofacial growth, *Am J Orthod Dentofac Orthop* 101:449, 1992.
142. Spalding PM, Vig PS: Respiration characteristics in subjects diagnosed as having nasal obstruction, *J Oral Maxillofac Surg* 46:189, 1988.
143. Staggers JA: A comparison of the results of second molar and first premolar extraction treatment, *Am J Orthod Dentofac Orthop* 98:430, 1990.
144. Steedle JR, Proffit WR: The pattern and control of eruptive tooth movements, *Am J Orthod* 87:56, 1986.
145. Steiner CC: The use of cephalometrics as an aid to planning and assessing orthodontic treatment, *Am J Orthod* 46:721, 1960.
146. Stricher G et al: Psychosocial aspects of craniofacial disfigurement, *Am J Orthod* 76:410, 1979.
147. Stoller AE: The normal position of the maxillary first permanent molar, *Am J Orthod* 40:259, 1954.
148. Stockli P: Personal communication.
149. Strang RHW, Thompson WM: *A textbook of orthodontia,* ed 4, Philadelphia, 1958, Lea & Febiger.
150. Tanaka MM, Johnston LE: The prediction of the size of unerupted canines and premolars in a contemporary orthodontic population, *J Am Dent Assn* 88:798, 1974.
151. Tanner JM: *Growth at adolescence,* ed 2, Springfield, Ill, 1962, Charles C Thomas.
152. Tulloch JFC, Rogers L, Phillips C: Early results from a randomized clinical trial of growth modification in Class II malocclusion, *J Dent Res* 71:Special issue A, #523, 1992.
153. Turvey TA, Hall DJ, Warren DW: Alterations in nasal airway resistance following superior repositioning of the maxilla, *Am J Orthod* 85:109, 1984.
154. Tweed CH: A philosophy of orthodontic treatment, *Am J Orthod* 31:74, 1945.
155. Van Loon JAW: A new method for indicating normal and abnormal relations of the teeth to the facial lines, *Dent Cosmos* 57:973, 1093, 1229, 1915.
156. Vig PS, Cohen AM: Vertical growth of the lips: a serial cephalometric study, *Am J Orthod* 75:405, 1979.
157. Vig PS, Showfety KJ, Phillips C: Experimental manipulation of head posture, *Am J Orthod* 77:258, 1980.
158. Weed LL: *Medical records, medical education, and patient care: the problem-oriented record as a basic tool,* Cleveland, 1969, Case-Western Reserve Press.
159. Wei SHY: A roentgenographic cephalometric study of prognathism in Chinese males and females, *Angle Orthod* 38:305, 1968.
160. Weinberger BW: *Historical resume of the evolution and growth of orthodontics.* In Anderson GM: *Practical orthodontics,* ed 8, St Louis, 1955, Mosby.
161. Williams R: The diagnostic line, *Am J Orthod* 55:458, 1969.
162. Williamson EH, Steinke RM, Morse PK, Swith TR: Centric relation: a comparison of muscle-determined position and operator guidance, *Am J Orthod* 77:133, 1980.
163. Wylie WL: The assessment of anteroposterior dysplasia, *Angle Orthod* 17:97, 1947.
164. Wylie WL, Johnson EL: Rapid evaluation of facial dysplasia in the vertical plane, *Angle Orthod* 22:165, 1952.

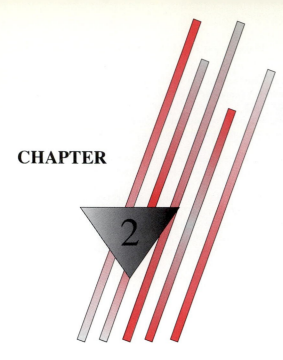

CHAPTER 2

Biomechanical Principles and Reactions

KAARE REITAN
PER RYGH

Histologic research in orthodontics has been performed partly on animal and partly on human material. To base as many conclusions as possible on observations of human tissues, two thirds of the experimental material in this chapter is taken from human structures. The main purpose of presenting a discussion on biophysical principles of tooth movement is to inform the reader of the facts and histologic findings that have a bearing on practical orthodontics. In addition, a discussion on some of the biological and histochemical observations made in present day investigations will be included. (See Chapter 3.)

There are general laws that may be applied to all types of tooth movement. The alveolar bone is resorbed wherever the root, for a certain length of time, causes compression of the periodontal ligaments (PDL); new alveolar bone is deposited wherever there is a stretching force acting on the bone. However, these seemingly obvious statements will be subject to numerous variations and exceptions when factors such as the *magnitude, direction,* and *duration* of the force are introduced.

SUPPORTING TISSUES

The tissue elements undergoing changes during tooth movement are primarily the periodontal ligament, with its cells, supporting fibers, capillaries, and nerves, and secondarily the alveolar bone.

Periodontal fibers. The arrangement of the periodontal fibers is well known. In humans many of the principal fibers have an oblique arrangement tending to withstand pressure during mastication (Fig. 2-1). In the marginal region some fibers are anchored to the alveolar bone crest. In addition, the free gingival fibers of the supraalveolar tissue constitute an independent group. In control nonorthodontic material

the supraalveolar fibers are not so conspicuous as those observed after tooth movement. In the latter case they appear stretched and can be readily distinguished, particularly those on the tension side of the tooth (Fig. 2-2, *A*). Anatomically one can distinguish between dentogingival, dentoperiosteal, transseptal, alveologingival, and circular fibers, all of which belong to the supraalveolar group. Gradual deterioration of

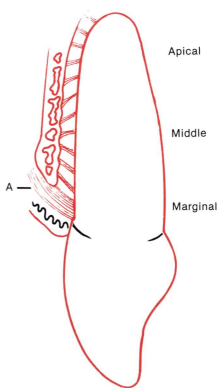

Fig. 2-1 Arrangement of the supporting fibers. *A*, Supraalveolar fibers.

some of these fiber bundles may, under special conditions, lead to pathologic tooth migration.

Several types of fibers exist in the periodontal ligament. Very thin tonofibrils are found in the cytoplasm of cellular elements. Fairly thin connective tissue fibers are observed in the interstitial spaces and in marrow spaces. However, the dense collagen fibers are the most important, because they are the supporting fibers of the teeth (Fig. 2-3). Fibers and fiber bundles of the periodontal ligament all consist of closely packed fibrils of an indefinite length.[152] During the formation of collagen, fibroblasts produce tropocollagen, which is macromolecules consisting of aggregated peptide

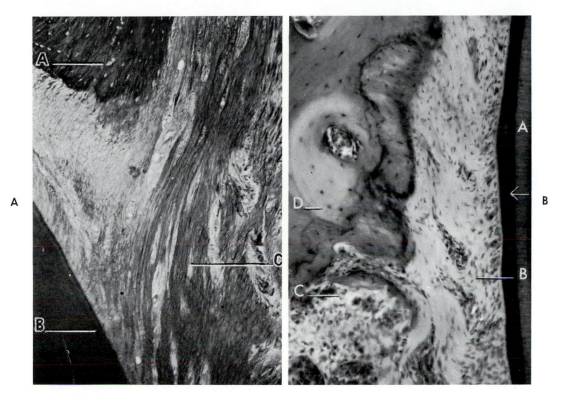

Fig. 2-2 **A,** Supra-alveolar tissue of a 12-year-old patient. *A,* Alveolar bone crest; *B,* root; *C,* free gingival fibers running from the root surface and terminating in fibrous structures of the gingiva and periosteum. **B,** Cross section of the tooth of a dog 11 months old. Slight degree of hyalinization after rotation. Force, 50 g. Note the persisting cellular elements in the periodontal ligament. *A,* Root; *B,* periodontal ligament; *C,* undermining resorption of bundle bone; *D,* haversian system with fine fibers in its matrix. (**A** from Reitan K: *Am J Orthod* 46:881, 1960.)

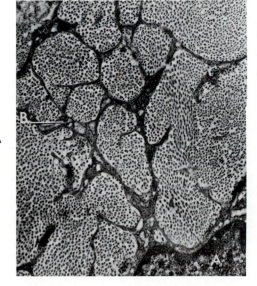

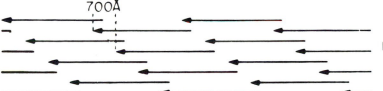

Fig. 2-3 **A,** Cross-sectioned periodontal fibers as seen by electron microscopy. (× 8900.) Black dots are uniformly wide collagen fibrils (thickness, 500 to 800 Å) here surrounded by a fine granular structure, the ground substance. Area close to the root surface. *A,* Cementoblast; *B,* protoplasmic processes. **B,** Overlapping arrangement of triple-stranded collagen molecules within the fibril. These molecules (length 2000 to 3000 Å) are polarized, exhibiting end portions *(arrowheads)* that produce the cross striation effect in the fibril. The distance between stippled lines represents a band and interband period of 700 Å length. (**A** courtesy K.A. Selvig; **B** from Olsen BR: *Z Zellforsch* 59:199, 1963.)

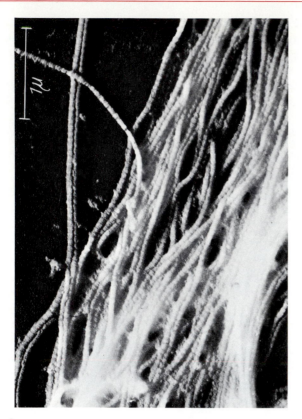

Fig. 2-4 Shadow casting of collagen fibrils as seen with the electron microscope. (× approximately 20,000.) Note the characteristic repetitive bands and interbands, which reflect the arrangement of the collagen molecules within the fibrils. (Courtesy G. Haim.)

chains of amino acids constructed as a helix.[100] These molecules will subsequently attain a so-called staggered array (Fig. 2-3, B), an arrangement that produces characteristic bands and interbands (Fig. 2-4). Under normal conditions the periodicity of collagen fibrils varies between 640 and 700 Å, and under other conditions 210 to 250 Å.* Electron microscopy may reveal structural details of the individual fibrils (Fig. 2-4).

The fibrils of the periodontal ligament are embedded in a ground substance, which is the amorphous structure left after all the cells, capillaries, and fibers have been removed.[14] It contains connective tissue polysaccharides (glycosylaminoglycans), salts, some other substances, and water. The polysaccharides are unipolyvalent electrolytes and are called polyelectrolytes. The connective tissue as well as the ground substance varies in different species. There is generally a more rapid turnover of the ground substance than of the collagen fibers. The ground substance constitutes the medium into which the connective tissue cells secrete soluble forms of collagen molecules that subsequently aggregate to form fibrils. Formation of fibrils occurs in the

ground substance more or less equidistant from the cells.[147] Compression of the periodontal ligament causes the tissue fluid to be squeezed out of the area, but the ground substance remains in the fibrous tissue.

During physiological conditions collagen turnover in the periodontal tissues is much higher than in most other connective tissues. Based on biochemical analyses in rats it has been found that collagen turnover in the PDL is about four times as high as that of the skin and twice that of the gingiva.[163] The high turnover has been attributed to the fact that forces on the PDL are multidirectional, having both vertical and horizontal components. Superimposed on the functional forces that act on the teeth are forces associated with functional drift, positional adaptation during growth of the jaw bone, and forces derived from the tongue, the cheeks, and the lips.[164] Functional forces may induce microtrauma known to involve rapid collagen turnover in wound repair of connective tissues. It is interesting to note that collagen remodeling in the PDL has many similarities in common with collagen behavior during wound repair. The lower turnover of collagen in the gingiva may be due to the lowered functional stress. The transseptal fibers function in a manner similar to tendons. The fibers provide a firm anchorage of the tooth, and are stable.[91] It is of note that cellular turnover of cementum is slow when compared to adjacent alveolar bone surface.[129]

During tooth movement the fiber bundles must elongate. It has been shown by Sicher[155,157] in his work on continuously erupting teeth that an intermediate plexus exists. During tooth movement a proliferation zone may be observed (Fig. 2-37, D). After the principal fibers have stretched and the periodontal space has widened, there is a definite increase in cellular elements.[112] A sort of intermediate plexus may exist in this proliferation zone where connective tissue cells are producing tropocollagen, thus ensuring production of fibrils and, subsequently, elongation of periodontal fibers with further movement of the tooth (Fig. 2-41, A). The interchange and production of collagen molecules are probably less marked in the area close to the root surface.[116,153]

With the electron microscope Kurihara and Enlow (1980) found that interfibrillar, strandlike, ground substance material may play an important role in adhesion onto resorbed bone surfaces and as a binding agent in connecting fibrils. It is not as yet determined whether collagen fibers join (1) in linear continuity, (2) as a splice between interdigitating filaments, or (3) as a splice between whole fibrils. During tooth movement the behavior of the principal and the supraalveolar fibers seems to be different.[114] In most instances there is a diminution in the number of cells of the supraalveolar fibers caused by compression of cellular elements between stretched fiber bundles (Fig. 2-28, B). They nevertheless appear to increase in thickness after tension (Fig. 2-2), an effect that does not seem unlikely since production of fibrils may occur some distance from the connective tissue cells.[88]

---

*Micrometer (μm) = 1/1000 mm; 1 Angstrom Unit (Å) = 1/10,000 μm. 1 nanometer (nm) = 1/1000.000 mm.

One of the important factors in collagen formation is ascorbic acid. It has been shown experimentally that absence of vitamin C may affect the fibroblasts and thereby the formation of collagen molecules. This should lead to the conclusion that a high intake of vitamin C is to be recommended for orthodontic patients. The question has been discussed by Avery,[4] who points out that vitamin C deficiency in the United States is slight.

Alveolar bone. In studies on physiologic and experimental tooth movement, little has been said about the anatomic variations of the alveolar bone. It may be of interest to look further into this question.

In histologic sections of adult alveolar bone the orthodontist may find large marrow spaces, notably in the apical region on the lingual side of the teeth (Fig. 2-5). The bone walls of the middle and marginal regions are often quite dense, with few marrow spaces.[118] It is in this latter area that the bone changes will occur when tooth movement is initiated. Lack of marrow spaces implies that bone resorption takes more time. Fig. 2-6 presents a section from the lingual side of an adult tooth. The alveolar bone is quite dense and devoid of any bone-forming cells on its surface. However, the bone wall shows an open channel—an anatomic detail that is characteristic of human periodontal structures, notably in young persons. Bone resorption may start at the inside of this channel because the periodontal fibers will not be directly compressed in this area as the root is moved against the bone surface.

Bone character. Marrow spaces are also seen in cross sections of adult teeth. The thin bone walls on the labial and lingual sides of these teeth are frequently dense (Fig. 2-6). This arrangement of the supporting bone will favor tooth movement in a mesial or distal direction more than in a labial or lingual direction. If the teeth are moved in a mesial or distal direction, the roots will be displaced to a great extent through the spongiosa of the alveolar bone as soon as the lamina dura has been eliminated by resorption.[120]

An alveolar bone as dense as that seen in Fig. 2-6 is not often found in the supporting tissues of young persons, who comprise the majority of our patients. The bone wall in the young human usually contains large marrow spaces, open clefts, and canals. However, there are variations and exceptions to this rule, as was seen in an investigation of normal supporting structures of teeth taken from 54 children aged 11 to 12 years.[118] Most of the alveolar bone areas of this material exhibited anatomic details that might have been characterized as typical of young supporting structures. There were large marrow spaces, canals, and openings communicating with the periodontal ligament. In other words a spongiosa frequently extended to the alveolar crest (Fig. 2-7, *A*).

Since tooth movement, (i.e., the progress of bone resorption) is facilitated by the formation of resorptive cells, whose number again increases according to the number of marrow spaces, the anatomic conditions can hardly be more favorable than in the supporting structures of the majority of young orthodontic patients.

In the material just mentioned[118] there were few exceptions. A tendency to bone density (i.e., fewer and smaller marrow spaces within the alveolar bone) was observed in only six cases. This form of bone density must be considered as an individual variation and has nothing to do with pathologic conditions such as marble bone disease. A dense bone plate was observed, notably on the labial side (Fig. 2-7, *B*). A corresponding density existed in the marginal and middle regions on the lingual side, but the lingual bone plate

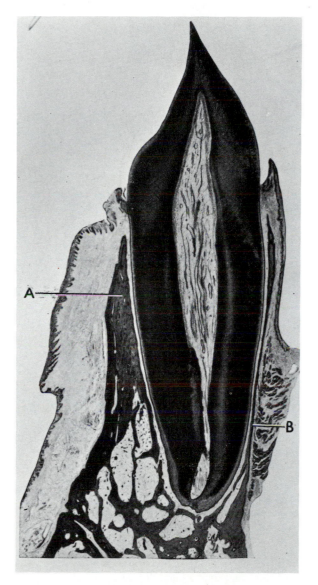

Fig. 2-5 Adult lower incisor. *A,* Dense alveolar bone; *B,* dense and thin alveolar bone wall on labial side, large marrow spaces are on the lingual side of the root. Note the muscles inserted on the periosteal side of the bony plate, *B,* a factor that tends to modify compensatory bone formation during movement of the root in a labial direction. (From Meyer WT: *Lehrbuch der normalen Histologie und Entwicklungsgeschichte der Zähne des Menschen,* Munich, 1951, Carl Hanser Verlag.)

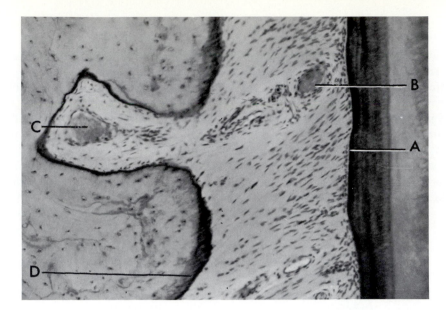

Fig. 2-6   Area from the alveolar crest of a 39-year-old patient. *A,* Chain of cementoblasts along a thick layer of cementum; *B,* interstitial space; *C,* widened capillary in a cleft, where bone resorption may start during the initial stage of tooth movement; *D,* darkly stained surface line containing connective tissue polysaccharides. Note the absence of osteoblasts along the bone surface.

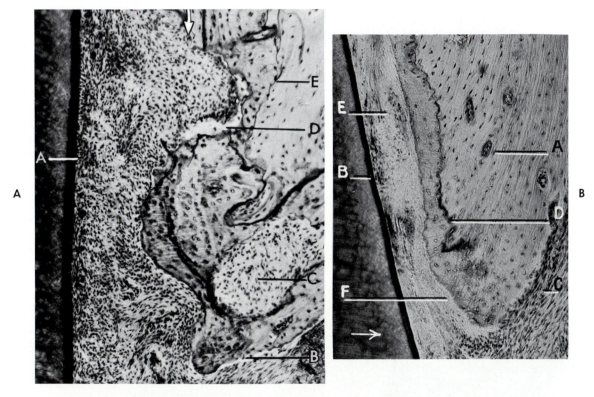

Fig. 2-7   **A,** Alveolar structures typical of young patients (here a 12-year-old child). *A,* Cementum; *B,* newly formed osteoid along the bone crest; *C,* marrow space containing a loose fibrous tissue; *D,* osteoid bordered by osteoblasts; *E,* demarcation line between old bone and bundle bone. Aplastic stretches along the protruding portion of the bone surface. Arrow indicates bone resorption. **B,** Dense alveolar crest in a 12-year-old child. *A,* Small marrow space in which no resorbing cells are formed during undermining bone resorption; *B,* root surface; *C,* periosteum with a chain of osteoblasts; *D,* reversal line between old bone and bundle bone; the periodontal ligament is hyalinized after tooth movement for 8 nights with an expanded activator; *E,* cellular elements in the hyalinized tissue; *F,* persisting osteoid layer compressed between the bone surface and hyalinized fibers. (**A** and **B** from Reitan K: *Acta Odontol Scand Suppl* 6, 1951.)

always contained marrow spaces in its thicker portion adjacent to the apical region (Fig. 2-5).

A limited number of cases exhibited an inner bone surface continuing as an unbroken line parallel to the root surface. On the other hand, even in the alveolar bone, which contained small marrow spaces, minor indentations and clefts

along the inner bone surface frequently occurred (Fig. 2-8, *A*). Another example of bone density is seen in Fig. 2-8, *B*. When tooth movement is initiated in such a case, a considerable length of time is required before the compact bone is eliminated by resorption. A similarly delayed initial tooth movement will take place where marrow spaces may

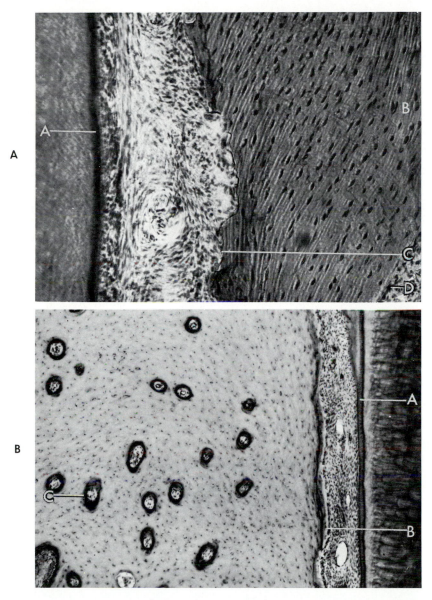

Fig. 2-8 **A,** A special type of dense bone in a 12-year-old patient. This was fairly recently formed and is readily resorbed despite lack of marrow spaces. It will be reconstructed into lamellated bone containing finer fibrils. *A,* Cementum of the root surface; note the even distribution of large osteocytes in the bone; *B* and *C,* indentation along the bone surface and also bone resorption; *D,* osteoblasts of the periosteum. **B,** Area from the interradicular septum of the upper first premolar in a 12-year-old child. This type of dense bone varies from that shown in **A.** *A,* Root surface; *B,* bone surface covered by a bundle bone layer and a thin line of osteoid; *C,* one of the marrow spaces, in which there will be no or an appreciably delayed formation of osteoclasts as a response to hyalinization of the periodontal ligament. Bone resorption takes place only along the inner bone surface. The dark lining of the marrow spaces, containing cementing substance, indicates that bone formation is terminated.*

---

*No mention of author's name indicates that the illustrations are derived from Reitan's work.

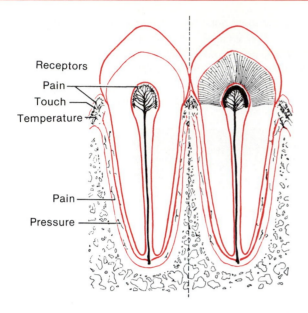

Receptors
Pain
Touch
Temperature

Pain
Pressure

Fig. 2-9 Innervation of teeth and periodontal structures. Many fine neurofibrils with myelinated or unmyelinated endings enter the periodontal ligament through the foramina in the alveolar bone. Compression of the periodontal ligament may cause pain, especially during the initial stage of tooth movement. (From Avery JK, Rapp R: *Dent Clin North Am* 499, July 1959.)

be present in the central part of the alveolar bone but where the lamina dura is thick and dense.

Bone in experimental cases. In a comparison of human alveolar bone with the alveolar bone of dogs and monkeys, it was shown that the bone in animals is frequently more dense. Relative bone density may be observed even in young animals. Human and animal alveolar bone contains osteons, or haversian systems, which consist of canals surrounded by concentric bone lamellae. In young human and animal structures the inner surface of the alveolus is normally covered by a layer of bundle bone, which is more readily resorbed than is lamellated bone[117] (Fig. 2-10). Density of the lamellated bone in animals is notably caused by the fact that the filling in of marrow spaces is more advanced than in humans. Even in young dogs, only a small aperture may be left of the central space of the haversian systems. This is less frequently observed in young human structures, in which the central spaces of the haversian systems are generally larger (Fig. 2-10).

A consideration of bone density is especially important in certain animal experiments of long duration, and in every case a careful comparison with the bone of control areas is necessary. Generally all animal experiments of short duration are fully comparable with those in humans.

The use of rat and mouse material permits an overview of the tissue reactions in the alveolar process as a whole by light microscopy (LM). The small size of the width of the PDL being about 100 μm in the rat permits detailed study in transmission electron microscope (TEM) of sections including alveolar bone, periodontal membrane, and root surface.[140] It is known that because the roots of rat teeth are short, the compression and tension effect may be located in

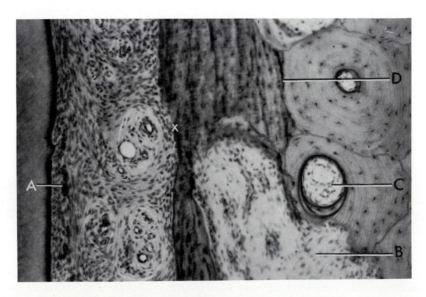

Fig. 2-10 Buccal area from slightly below the marginal third of the root in a 12-year-old patient. Note the reconstruction of bone layers. *A*, Epithelial remnants of Malassez; *B*, large marrow space containing a loose fibrous tissue; *C*, central aperture of the haversian system; *D*, resting line between old bone and bundle bone; *x* physiologic resorption process in bundle bone.

areas not exactly the same as those observed in other animals. These variations will be mentioned in the following discussion.

PHYSIOLOGIC TOOTH MOVEMENT

The term physiologic tooth movement hardly needs definition. It designates, primarily, the slight tipping of the functioning tooth in its socket and, secondarily, the changes in tooth position that occur in young persons during and after tooth eruption. The minor changes in tooth position observed in growing persons and adults are usually called tooth *migration*.

The functional movement of the tooth during mastication has a certain interest, because it also indicates how the tooth will be tipped in the initial stage of orthodontic tooth movement. A slight diversity of opinion has existed with regard to where the neutral axis is located in the root of a functioning tooth. The location of this point may, to some extent, be determined from what is observed in orthodontic experiments. When an adult tooth is tipped by an orthodontic force, bone will, in many cases, be resorbed almost up to

the apical region on the pressure side (Figs. 2-11 and 2-12). This indicates that there is but little movement of the apex, which is caused by the strong apical fibers restricting the movement of the apical portion of the root.[122] Likewise, in the functional movement of an adult tooth the neutral axis is frequently located between the middle and apical regions of the root. In younger persons the neutral axis will be located in the marginal region if the root is short, and somewhat closer to the middle portion if the root is fully developed (Fig. 2-13).

Tooth migration in both young and older persons is always related to definite tissue changes that may be readily observed in histologic sections.[112] In young persons, erupting teeth will migrate when assuming what is called a normal position. The new tissue added during eruption can also be observed on radiographs (Fig. 2-14). The opaque layer bordering the inner alveolar bone surface consists of not only the lamina dura but also recently calcified osteoid tissue. A similar layer may be formed as a result of orthodontic tooth movement, a favorable reaction that occurs in most young persons but less readily in some adults.

The new tissue deposited during tooth migration represents various stages of calcification. Bone formation always passes through three stages: osteoid, bundle bone, and lamellated bone.

Osteoid is the product of osteoblasts. It is found on all

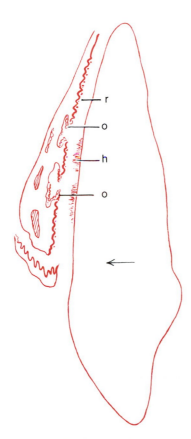

Fig. 2-11 Location of bone resorption adjacent to the apical third of an upper canine in a 39-year-old patient. The tooth was moved continuously for 3 weeks. *o,* Compensatory formation of osteoid in open marrow spaces; *h,* remnants of hyalinized tissue adhering to the root surface; *r,* direct bone resorption adjacent to the apical third of the root.

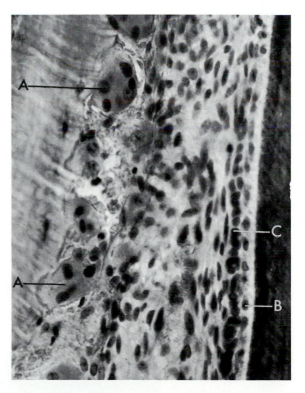

Fig. 2-12 Direct or frontal bone resorption (area marked *r* in Fig. 2-11). **A,** Osteoclasts along the bone surface; **B,** cementoblast with a line of cementoid; *C,* strand of epithelial remnants.

bone surfaces where new bone is deposited. In control material from 12-year-old humans, osteoid may appear as a white line or white outgrowth (Fig. 2-17). Unlike calcified bone, osteoid is not readily absorbed by osteoclasts. The periodontal fibers pass through this white layer but are not visible because the refractory index of the cementing substance in osteoid, which closely approximates that of the fibrils.

Generally bone consists of a matrix of collagen fibrils, cementing substance, and hydroxyapatite crystals.[183] It is also known to be formed only when the collagen fibrils have a 640 to 700 Å periodicity. There are different types of bone and various stages of bone formation. During growth and also during tooth movement, uncalcified osteoid will be formed around fairly thick fiber bundles.[112] The density of this new partly calcified tissue deposited on the lamina dura

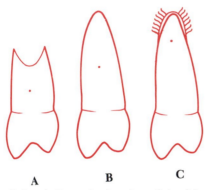

Fig. 2-13 Points indicate the location of the fulcrum in **A,** a young, **B,** a fully developed, and **C,** an adult tooth during initial tooth movement.

may explain why it is so conspicuous on radiographs (Fig. 2-14). A wider opaque line indicates that calcified tissue has been added.[149] Calcification of the deepest layers of the osteoid increases as the new tissue increases in thickness, with the superficial layer usually remaining uncalcified.

The newly calcified tissue, as well as that of longer existence, is called *bundle bone* (Fig. 2-10). It is basophilic and appears dark in sections stained with hematoxylin and eosin. The staining properties of bundle bone are related to its high content of cementing substance, consisting essentially of highly polymerized connective tissue polysaccharides.[147] The resting and reversal lines observed in lamellated bone also consist of cementing substance (Fig. 2-8, *B*).

Cells and fiber bundles will be incorporated in bundle bone during its life cycle. When it has reached a certain thickness and maturity, parts of the bundle bone will be reorganized into *lamellated bone,* with finer fibrils in its matrix (Fig. 2-10). The lamina dura will subsequently reappear as a somewhat thinner radiopaque line (Fig. 2-14). This sequence of events is, in principle, the same as that in bone formation after orthodontic tooth movement (Fig. 2-15).

Periodontal fibers. The fibrous tissue of the periodontal ligament, some of which will be incorporated into bundle bone, is usually considered to be of two kinds—Sharpey's fibers and undifferentiated tissue; the latter consists of thinner and less well-oriented fibrils. Some authors consider all fibers in the periodontal ligament to be Sharpey's fibers.

Using special staining methods, Fullmer[40] observed oxytalan fibers within the collagenous tissue of the periodontal ligament. The functional significance of these fibers, which are frequently anchored in the cementum, is still undergoing investigation. Electron microscopic studies have revealed

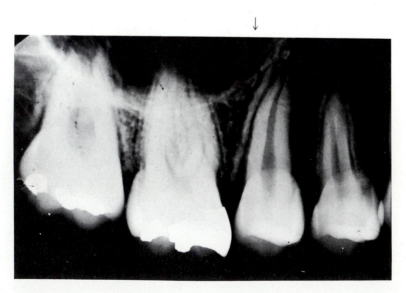

Fig. 2-14 Opaque layer *(A)* indicating bone formation along the inner bone surface of a second premolar after eruption.

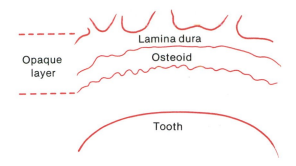

Fig. 2-15 Newly calcified bone layers, as seen in Fig. 2-14, tend to become conspicuous on the roentgenogram, since they are deposited on the lamina dura. Their presence indicates movement of the adjacent tooth.

that there is a morphologic similarity between the filaments of oxytalan fibers and those of elastic tissue; both lack the regular periodicity observed in collagen fibrils. New evidence has shown that a close connection exists between blood vessels and oxytalan fibers.[20]

How the periodontal fibers continue into the fibrous system of the bone may be demonstrated by special staining methods (Fig. 2-16, *A*). Although Sharpey's fibers in bundle bone appear fairly relaxed in physiologic tooth movement, they are more stretched to varying degrees when observed in the bundle bone that has been formed as a result of rapid orthodontic tooth movement (Fig. 2-16, *B*).

Physiologic tooth movement. The tissue reaction that occurs during physiologic tooth movement is a normal function of the supporting structures. This was pointed out for the first time by Stein and Weinmann[167] in 1925. They observed that the molars in adults would gradually migrate in a mesial direction, more or less corresponding to the wear of contact surfaces. Similar changes may be observed in animals. More recently (1955) Bjørk[17] described migration of erupting teeth in radiographic studies. The upper molars migrated chiefly in a mesial direction. In the lower jaw variations could be observed. Not infrequently the lower molars migrated more or less in a distal direction during eruption.

When the erupting tooth has been migrating in a lingual direction, bone resorption will be prevalent on the lingual side and bone deposition on the labial side. A study of teeth from 23 young persons[112] showed that in nine of these cases the premolars had been migrating in a lingual direction. It should be noted, however, that bone resorption may be observed in circumscribed areas even if the tooth erupts vertically. This is partly due to anatomic variations. A typical control area taken from the alveolar bone crest is seen in Fig. 2-17, *A*.

Tooth migration and eruption. It is generally recognized

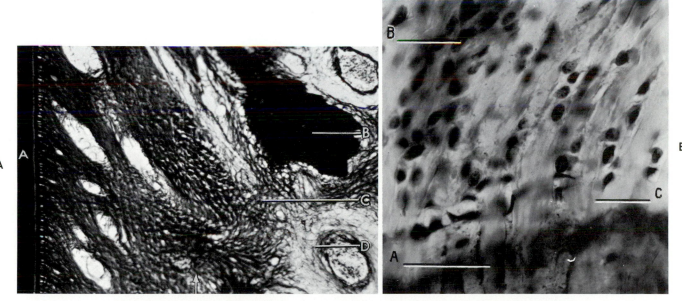

Fig. 2-16 **A,** The periodontal fibers interlace with the fibrous matrix of the bone, thus forming a fibrous system. In a physiologic state this system appears relaxed. *A,* Root surface; *B,* remaining calcified bone in which the fiber arrangement cannot be seen; *C,* Sharpey's fibers interlacing with fibers of the bone; *D,* loose fibrous tissue around a capillary; the bone surface is located along a line above arrow. (Silver impregnation.) **B,** Stretched periodontal fibers and bone surface after 4 days' tooth movement. The osteoblasts are partly located between the fiber bundles. *A,* Fiber bundle anchored in bundle bone; *B,* new connective tissue cells formed as a result of the tension of the fibers; *C,* osteoid layer.

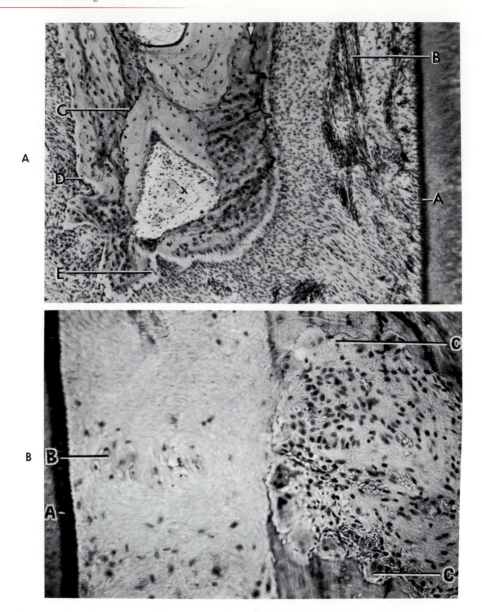

Fig. 2-17 **A,** Alveolar bone crest in a 12-year-old child. Circumferential lamellae consist of bundle bone bordered by a line of osteoid surrounded by many osteoblasts and fibroblasts. These findings indicate growth, particularly at the alveolar bone crest. *A,* Root surface; *B,* interstitial spaces cut longitudinally; *C,* reversal line between old bone and bundle bone; *D,* bone formation on the periosteal side; *E,* osteoid layer along the bone surface; *x,* marrow space containing a loose fibrous tissue. Arrow indicates reversal line. **B,** Hyalinized zone after reverse movement for 3 days in a 12-year-old boy. *A,* Root surface; *B,* capillary surrounded by a few cells; *C,* osteoclasts. Bone resorption usually persists for 8 to 10 days even if tension is exerted. Note the initial rearrangement of fibers and the reappearance of cellular elements in the periodontal ligament. (Similar area after 8 days' reverse movement is seen in Fig. 2-29.)

that the direction of tooth migration varies in different species. Thus in the rat the molars migrate in a distal direction whereas migration of human molars occurs in a mesial direction, especially in the maxilla (Fig. 2-18).[18,123] Compared with tooth eruption, migration is usually a slow movement. As discussed under "Extrusion" (p. 162), since tooth *erup-*

tion occurs quite readily it will be logical to perform such a movement with a comparatively light orthodontic force.

Ten Cate,[176] in his studies of erupting teeth, showed that fibroblasts under certain conditions may become active during elimination of fibrous tissue. It has been observed that the intrinsic forces causing the teeth to erupt still exist even

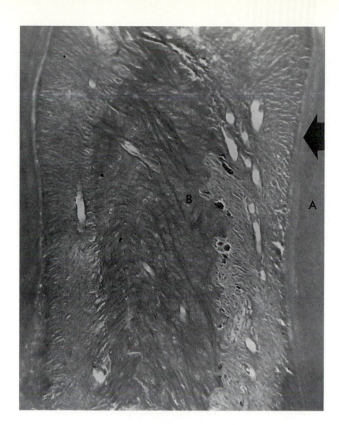

Fig. 2-18 Physiologic migration of first rat molar *(A)* in direction of arrow. Scattered osteoclasts, stained red, adjacent to the alveolar bone. *(B)* Tartrate resistant acid phospatase (TRAP) stain (Courtesy P. Brudvik.)

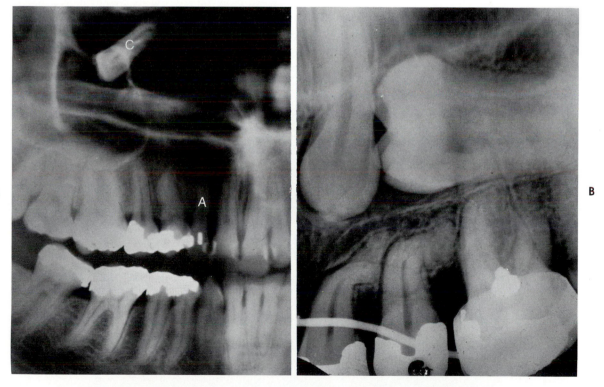

Fig. 2-19 **A,** Incidental finding in a patient 32 years of age. It had been assumed that the canine was missing. The tooth was located in the upper sinus wall and moved with it during vertical growth of the maxilla. *A,* Area where the tooth should have been located; *C,* impacted canine. **B,** Impacted teeth in 33-year-old immigrant who had not been examined roentgenographically in her home country. The second molar was subjected to *eruptional* movement until tooth movement was arrested when it made contact with the impacted canine. Note the curved roots of the premolars, which have migrated; the first one is almost in contact with the lateral incisor.

if the teeth remain impacted. Occasionally canines will be observed with their crown portions displaced close to the roots of the central incisors. In some cases the development of the maxillary sinus tends to determine further movement and location of impacted canines (Fig. 2-19, *A*). Although individual variations may be caused by hormonal factors, several observations seem to prove that tooth eruption is continued. If the tooth is located in spongy bone and in a horizontal position above the adjacent roots, it may be subjected to an *eruptional* movement for a long time and over a great distance (Fig. 2-19, *B*).

Cells of the periodontal ligament. The connective cells of the ligament comprise fibroblasts, osteoblasts, and cementoblasts. Some evidence indicates that fibroblasts and osteoblasts may descend from a common ancestral cell[3] and that the cells are born and die in the PDL. The cells that synthesize DNA before mitosis are predominantly located near blood vessels. Then they migrate away from that site. It is not known whether the cells that migrate to the surface of the alveolar bone and cementum originate paravascularly.[41,85] Roberts and Chase [129] observed that in mice, cells migrated in association with bone apposition incident to orthodontic tooth movement, and showed that the osteoblasts were derived solely from local precursor cells of the periodontal ligament. It should be noted, however, that the onset of tissue changes in physiologic and orthodontic tooth movement may, to some extent, be influenced by the preexisting conditions of the alveolar bone. As an example, we

might mention some of the variations that may influence bone formation in orthodontic movement.

If there is osteoid and a chain of osteoblasts along the bone surface on the tension side, formation of new osteoid will start shortly after tension has been exerted on the periodontal fibers.[112] If the bone surface is aplastic (i.e., devoid of osteoid and occasionally also of osteoblasts), there will be a time interval before new cells and osteoid are formed.

When there is bone resorption on the tension side, it may take 4 to 5 days before this resorption is converted into formative changes. Because the alveolar bone surface adjacent to adult teeth is frequently aplastic, the onset of the tissue changes is generally delayed in adults[122] (Fig. 2-6).

Osteolysis (i.e., bone resorption taking place in the absence of osteoclasts) is not observed during the active phase of tooth movement. As an exception, we might mention the rapidly enlarged lacunae of the osteocytes (formerly osteoblasts) of the bundle bone undergoing resorption during reverse tooth movement (*D* in Fig. 2-38, *A*).

ORTHODONTIC TOOTH MOVEMENT

Basically, there is no great difference between the tissue reactions observed in physiologic and those observed in orthodontic tooth movement. However, since the teeth are moved more rapidly during treatment, the tissue changes elicited by orthodontic forces are consequently more marked and extensive. As an example one might compare the re-

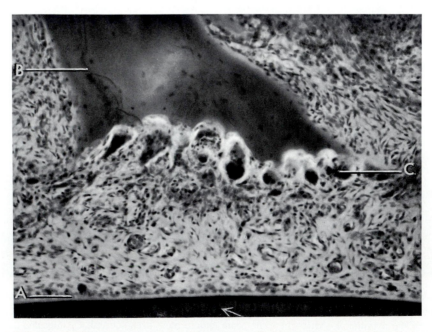

Fig. 2-20 Direct bone resorption during orthodontic movement. Animal experiment. The tooth was rotated as indicated by the arrow. *A*, Epithelial remnant adjacent to the root surface; *B*, protruding bone spicule; *C*, osteoclasts in Howship's lacunae (note spaces between the osteoclasts and the bone).

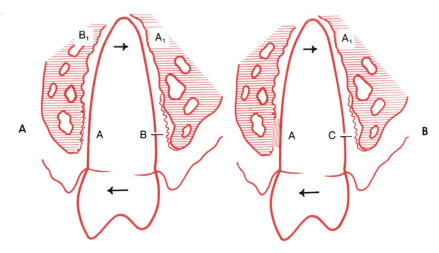

Fig. 2-21 **A,** Tipping, with direct bone resorption at *A* and formation of osteoid at *B*. **B,** In the majority of cases tooth movement is initiated by formation of a cell-free area at *A* and new osteoid formed at *C*. A_1 and B_1 represent corresponding pressure and tension sides in the apical region.

sorbed area in Fig. 2-8, *A*, with that shown in Fig. 2-20. This difference is also reflected in the longer time required for bone formation to start in areas previously resorbed following application of orthodontic forces.

It has been mentioned that a period of 4 to 5 days is needed before a stretching force can elicit bone formation in areas previously resorbed during physiologic tooth movement. If the preexisting bone resorption has been caused by orthodontic forces, it usually takes 8 to 10 days, occasionally longer, before a reverse movement will transform all the resorptive changes into bone formation.[117] This delay shows that there is, notable as to degree, a certain difference between physiologic and orthodontic tissue changes.

Bone resorption. It has been assumed that application of light orthodontic forces will result in direct bone resorption on the pressure side (Fig. 2-21, *A*). This is only partly true. Direct bone resorption implies that osteoclasts are formed directly along the bone surface in the area corresponding to the compressed fibers. If such a reaction is to be obtained, the periodontal fibers must be compressed only to a certain extent and must not cause hyalinization.*[35] As a rule this will not occur during the initial stage of tooth movement. A direct initial bone resorption is observed mainly under carefully controlled experimental conditions[121] (Fig. 2-24, *A*).

If the duration of the movement is divided into an initial period and a secondary one (Fig. 2-22), direct bone resorption, also called *frontal* resorption, is found notably in the secondary period—when the hyalinized tissue has disappeared after undermining bone resorption (Fig. 2-35).

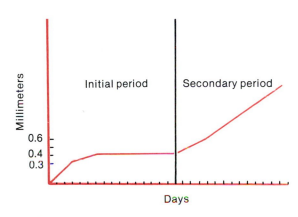

Fig. 2-22 Degree of tooth movement before and after hyalinization. Tooth movement occurring after hyalinization is termed secondary period.

Such direct bone resorption may, for instance, be observed during rotation of teeth. The root is then moved parallel to the bone surface without causing any marked compression (Figs. 2-22 and 2-23). There is also frontal bone resorption along the bone surface adjacent to a compressed hyalinized zone (Fig. 2-33).

Since the human periodontal ligament is frequently as narrow as 0.25 mm or less, obviously its fibers will be compressed between root and bone surface. Compression of the periodontal fibers so they become cell-free results in a standstill of the tooth moved. The tooth will not move again until the bone subjacent to the hyalinized tissue has been eliminated by undermining resorption from the rear and especially from the marrow space. Because the duration of this resorption will be more or less proportionate to the extent of the hyalinized zone, it is important to apply the initial forces in such a manner as to avoid formation of excessively widespread cell-free zones.

---

*In the present discussion, *hyalinization* indicates disappearance of cells with changes in the intercellular substance and not the type of hyalinization observed after irreversible pathologic changes, as for instance in the renal-glomeruli and the ovaries. In the latter cases these zones remain hyalinized for years without undergoing further changes.

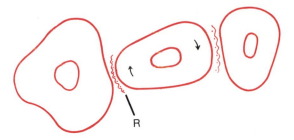

Fig. 2-23   Direct bone resorption after movement of the root parallel with the bone surface, as occasionally occurs during rotation. *R*, Bone resorption.

Formation of cell-free hyalinized zones may occur in other areas of the maxillary structures as well. Thus after widening of the median suture, not only are there cell-free zones in the periodontal ligament but hyalinization of collagen fibers also is observed in various sutures of the maxilla.[77]

The reaction by the osteoclasts as bone-resorbing cells constitutes a much discussed problem.[147] The osteoclast and the cementoclast in the PDL are believed to originate from the hemopoietic system in or before the differentiation of the monocyte series.[28,180] According to Kahn and Malone (1988)[61] there is agreement that the dissemination of osteo-

clast precursors occurs via the blood vascular system. It is furthermore assumed that progenitor osteoclasts are recruited to the sites of bone resorption through chemotaxis. Inductive interaction seems to exist between the bone matrix and the precursor cells resulting in the appearance of mature, multinucleated osteoclasts. Their cytoplasm is known to contain specific granules morphologically identifiable with primary lysosomes, tissue elements that could be carriers of acid phosphate and collagenolytic enzymes.[21] Although it is generally recognized that osteoclasts do not eliminate hyalinized collagen tissue, according to this last finding they obviously behave differently during bone resorption since they are capable of degrading and eliminating collagen fibers of the bone. After injection of parathyroid extract Roberts (1975) observed a ten-fold increase in the osteoclast number. These osteoclasts were most likely circulating cells that had migrated into the area. Dense lipidlike masses have been observed in the cytoplasm of osteoclasts,[150] as well as in hyalinized fibrous tissue.[25] Another unexpected finding in hyalinized tissue is the erythrocytic crystals that Rygh[134] observed in pressure zones of the rat but not in human tissue.

Hyalinization caused by strong forces. Most present-day orthodontists apply light forces in their daily work. Much stronger forces were used some years ago. In the description of tissue changes tooth movement by excessive forces, the

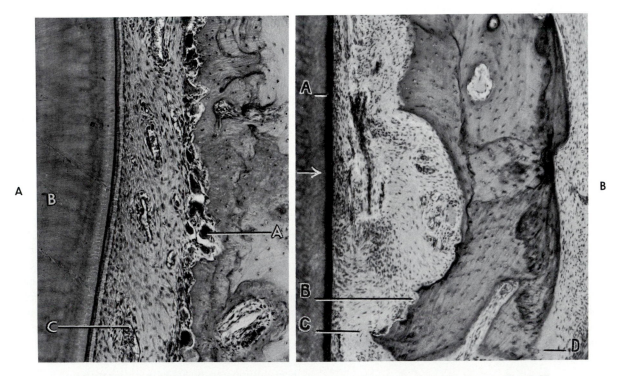

Fig. 2-24   **A,** Longitudinal section of an area corresponding to the resorption area in Fig. 2-23. Animal experiment. The root was rotated parallel with the bone surface. *A,* Direct bone resorption with numerous osteoclasts along the bone surface; *B,* root; *C,* capillary in the periodontal ligament. **B,** Initial hyalinization, alveolar crest area, in a 12-year-old child after 70 g of continuous force for 2 days. *A,* Root surface; *B,* incipient bone resorption with osteoclasts; *C,* area in which some cell nuclei are pyknotic, others have disappeared; *D,* new osteoid formed on the periosteal side.

terms *necrotic hyalinized tissue* and *necrotic alveolar bone* have been used. Necrosis of the alveolar bone has been reported by some investigators more or less as an incidental finding.[79,103]

A careful examination of a large number of hyalinized zones in experiments performed with moderate and strong forces on animal and human material revealed no necrotic changes in the cementum and only a few uncertain changes in the alveolar bone.[124] In new experiments on human structures the bone cells subjacent to hyalinized zones showed no signs of degenerative changes even in experiments of long duration[88] (Fig. 2-25, *B*). According to these and the authors' findings, it is therefore not likely that application of orthodontic forces used today will produce necrosis of the alveolar bone in human structures.

On the other hand, in experimental animals a hyalinization period lasting 60 to 70 days may lead to elimination of compressed fibrous tissue.[118] This phenomenon is due primarily to a high bone density, as shown in Fig. 2-102, *A*, which shows a circumscribed area of the root remaining nearly in contact with the bone surface. Thus it has been proved that compression of long duration may result in elimination and disintegration of the collagen fibers. Until now, similar extensive elimination of periodontal fibers as a result of orthodontic pressure has not been observed in histologic sections of human structures, although it is likely to occur in some cases after extraoral treatment (Fig. 2-90).

Hyalinization caused by light forces. Hyalinization is caused partly by anatomic and partly by mechanical factors. One of the anatomic factors is the form and outline of the bone surface. If there are open channels and spaces, there will be a short period of hyalinization.[115] The protruding bone spicule in Fig. 2-24, *B*, will soon be eliminated by resorption from the rear, and direct bone resorption will prevail in the following secondary period. An enlarged view of the area shown in Fig. 2-26, *A*, will disclose that the cellular structures are indistinct; some nuclei have disappeared, and others have become smaller (pyknosis). This is the first indication of hyalinization. The compressed collagenous fibers will gradually unite in a more or less cell-

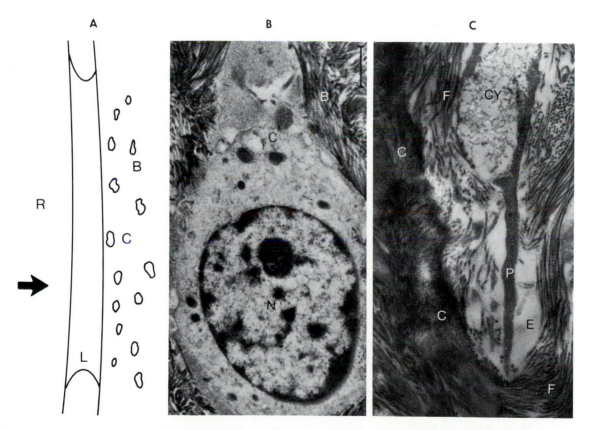

Fig. 2-25   **A,** Findings in human tissue of a 12-year-old. *L,* Hyalinized zone; *R,* root of the tooth; *B,* alveolar bone; *C,* bone cell subjacent to the hyalinized tissue. **B,** Bone cell located as seen at *C* in **A.** *N,* Nucleus; *C,* cytoplasm exhibiting normal structure; *B,* fibrous tissue of decalcified alveolar bone. Force, 120 g; duration, 21 days. (× 10,000. Bar, 1 μm.) **C,** Pioneer connective tissue cell invading the eliminating periodontal fibrils, *F,* inserted into cementum, *C.* Enzymatic dissolution of filaments, *E,* around a pseudopod-like extension, *P.* Human tissue, same age. *CY,* Cytoplasm; the nucleus is located some distance above this point and is not seen here. Force, 60 g; duration, 22 days. (× 20,000.) (From Rygh.)

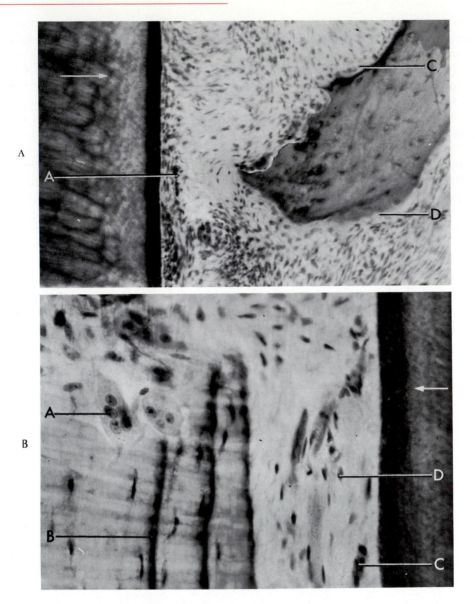

Fig. 2-26   A, Enlarged area seen at *C* in Fig. 2-24, *B.* Disappearance of connective tissue cells adjacent to a persisting epithelial remnant at *A* with formation of osteoclasts at the bone surface; *D,* layer of recently formed osteoid along the alveolar bone crest; *C,* osteoid layer bordered by osteoblasts. **B,** Hyalinized tissue with persisting cell nuclei, part of the compressed area of periodontal ligament from the marginal third of an upper premolar in an adult. Force, 60 g; duration 2 weeks. *A,* Undermining resorption with large osteoclasts; *B,* resting line in dense bone; *C,* persisting epithelial remnant, which will soon disappear; *D,* connective tissue cells and capillaries. The location of the hyalinized zone corresponds to that shown at *A* in Fig. 2-21, *B.*

free mass. Similar cell-free zones have occasionally been observed during physiologic migration of teeth.[68] It should be noted that hyalinized zones elicited by light forces are frequently small, covering not more than 1 or 2 mm² of the root surface.

The uniform hyaline appearance of a compressed zone is caused primarily by certain changes in the ground substance. Gradually the collagen fibers tend to become more or less masked and confluent with the surrounding jellylike ground substance. Phase-contrast and electron microscopy reveals

that in some cases the fibrils remain fairly unaltered (Fig. 2-27, *A*). As a result of the cell destruction and the injury of capillaries, there is a mild inflammatory reaction followed by the production of new capillaries and connective tissue cells in areas around the hyalinized zone. Electron microscopic studies[88] have revealed that masses of irregularly shaped erythrocytes tend to accumulate in the dilated vessels, but these masses will gradually disappear (Fig. 2-28). No polymorphonucleated leucocytes are found in the PDL around the hyalinized zone. There is a mild inflammation,

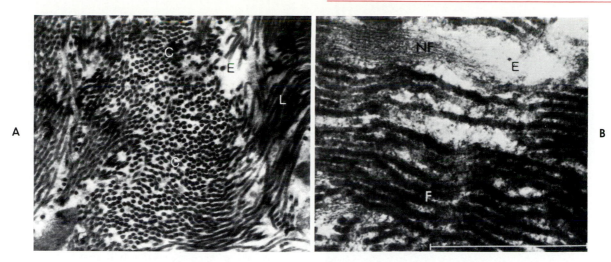

Fig. 2-27   Variations in reaction of hyalinized zones. **A,** Relatively unaltered tissue. *C,* Cross sectioned fibrils; *L,* fibrils cut longitudinally; *E,* eliminated area. (× 20,000.) Tissue from a 12-year-old patient. Force, 70 g; duration, 21 days. **B,** *F,* Fibrils of a more irregular contour and arrangement; *NF,* transformation of fibrils into filaments; such degradation constitutes the prerequisite for enzymatic elimination of fibrils; *E,* eliminated area. (× 41,000; bar, 1 μm.) (From P. Rygh.) (See Figs. 2-25 and 2-28.)

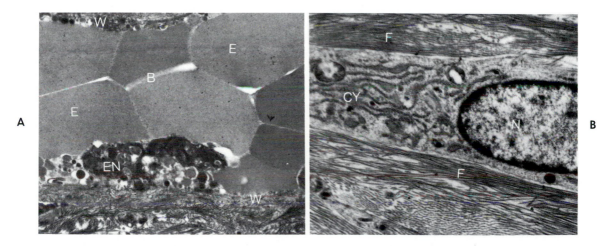

Fig. 2-28   **A,** Early capillary changes in the hyalinized zone (human tissue) as seen with the electron microscope, findings usually not visible by light microscopy. *E,* Stasis with packing of erythrocytes; *B,* borderline between red blood cells; *W,* disappearance of the capillary wall; *EN,* endothelial cell undergoing disintegration. Age, 12 years; force, 70 g; duration, 2 days. (× 6000.) **B,** Principal fibers on the tension side in the rat. *F,* Fibrils subjected to moderate tension and located on both sides of a fibroblast; *N,* nucleus; *CY,* cytoplasm with well-developed endoplasmic reticulum. Force, 10 g; duration, 28 days. (× 9000.) It is not unlikely that prolonged stretching of supraalveolar fibers may cause disappearance of similarly located cellular elements as a result of compression. Compare with Figs. 2-2, *A,* and 2-83, *A.* (From P. Rygh.)

and, as observed by Rygh[136,138] in TEM studies, macrophages play an important role in the latter stage of the reaction (Fig. 2-30).

Many authors would term all types of hyalinized zones *necrotic.* It is true that the cells and the capillaries disappear; but, varying with the magnitude of the force, there will be various degrees of hyalinization. TEM studies have revealed

that isolated cell nuclei may persist for a period while undergoing disintegration[135,136] (Figs. 2-2, *B,* and 2-57, *A*). In addition, unlike necrotic bone, hyalinized fibrous tissue will soon be reconstructed as new collagen fibrils are formed by connective tissue cells, which, together with capillaries reappear in the formerly cell-free tissues[117] (Figs. 2-17, *B,* and 2-29). The only cellular elements that disappear per-

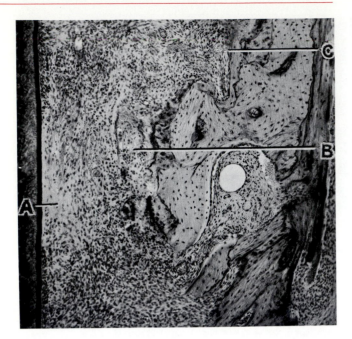

Fig. 2-29 Area corresponding to *A* in Fig. 2-21, *B*, of the upper first premolar in a 12-year-old patient. Hyalinized tissue created during 8 days' compression has been rapidly reconstructed with cells and capillaries as a result of the 8 days of reverse tooth movement. *A*, Central area of the formerly hyalinized zone; note the absence of epithelial remnants; *B*, persisting osteoclasts in resorption lacunae; *C*, incipient bone formation; an empty capillary is plainly evident in the marrow space below line *B*. (Similar area after 3 days' reverse movement is seen in Fig. 2-17, *B*.)

manently are the epithelial remnants of Malassez.[116]

Elimination and reconstruction of hyalinized zones. These processes occur more or less simultaneously, as also observed in electron microscopic studies of human structures.[136,138] In the circumscribed hyalinized area, the connective tissue cells will undergo early loss of the cytoplasm with incipient shrinkage of the nucleus even after a few hours. This autolytic process is caused by various enzymes. At the same time new connective tissue cells accumulate around the compressed area. Fibroblasts appear quite soon after compression has started, macrophages a little later (Fig. 2-29). (See Chapter 3.)

Changes in the compressed fibrous tissue vary and are largely influenced by the duration of the experiment and the magnitude of force. After compression of 2 days' duration, periodontal fibrils remained more or less intact, with a normal cross-striation. After a longer period there was marked packing of fibrils, some of which exhibited frayed ends, and longitudinal splitting of individual fibrils (Fig. 2-27, *B*). It is known that randomly coiled chains of collagen may undergo hydrolysis by enzymes such as acid hydrolase, a process that may explain how periodontal fibers can be gradually eliminated in animal experiments of long duration

(Fig. 2-61, *A*). Degraded fibrous tissue as well as remnants of cellular elements seem to be removed mainly by macrophages[69,138] (Figs. 2-25, *C*, and 2-30). Fibroblasts may also act as tissue-removing cells.[176] It is likely that in the majority of cases gradual and total exchange of fibrous tissue occurs in the central area of the hyalinized zone. In humans this represents only a small fraction of the periodontal fibers on the pressure side of the tooth.

The location of the hyalinized tissue, as well as its extent, is determined largely by mechanical factors such as the nature of the movement. In a tipping movement the hyalinized zone will be located near the alveolar crest; in a bodily movement, closer to the middle portion of the root.[115] In a rotating movement there are nearly always two compressed zones[114] (Fig. 2-103, *A*). A tipping movement performed by an excessive force will also result in two compressed zones, one in the marginal and one in the apical region (Fig. 2-63). If several spicules protrude along the bone surface, two or more minor hyalinized zones may be observed along the same pressure side (Fig. 2-31). As a rule there is only one hyalinized zone, whose extent is largely determined by the form and outline of the bone surface. If this is flat and even, there will be a fairly large cell-free zone.[113] Its extent is moreover, influenced by the magnitude of the force. When a strong initial force is applied against a flat bone surface, the hyalinized zone is bound to be extensive.

Initial tissue reaction. These observations are all related to the initial tissue changes. Elimination of the bone subjacent to the hyalinized tissue is included in the initial period of tooth movement (Fig. 2-22). The duration of this initial phase may vary considerably, from a few days in humans up to 80 days in animals when the anatomic and mechanical conditions are unfavorable. What happens during an initial movement may be observed by periodic measurement of the distance between the tooth moved and the control tooth (Fig. 2-32). On the average it takes 5 to 6 days before the periodontal fibers are compressed enough to produce a standstill of the tooth moved. This period is shorter if the force is excessive. The duration of the subsequent undermining bone resorption is indicated by a horizontal line on the graph. Because the measurements are taken from the crown portion of the tooth, the numbers given are only relative. They will, nevertheless, illustrate the sequence of events during the initial phase of tooth movement. Measurements during the hyalinization period will occasionally reveal minor changes in the position of either the tooth moved or the control tooth. In most cases no perceptible changes in tooth position are evident during the hyalinization period.

It is possible to verify these measurements by removing the tooth and examining the supporting tissues histologically. An example is shown in Fig. 2-33. The tooth was removed before the underlying bone had been eliminated by indirect bone resorption (Fig. 2-34). The relatively long duration of this indirect bone resorption was caused by the

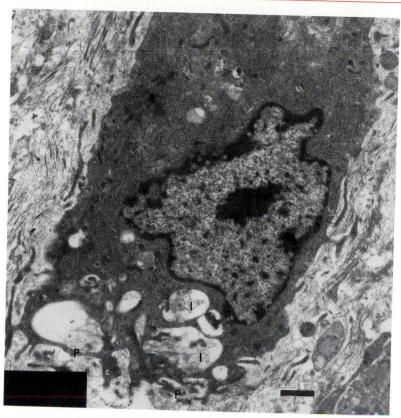

Fig. 2-30 Pressure area in the PDL. Macrophage adjacent to hyalinized zone. Pseudopodia, *P*, delimit inclusions, *I*, of phagocytosed material. Bar is 1μm (original magnification × 10000). (From Rygh.)

bone density and the flat inner bone surface. In humans the hyalinization period usually lasts about 2 or 3 weeks. When there is a high bone density, the duration is longer (Fig. 2-34). A typical hyalinization period in a 12-year-old patient is shown in Fig. 2-35, in which elimination of the underlying bone was followed by further tooth movement (Fig. 2-36).

The changes observed during formation of hyalinized zones may be summarized as follows:

1. There is a gradual compression of the periodontal fibers leading to shrinkage and disappearance of cell nuclei and, subsequently, an exchange of degraded capillaries and fibrils as well.[136,138,140]

2. Osteoclasts are formed in marrow spaces and adjacent areas of the inner bone surface after a period of 20 to 30 hours. It has been assumed that multinucleated cells do *not* attack the cell-free fiber bundles of the hyalinized tissue.

3. There is a gradual increase in the number of young connective tissue cells around the osteoclasts and in areas where the pressure is relieved by undermining bone resorption (Fig. 2-29). This change in appearance before and after hyalinization is especially marked in the adult periodontal ligament, where there are comparatively few cells under a physiologic en-

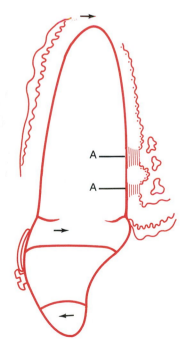

Fig. 2-31 Formation of hyalinized zones against two protruding bone spicules. The tooth was subjected to a torquing movement.

Tooth moved   **Control**

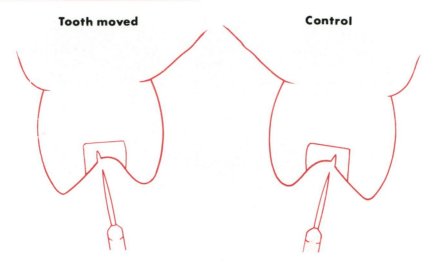

Fig. 2-32 Methods for the measurement of experimental tooth movement. Tiny holes are prepared in amalgam fillings.

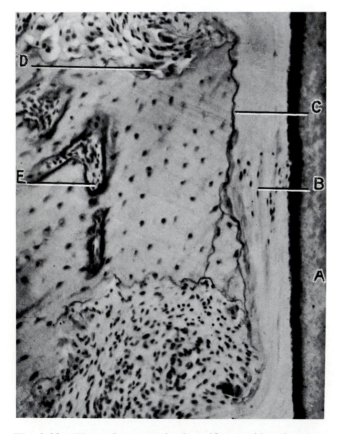

Fig. 2-33 Upper first premolar in a 12-year-old patient (area *A* in Fig. 2-21, *B*). Hyalinization of fairly long duration, here mainly caused by high bone density. There is no formation of osteoclasts in the marrow spaces. *A*, Root surface; *B*, remaining pyknotic cell nuclei in hyalinized tissue; *C*, reversal line.

vironment (Fig. 2-37, *A*). The general increase in cell number will facilitate bone resorption during the secondary stage of tooth movement.

Investigators agree that the osteoclasts, by their chemical action, will remove organic and inorganic substances of the bone more or less simultaneously.[43] Artifacts in the form of spaces between the osteoclasts and Howship's lacunae are readily produced on histologic sections (Fig. 2-20). When tension is exerted on a bone surface undergoing resorption, occasionally the osteoclasts are moved out of their lacunae with the fibrous tissue[117] (Fig. 2-37, *B*).

In autoradiographic studies Young[190] observed that osteoclasts are formed by fusion of precursor cells. Although the cells incorporated in the bone (the osteocytes) will survive until reached by resorption, the life span of the original osteoclasts is relatively short. Their function is nevertheless maintained (Fig. 2-38, *A*). In addition, as observed in Reitan's experiments,[117] there is a tendency to overreaction after the application of orthodontic forces. *Once started, bone resorption tends to continue for up to 10 or 12 days even if no pressure is exerted.* A similar overreaction of the osteoclasts is not observed in physiologic bone resorption.

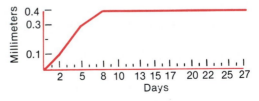

Fig. 2-34 Movement of the tooth in Fig. 2-33. Note 8 days' movement before the tooth came to a standstill, partly because of the light force applied. Duration of hyalinization, which might have lasted longer, was 19 days. Force, 30 g.

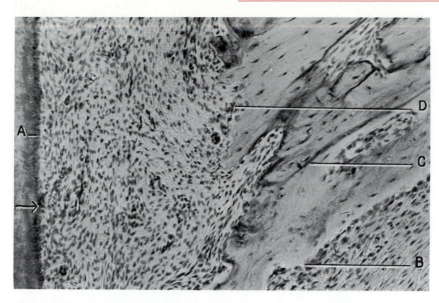

Fig. 2-35   Upper first premolar in a 12-year-old patient (area corresponding to *A* in Fig. 2-21, *A*). Continuous force, 30 g. Alveolar crest with clefts and indentations. This is the secondary period of tooth movement, hyalinization terminated. *A,* Absence of epithelial remnants in adjacent periodontal tissue, center of the formerly cell-free zone; note the widening of periodontal space; *B,* periosteal structures with compensatory bone formation; *C,* resting line; *D,* direct bone resorption with osteoclasts.

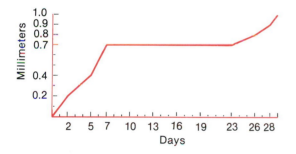

Fig. 2-36   Movement of the tooth in Fig. 2-35. Prehyalinization movement 0.7 mm during 7 days, a result caused mainly by the favorable anatomic environment. Duration of hyalinization, 16 days; force, 30 g. A similar graph was obtained by Storey (1955), who measured the degree of tooth movement in guinea pigs by means of histologic sections.

The enzymatic messenger mechanisms that cause formation of osteoclasts around the hyalinized tissue are not fully understood. The various types of indirect bone resorption are to a large extent, influenced by the anatomic environment. If the bone is dense, osteoclasts are not readily formed in the small marrow spaces subjacent to the hyalinized area (Fig. 2-33). Instead, *frontal resorption* will prevail along the periodontal surface. In the majority of young patients, however, the alveolar bone contains channels and marrow spaces that will be readily reached by the enzymatic messengers, the effect of which will be formation of osteoclasts and typical *undermining resorption* (Fig. 2-38, *B*).

Periosteal undermining resorption has been observed only in the rat and not in other experimental animals or in humans.[123]

Force application during initial tooth movement. If the force is applied only once a week and not reactivated much, the final graph will be similar to those shown in Figs. 2-34 and 2-36. If the force is strictly maintained and even reactivated once a week, additional tipping of the tooth may be obtained (Fig. 2-39) and possibly also bone deformation if the force is excessive. In such cases the duration of the initial undermining bone resorption cannot be observed on the final graph, on which there will be no distinct horizontal line.[115] Instead, various steps along an ascending line will be observed. Frequent reactivation of the force tends to increase the extent and duration of the hyalinized zone. In young persons there may be some increase in the degree of tooth movement but no marked increase in bone resorption.[120] In adult patients frequent reactivation of the force tends to prolong the duration of the undermining resorption period.

Secondary period of tooth movement. In the secondary period of tooth movement (Fig. 2-22) the periodontal ligament is considerably widened (Fig. 2-37, *B*). The osteoclasts will attack the bone surface over a much wider area and, provided the force is kept within certain limits, further bone resorption will be predominantly of the direct type. Notably in a tipping movement, however, a sudden increase in the magnitude of force may cause formation of new hyalinized zones.[115] As a rule these are of relatively short

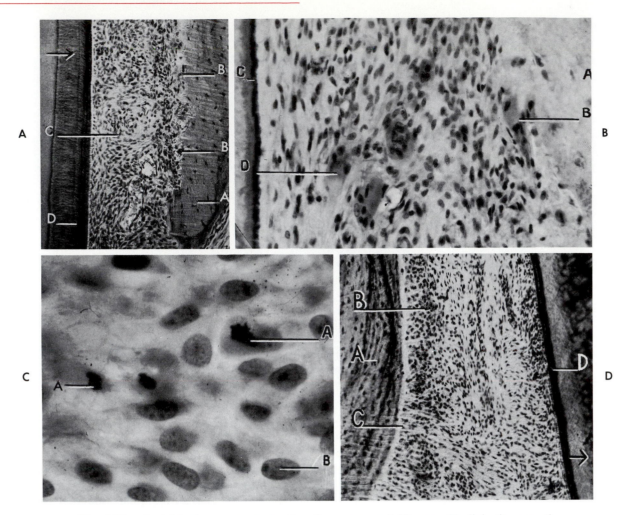

Fig. 2-37   A, Adult tissue, upper premolar of a person aged 39 years. Hyalinization recently terminated. *A,* Alveolar bone crest; *B,* direct bone resorption; *C,* center of formerly hyalinized tissue; *D,* thick cementum layer. Compare the cell number with that shown in the control area of the same individual (Fig. 2-6). **B,** Human material. Migrating osteoclasts after reverse tooth movement. *A,* Bone close to the alveolar crest; *B,* osteoclasts at the bone surface; *C,* root surface; *D,* osteoclasts close to the root surface, a result of tension exerted on periodontal fibers. **C,** Human material. *A,* Mitotic cell division on the tension side during the initial stage of tooth movement; *B,* nucleus of connective tissue cell. **D,** Tension side of an upper premolar in a 12-year-old patient. Continuous force, 70 g; duration, 4 days. *A,* Bundle bone; *B,* increase in the number of connective tissue cells, a proliferation zone where new collagen fibrils are formed (compare with Fig. 2-41, *A*); *C,* newly formed osteoid; *D,* root surface; note the stretched fiber bundles anchored in the bundle bone at the alveolar crest.

duration. Experimental bodily tooth movement performed with measured forces has shown less of a tendency to such formation.[111]

Bone formation. Simultaneously with the changes taking place on the pressure side, formative changes may be observed on the tension side. As a forerunner to bone formation the number of fibroblasts and osteoblasts increase. This increase in cell number occurs by mitotic cell division, first described by Reitan[112] and later by Macapanpan et al.[79] In animal tissue labeled with tritiated thymidine Roberts et al. (1974) observed that initially cells of the periodontal ligament undergo two periods of mitotic division, the first one lasts between 2 and 16 hours and the second, between 36 and 50 hours. In humans an incipient cell proliferation may be observed in the marginal tension area after 30 to 40 hours. The newly formed cells—osteoblasts with darkly stained nuclei—have a characteristic appearance (Fig. 2-37, *D*). They may be observed along stretched fiber bundles; however, because of the tension exerted, some of them will be moved slightly apart. This arrangement is frequently observed during the initial stage of bone formation in humans as well as in animals (Fig. 2-40, *B*) (Chapter 3).

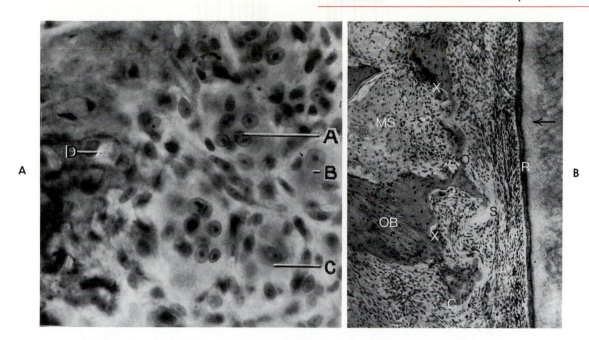

Fig. 2-38   Experimental reverse tooth movement has shown that recently calcified bundle bone is more readily resorbed than old bone. **A,** Rapid formation of osteoclasts. *A,* Typical osteoclast containing eight or nine nuclei; *B* and *C,* osteoclasts in a transitional stage; *D,* rapid resorption of bundle bone with formation of large lacunae. **B,** Four days' reverse movement in one of two brothers with identical alveolar bone. Rapid tooth movement in this case was caused by favorable anatomic characteristics (i.e., large marrow spaces in which undermining bone resorption started quite readily). *R,* Root surface; *O,* osteoid formed during the first 8 days' movement in the opposite direction; to some extent, this new osteoid layer prevents formation of osteoclasts and thus the onset of frontal bone resorption; *S,* semihyalinized periodontal fibers; *X,* osteoclasts, undermining resorption; *OB,* old bone; *C,* alveolar bone crest; *MS,* large marrow spaces.

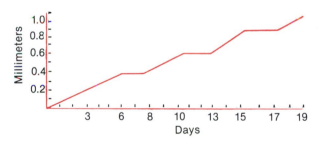

Fig. 2-39   Movement of a tooth subjected to frequent reactivation. Initial force between 150 and 200 g. The hyalinization period is not terminated, so its duration cannot be shown in the graph.

Shortly after the cell proliferation has started, osteoid tissue will be deposited on the tension side. The formation of this new osteoid is to some extent dependent on the form and thickness of the fiber bundles. If they are thick, the newly formed osteoid will be deposited along stretched fiber bundles, resulting in the formation of bone lamellae[112] (Fig. 2-41, *A*). If the fiber bundles are thinner, a more uniform layer of osteoid will be formed along the bone surface. Age may influence the type and amount of bone formed as shown by Reitan[112,122] and by Storey.[170] Bone formation in humans

may also be observed in the form of osteoid bridges, layers extending into the periodontal ligament more or less parallel to the bone surface[117] (Fig. 2-42).

This rapid formation of osteoid is especially marked during the secondary period after the undermining bone resorption on the pressure side is completed (Fig. 2-22). The numerous new cells on the tension side are then conspicuous and are frequently arranged in a proliferation zone containing chains of osteoblasts (Fig. 2-41). These observations illustrate that bone formation is the result of tension exerted

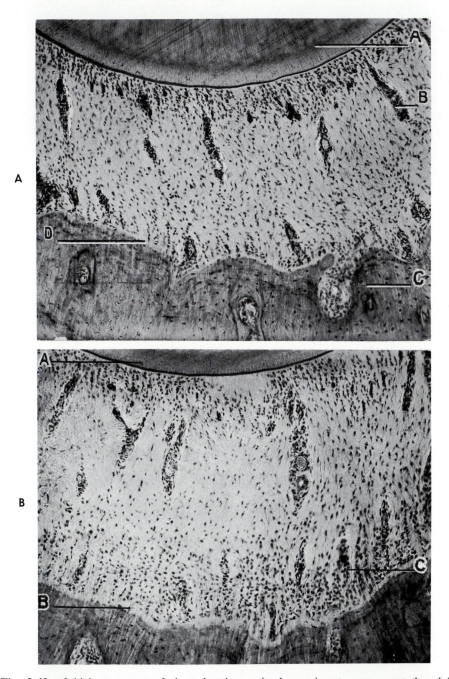

Fig. 2-40   Initial movement of short duration, animal experiment, upper central and lateral incisors. **A,** Control. *A,* tooth root; *B,* interstitial space, *C,* bundle bone; *D,* undecalcified osteoid layer. **B,** Experimental second incisor, tension side. Continuous force, 45 g; duration, 36 hours. Note the increase and spreading of new cells, particularly in areas close to the bone surface and adjacent to stretched fiber bundles. *A,* Tooth root; *B,* increase in osteoid tissue; *C,* proliferating osteoblasts between fiber bundles. Compare with Fig. 2-37, *D.* (From Reitan K; *Acta Odontol Scand Suppl* 6, 1951.)

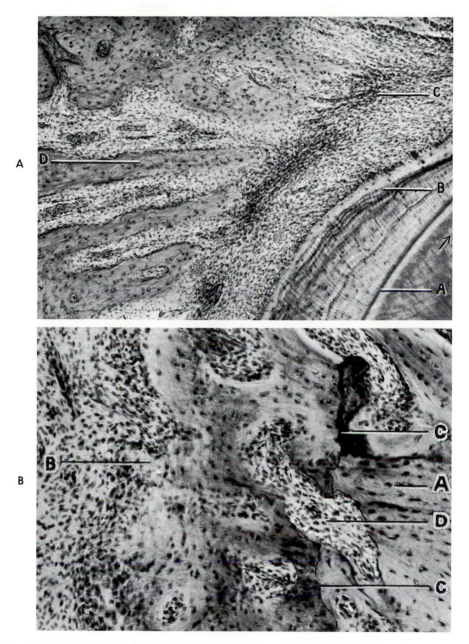

Fig. 2-41   Effect of the fiber bundle thickness on bone formation. **A,** Tension side, middle third of an upper second incisor rotated in the dog. *A,* Line indicating thickness of cementum layer; *B,* new cementum formed as a result of the experiment; *C,* new connective tissue cells, a proliferation zone where new collagen fibrils are formed, thus ensuring elongation of the periodontal fibers; *D,* bone lamellae formed along the stretched fiber bundles. Arrow shows the direction of movement. **B,** Tissue from a 12-year-old child. Tension side (area *B* or *C* in Fig. 2-21). Continuous movement for 14 days of an upper premolar. Force, 70 g. Note the different arrangement of new bone layers as compared with the experiment in *A,* a result of the thinner fiber bundles in this patient. *A,* Old bone; *B,* osteoid tissue bordered by osteoblasts; *C,* reversal line indicating where the bone formation started during the experimental period; *D,* marrow space; the new bone is already partly calcified; only the superficial layer, seen at *B,* remains uncalcified. Root surface to the left not seen here.

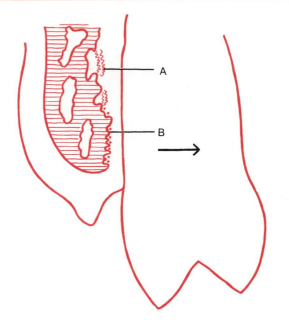

Fig. 2-42 Tension side, reverse movement. *A,* Osteoid formed in the proliferation zone parallel with the bone surface; *B,* persisting bone resorption.

on the periodontal fibers and that such changes are closely related to the distance through which the force is active.

As previously described, calcification of the osteoid layers that were deposited first on the tension side starts quite soon; however, the superficial layer remains uncalcified and will not be visible radiographically. This uncalcified tissue, together with the space created as the tooth is moved away from the bone surface, will appear as a dark line on the radiograph, a space not unlike the widening of the periodontal ligament seen in pathologic conditions. It is, nevertheless, a perfectly normal reaction, notably observed after special types of tooth displacement, such as extrusion or bodily movement (Figs. 2-64 and 2-108, *A*).

When the new bundle bone layers have attained a certain thickness, a reorganization of the new bone will take place, to some extent influenced by the physiologic movement of the tooth. This phase of bone changes is dealt with in greater detail under the discussion of relapse tendencies.

BIOLOGIC CONTROL MECHANISMS IN TOOTH MOVEMENT
Transformation of Mechanical Stimuli into Bone and Connective Tissue Remodeling

For a long time it has been a general agreement that the most dramatic remodeling changes incident to orthodontic tooth movement occur in the PDL. More recently it was found that simultaneously important reactions take place in marrow spaces of the alveolar bone and in the gingival periosteum at some distance from the tooth root.[112]

In a bodily movement over a greater distance the tooth is usually moved through spongy interseptal bone which contains many large marrow spaces. The content of these spaces is either loose fibrous tissue (frequently observed in young persons) or fatty marrow. If a tooth is moved against a marrow space of the latter type, one may observe how the fatty tissue is gradually transformed into loose fibrous tissue. Different bone reactions occur: direct resorption of the alveolar bone bordering the compressed periodontal space, apposition on the marrow side, and compensatory formation of a new bone lamina within the marrow space (Fig. 2-43).

What makes the tissues respond? What are the control elements that transform application of sustained mechanical loads into the cell reaction that are necessary for remodeling of the tooth-supporting tissues? Two mechanisms have been proposed. The pressure-tension theory relates tooth movement to *biochemical-responses* by the cells and extracellular components of the PDL and alveolar bone. The other theory deals with tooth movement as *bioelectric* phenomena that may occur as a result of mechanical distortion of collagenous matrices, mineralized or nonmineralized, in the alveolar bone, the PDL, and the teeth. It appears that both mechanisms are involved.

Much information on cellular signaling which is directly related to the understanding of orthodontic reactions has been presented during the last few years. It is generally accepted that cells respond to signals from other cells and to changes in the environment. Extracellular signals can be classified as endocrine, paracrine, or autocrine based on the distance over which the signal must act. In *endocrine* signaling the cells of the endocrine organs release hormones which are signaling substances usually carried by the blood to the distant target cells. In *paracrine* signaling the cell is close to the target cell and the compound that is released (local mediator) affects only a group of cells adjacent to it. The conduction of an electric impulse from a nerve cell to another or to a muscle cell involves signaling by extracellular chemicals called neurotransmitters. In *autocrine* signaling cells respond to substances that they themselves release.

Some hormones bind to receptors within the cell; others bind to cell surface receptors:

1. Intracellular receptors. Steroids, retinoic acid and thyroxine, being hydrophobic, enter the cell and bind to specific receptors in the cytosol or nucleus and act on nuclear DNA to alter transcription of specific genes. At present it is unclear whether cells being affected by mechanical forces react via these mechanisms.
2. Cell surface receptors. Peptide and protein hormones, prostaglandins, aminoacids, epinephrine, and other water-soluble signaling molecules called ligands act as *first messengers* and bind to cell surface receptor proteins and thereby activate enzymes that generate an increase (or decrease) in the concentration of intracellular signaling compounds termed *second messengers*. These include adenosine 3',5'-monophos-

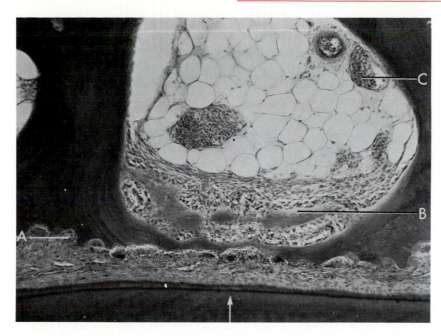

Fig. 2-43 Bodily movement of an upper second incisor in a dog. Arrow indicates the tooth and the direction of movement. The root was moved against a space containing fatty marrow, which was transformed into loose fibrous tissue in advance of the movement. Note the compression of the periodontal ligament (*arrow*). The periodontal space is narrower in this area because the uncalcified bone layer along the inside of the marrow space is less readily resorbed by osteoclasts. *A,* Direct bone resorption, one of the many Howship's lacunae with osteoclasts; *B,* compensatory bone formation, osteoid layer bordered by osteoblasts; *C,* capillary surrounded by fatty marrow.

phate (cyclic AMP or cAMP)[174]; guanosine 3', 5'-monophosphate (cGMP)[130]; 1, 2-diacylglycerol and inositol 1, 4, 5-triphosphate. So far these second messengers cAMP and cGMP have been identified as mediators of external stimuli on bone cells. Fluctuations in the level of these two mediators have been found to occur also in bone treated by parathyroid hormone (PTH),[158] calcitonin, vitamin D_3;[109] and electric currents.[65] The use of cAMP as the second messenger in signaling systems is widespread, in fact it operates in all eukaryotic (plant and animal) cells.[26] The other way in which extracellular signals are generated into intracellular signals lies inherent in the fact that surface receptors may open or close gated ion channels in the plasma membrane and in turn change the flux of ions into the cell. Particularly important is the influx of Ca^{2+}, which also acts as a second messenger.[52] The elevated intracellular concentration of one or more such second messengers triggers a rapid alteration in the activity of one or more enzymes or nonenzymatic proteins which effectuate the cellular response requested by the receptor ligand.[48] The use of the Ca^{2+} ions as signal transducers is widespread in animals.

Prostaglandins are lipid soluble, hormone-like chemicals that are produced by many types of mammalian cells and that bind to surface receptors. Several prostaglandins act as local mediators during paracrine signaling and are rapidly destroyed near the site of their synthesis. They modulate the responses of other hormones and have profound effects on many cell processes. Prostaglandins cause contraction of smooth muscle, as well as inflammation development.[145] Generally prostaglandins are vasoactive and influence the Ca^{2+} concentration in the cellular cytosol. Another important effect of prostaglandins is regulation of the intracellular concentration of cAMP through an effect on the enzyme adenylate cyclase. On the other hand Ca^{2+} liberation in cells may influence prostaglandin synthesis directly or through cAMP. (See Chapter 3.)

Synthesis of prostaglandins takes place in cellular membranes where fatty acids are cleared from membrane phospholipids by enzymes (phospholipase) into arachidonic acids.[19] By a change of arachidonic acid from an extended into a folded conformation and by further oxidation steps by different enzymes (cyclo-oxygenases) one of the prostaglandins will be produced.

Many anti-inflammatory agents used in everyday medicine seem to work by inhibiting phostaglandin biosynthesis.[90] Whereas the corticosteroids inhibit the phospholipase activity, indomethacin inhibits the cyclo-oxygenase and may also inhibit the total hemostasis in the body, provided the doses are high enough. Aspirin and other acetylsalicylic acids inhibit the cyclo-oxygenases irreversibly.

The concentration of prostaglandins on the receptor site,

which decides the binding to receptors and the effect on the cells, is dependent on the speed of the synthesis. Many hormones are believed to influence prostaglandin synthesis: epinephrine, angiotension, prolactin, and histamine.

Tissue trauma stimulates prostaglandin release. Even gentle tissue manipulation increases the local concentration of prostaglandins. Ischemia seems to be a potent stimulus for prostaglandin synthesis.[54] These observations may be particularly interesting from an orthodontic viewpoint as are the findings that local concentration of prostaglandins is related to the mild and sterile inflammation process that develops.

Orthodontic/Experimental Tooth Movement as Related to Biochemical Reactions

When orthodontic stress is applied to the tooth, and thereby to the PDL and the bone as well, the extracellular fluids of the PDL shift and the cells and matrix are distorted. Vascular changes with dilation of vessels and stasis and disintegration of vessel walls is seen in sites of compression.[133] Changes in blood flow with migration of leucocytes into the extra vascular space can be observed in areas of tension as well, indicating that there is a mild inflammatory reaction.[140,141]

Experimental evidence proves that the open state of ion channels seen in most cells depends on stress exerted at the membrane,[93] a finding which again is influenced by the maintenance and composition of the extracellular matrix.[29,59] It is therefore assumed that when an orthodontic force displaces the periodontal ligament, such a movement may result in cell perturbation, altering the influx of Ca^{2+} and other ions, which in turn has been believed to alter the synthesis of cAMP.[29]

Davidovitch and Shanfeld (1975)[32] reported findings indicating that levels of cAMP and cGMP increased in alveolar bone and PDL cells following the application of orthodontic forces to teeth.

Somjen et al (1980)[165] demonstrated that the synthesis of cAMP coincident with the stretching of the cells is prostaglandin dependent. This report and others led to the assumption that what happens to the cellular structures during transduction of orthodontic mechanical forces consists in physical deformation of cell membranes with resultant prostaglandin synthesis.[15,131] This would result in activation of membrane-bound adenylate or guanylate cyclases responsible for converting the respective substrates to cAMP and cGMP.

In a histochemical study it was found that the macrophages of the new blood vessels that penetrate the tissues of a hyalinized area could be identified by their high arylsulfatase and aminopepidase-M activity, enzymes known as markers of macrophage activity.[74] These cells also revealed high prostaglandin synthetase (PgS) activity (PgS being an enzyme complex that converts arachidonic acid to prostaglandins). It has been assumed that macrophages, while invading and removing hyalinized tissue, may release prostaglandins and also stimulate the formation of osteoclasts. On the other hand osteoclast-like cells showed typical high acid phosphatase activity and, in contact with bone surfaces, revealed no PGS activity. Whereas these authors demonstrated prostaglandin synthetase associated with macrophages invading hyalinized tissue, Davidovitch and Shanfeld (1980) showed a rise of prostaglandin E_2 (PGE$_2$) levels in the PDL and alveolar bone, both in sites of tension and compression in orthodontically treated cats.[32]

Yamasaki et al (1980)[187] have shown that prostaglandins that were produced during orthodontic tooth movement may increase bone resorption activity. These authors performed a series of experiments in rats, monkeys, and humans; PGE was injected in the gingiva of the teeth to be moved.[188] They reported an enhanced rate of tooth movement. However, new evidence indicates that the effect of PGE on bone cells differs, depending on location.[99] Bone growth may even be influenced.[82] When root resorption was quantified after experimental tooth movement with local PGE$_2$ injections in rats, the trend was toward more root resorption in the injection group.[24]

Now, increasing evidence proves that although PGE is involved in the transduction of mechanical stress on the PDL and alveolar bone during orthodontic tooth movement, several other inflammatory mediators are active. It appears that orthodontic forces may activate the *nervous* as well as the *immune* systems. Results of experiments performed by Davidovitch et al (1988)[31] and Kvinnsland and Kvinnsland (1990)[73] indicate that the increases in second messengers (cAMP, cGMP) in periodontal cells do not result solely from the direct effects of the mechanical forces but are also caused by endogenous signaling agents. Mechanical stress would alter the level and distribution of the *neurotransmitter* substances in the PDL. Neuropeptides: substance P (SP), vasoactive intestinal polypeptide (VIP), calcitonin gene related peptide (CGRP) and others act as neurotransmitters from sensory nerve fibres in the PDL and supply a link between physical stimulus and the biochemical response. Pain sensitive nerve endings release stored SP into the PDL, leading to binding of SP to specific cellular receptors. Through interaction with endothelial cells there will be a rapid vasodilation and migration of leucocytes from blood vessels.

Also immune systems play a regulatory part in orthodontic tissue reactions. Pronounced vasodilation has been reported in areas of tension and in the periphery of compressed sites of the PDL in experimental tooth movement.[63,141] Macrophages have been identified near the blood vessels.[48,141] It is generally accepted that vasodilation leads to migration of macrophages, lymphocytes, proteins, and fluid into the extracellular space. These inflammatory cells as well as fibroblasts and osteoblasts, produce signal molecules, *cytokines:* interleukins 1α and 1β (IL-1α and IL-1β) that attract leucocytes, stimulate fibroblast proliferation and enhance bone resorption and a so-called tumor necrosis factor-α (TNF-α) which induces IL-1 production by monocytes, enhances PGE_2 and collagenase production, and increases the number of osteoclasts. Lymphocytes produce gamma interferon (γIFN) which inhibits IL-1-induced bone resorption and seems to favor tissue repair.

It has been reported in experimental studies that stress produced by orthodontic forces would cause a marked increase in the staining intensity of IL-1α in all cell types of the PDL, in particular osteoblasts in tension sites and PDL cells and osteoclasts at compression sites. Similarly, orthodontic forces would produce a marked increase in cellular staining intensity of IL-1β, particularly in the osteoblasts at PDL tension sites and osteoclasts at compression sites. Even TNF-α and γIFN were observed in the PDL in experimental tooth movement.[31]

Many questions concerning the interplay between cellular regulators, hormones, neurotransmitters, prostaglandins and cytokines and mechanical stress remain unanswered.[144] Biological consideration should influence treatment planning. There is evidence that pharmacological agents used for pain control may influence cellular activity that is vital for the remodeling of the tooth supporting tissues.

As was discussed previously many agents used in today's medicine may work by inhibiting prostaglandin biosynthesis.[90] Nonsteroidal anti-inflammatory drugs: aspirin and other acetylsalicylic acids, as well as ibuprofen and related agents, slow down orthodontic tooth movement. Patients treated for other purposes by corticosteroids or indomethacin-related agents may also expect a slower orthodontic tissue reaction. Epileptic patients in anti-convulsive treatment may show abnormal bone resorption patterns.[89]

Since drugs can affect prostaglandin levels, as well as other messenger compounds, it would be natural to keep these findings in mind during orthodontic procedures. It is not unlikely that drugs may be used to enhance orthodontic treatment results in the future.

Orthodontic Tooth Movement as Related to Bone Deformation; Bioelectricity

So far in this discussion cAMP proliferation kinetics has been related only to cellular changes induced by chemical messengers. However, it has been shown that distortion of cells and extracellular matrix is associated with alteration in tissue and cellular electric potentials.

Bones have a remarkable ability to remodel their structure in such a way that stress is optimally resisted (Wolff's law). Deposition and resorption are somehow controlled by mechanical influence. It is well known that the maintenance of bone structure is dependent upon exercise. Without any mechanical stress (e.g., in elderly bedridden persons or in astronauts in space flights without gravitational forces), there is loss of bone mineral and skeletal atrophy.[80,162] It has been hypothesized that mechanical deformation of the crystalline structure of hydroxyapatite and the crystalline-like structure of collagen induce migration of electrons that generate local electrical fields. This phenomenon is called

piezoelectricity. Such signals die away quickly even though the force is maintained. But when the force is released and the crystal lattice returns to original shape, a reverse flow of electrons occurs. Rhythmic activity would cause a rhythmic flow of electrons in both directions. Cells are sensitive to these strain-generated potentials (piezoelectric effect). It has been assumed that bending of bone may create negative fields occurring in the concave aspect of the bone surface leading to deposition.

It has been suggested that ions in the fluids surrounding living bone interact with the electrical fields generated when the bone is bent. These currents of small voltages are called *streaming potentials*. In their in vivo experiments, Zengo et al. (1973)[192] observed the highest electrical potentials at the enamel surface of the tooth moved, less in the cementum and dentin and least in the alveolar bone. At the same time a bioelectric effect could be observed in the gingiva as well as in the proximal teeth and their supporting tissues.

Recent observations have shown that not only bone deformation but also tension may create bioelectrical signals. Thus in vivo experiments conducted by Roberts et al (1981)[129] have revealed that a negative electrical field is created in areas where the periodontal ligament is widened.

Reports on the bone changes created by electric currents have led to the use of local application of weak electric currents in therapeutic procedures during healing of bone fractures. The treatment results were good.[38,81] Application of weak electric currents in combination with experimental tooth movement in cats gave different results.[11,30] Although acceleration of tooth movement has been reported, use of the method in therapeutic treatment of patients does not seem to have been reported. The possibility of unwanted effects cannot be disregarded (Chapter 3).

Some investigators have reached highly diverging conclusions as regards the stimulus required for producing bone deformation. Baumrind,[8] conducting experiments on 99 rats, concluded that "bone deflection can be produced by forces lower than those required to produce consequential changes in the periodontal ligament width." Contrary to this statement, Murphy,[98] using the oxytetracycline microfluorescent technique, observed no bending of the alveolar bone during retraction of teeth in the monkey. Obviously deflection of thin bone lamellae occurs quite frequently during treatment, but in most cases deformed bone walls tend to move back to their former position as a result of bone elasticity and fiber contraction as soon as space has been created by resorption[123] (Fig. 2-75).

The initial changes in the periodontal ligament have also been included in these studies. Baumrind and Buck[9] investigated the changes in the rat periodontium at varying periods up to 72 days by injecting radioactive precursors that labeled individual cellular and connective tissue elements to be investigated: tritiated thymidine for observation of cell replication as indicated by the presence of deoxyribonucleic acid (DNA), tritiated uridine for ribonucleic acid (RNA) assessment, and tritiated proline for observation of collagen formation. The autoradiographic findings indicated that there was a significant increase in cell division adjacent to the roots of the experimental teeth as compared with those of the nondisplaced control teeth. Collagen synthesis seemed to decrease in areas adjacent to the experimental teeth. On the pressure side there was an increase in the number of labeled cells fairly similar to that on the tension side. It was suggested that the major physiologic and mechanical changes might occur not in the periodontal ligament but rather in the alveolar bone.

Fiber Remodeling in the Rat

When Ten Cate (1971)[176] demonstrated that the fibroblast is capable of degrading and synthesizing collagen simultaneously and thereby being able to control collagen remodeling, it was inferred that in the healthy PDL all collagen degradation was intracellular.[178] It was therefore assumed that rapid remodeling of the periodontal connective tissue during experimental/therapeutic tooth movement would be characterized by a high ratio of internalized collagen/fibroblast volume. The hypothesis was supported by the observation that macrophages cells, which under certain circumstances ingest and degrade collagen (the classical example being the rapid removal of collagen from the uterine wall after pregnancy), are not numerous in the normal functioning PDL.

In experimental tooth movement in rats conducted by Rygh et al (1986)[141] the PDL revealed a marked widening of blood vessels especially in the middle areas and adjacent to the bone wall in areas of tension. This was not a new observation. Khouw and Goldhaber (1970)[63] using light microscopy (LM) had reported PDL vasodilation incident to orthodontic tooth movement. In transmission electron mi-

croscope (TEM) studies, however, it was found that a great number of cells located near the blood vessels during vascular infiltration in reality were macrophages (Fig. 2-44). These cells and other leucocytes which migrate out of the PDL blood vessels simultaneously with proteins and fluid are known to be capable of producing and releasing factors that interact with target cells in the PDL. They may also initiate an acute response in the alveolar bone. The local areas of tension revealed that the volume of the collagen fibers running from tooth to alveolar bone was reduced as the volume of blood vessels increased. In TEM, collagen fibrils and other formed structures were more sparse in the intercellular spaces in areas of tension after 5 days. Not many fibroblasts containing collagen profiles could be observed except in the experimental periods between 2 and 5 days. In experiments lasting longer, the amount of intracellular collagen profiles in the fibroblasts was limited. Therefore the extensive fibrous breakdown and remodeling that was observed in experimental tooth movement in the rat was not associated with intensive phagocytic activity by ligament fibroblasts.

The evidence indicated that in orthodontic tooth movement the remodeling of PDL is related to inflammation-like phenomena, vasodilation and migration of macrophages, and other leucocytes into the extravascular space in addition to phagocytosis. On the basis of the observed inflammation-like reactions involving the hematogenous system, other changes seemed more likely to occur, such as extracellular breakdown of collagen by collagenases effected by macrophages or fibroblasts through macrophage/fibroblast interaction.[66] Ten Cate and Anderson (1986)[177] observed that in the physiologic situation of tooth shedding in kittens the removal of collagen from the PDL constitutes an extracellular occurrence that does not involve phagocytic activity by fibroblasts.

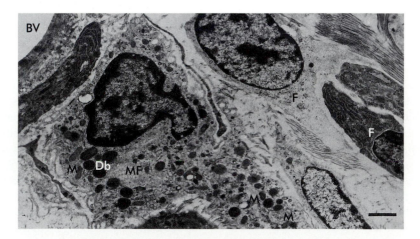

Fig. 2-44   Area of tension in the middle of the periodontal membrane, experimental time: 14 days. Macrophage *(MF)* shown with many dense bodies *(Db)* of varying size and stainability and mitochondria *(M)* near blood vessel *(BV)*. *F,* Fibroblast. Bar is 1 μm (original magnification × 10,000). (From Rygh P et al: *Am J Orthod* 89:453, 1986.)

The term *inflammation* has not been used by many of the earlier investigators using the light microscope, and the reaction in the compressed area would be called a mild inflammation by most pathologists. In orthodontics it should be regarded as a process that occurs in the PDL as a rapid response to stress transiently felt by the cells as being too heavy. As long as the local sterile necrotic spots or limited area is of short duration and is not complicated by infection, there will not be any unwanted sequelae in the average patient. However, a few patients (for reasons not fully clarified) exhibit an individual tissue reaction that may lead to loss of periodontal support and root resorption, even in cases where the tissue injuries are small.

Reactions to Heavy Loads in Tension Areas of the Rat

It is generally known that parallel movement of teeth causes little or no overstretching of the PDL in areas of tension.[139] However, during continuous tipping such a reaction may well occur. In order to study reactions to heavy, continuous loads (50 g) experimental tipping of first molars in rats were performed. During a tipping movement in the rat there seems to be a pattern in the reaction of the PDL and bone to tensional stress: (1) up to a certain level of stress/duration the reactions occur mainly in the periodontal membrane; increasing vascularization, cell proliferation, fiber formation, and osteoid application on the bone surface; (2) beyond a certain level of stress/duration there is decreased vascular supply in the periodontal membrane (PDM) and destruction of cells between stretched fibers; then the reactions become more marked within the alveolar bone with removal and resorption of Sharpey's fibers from the rear (Fig. 2-45), subsequently permitting vascular invasion of cells into the periodontal membrane from the alveolar bone; in certain areas the alveolar bone may become resorbed from both sides of the alveolar lamina; (3) when the force is strong and of long duration, there is a temporary increase in the periodontal membrane width. A vertical reduction of the height of the approximal alveolar bone may occur. There is reason to assume that the pressure exerted on the alveolar crest by the stretched transseptal fibers contributes to this bone resorption. A tipping tooth movement accentuates the vertical reduction. A similar resorption of

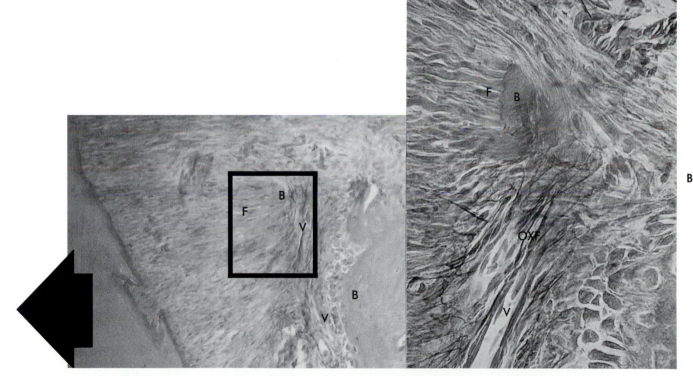

Fig. 2-45 **A,** Area of tension of 28-day duration in the rat. Tooth moved in direction of arrow. Interface between Sharpey's fibers *(F)* and alvolar bone *(B)* near the alveolar crest. Note the proliferation of blood vessels *(V)* in the alveolar bone, detaching periodontal membrane fibers from the bone surface from the rear. **B,** Area corresponding to box in **A.** Sections 6 μm apart. Blood vessels have infiltrated the alveolar bone plate *(B)* from the rear. Sharpey's fibers and parts of the alveolar bone have disappeared—Oxytalen fibrils *(OXF)* stained violet by Aldehyde–fuchsin–Halmi after oxidation. (From Rygh P et al: *Am J Orthod* 89:459, 1986.)

the alveolar bone crest by fiber pressure seldom occurs in humans (see Fig. 2-67). In humans, inner root resorption may be caused by compression of fibrous tissue (Figs. 2-183 and 2-184).

Bone deformation in the rat, with deposition of maxillary bone layers, has been observed in all cases after an experimental period of 2 days. It is not unlikely that this bone deposition can be considered a result of bioelectric changes[123] (Figs. 2-46 and 2-47). Similar periosteal and endosteal bone deposition has been observed in the monkey.[77,87] Whether periosteal bone deposition occurs in young children undergoing extraoral treatment or after widening of the median suture has not yet been determined.

As pointed out by Picton,[106] distortion of the root would

be minimal during orthodontic treatment. An exception to this rule is observed in teeth with undeveloped roots (Fig. 2-48). It is found that formation of uncalcified cementoid will be controlled and even diminished by compression against fibrous tissue.[124] In addition, new cementoid is added on the tension side. According to Shamos and Lavine[154] the electromechanical effect is related solely to the organic components of mineralized tissue—in other words, to the altered arrangement of collagen fibers. If this theory is correct, the possibility exists that tension transformed into bioelectric signals along fibers incorporated in cementum could result in the formation of new cementoid.

More than the effect caused by these bioelectric changes, intrinsic factors seem to be important during bone formation.

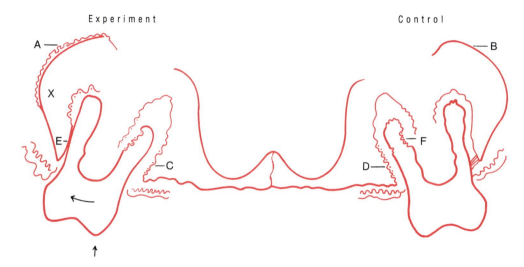

Fig. 2-46   Experimental tooth and a nondisplaced control tooth in the rat. *E,* Hyalinized zone; *X,* bone wall possibly deformed during tooth movement; *A,* periosteal bone deposition observed in all cases after 2 days' tooth movement; *B,* aplastic bone surface on the control side.

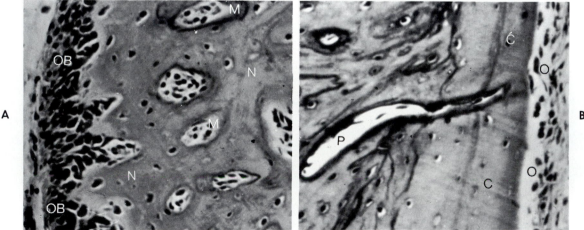

Fig. 2-47   **A,** Area corresponding to *A* in Fig. 2-46. *OB,* Proliferating osteoblasts bordering thick new bone layer; *M,* marrow spaces in new bone. **B,** Control side, corresponding to *B* in Fig. 2-46. *O,* Osteogenic layer of periosteum with some osteoblasts; *C,* dense circumferential bone layer with *P,* a perforating canal. (From Reitan K, Kvam E: *Angle Orthod* 41:1, 1971.)

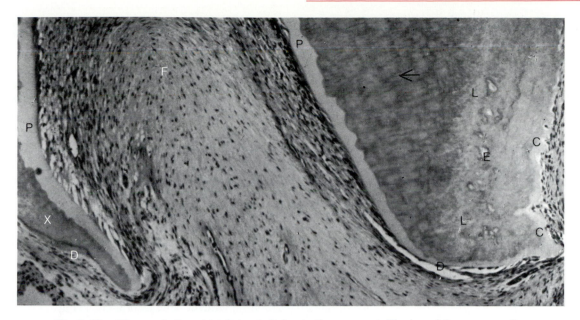

Fig. 2-48 Changes in the root substance during tooth movement. Tipping of the crown portion of a lower first premolar in a direction opposite that indicated by the arrow. Developmental stage of the root. *F,* Fibrous tissue located in the apical foramen; *P,* predentin layers; note the difference in thickness of the walls of the root, with some deformation of the thin wall on the left side, *X,* and slight increase in the thickness of predentin; new cementum has been formed on the right side of the root; *L,* demarcation line indicating thickness of newly formed cementum; *C,* cementoid bordered by cementoblasts; *E,* lacunae in the new cementum partly empty, partly containing cementoblasts; *D,* diminution in the thickness of cementoid and predentin layers as a result of compression by fibrous tissue. No root resorption occurred because the force applied was moderate and the uncalcified cementoid and predentin layers protected the calcified surfaces. Age, 12 years; force, 80 g; duration, 47 days.

Their influence has been noted in various types of experimental work. Thus variations in the onset of the major growth period were demonstrated by Bjørk[18] in his diagrams of patients undergoing observation. Likewise, histologic studies have revealed that rapid bone formation is caused primarily by the presence of growth hormones, as shown in Figs. 2-58 and 2-67, *B.* These patients were more or less of the same age; but whereas the amount of new bone was extensive in one patient, it was negligible in the other.

CONTINUOUS VERSUS INTERMITTENT TOOTH MOVEMENT

Variations in the tissue reaction are caused by several factors. One of them is the duration of the force and to some extent the character of this force. Thus certain variations occur when a continuous force acts only for a short time. An even greater difference exists between the tissue elicited by fixed as compared to removable appliances. Based on these external influences, tooth movement in general may conveniently be divided into two types, each with one subdivision:

1. Continuous movement (fixed appliances)
   (a) Interrupted type

2. Intermittent movement (removable appliances)
   (a) Functional type

The nomenclature used here may need to be explained. Some practitioners would probably apply the word *intermittent* to a tooth movement of short duration as obtained with fixed appliances. However, this term could be confusing especially since the word *intermittent* was chosen many years ago to describe the use of removable appliances. It must be admitted that *intermittent* and *interrupted* are more or less synonymous, but in the following, they will be used for different types of tooth movement: the word *interrupted* designates movement of short duration elicited by fixed appliances; *intermittent* is used mainly to designate removable appliances.

Continuous Tooth Movement

A description of the tissue changes observed after application of a typical continuous force has been given under the headings "Bone resorption" and "Bone formation" (pp. 109 and 118).

Although it is not always possible to distinguish between a continuous movement and an interrupted movement, the latter will, under certain conditions, cause definite variations

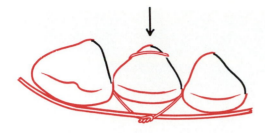

Fig. 2-49   Interrupted movement, a continuous force acting over a short distance. After movement there is a resting period.

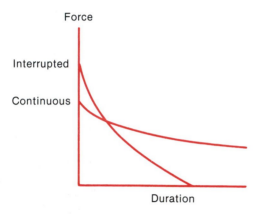

Fig. 2-50   Difference in magnitude and duration of force between continuous tooth movement and interrupted movement.

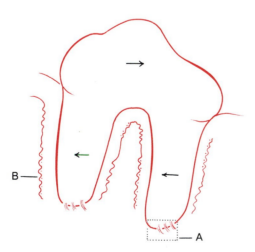

Fig. 2-51   Distal tipping of a lower premolar in a dog. *B*, Bone resorption. The boxed area *(A)* is shown in Fig. 2-52, *B*.

in the tissue response. These changes have a bearing on the phases of clinical orthodontics.

Interrupted type. Although the typical continuous force acts for longer periods, the interrupted force is of comparatively short duration (3 to 4 weeks on the average). An example of interrupted force is the movement that occurs when a tooth is ligated to a labial arch, the tooth being held in position after the force is no longer acting (Fig. 2-49). Torque performed with the edgewise arch is, in many instances, an interrupted movement (Fig. 2-50).

Varying with the force exerted, the bone resorption may be of either the direct or the indirect type. Compression and hyalinization of fibrous tissue may frequently occur on the pressure side during the initial phase of an interrupted movement; as the force rapidly decreases, however, the tissues will soon be reorganized after the hyalinized zone is undermined. Certain interrupted movements, such as small increments of torque performed with measured forces, may result in a direct bone resorption[113] (Fig. 2-99).

Because of the increase in the number of cells, osteoid tissue will be deposited in open marrow spaces on the pressure side and in other areas not undergoing direct resorption (Figs. 2-51 and 2-52, *A*). On the tension side there will be a gradual calcification and reorganization of newly formed tissue during the rest period. Hence the tissues are given ample time for reorganization, and the cell proliferation is favorable for further tissue changes when the appliance is again activated.

In actual practice an interrupted tooth movement may have certain advantages—as noted, for instance, when impacted canines are brought into position by orthodontic forces. In a good many cases disturbances of the pulp tissue may result from prolonged continuous traction exerted on the impacted tooth. A sudden movement of the apical portion of the impacted tooth may occur after undermining bone resorption around hyalinized tissue, by which the blood vessels that supply the pulp tissue are compressed and give rise to stasis and subsequent disturbances within the pulp (Fig. 2-52, *B*). A typical interrupted movement may be obtained with a force acting through a distance of 1 to 1.5 mm (Fig. 2-53). By reactivating according to the interrupted principle, the orthodontist can bring the tooth into position without causing much disturbance to the pulp tissue.

The advantage of using an interrupted force may be found in certain areas of tooth rotation. A planned interrupted rotating movement may, to some extent, lessen the relapse tendencies after treatment. Interrupted movement by light forces may also be considered a recommended method in adult open bite cases (Fig. 2-107).

Intermittent Tooth Movement

Various types of removable plates exerting an intermittent action are among the oldest appliances used. The typical intermittent action is produced by a force that acts as either an impulse or a shock of short duration or for short periods

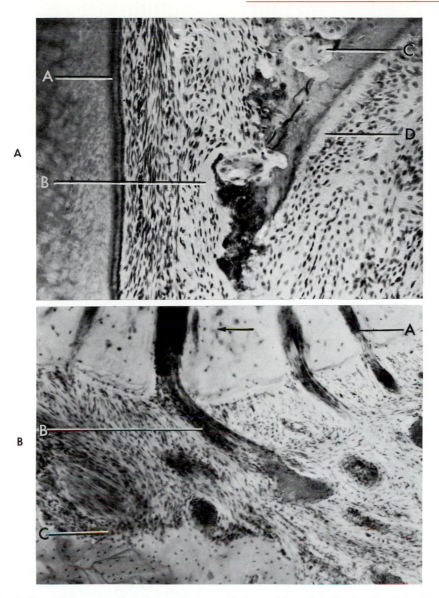

Fig. 2-52   A, Pressure side of an upper premolar moved interruptedly. Semihyalinization (i.e., no complete hyalinization between the root surface and the protruding bone spicule). *A,* Root surface; *B,* cell-free fibers close to the bone with direct resorption of subjacent bone areas; *C,* numerous osteoclasts, a typical bundle bone resorption; *D,* compensatory bone formation, wide layers of newly formed osteoid bordered with osteoblasts. **B,** Area *A* in Fig. 2-51. Note the capillary and nerve, *A,* entering one of the root canals of a second premolar in a dog. *B,* Stretched and slightly compressed capillary; a similar compression may cause obstruction of circulation during continuous movement of impacted canines; *C,* bone resorption at the alveolar fundus.

with a series of interruptions. These breaks occur when the force becomes gradually more active or more passive in turn as the appliance moves. Hence the intermittent action is not necessarily always related to plate construction. Removable appliances of the Crozat type and certain types of fixed appliances may periodically produce forces that are partly of the intermittent type. This applies to spurs or springs resting on the tooth surface that produce impulses and stimuli of short duration as the appliance moves during speech

and mastication. The intermittent action may then, to a varying extent, result in less compression on the pressure side and shorter hyalinization periods.

The most important variation in tissue reaction is produced when the appliance is removed intermittently and thus no longer contacts the teeth to be moved. During the rest period the teeth will move slightly toward the tension side and remain in normal function for the major part of treatment.[112] For the same reason the periodontal fibers will

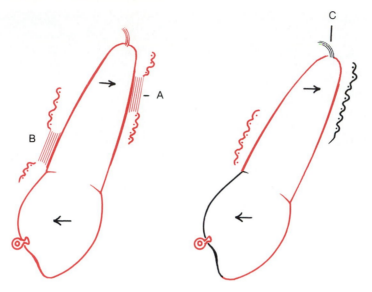

Fig. 2-53   Two stages in the movement of an impacted canine. *A* and *B*, Localization of hyalinized zones during initial movement; *C*, stretching of capillaries after undermining bone resorption. Compare with Fig. 2-52, *B*.

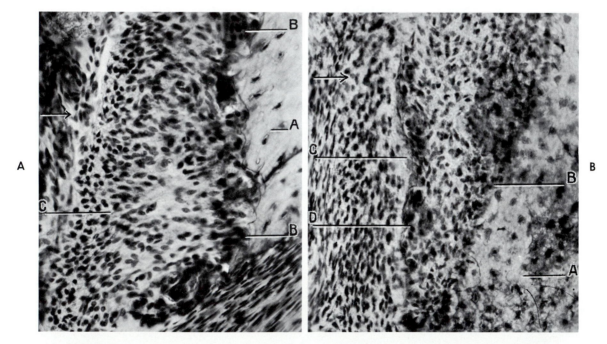

Fig. 2-54   A, Upper premolar of a 12-year-old patient. Effect on the pressure side after tooth movement with an attached removable plate that was gradually expanded and worn every night for 2 weeks. The tooth was moved as indicated by the arrow. The root surface is not seen. Direct bone resorption is apparent in the area of the alveolar crest. Note the increase in number of connective tissue cells. *A,* Alveolar bone; *B,* large osteoclasts along the bone surface; *C,* cell proliferation; mitotic cell division was noted in several areas. This area corresponds to *A* in Fig. 2-21, *A.* **B,** Upper premolar of another 12-year-old. Gradually expanded loose activator worn every night for 2 weeks. Pressure side; the root, which was moved as indicated by arrow, is not visible. The alveolar bone was bordered by an osteoid layer that persists. Extensive bone resorption has occurred in the area subjacent to this osteoid tissue. *A,* Alveolar bone; *B,* bone surface lined with osteoclasts; *C,* persisting layer of osteoid; *D,* chain of osteoclasts close to the osteoid layer. Note the increase in cellular elements, which was similar to that in **A.**

usually retain a functional arrangement. This results in an improved circulation, and there is frequently an increase in the number of cells in the periodontal ligament (Fig. 2-54). An intermittent-pressure may act as an irritant and will often elicit formative changes, especially in young persons. Osteoid will then be deposited in areas of the bone surface not subjected to pressure. The increase in cellular elements is largely dependent on the individual reaction; thus one may find cases in which there is only a moderate increase in the cell number (Fig. 2-58).

Experiments have shown that the movement effected by an intermittent force is dependent on the length of time of application and on the magnitude of the force. Since the teeth are displaced by a tipping movement, hyalinized tissue may form on the pressure side during the initial phase of treatment. Because of the force factor, hyalinization will occur more readily when the appliance is rigid and unyielding (Fig. 2-7, *B*). If the force has an elastic action, one will occasionally observe semihyalinization on the pressure side (Fig. 2-57, *A*), a term denoting that not all the fibers in the compressed area have become cell free.[113] In such cases osteoclasts may be formed directly along the bone surface subjacent to the hyalinized tissue. This implies that the bone resorption is less disturbed by the hyalinization. Because of these factors, it is found that a smooth and uniform movement can be effected with a removable appliance that exerts a fairly small force and is used as regularly as possible.

The disadvantage of intermittent tooth movement is the mode of displacement, which always occurs in the form of tipping. Unsatisfactory results are not infrequently observed when some of the teeth, moved over a certain distance, end up in an inclined position. There are nevertheless exceptions to this rule. Some persons in a growth period react more favorably than others in this respect, and gradual reuprighting of inclined teeth may occur.

Another difficulty can be caused by the periodontal fiber system, whose reaction is highly individual. Thus transformation of fibrous tissue will occur less readily in some persons than in others, the effect of which occasionally tends to restrict movement that is based on the intermittent principle. In addition, since treatment with intermittent appliances frequently involves a widening of the dental arches, this may cause a general stretching of the supraalveolar fibrous system. As in other types of tooth movement, stretched periodontal fibers tend to contract. This contraction may lead to relapse, especially when the dental arches have been expanded. The degree of relapse is appreciably dependent on the individual tissue reaction. After a prolonged retention period it has been observed that even a certain number of the expansion cases may remain stable, particularly those in which the third molars are absent.

Functional type of intermittent forces. Functional plates, such as the activator,[16] remain loose in the mouth and will, theoretically, move during treatment more or less in accordance with the movement of the lower jaw.[51,112] It has been observed experimentally that a typical intermittent action in

the form of impulses and shocks occurs more frequently when the plate is worn during the day. This occurs notably as a result of swallowing, which always entails a reflex movement of opening and closing the lower jaw.[74] Since swallowing occurs less frequently when the patient is asleep, it is found that during the night the appliance may remain immobile in the mouth for fairly long periods.

The tissue changes brought about by an activator are therefore due less to intermittent shocks and impulses than to the pressure exerted during certain periods as the appliance remains in contact with the tooth surfaces. These observations are verified in studies on the tissue reaction. Hence it is not always possible to distinguish between the reactions evoked by loose and fixed removable appliances solely on the basis of the histologic findings (Fig. 2-54).

Functional plates may frequently give rise to direct bone resorption on the pressure side, even during the initial stage. This occurs when the plate exerts a light pressure on the teeth. Osteoclasts are then observed along the bone surface after a period of 3 to 4 days. Since a resorption process, once started, will continue for 8 to 10 days,[117] conditions are provided for a favorable tissue reaction even if the plate is worn only at night. The intermittent action stimulates the circulation and a considerable increase in the cell number is frequently observed on the pressure side, as well as on the tension side. If the force is increased, hyalinization may occur on the pressure side (Fig. 2-7, *B*). In experiments conducted with Bimler's elastic plate the expanding force ranged between 70 and 100 g (Fig. 2-55). The plates were worn during the afternoon and at night. Fig. 2-56 shows the degree of movement and the duration of the hyalinization. In *B* the plate remained passive for 6 days, whereupon the force was gradually increased. At the end of the experiment semihyalinization was observed on the pressure side (Fig. 2-57, *A*). These observations tend to prove that an intermittent appliance will move the teeth more rapidly

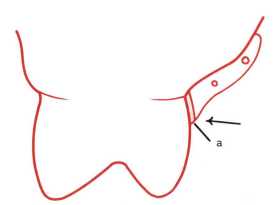

Fig. 2-55 Arrangement for experimental movement of upper premolars with Bimler's appliance. *a*, Layer of gutta-percha increasing the force as desired. The plate does not contact the corresponding premolar of the opposite side. The force is measured at various intervals by placing the plate in a specially constructed device.

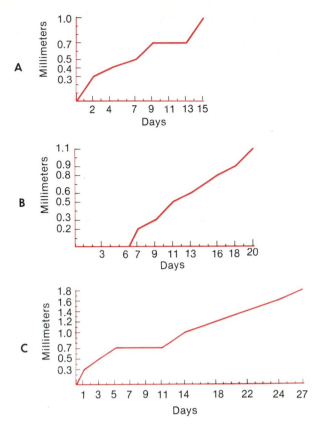

Fig. 2-56 Movement of upper premolars with Bimler's removable appliances. Force, between 70 and 100 g. Note the short hyalinization periods. **A,** A cell-free zone lasted for about 4 days. **B,** The appliance remained passive during the first 6 days. Tooth movement, 1.1 mm during 14 days, started after a layer of gutta-percha had been added (see Fig. 2-55). **C,** A cell-free area existed from the fifth to the eleventh day. (From Reitan K: *Am J Orthod* 43:32, 1957.)

provided the force is light and is also acting during the day (Fig. 2-58).

This principle also applies to the tension side. Formation of osteoblasts and osteoid tissue is dependent largely on the length of time the appliance is functioning. When a functional appliance is used only at night, osteoid will be formed on the tension side after 2 to 3 days. During the day, after the appliance has been removed, the tooth slips back toward the tension side. However, since osteoid is resistant to resorption and because the tooth moves back only slightly, exerting no direct pressure, new osteoid tissue will be formed every time the plate is used (Fig. 2-57, *B*). This gradual addition of new tissue on the tension side will lead to a less extensive reorganization of new bone layers than after a movement performed with continuous forces. Because the teeth are left in normal function during the major period of treatment, there is a gradual functional adaptation of the newly formed structures. On the other hand, over-expansion may lead to relapse of the teeth moved.

During experiments performed with the Fränkel appli-

ance, Stutzmann and Petrovic (1981) did not observe any increased tissue changes on the pressure or tension sides of the experimental teeth. They concluded that its action might consist of an alteration of the growth changes in the temporomandibular joint *(TMJ)* area, an effect not likely to be observed in adult tissues.

Changes in the temporomandibular joint. A controversial issue is whether functional appliances may cause transformation of the osseous structures of the TMJ. During treatment of Class II malocclusions the mandible is brought forward about 2 mm, so the head of the condyle is moved out of its postural area. Experiments have purported to show that such a stretching force may lead to bone apposition in the glenoid fossa and on the posterior part of the condylar process, with corresponding bone resorption of the anterior side.[23] Animal experiments of fairly long duration have apparently disclosed that these changes occur notably within the condylar cartilage, the distal portion of which increases in thickness as a response to mandibular displacement.[7] There is simultaneous deposition of bone on the distal border of the condyle, with remodeling resorption on the mesial border.

In the majority of cases, however, analysis of cephalometric radiographs taken before and after treatment indicate that the tissue response of the bony structures of the condylar head is highly variable. It is thus likely that the changes occurring during treatment can, in many cases, be regarded as variants of normal growth.[16] In practice the ultimate result of the changes taking place in the TMJ will be largely influenced by the muscle function.[94,112] If the muscular pattern remains unchanged, the condyle tends to return to its original postural position. This return, which occurs during rest periods and after treatment, may lead to reverse tissue changes. Reverse bone changes have been observed after application of continuous extraoral forces[60] and such daily relapse obviously occurs even during routine treatment of patients.[118]

Most investigators agree that the age factor is important. It is also logical to assume that the changes in the TMJ occur more readily during a growth period, an observation that has been corroborated in experiments on intermittent forces acting for several days.[86] Radiographic investigations with the implant method revealed that, in boys, the major growth period is centered around the age of 14 years.[17] The final result of the tissue changes in the TMJ is further influenced by whether a stable intercuspation has been obtained between the dental arches. Any forward displacement of the mandible may be contraindicated in some cases in which there is overclosure of anterior teeth. The result of the treatment may be increased hypermobility of the TMJ and persisting malocclusion.[112]

Myofunctional observations. One important aspect of functional treatment ought to be considered—correction of habits and abnormal muscular function. During treatment with an activator, the muscles are subjected to what may be termed a myofunctional therapy.[112] This may lead to a

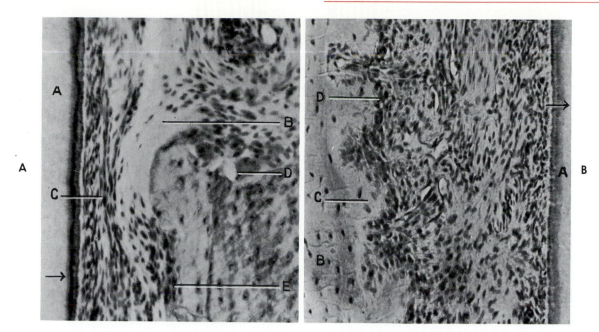

Fig. 2-57   A, Pressure side of experiment *B* in Fig. 2-56. As a result of new gutta-percha added, a semihyalinized zone was created. *A,* Root surface; *B,* cell-free fibers adjacent to protruding bone spicule; *C,* compressed periodontal fibers; *D* and *E,* osteoclasts in resorption lacunae; *E,* resorption along the inner bone surface. This area corresponds to that in Fig. 2-21, *A.* **B,** Tension side of the experiment with Bimler's removable appliance. Area slightly above the alveolar bone crest. *A,* Root surface; *B,* old bone; *C,* new osteoid; *D,* chain of osteoblasts. The periodontal fibers are relaxed, and there is an increased number of connective tissue cells. (From Reitan K: *Am J Orthod* 43:32, 1957.)

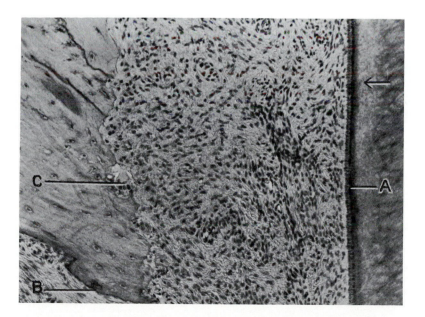

Fig. 2-58   Pressure side of experiment *C,* in Fig. 2-56. Note the moderate increase in cellular elements, a result of the individual tissue character. *A,* Root surface adjacent to which epithelial remnants are absent because of the hyalinization; *B,* periosteal side of the alveolar bone, with little growth activity; *C,* direct bone resorption with osteoclasts. The fiber bundles are relaxed, and there is a slightly increased number of connective cells. (From Reitan K: *Am J Orthod* 43:32, 1957.)

change in the contraction pattern of the masticatory muscles, which is, in some cases, conspicuous. Investigators have also observed a change in position of the condyle as a result of the altered muscle function. In an electromyographic study Ahlgren[1] stated that "it seems possible to permanently change the basic contraction pattern of the jaw muscles and reposition the mandible in a forward position." It is not as yet known whether this new position of the condyle will be a permanent one in all cases or whether secondary changes may occur. It may thus be shown that in a good many cases the correction of a postnormal jaw relationship by functional appliances occurs mainly by tooth movement and by the elimination of functional retrusions and overclosure.[16] The premolars and molars will move distally in the upper jaw, mesially in the lower jaw. This change in direction of movement can be verified by examining histologic sections. The teeth are displaced by a tipping movement.

Changes in the growth pattern of the condylar head and compensatory migration of the dentition were observed after application of continuously acting intermittent appliances in an extensive experimental series conducted by McNamara.[86] As recorded electromyographically, hypertonic discharges from the suprahyoid muscles were observed shortly after the experiments were started. Later the anterior portion of the temporal muscle gradually reassumed the most active role during posture and the most pronounced adaptation observed after a certain experimental time occurred in the function of the superior portion of the lateral pterygoid muscle. There was a marked variation in the tissue reaction, obviously caused by the age factor. Although the growth changes in the ramus and condylar structures were extensive in the monkeys aged 5 to 8 months, the corresponding changes observed in 4-year-old animals were insignificant. It was suggested that the mesial displacement of the mandible would result in an altered neuromuscular function. The extensive tissue alterations observed in the younger group of animals may, to some extent, be attributed to the time factor, since the functional adaptation of the structures involved occurred without any interruption (Fig. 2-59).

Treatment with functional plates may cause an inclined position of individual teeth or groups of teeth. This is noted, for example, in some Class III occlusions in which the labial arch has been exerting pressure against the lower anterior teeth. The result may be a lingually inclined position of the lower incisors. Undesirable side effects are also caused in some Class II cases. Since the lower molars and premolars are moved in a mesial direction during treatment, crowding may take place in the lower dental arch, especially when the tendency is toward space inadequacy before the treatment.

EVALUATION OF ORTHODONTIC FORCES

It is the aim in all types of orthodontic treatment to complete the necessary tooth movements within a reasonably short time. In the "good old days," too much time obviously was spent on many phases of orthodontic treatment, with tooth movement that could have been completed more rapidly by applying present-day methods. As will be discussed later, however, moving the teeth fairly rapidly may have its disadvantages as well as its advantages.

The reactions of supporting tissues will, in most instances, be typical of what has been observed in experimental studies.* This applies notably to a tipping movement performed with continuous forces. Also intermittent movement elicited by removable appliances is largely dependent on the force factor and the duration of action. However, other types of tooth movement that depend on anatomic factors other than those previously mentioned include rotation and extrusion of teeth. These types of movement will be discussed under separate headings.

Alveolar bone density. In experiments conducted with continuous forces it has been observed that application of special mechanical arrangements, exerting an extraordinar-

---

*An exception to this rule is observed in cases of hypercementosis[58] and bony ankylosis, which tend to restrict or prevent orthodontic tooth movement.

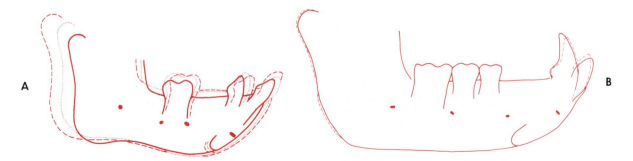

Fig. 2-59 Intermittent forces acting over a long period. **A,** Note the growth of the mandible in an infant monkey as enhanced by the inclined plane action of the bite plate. **B,** Mandible of an adult monkey after treatment with a similar appliance acting for a corresponding period (26 weeks). (From McNamara JA: *Am J Orthod* 64:578, 1973.)

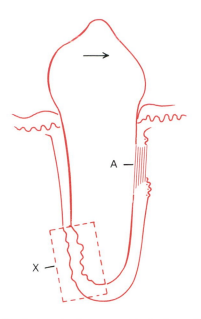

Fig. 2-60   Continuous tooth movement of a lower first premolar in a dog. Force, 40 g acting as indicated by the arrow. A fulcrum was established close to the hyalinized zone at *A*. Pressure was thus exerted in the area marked *X*. Duration of the experiment, 40 days. (From Reitan K: *Acta Odontol Scand* 6:115, 1947.)

ily light force, may result in hyalinization periods as short as 8 to 10 days. However, there are experimental cases in which the duration of the hyalinization may be caused by a high density of the alveolar bone.

An example may illustrate what occurred when a dog's lower first premolar (which is a small tooth) was tipped mesially with a force of 40 g over a period of 40 days. On the pressure side the periodontal ligament was gradually eliminated, and the root nearly contacted the bone surface after some 5 to 7 days (Fig. 2-60). It is of interest to note that no resorption occurred in the root surface adjacent to the compressed zone. By contrast, three minor resorbed lacunae were seen in the root surface adjacent to the pressure zone of the apical region (Fig. 2-61, *B*).

These observations tend to indicate that resorption does not always occur in the root surface adjacent to a compressed hyalinized zone formed against a dense alveolar bone wall. In a great number of cases root resorption is elicited as readily when the bone is only moderately dense. This is of great clinical significance to the orthodontist. The problem is discussed further under "Torque" (p. 155) and "Root Resorption" (p. 169).

Although the dense bone type is encountered only in certain areas of the alveoli of experimental animals, such as the dog,[118] a dense bone may exist in humans as well (Fig. 2-7, *B*); but the texture of the human alveolar bone is always more favorable, and the bone resorbed more readily.

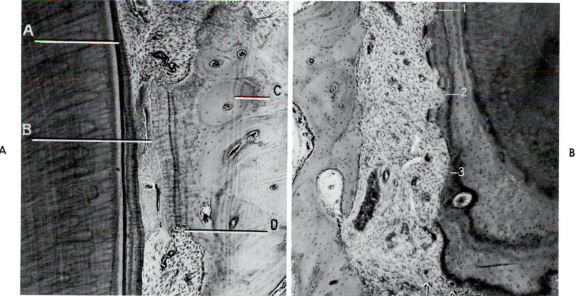

Fig. 2-61   **A,** Animal experiment (area *A* in Fig. 2-60). Note the dense alveolar bone. *A,* Root surface; *B,* hyalinization and elimination of fibrous tissue, contact has been established between the bone and the root surface, caused by the dense bone; no further movement will occur for a long time; *C,* haversian system; *D,* bone resorption. **B,** Apical region of the tooth shown at area *X* in Fig. 2-60. Root resorptions marked *1, 2,* and *3*. Several marrow spaces in alveolar bone to the left. Arrows at the bottom indicate epithelial remnants close to the apex. (From Reitan K: *Acta Odontol Scand* 6:115, 1947.)

Hyalinization related to the force factor. If a tooth is moved by muscular impulses exerting a light intermittent force, hyalinization will not occur.[184] Intermittent forces elicited by removable appliances may produce either hyalinization of fairly short duration or no hyalinization at all.[112,113] Light intermaxillary elastics, as applied in some present-day techniques, may produce short hyalinization periods or semihyalinization.

The tendency is more toward an initial hyalinization of some duration when the teeth are moved by fixed labial or lingual arches. This reaction is frequently caused not by the orthodontic force itself but by occlusal pressures, which tend to increase the active force as a result of a change in the relationship between occluding tooth surfaces.

Generally, it is the magnitude of the force that will determine the duration of the hyalinization. This will be shorter within the light force level, although the tendency is toward a longer initial hyalinization period, and also formation of secondary hyalinized zones, when excessively strong forces are applied.[115] As demonstrated by Joho,[60] extraoral forces applied continuously on the mandibular first molars of the monkey cause formation of fairly large resorption lacunae in the experimental teeth and also in the osseous structures of the TMJs. Radiographs of the effects caused by this type of tooth movement in humans have shown that the size of the teeth, as well as the interruption of the forces during the day, may explain why there is less resorption in human roots.

The amount of force exerted by the appliances used today can, in many instances, be measured. It has been shown experimentally that the optimal force required for certain types of tooth movement varies considerably. For instance, a force as light as 25 to 30 g is preferable for extrusion of teeth (Fig. 2-108).[113] To avoid formation of extensive hyalinized zones, even a lesser initial force is favorable for intrusion of teeth.

The purpose of applying a light initial force is to increase cellular activity without causing undue tissue compression and to prepare the tissues for further changes. The size of the teeth and the type of movement may necessitate a slight variation in the magnitude of force; however, it is nevertheless possible to indicate certain force values. Observation of a great many experimental cases has revealed that formation of extensive hyalinized zones can be avoided by applying a force below a 50- to 70-g threshold. Histologically this is the optimal force to be exerted in a tipping movement of incisor teeth and premolars. A tipping movement of canines and molars would not require a much stronger force. It is frequently noted that a tipping movement of these teeth will occur even with a force of, for instance, 30 g (Fig. 2-62). In practice this light force reaction may lead to mesial drift of molar teeth if not counteracted by establishing prepared anchorage.

For movement of a small tooth it would be favorable to apply an initial force as light as 20 to 30 g. Similar force values were given by Burstone and Groves,[27] who stated

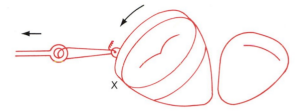

Fig. 2-62 Experimental uprighting movement of a canine. Force, 30 g. The crown portion of the tooth will usually be moved quite readily and may even become rotated if the staple is not placed correctly at *X*.

that "optimal rate of tooth movement" (maxillary anterior teeth) was observed in groups of children in whom 50 to 75 g was applied. Increasing the magnitude of the force did not increase the rate of tooth movement.

As shown in this investigation and in other experimental studies, there are two sides of the force problem: the *amount* of force acting at the moment that tooth movement is initiated and the *working range* of this force. Both are equally important. A fairly heavy arch may be adjusted so it delivers a small force, whereby the tooth will move over only a short distance. More stretch of fiber bundles on the tension side and shorter hyalinization periods are elicited by a lighter archwire. Various arch configurations (e.g., the box loop) are examples of how the two prerequisites, light force and favorable working range, can be combined.

Pain caused by tooth movement. There are several reasons for avoiding too much compression of the periodontal ligament during the initial stage. The favorable effect obtained by applying light forces is enhanced by the fact that there will be less discomfort and pain to the patient. It is noted in Figs. 2-26, *B*, and 2-33 that several cell nuclei persist in the hyalinized tissue. Likewise unmyelinated nerve endings are within the hyalinized tissue (Fig. 2-9). These are visualized by special staining methods. The nerve endings will be more or less compressed during the initial period.[4]

As shown experimentally, it is likely that mechanical vibration of the tooth moved[166] and possibly also applications of heat[179] may alter the effect of hyalinization and thereby also the feeling of pain. In practice a slight feeling of pain can hardly be avoided in most cases; yet there is certainly a great difference between a slight discomfort and the intense pain caused by application of an initial force of 300 to 400 g. Some patients react more intensely than others to an initial compression of the periodontal ligament.

Duration of force, whether light or heavy, conditions the amount of pain. Quite considerable amounts of force may be directed against the maxillary arch by extraoral orthopedic appliances, for example, and yet produce relatively little pain because the force is interrupted—8 to 12 hours application, 12 to 6 hours rest.

Pain is the result of compression. It may indicate that hyalinized zones are about to be formed in the periodontal ligament. Evidence proves, however, that after the periodontal space has become widened by bone resorption, new hyalinized zones may be formed without appreciable discomfort to the patient. In the further course of treatment, even extensive root resorption may occur without much complaint on the part of the patient. Root resorption causes widening of the periodontal ligament and thereby less compression. This fact illustrates that the patient's subjective feeling, as a safeguard against too rapid a tooth movement, can be relied on only during the short initial period of treatment.

These observations also explain why extensive root resorption is frequently observed after a rapid tipping movement by light continuous forces. The resorbed lacunae are located particularly in the apical region of the root (Fig. 2-61, *B*). Examination of radiographs taken at intervals during the treatment period may enable the practitioner to plan how to move the teeth without producing any undesirable shortening of the roots as a result of too rapid movement.

Occlusal stress. During orthodontic treatment there is always a certain tooth mobility. This occurs primarily as a result of widening of the periodontal space by bone resorption. Mobility may also become manifest during mastication when the tooth moves against an alveolar bone wall that is covered by a layer of recently formed elastic osteoid. This effect disappears gradually as new bone layers calcify. In his experiments on human material Hotz[56] observed increased tooth mobility during the period of tooth movement. After retention periods of 3 months' duration the teeth were approximately as stable as before the experiments started. Bien[14] stated that "with repetitive intrusive thrusts at short intervals the restoration toward the original equilibrium position decreases with each repeated application of force, accompanied by a concomitant reduction of tooth mobility. With thrusts at longer intervals, an increase in mobility is observed." These remarks deal with some of the factors related to the mobility problem. In addition, the direction of tooth movement is of importance. Thus when under physiologic conditions a repetitive occlusal force is dissipated in the long axis of the tooth, the tooth will not only remain stable but even acquire greater stability. On the other hand, lateral force components acting on a slightly mobile tooth may produce jiggling and increased mobility.

Still other factors are important during orthodontic tooth movement. When occlusal stress is absent, one may observe that a tooth being moved bodily will remain stable even after a prolonged treatment period. On the other hand, a tooth being rotated will become mobile because fiber bundles all around the root have elongated. In practice it is usually not the orthodontic force per se but occlusal interference during fixed appliance treatment that produces any marked tooth mobility. As we know, such untoward effects caused by occlusal stress may be avoided by spot grinding or by insertion of a bite plate.

Tipping Movement

Tipping was for many years considered the safest, most *biologic* type of tooth movement. This notion was probably derived from the fact that physiologic tooth movement takes place mainly in the form of a tipping action. During orthodontic treatment a tooth may be tipped with some variations in either a mesiodistal or a labiolingual direction. It is characteristic that a tipping nearly always results in the formation of a hyalinized zone slightly below the alveolar crest. This is the location of the hyalinized zone, particularly when the tooth has a short undeveloped root.[115] If the root is fully developed, the hyalinized zone will be located a short distance from the alveolar crest. During the initial period a fulcrum is formed between root and alveolar bone in the area of the hyalinized tissue, whereby the apical portion of the root will move in the opposite direction.

The time factor may influence the resorption process. A prolonged tipping movement may result in apical root resorption even if the force is light (Fig. 2-61, *B*). In some cases after elimination of the marginal hyalinized zone, the fulcrum will shift to the middle region of the root[103] (Fig. 2-63). After a prolonged tipping movement the resorbed lacunae of the root may be observed radiographically in areas that correspond to the location of the initial hyalinized zones (Fig. 2-64).

Tipping of a tooth by light continuous forces will result in a greater movement within a shorter time than obtained by any other method. It is, however, chiefly the coronal

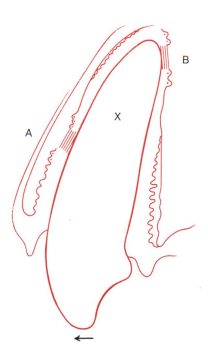

Fig. 2-63 A prolonged tipping movement may result in formation of a secondary hyalinized zone, *A*, after the first hyalinized zone has been eliminated. Compression of the periodontal ligament is maintained in the apical region, *B*.

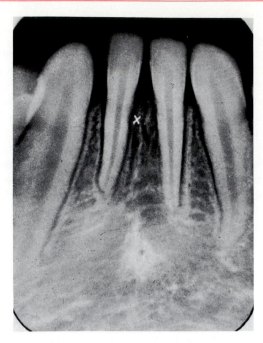

Fig. 2-64   Mesial movement of two lateral incisors. The left tooth was tipped resulting in root resorption at *x* and in the apical portion. The right tooth was moved bodily. No perceptible root resorption occurred. Note the widened space and opaque bone layer on the tension side. The root was moved bodily by a force of 40 g that was gradually increased to 140 g. (From Reitan K: *Am J Orthod* 48:881, 1960.)

portion of the tooth that is moved. This rapid displacement is partly because there are relatively few fiber bundles on the tension side to resist movement. During tipping a certain number of free gingival and alveolar crest fiber bundles will be stretched (Figs. 2-65 and 2-66). After further bone resorption on the pressure side the tooth will gradually assume a tilted position. If the tooth is prevented from slipping back toward the tension side, it may be reuprighted and will thus move in toto over a considerable distance within a fairly short time.

A tipping movement in either a labial or a lingual direction will frequently lead to relapse, whereby the tooth moves gradually back toward the tension side. This tendency to relapse may be compensated for partly by overelongating the fiber bundles while tipping the tooth over a greater distance than considered necessary for precise positioning. The final tooth position after relapse may then be approximately as intended. However, several reasons are apparent for avoiding such a procedure. The principle will hardly be as effective if several contiguous teeth are tipped in a labial direction. Relapse is then more likely to occur. The reaction of the alveolar bone must also be deemed unfavorable.

Tipping of adult teeth in a labial direction may result in bone destruction of the alveolar crest, with little compensatory bone formation. Such undesirable bone resorption has been observed even in young patients (Fig. 2-67, *A*). In addition, after a prolonged movement of the apical root portion in the opposite direction, resorption of the bone plate

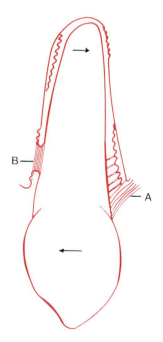

Fig. 2-65   Location of the limited number of fiber bundles to resist movement during tipping. If the force is light, the hyalinization period will be of short duration and the coronal portion will move quite readily. *A*, Supraalveolar fibers; *B*, hyalinized zone on the pressure side. Compare with Fig. 2-62.

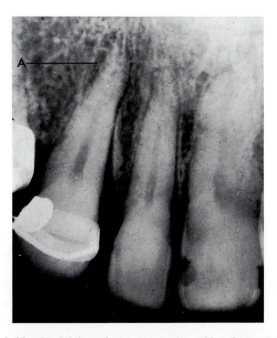

Fig. 2-66   Uprighting of an upper canine with a force of 50 g before bodily movement in a patient aged 40 years. The tissue reaction was similar to that shown in Fig. 2-65. *A*, Tension side of the apical region. Note the widened periodontal space on the opposite marginal tension side where the new uncalcified bone layers cannot be seen on the radiograph.

in the apical region may occur so rapidly that the root is finally moved through the bone.[118] This has also been observed as a result of a prolonged expansion with removable plates, whereby the lingual roots of first molars may become denuded. Experimental torque of teeth in the dog has shown that resorption of roots moved outside of the PDL area will not become repaired by secondary cementum.

The PDL may to a certain extent be regarded as a specialized organ. If bone tissue is absent, the tooth cannot be moved. This explains why an impacted tooth will move or can be moved by orthondontic force into the previously open cleft following transplantation (grafting) of bone in a patient with total cleft lip, alveolus, and palate (Fig. 2-68). During tooth eruption a space is always present between the incisal edge of the erupting tooth and the resorbed hard tissue, (Fig. 2-117, *A*). A similar space will be created by resorption of transplanted bone packed around the crown portion

of the impacted tooth. Since so many canines start to erupt as a result of this procedure, it does not seem unlikely that a connection will be established between the resorbed area and the unerupted tooth. According to one theory, the resorption process will lead to information of enzymatic messengers that may be able to activate the mechanism causing eruption of the impacted tooth. At present, it may be stated that bone transplantation is the important factor in this reaction.

Compensatory bone resorption. It was observed in Reitan[114] animal experiments performed by the author that remodeling of the labial bone plate sometimes occurred after rotation of teeth[114] (Fig. 2-69). Such compensatory bone resorption became manifest in some experimental cases. Remodeling by resorptive changes has also been observed in humans, especially after tipping of canines in patients who were past the major growth period. After extensive

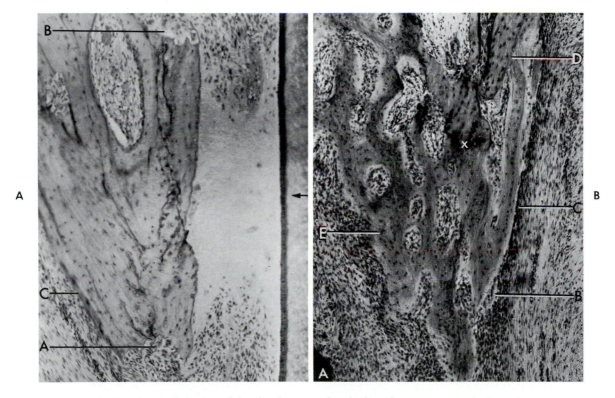

Fig. 2-67 **A,** Hyalinization of the alveolar crest after tipping of an upper premolar in a 12-year-old patient. Force, 60 g. Height of the alveolar crest reduced by undermining resorption, a phenomenon that may also occur after tipping of adult teeth and then without any appreciable reconstruction of the resorbed bone. *A,* Resorption at the alveolar crest; *B,* corresponding undermining bone resorption; *C,* periosteal side of the alveolar plate with a thin chain of osteoblasts. Arrow indicates the direction of movement and the central portion of the hyalinized zone. **B,** Extensive periosteal bone deposition in an individual aged 12. This area is from the alveolar crest. The tooth, an upper premolar, was initially moved against the bone surface, then away from it. *A,* The tooth; *B,* periosteal formation of osteoid; *C,* osteoblast chain of the periosteum (amount of new bone formed on the periosteal side indicated by *D* and *x*); *E,* new bone formed along the inner bone surface during the reversal period of tooth movement. The result illustrates the importance of the hormonal factor in tooth movement. Compare with Fig. 2-58.

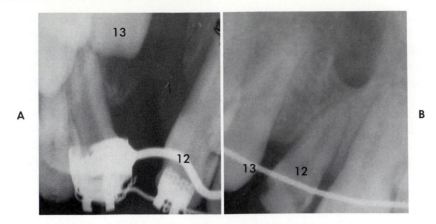

Fig. 2-68 **A,** Cleft palate patient before bone-grafting at 10 years. Note position of cuspid *(13)*. **B,** Same patient at 15 years shows development of bone, cuspid *(13)* and lateral *(12)* in position after bone grafting. (From Rygh P: *Den norske tannlegeforenings tidende* 100:377, 1990.)

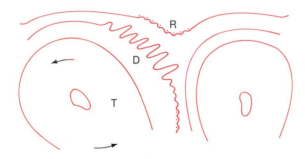

Fig. 2-69 Bone remodeling during rotation of teeth in the dog. *R,* Compensatory bone resorption; *D,* deposition of new bone layers along stretched fiber bundles; *T,* experimental tooth.

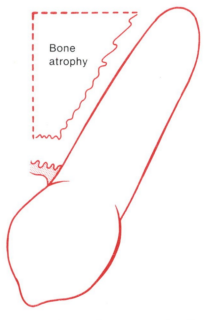

Fig. 2-70 Location of resorptive changes after distal tipping of canines in an adult.

distal tipping of an adult canine, bone covering the root may be felt as a marked ridge in front of a deep groove on the distal side of the root (Fig. 2-70). This observation has appreciable practical significance (Fig. 2-71).

During uprighting of such a tooth the thin distal bone plate may soon disappear by bone resorption; since the root is largely moved against fibrous tissue, further movement may become difficult. Extensive apical resorption may occur or the root tip may end up outside the bony area.[118] Initial uprighting and bodily movement would be the recommended method in adult cases.

Similar resorptive changes occasionally cause difficulties during mesial movement of lower second molars when the first molar has been extracted. Resorption with bone atrophy may occur in the area where the first molar was located. Starting movement of the second molar shortly after first molar extraction may solve this problem.

Compensatory bone deposition. In most young orthodontic patients bone resorption resulting from a moderate tipping movement is usually followed by compensatory bone formation. Such bone formation has been found in histologic experiments.[44,113] In a group of 12 human premolars tipped by a force of 60 to 70 g, compensatory bone formation occurred more readily in some persons than in others. In Fig. 2-67, *B,* extensive new bone layers have been formed on the periosteal side as a result of resorptive changes along the inner bone surface adjacent to the tooth that has been moved.

The degree of such compensatory bone formation varies individually and depends primarily on whether bone-forming osteoblasts are present in the periosteum (Fig. 2-67). In the adult periosteum the fibrous layer and the cambium layer may be observed, whereas the osteoblast chain may

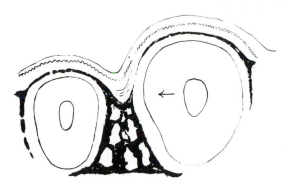

Fig. 2-71 Cross section of the tooth in Fig. 2-70. Rapid bone resorption tends to diminish thickness of the marginal bone layer. The root will be displaced against fibrous tissue.

be absent.[157] Some variations in this respect have been found in young persons as well. Fig. 2-58 shows the periosteal bone surface to be fairly aplastic, although resorption prevails along the inner bone surface. Usually, however, there is formation of osteoblasts and subsequent periosteal bone formation in the young person, particularly after bone resorption has started in the marrow spaces next to the hyalinized PDL.

Observation of the inner bone surface of the periodontal ligament may show that it usually takes some time before new osteoblasts appear along an aplastic bone surface. This delay in the formation of osteoblasts is even more marked in the periosteum than it is in the periodontal tissue.

A rapid tipping movement in an adult may, in many instances, cause a considerable diminution in the height of the alveolar crest and delayed or absent reconstruction of the resorbed area. Again individual variations exist.

Compensatory periosteal bone apposition in the apical region is also subject to some variation. Such bone formation may be observed on the radiograph (Fig. 2-72). It has been observed, experimentally, that bone resorption caused by a tipping movement of as short as 4 weeks' duration may result in periosteal bone formation (Figs. 2-73 and 2-74). Also in this respect the onset of bone formation varies according to whether osteoblasts are present or absent in the periosteum.

According to Young[190] a generally slower division and production of cellular elements may be observed in the periosteum than in other areas of the bone. Furthermore, individual variations exist. Under favorable circumstances a tipping of lower incisors may lead to tissue changes, as shown in Fig. 2-75. However, a tipping of lower incisors does not always lead to formative changes; in some instances only a little compensatory bone formation may be expected in the apical region of the lower jaw, especially in older patients.

Simultaneous with an increase in the thickness of new bone layers formed on the tension side adjacent to the tooth moved, resorption of the old bone will occur on the corresponding periosteal side (Fig. 2-75). Such a secondary resorption process has been observed as a result of physiologic tooth movement and particularly after orthodontic treatment[111]; it illustrates that the alveolar plate tends to maintain its original thickness.

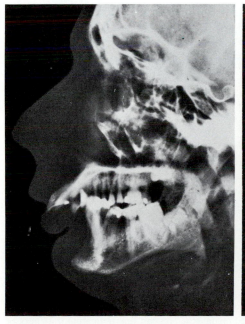
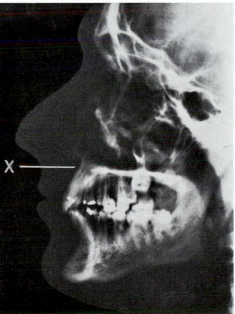

Fig. 2-72 Compensatory bone deposition has occurred in the area marked *X*. The patient was 19 years of age when treatment started.

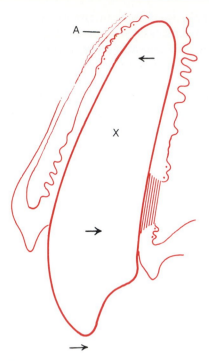

Fig. 2-73 Compensatory bone formation on the periosteal side after tipping of an upper second incisor in the dog. *A*, Compensatory bone deposition shown in Fig. 2-74.

Bodily Movement

Bodily tooth movement implies that the root is moved more or less parallel to the inner bone surface of the alveolus.[111] It has been shown experimentally that this is a favorable method of displacement, provided the force does not exceed a certain limit (Fig. 2-76). Movement of second and third lower premolars in the dog with a force of 40 g revealed no compressed areas, and direct bone resorption occurred along the bone surface on the pressure side (Fig. 2-77). It should be noted, however, that this was a carefully controlled experiment that could hardly be reproduced in an orthodontic practice. Application of a light continuous force on human teeth has resulted in small compressed areas shortly after the movement began. Hyalinization lasted for only a few days and was followed by direct bone resorption. If the initial force is increased to 150 g, there is always a period of hyalinization. The hyalinized zone is usually located as seen in Fig. 2-78, *A*. It is characteristic of the initial bodily movement that the hyalinization periods are of shorter duration than in a tipping movement.

Hyalinization during an initial bodily movement occurs largely as a result of mechanical factors. Shortly after the movement is initiated, no bodily movement of the tooth in a mechanical sense is observed, but instead a slight tipping is noticed. The tooth will be subjected to what in mechanics is termed a *couple* (i.e., a pair of forces acting in opposite directions along parallel lines). The degree of initial tipping produced by these forces varies according to the size of the arch and the width of the brackets. The result is compression on the pressure side with formation of a hyalinized zone between the marginal and middle regions of the root.

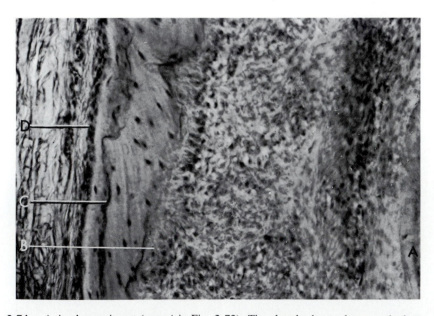

Fig. 2-74 Animal experiment (area *A* in Fig. 2-72). The alveolar bone plate resorbed as a result of tipping of the tooth for 4 weeks. *A*, Root surface moved away from the bone surface as a result of relapse; *B*, bone formation in formerly resorbed lacunae; *C*, resting line indicating thickness of the compensatory bone layer; *D*, osteoblast chain of the periosteum covering new partly calcified bone layer.

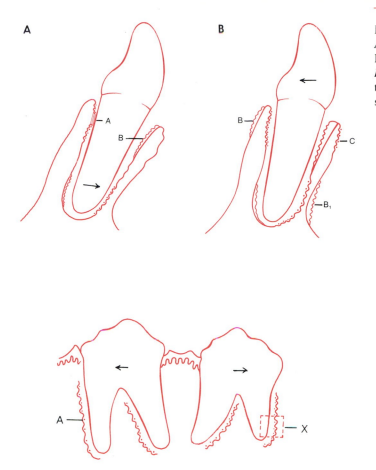

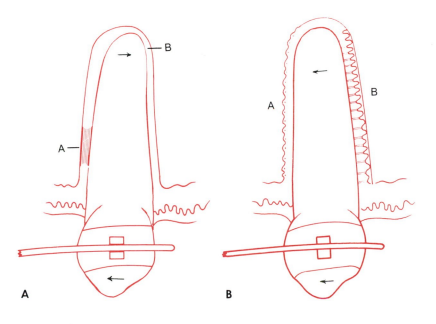

Fig. 2-76 Bodily movement of second and third premolars in a dog. Continuous force, 40 g. Note the difference in root length of the second and third premolars. Direct bone resorption on the pressure sides. Compare with the experiment of torque performed using an interrupted force on human premolars (Fig. 2-99).

Fig. 2-75   **A,** Initial movement of a lower incisor lingually. *A,* Hyalinized bone; *B,* initial bone deposition on the tension side. **B,** Tissue changes during the secondary stage of movement. *B₁* Compensatory bone formation in the apical region, a finding that is subject to individual variations; *C,* compensatory bone resorption.

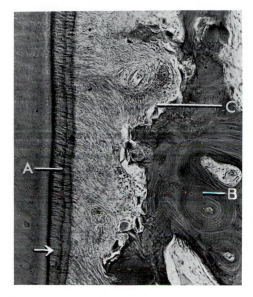

Fig. 2-77   Area *X* in 2-76. Bodily movement has resulted in direct bone resorption. *A,* Cementum of the root surface; *B,* haversian system of the bone; *C,* one of the osteoclasts lining the bone surface. (From Reitan K: *Acta Odontol Scand* 6:115, 1947.)

Fig. 2-78   Two stages of bodily tooth movement. **A,** Effect of a couple as observed during the initial stage of a continuous bodily tooth movement. *A,* Hyalinized tissue; *B,* slight initial compression as a result of tipping of the tooth. **B,** Undermining bone resorption terminated. Gradual uprighting of the tooth caused increased bone resorption adjacent to the middle and apical thirds of the root. Further movement is largely controlled by stretched fiber bundles. *A,* Bone resorption on the pressure side; *B,* bone deposition along the stretched fiber bundles.

The short duration of the hyalinization is due to an increased bone resorption on both sides of the hyalinized tissue, especially in the apical region of the pressure side. This leads to a rapid elimination of the hyalinized zone. The periodontal ligament on the pressure side is usually considerably widened by the resorption process. Further tooth movement will in most cases produce only minor hyalinized zones of short duration. This favorable reaction on the pressure side is partly caused by gradually increased stretching of fiber bundles on the tension side, which tends to prevent the tooth from further tipping (Fig. 2-78, *B*). New bone layers are formed on the tension side along these stretched fiber bundles (Fig. 2-37, *D*).

It has been found that by varying the type of brackets used and by the size of the archwire a tooth can be moved further in the slightly tilted position that it assumed during the initial period of movement. This frequently occurs in a bodily displacement performed with a light wire arch placed in conventional edgewise brackets. Bone resorption and apposition will then take place in accordance with the position of the root. It has also been demonstrated experimentally that the tooth will move as readily when the arch fits more exactly in the bracket slots, provided there is no marked interference caused by friction in the bracket areas.[96] Occasionally, the tooth will move more or less sporadically if

such friction exists. The mechanics involved are therefore of great importance.

We also know that some of the more recent thin edgewise configurations may retract canines bodily with a light force (Fig. 2-79). Friction is entirely avoided, since the end of the sectional arch is fixed in the bracket of the tooth to be retracted. Earlier investigations have shown that the hyalinization period[111] is short, but the force must simultaneously be strong enough to produce elongation of fiber bundles on the tension side. The effect on the tissues is similar to that of a light wire torque movement[118] (Fig. 2-102, *B*).

As in other types of tooth movement a light initial force is preferable in bodily movement, especially during the first 5 or 6 weeks. The optimal magnitude of the force to be applied depends on the resistance exerted by the stretched fiber bundles.

During closure of extraction spaces, one must also consider the resistance exerted by fibrous gingival tissue accumulated between the anchor tooth and the tooth being moved.[37] Surgical removal of hypertrophic gingival tissue is therefore indicated in some cases.

During the secondary period a force within the range of 150 to 200 g has proved favorable for bodily movement of premolars and canines. As pointed out by Storey and Smith[171] a force exceeding 300 g is unnecessary and tends to delay the movement as a result of formation of new hyalinized zones. It may, however, become necessary to apply a force of about 300 g during the final closure of spaces to bring the tooth being moved into contact with the anchor tooth.

Bodily tooth movement with light continuous forces is especially indicated for displacement of adult teeth. A tip-

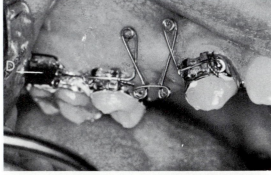
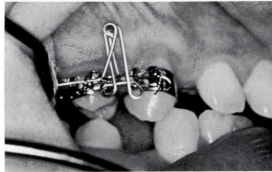

Fig. 2-79 Retraction of a canine in an adult before and after tooth movement. With adjustments of the mesial end of the light sectional arch to counteract the tendency to tipping, the tooth will be moved bodily with force ranging between 80 and 120 g. The first molar band is provided with a tube for a facebow. (Courtesy H. Lager.)

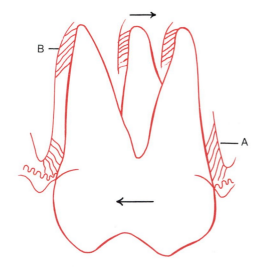

Fig. 2-80 Distal tipping of an upper molar causes stretching of the marginal fiber bundles, *A*. After a short time the apical fibers also stretch, *B*. Physiologic migration of the tooth does not occur as long as the stretching continues.

ping movement of adult teeth may lead to destruction of certain areas of alveolar crest (Fig. 2-67, *A*). This undesirable bone resorption may be largely avoided by moving the teeth bodily.

Prepared anchorage. An important factor in a bodily movement is the inclination of the tooth moved.[120] Distal movement of a canine that is in a mesially inclined position before treatment may be more or less delayed if the tooth is to be moved bodily. This slow movement of the tooth to be retracted is noted especially when the mesially inclined tooth has a long and firmly anchored root. Uprighting the tooth by a light tipping force before bodily movement is started may therefore be indicated (Fig. 2-65).

This well-known observation touches on the principle of prepared anchorage. It is a fact that a tooth, such as a first molar, will remain in a fairly stabilized position as long as it is tipped distally. Stretch of the marginal and apical fiber bundles will overlap any tendency to physiologic migration (Fig. 2-80). The question may then arise, to what extent will such a distally tipped anchor tooth resist movement when a force is acting in a mesial direction?

Experiments on mesial movement of second and third premolars in the dog revealed that the size of the tooth would determine the degree of movement (Fig. 2-76). In this series of experiments a double bracket on the left side tooth was ligated to a sectional arch, while the right side premolar was tipped distally before mesial movement. The distally tipped tooth was maintained in that position during mesial movement by an extension soldered to the lingual side of the band (Fig. 2-81).

When forces ranged between 70 and 90 g, no perceptible variation in the degree of movement of the left and right side second premolars could be observed. A slight retardation was noted in the mesial movement of the distally tipped right third premolars as compared to the left ones. This result could be ascribed to the longer and more firmly anchored roots of these teeth.

During mesial movement of the teeth subjected to prepared anchorage, a minor hyalinized zone was created between the middle and apical thirds on the pressure side of the mesial root (Fig. 2-82). In some instances such hyalinization occurred on the mesial side of both roots. The hyalinization lasted for 12 to 15 days, whereupon mesial movement started. The resistance to mesial movement is therefore due to the tension exerted by stretched fiber bundles and to the bone changes.

Tipping Versus Bodily Movement

A tooth that is moved by tipping will also frequently be somewhat extruded, which is a direction of fiber stretching that facilitates further tipping (Fig. 2-83). Even a tooth moved bodily may become slightly extruded unless the archwire has been adjusted to compensate for any tendency to extrusion. If traction is exerted on a tooth subjected to prepared anchorage, the tooth shows less tendency to extrude. On the contrary, in some cases a certain degree of intrusion may be observed. Owing to the distally tipped position of the tooth, all the fiber bundles on the tension side, especially the apical fibers, will be stretched and for certain periods immobilized (Fig. 2-84). The resisting effect will be significantly greater if several teeth have been subjected to prepared anchorage (Fig. 2-84). If, for instance, all the lower teeth have been tipped distally and are maintained in that position—a well-known procedure in the

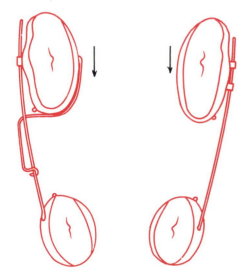

Fig. 2-81 Experimental arrangement for observation of the effect of distal tipping during mesial movement of second and third premolars in the dog. The difference in approximate root length is seen in Fig. 2-76. The extension placed on the right side bands acts similarly to that shown in Fig. 2-94.

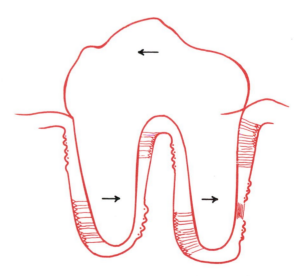

Fig. 2-82 Stretch of apical fibers during distal tipping. The duration of hyalinization on the pressure side was between 12 and 15 days.

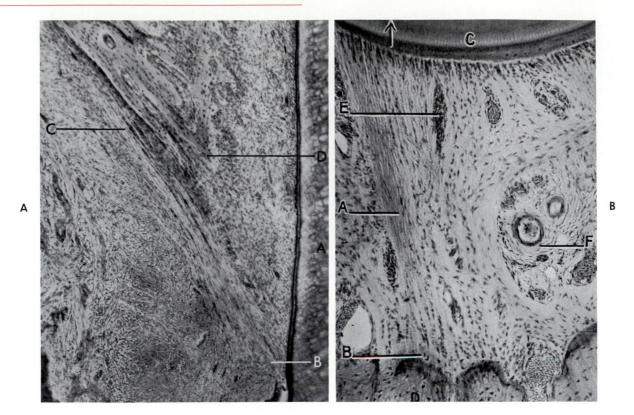

Fig. 2-83   **A,** Lingual bone crest of a first premolar tipped labially in a 12-year-old patient. Note the relaxed fibers of the periodontal ligament and the stretched supraalveolar fibers. *A,* Tooth; *B,* attachment of supraalveolar fiber bundles which intertwine with the periosteal structures, where they also appear stretched, *C; D,* osteoid layer bordering the newly formed bundle bone. Similar stretch of free gingival fibers occurs during extrusion of teeth; Area corresponding to *A* in Fig. 2-106. **B,** Stretch and temporary immobilization of individual fiber bundles in an animal experiment. The fibers must elongate before further tooth movement can take place. *A,* Stretched fiber bundles; *B,* increased formation of osteoid, a result of the fiber tension; *C,* tooth cut horizontally; *D,* old bone bordered by a dark layer of bundle bone; *E* and *F,* interstitial spaces.

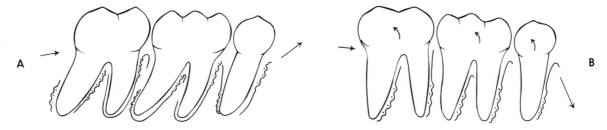

Fig. 2-84   Location of resorbed lacunae during tipping, **A,** and after mesial movement of teeth that are tipped distally, **B.**

edgewise technique—no perceptible degree of movement will occur when a mesially directed force is exerted by intermaxillary elastics. This occurs because the degree of resistance is proportionate to the number of periodontal fiber bundles engaged in withstanding mesial movement. Histologically, however, a slight degree of mesial movement is always apparent after application of a mesially directed force, even when all the teeth of the dental arch have been subjected to prepared anchorage.

As observed clinically, prepared anchorage established by distal tipping may not always provide any great stabilizing effect if there is only one anchor tooth. If it is not maintained in a distally tipped position, the tooth may be gradually uprighted and even moved in a mesial direction

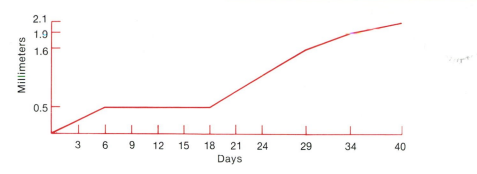

Fig. 2-85   Bodily movement of a premolar by a force of 120 g. A hyalinized zone existed from the sixth to the eighteenth day.

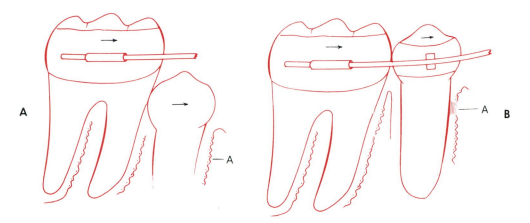

Fig. 2-86   Difference in tissue reaction between teeth that are undergoing eruption and those that are fully erupted. **A,** Second premolar moved indirectly. The force exerted by intermaxillary elastics results in direct bone resorption on the pressure sides of both the first molar and the second premolar. **B,** Tooth movement of fully erupted teeth occurs more readily if the second premolar is moved separately. Moving the second premolar first by a continuous force of, for instance, 70 to 150 g and then the first molar will be the fastest method of mesial displacement of these teeth. *A,* Pressure side with initial hyalinized zone.

by intermaxillary elastics exerting a force as light as 60 to 90 g. Intermaxillary elastics tend to elicit a favorable tissue reaction. The force is usually interrupted several times during the day, which will lead to shorter periods of hyalinization.

Influence of the growth factor. Another observation may be of interest in this connection. If a lower molar, whether subjected to prepared anchorage or not, remains in contact with an erupting or recently erupted second premolar while being moved mesially, both teeth will move quite readily (Fig. 2-86, *A*). This reaction is caused partly by the fact that the supporting tissues of the premolar are in a proliferation stage because of the eruption. In such a case, application of light intermaxillary elastics may result in short periods of hyalinization adjacent to the first molar and only direct bone resorption on the mesial side of the root of the premolar. Under these circumstances the tissue reaction is favored by the growth changes that occur in the supporting tissues around the premolar.

In older or adult patients the histologic picture is quite different. In the latter case, closure of a first lower premolar space by an intermaxillary elastic, exerting mesial traction on the first molar, will cause relatively little movement of the molar and second premolar because the tissues in the not-so-young patient are in a static phase. Light continuous forces, such as those exerted by coil springs, must be applied to elicit cell proliferation, and further movement of the teeth will start only after a period of 8 to 10 days, when the tissues have reached the proliferation stage (Fig. 2-86, *B*).

In addition, if the aim of the treatment is mesial movement of the second premolar and first molar, this will occur more readily by moving the second premolar first and then the first molar. The reason is that a fully developed fiber system tends to withstand displacement of teeth that are to be moved bodily and simultaneously. This rule exists regardless of whether the force is continuous or of the interrupted type, such as that exerted by intermaxillary elastics.

EXTRA-ORAL FORCE

The extra-oral principle of treatment has been known for many years. Generally extra-oral forces can be divided into two categories. In the first group strong extra-oral forces are applied for early control of facial bone growth.

Orthopedic forces. One example of orthopedic force is the strong vertical traction exerted by means of a chin cap for correction of open bite or mandibular prognathism in the deciduous or mixed dentition.[47] This method implies that not only the tooth position but also the direction of bone growth is influenced during treatment. Unlike what may occur initially when individual teeth are moved by conventional forces in a lingual or labial direction, not much pain is associated with this type of extra-oral treatment, even if the forces are excessively strong. The explanation is that the forces are acting on the jaw bone as a whole or on groups of teeth. For the orthopedic type of treatment just mentioned the force on each side may range up to 1400 g without causing pain or undesirable side effects.

Although extra-oral forces act according to the interrupted principle, the time factor is nevertheless important.[60] As observed when teeth are moved with conventional forces, extraoral treatment is also influenced by the duration of the treatment. Thus, heavy orthopedic forces that act uninterruptedly (e.g., those produced by the Milwaukee brace for

treatment of scoliosis) may cause side effects in the form of jaw deformities and malocclusions.[47]

Tooth movement by extra-oral forces. In the second type of extra-oral treatment, consisting of movement of individual teeth, it is impractical to apply forces that are too strong.

A change in the direction of the force applied may alter and modify the reaction of the tissues involved. Such a variation in the tissue response occurs after distal movement of upper first molars by facebow and occipital anchorage.[45,64] During this type of tooth movement the first molar usually remains in contact with the second molar, and both molars frequently undergo a degree of distal movement. Measurement reveals that the force exerted on each first molar ranges from 300 to 900 g. According to observations in experiments on tipping and bodily movement, this force must be considered inadmissibly strong. However, several factors will explain why such strong forces may be applied.

The mechanics involved in an extra-oral force treatment were duplicated in animal experiments.[118] Elastics that exerted forces of about 400 g during the night were placed between hooks on the upper canine and second incisor bands in the dog (Fig. 2-87). Stabilizing wires were provided with a sleeve arrangement, one on each side, that allowed distal movement but prevented rotation or tipping of the teeth being moved. During experimental periods ranging between 16 and 40 days, it was observed that the two second incisors were partly tipped and moved bodily in a distal direction. It was also noted that the experimental teeth slipped mesially toward the tension side during the day, after the elastics were removed. In all instances the tissue reaction was similar. Direct bone resorption was observed on the distal side of the third incisor whereas semihyalinization occurred on the pressure side of the tooth moved (Fig. 2-88). Semihyalinization implies that osteoclasts are formed subjacent to the hyalinized fibers, so this resorption process occurred rapidly and the second as well as the third incisors were considerably displaced. On the tension side of the second incisor a slight curving of a new bone lamellae was observed (Fig. 2-87). The bone lamellae had been curved by the pressure exerted when the experimental tooth slipped back toward the tension side during the day.

Since the interseptal bone in the dog is predominantly spongy and therefore similiar to interseptal areas of human alveolar structures, these experiments may have illustrated fairly well what happens in tooth movement performed with extra-oral forces. Apparently, the facebow exerts a certain type of interrupted force that may cause a considerable movement of the banded tooth as well as the contiguous teeth.[98] This force may be indicated graphically approximately as seen in Fig. 2-89. An equally strong force is exerted every time the appliance is used. Considering the size of the second incisor in the dog, the force exerted in the experimental series was proportionately as strong as that applied during orthodontic treatment.

The question arises why only semihyalinization occurs after application of such strong forces. There are several

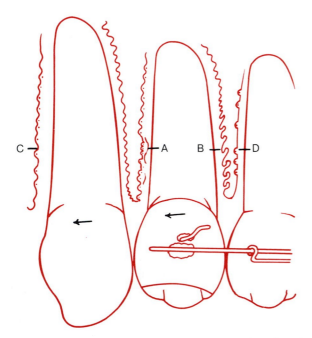

Fig. 2-87   Right side, first, second, and third incisors in a dog. Light wire sleeves prevented rotation of the second incisor. Elastics exerting a force of 400 g were placed between hooks on the second incisor and canine. *A,* Semihyalinization on the pressure side; *B,* curved bone spicules on the tension side; *C* and *D,* bone resorption adjacent to the distal surfaces of the third and first incisors. (From Reitan K: *Angle Orthod* 34:244, 1964.)

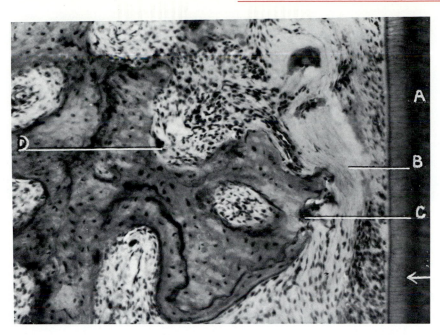

Fig. 2-88 Pressure side in an animal experiment duplicating the mechanics of extraoral force treatment (area *A* in Fig. 2-87). Note the large marrow spaces of the interseptal bone. *A*, Root; *B*, semihyalinized tissue; *C*, direct bone resorption subjacent to the semihyalinized fibers; *D*, osteoclast with undermining bone resorption. Arrow indicates the direction of movement.

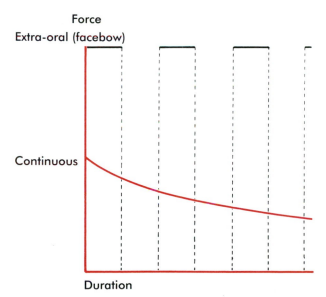

Fig. 2-89 Magnitude of force exerted in facebow and extraoral force treatment as compared with an average continuous force. The strong extra-oral force is of the interrupted type and acts only during the night.

reasons why an extra-oral force may produce such a reaction. The interseptal bone contains a system of marrow spaces whereby osteoclasts are formed in many areas. The additional thickness of the band material and the fact that the tooth that was moved remained in firm contact with the proximal tooth also tended to prevent complete hyalinization. Finally, after removal of the elastics during the day, the tissues are temporarily relieved from compression so the circulation on the pressure side is increased. Similar tissue changes were observed in other experiments in which the force was interrupted during the day.[112]

In practice, however, variations are frequent in the degree of first molar displacement. Some patients react more readily than others to an extraoral force. It also appears that the magnitude of force will influence the degree of movement. Although forces around 300 g may move the first molar distally in some, a stronger force has proved to be more effective in other cases. This observation also involves the position of the teeth moved. Slightly mesially inclined upper first and second molars tend to resist distal movement by an interrupted force, notably because two teeth are moved simultaneously.

The extent to which the position of the second molar may restrict the degree of tooth displacement in an extra-oral force treatment has been partially explored in experiments by the author. As shown by Graber[45,46] erupted molars, even in 16- to 17-year-old patients, may be moved over a considerable distance within a relatively short time. By contrast, 9- or 10-year-old patients occasionally reveal less tooth movement, regardless of whether the force exerted on each first molar is 400 or 800 g. Not infrequently the second molar in young patients is located as seen in Fig. 2-90. The crown of the second molar remains in contact with the root of the first molar and prevents further movement.

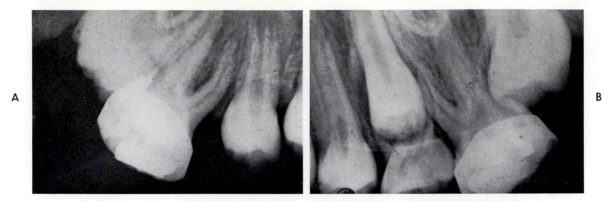

Fig. 2-90 Facebow extra-oral force treatment in a 12-year-old patient. Difference in degree of right side, **A,** and left side, **B,** movement possibly caused by the tooth position. On the right, note that the mesial root of the first molar remains in contact with the erupting second premolar while the distal root rests against the crown of the second molar. In young individuals the eliminated bone lamellae between the roots of the first and second molars will be gradually reconstructed during the posttreatment period.

As just mentioned, the fact that the forces are acting interruptedly and that large first molars are moved against second molars seems to play an important part in the tissue reaction in humans. A variation is also caused by the tissue characteristics of various experimental animals. Less root resorption occurs in the dog as compared with the monkey. As shown by Joho[60] in the studies of the monkey, extraoral forces acting continuously may cause appreciable root resorption between the middle and apical thirds of the root, but no definite shortening of the apical portion is evident. This lack of apical shortening is usually observed in most cases of extra-oral tooth movement.

Tooth movability. Some authors (Roberts, 1975; Midgett et al., 1981) have examined the effect caused by hormonal factors on the degree of tooth movement. Roberts (1975) observed a certain diurnal periodicity in animal experiments. Stutzmann and Petrovic (1980) moved a great number of human premolars, mostly interruptedly with intermaxillary elastics, 14 hours per day, each experiment lasting 21 days. The force varied between 50 and 275 g. Control and experimental teeth were removed, and some of the supporting bone from the pressure and tension sides was placed in tissue culture. Bone formation was determined by examining the osteoblast function as revealed by phenylphosphatase activity, bone calcification by the uptake of ^{45}Ca. Likewise, bone resorption on the pressure side could be evaluated by determining the degree of β-glucuronidase and acid phenylphosphatase activity. Diverse observations were made: (1) an annual periodicity—a higher tissue activity during the spring season than during the fall; (2) a higher rate of bone formation in patients with an anterior growth rotation than in patients with a posterior growth rotation; and (3) more bone formation obtained by moving the teeth with interrupted forces rather than with continuous forces (Stutzmann et al., 1979).

These observations were based on an evaluation of the bone changes. During treatment conducted over a period of 6 to 12 months, however, the degree of tooth movement is largely influenced by the quality of bone and fibrous tissue. In an experimental series it was found that persons of the same family tended to react similarly. Thus, inherited characteristics creating a favorable bone and fibrous tissue reaction might be expected to exist in several members of the same family (Fig. 2-38, *B*). This hereditary influence was especially noted in brothers and sisters who reacted favorably, occasionally revealing an identical distal displacement of molars greater than that required for further alignment of the teeth (Fig. 2-91). Although it would be logical to apply a moderate force for individual molar displacement, the conclusions of this study indicated that tooth movability during interrupted extra-oral treatment was influenced more by inherited tissue characteristics than by the force factor. Similar effects caused by individual hormonal factors are observed in other types of tooth movement as well (Fig. 2-58 as compared with Fig. 2-67, *B*).

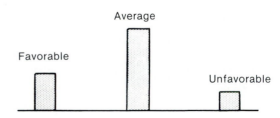

Fig. 2-91 Degree of tooth movement in a group of patients treated with moderately strong extra-oral forces. In the group termed *Favorable,* some of the patients were brothers or sisters exhibiting a similar tissue reaction. The bone characteristics that influence the degree of tooth movability in the *Favorable* group are exemplified in Fig. 2-38, *B*.

The influence exerted by extra-oral forces on the position of the maxilla has been frequently discussed.[45-47,64,92,125] In some cases in which the first molars are not displaced appreciably during treatment, it is likely that a strong extra-oral force may nevertheless influence the growth of the maxilla. This can occur when an extra-oral force, applied regularly for a certain period, is strong enough to change the direction of growth. Sutural growth is not inhibited; however, the force applied may tend to change its direction, whereby a certain control of the position of the maxilla as related to the surrounding facial structures is attained.[47]

In an extensive radiographic study on young patients treated by extra-oral force as compared with nontreated cases, Wieslander[186] observed changes proving that not only is the dentoalveolar area of the face influenced by extraoral treatment but even the craniofacial complex undergoes significant changes. Hence this is the type of treatment that may be termed *jaw orthopedics.*

Apparently one effect attained by an extra-oral treatment consists of an alteration of the relationship of the sphenoid bone to the other bones of the craniofacial complex. Wieslander[186] found that the anterior part of the palatal plane had been tipped in a downward direction. A posterior change in the position of the pterygomaxillary fissure also was evident. In the treated patients the anterior nasal spine revealed a smaller amount of anterior growth than in the control group, indicating that the position of the maxilla had been influenced during treatment. The findings of this experimental series have been corroborated in other observations of patients treated by extra-oral force.

As shown in more recent experiments,[77] widening or contraction of the median suture may also cause hyalinization of sutural tissue, undermining bone resorption, and some displacement of maxillary bones.

Combination of extra-oral force and light wire tooth movement. A light force will always move a tooth more rapidly than a strong force. The hyalinization period is shorter, and the continuous tension on the periodontal fiber bundles will result in tooth movement after only a few weeks. This effect may be observed after insertion of light wire springs for early distal movement of upper molars.

An arrangement similar to that shown in Fig. 2-92 may be applied, although other technical variations are available. Bands on the upper second deciduous molars are provided with buccal tubes for facebow treatment. In addition, springs are attached to twin tie brackets that are welded on the lingual side of the bands. A removable plate, to be worn almost constantly, is provided with horizontal spurs that will add to the stabilization of the deciduous teeth. This type of appliance has been useful for early treatment in Class II borderline cases. When the second deciduous molars are about to shed, bands may be placed on the first permanent molars for further facebow treatment.

Protraction of maxillary structures by extra-oral forces. As described by Rygh and Tindlund (1982)[143], extra-oral force can be used not only during distal movement of molars but also as a method for protracting the dentoalveolar system as a whole, thus influencing the growth direction of the basal maxillary structures. The method can be used for early treatment of severe Class III malocclusions and especially in cleft palate cases (Delaire, 1976).

Rygh and Tindlund (1982)[143] combined three methods by which surface bone deposition might be enhanced during the growth period of 5- to 6-year-old patients. The treatment stages of such cleft palate cases consisted of the following:

1. Correction of the crossbite in the molar region by applying the appliance seen in Fig. 2-93, *F.* (Bodily movement of second deciduous molars and canines is obtained during this treatment period, which lasts 2 to 3 months.)
2. Protraction of the teeth and maxillary structures by placing rubber bands from hooks on the lingual appliance to the facial mask, an appliance devised by Delaire et al., 1972. (Even an increase in the vertical dimension can be achieved during this protraction period, which lasts 6 to 7 months on the average [Fig 2-93].)
3. Alignment of the erupted anterior teeth by using a

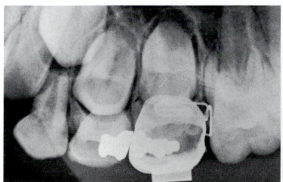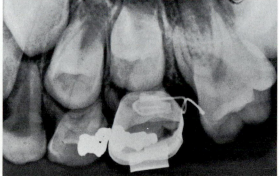

Fig. 2-92   Tooth position before and after 7 weeks' treatment with combined light wire and an extra-oral appliance. (Courtesy A. Hasund.)

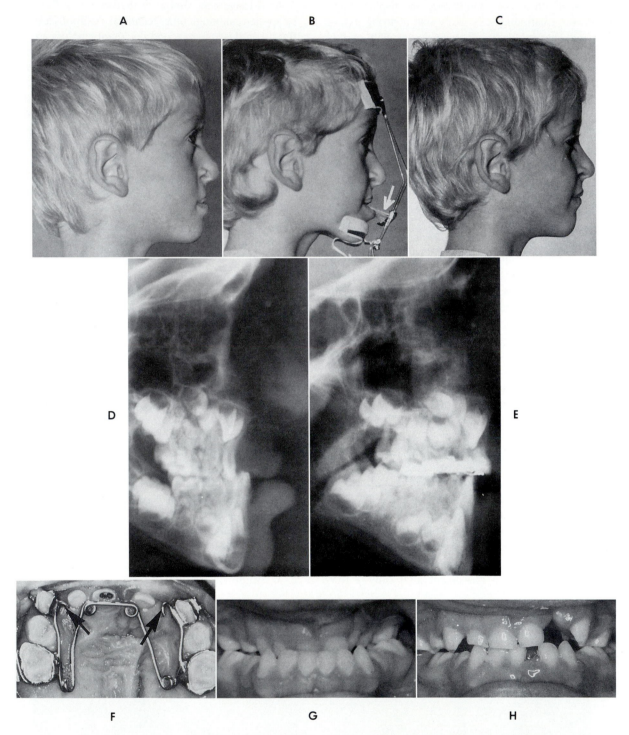

Fig. 2-93 Patient with unilateral total cleft lip and palate. At control 6 years there is underdevelopment of midface and full Class III malocclusion **(A, D, G).** Facial mask type Delaire with anteriorly directed pull (*white arrow,* **B**) from elastics to hooks (*black arrow,* **F**) in cuspid region of cemented Quad-helix expansion appliance **(G).** Profile and occlusion after 12 months' treatment **(C, E, H).** (From Rygh P: *Den norske tannlegeforenings tidende* 100:377, 1990.)

conventional multiband technique also comprising extrusion and bodily uprighting of malposed incisor teeth. (By this method a stable vertical overbite is obtained, as well as a stimulation of bone deposition in the cleft area.)

The effect of protraction of the maxilla by the Delaire facial mask in a patient with total cleft lip/palate and midfacial underdevelopment is seen in Fig. 2-93, *D* and *E*.

The ideal time for such treatment is considered to be during the growth period before the age of 7 years. Retention is obtained by placing an upper lingual arch soldered to bands cemented on the first permanent or second deciduous molars.

TORQUE

It is generally assumed that torque movement in a labial or lingual direction essentially causes displacement of the root portion of the tooth while a fulcrum is established somewhere close to the bracket area. It may be shown mechanically, however, that there is always a tendency for the crown portion to move in the opposite direction. This tendency toward a reactive movement of the marginal portion of the root is fairly similar to that observed during re-uprighting or distal tipping of a tooth in the buccal segments (Fig. 2-94). When the open eyelet of the spring in Fig. 2-94 is lifted to the archwire, it causes the apical portion of the root to move in a mesial direction and the crown portion in a distal direction. This is also what may be expected according to the laws of mechanics. Theoretically, the strongest force will be exerted on opposite sides in the

marginal and apical thirds of the root. Because of anatomic factors; however, certain variations in this type of movement may be observed.[118]

The position of the tooth and the narrowness of the dental arch will largely determine the degree of movement of the crown portion. Provided that the tooth to be uprighted does not remain in contact with the proximal tooth on the distal side, pressure will be exerted in two areas: a small circumscribed area on the distal side and a wider area on the mesial side (Fig. 2-95). On the other hand, it has been shown experimentally that if the tooth to be reuprighted is maintained in position by a ligature tied from bracket to bracket, then little or no pressure will be exerted in the small circumscribed area on the distal side. There will be movement of the root portion of the tooth only (Fig. 2-96).

Similar observations are manifest in experiments on torque force. If the labial arch is tied back to the posterior anchor teeth, there will be no perceptible degree of pressure exerted on the opposite side in the marginal region.

The fact that the force is distributed over a greater surface area on the pressure side of the middle and apical thirds would imply that less force is exerted per square millimeter. During the initial movement of torque, however, the pressure area is usually located close to the middle region of the root. This occurs because the periodontal ligament is normally wider in the apical third than in the middle third. After resorption of bone areas corresponding to the middle

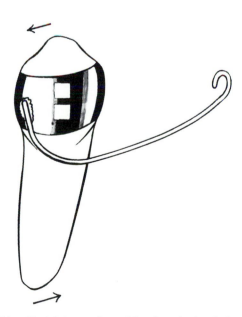

Fig. 2-94 Uprighting spring soldered to the band. Its action is similar to that of the uprighting spring soldered to the lingual side of the band in Fig. 2-81, and also similar to that of the uprighting light wire springs usually inserted in the brackets. (From Reitan K: *Am J Orthod* 46:881, 1960.)

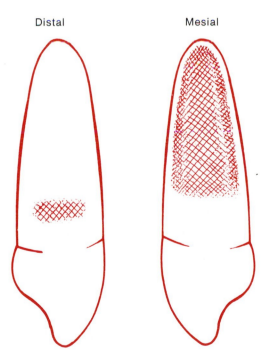

Distal   Mesial

Fig. 2-95 Surface areas where pressure will be exerted during distal tipping. Because the periodontal space is narrower adjacent to the middle third of the root, the pressure area on the mesial side will only gradually become as wide in the apical region as shown here. (From Reitan K: *Am J Orthod* 46:881, 1960.)

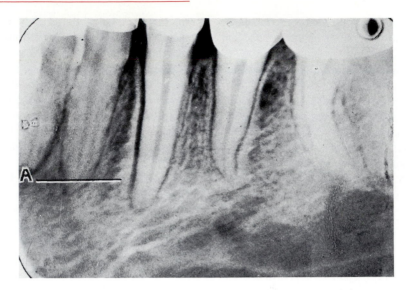

Fig. 2-96 Canine and second premolar reuprighted by springs acting as shown in Fig. 2-94. Ligature was placed from bracket to bracket, thus preventing the coronal portion of the teeth from moving in an opposite direction. *A,* New bone layers formed along stretched fiber bundles. (From Reitan K: *Am J Orthod* 46:881, 1960.)

third, the apical surface of the root will gradually begin to compress adjacent periodontal fibers and a wider presssure area (similar to that shown on the mesial side in Fig. 2-95) will be established.

In current orthodontic techniques two methods can be distinguished: torque performed with the edgewise mechanism and light wire torque.

Edgewise torque. In a series of experiments by the author on human structures using rectangular wire,[113] it was found that favorable movement could be induced. Because the tooth was moved bodily, direct bone resorption was frequently found in these cases, provided the magnitude of the force was kept within certain limits. In practice a better working range can be obtained when the torquing force is exerted by an arch configuration as shown in Fig. 2-97, notably when a thin rectangular arch is used.

In experimental work it is possible to measure the force exerted in the apical region. By determining the root length from the radiograph and by placing a device (Fig. 2-98) on the arch before the band is cemented, the force may be measured at the end of the section and thus obtain information about the magnitude of force exerted in the apical region. Fig. 2-99 shows the reaction observed in the middle third of the root of an upper first premolar in a 12-year-old patient after application of a torque force for 2 weeks to move the root in a buccal direction. The area corresponds to *X* in Fig. 2-98. The initial force exerted in the apical region was 120 to 130 g. Direct bone resorption was observed on the pressure side. By contrast, after a tipping movement, compressed cell-free tissue would have been found on this side of the root.

The favorable reaction occurs because of the interrupted

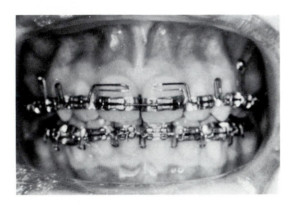

Fig. 2-97 If the rectangular wire is thin, there may be an advantage in constructing special arch configurations to obtain a gentle torquing force on teeth such as central incisors.

type of force, which acts over a fairly short distance (Fig. 2-50). It should be noted, however, that if more torque is incorporated in the archwire, there may be a considerable increase in the magnitude of force. A cell-free area of fairly short duration may then be created adjacent to the middle third of the root. The ensuing tissue reaction will be either similar to that resulting from an interrupted type of force or, in some cases, more like that from a continuous force.

The magnitude of the force in a torque movement is largely dependent on the physical properties and the thickness of the edgewise arch. It has been found that a thin arch and also a laminated arch may deliver a force that will act over a slightly longer distance without having an unfavorable strong effect.

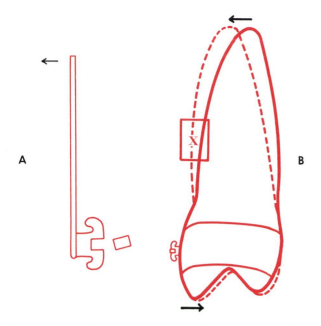

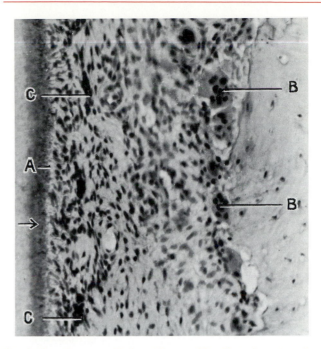

Fig. 2-98 **A,** Device for measuring the force exerted in experimental torquing of an upper first premolar. **B,** Area *X* in Fig. 2-99.

Fig. 2-99 Pressure side in a 12-year-old patient after a torquing movement performed by a 0.021 by 0.025 inch edgewise arch (area *X* in Fig. 2-98). Duration, 2 weeks. Force, 120 to 130 g exerted in the apical region. As indicated by the presence of epithelial remnants, there has been no hyalinization of the periodontal ligament. *A,* Root surface; *B,* osteoclasts along the bone surface; *C,* epithelial remnants.

Light wire torque. This type of movement is usually performed by an additional arch *(piggyback)* that in most cases is inserted for moving the root portions of the teeth in a lingual direction after the crown portions have been tipped lingually. From what has been observed in experimental work on root resorption problems, a prolonged tipping of anterior teeth will occasionally cause undesired effects in the root substance.[124] For this reason it would be an advantage in some cases to insert fairly early a stabilizing light wire configuration similar to that seen in Fig. 2-97 and thus obtain a modified type of bodily movement.

The force exerted during light wire torque is of the continuous type (Fig. 2-50). This method of torque has been investigated by Reitan, partly on human and partly on canine material.[118] The arrangement used for the experiments is seen in Fig. 2-100. The pressure exerted by the loop extending from the coil was measured before the arch was inserted.

It was found that the tissue reaction was largely influenced by variations in the magnitude of force exerted at point *A* (Fig. 2-100). On maxillary second incisors in the dog, forces between 100 and 200 g caused hyalinization and root resorption in two areas. The first was in the middle third of the root; the second, which was formed after the first undermining resorption had terminated, was all along the apical third of the root (Fig. 2-101, *B*). A force of 70 g caused formation of a minor resorbed area in the middle third of the root and subsequent direct bone resorption all along the middle and apical thirds. Bone formation along stretched fiber bundles was observed on the tension side (Fig. 2-113).

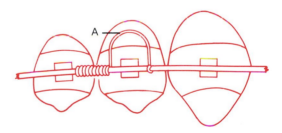

Fig. 2-100 Experimental torquing movement performed on upper human premolars and on upper second incisors in a dog. The force exerted at point *A* in human experiments ranged between 50 and 60 g.

In experiments performed on human first premolars with a force of 50 g acting at point *A*, the bone resorption was predominantly of the direct type. In an experiment lasting 30 days a minor resorption lacuna in the middle third of the root was repaired by cellular cementum, a finding which indicates that the hyalinization period had been of short duration (Fig. 2-102, *B*). These observations reveal that a force of 50 to 60 g exerted at point *A* on human anterior teeth (Fig. 2-100) causes a favorable tissue reaction.

If the labial arch is not tied back to the anchor teeth during light wire torque, the tissue changes will be approximately as seen in Fig. 2-101, *A*. In some cases new bone layers

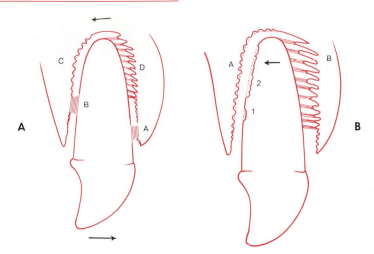

Fig. 2-101 Pressure areas and resorption lacunae formed during experimental light wire torque in the dog. **A,** Location of hyalinized zones, *A* and *B,* where the labial arch was not tied securely back to the anchor teeth. **B,** Result of an increase in the force exerted at point *A* (Fig. 2-100). Two resorbed lacunae of the root surface. This type of root resorption is usually repaired by cellular cementum and will not imperil the stability and function of the tooth. *A,* Bone resorption; *B,* bone deposition along the stretched fiber bundles.

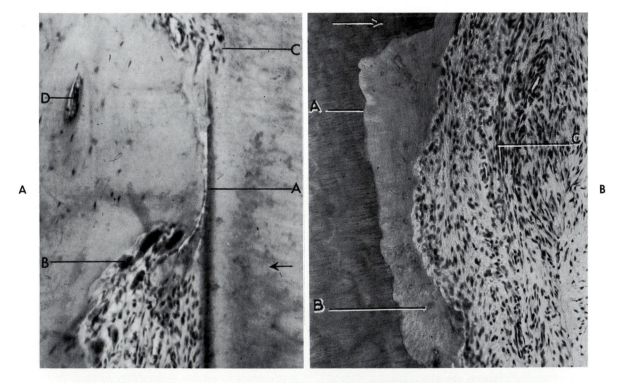

Fig. 2-102 **A,** Pressure side in an animal experiment with light wire torque. *A,* Shrinkage of the periodontal ligament after a torque movement lasting 67 days; the long duration of the undermining resorption is caused by the high bone density; *B,* undermining bone resorption; *C,* minor root resorption; *D,* small marrow space, no formation of osteoclasts; Force exerted at *A,* Fig. 2-100, 100 g. **B,** Enlarged view of the upper first premolar in a 12-year-old patient. Torque exerted as shown in Fig. 2-100. Force at point *A,* 50 g; duration, 30 days. Small root resorption repaired by cellular cementum. *A,* Demarcation line between dentin and cellular cementum; *B,* incorporated cementoblast; *C,* periodontal ligament. Note the absence of epithelial remnants. This case illustrates that hyalinization, root resorption, and repair by cellular cementum all may be completed within a period of only 30 days.

may be formed close to point B_1 of the lower jaw as a result of bone resorption elicited by movement of the root in a labial direction (Fig. 2-75, *B*). As observed in other experiments, this bone formation may depend on individual variations of the periosteum. Less periosteal bone deposition occurs in older or adult patients.

ROTATION

Correction of a rotated tooth position is usually considered to be a fairly simple and mechanical procedure. Histologically, however, the tissue transformation that occurs during rotation is largely influenced by the anatomic arrangement of the supporting structures. In experimental work on rotation of teeth, the marginal, middle, and apical thirds of the root are distinguishable[114,159] (Fig. 2-1). In the marginal region most of the periodontal fiber bundles consist of the free gingival and transseptal fiber group (Fig. 2-144). Although the principal fibers of the middle and apical thirds are anchored to the root surface and the alveolar bone, the supraalveolar fibers are connected to the whole fiber system of the supraalveolar structures.[114] This difference in the attachment of the fiber bundles has proved to be of great importance, particularly during the retention period. After rotation of teeth the stretch of free gingival tissue may cause displacement of collagen, elastic, and oxytalan fibers lo-

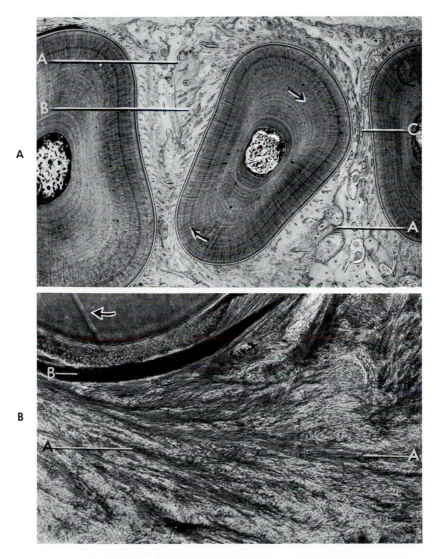

Fig. 2-103   A, Experimental rotation of an upper second incisor in a dog. Formation of two pressure sides and two tension sides. *A,* Demarcation line between old and new bone layers *(B); C,* pressure side with direct bone resorption. **B,** Animal experiment, horizontal section. The supraalveolar fibers, appear stretched and displaced even at a distance from the rotated tooth. Supraalveolar structures contain elastic fibers, a factor that increases their tendency to contract during the retention period. *A,* stretched free gingival fibers; *B,* artifact caused by folding of the section, a phenomenon observed especially on the pressure side. The tooth was rotated approximately 160°.

cated even some distance from the tooth being moved.[114]

Various factors are involved in the movement of rotation. The anatomic factor is primarily related to the position of the tooth, its form, and its size. Except for the upper central incisors and, to some extent, the lower first and second premolars in humans, most roots, seen in cross section, have an oval form. This fact implies that during rotation a parallel movement between the root and bone surface takes place mainly on the buccal and lingual sides of the root (Fig. 2-23). In practice most teeth to be rotated will create two pressure sides and two tension sides (Fig. 2-103, *A*).

A movement of rotation may cause certain variations in the type of tissue response observed on the pressure sides. Occasionally hyalinization and undermining bone resorption take place in one pressure zone while direct bone resorption occurs in the other. These variations are caused chiefly by the tooth position, as related to proximal teeth, and also the magnitude of the force. As in other types of tooth movement, it is favorable to apply a light force during the initial period. After rotation for 3 to 4 weeks, the undermining

resorption is usually completed and direct bone resorption prevails on the pressure sides.

Root resorption may occur on one of the pressure sides and frequently on both pressure sides in cases of extensive rotation; however, the resorbed lacunae of the root will be repaired over a retention period of 6 to 8 weeks. In animal experiments even quite large lacunae are completely filled in by cellular cementum after a retention period of 6 months. A similar tendency in the repair of resorbed lacunae of the root surface has been observed in humans (Fig. 2-102, *B*).

In the marginal region a movement of rotation usually causes a marked displacement and stretch of fibrous structures (Fig. 2-104). The free gingival fibers that tend to be displaced are especially those located on the labial and lingual sides of the root. The free gingival fiber groups are arranged obliquely from the root surface. Because these fiber bundles interlace with the periosteal structures and with the whole supraalveolar fibrous system, rotation also causes displacement of the fibrous tissue located some distance from the rotated tooth (Fig. 2-103, *B*).

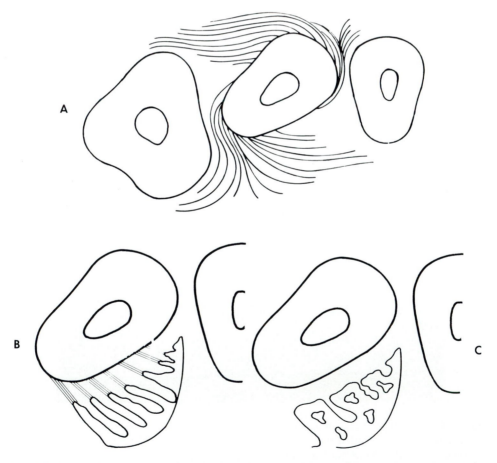

Fig. 2-104   **A,** Arrangement of free gingival fibers after rotation. **B,** Arrangement of new bone layers formed on the tension side along stretched fiber bundles following rotation. **C,** Same area after a retention period of 3 to 4 months. The bone and the principal fibers are rearranged much sooner than the displaced supraalveolar structures. (From Reitan K: *Angle Orthod* 29:105, 1959.)

On the tension side of the middle third new bone spicules will be formed along stretched fiber bundles arranged more or less obliquely (Fig. 2-104). This stretch of the periodontal fibers coincides with the formation of cellular cementum along the root surface, as seen in Fig. 2-41, *A*. In some cases a marked increase in the thickness of the cementum layer may be found on the tension side. Little cementum will be deposited on the pressure side. In the apical region less new bone will be formed during rotation, but some fiber groups are frequently elongated and arranged obliquely.

The elongation and oblique arrangement of the supporting fiber bundles will necessitate a retention period after treatment has been completed. It should also be noted that the periodontal space is considerably widened by bone resorption after rotation. In addition, the new bone on the tension side consists partly of uncalcified bone spicules. This new bundle bone may be readily rearranged after the appliances have been removed, as a result of contraction of displaced and stretched fiber bundles. The presence of elastic and oxytalan fibers in the marginal region tends to increase the

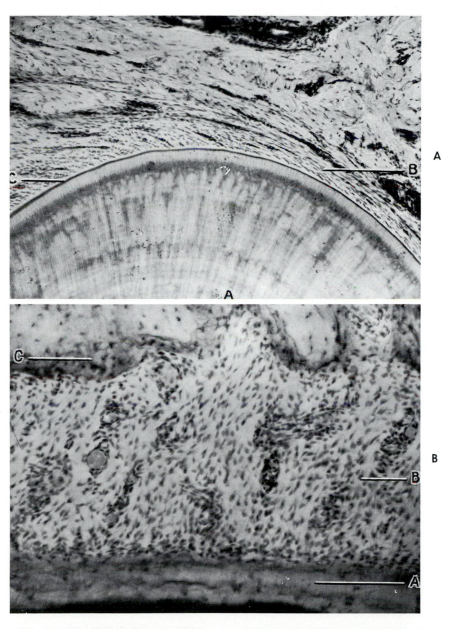

Fig. 2-105 **A,** Free gingival fibers as seen in a cross section of a rotated tooth, *A,* retained for 232 days; *B,* elongated and stretched fiber bundles; *C,* thin cementum layer along the root surface. **B,** Apical region as seen in the cross section of a tooth retained for 147 days. *A,* Cementum layer of the root surface; *B,* rearranged fiber bundles of the periodontal ligament; *C,* rearranged alveolar bone tissue. (From Reitan K: *Angle Orthod* 29:105, 1959.)

contraction of the supraalveolar structures, leading to a relapse tendency.[114]

It has been shown experimentally that the fiber bundles and the new bone layers of the middle and apical thirds rearrange themselves after a fairly short retention period. However, the free gingival fibers remain stretched and displaced for as long as 232 days and possibly longer (Fig. 2-105). According to these observations overrotation must be recommended. Experiments have shown that relapse after rotation occurs in all cases.[35]

It is therefore necessary to continue rotation through a few degrees more than considered necessary for exact positioning of the tooth moved. This degree of overrotation should, as far as possible, be proportionate to the degree of malposition of the tooth to be rotated.

Evidence indicates that the method of treatment may influence the final result of a rotating movement. If the tooth to be rotated is moved interruptedly with a fairly light force that acts over a certain distance, and afterwards, if it is held in position by the appliance until reactivation, more fiber bundles will be rearranged during the treatment period. Furthermore, the supporting fiber bundles of a tooth that has undergone a certain degree of physiologic movement during the treatment and retention periods will be more readily rearranged. The degree of relapse is especially pronounced when the tooth is rotated rapidly with a typical continuous force.

EXTRUSION

Extrusion of teeth is usually necessary in cases in which an anterior open bite exists.

Young patients. In young persons various types of labial arches, equipped with spurs for vertical elastics, have been used for closure of an open bite. When this method is applied, not only are individual teeth extruded, but also, simultaneously, growth processes are stimulated in the surrounding alveolar structures. Varying with the individual tissue reaction, the periodontal fiber bundles will elongate and new bone will be deposited in areas of the alveolar crest as a result of the tension exerted by these stretched fiber bundles[102,113] (Fig. 2-106).

Successful extrusion of teeth is largely dependent on whether the treatment is peformed during a favorable growth period. The onset and duration of growth periods may vary for each individual, but usually a major growth period occurs after the age of 13 or 14 years. Similar observations were made by Graber,[45] who found a later onset of this growth period in boys than in girls.

On the other hand, the specific supporting structures of an individual tooth reveal a period of increased growth during eruption. It has been shown that extrusion in a mass movement may result in complete and permanent closure of the bite, provided the treatment is performed shortly after the teeth have erupted. Such a favorable result is due to the readiness by which young persons' supporting tissues are

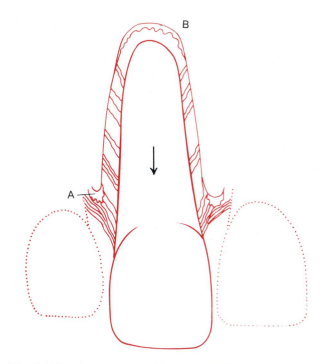

Fig. 2-106 Arrangement of fiber bundles during or after extrusion of an upper central incisor. *B,* New bone layers at the fundus alveolaris. The fiber bundles anchored in area *A* are arranged approximately as seen in Fig. 2-83, *A.*

transformed and rearranged after tooth movement. However, even young patients reveal certain variations in the degree of transformation of the supporting fibers. These tissue changes are not unlike those observed during rotation.

It may be seen experimentally that extrusion of a tooth involves a more prolonged stretch and displacement of the supraalveolar fiber bundles than of the principal fibers of the middle and apical thirds (Fig. 2-106). Some of the principal fiber groups may be subjected to stretch for a certain time as the tooth is moved, but these will be rearranged after a fairly short retention period. There is usually an essentially complete rearrangement of the principal fibers of the middle and apical thirds after a retention period of 4 to 5 months. Only the supraalveolar fiber bundles remain stretched for a longer time (Fig. 2-83, *A*). For this reason a certain degree of relapse may occur and it may be advisable to overcorrect the tooth position during closure of an open bite to avoid reopening.

A factor of importance is the method of treatment. If the labial arch is fairly heavy, application of several vertical elastics may result in jiggling of the teeth moved, with subsequent widening of the alveoli. The result may be a relapse of the extruded teeth every time the elastics are removed. Relatively little tooth movement will be seen. A light archwire that permits a certain degree of physiologic tooth movement may largely prevent such relapse tendencies in young patients. Light vertical elastics must be worn to obtain complete closure of the bite.

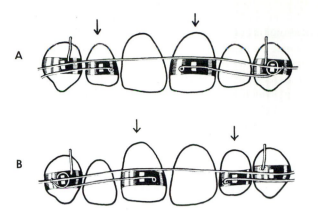

Fig. 2-107 Arrangement for individual extrusion of anterior teeth, a type of light-force interrupted movement. **A,** In some cases the spring acting on the right lateral may be attached to the first premolar bracket. **B,** After 4 or 5 weeks the arrangement may be reversed so the proximal incisor teeth are extruded while the two teeth moved are released. A similar arrangement may be applied for the lower anterior teeth. The springs should be preferably around 0.3 mm thick. Vertical elastics must be worn between upper and lower canines. This is the recommended method for closure of an open bite in adult patients. (From Reitan K: *Am J Orthod* 53:721, 1967.)

Adult patients. After the age of 18 to 20 years growth activity slows. The periodontal fiber bundles will become stretched after extrusion; however, they are less readily elongated and rearranged. Also more distant fibers along the alveolar crest tend to stretch. Extrusion of adult teeth in a mass movement may thus result in relapse after displacement and subsequent contraction of the whole free gingival fiber system. In such cases it has been observed that closure of an open bite may be performed with greater success if the anterior teeth are extruded individually and not in a mass movement.[113]

An example of how to place the springs to be used for closure of an open bite in patients aged 20 to 30 years is seen in Fig. 2-107. The individual springs exerting an extruding force are usually placed around the canine bracket or, occasionally, on the first premolar. The force exerted must not exceed 25 to 30 g because extrusion constitutes the type of movement that requires a minimal force. Disturbance of the pulp structures may occur if a stronger force is used. Thus it is evident that this is no routine physiologic method. On the other hand, it has been found that if the force is carefully measured no perceptible root resorption will occur in humans, although small resorbed lacunae have been observed in a few experimental cases.[124] It has not

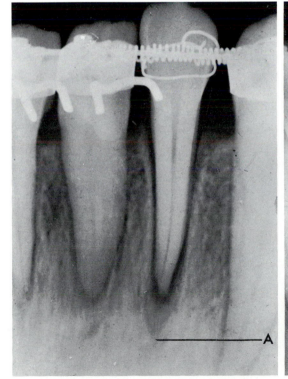
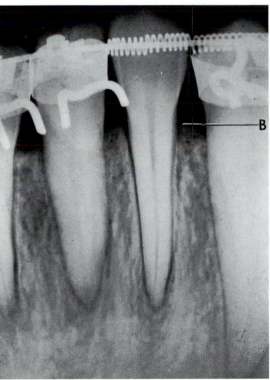

Fig. 2-108 Two stages of individual extrusion of a lateral incisor in a 20-year-old patient recently treated periodontically. **A,** Note the degree of extrusion of the tooth. *A,* Bone wall at the fundus alveolaris. (Compare with Fig. 2-109.) **B,** Released and left free for 7 weeks. There is only a slight degree of relapse. Note the calcification of bone in the apical region. *B,* Some formation of new bone layers at the alveolar bone crest. (From Reitan K; *Am J Orthod* 53:721, 1967.)

been possible, however, to reproduce such apical root resorption in the dog or monkey. After a few weeks the two teeth moved are released, and a similar force is applied to the two proximal teeth. In this way the structures around the first two teeth will have time to be rearranged and new osteoid tissue will become calcified. Two stages of extrusion of an individual tooth are seen in Fig. 2-108.

Relapse of the recently moved and free incisor teeth is only slight, because individual fiber bundles have become elongated and the whole area is stimulated to added growth as extrusion of the proximal teeth continues. It may be necessary to reverse this arrangement after a certain period until desirable extrusion is obtained. Usually a similar arrangement with springs anchored to the canines and premolars is used in both jaws.

An important technical detail demands the placing of vertical elastics between the upper and lower canines, to which the springs are anchored. If vertical elastics are not worn, root resorption will soon appear in the apical portion of the anchor teeth. This occurs because the intruding force exerted on the canines is much stronger than the extruding force acting on the anterior teeth. Periodic radiographic ex-

amination is desirable and may reveal what happens in the apical regions of the anchor teeth and the teeth moved. The histologic picture corresponding to the apical region in Fig. 2-108 is shown in Fig 2-109. The open space in the apical region, seen in Fig. 2-108, consists partly of uncalcified osteoid, which is not perceptible on the radiograph. After 4 to 5 weeks calcified bone starts to become visible in the apical area. New calcified bone at the alveolar crest may also be observed.

In addition to the mechanical arrangement just described, application of a chin cap, combined with vertical extra-oral traction, may shorten the treatment period required for closure of an open bite.

The methods described indicate that it is less complicated to close an open bite in young patients. It has also been shown that, if necessary and desirable, an open bite may be closed even in adult patients. The final closure of the bite requires that light wire labial arches, combined with light vertical elastics, should be used for stabilization of the tooth position.

An important phase of an open bite treatment is effective control of muscle habits, such as overactive tongue function. In many cases it may become necessary to place vertical spurs extending from the linguo-incisal aspects of the bands or lingual arches to prevent the tongue from resting between the dental arches.

Deformed Roots

Although extrusion of teeth can usually be performed quite readily by application of light forces, dilaceration or curvature of the root may delay movement of certain teeth. Occasionally, a single tooth will remain below the occlusal plane because its root is deformed (Fig. 2-110). Such an anatomic defect may cause difficulties when force is applied for extrusion of the tooth (Fig. 2-111). Increasing the magnitude of force to obtain a more rapid movement will only

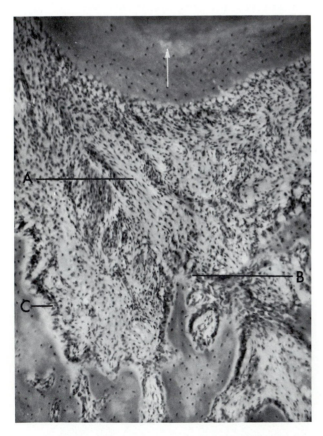

Fig. 2-109 Extrusion of a lower second incisor in the dog (area B in Fig. 2-106). Continuous force; 30 g. *A*, Stretched fiber bundles; *B*, newly formed osteoid; *C*, osteoblast chain along an osteoid layer. As in other areas of the periodontal ligament, the new bone is laid down along stretched fiber bundles. Arrow indicates the direction of movement.

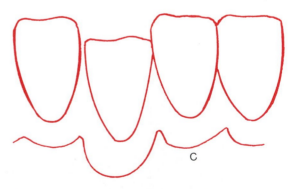

Fig. 2-110 Lower incisor not fully erupted because of curvature of the root. *c*, Undeveloped alveolar bone crest is due to the position of the tooth and its marginal structures. The crest cannot develop since there exists a strong antagonism between epithelial tissue and bone. This antagonism will also become manifest in cases of persisting ankylosed deciduous molars that tend to cause arrested development of the alveolar bone.[100]

increase the resistance and lead to a standstill of the tooth because fibrous tissue may be completely eliminated with contact between root and bone surface.

By application of a light force, frequently interrupted, the orthodontist may be able to extrude the tooth. Surgical resection of the curved end and subsequent root filling may also facilitate the ensuing orthodontic movement. Likewise, surgical removal of bone and application of a light force by insertion of a spring similar to those seen in Fig. 2-107 may solve the problem.[55]

INTRUSION

Intrusion of teeth is an important part of the technical procedures performed during orthodontic treatment. The movement of intrusion has been widely discussed in the literature. In the majority of cases intrusion of anterior teeth is undertaken during active growth periods. As a result there is, simultaneously and to a varying extent, extrusion of the posterior teeth. If the growth period is active, cephalometric radiographs taken before and after treatment may reveal a general increase in the vertical dimensions of the facial structures. This change in the facial dimensions may cause uncertainty about whether an actual intrusion of the anterior teeth has occurred. A study of the effect caused by an intruding force can therefore be conducted with greater accuracy in persons whose major growth period is over. During such treatment it is important to consider the differences in tissue reaction between young and adult structures.

Adult patients. Some practitioners state that intrusion of adult teeth cannot be undertaken without a corresponding

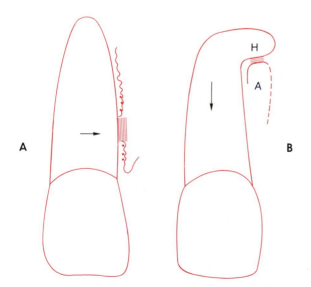

Fig. 2-111 **A,** Bodily movement of a tooth with a hyalinized zone in the middle third of the root and frontal bone resorption, a type of tooth movement that requires a moderately strong force. **B,** Extrusion of a tooth with a curved root. Since minimal force is required for extrusion, there will be a recurrent form of hyalinization *(H)* and a slow movement. *A,* Bone layer that must be removed by resorption.

shortening of the apices by root resorption. It is a fact that routine treatment by conventional appliances may frequently result in root resorption. If carefully measured forces are applied, however, there will be less tendency to such shortening of the roots. In many instances a principle similar to that described under "Extrusion" may be applied, with the exception that for intrusion of teeth the spring shown in Fig. 2-107 must be placed so it acts in the opposite direction. Such a light force will cause bone resorption, and the apex of the tooth will be moved against the bone without causing extensive root resorption. This proves that the problem of intrusion is largely dependent on a careful planning of the technical procedures. Since the treatment is based on a corresponding extrusion of posterior teeth, it is essential to relieve occlusal pressure by inserting a bite plate. Even for intrusion of teeth, it has proved practical to release the tooth moved for certain periods and to apply the intruding force temporarily to the proximal teeth.

Investigation of nine adult patients treated by the author revealed that the incidence of apical root resorption was highly individual. It was found that by examining the intruded teeth radiographically and releasing the intruded teeth periodically, there would be no marked apical root resorption. In a certain number of cases no perceptible root resorption was observed. Hence, this problem is related as much to the technical method as to the individual tissue reaction.

It is characteristic of the treatment of adults with deep bite that the lower anterior teeth are intruded more readily than the upper. Radiographic examination after intrusion revealed that the vertical dimension, which is dependent on the height of the existing free way space, could increase by as much as 7 or 8 mm. Of this increase, 3 to 4 mm was caused by intrusion of the lower anterior teeth while extrusion of lower premolars and first molars would range between 2 and 4 mm. Only 1 or 2 mm of increase in the vertical dimension could be traced back to an intrusion of the upper anterior teeth. The reason for such difference in the degree of tooth movement is partly because of the size of the teeth. Stabilization of the tooth position after intrusion of adult teeth can be attained only by establishing a correct mesiodistal relationship between the dental arches. In addition, the anterior teeth must be moved so the position of the upper and lower canines, and partly the incisor teeth, is maintained by well-established occluding surfaces. Spot grinding of the occluding surfaces is therefore necessary during treatment, and retention plates must be worn. If these precautions are not taken, relapse may occur (Fig. 2-112).

Young patients. As stated, where intrusion is necessary, it is primarily the anterior teeth of the upper and lower jaws that must be intruded. Various methods have been applied for this type of movement. Some present-day appliances intrude teeth more readily than others.

Experiments have shown that more rapid intrusion is obtained by light continuous forces than by other types of tooth movement. There are times, however, when the forces

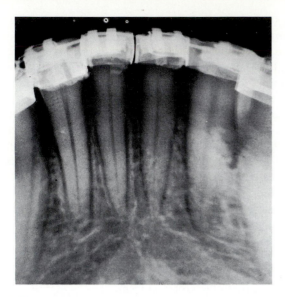

Fig. 2-112   Intrusion at the end of active treatment in an adult. There is definitely root resorption but no shortening of the apical portion.

applied must not act for excessively long periods if shortening of the roots is to be avoided. As already mentioned, this applies primarily to adult patients. A carefully measured intruding force may cause root resorption, even in young patients; however, radiographically no visible shortening of the roots may be evident.

As an example of a small magnitude of force, the intruding movement exerted in the light wire technique may

be mentioned. The molars are tipped distally while an intruding force is exerted on the six anterior teeth. Since the total force acting on the anterior teeth is frequently not stronger than 80 to 120 g, each anterior tooth will be intruded by a force as light as 20 to 30 g. This light force produces short hyalinization periods, and the anterior teeth will be intruded quite rapidly.

Minor hyalinized areas may be formed even with this light force, and small resorbed lacunae of the root surface may also be observed. This root resorption is frequently located between the middle and apical thirds. It occurs as a result of a tipping of the individual tooth during intrusion. If the force is extremely light, however, there is less tendency to shortening of the apical portion of the root.[34]

Anatomic variations.   Apical root resorption after intrusion depends to a large extent on the anatomic environment of the root. Examination of radiographs taken before treatment may provide information about the form and character of the bone adjacent to the apices of the teeth to be intruded. In young patients the apex is often surrounded by spongy bone and large marrow spaces. A light continuous force, such as that obtained in the light wire technique, has proved to be favorable for intrusion of teeth in young patients. In other cases, the alveolar bone may be closer to the apex (Fig. 2-113). If the bone of the apical region is fairly compact, as it is in some adults, a light interrupted force may be preferable. This will provide time for cell proliferation to start, and direct bone resorption may prevail when the labial arch is reactivated after the rest period.

As in other types of tooth movement, the force applied during the *initial* period of intrusion may determine the

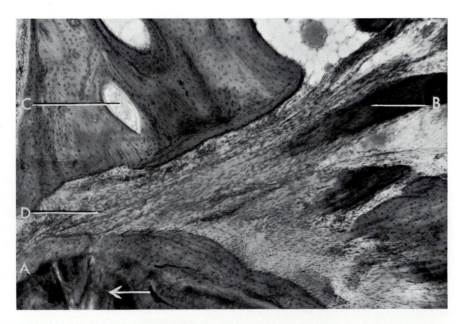

Fig. 2-113   Apical region in a dog during an experimental torquing movement, upper second incisor. Note the short distance between the root surface and fundus. *A,* Root surface; *B,* new bone spicule formed as a result of the tooth movement; *C,* marrow space in fairly dense alveolar bone; *D,* stretched fiber bundles. During intrusion, care must be taken to apply a light initial force.

ultimate degree of root resorption. If a definitely light force is exerted for a period of 5 to 6 weeks, there is less tendency for root resorption to occur during the later period of intrusion. The factors related to this problem are discussed more extensively under "Root Resorption" (p. 169).

The behavior of intruded teeth may also be observed in experimental work. The author's experiments have revealed that strong forces—100 to 200 g—produce root resorption in the apical region of maxillary anterior teeth in the dog. Insignificant apical resorption with no shortening of the roots was produced with forces ranging between 15 and 50 g in the lower anterior teeth of the dog. In some cases, however, resorption took place along the middle third of the roots. The resorbed lacunae were produced as a result of a tipping of the intruded teeth. The form of the resorption was similar to that seen in the middle third of the root in Fig. 2-101, *B*. Repair of the resorbed lacunae by secondary cementum was observed in all cases in which the teeth had been retained. Dellinger[34] also observed insignificant apical root resorption in animal experiments after application of forces below 50 g.

These observations reveal that intruded teeth vary in their reaction according to the magnitude of the force exerted. However anatomic details such as the width of the periodontal ligament and the existing type of the alveolar bone surrounding the apical portion of the roots may largely influence the tissue reaction after a movement of intrusion (Fig. 2-114). Generally teeth in young patients may be intruded more readily and with less tendency to shortening of the apical portion of the roots.

Occasionally, intrusion occurs in conjunction with other types of tooth movement. Fig. 2-115 illustrates how the apical third of an upper first premolar in a 12-year-old has become slightly curved as a result of compression during bodily movement. Curving of the root occurred as uncalcified predentin developed in the apical third of the root. Since odontoclasts do not attack uncalcified tissue, only the calcified structures exhibit root resorption. A similar sequence of events occurs in the majority of autotransplantation cases[161] (Fig. 2-116). Deformation of the root is fre-

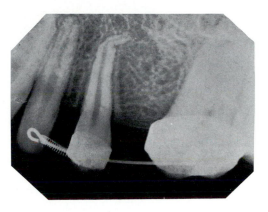

Fig. 2-115 Congenitally absent canine and first premolar in a young patient. Mesial movement of the second premolar. There has been a slight intrusion of the tooth. Curvature of the root is partly a result of further development of the root. No root resorption of the uncalcified apical portion has occurred.

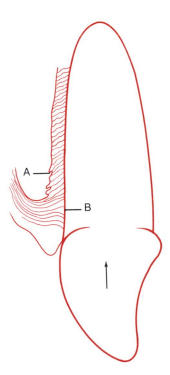

Fig. 2-114 Relaxation of the free gingival fibers during intrusion. *A*, Bone spicules laid down according to the direction of the fiber tension; *B*, relaxed supraalveolar tissue. In young patients no marked relapse tendency becomes manifest, provided retention plates are worn after the intrusion.

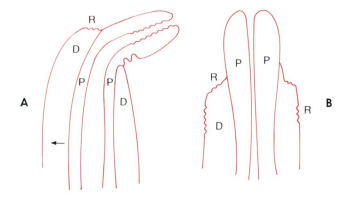

Fig. 2-116 According to what has been observed in recent experiments, the thickness of the predentin layer plays an important role during root development (Figs. 2-48 and 2-128). The structures seen in Fig. 2-115 would be arranged as in **A.** *D*, Dentin slightly resorbed and diminished at *R*, *P*, predentin forming the major part of the curved apical portion. From what has been observed in cases of autotransplantation of teeth, **B,** the tissue changes are fairly similar. *D*, Dentin being resorbed at *R*; *P*, predentin layers forming the main part of the root during its further development.

quently observed after physiologic tooth movement (Fig. 2-117, *B*).

Relapse tendency. Unlike extruded teeth, intruded teeth in young patients will undergo only minor positional changes after intrusion. Relapse doesn't occur often partly because the free gingival fiber bundles become slightly re-laxed (Fig. 2-114). Stretch is primarily exerted on the principal fibers. An intruding movement may thus cause formation of new bone spicules in the marginal region. These new bone layers occasionally become slightly curved as a result of the tension exerted by stretched fiber bundles (Fig. 2-114). Such tension is also seen in the middle third of the

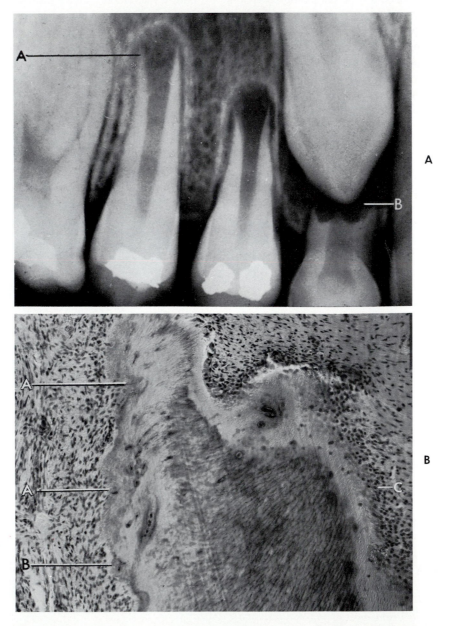

Fig. 2-117 **A,** Developmental stage of the root portion of recently erupted premolars. *A,* Distal wall of the root; *B,* a certain distance is maintained between the crown of the erupting canine and the resorbed deciduous tooth. Dentinoclasts are formed as pressure is exerted on the fibrous layer situated between the erupting canine and the deciduous tooth. A similar process may occur if an erupting canine has started resorption in the apical portion of a lateral incisor. **B,** Area of the distal wall of the premolar root corresponding to that in **A.** The indentations *(A)* are fairly well calcified cementum; in such indentations pressure exerted by the crown (or the root) of a proximal tooth may lead to formation of cementoclasts and root resorption. The cementoid layer *(B)* is not as readily resorbed as calcified tissue. Many odontoblasts cover the thick layer of predentin on the pulpal side of the root wall *(c).*

roots. Rearrangement of the principal fibers occurs after a retention period of 2 to 3 months. In the young patient the intruded tooth will then remain fairly stable with comparatively little tendency to relapse. More relapse after intrusion may occur in adults, particularly those in whom a correct relationship between the upper and lower canines has not been established or when the retention period has been too short.

Removable appliances. Although intrusion of individual teeth occurs in nearly all cases after application of light continuous forces, the supporting tissues respond less readily to an intruding force exerted by removable appliances. The effect exerted during treatment by a bite plate consists largely of preventing the anterior teeth from further eruption. The position of the anterior teeth may be improved and maintained with no significant intrusion. In patients with deep bite an improved plane of occlusion can be attained only as a result of eruption of molars and premolars and simultaneous vertical growth of the supporting structures. This fact implies that correction of an exaggerated curve of Spee by means of a removable appliance should preferably be performed during a favorable growth period.

INJURIES OF THE SUPPORTING TISSUES DURING TOOTH MOVEMENT

Histologic investigations of the periodontal structures have from time to time indicated the possibility that orthodontic treatment may cause more damage to the root substance and the supporting tissues than is generally assumed.[101] When considering the advances in appliance construction and treatment procedures in recent decades, it should be unnecessary to discuss the side effects produced by orthodontic appliances. In light of what is known today about fixed appliances, it seems more likely that the unfavorable side effects were caused essentially by the less well-developed technical procedures of the time and, in some areas, the lack of personal dental care.

Removable appliances. From a periodontal point of view it is obvious that the absence of bands, arches, and ligatures during orthodontic treatment seems preferable. Nevertheless, the premature conclusion that every patient should be treated by removable appliances to maintain ideal periodontal conditions appears shortsighted in many respects.

Those who have had an opportunity to observe the beneficial physiologic effect of establishing what has been termed an *upright tooth position* may be convinced that it is preferable to perform many types of treatment with fixed appliances. The supporting structures are far more resistant to periodontal disorders when the tooth has been moved to an upright position, and stress is dissipated in the long axis of the tooth.

Fixed appliances. The method of tipping teeth and subsequently reuprighting them has been stressed especially in the movement of canines by the light wire technique. Overdoing this initial tipping, which has occasionally hap-

pened, can hardly be considered a recommended method. Again, a distinction must be drawn between young and adult patients. The supporting structures of recently erupted canines are in a favorable growth period, and after reuprighting, few if any traces of the drastic initial procedures that might have been undertaken will be evident. In older children and in adults various disturbances may ensue from too extreme a tipping of the canines. The apical portion of the tooth may be moved through the bone.[118] Destruction of bone in the marginal areas similar to that previously described may also be the result (Fig. 2-71).

As stated, bodily movement of adult teeth is preferable in most cases. Undesirable alveolar bone destruction is prevented by using this method. The resorption process may be readily observed by requiring that radiographs be taken at various intervals during the treatment period. These should be checked carefully and compared with the original radiographs. The litigious benefits are obvious.

ROOT RESORPTION

In discussions of tissue injuries caused by orthodontic tooth movement, root resorption has always been one of the central problems. Schwarzkopf demonstrated root resorption on extracted teeth as early as 1887. Ketcham (1929), Rudolph (1940), and others reported resorbed lacunae of the root surface visible on radiographs.[62,132] Root resorption has been observed in histologic investigations by many authors.*

Comparisons between radiographic and histologic studies have revealed that minor resorbed lacunae of the root surface remain undetected as a rule on the radiograph. This is natural, since most resorbed lacunae in the root surface are very small and cannot be visualized by radiographic methods. A distinction must therefore be drawn between the minor resorbed lacunae and those that can be clearly seen radiographically.

Root resorption not related to orthodontics. New cementoid layers are constantly being deposited along the root surface after the root of the erupting tooth has fully developed. As seen in Fig. 2-48, the changes observed in the apical portion of teeth with undeveloped roots are conspicuous, especially after intrusion or a tipping movement. Examination of histologic sections of teeth in young persons reveals that formation of cementum during this period is not the sole phenomenon. The newly calcified secondary cementum will occasionally resorb. As a result of pressure, resorption may start in depressions of the root surface, notably in the apical third (Fig. 2-117, *B*). The lacunae resulting from such a resorption process are not visible radiographically. In this physiologic type of root resorption the small resorbed lacuna soon fill in and are repaired by cementoid tissue (Fig. 2-102, *B*). The cause of this type of root resorption is essentially compression of the periodontal

---

*References 49, 56, 84, 100, 103, 173.

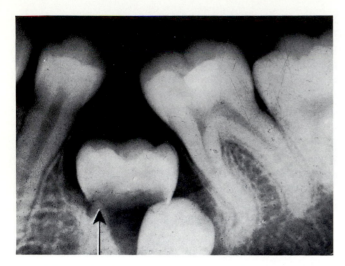

Fig. 2-118   Ankylosed second deciduous molar. No further resorption of the deciduous tooth occurs, primarily because of the contact established between the deciduous tooth and the crown of the premolar. Arrow indicates the area with union between alveolar bone and tooth substance.

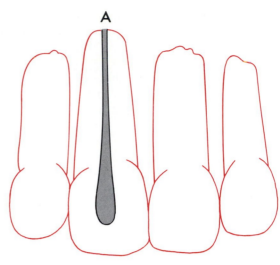

Fig. 2-119   Case in which the anterior teeth have been subjected to rapid tipping by light forces. Note that there is less root resorption of one tooth *(A)* whose dentin has acquired an increased hardness after root canal treatment.

ligament resulting from an increased occlusal load. As a rule such resorption is preceded by a short hyalinization period. The resorbing dentinoclasts in these lacunae soon disappear and cementoblasts resume the formation of cementoid. It is thus, to some extent, the quality of the root substance that, facilitates the formation of resorption lacunae in the recently developed root.

On the other hand, the density and hardness of the cementum and dentin may cause retardation of root resorption. An example is the resorption occurring in deciduous teeth during tooth eruption.[142] The hardness of the deciduous tooth substance may cause a slow and retarded resorption process. Thus ankylosed deciduous teeth tend to prevent eruption of permanent premolars. In Fig. 2-118 the bony union between root and alveolar bone on one side of the deciduous root is strong enough to retain the second deciduous molar and maintain the premolar in position. Even if the deciduous tooth is ankylosed, the erupting tooth should be able, at least theoretically, to cause further resorption of the deciduous root; but this does not occur. The resorption process has more or less terminated partly because of the hard unresorbable dentin of the deciduous molar. This type of dentin is found particularly when the pulp tissue of the deciduous tooth is deteriorated or infected.[185] From a practical point of view it is important to remove a deciduous molar at the time it is ascertained that its crown remains definitely at a level below the proximal teeth.

The effect of increased density of the dentin in devitalized teeth has occasionally been observed during tooth movement. Thus delayed resorption of root-filled teeth has become manifest in some cases in which the apical portion of

several teeth had been shortened after rapid tipping by light forces (Fig. 2-119).

An erupting canine may cause root resorption on the distal surface of the lateral incisor to occur rapidly. This resorption is partly due to the texture of the newly formed cementum of the lateral. Extensive root resorption occurs, particularly when the canine erupts in the direction of the long axis of the lateral incisor. Broadbent has called attention to this canine position in his *ugly duckling pattern*. Once an initial resorption lacuna has been formed, it will soon be enlarged as the canine moves. In some cases the canine erupts more or less continuously, so the resorption process is maintained and gradually increased. The lateral root is resorbed directly as odontoclasts are formed by compression of the fibrous tissue surrounding the apex of this tooth (Fig. 2-117, *A*). Occasionally, the whole lateral root is completely eliminated during a period as short as 2 months. If the initial resorption is observed on the radiograph, the orthodontist may be able to intervene. The canine may be moved distally or lingually and further resorption of the lateral root prevented.

In addition to the resorption caused by erupting teeth, several other causes have been observed. Root resorption appears to be a fairly common occurrence during physiologic tooth movement, as shown by Gottlieb and Orban,[44] Orban,[105] Kronfeld and Weinmann,[68] and others. If parts of the periodontal ligament have been transformed into granulation tissue, odontoclasts may form with resorption of the root surface. Replantation of teeth invariably results in root resorption and bony ankylosis. Excessive occlusal stress of some duration may cause resorption and shortening of the root of the involved tooth.

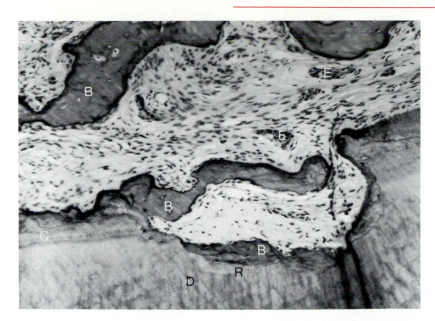

Fig. 2-120   Resorbed lacunae of unknown origin at the root surface of an impacted lower second premolar in a 19-year-old patient. The cementum *(C)* reveals increased thickness. *D*, Dentin; *R*, resorbed lacunae partly repaired by cellular cementum, which is covered by bone *(B); E*, epithelial remnants.

Of special interest are such metabolic anomalies as hypothyroidism, a condition that some authors assume may predispose to root resorption during orthodontic treatment. Factors related to this endocrine problem have been discussed by Marshall,[83] Becks,[10] and others.

Resorbed lacunae of unknown etiology, the so-called idiopathic resorption, may become manifest in certain cases. Some impacted teeth subjected to root resorption are on the borderline of being hypercementotic.[58] The impacted second premolar shown in Fig. 2-120 revealed thick layers of cementum and at the same time resorbed lacunae all along its root surface, a few of which were repaired with secondary cementum and bone. In other patients one or more teeth will occasionally appear to be shortened by root resorption before orthodontic treatment. If the practitioner is aware of this anomaly before treatment is started, further resorption may be largely avoided. Moving the teeth interruptedly by light forces, relieving the bite by using a plate, and examining the teeth radiographically at intervals are some of the measures that may enable the orthodontist to prevent any extensive root resorption of such teeth.

Functional disturbances. Although many types of root resorption exist in which the genetic origin is obscure, it has been observed that where a general tendency to root injuries exists, resorption may increase appreciably in certain cases as a result of malfunction. Two types of such root resorption are seen in Fig. 2-121. The radiograph of a functional case of resorption (Fig. 2-122) shows an open bite in the anterior region where a tongue habit may have increased the tendency to apical resorption of the central incisors.

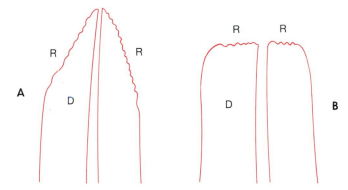

Fig. 2-121   Two types of apical root resorption caused by functional disorders of the dental mechanism. **A,** Shortening of the root due to muscular dysfunction, an open bite caused by tongue pressure, and torque. Compare with Fig. 2-122. **B,** Root of a premolar in a Class III case in which the occlusal load was dissipated in the long axis of the first premolars, three teeth being shortened as seen at *R*. Dentin, *D*.

Root resorption caused by orthodontics. Bien (1967) is of the opinion that root resorption is caused less by the magnitude of the forces than by the rate of application of those forces. If this mechanical principle is neglected, disturbances will occur in the complicated drainage system of the periodontal ligament, a basket-shaped rete enveloping the root. He states that "tiny bubbles of carbon dioxide are liberated at the tooth apex." The local drop in pH that occurs causes decalcification of the root between the apertures, showing up grossly as root resorption. In tissue culture

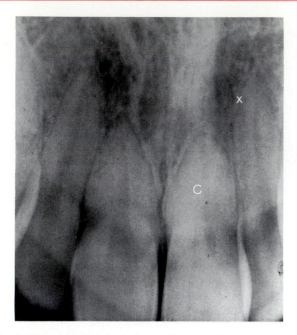

Fig. 2-122 Functional root resorption in a 19-year-old patient. There was contraction, especially of the upper dental arch, along with an open bite and tongue habit. *C,* Central incisor, which was mobile and shortened as seen in Fig. 2-121; *x,* resorbed area of the lateral incisor root. The patient had not been treated orthodontically.

experiments Goldhaber (1965) has also listed carbon dioxide as a bone-resorbing factor.

The type of root resorption that occurs during orthodontic treatment is nearly always preceded by hyalinization of the periodontal ligament. As a result of the undermining resorption process, even the root surface may become involved. Root resorption would then occur around this cell-free tissue, starting at the border of the hyalinized zone (Fig. 2-102, *A*).[140] Superficial root resorption in the rat is shown in Fig. 2-123.

From a practical point of view it is of interest to determine which is the type or degree of root resorption that can be injurious—i.e., leading to a weakening of the stability and normal function of the individual tooth. The main factors related to this problem have already been discussed. A summary of these observations will be given here.

General considerations. As stated by Gianelly and Goldman,[42] root resorption, unlike alveolar bone resorption, is unpredictable. However, in general root resorption depends on the mechanics involved. Thus x-ray examination has shown that only insignificant root resorption occurs during bodily tooth movement with frictionless appliances of the type shown in Fig. 2-39.

Earlier experiments have shown that in the middle portion of the root, resorption tends to start close to or around the hyalinized zone (Fig. 2-104, *A*); but many exceptions are discovered by scanning and electron microscopy. In an ex-

Fig. 2-123 Migrating multinucleated cells in the middle of rat PDL close to remnants of hyalinized tissue, *H,* during the stage of elimination of necrotic tissue. (Courtesy P. Brudvik.)

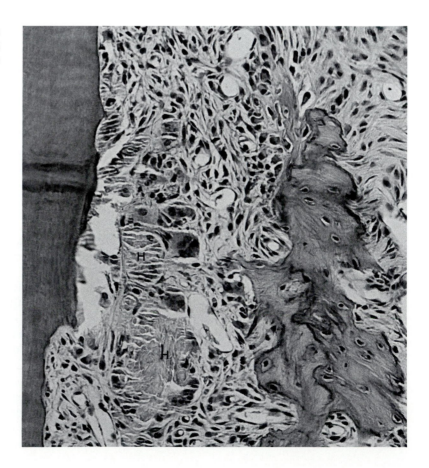

tensive collection of animal material, initial root resorption subjacent to the hyalinized tissue was observed in only a few cases[112] (Fig. 2-124). The majority of resorption lacunae are small and insignificant.[53] They will soon be repaired by cellular cementum. Periodontal fibers are incorporated in the new cementum layer, and the tooth will remain in normal function.

It is known that cementum is a fairly independent tissue and, unlike bone, is not involved in metabolic processes such as calcium homeostasis. However, certain changes in cementum resemble those that take place in bone. Like osteoid, cementoid tends to decrease in thickness on the side of compression (Fig. 2-48). If the pressure continues for a longer period, root resorption may start even if the root was initially protected by uncalcified tissue.

It was shown in Fig. 2-104, *B*, that hyalinization, root resorption, and repair occur within a period of 30 days. Several of these small resorption lacunae are visible only by the scanning electron microscope. According to Kvam[71] organic tissue tends to remain in the resorbed area, which can be exposed more clearly by removing the organic components (Fig. 2-125). Another interesting observation is the difference in size of the resorption lacunae of cementum and dentin (Fig. 2-126).

These initial injuries are all small and insignificant. It is the extensive type of apical root resorption that must be regarded as deleterious to the function and stability of the tooth moved. The root resorption of the tipped tooth in Fig. 2-64 can hardly be regarded as a lessening of the tooth stability. By contrast, a resorption whereby one third or up to one half of the root length is eliminated must be avoided.

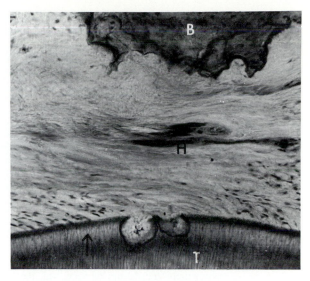

Fig. 2-124   Continuous tooth movement in a dog. Force, 200 g; duration, 36 hours. *B*, Alveolar bone; *H*, blood vessels in the hyalinized zone. Resorption lacunae with cellular elements are seen between the arrow and *T*. Such initial lacunae may appear subjacent to hyalinized zones where the compression is increased (e.g., in the apical portion of human teeth).

If the tendency is toward extensive root resorption, a period of rest may be of great value. The resorbed lacunae are usually covered by fibrous tissue in which secondary cementum layers will be formed on the resorbed root surface (Fig. 2-127). When tooth movement is resumed, the ortho-

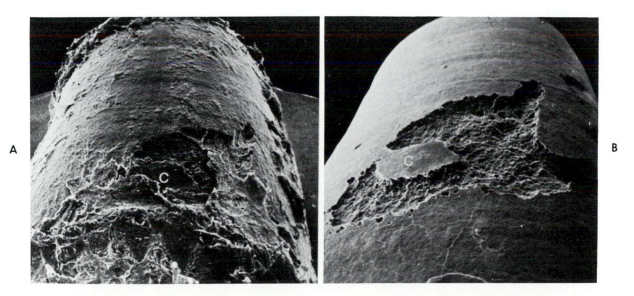

Fig. 2-125   **A,** Resorbed lacunae in the middle third of a root as seen with the scanning electron microscope. *C,* Denuded root surface. Organic tissue components cover the major portion of a lacuna. **B,** Same root surface, previously covered by hyalinized tissue, after removal of organic tissue by NaOCl. Force, 50 g; duration, 35 days. ($\times$ 30.) This type of root resorption never causes any reduction of tooth stability. (Courtesy E. Kvam.)

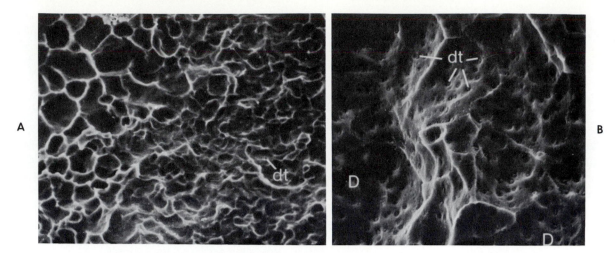

Fig. 2-126 Lacunae in the middle third of the root surface, the effect of resorbing cells on cementum and dentin, as seen with the SEM. **A,** Effect on cementum. The lacunae or cavities produced by cementoclasts are smaller than those observed in the dentin. *S,* Root surface; *dt,* dentinal tubule at the bottom of a lacuna. Removal of organic tissue by 5% NaOCl for 25 hours. Force, 50 g; duration, 35 days. (× 560.) **B,** Remnants of odontoblast processes at *dt. D,* Larger resorbed lacunae produced by dentinoclasts. Force, 50 g; duration, 30 days. Pretreatment by 5% NaOCl for 42 hours. (× 650.) (From Kvam E: *Scand J Dent Res* 80:297, 1972.)

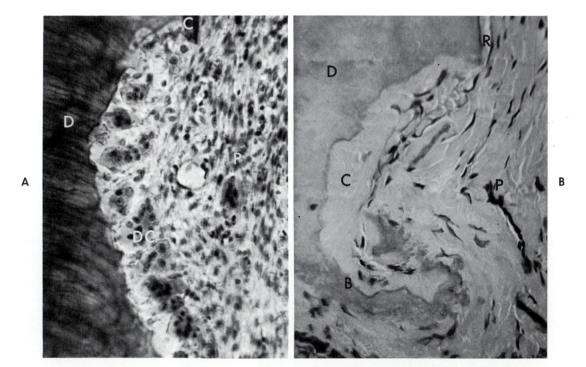

Fig. 2-127 Incidental findings in two 12-year-old patients. **A,** Resorbed lacuna between the marginal and middle thirds of a root. *C,* Cementum; *D,* dentin; *DC,* dentinoclasts. Force, 70 g; duration, 15 days. **B,** Repaired lacuna, apical side resorption. Compare with Fig. 2-122. Force, 70 g, tipping movement for 3 weeks. *A,* Apical portion of the root; *B,* demarcation line; *C,* secondary cementum; *D,* dentin; *P,* periodontal ligament. Repair of the resorbed lacunae may occur rapidly as a result of widening of the periodontal space after bone resorption. Compare with Fig. 2-102, *B.*

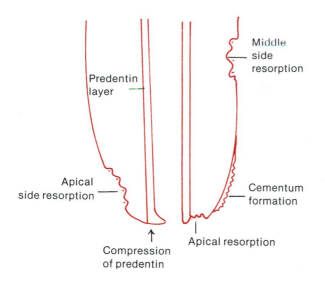

Fig. 2-128 Effects of tooth movement on the root surface of a partly undeveloped tooth. Hyalinization may lead to middle side resorption, which will not interfere with tooth stability. Compression of predentin layers does not prevent further development of the root, provided the pressure is discontinued. Apical side resorption may be reconstructed if it is located only on one side of the root. Small apical resorption lacunae produced in well-calcified tissue are always repaired during the retention period. (From Reitan K: *Angle Orthod* 44:68, 1974.)

dontist may be able to change the method of treatment so that further apical resorption is essentially avoided.

The various reactions on the root surface that may occur during tooth movement are shown in Fig. 2-128. As mentioned, root resorption is usually preceded by a period of hyalinization. In many instances (e.g., after tipping by intermittent forces) there will be insignificant root resorption or none at all. Prolonged tipping or intrusion of the tooth may result in compression of the predentin layers and also in apical root resorption. In practice certain factors tend to determine the degree of root resorption.

Force exerted during tooth movement. The root most frequently resorbed after orthodontic treatment is that of the maxillary lateral incisor. This is occasionally a small root and is frequently located in a lingual position. Bringing such a tooth into alignment by forcing a rectangular arch into bracket engagement may be effective mechanically, but the force may be too strong for the tissue. When the hyalinized zone has been undermined, the apex will be forced against the alveolar bone and the result is a fairly extensive root resorption.[185] Moving the tooth by temporarily inserting one of the light wire configurations used for torque control may prevent such an occurrence. The root may still be resorbed more or less, as shown in Fig. 2-101, *B*, but extensive shortening is less likely to occur.

The tooth movement described exemplifies how root resorption may be stimulated by a bodily movement when the force acting on the tooth is too strong. Contrary to this, it

has been stated previously that a lighter force of the interrupted type is favorable with regard to avoidance of root resorption. Magnitude is thus the critical factor. It has also been shown in several experiments that moving the teeth bodily by light continuous forces may cause less root resorption than a tipping movement.[111,113]

Experiments in the monkey revealed that bodily movement in a distal or mesial direction by light continuous forces may cause an initial hyalinized zone, occasionally followed by a corresponding resorbed lacuna in the middle third of the root[96] (Fig. 2-143). This type of root resorption is insignificant and may be regarded as a normal side effect.[56,110] Further tooth movement may result in the formation of minor resorbed lacunae that will be repaired when the movement is discontinued (Fig. 2-129, *A*).

Size and location of the teeth. It has been shown experimentally that less hyalinization and less root resorption occur after bodily tooth movement.[111] In this respect, one must also consider the size of the teeth. The appliance shown in Fig. 2-130 may move the first molars in either a lateral or a lingual direction. Examination of extracted teeth has shown that root resorption occurs notably in the middle portion of the root and there is also some apical side resorption. Up to the present time, no complete apical shortening has been detected in the teeth being moved. Similar resorption of anchor teeth was observed by Rinderer[127] after widening of the median suture. These observations reveal that there is generally less tendency to apical shortening of molar and premolar teeth (Fig. 2-131).

Duration and direction of tooth movement. The influence of the duration of movement has been recorded in Reitan's experiments. As a rule no root resorption was observed adjacent to the hyalinized zone in short-term experiments. With reference to anterior teeth a distinction must be drawn in this respect between the marginal and middle thirds as compared to the apical region of the root. It was stated previously that frequently more root resorption occurs in the apical third. As shown in Figs. 2-60 and 2-61, a tipping movement of some duration can cause apical resorption even if the force applied is light. In addition, hyalinization in the apical third is of comparatively short duration. If minimal resorption already exists, pressure exerted on the fibrous tissue adjacent to the initially resorbed lacunae tends to maintain and increase the resorption. It can be compared with the continuous resorption process elicited in the root of a lateral incisor by an erupting canine. The pressure exerted is fairly light, but it is acting constantly. If such a tendency exists, the only method for avoiding an extensive resorption is to discontinue tooth movement until the resorbed lacunae have been repaired by cellular cementum. Moving the tooth bodily rather than by tipping may also prevent further root resorption.

It has been emphasized that a light tipping force will move a tooth rapidly. In some cases this can be done without much root resorption. It should be noted, however, that there is more root resorption in some patients than in others.

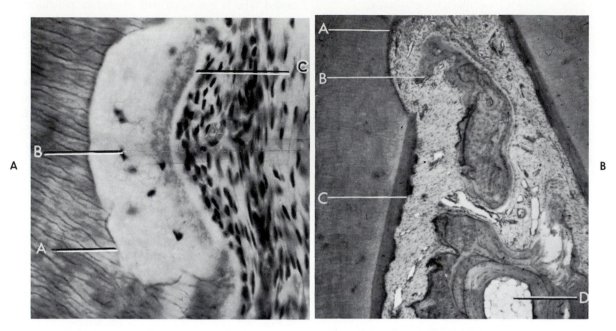

Fig. 2-129 **A,** Minor resorbed lacunae of the root surface are reconstructed by cellular cementum. *A,* Demarcation line between dentin and new cementum containing mucopolysaccharides; *B,* cementoblasts incorporated in newly formed cementum; *C,* cementoid line bordered by a chain of cementoblasts. **B,** Bifurcation area of the anchor tooth (a lower first molar) in a monkey. *A,* Root resorption partly repaired but less than usual because new bone, *B,* has been formed earlier than the cellular cementum, which accounts for the irregular outline of the periodontal space; *C,* a series of minor resorbed lacunae in the root surface, frequently observed in the roots of monkey teeth used for anchorage; *D,* space containing fatty marrow.

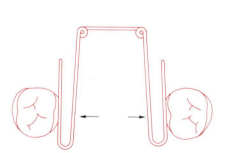

Fig. 2-130 Appliance for continuous bodily movement of molars (and occasionally also second premolars), either as initial treatment of a crossbite or combined with conventional labial arch treatment. Initial force acting on each molar is 150 to 200 g, which may be increased when the bands are recemented. It is an advantage to perform spot grinding of interfering cusps. The appliance can also be used for lingual movement of teeth in the upper as well as lower jaw.

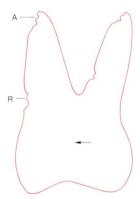

Fig. 2-131 Resorbed areas in a molar subjected to continuous bodily movement. Lacunae will be repaired during the retention period. Limiting the initial force to 150 to 200 g may prevent shortening of the apical portion. *A,* Apical side resorption; *R,* side resorption.

Once an apical resorption is started, the process may be rapidly increased as the tooth is constantly tipped. In such cases the patient cannot discern the difference between root resorption and bone resorption. Any feeling of pain is absent, since the periodontal ligament is less compressed and has become widened by the resorption process.

If apical resorption is started and the tipping movement is acting constantly, the root may be shortened appreciably within 2 to 3 months. It may thus be stated that the fairly painless and rapid tipping movement really constitutes the type of tooth displacement that may cause a considerable degree of root resorption. However, this is also the type of root resorption that may be clearly observed radiographically. Systematic radiographic examination is important and may enable the orthodontist to modify the technique so any extensive apical root resorption is avoided.

The time factor. The time during which the appliances are acting may influence root resorption also in other respects. The orthodontist may occasionally note that root resorption has increased appreciably after an active treatment period of several months. This may be explained by the fact that the periodontal fibers surrounding the apical portion of the roots will become gradually more compressed or stretched (Fig. 2-113). Pressure is then exerted against any existing resorbed areas of the root, accelerating the resorption process.[118]

This type of root resorption can be observed particularly when teeth (e.g., upper lateral incisors) are moved bodily and continuously over a large distance. Again the rest periods may be valuable if the definite tendency is toward a shortening of the apical root portion. It has also been observed that formation of new cementum occurs more rapidly when the resorbed tooth is left in such a position that a certain degree of physiologic movement is provided. Occasionally, this reconstruction will lead to an irregular outline of the periodontal space. Since the periodontal ligament has a tendency to maintain its physiologic width, it may be observed, particularly in the bifurcation areas of molars, that relatively little secondary cementum is formed after root resorption. As shown in Fig. 2-129, *B*, a protruding bone spicule has been formed whereby the width of the periodontal space is maintained. This end result of bone and cementum formation will in no way cause any reduction of the functional stability of the tooth.

Practical significance of root resorption. No weakening in the function and stability of the individual tooth occurs as long as the resorbed lacunae are confined to the marginal and middle thirds of the root. Only apical root resorption is an injury that can imperil the stability and normal function of the tooth. The problem is to avoid any increase in the resorption process that may shorten the root. This can be done by periodic radiographic examination of such types of tooth movement in which the orthodontist may expect an increased likelihood of apical root resorption. The following are some of the types of tooth movement that may lead to apical root resorption:

1. Prolonged tipping, notably of anterior teeth
2. Distal tipping of molars, causing resorption particularly of the distal roots of the molars (Gradual tipping of these teeth by light interrupted forces may reduce the tendency to root resorption.)
3. Prolonged continuous bodily movement of small teeth, such as upper lateral incisors (Interrupted movement, or continuous movement with rest periods, may diminish the occurrence of this type of root resorption.)
4. Intrusion (It is important to initiate the intruding movement by forces as light as 25 g. Frequent rest periods will prevent any extensive resorption.)
5. Extensive edgewise torque of anterior teeth in the more mature young and adult patients (This question is discussed further under "The age factor.")

Apical root resorption. Experiments have revealed that the anatomic environment constitutes an important factor during tipping movement and intrusion.[124] If the cementoid and predentin layers are fairly thick, there will be no apical root resorption following an experimental period of three or four weeks' duration (Fig. 2-48). If the root surface is well calcified and the predentin layer is thin, tipping movement may lead to resorption of the outer side of the apical portion as well as along the inside of the root canal (Fig. 2-132). The apical side resorption is preceded by a short hyalinization period. In some individuals this type of resorption occurs rapidly. Repair and reconstruction of the resorbed root substance will occur provided the apical area (marked *A*) is preserved and further movement is performed in a different way (e.g., a bodily movement).

The internal type of apical resorption is initiated after pressure is exerted by foraminal soft tissue against the root canal wall, notably when the foramen is fairly wide and more or less devoid of predentin layers. Whether the internal resorption is preceded by a hyalinization period has not been determined experimentally, but it is not unlikely that some fibers along the foraminal wall will become cell free as a result of prolonged compression. Resorption occurs by dentinoclasts located in fairly shallow lacunae.

As shown in Fig. 2-48, the root substance of developing teeth is liable to undergo tissue changes not unlike those observed in bone. Resorption and deposition of uncalcified tissue occur during tooth movement (Fig. 2-133).

In the age group up to 16 to 17 years, the anatomic environment, as well as the duration and direction of the movement, constitutes the determining factor in apical root resorption (Fig. 2-134). Experimental evidence has shown that the tissue reaction in adults is different in some respects.

The age factor. It is generally assumed (but only partly true) that adult patients will experience more root resorption after treatment than will younger patients. The adult supporting structures react somewhat differently when compared with young tissues because the anatomic environment (e.g., the type of alveolar bone) in adults is different.

The periodontal structures of adults, particularly the labial and lingual bony plates (Fig. 2-6), are composed of a dense lamellated bone tissue with relatively small marrow

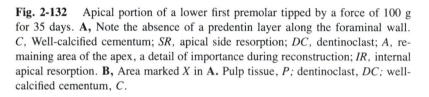
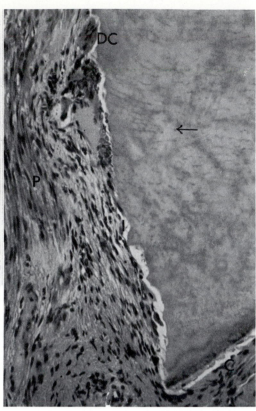

Fig. 2-132   Apical portion of a lower first premolar tipped by a force of 100 g for 35 days. **A,** Note the absence of a predentin layer along the foraminal wall. *C,* Well-calcified cementum; *SR,* apical side resorption; *DC,* dentinoclast; *A,* remaining area of the apex, a detail of importance during reconstruction; *IR,* internal apical resorption. **B,** Area marked *X* in **A.** Pulp tissue, *P;* dentinoclast, *DC;* well-calcified cementum, *C.*

spaces.[122] Spongy bone exists in the interseptal areas; therefore tooth movement in a mesiodistal direction within the "alveolar trough" is more favorable than that in a labiolingual direction. Along the inner alveolar bone surface of adults are a series of darkly stained resting lines, indicating that only minor tissue changes have occurred over a long time (Fig. 2-6). In the periodontal ligament the cells are mostly fibrocytes with small nuclei. There are few osteoblasts along the bone surface. The root exhibits a thick layer of cementum with some cementoblasts.

This last observation, the thick cementum layers and strong apical fibers of the root, will also influence the tooth movement. The apical third of the root is more firmly anchored in adult patients than it is in young patients (Fig. 2-13). Hence, when an adult tooth is tipped over a short distance, there is comparatively little movement of the apical third of the root. On the other hand, if the tipping is prolonged, the tooth will begin to act as a two-armed lever. There may be apical resorption, and there is frequently destruction of the alveolar bone wall as well.

It has been observed in Reitan's adult material[122] that the alveolar bone surface was predominantly aplastic before the experiments, indicating that the periodontal structures were in a state of rest. This was substantiated by the moderate number of cells (Fig. 2-6). Also the fibrous tissue reacted more slowly. Thus the turnover rate of collagen molecules are, in general, slower in adults than in growing children,[147] which difference is also reflected in the delayed onset of

tissue changes in adults during tooth movement. In these experiments it took more than 8 days for the tissues to attain what has been termed *the proliferation stage.* This cell proliferation is elicited by applying light forces, preferably 30 to 40 g, during the initial movement of individual teeth.[122]

In one experimental series a tipping force of 50 g caused hyalinization on the pressure side in a zone between the marginal and middle thirds of the root that lasted for approximately 2 weeks. A significant change also occurred on the pressure side at the end of the initial period, when the hyalinized tissue had been eliminated by undermining resorption. A great number of connective tissue cells had been formed in and around the formerly hyalinized area (Fig. 2-37, *A*). No root resorption occurred. The periodontal ligament on the pressure side was fairly wide, a finding that might be attributable to the resistance exerted by stretched fiber bundles on the tension side. As a result of the firm anchorage of the apical root portion, direct bone resorption was observed all along the root surface (Fig. 2-12).

These findings indicate that the apical third of the adult root does not move in the opposite direction after a short-term tipping movement. Although supporting structures of adult teeth are in a state of rest before the experiment, they will attain a proliferation stage at the end of the first 2 weeks of tooth movement. The proliferation stage is manifested by an increase in cellular elements on the pressure side, as well as on the tension side. It is the application of a light force that leads to this significant change in the anatomic

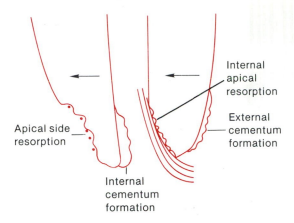

Fig. 2-133   Various types of resorption and apposition that may occur in the apical third of the root during experimental tipping of a tooth. The coronal portion was moved in the opposite direction.

environment (Fig. 2-135). It was, furthermore, shown that an adult tooth may be moved as readily, even when its pulp structures have been removed.

Application of a light force also constitutes the important step as regards avoidance of root resorption. Adult teeth must be moved carefully during the initial stage. Occlusal stress must be prevented. If these precautions are taken, tooth movement in an adult does not necessarily lead to root resorption.

It was observed in a 35-year-old patient that the right upper premolar had been shortened by malfunctional oc-

clusal stress. The patient had an unfavorable occlusion of long duration. On the left side the corresponding premolar was moved bodily and interruptedly by orthodontic forces over a distance of 5 mm to create space for the subsequent construction of a bridge. No resorption of this root could be observed on the radiograph (Fig. 2-136). The initial force was 40 g, which was gradually increased to the range of 100 to 150 g. This illustrates that, after a carefully planned initial period, adult teeth may be moved almost as readily as those of children. On the other hand, a persisting occlusal load may cause shortening of the root, even if the tooth is not moved orthodontically.

Apical root resorption in adults. One of the anatomic characteristics of adult teeth is the thick cementum layers of the apical third of the root. This cementum is in many respects more resistant to root resorption than that of children.

Nevertheless, this rule has exceptions. Although canines and premolars may be moved bodily without any perceptible tendency to root resorption, incisor teeth may react differently. In particular, a movement of intrusion must be performed carefully in adults. Rest intervals are important. The lamina dura of the apical region in adult teeth is frequently denser and the periodontal ligament somewhat narrower than in children's teeth (Fig. 2-5). A careful examination of the radiographs is always important during intrusion of adult teeth. It is frequently observed that after a successful initial period, adult teeth may be intruded without any perceptible shortening of the roots. The intruding force must then be light and frequently interrupted by rest periods.

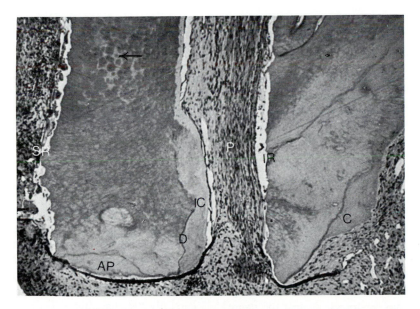

Fig. 2-134   Apical portion of a premolar during tipping in a 16-year-old patient. Force, 100 g; duration, 40 days. The crown of the tooth was moved in the opposite direction. *SR*, Side resorption; *IR*, internal resorption; *P*, pulp tissue; *IC*, internal cementum formed during the experimental period; *AP*, cementum formed in the apical portion of the root; *C*, cementum formed on the tension side of the root; *D*, demarcation line between dentin and the new cementum.

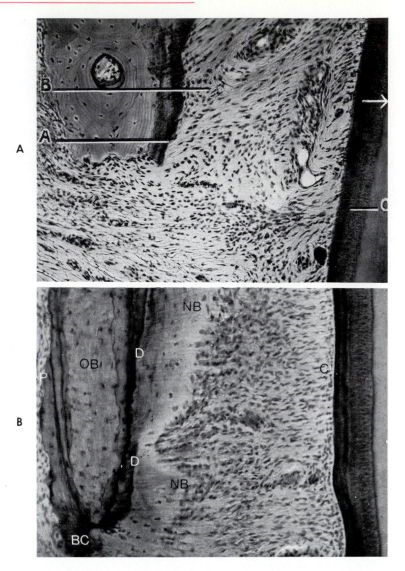

Fig. 2-135   Tension side; tipping movement in a 39-year-old patient. **A,** Force, 50 g; duration 4 days. *A,* Bone surface still devoid of osteoblasts and osteoid; *B,* slight increase in the number of cells; *C,* cementum surface with few cementoblasts. Note the dense bone with a large haversian system. Resorption at the alveolar bone crest is a finding characteristic of many adult cases. **B,** Force, 50 g; duration, 3 weeks. As compared with young tissues (Fig. 2-41, *B*), the new bone layer is more dense because it is laid down along thick fiber bundles of the periodontal ligament. *C,* Formation of cementoblasts; *NB,* new bone layer with osteoid laid down along stretched fiber bundles; *BC,* alveolar bone crest; *OB,* old bone; *P,* periosteal bone surface; *D,* demarcation line between old and new bone.

Torque in adults. A similar method may be applied for torque of anterior teeth in adults. A routine torque by conventional edgewise arches is not always the recommended method. In the anterior region of adult teeth the labial and lingual bony walls are frequently thin and dense (Fig. 2-5). If the movement of torque is not performed carefully, the apices of these teeth may be forced against the dense alveolar bone, with shortening of the roots as the result. It is essential that the initial period of tooth movement be carried out with light force and rest intervals. Thus a thin edgewise arch is preferable for torque movement in adults.

Light wire torque may lead to root resorption as well if the force is acting over too long a period. To avoid root resorption, the best technical solution would be to apply a light torquing force that acted interruptedly (i.e., over a short distance). No routine method is available. Every patient must be treated individually. It is necessary to examine carefully the anatomic environment as revealed on the radiographs. The subsequent technical procedures must be based on these observations. Radiographic examination must be undertaken at intervals as long as the torque movement is active.

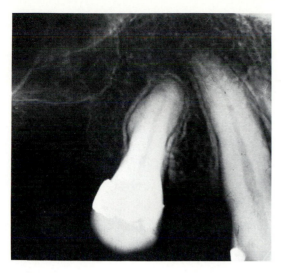

Fig. 2-136 First premolar moved bodily in an adult before construction of bridgework. No perceptible shortening of the apical portion. Note the rearrangement of the bone with the formation of new lamina dura.

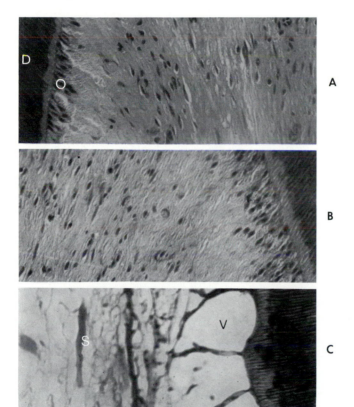

Fig. 2-137 Pulp reactions during tooth movement. **A,** Premolar intruded in a 12-year-old patient. Force, 30 g interrupted after 2 weeks. *O,* Slight reaction of the odontoblast layer, no marked vacuolization; *D,* dentin. **B,** Premolar with a fully developed apical portion in a 16-year-old patient. Extrusion for 4 weeks; force, 25 g. No definite changes occurred in the pulp tissue. **C,** Premolar with open apical foramen force, 80 g in an 11-year-old patient. Intrusion for 5 weeks; *V,* Vacuolization of osteoblast layer; *S,* stasis of the capillaries.

Pulp changes during tooth movement. It has been known for many years that cavity preparation and orthodontic treatment will cause certain changes in the pulp tissue—alterations that cannot be reproduced as readily in teeth of experimental animals. As demonstrated by Stenvik[168] and Stenvik and Mjør,[169] vacuolization of the odontoblast layer constitutes the most characteristic tissue alteration. After intrusion of teeth in young individuals, it was shown that a force of 90 g would cause a marked reaction with apical resorption as well as pulp alterations.

In Reitan's material it was found that a certain difference existed when the apical root portion was fully developed. Less vacuolization occurred in these cases and less marked pulp reactions were observed after tooth movement with interrupted forces (Fig. 2-137). These teeth were all moved with fixed appliances for a certain period.

On the basis of what has been observed experimentally, it is likely that all teeth moved with fixed appliances will undergo certain pulp alterations. The importance of the time factor is stressed by the fact that pulp injuries are absent during tooth movement with removable appliances. In all instances a borderline may be drawn between the small group of teeth that will become devitalized and all the other teeth that in spite of pulp alterations remain vital. Devitalization may occur when the pulp structures have become degraded after insertion of deep cavity fillings or when the teeth moved orthodontically have been subjected to trauma or severe pressure before the treatment period. Examination of the pulp status by electric testing may be indicated in such cases.[108]

RELAPSE AND RETENTION

Up to the present, histologic studies in orthodontics have been based essentially on observations of the tissue response that occurs during orthodontic treatment. The other side of the problem, the reaction of the supporting tissues that becomes manifest at various periods after the appliances have been removed, has not been investigated to a similar extent. Most of the authors of orthodontic textbooks, from Angle's time to the present, have not included chapters on relapse and retention in their publications. More recent discussions of the relapse problem,[37,46,78] however, have been published. (See Chapter 16.)

Interesting facts were shown by Krebs[67] regarding relapse movement after the widening of the median suture (Fig. 2-138). Likewise, Joho[60] observed remodeling of bone surfaces and relapse changes after application of a continuous extraoral force on the mandible in young monkeys (Fig. 2-139). Riedel[126] stated, "We find that orthodontists have come to realize that retention is not an item apart from treatment, but that it is a part of treatment itself and must be included in the treatment planning." Thus histologic investigation of the relapse and retention problem must be considered so that some factors that were previously discussed on the basis of practical observations can be elucidated.

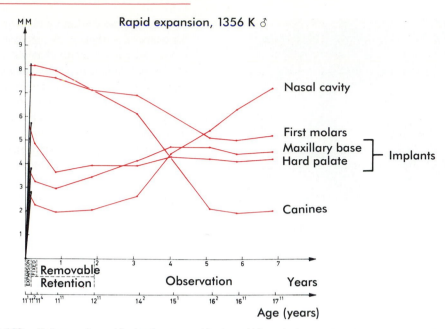

Fig. 2-138 Relapse after midpalatal suture widening. Although the nasal cavity has increased in width, the canines reveal the greatest degree of relapse movement. (From Krebs A: *Eur Orthod Soc Trans* 40:131, 1964.)

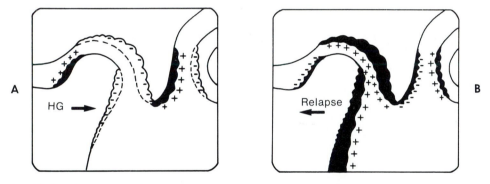

Fig. 2-139 Relapse and bone remodeling after continuous extraoral movement of the mandible in a young *Macaca mulatta*. **A,** Extensive bone resorption in the glenoid fossa. *HG* indicates the direction of extraoral movement during the experimental period; plus symbols indicate bone deposition, minus symbols bone resorption. **B,** Bone remodeling during the postexperimental period, with reverse changes possibly caused by the reaction of ligaments and muscles. (From Joho JP: *Am J Orthod* 64:555, 1973.)

In clinical studies dealing with stabilization of tooth position during the posttreatment period, it has become customary to enumerate certain factors, some of which have been considered essential in the prevention of relapse. Not all these factors, however, can be regarded as equally important, at least not under all circumstances. Thus if muscular imbalance is absent, it is definitely true that a well-established intercuspation may greatly assist in maintaining the end result of tooth movement. In other cases establishing the most precise intercuspal relationship between the dental arches will not prevent relapse from occurring if a strongly adverse muscular pressure exists. Muscle function, therefore, must be regarded as a dominant factor; however, the ensuing discussion will demonstrate exceptions to this rule.

Muscle behavior. In a chapter on the periodontal tissue reaction, muscle function should be dealt with only briefly as an introduction to the posttreatment reaction of the periodontal structures. (See Chapter 13.)

To what extent can increased muscle pressure influence tooth position? According to investigations by Weinstein et al.,[184] even a moderate increase in the thickness of the buccal or lingual surfaces of a tooth can lead to a certain degree of tooth movement. These authors attached gold onlay extensions, 2 mm thick, to the buccal or lingual surfaces of premolars, thus increasing their thickness. After 8 weeks the premolars had moved respectively either lingually or buccally. In one instance a lower premolar moved as much as 0.033 inch (0.84 mm) in a lingual direction. It is interesting to note that the estimated muscle force acting on the protruding onlay extensions ranged only between 3 and 7 g. This therefore constituted a type of gentle intermittent force that could hardly be duplicated by any appliance construction.

As shown in the graphs by Weinstein et al.[184] direct bone resorption occurred on the pressure side of the experimental teeth. The experiments thus demonstrated that, in children, a minor increase in the muscle tension may influence the tooth position more or less in the form of a gradual migration, not unlike that observed in physiologic tooth movement.

The importance of the muscle balance that exists between the tongue on one side and the muscles surrounding the dental arches on the other side has been emphasized by Ballard,[5] Graber,[45,46] Gwynne-Evans and Tulley,[50] Müller,[95] Rix,[128] and others. Observations of tongue function have disclosed that the posttreatment position of the tongue may be appreciably altered according to how thoroughly the orthodontic treatment has been carried out. This applies particularly to teeth of the buccal segments. No halfway measures are sufficient if a lasting change in tongue position is to be obtained. It is also important to insert a removable retention plate to be used for a certain period.

Generally the anterior teeth will react differently.[46,50] In spite of a precise positioning by fixed appliances and even after a retention period, these teeth will frequently tend to migrate toward their original positions when adverse muscular pressure exists. This untoward effect is caused partly by the smaller size of the teeth and partly by the fact that upper anterior teeth that were previously protruding are not maintained in position by the intercuspation. It is well known that relapse occurs particularly where strong tongue function and a weak orbicularis muscle complex are present.

It has been pointed out under "Functional type of intermittent forces" (p. 133) that the muscles may be subjected to a certain degree of myofunctional therapy after application of appliances such as the activator, which will control the tongue function. The favorable effect of this myofunctional therapy may become manifest when such an appliance is used for retention after treatment with fixed appliances. A similar type of appliance may be applied for the control of muscle function during retention of an open bite. In certain difficult cases it may be advisable for the patient to wear the appliance every night for 2 or 3 years.

The time factor. As already mentioned, a persistent muscular imbalance combined with rearrangement of displaced fibrous tissue may change the tooth position rapidly (Fig. 2-139). In many cases it is therefore important to insert the retention appliances as soon as possible. A clear acrylic plate may be constructed on the model and inserted within a few hours after removal of the fixed appliances. It will be necessary to grind the interior surfaces of the plate contiguous to teeth and tissues in certain places to prevent spacing of the teeth and leave space for further alignment of individual teeth. If necessary, a stronger type of *invisible* retention plate may be constructed later on.[107]

Reaction of the periodontal structures. The eruptional force exerted by mesially inclined third molars on the second and first molars and on other teeth of the lower jaw constitutes another problem. It has been found that this migration may cause post-treatment crowding of the anterior teeth in patients aged 20 to 30 years. On the other hand, observation of adult extraction cases has revealed that first and second molars continued to migrate mesially, while lower third molars, and notably those in a horizontal position, moved less. Thus, in adult patients examined 20 years after treatment (age 50 or more), the eruptional force was decreased. The third molars were no longer in contact with the second molars.

Although our concept of relapse caused by muscle function is based essentially on clinical observations, the posttreatment reaction of the periodontal fiber system has been demonstrated by experimental evidence. Reitan's experiments, conducted on human and animal material, showed that a certain contraction and rearrangement of fibrous structures occurs in every case and varies according to the type and degree of tooth movement. Investigations of this difference in fibrous tissue reaction have been based partly on measurement of the posttreatment changes in tooth position and partly on histologic examination of the structures involved. The contraction of displaced and stretched fibrous structures is less pronounced in some areas of the supporting tissues than in others. A marked reaction occurs in two areas: (1) the fibrous structures of the newly formed bone, including the principal fibers of the periodontal ligament; and (2) the supraalveolar and transseptal fibrous system (Figs. 2-1 and 2-144). (See Chapter 13.)

Posttreatment changes in new bone layers. It has been found that the reactive changes after tooth movement vary according to the anatomic environment. For example, consider an erupting second premolar that is brought gradually into position after extraction of the first premolar. In this case the fibrous structures of the bone will remain relaxed and rearranged according to the new position of the tooth that is moved. After treatment the three teeth—canine, second premolar, and first molar—will remain in contact and there will be little or no tendency to secondary migration. Thus relapse of the teeth approximated after extraction may be largely avoided by early treatment during tooth eruption and alveolar bone growth (Fig. 2-86, *A*).

However, when fully erupted teeth have been approximated after extraction, a certain tendency to secondary changes in tooth position is always present. The cause of this relapse is contraction of stretched fibrous structures, which occurs not only in the supraalveolar tissue but also as a result of early rearrangement of Sharpey's fibers in the newly formed bundle bone, as well as the principal fibers in the periodontal ligament. Unlike the supraalveolar structures, however, the fibrous tissue of the new bone and the periodontal ligament will be rearranged after a fairly short retention period (Fig. 2-105).

Removable appliances. During treatment with removable appliances a tooth that is moved always has a minor daily relapse. The new bone is laid down as a layer parallel to the old bone, and the periodontal fiber bundles remain relaxed (Fig. 2-57). Relapse after extensive expansion with removable appliances is caused by gradual contraction of various tissue elements, the effect of which may not become manifest for 1 or 2 years. Secondary changes in the new bone then occur as a result of this tissue contraction.

Fixed appliances. Relapse caused by immediate contraction of fibrous structures adjacent to the middle and apical thirds of the root is observed notably after a rapid and extensive movement of the tooth.

It has been found that stretched fiber bundles on the tension side tend to become functionally arranged (i.e., relaxed and rearranged according to the physiologic movement of the tooth). Fig. 2-17, A, illustrates the physiologic arrangement of the principal fibers and the fibrous structures of the adjacent bone layers in a control specimen. Since Sharpey's fibers of the periodontal ligament are incorporated in the bundle bone, these constitute a more or less continuous fibrous system (Fig. 2-16, A). Comparison with the arrangement of the stretched fibrous tissue of newly formed

spicules reveals why it will become necessary to retain a tooth until rearrangement of the structures involved has occurred (Figs. 2-41, A, and 2-135, B).

During retention, which also occurs when the fixed appliances are left passively in situ, new bone will fill in the spaces between the bone spicules (Fig. 2-104, C). Experiments on rotation have shown that rearrangement of principal fibers and new bone layers occurs quite rapidly. Most of the periodontal fibers and the fibers of the adjacent bone will become rearranged after a retention period of only 2 to 3 months. It has been shown in animal experiments that this newly rearranged bone layer may attain a texture more dense than that of the bone in a physiologic state[119] (Fig. 2-143, B). For a certain period this new dense bone will prevent further relapse of the tooth moved. The effect of the retention is noted particularly after reuprighting of teeth that were previously tipped (Fig. 2-140, B). Relatively little relapse tendency exists in the area adjacent to the middle and apical third of teeth that have been reuprighted and maintained in that new position for 5 to 6 months.

The degree of relapse of the marginal and apical portions of the root, when a tooth was tipped and not retained, is shown in Fig. 2-141. A different relapse movement was observed after a lower canine was retracted bodily and then left without retention.[96] As a result of the ensuing contraction of all the tension side fibers, a new bone layer was formed on the pressure side (Fig. 2-142). The amount of new bone indicates how far the tooth was moved as a result of this reactive movement. The even thickness of the new bone layer all along the apical third of the root indicates that contraction of the middle and apical fibers also contributed to the reactive movement (Fig. 2-143). Not infrequently this contraction of principal fibers results in the formation of a hyalinized zone on the tension side between the middle and apical thirds of the root. To attain rearrangement of the structures involved and to prevent relapse, the tooth must be retained for a certain time. In most cases the retention can be effected partly by leaving the fixed appliances passive on the teeth.

In some cases it may be practical to retain certain teeth by bonded wire sections, such as the lower second premolars (particularly in patients who are in a higher age range) after closure of spaces left by extraction of first premolars. If the second premolars have been in infraclusion before treatment, there is usually a strong tendency to a fibrous tissue contraction after extrusion.

The apical base. Several authors[13,151] have called attention to the anatomic and morphologic arrangement of the alveolar structures. The circumferential lamellae of the bone and the supporting fibrous tissues are so arranged as to withstand any greater tooth movement in a labial or lingual direction. When moved into imbalance, these structures tend to contract and relapse occurs.[78] This reactive movement of the teeth that are moved becomes dominant, particularly after expansion of the dental arches. In this connection *the apical base* concept has given rise to a cardinal principle of ortho-

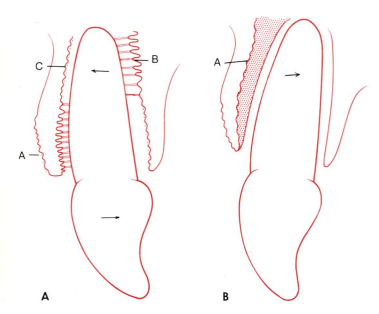

Fig. 2-140   Two stages of light wire treatment. **A,** Lingual tipping of an anterior tooth. *A,* Compensatory bone resorption; *B,* new bone formed adjacent to the middle and apical thirds of the root; *C,* bone resorption. **B,** After uprighting and retention a new bone layer may largely prevent any tendency to initial relapse of the tooth moved. *A,* Reversal line between old bone and the new bone layer.

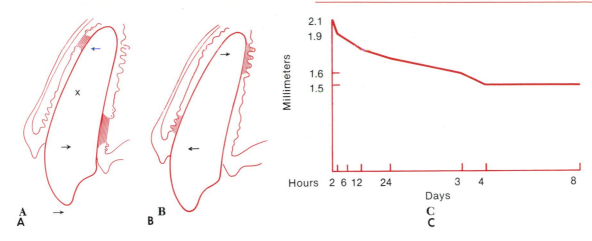

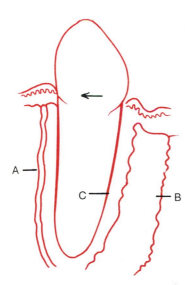

Fig. 2-141   **A,** Formation of hyalinized areas during tooth movement of an upper second incisor in a dog. Duration, 40 days. **B,** Formation of hyalinized areas during the relapse period. The tooth was not retained after movement. **C,** Relapse movement during a period of 8 days (tooth **B**). Hyalinization occurred after 4 days. (From Reitan K: *Am J Orthod* 53:721, 1967.)

dontic philosophy—if relapse is to be avoided, the treatment of malocclusion must not be based on expansion. The apical base concept is correct as a principle. However, a detailed observation of the behavior of the structures involved may disclose that after retention the tendency to relapse is less in the apical base area than in the structures of the marginal third of the root.

Torque of the root may be performed in either a labial or a lingual direction. A gradual torque movement, and also tipping of the tooth, may result in compensatory bone for-

Fig. 2-142   Tissue changes after bodily retraction of a lower canine in a monkey. Continuous force, approximately 120 g. *A,* New bone layer formed during the relapse period; *B,* resting line indicating the amount of new bone formed as a result of the movement; *C,* area of the periodontal ligament in which traces of a hyalinized zone were observed in some of the sections caused by the relapse movement. (From Mulligan W, Niewold BDL: Thesis, University of Texas, 1962.)

mation along the outer bone surface corresponding to the apical third of the tooth (Figs. 2-73 and 2-74). If the torque or tipping movement is carried out rapidly, the apical portion of the root may be moved through the bone and partly outside of the apical bone.[118] A root that has been moved through the bone tends to remain outside the bony area. As in a bodily movement, rearrangement and calcification of the new bone spicules on the tension side will result in a fairly dense bone tissue, which initially resists any appreciable degree of relapse (Fig. 2-143). The most persistent relapse tendency is caused by the structures related to the marginal third of the root.

From a practical standpoint it may thus be stated that only when retention is omitted does any appreciable relapse tendency exist in the bone adjacent to the apical base area.

Posttreatment changes in the supraalveolar structure. The free gingival and transseptal fibers, which some decades ago were termed the *circular ligament*, seem to have a special function. They are more active than other fibers in maintaining the tooth in its proper position (Fig. 2-144). The free gingival fibers interlace with the supraalveolar soft tissues of the proximal teeth and thus form a continuous fibrous system (Fig. 2-2). In addition, elastic and oxytalan fibers are present in the supraalveolar tissue. These elastic fibers will add to the contractive force of the fibrous system after displacement or stretch.[113]

The effect of this contraction is observed on the tension side of the tooth, particularly when the tooth is tipped or rotated. If a tooth is tipped and not retained at all, even surgical removal of the supraalveolar tissue does not prevent some relapse from occurring. Fiber bundles of the middle and apical thirds of the root will then enter into action.[114] The effect caused by contraction of the principal and the supraalveolar fibers is shown in Fig. 2-141. The crown of the experimental tooth was moved 2 mm by tipping during a period of 40 days. After the tooth had been released, the

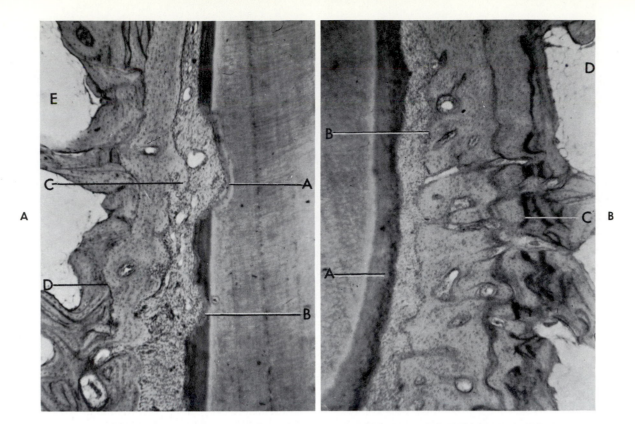

Fig. 2-143 Animal experiment seen in Fig. 2-142. **A,** Pressure side. *A* and *B,* Root resorption lacunae partly repaired by cellular cementum; *C,* osteoid formed during the relapse period; *D,* reversal line, indicating thickness of the new bone layer formed during the relapse period; *E,* marrow space. **B,** Tension side. *A,* Cementum of the root surface; *B,* resorption in circumscribed area of the newly formed bone layer; in some sections, traces of hyalinized tissue were observed slightly below area *B; C,* darkly stained resting line indicating thickness of the new bone layer; *D,* space containing fatty marrow. Further relapse is prevented by the fairly dense bone layer formed on the tension side. (From Mulligan W, Niewold BDL: Thesis, University of Texas, 1962.)

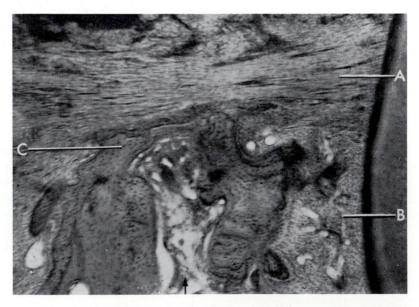

Fig. 2-144 Area of the alveolar crest in a monkey. **A,** Transseptal and free gingival fibers; note the difference in texture of these fibers as compared with the more relaxed principal fibers *(B); C,* alveolar crest bone; arrow indicates the marrow spaces. Similar supraalveolar fibers may be observed in humans (Figs. 2-2 and 2-83, *A*).

degree of relapse movement was recorded graphically (Fig. 2-141). It was noted that some relapse occurred even after 2 hours. This was partly caused by the tooth's regaining a more upright position within the periodontal space. Still more relapse occurred on the following days—in all, approximately 0.5 mm during 4 days. At this moment the tooth had apparently come to a standstill. Histologic examination revealed that this was caused by hyalinization on the tension sides. The experiment shows that fiber contraction may be strong enough to produce hyalinization.

Similar hyalinized areas may be observed as a result of tipping of human teeth without subsequent retention. An example is shown in Fig. 2-145. It is noted again that most of the relapse occurred during the first 5 hours after the appliances had been removed. This relapse tendency constitutes a challenge to the practitioner. Rearrangement of the alveolar bone and the principal fibers occurs when the fixed appliances are left on the teeth for at least 2 months. The supraalveolar structures, however will not become rearranged until the tooth has regained its physiologic equilibrium.

Overcorrection of the tooth position. Retention of rotated teeth may illustrate the effect of the persistent displacement of the supraalveolar fibrous tissue (Fig. 2-100). Rearrangement of the bone and principal fibers occurs adjacent to the middle and apical thirds of the root, but not in the supraalveolar region. Clinical experience has shown that overcorrection may partly solve this problem. Because of the tendency to relapse, certain precautions may be recommended even if the tooth involved has been overrotated.[35,119] Insertion of an *invisible* acrylic plate would be one of these

alternatives. Such plates can be worn in the upper and lower jaw. They cover all the teeth: the lingual and the buccal side. When used regularly for a long time, they will add appreciably to the stabilization of the tooth moved.

It would also be an advantage to perform the treatment while the patient is young. New fibers developed in the apical portion of the root would then assist in maintaining the teeth in its new position.

REFERENCES

1. Ahlgren J: An electromyographic analysis of the response to activators (Andresen-Häupl therapy), *Odontol Rev* 11:125, 1960.
2. Atherton JD: The gingival response to orthodontic tooth movement, *Am J Orthod* 58:179, 1970.
3. Aubin JE, Heersche JNM et al: Isolation of bone cells clones with differences in growth, hormone responses, and extracellular matrix production, *J Cell Biol* 92:452, 1982.
4. Avery J: *Histology and embryology.* In Shapiro M: *The scientific bases of dentistry,* Philadelphia, 1966, WB Saunders, p. 57.
5. Ballard CF: A consideration of the physiological background of mandibular posture and movement, *Dent Prac* 6:80, 1955.
6. Bassett CF, Pawluk RJ, Becker RO: Effects of electric currents on bone in vivo, *Nature* 204:652, 1964.
7. Baume LL, Derechsweiler H: Is the condylar growth center responsive to orthodontic therapy? An experimental study in *Macaca mulatta, Oral Surg* 14:347, 1961.
8. Baumrind S: A reconsideration of the propriety of the "pressure-tension" hypothesis, *Am J Orthod* 55:12, 1969.
9. Baumrind S, Buck DL: Rate changes in cell replication and protein synthesis in the periodontal ligament incident to tooth movement, *Am J Orthod* 57:109, 1970.
10. Becks H: Root resorption and its relation to pathologic bone formation, *Int J Orthod* 22:445, 1936.
11. Beeson DC, Johnston LE, Wisotzky J: Effect of constant currents on orthodontic tooth movement in the cat, *J Dent Res* 54:251, 1975.
12. Bélanger L, Migicovsky BB: Histochemical evidence of proteolysis in bone: the influence of parathormone, *J Histochem Cytochem* 11:734, 1963.
13. Benninghoff A: Die Architektur der Kiefer und ihre Weichteilbedeckung, *Paradentium* 6:48, 1934.
14. Bien SM: Fluid dynamic mechanisms which regulate tooth movement, *Adv Oral Biol* 2:173, 1966.
15. Binderman I, Zor U et al: The transduction of mechanical force into biochemical events in bone cells may involve activation of phospholipase A_2, *Calcified Tissue Int* 42:261, 1988.
16. Bjørk A: The principles of the Andresen Method of orthodontic treatment, *Am J Orthod* 37:437, 1951.
17. Bjørk A: Bite development and body build, *Dent Rec* 75:8, 1955.
18. Bjørk A: Sutural growth of the upper face studied by the implant method, *Europ Orthod Soc Trans* 40:49, 1964.
19. Bosch HVD: Intracellular phospholipases, *Biochem Biophys Acta* 604:191, 1980.
20. Bowling K, Rygh P: A quantitative study of oxytalan fibers in the transseptal region and tension zones of rat molars following orthodontic movement, *Eur J Orthod* 10:13, 1988.
21. Boyle PE, editor: *Kronfeld's histopathology of the teeth and their surrounding structures,* ed 4, Philadelphia, 1955, Lea & Febiger, p. 16.
22. Brain WE: The effect of surgical transsection of free gingival fibers on the regression of orthodontically rotated teeth in the dog, *Am J Orthod* 55:50, 1969.
23. Breitner C: Experimentelle Veranderung der mesiodistalen Beziehungen der oberen und unteren Zahnreihen, *Z Stomatol* 28:134 1930; 29:343, 1931.

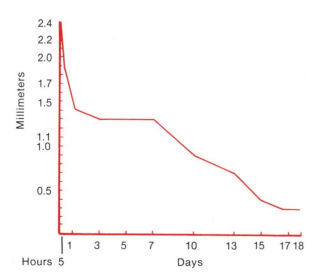

Fig. 2-145 Degree of movement after labial tipping and the subsequent relapse movement after the tooth had been released. Upper lateral incisor of a 12-year-old patient. Force, 40 g. Most of the relapse movement occurred during the first 5 hours. A hyalinized zone existed from the third to the seventh day. Part of this relapse movement may have been caused by the muscle function. (From Reitan K: *Am J Orthod* 53:721, 1967.)

24. Brudvik P, Rygh P: Root resorption after local injection of prostaglandin E_2 during experimental tooth movement, *Eur J Orthod* 13:225, 1991.
25. Buck DL, Griffith DA, Mills MJ: Histologic evidence for lipids during human tooth movement, *Am J Orthod* 64:619, 1973.
26. Burregde M: The molecular basis communication within the cell, *Sci Am* 253(4):142, 1985.
27. Burstone CJ, Groves MH: Threshold and optimum force values for maxillary anterior tooth movement, *J Dent Res* 39:695, 1961.
28. Chambers JJ, Horton MA: Osteoclasts: putative surrogate and authentic, *J Pathol* 144:295, 1984.
29. Davidovitch Z: Tooth movement, *Crit Rev Oral Biol Med* 2(4):411, 1991.
30. Davidovitch Z, Finkelson MD et al: Electric currents, bone remodeling and orthodontic tooth movement, II: increase in rate of tooth movement and periodontal cyclic nucleotide levels by combined force and electric current, *Am J Orthod* 77:33, 1980.
31. Davidovitch Z, Nicolay DF et al: Neurotransmitters, cytokines and the control of alveolar bone remodeling in orthodontics, *Adult Orthod Dent Clin North Am* 32(3):411, 1988.
32. Davidovitch Z, Shanfeld JL: Cyclic AMP levels in the alveolar bone of orthodontically treated cats, *Arch Oral Biol* 20:567, 1975.
33. DeAngelis V: Observations on the response of alveolar bone to orthodontic force, *Am J Orthod* 58:284, 1970.
34. Dellinger EL: A histologic and cephalometric investigation of premolar intrusion in the *Macaca speciosa* monkey, *Am J Orthod* 53:325, 1967.
35. Edwards JG: A study of the periodontium during orthodontic rotation of teeth, *Am J Orthod* 54:441, 1968.
36. Epker BN, Frost HM: Correlation of bone resorption and formation with the physical behavior of loaded bone, *J Dent Res* 44:33, 1965.
37. Erickson EM, Kaplan K, Aisenberg MS: Orthodontics and transseptal fibers, *Am J Orthod* 31:1, 1945.
38. Friedenberg ZB, Brighton CT: Bioelectricity and fracture healing, *Plast Reconstr Surg* 68:435, 1981.
39. Fukada E, Yasaka I: On the piezoelectric effect of bone, *J Physiol Soc Japan* 12:1158, 1957.
40. Fullmer HM: Observations on the development of oxytalan fibers in the periodontium of man, *J Dent Res* 38:510, 1959.
41. Garant PR, Cho MI: Cytoplasmic polarization of periodontal ligament fibroblasts: implications for cell migration and collagen secretion, *J Periodont Res* 14:95, 1979.
42. Gianelly AA, Goldman HM: *Biologic basis of orthodontics*, Philadelphia, 1971, Lea & Febiger.
43. Gonzales F, Karnovsky MJ: Electron microscopy of osteoclasts in healing fractures of rat bone, *J Biophysiol Biochem Cytol* 9:299, 1961.
44. Gottlieb B, Orban B: *Die Veranderungen der Gewebe bei übermässiger Beanspruchung der Zähne*, Leipzig, 1931, Georg Thieme Verlag.
45. Graber TM: Extraoral force-facts and fallacies, *Am J Orthod* 41:490, 1955.
46. Graber TM: The "three Ms": muscles, malformation, and malocclusion, *Am J Orthod* 49:418, 1963.
47. Graber TM, Chung DDB, Aoba JT: Dentofacial orthopedics versus orthodontics, *J Am Dent Assoc* 75:1145, 1967.
48. Greengaard P: Phosphorylated proteins as physiological effectors, *Science* 199:146, 1978.
49. Gubler W: Zur Frage der orthodontisch verusachten Wurzelresorptionen, *Schweiz Monatsschr Zahnheilkd* 49:917, 1939.
50. Gwynne-Evans E, Tulley WJ: Clinical types, *Dent Pract* 6:222, 1956.
51. Häupl K: *Gewebsumbau und Zahnverdrängung in der Funktions-Kieferorthopädie*, Leipzig, 1938, Johan Ambrosius Barth.
52. Heilbrunn LV, Wiercinski FJ: The action of various cations on muscle protoplasm, *J Cell Comp Physiol* 29:15, 1947.
53. Henry J, Weinmann JP: The pattern of resorption and repair of human cementum, *J Am Dent Assoc* 42:270, 1951.
54. Hirsch PD, Campbell WB et al: Prostaglandins and ischemic heart disease, *Am J Med* 71:1009, 1981.
55. Holland DJ: Surgical positioning of unerupted impacted teeth, *Oral Surg* 9:130, 1956.
56. Hotz R: Periodontal reaction to strong forces following treatment with fixed appliances, *Fortschr Kieferorthop* 27:220, 1966.
57. Huettner RJ, Young RW: The movability of vital and devitalized teeth in the *Macacus rhesus* monkey, *Am J Orthod* 41:594, 1955.
58. Humerfelt A, Reitan K: Effects of hypercementosis on the movability of teeth during orthodontic treatment, *Angle Orthod* 36:179, 1966.
59. Ingber DE, Folkman J: *Tension and compression as basic determinants of cell form and function: utilization of a cellular tensegrity mechanism*. In Stein WD, Bronner F, editors: *Cell shape: determinants, regulation and regulatory role*, San Diego, 1989, Academic Press.
60. Joho JP: The effects of extraoral low-pull traction to the mandibular dentition of *Macaca mulatta*, *Am J Orthod* 64:555, 1973.
61. Kahn AJ, Malone JD: *Lineage of bone resorbing cells: status and prospects for future research*. In Davidovitch Z, editor: *The biological mechanisms of tooth eruption and root resorption*, Birmingham, Ala, 1988, EBSCO Media, p. 313.
62. Ketcham AH: A progress report of an investigation of apical resorption of vital permanent teeth, *Int J Orthod* 15:310, 1929.
63. Khouw FE, Goldhaber P: Changes in vasculature of the periodontium associated with tooth movement in the rhesus monkey and dog, *Arch Oral Biol* 15:1125, 1970.
64. Kloehn SJ: Orthodontics, force or persuasion, *Angle Orthod* 23:56, 1953.
65. Kornstein R, Somjen D et al: Pulsed capacitive electric induction of cyclic AMP changes, Ca^{45} uptake and DNA synthesis in bone cells, *Trans Bioelectr Repair Growth* 1:34, 1981.
66. Krane S: Collagen degradation, *Connect Tissue Res* 10:51, 1982.
67. Krebs A: Midpalatal suture expansion studied by the implant method over a seven-year period, *Eur Orthod Soc Trans* 40:131, 1964.
68. Kronfeld R, Weinmann JP: Traumatic changes in the periodontal tissue of deciduous teeth, *J Dent Res* 19:441, 1940.
69. Kvam E: A study of the cell-free zone following experimental tooth movement in the rat, *Eur Orthod Soc Rep Congr* 45:419, 1970.
70. Kvam E: Preparation of human premolar roots for scanning electron microscopy, *Scand J Dent Res* 79:295, 1971.
71. Kvam E: Scanning electron microscopy of organic structures on the root surface of human teeth, *Scand J Dent Res* 80:297, 1972.
72. Kvam E: Topography of principal fibers, *Scand J Dent Res* 81:553, 1973.
73. Kvinnsland I, Kvinnsland S: Changes in CGRP-immunoreactive nerve fibers during experimental tooth movement in rats, *Eur J Orthod* 12:320, 1990.
74. Lear CSC, Flanagan JB, Moorrees CFA: The frequency of deglutition in man, *Arch Oral Biol* 10:83, 1965.
75. Lila E, Lindskog S, Hammarström L: Histochemistry of enzymes associated with tissue degradation incident to orthodontic tooth movement, *Am J Orthod* 83:62, 1983.
76. Lind V: Short root anomaly, *Scand J Dent Res* 80:85, 1972.
77. Linge L: "Tissue changes in facial sutures incident to mechanical influences." Thesis, University of Oslo, 1973.
78. Lundström AF: Malocclusions of the teeth regarded as problem in connection with the apical base, *Sven Tandläk Tidsskr* 16:147, 1923.
79. Macapanpan LC, Weinmann JP, Brodie AG: Early tissue changes following tooth movement in rats, *Angle Orthod* 24:79, 1954.
80. Mack PB, LaChance PA et al: Bone demineralization of foot and hand of Gemini-Tital IV, V and VII astronauts during orbital flight, *Am J Roentgenol* 100:503, 1967.
81. Marino AA: Electrical stimulation in orthopedics: past, present and future, *J Bioelect* 3:235, 1984.
82. Marks SC Jr, Miller SC: Local infusion of prostaglandin E_1 stimulates mandibular bone formation *in vivo*, *J Oral Pathol* 17:500, 1988.

83. Marshall JA: Root absorption of permanent teeth, *J Am Dent Assoc* 17:1221, 1930.

84. Massler M, Malone AJ: Root resorption in human permanent teeth, *Am J Orthod* 40:619, 1954.

85. McCulloch CAG, Melcher AH: Cell migration in the periodontal ligament of mice, *J Periodontal Res* 18:339, 1983.

86. McNamara JA: Neuromuscular and skeletal adaptations to altered function in the orofacial region, *Am J Orthod* 64:578, 1973.

87. Meikle NC: The effect of Class II intermaxillary force on the dentofacial complex in the adult *Macaca mulatta* monkey, *Am J Orthod* 58:323, 1970.

88. Melcher AH, Eastoe JE: *Synthesis of connective tissues*. In Melcher AH, Bowen WH: *Biology of the periodontium*, New York, 1969, Academic Press.

89. Melsen B, Melsen F, Mosekilde L: Bone changes of importance in the orthodontic patient with epilepsy, *Trans Europ Orthod Soc* p. 17, 1976.

90. Metz SA: Anti-inflammatory agents as inhibitors of prostaglandin synthesis in man, *Med Clin North Am* 65(4):713, 1981.

91. Minkoff R, Engström TG: A long-term comparison of protein turnover in subcrestal vs. supracrestal fiber tracts in the mouse periodontium, *Arch Oral Biol* 24:817, 1979.

92. Moore AW: Observations on facial growth and its clinical significance, *Am J Orthod* 45:399, 1959.

93. Morris CE: Mechanosensitive ion channels, *Membr Biol* 113:93, 1990.

94. Moyers RE: An electronmyographic analysis of certain muscles involved in temporomandibular joint movement, *Am J Orthod* 36:481, 1950.

95. Müller G: Function und Volumen, *Fortschr Kieferorthop* 24:276, 1963.

96. Mulligan W, Niewold BDL: "Differential forces in retracting cuspids in the monkeys (*Macaca mulatta*)," Master's thesis, University of Texas, 1962.

97. Murad F, Brewer B Jr, Vaughn M: Effect of thyrocalcitonin on adenosine, 3',5'-cyclic phosphate formation by rat kidney and bone, *Proc Natl Acad Sci USA* 65:446, 1970.

98. Murphy WH: Oxytetracycline microfluorescent comparison of orthodontic retraction into recent and healed extraction sites, *Am J Orthod* 58:215, 1970.

99. Nefussi JR, Baron R: PGE_2 stimulates both resorption and formation of bone *in vitro*: differential responses of the periosteum and the endosteum in fetal rat long bone cultures, *Anat Rec* 211:9, 1985.

100. Olsen BR: Electron microscope studies on collagen, II: mechanism of linear polymerization of tropo-collagen molecules, *Z Zellforsch* 59:199, 1963.

101. Oppenheim A: Die Krise in der Orthodontie, *Z Stomatol* 31:447, 1933.

102. Oppenheim A: Human tissue response to orthodontic intervention of short and long duration, *Am J Orthod* 28:263, 1942.

103. Oppenheim A: Possibility of orthodontic physiologic movement, *Am J Orthod* 30:277, 1944.

104. Orban B: Beziehungen zwischen Zahn und Knochen: Bewegung der Zahnkeime, *Z Anat Entw Gesch* 83:804, 1927.

105. Orban B: Tissue changes in traumatic occlusion, *J Am Dent Assoc* 15:2090, 1928.

106. Picton DCA: On the part played by the socket in tooth support, *Arch Oral Biol* 10:945, 1965.

107. Ponitz RJ: Invisible retainers, *Am J Orthod* 59:266, 1971.

108. Poulton DR: Electric pulp testing in orthodontic patients, *J Dent Child* 28:308, 1961.

109. Rasmussen H, Bordier P: Vitamin D and bone, *Metab Bone Dis Relat Res* 1:7, 1978.

110. Rateitschack KL, Herzog-Specht FA: Reaction and regeneration of the periodontal structure following orthodontic treatment with fixed appliances, *Schweiz Monatsschr Zahnheilk* 75:741, 1965.

111. Reitan K: Continuous bodily tooth movement and its histological significance, *Acta Odontol Scand* 7:115, 1947.

112. Reitan K: The initial tissue reaction incident to orthodontic tooth movement as related to the influence of function, *Acta Odontol Scand* (suppl 6), Dissertation 1951.

113. Reitan K: Some factors determining the evaluation of forces in orthodontics, *Am J Orthod* 43:32, 1957.

114. Reitan K: Tissue rearrangement during retention of orthodontically rotated teeth, *Angle Orthod* 29:105, 1959.

115. Reitan K: Tissue behavior during orthodontic tooth movement, *Am J Orthod* 46:881, 1960.

116. Reitan K: Behavior of Malassez' epithelial rests during orthodontic tooth movement, *Acta Odontol Scand* 19:443, 1961.

117. Reitan K: *Bone formation and resorption during reversed tooth movement*. In Kraus BS, Riedel RA, editors: *Vistas in orthodontics*, Philadelphia 1962, Lea & Febiger, p. 69.

118. Reitan K: Effects on force magnitude and direction of tooth movement on different alveolar bone types, *Angle Orthod* 34:244, 1964.

119. Reitan K: Principles of retention and avoidance of posttreatment relapse, *Am J Orthod* 55:776, 1969.

120. Reitan K: Evaluation of orthodontic forces as related to histologic and mechanical factors, *Schweiz Monatschr Zahnheilkd* 80:579, 1970.

121. Reitan K: Orthodontic treatment on patients with psychogenic, muscular and articulation disturbances, *Tandlaegebladet* 75:1182, 1971.

122. Reitan K: Tissue reaction as related to the age factor, *Dent Res* 74:271, 1954.

123. Reitan K, Kvam E: Comparative behavior of human and animal tissue during experimental tooth movement, *Angle Orthod* 41:1, 1971.

124. Reitan K: Initial tissue behavior during apical root resorption, *Angle Orthod* 44:68, 1974.

125. Ricketts RM: Various conditions of the temporomandibular joint as revealed by cephalometric laminography, *Angle Orthod* 22:98, 1952.

126. Riedel RA: Review of the retention program, *Angle Orthod* 6:179, 1960.

127. Rinderer L: The effects of expansion of the palatal suture, *Eur Orthod Soc Rep Congr* 42:1, 1966.

128. Rix RE: Deglutition and the teeth, *Dent Rec* 66:105, 1946.

129. Roberts WE, Chase DC: Kinetics of cell proliferation and migration associated with orthodontically-induced osteogenesis, *J Den Res* 60:174, 1981.

130. Rodan GA, Bourret LA et al: Cyclic AMP and cyclic GMP: mediators of the mechanical effects on bone remodelling, *Science* 189:467, 1975.

131. Rodan GA, Martin TJ: Role of osteoblasts in hormonal control of bone resorption—a hypothesis, *Calcif Tissue Int* 33:349, 1981.

132. Rudolph CE: An evaluation of root resorption occurring during orthodontic treatment, *J Dent Res* 19:367, 1940.

133. Rygh P: Ultrastructural vascular changes in pressure zones of rat molar periodontium incident to orthodontic tooth movement, *Scand J Dent Res* 80:307, 1972.

134. Rygh P: Erythrocytic crystallization in rat molar periodontium incident to tooth movement, *Scand J Dent Res* 81:62, 1973.

135. Rygh P: Ultrastructural cellular reactions in pressure zones of rat molar periodontium incident to orthodontic tooth movement, *Acta Odont Scand* 30:575, 1973.

136. Rygh P: Ultrastructural changes in pressure zones of human periodontium incident to orthodontic tooth movement, *Acta Odont Scand* 31:109, 1973.

137. Rygh P: Ultrastructural changes of the periodontal fibers and their attachment in rat molar periodontium incident to orthodontic tooth movement, *Scand J Dent Res* 81:467, 1973.

138. Rygh P: Elimination of hyalinized periodontal tissue associated with orthodontic tooth movement. *Scand J Dent Res* 82:57, 1974.

139. Rygh P: Ultrastructural changes in tension zones of rat molar peri-

odontium incident to orthodontic tooth movement, *Am J Orthod* 70:269, 1974.

140. Rygh P: Orthodontic root resorption studied by electron microscopy, *Angle Orthod* 47:1, 1977.

141. Rygh P, Bowling K et al: Activation of the vascular system: a main mediator of periodontal fiber remodeling in orthodontic tooth movement, *Am J Orthod* 89:453, 1986.

142. Rygh P, Reitan K: Changes in the supporting tissues of submerged deciduous molars with and without permanent successors, *Odontol Tidsskr* 72:345, 1964.

143. Rygh P, Tindlund R: Orthopedic expansion and protraction of the maxilla in cleft palate patients—a new treatment rationale, *Cleft Palate J* 19:104, 1982.

144. Saito M, Saito S et al: Interleukin 1 beta and prostaglandin E are involved in the response of periodontal cells to mechanical stress in vivo and in vitro, *Am J Orthod Dentofac Orthop* 99:226, 1991.

145. Samuelson B, Granström E et al: *Prostaglandins Annu Rev Biochem* 44:669, 1975.

146. Sandstedt C: Einige Beiträge zur Zahnregulierung, *Nord Tandl Tidssk* 5:236, 1904; 6:1, 1905.

147. Schubert M, Hamarman D: *A primer on connective tissue biochemistry*, Philadelphia, 1968, Lea & Febiger.

148. Schwarz AM: Ueber die Bewegung Belasteter Zähne, *D Stomatol* 26:40, 1928.

149. Schwarz AM: Tissue changes incident to tooth movement, *Int J Orthod* 18:331, 1932.

150. Scott BL: The occurrence of specific cytoplasmic granules in the osteoclast, *J Ultrastruc Res* 19:417, 1967.

151. Seipel CM: Trajectories of the jaws, *Acta Odontol Scand* 8:81, 1948.

152. Selvig KA: An ultrastructural study of cementum formation, *Acta Odontol Scand* 22:105, 1964.

153. Selvig KA: The fine structure of human cementum, *Acta Odontol Scand* 23:423, 1965.

154. Shamos MH, Lavine LS: Piezoelectricity as a fundamental property of biological tissues, *Nature* 213:267, 1967.

155. Sicher H: Bau und Funktion des Fixations apparates der Meerschweinchenmolaren, *Z Stomatol* 21:580, 1923.

156. Sicher H: Tooth eruption, the axial movement of continuously growing teeth, *J Dent Res* 21:201, 1942.

157. Sicher H, editor: *Orban's oral histology and embryology*, ed 5, St Louis, 1962, Mosby.

158. Silve CM, Hradek GT et al: Parathyroid hormone receptor in intact embryonic chicken bone: characterization and cellular localization, *J Cell Biol* 94:379, 1982.

159. Skillen W, Reitan K: Tissue changes following rotation of teeth in the dog, *Angle Orthod* 10:140, 1940.

160. Skogborg C: The use of septotomy in connection with orthodontic treatment, *Int J Orthod* 18:659, 1932.

161. Slagsvold O: Autotransplantation of premolars in cases of missing anterior teeth, *Eur Orthod Soc Rep Congr* 46:473, 1970.

162. Smith EL, Smith PE et al: Bone involution decrease in exercising middle-aged women, *Calcif Tissue Int* 36:129, 1984.

163. Sodek J: A comparison of the rates of synthesis and turnover of collagen and noncollagen proteins in adult rat periodontal tissues and skin using a microassay, *Arch Oral Biol* 22:655, 1977.

164. Sodek J: *Collagen turnover in periodontal ligament.* In Norton LA, Burstone CJ, editors: *The biology of tooth movement*, Boca Raton Fla, 1989, CRC Press, p. 177.

165. Somjen D, Binderman E et al: Bone remodeling induced by physical stress is prostaglandin E_2 mediated, *Biochem Biophys Acta* 627:91, 1980.

166. Spaulding FW: Obtundant effect of vibration, *Am J Orthod* 45:917, 1959.

167. Stein G, Weinmann J: Die physiologische Wanderung der Zähne, *Z Stomatol* 23:733, 1925.

168. Stenvik A: Pulp and dentine reactions to experimental tooth intrusion (a histologic study of long-term effects), *Eur Orthod Soc Rep Congr* 45:449, 1970.

169. Stenvik A, Mjør IA: Pulp and dentine reactions to experimental tooth intrusion: a histologic study of the initial changes, *Am J Orthod* 57:370, 1970.

170. Storey E: Bone changes associated with tooth movement: a histological study of the effect of force for varying durations in the rabbit, guinea pig and rat, *Aust J Dent* 59:209, 1955.

171. Storey E, Smith R: Force in orthodontics and its relation to tooth movement, *Aust J Dent* 56:11, 1952.

172. Strang HW: Factors associated with successful orthodontic treatment, *Am J Orthod* 38:790, 1952.

173. Stuteville OH: Injuries to the teeth and supporting structures caused by various orthodontic appliances and methods of preventing these injuries, *J Am Dent Assoc* 24:1494, 1937.

174. Sutherland EW: Studies on the mechanisms of hormone action, *Science* 177:401, 1972.

175. Tashjian AH Jr, Voelkel EF et al: Evidence that the bone resorption-stimulating factor produced by mouse fibrosarcoma cells is prostaglandin E_2, *J Exp Med* 136:1329, 1972.

176. Ten Cate AR: Physiological resorption of connective tissue associated with tooth eruption, *J Periodont Res* 6:168, 1971.

177. Ten Cate AR, Anderson R: An ultrastructural study of tooth resorption in the kitten, *J Dent Res* 65:1087, 1986.

178. Ten Cate AR, Deporter DA, Freeman E: The role of fibroblasts in the remodeling of the periodontal ligament during physiologic tooth movement, *Am J Orthod* 69:155, 1976.

179. Tweedle JA: The effect of local heat on tooth movement, *Angle Orthod* 35:219, 1965.

180. Underwood JCE: From where comes the osteoclast? *J Pathol* 144:225, 1984.

181. Utley RK: The activity of alveolar bone incident to orthodontic tooth movement as studied by oxytetracycline induced fluorescence, *Am J Orthod* 54:167, 1968.

182. Waerhaug J: Tissue reaction to metal wires in healthy gingival pockets, *J Periodontol* 28:239, 1957.

183. Weinmann JP, Sicher H: *Bone and bones*, St Louis, 1947, Mosby.

184. Weinstein S, Haack DC et al: On an equilibrium theory of tooth position, *Angle Orthod* 33:1, 1963.

185. Wentz FM, Jarabak JR, Orban B: Experimental occlusal trauma imitating cuspal interferences, *J Periodontol* 29:117, 1958.

186. Wieslander L: The effect of orthodontic treatment on the concurrent development of the craniofacial complex, *Am J Orthod* 49:15, 1963.

187. Yamasaki K, Miura F, Suda T: Prostaglandin as a mediator of bone resorption induced by experimental tooth movement in rats, *J Dent Res* 59:1635, 1980.

188. Yamasaki K, Shibata Y, Fukuhara T: The effects of prostaglandins on experimental tooth movement in monkeys (*Macaca fuscata*), *J Dent Res* 61:1444, 1982.

189. Yamasaki K, Shibata Y et al: Clinical application of prostaglandin E_1 (PGE$_1$) upon orthodontic tooth movement, *Am J Orthod* 85:508, 1984.

190. Young RW: Cell proliferation and specialization during endochondral osteogenesis in young rats, *J Cell Biol* 14:357, 1962.

191. Zachrisson BU: Gingival condition associated with orthodontic treatment, II: histologic findings, *Angle Orthod* 42:352, 1972.

192. Zengo AN, Pawluk RJ, Bassett CAL: Stress-induced bioelectric potentials in the dentoalveolar complex, *Am J Orthod* 64:17, 1973.

ADDITIONAL READING

Ahlgren JGA, Ingervall BF, Thilander BL: Muscle activity in normal and postnormal occlusion, *Am J Orthod* 64:445, 1973.

Andreasen G, Naessig C: Experimental findings on mesial relapse of maxillary first molars, *Angle Orthod* 38:51, 1968.

Armstrong MM: Controlling the magnitude, direction, and duration of extraoral force, *Am J Orthod* 59:217, 1971.

Avery JK, Rapp R: Pain conduction in human dental tissues, *Dent Clin North Am*, p. 489, July 1959.

Bassett CAL, Becker RO: Generation of electric potentials by bone in response to mechanical stress, *Science* 137:1063, 1962.

Bien SM: Difficulties and failures in tooth movement: responses to mechanotherapy, *Eur Orthod Soc Trans* p. 52, 1967.

Björk A, Skieller V: Facial development and tooth eruption: an implant study at the age of puberty, *Am J Orthod* 62:339, 1972.

Brescia NJ: *Applied dental anatomy*, St Louis, 1961, Mosby.

Brodie AG: Muscular factors in diagnosis, treatment, and retention, Angle Orthod 23:71, 1953.

Buck DL, Church DH: A histologic study of human tooth movement, *Am J Orthod* 62:507, 516, 1972.

Carmichael GG, Fullmer HM: The fine structure of the oxytalan fiber, *J Cell Biol* 28:33, 1966.

Clark AB, Sims MR, Leppard PI: An analysis of the effect of tooth intrusion on the microvascular bed and fenestrae in the apical periodontal ligament of the rat molar, *Am J Orthod Dentofac Orthop* 99:21-29, 1991.

Crumley PJ: Collagen formation in the normal and stressed periodontium, *Periodontics* 2:53, 1964.

Cunat JJ: Activators: an orthopedic puzzle, *Am J Orthod* 65:16, 1974.

Davidovitch Z, editor: Biological mechanisms of tooth eruption and root resorption: an international conference, Columbus Ohio, 1988, Ohio State University, pp. 293, 401.

Delaire J: Le syndrome prognathique mandibulaire, *Orthod Fr* 45:203, 1976.

Delaire J, Verdon P, Lumineau JP, et al: Quelques résultates des tractions extra-orales à l'appui fronto-mentonnier dans le traitement orthopédique des malformations maxillo-mandibulaires de classe III et des séquelles osseuses des fentes labio-maxillaires, *Rev Stomat* 73:633, 1972.

Edwards JG: The prevention of relapse in extraction cases, *Am J Orthod* 60:128, 1971.

Enlow DH: Functions of the haversian system, *Am J Anat* 110:269, 1962.

Fortin JM: Translation of premolars in the dog by controlling the moment-to-moment force ratio on the crown, *Am J Orthod* 59:541, 1971.

Frank FM: Apposition et resorption de l'os alvéolaire, *Orthop Dentofaciale* 6:201, 1972.

Furseth R: Studies of normal and of clinically and experimentally altered dental cementum. Master's thesis, University of Oslo, 1970.

Furstmann L, Bernick S, Aldrich D: Differential response incident to tooth movement, *Am J Orthod* 59:600, 1971.

Gaudet EL: Tissue changes in the monkey following root torque with the Begg technique, *Am J Orthod* 58:164, 1970.

Gianelly A: Mandibular cervical traction in the treatment of Class I malocclusions, *Am J Orthod* 60:257, 1971.

Goldhaber P: *Bone-resorption factors, cofactors, and giant vacuole osteoclasts in tissue culture*. In Gaillard J, Talmage TV, Budy AM, editors: *The parathyroid glands*, Chicago, 1965, University of Chicago Press, p. 1953.

Goldie RS, King GJ: Root resorption and tooth movement in orthodontically treated, calcium deficient and lactating rats, *Am J Orthod* 85:424-430, 1984.

Haim G: Elektronenmikroskopische Untersuchungen der kollagenen und elastichen Fasern, *Dtsch Zahn Mund Kieferheilkd* 41:196, 1965.

Halderson H, Johns EE, Moyers R: The selection of forces for tooth movement, *Am J Orthod* 39:25, 1953.

Harris EF, Baker WC: Loss of root length and crestal bone height before and during treatment in adolescent and adult orthodontic patients, *Am J Orthod Dentofac Orthop* 98:463, 1990.

Harvold EP, Vargevik K, Chierici G: Primate experiments on oral sensation and dental malocclusions, *Am J Orthod* 63:494, 1973.

Hodel C, Meier-Ruge W: Enzyme histochemical investigations on giant cells of specific and nonspecific granulation tissue, and of malignant tumours, *Pathol Eur* 1:425, 1966.

Hovell JH: Recent advances in orthodontics, *Br Dent J* 98:114, 1955.

Janzen EK, Bluher JA: The cephalometric, anatomic, and histologic changes in *Macaca mulatta* after application of a continuous-acting retraction force on the mandible, *Am J Orthod* 51:823, 1965.

Jarabak JR: The adaptability of the temporal and masseter muscles; an electromyographical study, *Angle Orthod* 24:193, 1954.

Kaplan RG: Mandibular third molars and postretention crowding, *Am J Orthod* 66:411, 1975.

Kloehn SJ: An appraisal of the results of treatment of Class II malocclusions with extra-oral forces, *Eur Orthod Soc Trans*, p. 112, 1961.

Koski K: Cranial growth centers: facts or fallacies? *Am J Orthod* 54:566, 1968.

Kurihara S, Enlow DH: An electron microscopic study of attachments between periodontal fibers and bone during alveolar remodeling, *Am J Orthod* 77:516, 1980.

Kvam E: Scanning electron microscopy of tissue changes on the pressure surface of human premolars following tooth movement, *Scand J Dent Res* 80:357, 1972.

Langeland K: "Tissue changes in the dental pulp: an experimental histologic study." Thesis, University of Oslo, 1957.

Lemoine C, Petrovic A, Stutzmann J: Inflammatory process of the rat maxilla after molar auto transplantation, *J Dent Res* 49:1175, 1970.

Levander E, Malmgren O: Evaluation of the risk of root resorption during orthodontic treatment: a study of upper incisors, *Eur J Orthod* 10:30, 1988.

Lind V: Short root anomaly, *Scand J Dent Res* 80:85, 1972.

Lindskog S, Blomhof L, Hammarström L: Cellular colonization of denuded root surfaces in vivo: cell morphology in dentin resorption and cementum repair, *J Clin Periodontol* 14:290, 1987.

Linge BO, Linge L: Patient characteristics and treatment variables associated with apical root resorption during orthodontic treatment, *Am J Orthod Dentofac Orthop* 99:35, 1991.

Löe H: Bone tissue formation: a morphological and histochemical study, *Acta Odontol Scand* (suppl 27):1, 1960.

Magnusson B: Tissue changes at erupting molars in germ free rats, *J Periodont Res* 4:181, 1969.

Massler M: Changes in the lamina dura during tooth movement, *Am J Orthod* 40:364, 1954.

Melcher AH: Presence of histologically demonstrable bound lipid in gingival connective tissue and loss during collagenolysis, *J Periodont Res* 1:237, 1966.

Midgett RJ, Shaye R, Fruge JF: The effect of altered bone metabolism on orthodontic tooth movement, *Am J Orthod* 80:256, 1980.

Moss ML, Salentijn L: Differences between the functional matrices in anterior open-bite and in deep overbite, *Am J Orthod* 60:264, 1971.

Moyers RE, Bauer JL: The periodontal response to various tooth movements, *Am J Orthod* 36:572, 1950.

Mühlemann HR: Periodontometry: a method for measuring tooth mobility, *Oral Surg* 4:1220, 1951.

Mühlemann HR: Ten years of tooth mobility measurements, *J Periodontal* 31:10, 1960

Nakamura M: In vitro study on the cellular responses to the compressive force in orthodontics, *J Osaka Dent Univ* 2:1, 1968.

Nordenram Å, Bang G, Anneroth G: A histopathologic study of replanted teeth with superficially demineralized root surfaces in Java monkeys, *Scand J Dent Res* 81:294, 1973.

Oppenheim A: Die Veränderungen der Gewebe insbesondere des Knochens bei der verschiebung der Zähne, *Oester Ung Vjschr Zahnheilkd* 27:302, 1911.

Oppenheim A: Biologic orthodontic therapy and reality, *Angle Orthod* 6:69, 1936.

Oppenheim A: Artificial elongation of teeth, *Am J Orthod* 26:931, 1940.

Parker GR: Transseptal fibers and relapse following bodily retraction of teeth: a histologic study, *Am J Orthod* 61:331, 1972.

Perez-Tamayo R: *Mechanisms of disease: an introduction to pathology*, Philadelphia, 1961, WB Saunders.

Perry HT: Functional electromyography of the temporal and masseter muscles in Class II, division I, malocclusion and excellent occlusion, *Angle Orthod* 25:49, 1955.

Perry HT: Adolescent temporomandibular dysfunction, *Am J Orthod* 63:517, 1973.

Posselt U: Occlusal rehabilitation, *Dent Pract* 9:255, 1959.

Roberts WE: Cell kinetic nature and diurnal and periodicity of the rat periodontal ligament, *Arch Oral Biol* 20:465, 1975.

Roberts WE: Cell population dynamics of periodontal ligament stimulated with parathyroid extract, *Am J Anat* 143:263, 1975.

Roberts WE, Chase DC: Kinetics of cell proliferation and migration associated with orthodontically induced osteogenesis, *J Dent Res* 60:174, 1981.

Roberts WE, Chase DC, Jee WSS: Counts of labelling mitoses in the orthodontically stimulated periodontal ligament in the rat, *Arch Oral Biol* 19:665, 1974.

Roberts WE, Goodwin WC, Heiner SR: Cellular response to orthodontic force, *Dent Clin North Am* 25:3, 1981.

Roberts WE, Smith RK, Cohen JA: *Change in electrical potential within the periodontal ligament of a tooth subjected to osteogenic loading.* In Dixon AD, Sarnat BG, editors: *Factors and mechanisms influencing bone growth*, New York, 1982, Alan R. Liss.

Robinson QC, Woods MA, Harris EF: External root resorption: an epidemiologic study of causes. *J Dental Res* 70A:419, 1991.

Rosenstein SW, Jacobsen BN: Retention: an equal partner, *Am J Orthod* 59:323, 1971.

Rygh P: *Periodontal responses to orthodontic forces.* In McNamara JA, Ribbens KA, editors: *Malocclusion and the periodontium*, Monograph 15, Craniofacial Growth Series, Center for Human Growth and Development, Ann Arbor, Mich, 1984, University of Michigan, p. 17.

Rygh P: *Periodontal response to tooth-moving force: is trauma necessary?* In Graber LW editor: *Orthodontics: state of the art, essence of the science*, St Louis, 1986, Mosby, p. 100.

Rygh P: *The periodontal ligament under stress.* In Norton LA, Burstone CJ, Editors: *The biology of tooth movement.* Boca Raton, Fla, 1989, CRC Press, p. 9.

Rygh P, Moyers RE: *Force systems and tissue reactions to forces in orthodontics and facial orthopedics.* In Moyers RE, editor: *Handbook of orthodontics*, Chicago, 1988, Year Book Medical, p. 306.

Sharpe W, Reed B, Subtelny J, Polson A: Orthodontic relapse, apical root resorption, and crestal alveolar bone levels, *Am J Orthod Dentofac Orthop* 91:252, 1987.

Slagsvold O, Bjercke B: Autotransplantasjon av premolarer, *Göteborgs Tandlak Sallsk Arsbok* p. 45, 1967.

Smith R, Storey E: The importance of force in orthodontics: the design of cuspid retraction springs, *Aust Dent J* 56:291, 1952.

Spiegel RN, Sather AH, Hayles AB: Cephalometric study of children with various endocrine disease, *Am J Orthod* 59:362, 1971.

Stenvik A: The effect of extrusive orthodontic forces on human pulp and dentin, *Scand J Dent Res* 79:430, 1971.

Stöckli PW, Willert HG: Tissue reactions in the temporomandibular joint resulting from anterior displacement of the mandible in the monkey, *Am J Orthod* 60:142-154, 1971.

Storey E: Bone changes associated with tooth movement: a radiographic study, *Aust Dent J* 57:57, 1953.

Storey E: The nature of tooth movement, *Am J Orthod* 63:292, 1973.

Storey E: Tissue response to the movement of bones, *Am J Orthod* 64:229, 1973.

Stutzmann J, Petrovic A: La vitesse de renouvellement de l'os alvéolaire chez l'adulte avant et pendant le traitement orthodontique, *Rev Orthop Dentofaciale* 14:437, 1980.

Stutzmann J, Petrovic A: Die Umbaugeschwindigkeit des Alveolarknochens beim Erwachsenen vor und nach orthodontischer Behandlung, *Fortschr Kieferorthop* 42:386, 1981.

Stutzmann J, Petrovic A, Shaye R et al.: Analyse en culture organotypique de la vitesse de formation-résorption de l'os alvéolaire humain prélevé avant et pendant un traitement comprenant le déplacement de dents: nouvelle voie d'approche en recherche orthodontique, *Orthod Fr* 50:399, 1979.

Tayer BH, Gianelly AA, Ruben MP: Visualization of cellular dynamics associated with orthodontic tooth movement, *Am J Orthod* 54:515, 1968.

Thompson HF, Meyers HI, Waterman JM, Flanagan VD: Preliminary macroscopic observations concerning the potentiality of supraalveolar collagenous fibers in orthodontics, *Am J Orthod* 44:485, 1958.

Thompson JR: Function—the neglected phase of orthodontics, *Angle Orthod* 26:129, 1956.

Tronstad L: *Root resorption—a multidisciplinary problem in dentistry.* In Davidovitch Z, editor: *The biological mechanisms of tooth eruption and root resorption*, Birmingham, Ala, 1988, EBSCO Media, pp. 293-301.

Tulley W: Methods of recording patterns of behaviour of the orofacial muscles using the electromyograph, *Dent Rec* 73:741, 1953.

Turpin DL: Growth and remodeling of the mandible in the *Macaca mulatta* monkey, *Am J Orthod* 54:251, 1968.

Valderhaug JP, Nylen MU: Function of epithelial rests as suggested by their ultrastructure, *J Periodont Res* 1:69, 1966.

Van der Linden FPGM: The removable orthodontic appliance, *Am J Orthod* 59:376, 1971.

Vardimon AD, Graber TM, Voss LR, Lenke J: Determinants controlling iatrogenic external root resorption and repair during and after palatal expansion, *Angle Orthod* 61:113-122, 1991.

Wainwright WM: Faciolingual tooth movement: its influence on the root and cortical plate, *Am J Orthod* 64:278, 1973.

Woods MA, Robinson QC, Harris EF: The population distribution of cases with root resorption, *J Dent Res* 71A:214, 1992.

Wylie WL: Overbite and vertical dimension in terms of muscle balance, *Angle Orthod* 14:13, 1944.

Zander HA, Mühlemann HR: The effect of stresses on the periodontal structures, *Oral Surg* 9:380, 1956.

Zengo AN, Bassett CAL, Pawluk RL, Prountzos G: In vivo bioelectric potentials in the dentoalveolar complex, *Am J Orthod* 66:130, 1974.

Zengo AN, Pawluk RJ, Bassett CAL: Stress-induced bioelectric potentials in the dentoalveolar complex, *Am J Orthod* 64:17, 1973.

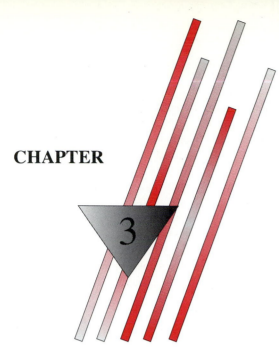

CHAPTER

3

Bone Physiology, Metabolism, and Biomechanics in Orthodontic Practice

W. EUGENE ROBERTS

The skeletal system is composed of highly specialized mineralized tissues, with both structural and metabolic functions. Structurally, lamellar, woven, composite, and bundle bone are unique types of osseous tissue adapted to specific functions. Bone *modeling* and *remodeling* are distinct physiological responses to integrated mechanical and metabolic demands. Biomechanical manipulation of bone is the physiological basis of orthodontics and facial orthopedics. However, before dentofacial considerations, an orthodontist must assess the overall health status of a patient. Orthodontics is bone manipulative therapy. Favorable calcium metabolism is an important consideration. Because of the interaction between structure and metabolism, a thorough understanding of osseous structure and function is fundamental to patient selection, risk assessment, treatment planning, and retention of desired dentofacial relationships.[70,82]

The physiological mediator of orthodontic therapy is the periodontal ligament (PDL): the osteogenic bone/tooth interface. It is a modified periosteum, with remarkable bone resorptive and formative capability. Via the teeth, alveolar bone can be loaded in a noninvasive and relatively atraumatic manner. Clinical therapy is a combination of orthodontics (tooth movement) and orthopedics (relative repositioning of bones), depending on the magnitude, the direction, and the frequency of applied mechanics. Cell kinetic studies of the PDL have helped define the proliferation and differentiation events of the orthodontic reaction, providing a fundamental basis for mechanically-induced osteogenesis.[66,78] The sequence of proliferation and differentiation events involved in the histogenesis (formation) of osteoblasts was first described in rat PDL.[78] Some aspects of the osteoclastic reaction of the PDL have been described,[59,67] but little is known about the cellular mechanism of orthopedic changes in the sutures.

A major problem in orthodontics and facial orthopedics is anchorage control.[72] Undesirable movement of the anchorage units is a common problem that limits the therapeutic range of biomechanics.[2] An important application of the basic principles of bone physiology is the use of rigid endosseous implants for orthodontic and orthopedic anchorage. Both animal studies[74] and clinical trials of custom orthodontic devices[77] have established that rigidly integrated implants do not move in response to conventional orthodontic and orthopedic forces. These devices are opening new horizons in the management of asymmetry, mutilated dentitions, severe malocclusion and craniofacial deformity.

BONE PHYSIOLOGY

Morphology of bone is well described, but its physiology is elusive because of the technical limitations inherent in the study of mineralized tissues. Accurate assessment of the orthodontic or orthopedic response to applied loads requires time markers (bone labels) and physiological indices (DNA labels, histochemistry, and in situ hybridization) of bone cell function. Systematic investigation with these advanced methods have defined new concepts of clinically relevant bone physiology.*

Specific Assessment Methodology

Physiologic interpretation of the response to applied loads requires specially adapted methods: (1) *mineralized sections* are an effective means of accurately preserving structure and function relationships[84]; (2) *polarized light birefringence* detects the preferential orientation of collagen fi-

---

*References 61, 63, 67, 69-71, 74, 77, 85.

bers within bone matrix[85]; (3) *fluorescent labels,* such as tetracycline, permanently mark all sites of bone mineralization at a specific point in time (anabolic markers)[85]; (4) *microradiography* assesses mineral density patterns in the same sections[61]; (5) *autoradiography* detects radioactively tagged precursors (nucleotides; amino acids) used to mark physiologic activity[58,66,75]; (6) *nuclear volume morphometry* differentially assesses osteoblast precursors in a variety of osteogenic tissues[79]; (7) *cell kinetics* is a quantitative analysis of cell physiology based on morphologically distinguishable events in the cell cycle (i.e. DNA synthesis (S) phase, mitosis, and differentiation-specific change in nuclear volume)[67,79]; (8) *finite element modeling* is an engineering method for calculating stresses and strains within all ma-

terials, including living tissues[51,62,71,93]; and (9) *microelectrodes* inserted in living tissue such as PDL can detect electrical potential changes associated with mechanical loading.[67,83]

Mineralized sections. Fully mineralized specimens are superior to routine demineralized histology for most critical analyses of teeth, periodontium, and supporting bone.[61,81,84,85] There is less processing distortion. Both the inorganic mineral and organic matrix can be studied simultaneously. For tissue-level studies, 100 μm thick sections are appropriate because they can be studied with multiple analytical methods. Even in the absence of bone labels, microradiographic images of polished mineralized sections provide substantial information about the strength, matu-

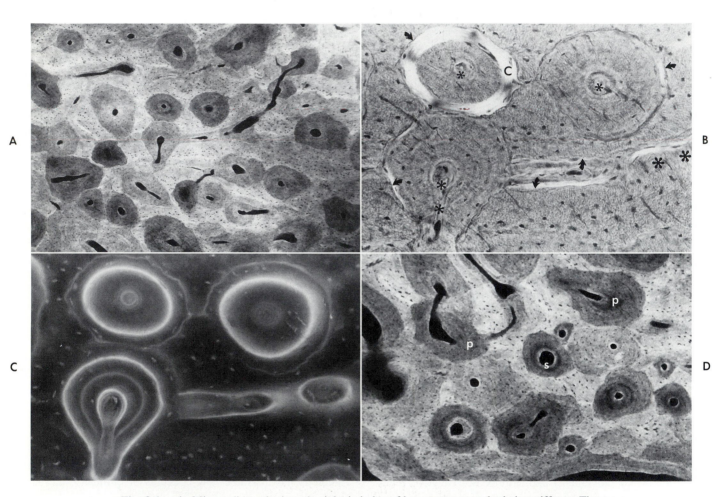

Fig. 3-1   A, Microradiography is a physiologic index of bone turnover and relative stiffness. The more radiolucent *(darker)* osteons are the youngest, the least mineralized, and the most compliant. Radiodense *(white)* areas are the oldest, most mineralized, with rigid portions of the bone. **B,** Polarized light microscopy reveals collagen fiber orientation within bone matrix. Lamellae with a longitudinally oriented matrix *(bright)* are particularly strong in tension while horizontally oriented matrix *(dark)* has preferential strength in compression. (From Roberts WE et al: *Calif Dent Assoc J* 15(10):58, 1987.) **C,** Multiple fluorochrome labels administered at 2-week intervals demonstrate the incidence and rates of bone formation. (From Roberts WE et al: *Calif Dent Assoc J* 15(10):58, 1991.) **D,** This microradiographic image demonstrates an array of concentric secondary osteons (Haversian systems) characteristic of rapidly remodeling cortical bone. Primary *(p)* and beginning secondary *(s)* mineralization are more radiolucent and radiodense respectively. (From Roberts WE et al: In *Bone biodynamics in orthodontic and orthopedic treatment,* ed 27, Ann Arbor, 1991, University of Michigan Press, pp 189–255.)

ration, and turnover rate of cortical bone (Fig. 3-1, *A*). Cellular detail and resolution of bone labels are considerably enhanced by reducing the thickness of the section to <25 μm. Specific stains are useful for enhancing contrast of both cellular and extracellular structures. The disadvantages of thin mineralized sections are that bone labels quench more rapidly and that there is inadequate tissue density for microradiographic analysis.

Polarized light. Birefringence of polarized light (Fig. 3-1, *B*) has particular biomechanical significance. The lamellar fringe patterns revealed with polarized light indicate the preferential collagen orientation within the matrix.[3] Most lamellar bone displays alternating layers of collagen fibers at right angles, resulting in the lamellae multiplying. However, two specialized collagen configurations are noted in the same or adjacent osteons: (1) longitudinally aligned collagen efficiently resist tension; and (2) transverse or circumferential collagen fibers are preferential support for compression.[43] It appears that loading conditions at the time of bone formation dictate the orientation of the collagen fibers to best resist the loads to which the bone is exposed. The important point is that bone formation can adapt to different loading conditions by changing the internal lamellar organization of mineralized tissue.

Fluorescent labels. Administered in vivo, calcium binding labels are anabolic time markers of bone formation. Histomorphometric analysis of label incidence and interlabel distance is an effective method for determining the mechanisms of bone growth and functional adaptation (Fig. 3-1, *C*). Because they fluoresce at different wavelengths (colors), six different bone labels can be used: (1) tetracycline (10 mg/kg, bright yellow); (2) calcein green (5 mg/kg, bright green); (3) xylenol orange (60 mg/kg, orange); (4) alizarin complexone (20 mg/kg, red); (5) demeclocycline (10 mg/kg, gold); and (6) oxytetracycline (10 mg/kg, dull or greenish yellow). The multiple fluorochrome method, sequential use of a variety of different color labels,

is a powerful method for assessing bone growth, healing, functional adaptation, and response to applied loads.[74,85]

Microradiography. High resolution images require polished sections that are approximately 100 μm thick. Differential x-ray attenuation reveals that new bone is less mineralized than mature bone. Newly formed bone matrix requires approximately 1 week of maturation to become mineralizable *osteoid*. Depending on the collagen configuration of the bone matrix, osteoblasts deposit 70% to 85% of the eventual mineral complement by a process called primary mineralization.[43,85] Secondary mineralization (mineral maturation) completes the maturation process in about 8 months by a crystal growth process (Fig. 3-1, *D*). Since strength of bone tissue is directly related to mineral content, the stiffness and strength of an *entire* bone depends on the distribution and relative degree of mineralization of its osseous tissue.[17] The initial strength of new bone is due to the cell-mediated process of primary mineralization, but its ultimate strength is dictated by secondary mineralization: the physiochemical process of crystal growth. This concept has important clinical value in orthodontics. Fully mineralized lamellar bone (in steady-state with respect to modeling and remodeling) is expected to be less susceptible to relapse tendencies than are its woven and composite bone predecessors.[60,84] Following active orthodontic therapy, it is important to retain dental corrections for at least 6 to 8 months to allow for mineral maturation of the newly formed bone (Fig. 3-2).

Autoradiography. Radioactive precursors for structural and metabolic materials are detected within tissue by coating histological sections with a nuclear track emulsion. Localization of radioactive disintegrations reveals the location of the radioactive precursors (Fig. 3-3). Specific radioactive labels for proteins, carbohydrates, or nucleic acids are injected at a known interval before tissue sampling. Qualitative and quantitative assessment of label uptake is a physiologic index of cell activity. The most common autora-

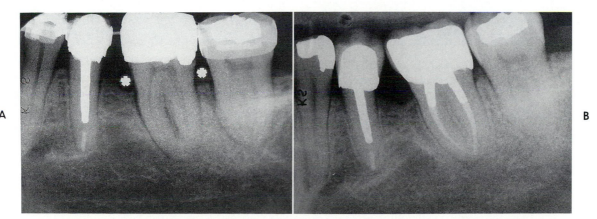

Fig. 3-2   Compare bone maturation in a periapical radiograph from the end of active orthodontic treatment (**A**) to the same area 2 years later (**B**). At the end of treatment there are large amorphous areas of relatively immature bone. After retention and restorative treatment, including endodontics, distinct definition of cortices and trabeculae are evident. (From Roberts WE et al: In *Bone biodynamics in orthodontic and orthopedic treatment,* ed 27, Ann Arbor, 1991, University of Michigan Press, pp 189-255.)

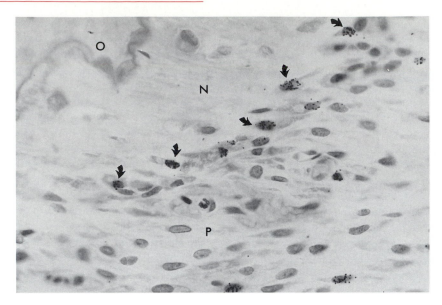

Fig. 3-3 At 56 hours after initiation of orthodontic force, new bone *(N)* is forming on the original *(O)* alveolar bone surface. The ³H-thymidine labeled osteoblasts *(arrows)* are derived from preosteoblasts in the periodontal ligament *(P).* (×450.) (From Roberts WE et al: In *Bone biodynamics in orthodontic and orthopedic treatment,* ed 27, Ann Arbor, 1991, University of Michigan Press, pp 189-255.)

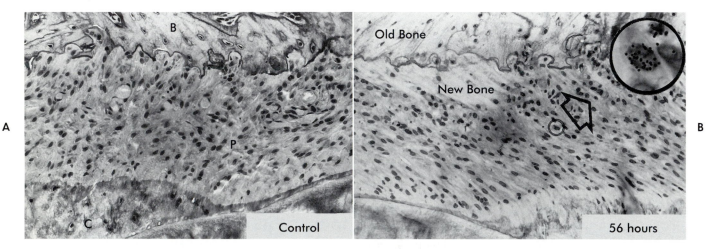

Fig. 3-4 **A,** Bone *(B),* periodontal ligament *(P),* and cementum *(C)* are shown in control periodontum of a young adult rat (6 to 8 weeks of age). (×100.) **B,** At 56 hours, following application of force, new bone is noted; a ³H-thymidine labeled preosteoblast is selected from the periodontal ligament and magnified to ×1000 in the upper right hand corner. (×100.) (From Roberts WE et al: In *Bone biodynamics in orthodontic and orthopedic treatment,* ed 27, Ann Arbor, 1991, University of Michigan Press, pp 189-255.)

diographic labels used in bone research are ³H-thymidine labeling of cells synthesizing DNA (S-phase cells) and ³H-proline labeling of newly formed bone matrix. Bromodeoxyuridine (BDU) immunocytochemistry, a nonradioactive method for labeling S-phase in vivo, shows promise as an important bone cell kinetic method of the future.[62]

Nuclear volume morphometry. Measuring nuclear size is a cytomorphometric procedure for assessing the stage of differentiation of osteoblast precursor cells. This method has been particularly useful for assessing the mechanism of osteogenesis in orthodontically activated PDL (Fig. 3-4). Preosteoblasts (C and D cells) have significantly larger nuclei than committed osteoprogenitor (A′) cells or their less-differentiated precursors (A cells). The B cell compartment is a group of fibroblast-like cells that appear to have little or no osteogenic potential.[78] Careful cytomorphometric as-

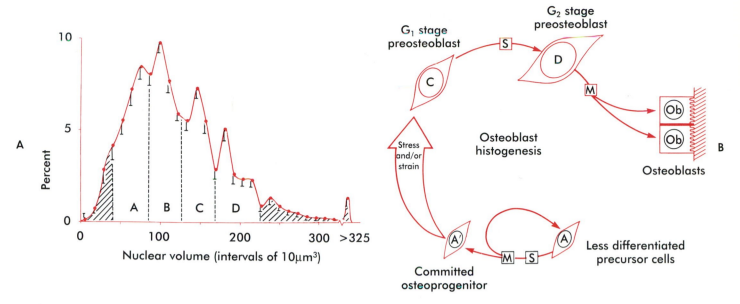

Fig. 3-5   **A,** Frequency distribution of nuclear volume for fibroblast-like cells in unstimulated rat
PDL. *A, B, C,* and *D* cells are a morphologic classification based on peaks in the distribution
curve. (From Roberts WE et al: *Am J Anat* 165:373-384, 1982.) **B,** The osteoblast histogenesis
sequence is a progression of five morphologically and/or kinetically distinguishable cells. There
are two DNA synthesis *(S)* phases and two mitotic *(M)* events. (From Roberts WE, Morey ER:
Am J Anat 174:105-118, 1985.)

sessment of nuclear size (Fig. 3-5, *A*) has proven to be an effective means for determining the relative differentiation of PDL and other bone lining cells.

Cell kinetics. The increase in nuclear size (A′ → C) that occurs as committed osteoprogenitor (A′) cells differentiate to preosteoblasts (C cells) is the rate limiting step in osteoblast histogenesis (Fig. 3-5, *B*).[78,79] Development of this morphometric method substantially expanded the scope of bone cell kinetics particularly in an easily manipulated osteogenic tissue like PDL. In general, metabolic stimuli like parathyroid hormone (PTH) have a systemic effect on *remodeling* (coordinated bone resorption and formation to achieve turnover) but are nonspecific with regard to *modeling* events, such as the bone resorption and formation that allows a tooth to move. For instance, PTH results in a short burst of DNA synthesis and mitosis[57] that depletes the preosteoblast census (Fig. 3-6, *A*) but does not initiate specific resorption and formation sites to achieve tooth movement. On the other hand, a localized mechanical stimulus (orthodontic force) creates a reciprocal pulse of A + A′ and C + D waves that generate huge numbers of osteoblasts (Fig. 3-6, *B*). Studies of control and orthodontically stimulated PDL[86] established the vascular dependence of osteogenesis. Less differentiated osteogenic cells (A + A′) are paravascular: within 20 μm of a blood vessel. A relatively cell free zone borders the paravascular compartment and preosteoblasts (C + D cells) are concentrated >30 μm away from blood vessels (Fig. 3-7).[86] Fig. 3-8 is a photomicrograph of a histologic section of human periodontium showing paravascular arrays in control (unstimulated) human PDL: a

gradient of small nuclei (A + A′ cells), a cell free zone, and a contravascular compartment of cells with large nuclei (C + D cells). The relatively cell free zone is less evident in orthodontically stimulated PDL because large numbers of cells are migrating away from the blood vessels to form new osteoblasts. Later in this chapter the cell kinetic methodology presently defined will be used to describe the physiology of tooth movement.

Finite element modeling (FEM). FEM is a powerful analytical technique for calculating stresses and strains within mechanically loaded structures. The method can be used to model intricate structures, consisting of various shapes and materials, under complex loading. By breaking the structure down into a group of appropriately connected small elements, of known mechanical behavior, the response of the entire structure to loading can be estimated (Fig. 3-9). For complex osseous tissues, such as periodontium, both solid and fluid mechanics must be modeled because most of the components are viscoelastic. Good estimates of *initial* stress levels can be derived by assuming linear elastic properties for periodontal tissues.[62,71] However, realistic estimates of periodontal stress and strain over time requires modeling of viscoelastic properties.[67,73] To date the latter has not been accomplished; however, estimates of initial stress have been useful for defining the mechanical conditions for initiating orthodontically induced bone resorption and formation.[62]

Microelectrodes. Thin tungsten or glass electrodes are inserted into the PDL via the gingival sulcus, providing relatively atraumatic access to osteogenic tissue in an intact animal. This methodology is to measure changes in electric

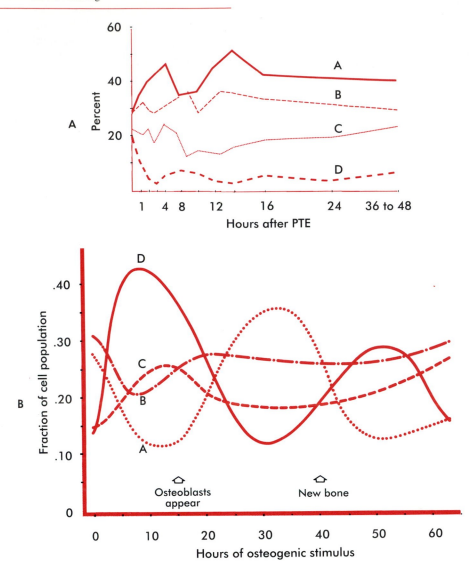

Fig. 3-6 A, Injection of parathyroid extract (PTE) results in a relative increase in *A* cells and a reciprocal decrease in *C* and *D* cells. These results are consistent with a nonspecific release of G_2 blocked preosteoblasts (mitosis of *D* cells during the first 4 hours). From 8 to 48 hours, differentiation of new *C* cells is slowly replenishing the preosteoblast population. **B,** In areas where the PDL is widened by applying orthodontic force, reciprocal waves of *D* and *A* cells generate a rapid and sustained supply of preosteoblasts. These data demonstrate that about half of the less differentiated precursor *(A)* cells are actually committed preosteoblasts (*A'* cells) that form preosteoblasts within about 8 hours. (From Roberts WE et al: *Am J Anat* 165:373-384, 1982.)

potential within the extracellular space of the PDL during the initial response to orthodontic force (Fig. 3-10, *A*).[83] In general, there is a more negative electrical potential in areas of the PDL that are widened and a more positive electrical potential where the PDL is compressed. These results are consistent with the time-honored principle that bone forms near the cathode and resorbs near the anode.[83] The electrical changes noted in orthodontically stressed PDL are apparently specific to living tissue because the electrical response is lost about 20 minutes after cessation of breathing (Fig. 3-10, *B*).

Classification of Bone Tissue

Orthodontic tooth movement results in rapid formation of relatively immature new bone (Fig. 3-11). During the retention period, the newly formed bone remodels and matures. To appreciate the biological mechanism of orthodontic therapy requires a knowledge of bone types.

Woven Bone

Woven bone is highly variable in structure: relatively weak, disorganized, and poorly mineralized. It serves a critical wound healing role by (1) rapidly filling osseous defects,

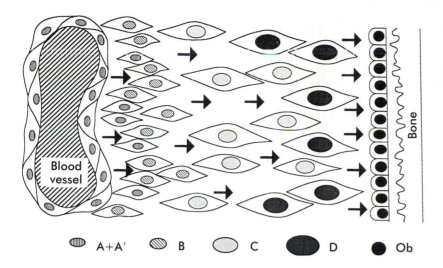

Fig. 3-7 Less differentiated precursor *(A)* cells are a paravascular population. They differentiate to committed osteoprogenitor *(A′)* cells which migrate away from the blood vessel. Traversing the low cell density zone the *A′* cells differentiate to G_1 stage preosteoblasts *(C cells)* that synthesize DNA and become G_2 stage preosteoblasts *(D cells)*. (Adapted from Roberts WE et al: *J Periodont Res* 22:461-467, 1987.)

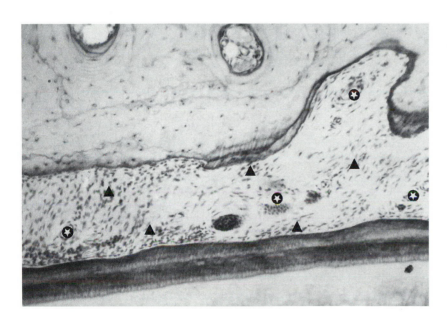

Fig. 3-8 A demineralized section of unstimulated human PDL shows paravascular arrays of osteoblast precursor cells similar to those previously described in the rat (Fig. 3-7). PDL blood vessel *(stars)* are surrounded by fibroblast-like cells with predominantly small nuclei (A + A′ cells). Cells with larger nuclei, preosteoblasts or C + D cells are concentrated away from blood vessels (▲). (Adapted from Roberts WE et al: In *Geriatric dentistry,* Munksgaard, 1986, Copenhagen.)

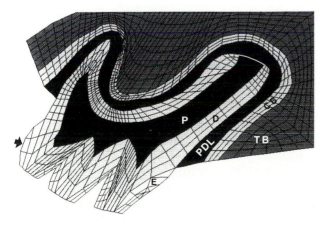

Fig. 3-9 Mesh for a two-dimensional finite element model of a rat maxillary first molar with adjacent periodontium is based on a histologic section in the midsagittal plane of the mesial root *(arrow:* orthodontic force; *P:* pulp; *D:* dentin; *CB:* cortical bone; *TB:* trabecular bone; *E:* enamel.) (From Katona TR et al: Submitted for publication, *J Biomechan.*)

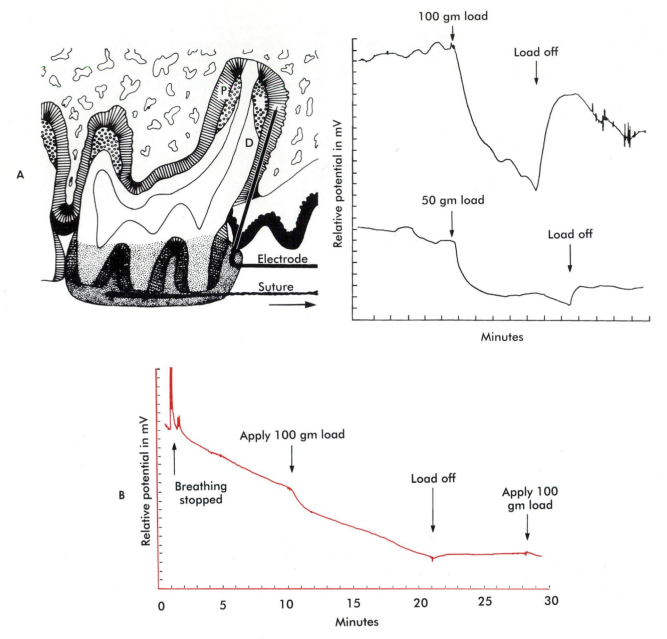

Fig. 3-10 **A,** A tungsten microelectrode is inserted on the mesial aspect of a rat maxillary first molar and stabilized to the tooth with composite resin. An orthodontic load, of 50 or 100 g (about 0.5 to 1.0 N) applied with a traction suture, results in a more negative electrical potential in the PDL where new bone formation will occur. (From Roberts WE et al: In Dixon A, Sarnat B, editors *Factors and mechanisms influencing bone growth,* New York, 1982, Alan R. Liss, pp 527-534.) **B,** Similar measurements of electrical potential were performed in orthodontically stimulated PDL of a rat terminated with an overdose of anesthetic. Following cessation of breathing the electrical response was lost after 20 minutes. (From Roberts WE, Ferguson DJ: In *The biology of tooth movement,* Boca Raton, Fla, 1989, CRC Press, pp 55-70.)

(2) providing initial continuity for fractures and osteotomy segments, and (3) strengthening a bone weakened by surgery or trauma. The first bone formed in response to orthodontic loading is usually of the woven type. Woven bone is not found in the adult skeleton under normal, steady-state conditions. It is either compacted to form composite bone, remodeled to lamellar bone, or rapidly resorbed if prematurely loaded.[37,61] Functional limitations of woven bone are an important aspect of orthodontic retention (Fig. 3-2) and the healing period following orthognathic surgery.[72]

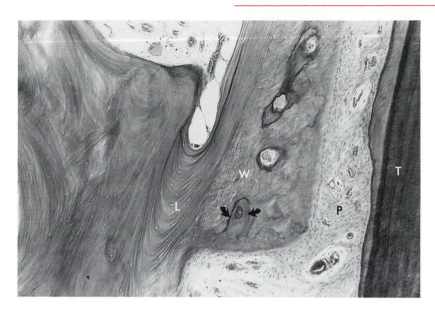

Fig. 3-11   A section of human periodontium from the lower first molar region documents a typical histologic response to orthodontic tooth movement. With respect to the mature lamellar *(L)* bone on the left, the tooth *(T)* is being moved to the right. The first bone formed adjacent to the periodontal ligament *(P)* is of the woven type *(W)*. Subsequent lamellar compaction forms primary osteons of composite bone *(arrows)*. (From Roberts WE et al: *Calif Dent Assoc J* 15(10):58, 1987.)

Lamellar Bone

Lamellar bone, a strong, highly organized, well-mineralized tissue composes >99% of the adult human skeleton. When new lamellar bone is formed, a portion of the mineral component (hydroxylapatite) is deposited by osteoblasts during primary mineralization (Fig. 3-1, *D*). Secondary mineralization, to complete the mineral component, is a physical (crystal growth) process that requires many months to develop. Within physiologic limits, strength of bone is directly related to mineral content.[17,43] The relative strengths of different histologic types of osseous tissue are: woven bone < *new* lamellar bone < *mature* lamellar bone.[72] The bone of adult humans is almost entirely of the remodeled variety: secondary osteons and spongiosa.[43,61,85] Full strength of lamellar bone supporting an orthodontically moved tooth is not achieved until approximately 1 year after completion of active treatment—an important aspect of the orthodontic retention process (Fig. 3-2) and the postoperative maturation period following orthognathic surgery.

Composite Bone

Composite bone is an osseous tissue formed by depositing lamellar bone within a woven bone lattice: cancellous compaction.[20,84] This process is the most rapid means for producing relatively strong bone.[17] Composite bone is an important intermediary type of bone in the physiologic response to orthodontic loading (Fig. 3-11) and is usually the predominant osseous tissue for stabilization during the early process of retention or postoperative healing. When it is formed in the fine compaction configuration, the resulting composite of woven and lamellar bone is also known as primary osteons. Although composite bone may be high quality, load bearing osseous tissue, it is eventually remodeled to secondary osteons.[72,85]

Bundle Bone

Bundle bone is a functional adaptation of lamellar structure for attachment of tendons and ligaments. The major distinguishing characteristic is perpendicular striations of bundle bone called Sharpey's fibers. Distinct layers of bundle bone are usually seen adjacent to PDL (Fig. 3-11) along physiological bone forming surfaces.[14] Bundle bone is the mechanism of ligament and tendon attachment throughout the body.

SKELETAL ADAPTATION

Skeletal adaptation to the mechanical environment occurs by alterations in: (1) bone mass; (2) geometric distribution; (3) matrix organization; and (4) collagen orientation of the lamellae. In addition to these adaptive mechanisms influencing bone formation, the mechanical properties of osseous structures are also influenced by maturation, function, aging, and pathologic processes. A few physiologic and pathologic examples are: (1) secondary mineralization; (2) mean

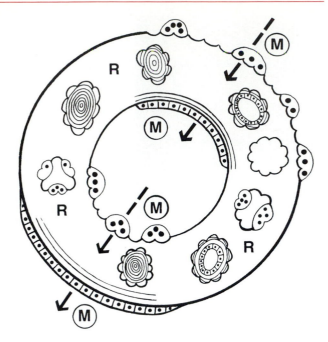

Fig. 3-12 A schematic cross-section of cortical bone shows surface modeling *(M):* uncoupled resorption and formation. Remodeling *(R)* is turnover of previously existing bone. (From Roberts WE et al: *Indiana Dent Assoc* 68:19-24, 1989.)

bone age; (3) fatigue damage; and (4) loss of vitality (pathologic hypermineralization).[69]

Modeling and remodeling. Both trabecular and cortical bone grow, adapt, and turnover by two fundamentally distinct mechanisms: *modeling* and *remodeling.* Bone modeling involves independent sites of resorption and formation that change the form (shape and/or size) of a bone. However, bone remodeling is a specific, coupled sequence of resorption and formation events to replace previously existing bone (Fig. 3-12). The mechanism for internal remodeling (turnover) of dense compact bone is via axially oriented cutting/filling cones (Fig. 3-13).[84] From an ortho-

dontic perspective, the biomechanical response to tooth movement involves an integrated array of bone modeling and remodeling events (Fig. 3-14, *A*). Bone modeling is the dominant process of facial growth and adaptation to applied loads, such as headgear, rapid palatal expansion, and functional appliances. We see *modeling* changes on cephalometric tracings (Fig. 3-14, *B*), but *remodeling* events, which are usually present at the same time, are only apparent at the microscopic level. True remodeling is not usually imaged on clinical radiographs.[77]

Constant remodeling (internal turnover) mobilizes and redeposits calcium by *coupled* resorption and formation events: bone is resorbed and redeposited at the same site. Osteoblasts, osteoclasts, and possibly their precursors are thought to communicate via chemical messages referred to as *coupling factors.* Transforming growth factor beta (TGF-β) has been implicated as a potential coupling factor.[46]

The rate of progression of cutting/filling cones through compact bone is an important determinant of turnover, and it is calculated by measuring the distance between initiation of labeled bone formation sites along the resorption arrest line in longitudinal sections.[84] Using two fluorescent labels administered 2 weeks apart in adult dogs, the velocity is $27.7 \pm 1.9 \, \mu\text{m/d}$ (mean $\pm$ SEM, n = 4 dogs, 10 cutting/filling cones sampled from each). At this speed, evolving secondary osteons travel about 1 mm in 36 days. Newly remodeled secondary osteons (formed within the experimental period of the dog study) contain an average of 4.5 labels (administered 2 weeks apart); the incidence of resorption cavities is about one third of the incidence of labeled osteons.[74] These data are consistent with a remodeling cycle of approximately 12 weeks in dogs[74] compared with 6 weeks in rabbits[84] and 17 weeks in humans.[61,85] This relationship is useful for extrapolating animal data to human applications.

Traumatic or surgical wounding usually results in intense but localized modeling and remodeling responses. Following osteotomy or placement of an endosseous implant, callus formation, and resorption of necrotic osseous margins are

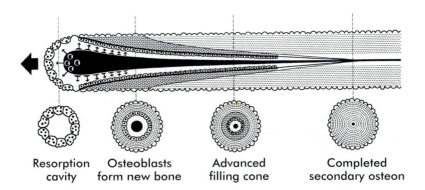

| Resorption cavity | Osteoblasts form new bone | Advanced filling cone | Completed secondary osteon |

Fig. 3-13 The cutting/filling cone has a head of osteoclasts that cut through the bone and a tail of osteoblasts that form a new secondary osteon. (Adapted from Roberts WE et al: *Am J Orthod* 86:95-111, 1984.)

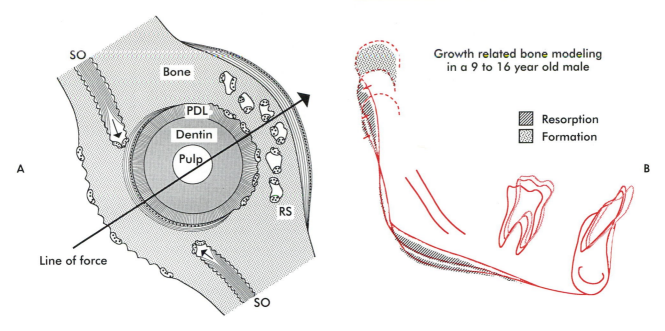

Fig. 3-14   A, Orthodontic bone *modeling,* site specific formation and resorption, occurs along PDL and periosteal surfaces. *Remodeling* (turnover) events occur within the alveolar bone along the line of force on both sides of the tooth. **B,** Orthopedic bone *modeling* related to growth in an adolescent male involves multiple, site specific areas of bone formation and resorption. Although extensive bone *remodeling* (internal turnover) is also occurring, it is not evident in cephalometric radiographs, superimposed on stable mandibular structures.

modeling processes. However, internal replacement of the devitalized cortical bone surrounding these sites is a *remodeling* activity. In addition, a gradient of localized remodeling disseminates through the bone adjacent to any invasive bone procedure. This process, referred to as a *regional acceleratory phenomenon* (RAP), is an important aspect of postoperative healing.[23,61] Orthodontists can take advantage of the intense postoperative modeling and remodeling activity to (1) orthopedically position a maxilla with headgear, occlusal biteplates, or cervical support within a few weeks following a Le Forte I osteotomy, and to (2) rapidly finish orthodontic alignment of the dentition following orthognathic surgery.[63,71]

Both modeling and remodeling are controlled by an interaction of metabolic and mechanical signals. Bone *modeling* is largely under the integrated biomechanical control of functional applied loads (see box p. 204). However, hormones and other metabolic agents have a strong secondary influence, particularly during growth and advanced aging. Paracrine and autocrine mechanisms, such as local growth factors and prostaglandins, are capable of temporarily overriding the mechanical control mechanism during wound healing.[68] *Remodeling* responds to metabolic mediators, like parathyroid hormone and estrogen, primarily by varying the rate of bone turnover (see box p. 204). Bone scans with [99]Te-bisphosphate, a marker of bone activity, indicate that the alveolar processes but *not* the basilar mandible have a high remodeling rate.[34,52] Uptake of the marker in alveolar

bone is similar to the trabecular bone in the vertebral column. The latter is known to remodel at a rate of about 20% to 30% per year compared with most cortical bone, which turns over at approximately 2% to 10% per year.[48] Metabolic mediation of continual bone turnover provides a controllable flow of calcium to and from the skeleton.

Structural and metabolic fractions. The structural fraction of cortical bone is the relatively stable outer portion of the cortex, while the metabolic fraction is the highly reactive inner aspect (Fig. 3-15, *A*). Metabolically, the primary calcium reserves of the body are located in trabecular bone and the endosteal half of the cortices. Analogous to orthodontic wires, the stiffness and strength of a bone are directly related to the bone's cross-sectional area. Diaphyseal rigidity is rapidly enhanced by adding circumferential lamella at the periosteal surface. Even a thin layer of new osseous tissue at the periosteal surface greatly enhances bone stiffness because it increases the diameter of the bone. In engineering terms, cross-sectional rigidity is related to the second moment of the area.[16] The same general relationship of round wire diameter and stiffness (strength) is well known to orthodontists. The rigidity of a wire increases as the fourth power of diameter.[47]

When new osseous tissue is added at the endosteal (inner) surface, it has little effect on overall bone strength. Structurally, long bones and the mandible are modified tubes—an optimal design for achieving maximum strength with minimum mass.[17] Within limits, loss of bone at the endosteal

CONTROL FACTORS FOR BONE MODELING

MECHANICAL*	Peak Load in Microstrain (με)†
Disuse atrophy	<200
Bone maintenance	200-2500
Physiological hypertrophy	2500-4000
Pathological overload	>4000

ENDOCRINE

Bone metabolic hormones—PTH, vitamin D, calcitonin
Growth hormones—somatotropin, IGF I, IGF II
Sex steroids—testosterone, estrogen

PARACRINE AND AUTOCRINE

Wide variety of local agents

*Frost's "mechanostat" theory.
†με is percent deformation × 10⁻⁴.

CONTROL FACTORS FOR BONE REMODELING

METABOLIC

PTH- ↑ Activation frequency
Estrogen- ↓ Activation frequency

MECHANICAL

<1000 με; more remodeling
>2000 με; less remodeling

A

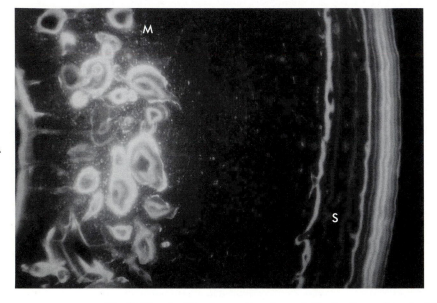

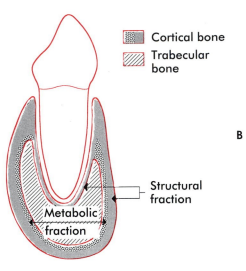

Cortical bone

Trabecular bone

Structural fraction

Metabolic fraction

B

Fig. 3-15 **A,** The structural and metabolic fractions of cortical bone are revealed by multiple fluorochrome labeling of a rabbit femur during the late growth and early adult periods. Continuing periosteal bone formation *(right)* contributes to structural strength while high remodeling of the endosteal half of the compacta provides a continual supply of metabolic calcium. (From Roberts WE et al: In *Bone biodynamics in orthodontic and orthopedic treatment,* ed 27, Ann Arbor, 1991, University of Michigan Press, pp 189-255.) **B,** Structural and metabolic fractions of bone in the mandible. (From Roberts WE et al: Submitted for publication to *Implant Dentistry,* 1993.)

surface or within the inner third of the compacta has little effect on bone rigidity. The inner cortex can be mobilized to meet metabolic needs without severely compromising bone strength (Fig. 3-15). This is the reason that osteoporotic patients have bones with normal diameter but thin cortices. Even under severe metabolic stress, the body follows a cardinal principal of bone physiology: *maximal strength with minimal mass.*[70]

BONE METABOLISM

Orthodontics and dentofacial orthopedics are bone manipulative procedures. The biomechanical response to altered function and applied loads depends on the metabolic status of the host. Bone metabolism is an important aspect of clinical medicine that is directly applicable to orthodontics and orthopedics. This section will discuss the fundamentals of bone metabolism with respect to clinical practice.

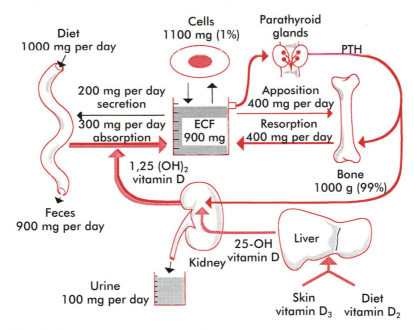

Fig. 3-16 Calcium metabolism is a complex physiologic process. Maintaining zero calcium balance requires optimal function of the gut, parathyroid glands, bone, liver, and kidneys. Parathyroid hormone (PTH) and the active metabolite 1,25 (OH)₂ vitamin D are the major hormones involved. (Adapted from Roberts WE et al: In *Bone biodynamics in orthodontic and orthopedic treatment,* ed 27, Ann Arbor, 1991, University of Michigan Press, pp 189-255.)

Bone is the primary calcium reservoir of the body (Fig. 3-16). Approximately 99% of the calcium in the body is stored in the skeleton. The continual flux of bone mineral responds to a complex interaction of endocrine, biomechanical, and cell-level control factors to maintain the serum calcium level at about 10 mg/dl (10 mg%).

Calcium Homeostasis

Calcium homeostasis is the process by which mineral equilibrium is maintained. Maintenance of serum calcium levels at about 10 mg/dl is an essential life support function. Life is thought to have evolved in the sea; calcium homeostasis is the body's mechanism for maintaining the primordial mineral environment in which cellular processes evolved.[70] Calcium metabolism is one of the most fundamental of the life support physiologic processes. When substantial calcium is needed to maintain the critical serum calcium level, bone structure is sacrificed (Fig. 3-16). The aveolar processes and basilar bone of the jaws are also subject to metabolic bone loss.[44] Even in severe skeletal atrophy, the outer cortex of the alveolar process and the lamina dura around the teeth is preserved. This condition is analogous to the thin cortices of osteoporosis. Calcium homeostasis is supported by three temporally related mechanisms: (1) rapid *(instantaneous)* flux of calcium from bone fluid (seconds); (2) short-term response of osteoclasts and osteoblasts (minutes to days); and (3) long-term (weeks to months) control of bone turnover (Fig. 3-17). Precise regulation of serum calcium levels at about

10 mg/dl is essential for nerve conductivity and muscle function. Low serum calcium can result in tetany and death. Sustained high serum calcium is often a manifestation of hyperparathyroidism and some malignancies. Hypercalcemia may lead to kidney stones and dystrophic calcification of soft tissue. Normal physiology demands precise control of serum calcium.[54,70,82]

Instantaneous regulation of calcium homeostasis is accomplished in seconds by selective transfer of calcium ions into and out of bone fluid (BF) (Fig. 3-17, *B*). BF is separated from extracellular fluid (ECF) by osteoblasts or relatively thin bone lining cells; the latter are thought to be atrophied remnants of osteoblasts.[43] A decreased serum calcium level stimulates secretion of parathyroid hormone (PTH). PTH enhances transport of calcium ions from BF into osteocytes and bone lining cells. The active metabolite of vitamin D (1, 25-Dihydroxycholecalciferol or 1, 25-DCC) enhances pumping of calcium ions from bone lining cells into ECF. This sequence of events transports calcium across the bone lining cells resulting in a net flux of calcium ions from BF to ECF. Within physiological limits, *it is possible to support calcium homeostasis without resorbing bone.* Radioisotope studies confirm that bone contains diffuse mineral component that can be mobilized or redeposited without osteoblastic and osteoclastic activity.[43] However, *sustained negative calcium balance can only be compensated by removing calcium from bone surfaces.*[70,82]

Short-term control of serum calcium levels affects rates of bone resorption and formation within minutes via the

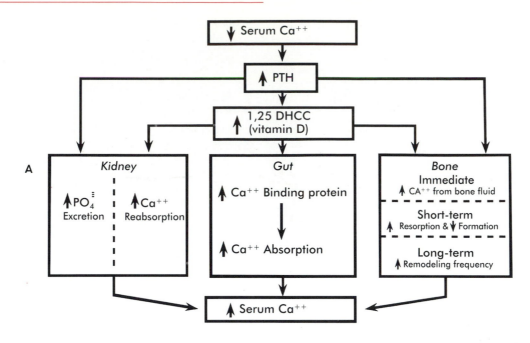

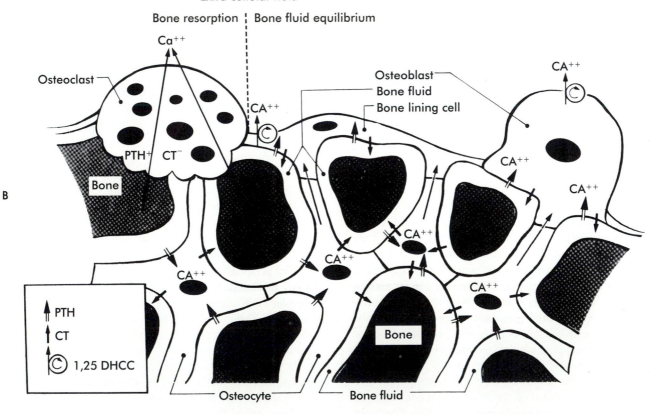

Fig. 3-17 **A,** A flowchart of calcium homeostasis demonstrates the roles of parathyroid hormone *(PTH)*, vitamin D, kidney, gut, and bone in the maintenance of serum calcium levels. Note that bone has immediate, short-term and long-term responses. **B,** Parathyroid hormone (PTH), the active metabolite of vitamin D *(1,25 DHCC)* and calcitonin (CT) play an active role in transferring ionic calcium *(Ca++)* between the bone fluid and extracellular fluid compartments. This is the mechanism of immediate homeostatic control for serum calcium levels. (From Roberts WE et al: *Implant Dentistry* 1:11-21, 1992.)

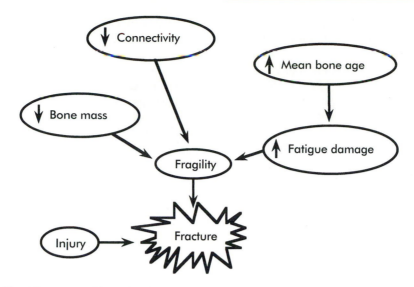

Fig. 3-18 The structural integrity (fracture resistance) of osseous tissue is affected by bone mass, connectivity (geometric distribution), mean bone age, and fatigue damage. Fragile bone may be fractured by normal functional loads or minor injuries.

three calcific hormones: PTH, 1, 25 DHCC and calcitonin (CT). CT, a hormone produced by interstitial cells in the thyroid, is believed to help control hypercalcemia by transiently suppressing bone resorption. PTH, in concert with 1, 25 DHCC, (1) enhances osteoclast recruitment from promonocyte precursors,[30] (2) increases the resorption rate of existing osteoclasts, and (3) may suppress the rate of bone formation by osteoblasts.[70,82]

Long-term regulation of metabolism has profound effects on the skeleton. Biomechanical factors (e.g., normal function, exercise, posture, and habits), noncalcific hormones (e.g., sex steroids and growth hormone) and the metabolic mechanisms previously discussed (Figs. 3-16 and 3-17) dictate mass, geometric distribution, and mean-age of bone (Fig. 3-18). Mass and geometric distribution of bone are strongly influenced by load history (biomechanics) and sex hormone status. PTH is the primary regulator of remodeling frequency: coupled turnover events within bone (see box p. 204). Since the adult skeleton is composed almost entirely of secondary (remodeled) bone, the PTH-mediated activation frequency determines mean bone age. Bone age is an important determinant of fragility because old bone has presumably been weakened by fatigue damage (Fig. 3-18).[70,82]

CALCIUM CONSERVATION

Calcium conservation is the aspect of bone metabolism that relates to preserving skeletal mass. A failure in calcium conservation because of one problem or a combination of metabolic and biomechanical problems may leave a patient with inadequate bone mass for reconstructive dentistry, including orthodontics and/or orthognathic surgery.

The kidney is the primary calcium conservation organ in the body. Through a complex series of excretion and endocrine functions, the kidney excretes excess phosphate, while minimizing the loss of calcium (Figs. 3-16 and 3-17, A). A patient with impaired renal function is often a high risk for osseous manipulative procedures, such as endosseous implants or orthognathic surgery. Because of secondary hyperparathyroidism and impaired vitamin D metabolism, kidney disease may result in poor bone quality, a condition often referred to as renal osteodystrophy.[41,70,82]

Absorption from the small intestine is the primary source of exogenous calcium and phosphate. Phosphate is passively absorbed and rarely deficient. On the other hand, optimal calcium uptake requires an active absorption mechanism. A unique factor involved in the gut absorption process is calcium binding protein, formed in response to the active metabolite of vitamin D. Common clinical profiles associated with poor calcium absorption include a diet deficient in dairy products, vitamin D deficiency, liver disease, and kidney problems.[70,71,82]

Under normal physiologic conditions, the body expends about 300 mg of calcium per day, primarily because of secretory processes in the intestines and kidneys. To maintain the serum calcium level, this 300 mg deficit must be recovered by absorption from the gut. However, absorption of calcium from the gut is vitamin D dependent and only about 30% efficient. If less than about 300 mg per day of calcium is absorbed from the intestine, the serum calcium level decreases, parathyroid hormone secretion turns on, and the necessary calcium is removed from the bones (Fig. 3-16).

Positive calcium balance normally occurs during the growing period and for about 10 years thereafter. The skeletal mass of *prepubertal* children can be enhanced with regular calcium supplements.[36] Peak skeletal mass is attained between 25 and 35 years of age. After the early adult years, natural aging is associated with a slightly negative calcium balance that progressively erodes bone volume throughout life. Zero calcium balance (Fig. 3-16) is the ideal metabolic state for maintaining skeletal mass. Preservation of bone requires a favorable diet, endocrine balance, and adequate exercise.[70,82]

Diet. Animal studies have documented endosteal bone loss of the alveolar processes of dogs maintained on a low calcium diet.[44] These data indicate that a low calcium diet may have severe effects on the bones of the oral cavity. In humans, the current recommended daily allowance (RDA)

of calcium for adults over 19 years of age is 800 mg calcium per day (Table 3-1). However, middle-aged adults probably need more like 1000 mg per day. Growing adolescents, pregnant or lactating women, and, in particular, pregnant teenagers need up to 1600 mg per day. It is suggested that postmenopausal women not maintained on estrogen replacement therapy consume 1500 mg of calcium per day. In the United States, dairy products supply about 70% of dietary calcium. As previously mentioned, dietary phosphate deficiency is rarely a problem.[60,70,71,82]

Obesity has few health benefits; however, it is a protective factor against osteoporosis. This is most probably a result of the high rates of mechanical loading needed to support an overweight body. On the other hand, slight stature is a risk factor for osteoporosis. Because weight control is a concern for the population at risk, the calcium to calorie ratio is an important consideration in dietary counseling (Table 3-2). The most favorable dairy products with respect to the calcium-to-calorie ratio are nonfat milk, part-skim mozzarella cheese, Swiss cheese, and plain, low-fat yogurt. Typical servings of these products have approximately 300 mg of calcium and 100 to 200 calories. Some adults avoid milk because of an intolerance to lactose. Often, these patients assume that they have a *milk allergy*, which should be distinguished according to symptoms. Lactose intolerance is usually manifest by an upset stomach rather than a classic anaphylaxis. Even patients intolerant of milk can usually tolerate cultured products like buttermilk, cheese, and yogurt. Calcium supplements are indicated if a patient is allergic to milk or fails to achieve a calcium sufficient

TABLE 3-1
Dietary Calcium Recommendations

Group	Age	Calcium (mg)
Infants	0 to 6 months	360*
	6 to 12 months	540*
Children	1 to 10 years	800*
Adolescents	11 to 18 years	1,200*
Young adults	19 years and over	800*
Pregnant or lactating women	Under 19 years	1,600*
	Over 19 years	1,200*
Postmenopausal women without estrogen replacement		1,500

*Recommended daily allowance (RDA) data provided by the American Dairy Association.

TABLE 3-2
Calcium and Calorie Content of Common Dairy Products*

	Calcium (mg)	Calories	Ratio
MILK			
Whole, 3.3% fat, 1 cup	291	150	1.9:1
Low-fat, 2% fat, 1 cup	297	120	2.5:1
Buttermilk, 1 cup	285	100	2.8:1
Skim milk, 0% fat, 1 cup	**302**	**85**	**3.6:1**
CHEESE			
American, pasteurized process, 1 oz	174	104	1.7:1
Cheddar, 1 oz	204	115	1.8:1
Cottage, creamed, 4% fat, 1 cup	135	235	0.6:1
Cottage, low-fat, 2%, 1 cup	155	205	0.8:1
Monterey Jack, 1 oz	212	106	2.0:1
Mozzarella, part-skim, 1 oz	**207**	**80**	**2.6:1**
Swiss, 1 oz	**272**	**105**	**2.6:1**
YOGURT			
Plain, low-fat, 8 oz	415	145	2.9:1
Plain, nonfat, 8 oz	**452**	**125**	**3.6:1**
Fruit, low-fat, 8 oz	345	230	1.5:1

*Most favorable calcium to calorie ratio in each category is highlighted. Data provided by the American Dairy Association.

diet for any other reason. Other foods, particularly green leafy vegetables (e.g., turnip greens and spinach) contain some calcium; however, it is difficult to consume adequate calcium in a diet excluding dairy products.[70,82]

Calcium supplements of many varieties are available in pharmacies and health food stores. Most will provide adequate calcium when used as directed. However, beware of toxic contaminants in some *natural* supplements, such as bone meal and dolomite. They may contain significant quantities of lead, arsenic, or other heavy metals. Among the least expensive, readily tolerated supplements are calcium carbonate antacids (e.g., Tums® and *Ca-rich* Rolaids®). When determining the elemental calcium in a supplement, remember to use the molecular weight. For instance, calcium carbonate is only 40% calcium. This means a 500 mg tablet provides only 300 mg of calcium.[70,82]

Endocrinology. Peptide hormones (e.g., PTH, growth hormone, insulin, and calcitonin) bind receptors at the cell surface and may be internalized with the receptor complex. Steroid hormones (e.g., vitamin D, androgens and estrogens) are lipid soluble and pass through the plasma membrane to bind receptors in the nucleus.[70,82]

PTH increases serum calcium by direct and indirect vitamin D mediated effects. Vitamin D was originally thought to be an essential dietary factor. However, it is not a vitamin at all; it is a hormone. Cholecalciferol (vitamin D) is synthesized in skin irradiated by ultraviolet (UV) light, hydroxylated in the liver at the #25 position, and then hydroxylated in the kidney at the #1 position to produce the active metabolite 1, 25 DHCC. This last step is feedback controlled; hydroxylation at the #1 position is induced by low serum calcium level, probably via PTH (Fig. 3-16). Clinically, a major effect of 1, 25 DHCC is inducing active absorption of calcium from the gut. Because of the complexity of the vitamin D synthesis and metabolic pathway, calcium adsorption may be inhibited at many levels: (1) lack of skin exposure to adequate sunlight of the proper wavelength; (2) failure to consume vitamin D through the diet, thereby not compensating for the lack of vitamin D synthesis; (3) genetic defect in skin; (4) liver disease; and (5) kidney failure.[70,82]

Sex hormones have profound effects on bone. Androgens (testosterone and other anabolic steroids) build and maintain musculoskeletal mass. The primary hypertrophic effect of androgens is to increase muscle mass. The anabolic effect on bone is a secondary biomechanical response to increased loads generated by the enhanced muscle mass. On the other hand, estrogen has a direct effect on bone; it conserves skeletal calcium by suppressing the activation frequency of bone remodeling.[22] At menopause, enhanced remodeling activation increases turnover. Since a slight negative calcium balance is associated with each remodeling event, a substantial increase in the turnover rate can result in rapid bone loss, leading to symptomatic osteoporosis. Even young women are susceptible to significant bone loss if the menstrual cycle (menses) ceases.[19] Bone loss is a common prob-

lem in women who have low body fat and who exercise intensely (e.g., running, gymnastics) or in women who are anorexic.[56] It is clear that estrogen protects the female skeleton from bone loss during the childbearing years. Lack of menses in women of any age presents a high risk factor for developing osteoporosis later in life.[70,82]

Estrogen replacement therapy is widely recommended for calcium conservation and prevention of osteoporosis in postmenopausal women.[15,21] A major concern of many patients and of some physicians is the relationship of estrogen therapy to incidence and progression of breast cancer. A number of recent studies around the world have failed to demonstrate an increased risk or progression of breast cancer in women who receive estrogen replacement therapy.[29] The anti-estrogen tamoxifen is used to treat some forms of breast cancer. Fortunately, tamoxifen has a beneficial bone effect in postmenopausal women similar to estrogen.[40]

SKELETAL COMPROMISE

Skeletal health is related to diet, exercise, life-style, and the proper function of numerous organ systems. To provide optimal support over a broad spectrum of conditions, the skeletal system has evolved complex mechanical, endocrine, and cell-level regulatory mechanisms. A failure of one or more of these homeostatic mechanisms can result in metabolic bone disease. Because of low skeletal mass and/or poor osteogenic capability, some patients may be a poor risk for orthodontic or orthognathic procedures. Skeletally compromised patients presenting for unrelated dental treatment provide dentists with unique diagnostic opportunities. Timely referral of individuals with high-risk profiles to appropriately trained physicians can result in substantial health benefits. If osteopenia is confirmed, it is then possible to initiate corrective medical therapy before the onset of the debilitating symptoms associated with osteoporosis.[70,82]

The concept of structural and metabolic fractions (Fig. 3-15) has considerable clinical significance. The dietary requirement for calcium increases during the growing years. High dietary calcium (1200 mg per day) is essential during the adolescent period (Table 3-1) to provide structural strength without compromising the metabolic reserve. Pregnancy and lactation before the age of 19 years may be a precipitating factor for osteopenia later in life. Multiple births during the teenage years are of particular concern. Under these circumstances, young women may fail to deposit sufficient skeletal reserves to withstand the sustained negative calcium balance that follows menopause.[70,82,95]

Although the metabolic fraction of cortical bone can make a substantial contribution, the major source of serum calcium under steady-state conditions is trabecular bone. The primary reason is differential remodeling rates. Cortical bone turns over about 2% to 10% per year, while trabecular bone is much more active, remodeling at 20% to 30% per year.[48] Because it is more labile, trabecular bone is more susceptible to loss under conditions of negative calcium

balance. For this reason, patients who have osteoporosis have a tendency for structural failure at sites primarily dependent on trabecular bone: the spine (compression fracture), wrist (Colles' fracture), and hip (femoral neck). Degenerative changes in the temporomandibular joint have not been directly related to skeletal atrophy. However, some relationship is probable because both problems preferentially affect the same high risk group: postmenopausal females.[26,70,82]

Aging. Women depend on estrogen to maintain skeletal mass. Lack of normal menses even in young women usually indicates an estrogen deficiency and probable negative calcium balance. Numerous national and international consensus conferences[13,15] have recommended that most postmenopausal Caucasian and Asian women be treated with estrogen to prevent osteoporosis. However, surveys indicate that many physicians fail to prescribe estrogen for their postmenopausal patients,[25] and many patients, for which estrogen has been prescribed, fail to take it. For these reasons many women in our society are estrogen-deficient. About 20% will develop frank osteoporosis, and up to 50% will demonstrate some signs or symptoms.[82] All health providers should be particularly concerned about the skeletal status of postmenopausal Caucasian and Asian women. However, even the low-risk groups, such as males and black American women, still demonstrate an incidence of osteoporosis that approaches 5%. Thus osteopenia and osteoporosis are a significant health risk for almost everyone. Bone metabolic evaluation is an important diagnostic consideration for all patients being considered for orthodontics or orthognathic surgery.[63,70,71]

METABOLIC BONE DISEASE

Osteoporosis is a generic term for low bone mass (osteopenia). The most important risk factor for developing osteoporosis is age: after the third decade, osteopenia is directly related to longevity. Other high risk factors are: (1) a history of long-term glucocorticoid treatment; (2) a slight stature; (3) smoking; (4) menopause or dysmenorrhea; (5) low physical activity; (6) low calcium diet; (7) excessive alcohol consumption; (8) vitamin D deficiency; (9) kidney failure; (10) liver disease (cirrhosis); and (11) a history of fractures. These osteopenic risk factors are effective in identifying 78% of those with the potential for osteopenia.[35,95] This is a particularly good screening method for skeletally asymptomatic dental patients. However, it is important to realize that over 20% of individuals that eventually develop osteoporosis present a negative history for known risk factors. Any clinical signs or symptoms of low bone mass, such as low radiographic density of the jaws, thin cortices, or excessive bone resorption, are grounds for referral. A thorough medical work-up, including a bone mineral density measurement, is usually necessary to establish the diagnosis of *osteopenia.* The term *osteoporosis* is usually reserved for patients with evidence of fracture or other osteoporotic

symptoms. Treatment of metabolic bone diseases, such as osteoporosis, depends on the causative factors. Medical management of these often complex disorders is best handled by physicians specifically trained in bone metabolism.[70,82]

Increasing numbers of adults are seeking orthodontic treatment. Because all orthodontic and facial orthopedic therapy requires bone manipulation, orthodontists should have a detailed knowledge of bone physiology. All health practitioners can play an important role in screening patients with high-risk life-styles. Arresting the progression of metabolic bone disease is preferable to treating the condition after debilitating symptoms appear. A carefully taken history is the best screening method for determining which patients should be referred for a thorough metabolic work-up. No age limit is specified for orthodontic treatment; however, the clinician must carefully assess the probability of metabolic bone disease.[70,82] In addition to osteoporosis, orthodontists should be particularly vigilant for *osteomalacia,* a poor bone mineralization disease associated with vitamin D deficiency,[48] and for *renal osteodystrophy,* a related condition in patients with compromised kidney function.[41]

Orthodontics is usually contraindicated in patients with active metabolic bone disease because of excessive resorption and poor bone formation. However, if the metabolic problems (particularly negative calcium balance) are resolved with medical treatment, these patients can be treated orthodontically, assuming sufficient skeletal structure remains. In fact, some osteoporotics retain near normal jaw and alveolar bone probably because they have healthy oral structures that are normally loaded. Apparently, under these circumstances the disease preferentially attacks bone in other parts of the body with a less optimal mechanical environment.[70,82]

BIOMECHANICS

Gravitational loads have a substantial influence on normal skeletal physiology. Osteoblast differentiation leading to new bone formation is stimulated by mechanical loading,[79] but is inhibited by weightlessness.[78,80] Space flight studies have established that gravity helps maintain skeletal mass.[45,94] A substantial portion of the physiological loading of the mandible is related to antigravity posturing. In erect posture, gravity tends to open the mouth. Muscular force is used to hold the mouth closed. Apparently, growth of the rat mandibular condyle may be inhibited during space flight because of less functional loading in weightlessness.[33] Gravity may prove to be an important factor in the secondary growth mechanism of the mandible.

Mechanical loading is essential to skeletal health. Control of most bone modeling (box p. 204) and of some remodeling processes (box p. 204) is related to strain history. Repetitive loading generates a specific response, which is determined by the peak strain.[39,55,89-91] In an attempt to simplify the often conflicting data, Frost[24] proposed the *mechanostat* theory.

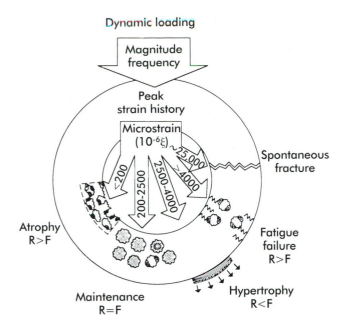

Fig. 3-19 Schematic drawing of the mechanostat concept of Frost[24a] as defined by Martin and Burr.[43] Bone formation *(F)* and resorption *(R)* are the modeling phenomena that change the shape and/or form of a bone. The peak strain history determines if atrophy, maintenance, hypertrophy, or fatigue failure occurs. (From Roberts WE et al: Submitted to *Implant Dentistry,* 1993.)

Reviewing the theoretical basis of the *mechanostat,* Martin and Burr[43] propose that: (1) subthreshold loading of <200 $\mu\epsilon$ results in disuse atrophy, manifest as decreased modeling and increased remodeling; (2) physiological loading of about 200 to 2500 $\mu\epsilon$ is associated with normal, steady-state activity; (3) loads exceeding the minimal effective strain (about 2500 $\mu\epsilon$) result in a hypertrophic increase in modeling and concomitant decrease in remodeling; but (4) once peak strains exceed about 4000 $\mu\epsilon$, structural integrity of bone is threatened: pathologic overload. Fig. 3-19 is a visual representation of the mechanostat. Although many of the concepts and $\mu\epsilon$ levels are based on experimental data,[43] the mechanostat has not been adequately verified under a variety of conditions. The strain range for each given response probably varies between species and may be site specific in the same individual.* However, the mechanostat provides a useful clinical reference for the hierarchy of biomechanical responses to applied loads.

Normal function helps build and maintain bone mass. Suboptimally loaded bones atrophy by increasing the remodeling frequency while inhibiting osteoblast formation.[24] Under these conditions, trabecular connections are lost and cortices are thinned from the endosteal surface. Eventually, the skeleton is weakened until it cannot sustain normal function. Increasing numbers of adults with a history of osteo-

---

*References 39, 43, 71, 89, 91.

penia caused by metabolic bone disease are seeking orthodontic treatment for routine malocclusions. Assuming the negative calcium balance is corrected and adequate bone structure remains, patients with a history of osteoporosis or other metabolic bone disease are viable candidates for routine orthodontic therapy. The critical factor is the residual bone mass in the area of interest after the disease process is arrested (Fig. 3-20).

When flexure (strain) exceeds the normal physiologic range, bones compensate by adding new mineralized tissue at the periosteal surface. Adding additional bone is an essential compensating mechanism because of the inverse relationship between load (strain magnitude) and the fatigue resistance of bone.[10] When loads are less than 2000 $\mu\epsilon$, lamellar bone can withstand millions of loading cycles: more than a lifetime of normal function. However, increasing the cyclic load to 5000 $\mu\epsilon$, approximately 20% of the ultimate strength of cortical bone, can produce fatigue failure in a thousand cycles, which is easily achieved in only a few weeks of normal activity. Repetitive overload at less than one fifth of the ultimate strength of lamellar bone (25,000 $\mu\epsilon$ or 2.5% deformation) can lead to skeletal failure, stress fractures, and shin splints.

From a dental perspective, occlusal prematurities or parafunction may lead to compromises in periodontal bone support. Localized fatigue failure may be a factor in periodontal clefting, alveolar recession, tooth oblation (cervical ditching), or temporomandibular arthrosis. Avoiding persistent occlusal prematurities, guarding against excessive tooth mobility, and achieving an optimal distribution of occlusal loads are important objectives for orthodontic treatment. The human masticatory apparatus can achieve a biting strength of over 2200 Newtons (more than 500 pounds of force).[6,7] Because of the high magnitude and frequency of oral loads, functional prematurities during orthodontic treatment could contribute to isolated incidence of alveolar clefting (Fig. 3-21, *A*) and root resorption (Fig. 3-21, *B*). It is recommended that excessive tooth mobility be carefully monitored during active orthodontic treatment and retention. Avoiding occlusal prematurities is a particular concern in treating periodontally compromised teeth.

ORTHODONTIC TOOTH MOVEMENT

Fig. 3-22 illustrates a typical tooth movement response following application of a moderate, continuous load (0.2 to 0.5 N or about 20 to 50 g). The orthodontic response is divided into three elements of tooth displacement: *initial strain, lag phase, progressive tooth movement.* Initial strain of 0.4 to 0.9 mm occurs in about 1 week[53,71,92] because of PDL displacement (strain), bone strain, and extrusion (Fig. 3-23). The initial deformation response varies with: PDL width, root length, anatomical configuration, force magnitude, occlusion, and periodontal health. Initial tooth displacement occurs within seconds,[9,44a,92] but actual compression of the PDL requires from 1 to 3 hours (Fig. 3-24).[67]

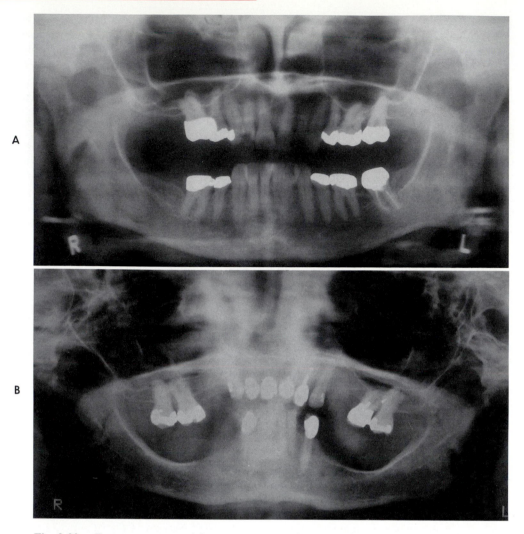

Fig. 3-20   Two postmenopausal females with systemic osteopenia present widely varying patterns of lower posterior bone loss: **A,** Alveolar bone in the buccal segments is well preserved by functional loading of natural teeth. **B,** Severe resorption of the alveolar process and basilar mandible has occurred in the absence of adequate functional loading. (From Roberts WE et al: Submitted to *Implant Dentistry,* 1993.)

Unfortunately, no studies have employed a broad range of invasive and noninvasive techniques to completely define the fluid and solid mechanics associated with initiating and sustaining tooth movement. Fig. 3-22 is an attempt to unify a broad range of data. The fluid mechanics of root displacement within the PDL probably accounts for about 0.3 mm of crown movement.[73] Assuming an average anatomical configuration and bone strain of ≤1% (about 40% of ultimate strength),[17] distortion of mineralized tissue caused by bending and creep[11,43] probably accounts for about another 0.3 mm of the initial movement.[73]

Extrusion in response to a horizontal load may be a component of initial displacement[9] depending on the direction of the force, point of application, and axial inclination of the root; however, varying amounts of extrusion are expected because of the inclined plane effect of the root apex being compressed against the alveolus (Fig. 3-23). The tendency toward extrusion and enhanced horizontal displacement during tooth movement varies directly with force magnitude and periodontal compromise of the dentoalveolar fibers at the alveolar crest. Extrusion and occlusal prematurities are distinct possibilities, particularly for periodontally compromised teeth, and depend on the vertical constraint of a clinically applied load (Fig. 3-21, *A*). If occlusal prematurity is a chronic periodontal trauma, root resorption may result because of catabolic cytokines in the PDL[18] or because of fatigue failure (Fig. 3-21, *B*).

Progressive displacement of the tooth relative to its osseous support ceases in about a week (Fig. 3-22) apparently because of areas of PDL necrosis *(hyalinization)*. This lag phase is highly variable—usually 2 to 3 weeks, but it may be as long as 10 weeks.[53] Clinical experience and histological studies[53,73] suggest the duration of the lag phase is directly related to the age of the patient, density of the alveolar

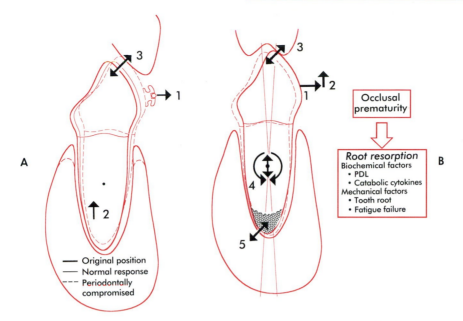

Fig. 3-21   A, A moderate load in the buccal direction *(1)* results in a tipping displacement of the crown. In the absence of vertical constraint, a normal healthy tooth is expected to extrude slightly because of the inclined plane effect of the root engaging the tapered alveolus *(2)*. Because of less bone support and destruction of restraining collagen fibers at the alveolar crest, a periodontally compromised tooth may tip and extrude considerably more. Depending on occlusion, this displacement may produce an occlusal prematurity *(3)*. **B,** Orthodontic tipping *(1)* with an extrusive component *(2)* may produce an occlusal prematurity *(3)* and mobility *(4)*. An individual tooth in chronic occlusal trauma is expected to continuously generate catabolic cytokines in the PDL, and the root apex is exposed to fatigue damage. This combination of physical failure in a catabolic environment may lead to progressive root resorption *(5)*.

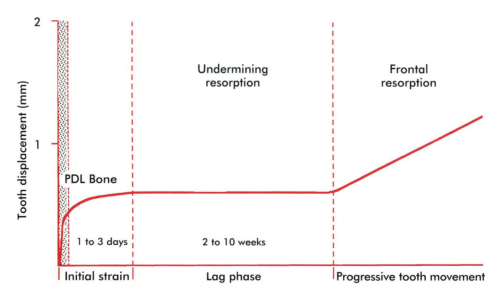

Fig. 3-22   Following application of a moderate orthodontic load (0.2 to 0.5 N or about 20 to 50 g), tooth displacement is divided into three phases: (1) initial strain for 1 to 3 days within PDL and supporting bone; (2) variable lag phase when undermining resorption removes bone adjacent to crushed areas in the PDL; and (3) progressive tooth movement when frontal resorption within the PDL limits the rate of orthodontic correction.

bone, and extent of PDL necrotic zones. Once undermining resorption restores vitality to the necrotic areas of the PDL, tooth movement enters the secondary[53,92] or progressive tooth movement phase (Fig. 3-22). Frontal resorption (modeling) in the PDL and initial remodeling events (resorption cavities) within cortical bone ahead of the advancing tooth (Fig. 3-14, *A*), allow for progressive tooth movement at a relatively rapid rate.(See Chapter 2.)

The mechanism of sustained tooth movement is a coordinated array of bone resorption and formation events (Fig. 3-14, *A*). Both fundamental mechanisms of osseous adaptation (modeling and remodeling) are involved. A *modeling* response is noted within the alveolus: bone resorption occurs where the PDL is compressed (in the direction of movement), and bone formation maintains the normal width of the trailing PDL. Via this coordinated series of surface modeling events, the alveolus drifts in the direction of tooth movement. The modeling events of tooth movement are

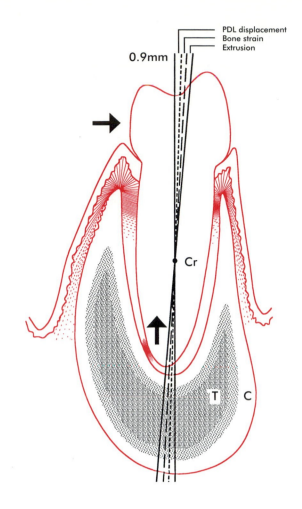

Fig. 3-23   Initial displacement (1 to 3 days) for a tooth exposed to a tipping (horizontal) load is usually about 0.5 mm but may be as much as 0.9 mm for teeth that are slightly mobile, periodontally compromised, or heavily loaded. There are three components: (1) displacement of the root within the PDL; (2) bone strain caused by bending and creep; and (3) extrusion caused by the inclined plane effect of the tooth root pressing against a tapered alveolus. (Adapted from Roberts WE et al: In *Bone biodynamics in orthodontic and orthopedic treatment,* ed 27, Ann Arbor, 1991, University of Michigan Press, pp 189-255.)

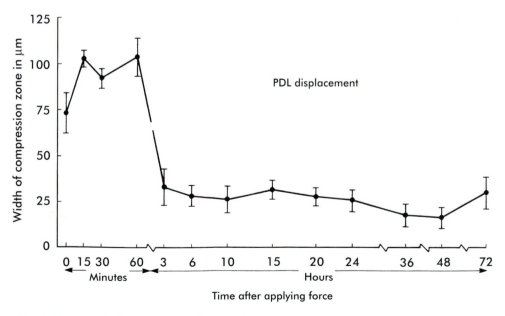

Fig. 3-24   Initial displacement of the mesial root of rat maxillary first molars within the PDL space is assessed by measuring the width of the maximum compression zone. This method is an index of PDL displacement that is relatively independent of bone deformation. Note the resistance to compression during the first hour followed by maximal compression at 3 hours, creating necrotic areas where undermining resorption will occur.

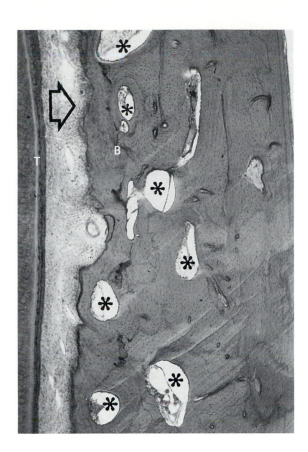

commonly referred to as *areas of compression and tension* within the PDL.[53,92] For small amounts of tooth movement (<1 mm) over 1 or 2 months, PDL modeling is probably the predominant mechanism of tooth movement. However, when teeth are moved greater distances over longer periods of time, the PDL response is supplemented by alveolar bone *remodeling* and periosteal *modeling* (Figs. 3-25 and 3-26).

Remodeling of dense alveolar bone (Fig. 3-25) enhances the rate of tooth movement[73] and replaces the less mature osseous tissue formed by rapid PDL osteogenesis (Fig. 3-26). Resorption cavities ahead of the moving tooth decrease the density of cortical bone (Fig. 3-25). These intraosseous cavities are the initial remodeling events that occur during

Fig. 3-25   A demineralized histologic section of human periodontium reveals the modeling and remodeling mechanisms of progressive tooth movement through dense cortical bone *(B)*. A tooth *(T)* is moving in the direction of the large arrow. The rate of translation is enhanced by frontal resorption in the PDL communicating with the extensive resorption cavities *(*)* created by initial remodeling events (cutting cones). Via this mechanism, teeth move through dense cortical bone at a rate of about 0.3 mm per month × 25. (From Roberts WE et al: In *Bone biodynamics in orthodontic and orthopedic treatment,* ed 27, Ann Arbor, 1991, University of Michigan Press, pp 189-255.)

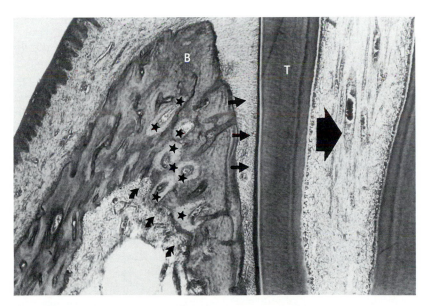

Fig. 3-26   A demineralized histologic section of human periodontium documents the bone modeling and remodeling aspects of alveolar bone *(B)* drift in the direction of tooth *(T)* movement *(large black arrow)*. Three major aspects of bone modeling are noted: (1) new bone formation within the PDL *(small horizontal arrows);* (2) periosteal resorption on the lingual alveolar bone surface *(left);* and (3) endosteal resorption in the direction of the curved arrows to maintain the cortical thickness of the alveolar crest as it drifts to the right. Bone *remodeling* replaces relatively immature bone with new secondary osteons *(stars)*. ×25. (From Roberts WE et al: In *Bone biodynamics in orthodontic and orthopedic treatment,* ed 27, Ann Arbor, 1991, University of Michigan Press, pp 189-255.)

the first month of the remodeling cycle (Fig. 3-1). With progressive tooth movement, it appears that these resorption cavities are truncated remodeling events.[73] Continuous force[8,42] or reactivation at approximately 1-month intervals[73] is expected to yield the maximal rate of tooth movement through cortical bone. The remodeling dependent concept of long-range tooth movement has important clinical implications. Efficient mechanics and regular reactivations at about 4-week intervals have long been associated with optimal rates of tooth movement.[73] However, breakage, distortion of appliances, and appointment failures substantially increase treatment time. One reason for slow tooth movement in uncooperative patients may be the tendency for resorption cavities initiated by orthodontic activation to complete the remodeling cycle by refilling with new bone if appropriate mechanics are not maintained. Repeatedly reinitiating force after periods of periodontal recovery requires one start-up period after the other (Fig. 3-22) to reestablish the modeling and remodeling mechanisms to move a tooth through dense cortical bone.

Secondary osteons are formed in new cortical bone trailing a moving tooth (Fig. 3-26). The major modeling and remodeling events associated with sustained buccal movement (controlled tipping) of a lower premolar are summarized in Fig. 3-27. Efficiency of bone resorption is the limiting factor in the rate of tooth movement. Bone removal ahead of the moving tooth occurs by two mechanisms: frontal resorption at the PDL interface and initial remodeling events (resorption cavities) within the cortical plate. In ad-

dition to PDL modeling of the alveolus (bone resorption in the *area of pressure* and bone formation in the *area of tension*), Fig. 3-27 demonstrates surface modeling on periosteal and endosteal surfaces. These coordinated modeling events maintain the structural relationship of the alveolar process as the tooth moves.[15]

PERIODONTAL LIGAMENT RESPONSE

Within a minute after application of a continuous orthodontic load to a rat maxillary first molar, a more negative electrical potential is noted where the PDL is widened and a more positive signal where it is compressed (Fig. 3-10). These bioelectrical changes are not piezoelectric signals but are probably streaming potentials.[83] Changes in electrical potential may drive the PDL osteogenic and osteoclastic responses or merely be physical manifestations of the intense cellular activities (ion flux across cell membranes) triggered by orthodontic stimuli.[67] Coordination of cellular reactions in the PDL to changes in electrical potential is a prime area for future investigation.

A cascade of cellular proliferation and differentiation events is initiated in the periodontal ligament (PDL) by application of orthodontic force. Maximal compression of the PDL occurs in 1 to 3 hours (Fig. 3-24), which is consistent with most clinical estimates for initial displacement following application of an orthodontic load (Fig. 3-22). As the root of the tooth is displaced, an array of nervous, immune and endocrine system responses, as well as local cytokines and intracellular messages, have been implicated in the osseous adaptive reaction.[18] These localized agents are probably mediators of the often painful, transient inflammatory events noted during the initiation of the orthodontic reaction. The role of local cytokines in the sustained bone modeling and remodeling events of tooth movement is unknown. However, prostaglandins are thought to be important factors in the control of mechanically mediated bone adaptation.[18,50,87,97]

Comparing control rat PDL (Fig. 3-28, *A*) to orthodontically stimulated PDL (Fig. 3-28, *B*) helps define the biologic mechanisms for mechanically induced bone formation and resorption (Fig. 3-28, *B*). The specificity of bone resorbing and forming sites is dictated by the physics of the applied force system.[8] Although the PDL histologic changes and cell kinetics associated with orthodontically induced osteoclasis and osteogenesis are well defined,* the actual cellular mechanisms effecting and controlling tooth movement are less clear. An interaction of metabolic, biomechanical, bioelectrical, and biochemical factors have been implicated.† The challenge is to determine the sequence or cascade of cybernetic events.[73]

Minimal proliferative activity is noted in areas of the PDL where bone resorption predominates. However, an intense

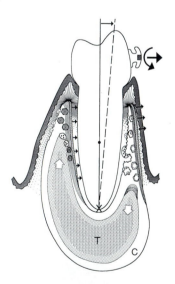

Fig. 3-27 A force and a moment produces a center of rotation *(X)* near the apex. Surface *modeling* is noted within the PDL, resorption on the right and deposition on the left, and on the periosteal surfaces, resorption on the left and apposition on the right. Bone remodeling assists with cortical bone resorption on the right and replaces immature bone on the left sides of the alveolar process. The mandible is composed of both trabecular (T) and cortical (C) bone. (From Roberts WE et al: In *Bone biodynamics in orthodontic and orthopedic treatment,* ed 27, Ann Arbor, 1991, University of Michigan Press, pp 189-255.)

---

*References 53, 66, 71, 73, 75, 92, 96, 98.
†References 18, 38, 67, 71, 73.

proliferative response is noted in PDL where new bone is destined to form.* For the first 12 hours after initiation of orthodontic stimulus there is a modest, *nonspecific* increase of cells in the mitotic and DNA synthesis (S) phases through-

out the PDL (Fig. 3-29, *A*). After 16 hours a specific osteogenic response is noted in the area of the PDL where new bone formation will initiate (Fig. 3-29, *B*). Over half of the fibroblastlike PDL cells in the widened area of the PDL enter the DNA synthesis (S) phase of the cell cycle[65] and subsequently divide.[73,78] Preosteoblasts then migrate

*References 66, 75, 96, 98, 99.

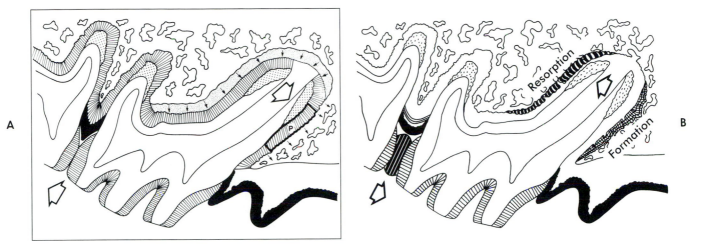

Fig. 3-28   **A,** Physiologic drift for the mesial root of a rat maxillary first molar involves a relative tipping of the tooth in the direction of the large arrows. Net resorption occurs adjacent to the area of the PDL *(P)* marked with bold outline. Bone formation is noted along PDL adjacent to the *stippled area.* (From Roberts WE, Morey ER: *Am J Anat* 174:105-118, 1985.) **B,** Inserting a latex elastic between the first and second molars reverses the direction of tooth movement resulting in resorption on a previously bone-forming surface *(above)* and vice versa *(below).* The area of *de novo* bone formation is the experimental model used to determine the osteoblast histogenesis sequence. (From Roberts WE et al: *Am J Anat* 165:373-384, 1982.)

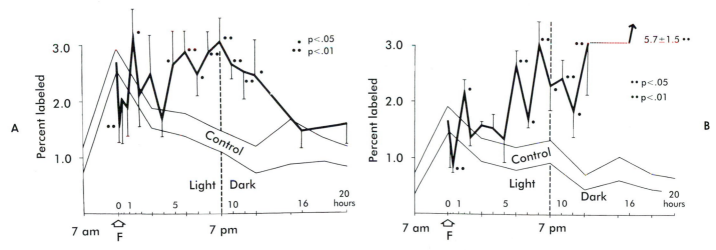

Fig. 3-29   **A,** Compared to the normal circadian range of DNA synthesis phase cells, orthodontic stimulus *(F)* results in a modest nonspecific increase in S phase cells throughout the PDL. This is a mechanically induced release of G_1 blocked cells. These data are from the alveolar crest area, where no new bone formation will occur. **B,** In the midroot area, where new bone formation is induced, a similar nonspecific response is followed by large proliferative reaction that specifically supports orthodontically induced osteogenesis. (From Smith RK, Roberts WE: *Calc Tiss Int* 30:51-56, 1980.)

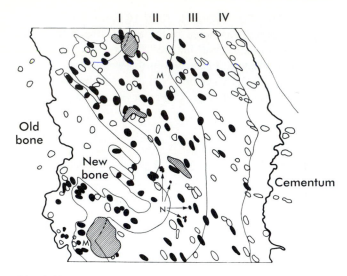

Fig. 3-30 During the first 70 hours of orthodontically induced osteogenesis PDL osteogenic cells migrate toward the bone surface from throughout the PDL. Cell migration patterns are tracked by repeated injection of the DNA precursor ³H-thymidine. Labeled cells have black nuclei. (From Roberts WE, Chase DC: *J Dent Res* 60:174-181, 1981.)

from throughout the PDL to the alveolar bone surface (Fig. 3-30),[96] form osteoblasts, and initiate new bone formation in about 40 to 48 hours.[66,73]

The orthodontic response in the PDL is an effective experimental model for determining the physiological mechanisms of mechanically induced bone modeling. Orthodontic stimulation of rat maxillary molars has been particularly useful for initiating a defined osteogenic reaction within the PDL on the mesial aspect of the mesial root (Fig. 3-28, *B*). Application of the finite element method (FEM) permits calculation of stresses within the tissue down to the cellular level. Because of the tissue complexity and diverse range of mechanical properties, orthodontically stressed periodontium is a relatively challenging application of the FEM method. The model simulates the experimental tipping of a rat maxillary first molar (Fig. 3-31, *A*). It was concluded that osteogenesis occurred where maximum principal stress was elevated within the PDL (Fig. 3-31, *B*). Bone resorption initiated where there were peaks in minimum principal stress, maximum shear, and strain energy density.[62]

OSTEOBLAST HISTOGENESIS AND BONE FORMATION

Osteoblasts are derived from paravascular connective tissue cells (Fig. 3-7). The less differentiated precursor and committed osteoprogenitor cells are closely associated with blood vessels. Their progeny (preosteoblasts) migrate away from the blood vessels. The major rate-limiting step in the histogenesis sequence occurs as the cells move through an area of low cell density about 30 μm away from the nearest

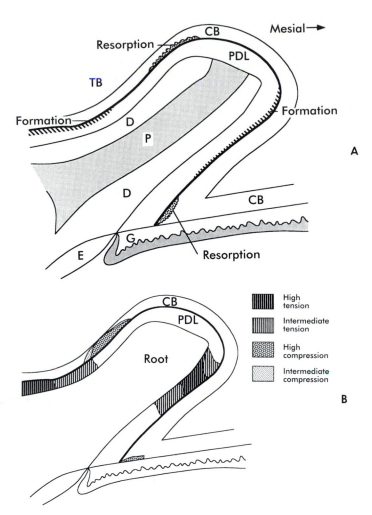

Fig. 3-31 **A,** The mesial tipping of the rat maxillary first molar results in a typical pattern of bone resorption and formation that produces tooth movement: gingiva *(G)*, enamel *(E)*, dentin *(D)*, trabecular bone *(TB)*, cortical bone *(CB)*, and pulp *(P)*. **B,** Finite element model (Fig. 3-9) stress analysis of orthodontic tipping indicates that areas of elevated maximum principal stress *(tension)* in PDL and minimum principal stress *(compression)* in the cortical bone of the lamina dura are associated with areas of bone formation and resorption respectively. (From Katona TR et al: conditionally accepted by *J Biomechan.*)

blood vessel.[86] The osteoblast histogenesis sequence (Fig. 3-5, *B*) was determined by in situ morphological assessment of three distinct events in cell physiology: (1) DNA synthesis (S) phase; (2) mitosis (M); and (3) the increase in nuclear volume (A'Æ C shift) to differentiate to a preosteoblast.[78]

Careful cell kinetic analysis of orthodontically induced osteogenesis[79] demonstrated the *initial mechanically mediated step* in osteoblast histogenesis is differentiation of preosteoblasts from less-differentiated precursor cells (Fig. 3-32). Subsequent studies further classified the less differentiated precursor cells into committed osteoprogenitor (A') cells and self-perpetuating precursor (A) cells.[78] The morphological marker for this key step in osteoblast differen-

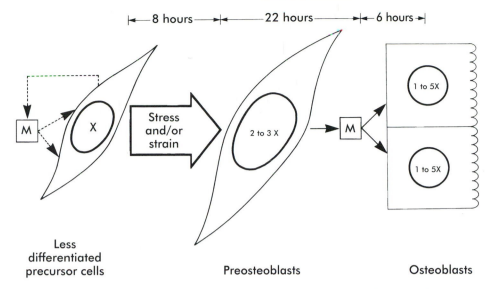

Fig. 3-32   Differentiation of less differentiated precursor cells to preosteoblasts involves a stress and/or strain mediated increase in nuclear volume. The increase in nuclear size is a morphologic manifestation of change in genomic expression *(differentiation).* (From Roberts WE et al: *Am J Anat* 165:373-384, 1982.)

tiation (change in genomic expression) is an increase in nuclear volume: preosteoblasts have larger nuclei than their precursors (Fig. 3-32). The FEM studies[62] suggest that the critical mechanical parameter initiating the rate-limiting step in the osteogenic response is probably maximum, principal stress within the PDL (Fig. 3-31). Cell kinetic analyses (DNA labeling; nuclear volume morphometry) coordinated with finite element modeling (FEM) of identical specimens, are powerful methods for elucidating the biomechanical control of bone cells in vivo. The use of these analytical methods is only in its infancy; however, it is already clear that *pressure* and *tension* in the PDL is far too simplistic an explanation to account for the complex mechanical control of the bone resorption and formation processes effecting orthodontic tooth movement.

The current sequence for kinetic control of orthodontically induced osteogenesis is depicted in Fig. 3-33. The stopcock labeled *1* shows that unstimulated PDL maintains a substantial fraction of preosteoblasts (C and D cells) by restricting cell flow before mitosis of D cells. This is a block in the G_2 stage of the cell cycle. With orthodontic stimulus, the stopcock (1) is opened, preosteoblasts (C and D cells) are depleted, new C cells are formed by A′ cells (2) and A cells produce more A′ cells.

In an unstimulated PDL, note that some cells tend to be blocked at the end of the G_1 and G_2 periods, but most osteogenic cells are held in reserve (G_0 phase) until the osteogenesis is mechanically induced (Fig. 3-34). Fig. 3-35 shows the cell kinetic sequence associated with orthodontic induction of new bone formation: (1) a peak of new preosteoblasts (increased A′ → C activation) is noted at 8 hours; (2) maximum levels of DNA synthesis are evident at about 20 hours; (3) a burst of mitotic activity is seen at about 30 hours; (4) new labeled osteoblasts progressively

accumulate after about 35 hours; and (5) new bone formation is initiated about 40 to 48 hours after application of the force.[66,75] Five compartments of PDL cells have been defined in the osteoblast differentiation sequence.[78] The rate-limiting step in the differentiation of osteoblasts is the formation of preosteoblasts from committed osteoprogenitor cells. Induction of preosteoblast formation (A′ → C) is mechanically mediated (Figs. 3-32 and 3-33). The photoperiod (circadian

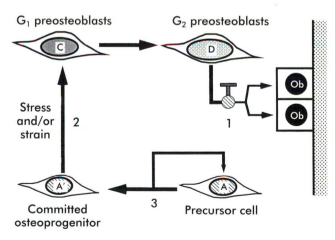

Fig. 3-33   The control scheme for osteogenic induction of a relatively quiescent PDL cell population involves: (1) release of G_2 block, allowing mitosis to form two osteoblasts *(Ob)*; (2) mechanically mediated differentiation to preosteoblasts *(A′ → C)*; and (3) increased proliferation of precursor cells to produce more committed osteoprogenitor cells *(A′)*. (From Roberts WE et al: In *Bone biodynamics in orthodontic and orthopedic treatment*, ed 27, Ann Arbor, 1991, University of Michigan Press, pp 189-255.)

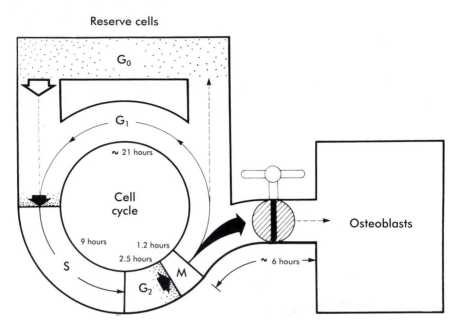

Fig. 3-34 This composite cell cycle diagram shows the approximate duration and the various phases of the cell cycle. The cells arrested at the end of the G_1 and G_2 phases are referred to as G_1 or G_2 blocked cells. These cells can be released by metabolic and/or mechanical stimuli (Fig. 3-31). (From Roberts WE et al: *Dent Clinics North Am* 25:3-17, 1981.)

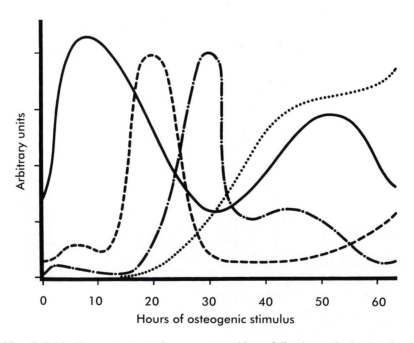

Fig. 3-35 Cell kinetic events to produce new osteoblasts following orthodontic stimulus are represented by peaks in the curves from left to right: (1) accumulation of preosteoblasts (A' → C); (2) DNA synthesis to form D cells; (3) mitosis of D cells; and (4) accumulation of mature osteoblasts. This sequence established D cells as the immediate proliferating progenitors of osteoblasts. (From Roberts WE et al: *Am J Anat* 165:373-384, 1982.)

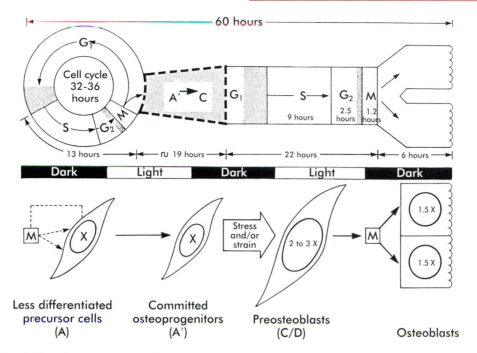

Fig. 3-36 Photoperiod (circadian rhythm) influence on physiologic osteoblast histogenesis in rat
PDL. Note that the $A' \to C$ increase in nuclear size occurs during the late resting and early arousal
phases. The overall osteoblast differentiation is 60 hours, five alternating dark/light cycles of 12
hours each. (From Roberts WE, Morey ER: *Am J Anat* 174:105-118, 1985.)

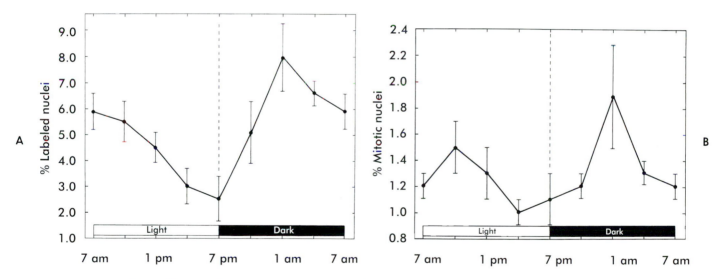

Fig. 3-37 **A,** Circadian rhythm (photoperiod) of S phase cells in unstimulated rat PDL along a
natural bone forming surface. **B,** Circadian rhythm (photoperiod) of mitotic cells in unstimulated
rat PDL along a natural bone forming surface. (**A** and **B** from Roberts WE, Morey ER: *Am J Anat*
174:105-118, 1985.)

rhythm) influence is strong on the 60 hour proliferation and
differentiation sequence. S phase, mitosis and the $A' \to C$
shift in nuclear size have specific photoperiod preferences
(Fig. 3-36). It requires five alternating 12 hour dark/light
cycles (total of 60 hours) for a G_1 stage A cell to progress
through the entire histogenesis sequence to form two os-

teoblasts. At least a portion of the photoperiod effect reflects
varying endocrine levels during the circadian cycle. For
instance, corticosteroids tend to enhance differentiation
($A \to C$), but suppress DNA synthesis of preosteoblasts
(C cells). The important point is that optimal osteoblast
histogenesis under physiological circumstances requires a

normal photoperiod (Fig. 3-37, *A* and *B*).[67,78] Disruption of circadian rhythm caused by physiological stress, traveling, or irregular sleep patterns may adversely affect osteoblast production.

OSTEOCLAST RECRUITMENT AND BONE RESORPTION

Bone resorption is the limiting factor determining the rate of tooth movement.[67,73] Removal of osseous tissue during progressive tooth movement is directly related to: (1) *bone porosity;* (2) *remodeling rate;* (3) *resorption rate;* and (4) *osteoclast recruitment.* Porous cortical and trabecular bone allows improved access for osteoclasts. The remodeling rate is directly related to resorption cavities and to the number of osteoclasts present at any time within resisting bone. The osteoclast resorption rate is largely controlled by metabolic factors, particularly PTH.[12,30] No direct evidence exists to suggest that osteoclasts are produced in the PDL or at any other bone surface. Preosteoclasts derived from the marrow enter the PDL and adjacent bone via the blood circulation.[59,67,73]

Roberts and Ferguson[67] compared the cell kinetics for metabolic and mechanical induction of PDL resorption. As shown in Fig. 3-38 the number of osteoclasts per mm bone surface is maximal about 9 hours after a single injection of parathyroid extract. Mechanical stimulation produces a slower but more sustained response requiring almost 50 hours to reach the same osteoclast density.[67] Preosteoclasts

are derived from the marrow via circulating promonocyte derivatives (Fig. 3-39).

Parathyroid hormone (PTH) is an established metabolic stimulus for recruiting preosteoclasts from the blood stream.[59] It produces a modest, nonspecific increase in PDL proliferation.[57] Contrary to the intense cell replication associated with osteogenesis,[73,75,96] neither PTH nor orthodontic induced resorption results in elevated cell proliferation in PDL or adjacent bone. These data are consistent with the marrow origin of osteoclasts. Metabolic stimulus of osteoclastic resorption may result in tooth mobility or in elevated turnover of alveolar bone. For instance, a low calcium diet in dogs results in elevated endogenous PTH levels; the resulting high turnover osteopenia contributes to an enhanced rate of orthodontic tooth movement[44] because of lower bone density and an elevated remodeling rate. Unfortunately, this approach is not acceptable for clinical use because of the large amount of systemic bone loss.

Since osteoclasts originate in the marrow, production of osteoclast precursor cells is under both systemic (metabolic) and local (hematopoietic) control. The reservoir of circulating osteoclast precursors is controlled systemically. However, the localization of resorptive sites in the PDL is regulated mechanically. Metabolic stimuli, such as PTH, produce a relatively nonspecific resorption response along previously resorbing surfaces.[57] Mechanical induction is a specific response and occurs only in the direction of tooth movement. The current challenge is to understand the mechanical and biological components of the resorptive mech-

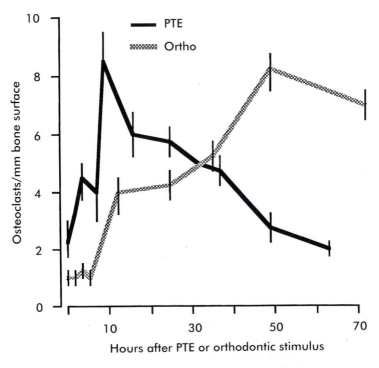

Fig. 3-38   Metabolic (parathyroid extract) vs. mechanical (orthodontic) stimulation of PDL osteoclastic activity. (From Roberts WE, Ferguson DJ: *The biology of tooth movement,* Boca Raton, Fla, 1989, CRC Press.)

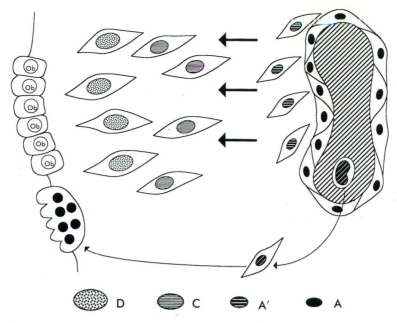

Fig. 3-39 Circulating osteoclast precursor cells, derived from the marrow, are the origin of the preosteoclasts in the PDL that form osteoclasts *(lower pathway).* The paravascular origin of osteoblasts from A, A', C, and D cells is an independent mechanism. At the local tissue level there are no common progenitors for osteoblasts and osteoclasts.

anism. Orthodontic force that results in elevated stress within the osseous cortex is followed by a specific resorptive response.[62] Prostaglandins, interleukins, neurosecretory agents and growth factors may be local mediators of the site specific resorption that is essential to the tooth movement response.[18]

Osteoclasts are relatively inert cells because they have few specific biochemical receptors. Calcitonin is the only receptor that is directly related to calcium homeostasis or bone adaptation. Since osteoblasts and their precursors have a more complete complement of bone related receptors: PTH, GH, and estrogen, they may play a role in controlling osteoclasts.[67,88] The intricate bone modeling and remodeling responses characterizing orthodontic tooth movement require close coordination of osteoblastic and osteoclastic function.

CLINICAL CORRELATIONS

Intermittent vs. continuous mechanics. Initiating and sustaining a coordinated bone resorptive response determines the rate of tooth movement.[73] The kinetics of continuous mechanics are relatively well known; however, the response to intermittent loads, such as headgear and removable appliances, is less clear. In general, tooth movement is directly related to the number of hours each day that force is applied. However, even when motivation and cooperation are optimal, the effectiveness of similar therapy between patients is inconsistent. This is a physiologic indication that additional variables are involved.

Reitan[53] reports that a short duration force (12 to 14 hours per day for 15 to 27 days) delivered by a functional appliance triggers a resorptive reaction that lasts a week or more. Apparently, this experience with functional appliances does not apply to cyclical intermittent mechanics, such as nighttime headgear wear. Otherwise, a headgear worn at night would be as effective as 24-hour wear. In the absence of specific experiments, interpolation from continuous force studies appears to be the best explanation available. Three hours of continuous loading is necessary to achieve maximal displacement of a tooth root within the periodontium (Fig. 3-24). If it is assumed that at least 3 hours are needed for PDL activation or recovery,[67] *continuous* wear of a headgear for 12 hours daily is expected to be more effective than a longer period of headgear *wear* with frequent release of force. It is recommended that the patient *not* remove the headgear at all during the daily interval of wear. If it is necessary to remove the device for meals or sports activities, the biomechanical activation of the periodontium is compromised. The complex biological response, associated with irregular force application, is probably the main factor in the unpredictable response to headgear or removable appliances.

Another potential variable in response to intermittent force is the circadian rhythm of PDL proliferation and differentiation (Figs. 3-36 and 3-37). Maximal cell proliferation in the PDL occurs during the resting hours[64,76]: daytime for rats; nighttime for humans. Differentiation to preosteoblasts, the key rate limiting step in osteoblast differentiation, occurs during the late resting and early arousal periods.[78] These data suggest that equal amounts of headgear or removable appliance wear at night will be more effective than during the day.[64]

Differential anchorage. Density of the alveolar bone and cross-sectional area of the roots in the plane perpendicular to the direction of tooth movement are the primary considerations for assessing anchorage potential. The volume of osseous tissue that must be resorbed for a tooth to move a given distance is its anchorage value. If all bone offered the same resistance to tooth movement, the anchorage potential of maxillary and mandibular molars would be about the same. However, clinical experience shows that maxillary molars usually have less anchorage value than mandibular molars in the same patient. A common example is space closure in a Class I four premolar extraction case; it is often necessary to use headgear on the maxillary first molars to maintain the Class I relationship. The relative resistance of mandibular molars to mesial movement is a well known principle of differential mechanics.

Why are mandibular molars usually more difficult to move mesially than maxillary molars? At least two physiologic factors can be considered: (1) the thin cortices and trabecular bone of the maxilla (Fig. 3-40, A) offer less resistance to resorption than the thick cortices and more coarse trabeculae of the mandible (Fig. 3-40, B); and (2)

the leading root of mandibular molars being translated mesially forms bone that is far more dense than the bone formed by translating maxillary molars mesially (Fig. 3-41). The reason mandibular molars form more dense bone than maxillary molars is unclear; however, it may be that new bone formed in the maxilla is remodeled more rapidly. In general, bones composed primarily of trabeculae remodel more rapidly than those composed primarily of cortical bone.[48,49]

Why is the alveolar process of mandibular molars more dense than maxillary molars? Functional loading dictates the osseous anatomy for the opposing jaws: (1) the maxilla is predominantly trabecular bone with thin cortices, similar to a vertebral body or an epiphysis (Fig. 3-40, A); and (2) the mandible has thick cortices like the diaphysis of a major long bone (Fig. 3-40, B). Although the forces of occlusion are distributed equally to the maxilla and mandible, the maxilla transfers a major fraction of functional loads to the rest of the cranium.

The loads (compression, tension, and torsion) to which the maxilla and the mandible are exposed are quite different.[4,32] The maxilla is loaded almost entirely in compression, while the mandible is subjected to substantial torsion and flexure caused by muscle pull and masticatory function.[4,32] Thick mandibular cortices are necessary to resist the tor-

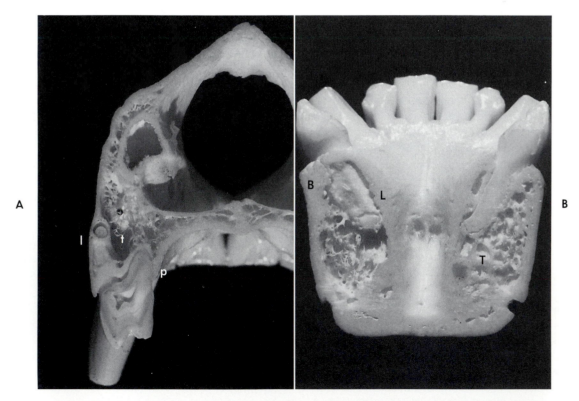

Fig. 3-40 **A,** A frontal section through a monkey maxilla shows the thin labial plate *(l)*, sparse trabeculae *(t)*, and somewhat thicker palatal plate *(p)*. **B,** A cross-section in the frontal plane of the mandible reveals thick buccal *(B)* and lingual *(L)* cortices. Trabecular bone *(T)* is usually more dense than in the maxilla. (From Roberts WE et al: In *Bone biodynamics in orthodontic and orthopedic treatment*, ed 27, Ann Arbor, 1991, University of Michigan Press, pp 189-255.)

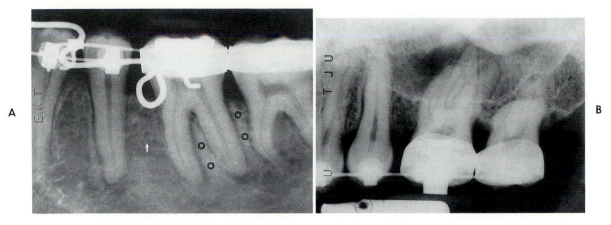

Fig. 3-41   **A,** Progressive mesial translation of second and third mandibular molars generates dense cortical bone *(stars)* that is more resistant to resorption than the trabecular bone *(t)* ahead of the first molar. (From Roberts et al: In *Bone biodynamics in orthodontic and orthopedic treatment,* ed 27, Ann Arbor, 1991, University of Michigan Press, pp 89-255.) **B,** Mesial movement of second and third molars in the maxilla of the same patient fails to demonstrate dense cortical bone distal to the moving roots.

sional and bending strain (Fig. 3-40, *B*). On the other hand, the maxilla is loaded predominantly in compression, there are no major muscle attachments and it transfers much of its load to the rest of the cranium. Because of its entirely different functional role, the maxilla is predominantly trabecular bone with thin cortices (Fig. 3-40, *A*). This anatomical configuration is similar to other bones loaded primarily in compression, such as proximal tibia and vertebral bodies of the spine.

Rate of tooth movement. The rate of tooth movement is the inverse of anchorage potential; the same physiological principles apply. Clinical studies using endosseous implants for anchorage[77] have provided an excellent opportunity to assess the rate of tooth movement through dense cortical bone in the posterior mandible (Fig. 3-41, *A*) compared with the less dense trabecular bone of the posterior maxilla (Fig. 3-41, *B*). The enhanced anchorage value of mandibular molars is related to the high density bone formed as the leading roots are moved mesially. After a few months of mesial translation, the trailing roots engage the high density bone formed by the leading root, and the rate of tooth movement decreases (Fig. 3-42).

Overall, the maximum rate for translation of the midroot area through dense cortical bone is about 0.5 mm per month for the first few months, and then the rate decreases to <0.3 mm per month, until the first molar extraction site is closed (Fig. 3-42). When teeth are moved continuously in the same direction, the remodeling rate increases in compact bone immediately ahead of the moving tooth (Figs. 3-25 and 3-27). This enhanced remodeling process is probably related to the regional acceleratory phenomenon (RAP) commonly noted in osseous wound healing. Cutting/filling cones are the means of osteoclast access to the inner portion of dense compacta (Fig. 3-13). This remodeling mechanism appears

to be particularly important for resorbing the dense cortical bone formed by the leading root during mesial movement of lower molars (Fig. 3-41). Note the radiolucent areas within the dense compact bone.

Fig. 3-43 is a summary of the relative rates of molar translation in the upper and lower jaws of growing children and adults. A maximal rate approaching 2 mm per month is possible with space closure mechanics or 24 hour per day headgear wear by a rapidly growing child (Child Mx). Similar mechanics in a nongrowing adult is capable of translating upper molars about 1 mm per month (Adult Mx). Mesial translation of lower molars in a child occurs at a rate of about 0.7 mm per month (Child Md). The slowest

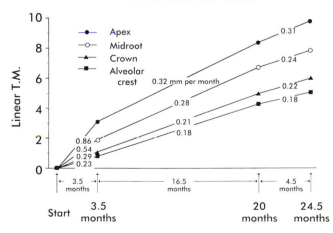

Fig. 3-42   Overall tooth movement curve for lower second and third molars demonstrate mesial root movement and translation of 8 to 10 mm in about 2 years. Note the rapid rate of movement (up to 0.86 mm per month) for the first 3.5 months slows to about 0.3 mm per month for the duration of space closure.

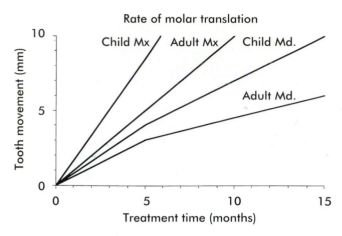

Fig. 3-43   Relative rates of molar translation in both jaws of rapidly growing children are compared to those of adults.

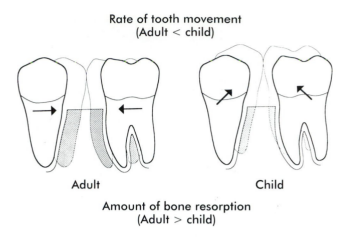

Fig. 3-44   The rate of molar translation is directly related to the amount and density of bone that must be resorbed. Because extrusion is associated with growth, there is relatively less bone to resorb when translating the molars of a child.

molar translation (0.3 mm per month) is in the lower arch of adults (Adult Md). Overall, the same teeth in growing children move about twice as fast as they move in adults. Certainly there are histological factors, such as less dense alveolar bone and more cellular PDL[53]; however, growth-related extrusion is the principal reason that space closure is almost twice as rapid in children. Fig. 3-44 demonstrates the considerably smaller volume of bone that is resorbed in a child as compared with that in an adult. In general, *the rate of tooth movement is inversely related to bone density and volume of bone resorbed.*

Rates for orthodontic tipping movements are usually higher but are more variable than for translation. There are no well-controlled studies of tipping in various intraoral sites of children and adults; however, some interesting theoretical considerations are offered. When teeth are moved rapidly, immature new bone can form at a rate of 100 μm per day or more (>3 mm a month). This rate of tooth movement is probably never achieved during routine treatment. However, premolar and cuspid tipping of approximately 2 mm per month may be achieved with removable appliances in the maxillary arch of growing children.

In brief, three principal variables determine the rate of tooth movement: (1) growth; (2) bone density; and (3) type of tooth movement. Alveolar bone of the maxilla is less dense than that of the mandible because it has a higher ratio of cancellous bone to cortical bone. Bone of children is generally less dense (more porous or cancellous) than bone of adults. Cancellous or trabecular bone has more surface area available for resorption, which is important because bone impeding tooth movement can be resorbed from all sides. Cortical bone is largely restricted to frontal and undermining resorption mechanisms within the periodontal ligament. In general, children have a higher rate of bone remodeling than adults. In simple terms, more osteoclasts are present within the bone that can help with the task of removing the osseous tissue impeding tooth movement.

Teeth of growing children extrude as they move through

bone. It is important to remember that it is not uncommon for the basilar bone of the jaws to separate 1 to 2 cm during 2 years of orthodontic treatment. This means that teeth of children move as much by differential apposition (guided eruption) as by resorption (Fig. 3-44). Tipping the teeth requires less resorption of bone adjacent to the middle of the root. This bone, which is farthest away from bone surfaces, is probably the most difficult for the osteoclasts to access. Eliminating the most difficult part of the resorptive process is probably the reason teeth move faster by tipping than by translation. Considering all the variables of age, arch and type of tooth movement, maxillary buccal segments in children move as much as 4 times faster than posterior mandibular segments in adults (Fig. 3-43).

Periodontitis and orthodontics. Osteoclasts are hardy cells that thrive in a pathological environment. On the other hand, osteoblasts are vascularly dependent cells whose histogenesis is easily disrupted.[67,78] Therefore most skeletal deficits probably are errors in bone formation rather than resorption. A good example of the fragility of bone formation is inflammatory suppression of osteoblast differentiation.[86]

Orthodontics is often a useful adjunct for enhancing periodontal health; however, moving teeth in the presence of progressive periodontal disease is inviting disaster.[86] Tooth movement within the alveolar process stimulates both resorption and formation. Osteoclasts thrive in an inflammatory environment because their origin is in the marrow, a protected site away from the localized lesion. Preosteoclasts are attracted to the inflammatory site by cytokine mediators.[18] On the other hand, the locally produced osteoblasts are strongly suppressed by inflammatory disease. So when teeth are moved in the presence of active periodontal disease, resorption is normal or even enhanced, while bone formation is inhibited. In the presence of periodontitis, orthodontics may exacerbate the disease process, resulting in a rapid loss of supporting bone (Fig. 3-45).

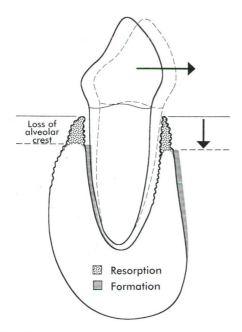

Loss of
alveolar
crest

☷ Resorption
▤ Formation

Fig. 3-45   Because of enhanced resorption and an inhibition of apposition, orthodontics in the presence of active periodontitis often results is a severe loss of alveolar bone support.

Endosseous implants.   Rigid orthodontic and orthopedic anchorage is opening new perspectives in mechanical therapy. A preclinical study in dogs tested the anchorage potential of two prosthetic-type titanium implants: (1) a prototype of an endosseous device with a cervical post, asymmetric threads, and an acid-etched surface; and (2) a commercially available implant with symmetrical threads (Fig. 3-46, *A* and *B*). Based on label incidence, (Fig. 3-47, *A*) and the relative number of new osteons in microradiographs (Fig. 3-47, *B*) there was a higher rate of bone

remodeling near the implant compared to basilar mandible only a few mm away.[28] Compared with titanium implants with a smooth surface, the degree of remodeling at the interface is greater for threaded implants placed in a tapped bone preparation.[72] This may be related to the increased resistance of threaded implants to torsional loads over time.[1]

Direct bone apposition at the endosseous interface results in rigid fixation *(osseointegration)*.[5] From an anchorage perspective a rigid endosseous implant is the functional equivalent of an ankylosed tooth. Complete bony encapsulation is not necessary for an implant to serve as a rigid anchorage unit. The critical feature is an indefinite maintenance of rigidity despite continuous orthodontic loads. Over time, orthodontically loaded implants achieve a greater fraction of direct osseous interface.[1,77] From an orthodontic and orthopedic perspective, titanium implants can resist substantial continuous loads (1 to 3 N superimposed on function) indefinitely. Histologic analysis with multiple fluorochrome labels and microradiography confirm that rigidly integrated implants do not move relative to adjacent bone (Fig. 3-47).[74] By definition, *maintaining a fixed relationship with supporting bone is true osseous anchorage.* Endosseous *(osseointegrated)* implants are well suited to many demanding orthodontic applications.[72,77]

Routine use of rigid implants for prosthetic or orthodontic applications requires placing fixtures between or near roots of teeth. Inadvertent impingement on the periodontal ligament and root of an adjacent tooth may still provide an acceptable result (Fig. 3-48). Cementum repair occurs where the root is cut; the PDL reorganizes, and the implant surface is rigidly integrated with osseous tissue. There is no evidence of ankylosis of the tooth.[74]

The isolated loss of a lower first molar with a retained third molar is a common problem. Rather than extract the

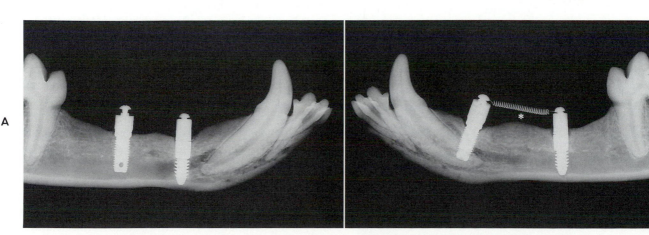

A   B

Fig. 3-46   **A,** Two titanium implants of different design were placed in the partially endentulous mandible of young adult dogs. **B,** After 2 months unloaded healing, a 3 N compressive load was applied between the implants for 4 months. Increased periosteal apposition *(*)* was noted between the implants of some dogs. None of the rigidly integrated fixtures was loosened by the continuous load superimposed on function. (Adapted from Roberts WE et al: *Angle Orthod* 59:247-256, 1989.)

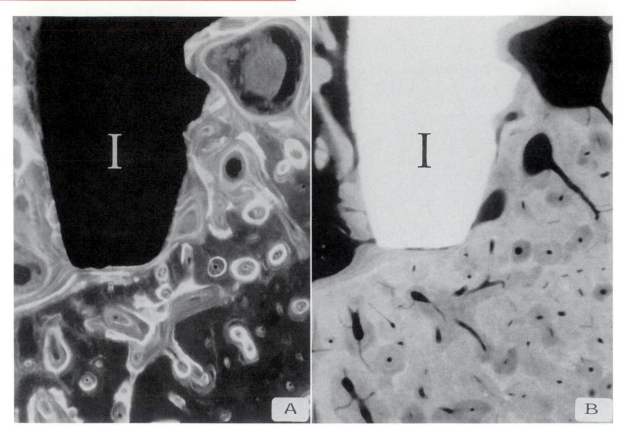

Fig. 3-47   **A,** Multiple fluorochrome labels in bone adjacent to the implant *(I)* demonstrate a high rate of remodeling at the bone/implant surface. **B,** Microradiographic image of the same section shows direct bone contact on the surface of the implant. (From Roberts WE et al: In *Bone biodynamics in orthodontic and orthopedic treatment*, ed 27, Ann Arbor, 1991, University of Michigan Press, pp 189-255.)

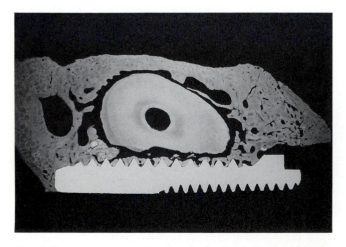

Fig. 3-48   An endosseous implant inadvertently impinged on the root of a cuspid *(B)*. The implant successfully integrated with bone and served as a rigid anchor for orthopedic loading. (From Roberts WE et al: *Angle Orthod* 1989.)

third molar and replace the first molar with a three unit bridge, mesial translation of second and third molars to close the edentulous space is often preferable (Fig. 3-49, *A* and *B*). The first case with long-term follow-up is published.[77] Because of the increasing incidence of progressive bone loss and of fatigue fracture associated with single tooth implants in lower first and second molar areas, the orthodontic option for mesially translating the molars to close the space is increasing in popularity. An anchorage wire that is secured to a retromolar implant can be used to intrude and protract mandibular second and third molars to close an atrophic first molar extraction site (Fig. 3-49, *B*).[71]

The tipping and extrusion of residual lower molars limits potential orthodontic repositioning. Rigid retromolar implants offer a unique capability for intrusion and alignment. Fig. 3-50, *A* through *C,* demonstrate the mechanics for achieving three-dimensional control to intrude the third molar to the plane of occlusion and to mesially translate both teeth. Cephalometric tracings (Fig. 3-51, *A* and *B*) document the >10 mm of mesial translation and its stability. Panoramic radiographs show the initial alignment (Fig. 3-

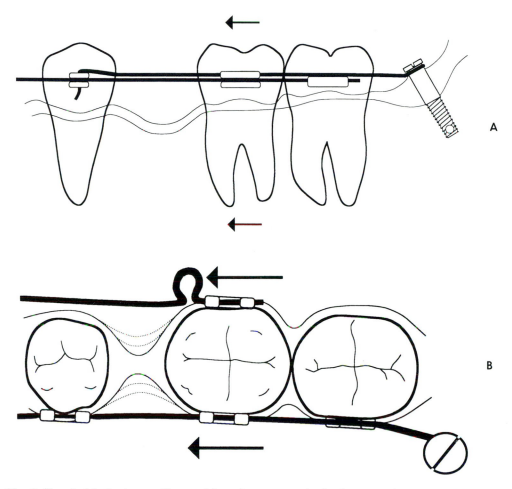

Fig. 3-49   A, Mechanics are illustrated for using a retromolar implant as anchorage to stabilize
the premolar anterior to an extraction site. **B,** Using buccal and lingual mechanics to balance the
load and shield the periosteum in the extraction site, the atrophic extraction site is closed without
periodontal compromise to any of the adjacent teeth. (From Roberts WE et al: In *Bone biodynamics
in orthodontic and orthopedic treatment,* ed 27, Ann Arbor, 1991, University of Michigan Press,
pp 189-255.)

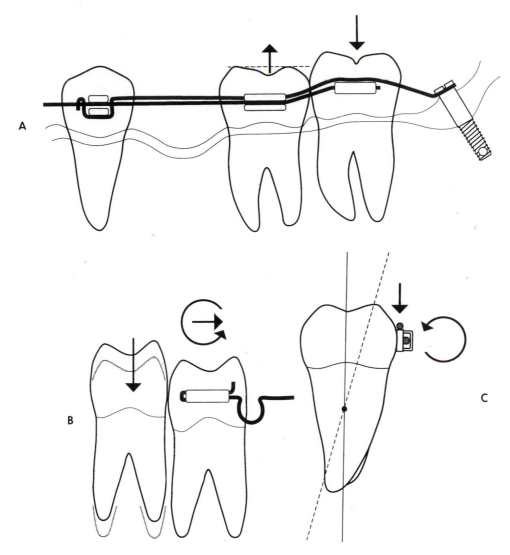

Fig. 3-50   A, Mechanics are illustrated for intruding a third molar with implant anchorage before space closure. **B,** Extrusion of the second molar is prevented with a removable lingual arch. **C,** Because the intrusive force on the third molar is buccal to the center of resistance, there is a tendency for the tooth to tip buccally. This problem is controlled by placing lingual crown torque in the rectangular wire inserted in the tube. (From Roberts WE et al: In *Bone biodynamics in orthodontic and orthopedic treatment,* ed 27, Ann Arbor, 1991, University of Michigan Press, pp 189-255.)

52, *A*) and the final space closure (Fig. 3-52, *B*). Clinical details are published.[77]

Histologic analysis of implants recovered after completion of treatment reveals important information on the continuous remodeling process that maintains the rigid integration and anchorage value of the endosseous device. Two intravital bone labels, administered within two weeks of implant recovery, reveal a continuing high rate of bone remodeling (>500% per year) within 1 mm of the implant surface (Fig. 3-52, *C* and *D*). This biologic mechanism is apparently the means for maintaining rigid osseous integration indefinitely.[61,77] In the absence of fracture at the implant interface or within its supporting bone, rigid implants are not moved by orthodontic loads.[74,77,84] Well-integrated endosseous implants remain rigid despite continued remodeling of bone supporting them because only a portion of the osseous resorbed interface is turned over at any given time.[77] Based on the long-term clinical success of the published case and histologic verification of a favorable bone reaction to the device, a 30-patient-prospective-clinical trial of rigid implants for orthodontic and orthopedic anchorage is now in progress. Fig. 3-53 demonstrates the mechanics for mesial translation of molars to close space when a premolar is congenitally missing. Rigid endosseous implants show great promise for considerably extending the therapeutic possibilities of orthodontics and dentofacial orthopedics.

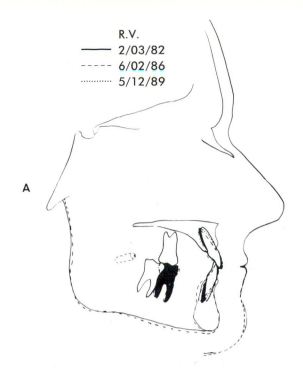

R.V.
—— 2/03/82
- - - - 6/02/86
··········· 5/12/89

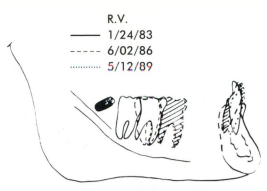

R.V.
—— 1/24/83
- - - - 6/02/86
··········· 5/12/89

Fig. 3-51 **A,** Pretreatment, finish and 3-year post-retention cephalometric tracings document 10 to 12 mm of molar translation to close an atrophic first molar extraction site. **B,** Mandibular superimposition shows the mesial movement of the second and third molars as well as lingual root torque of the lower incisors. (From Roberts WE et al: *Angle Orthod* 60:135-152, 1990.)

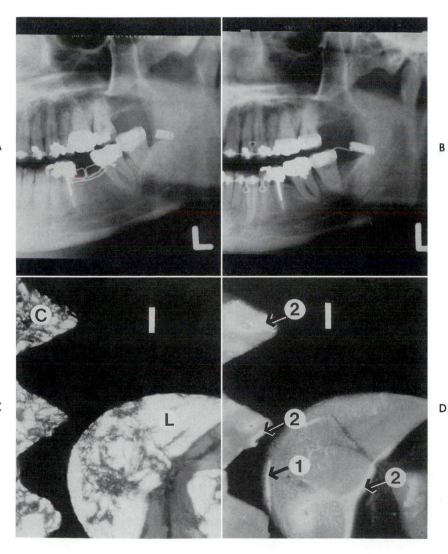

Fig. 3-52 **A,** Panoramic radiograph of the initial buccal alignment before uncovering the implant. **B,** Panoramic radiograph of the closed exraction site. **C,** Polarized light microscopy of bone around the implant recovered after the completion of treatment. **D,** Two demeclocycline labels in bone adjacent to the implant document the high rate of bone remodeling that is apparently the mechanism for long-term maintenance of rigid osseous fixation *(osseointegration).* (From Roberts WE et al: *Angle Orthod* 60:135-162, 1990.)

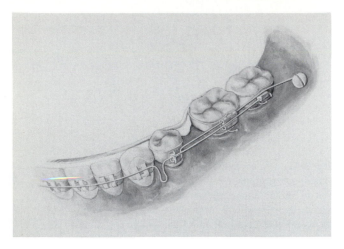

Fig. 3-53   Mechanics for mesial closure of an edentulous site, due to congenital absence of a lower second premolar, are anchored with a rigid endosseous implant.

Concluding Remarks

Bone physiologic, metabolic, and cell kinetic concepts have important clinical applications in orthodontics and dentofacial orthopedics. The application of fundamental concepts is limited only by the knowledge and imagination of the clinician. Modern clinical practice features a continual evolution of methods based on fundamental and applied research.

ACKNOWLEDGMENTS

This research was supported by the National Institute of Dental Research (NIH) Grants No. DE09237 and DE09822; NASA-Ames Grants No. NCC 2-594 and NAG 2-756; and private donors through Indiana University Foundation. The author gratefully acknowledges the assistance of faculty and staff at the University of the Pacific School of Dentistry and Indiana University School of Dentistry.

REFERENCES

1. Albrektsson T, Jacobsson M: Bone-metal interface in osseointegration, *J Prosthetic Dent* 60:75-84, 1987.
2. Arbuckle GR, Nelson CL, Roberts WE: Osseointegrated implants and orthodontics, *Oral Maxillofac Surg Clin North Am* 3:903-919, 1991.
3. Ascenzi A, Baschieri P, Benvenuti A: The bending properties of single osteons, *J Biomech* 8:763-771, 1990.
4. Atkinson SR: Balance—the magic word, *Am J Orthod* 50:189-202, 1964.
5. Brånemark P-I: Osseointegration and its experimental background, *J Prosthetic Dent* 50:399-410, 1983.
6. Brunski JB: *Forces on dental implants and interfacial stress transfer.* In Laney WR, Tolman DE, editors: *Tissue integration in oral, orthopedic and maxillofacial reconstruction,* Chicago, 1992, Quintessence, pp 108-124.
7. Brunski JB, Skalak R: *Biomechanical considerations.* In Worthington P, Brånemark PI editors: *Advanced osseointegrations surgery,* Chicago, 1992, Quintessence, pp 15-39.
8. Burstone CJ: *Application of bioengineering to clinical orthodontics.* In Graber TM, Swain BF, editors: *Orthodontics: current principles and techniques,* St Louis, 1985, Mosby, pp 193-227.
9. Burstone CJ, Pryputniewicz RJ, Bowley WW: Holographic measurement of tooth mobility in three dimensions, *J Periodont Res* 13:283-294, 1978.
10. Carter DR: Mechanical loading history and skeletal biology, *J Biomech* 20:1095-1109, 1987.
11. Carter DR, Smith DJ et al: Measurement and analysis of in vivo bone strains on the canine radius and ulna, *J Biomech* 13:27-38, 1980.
12. Chambers TJ, McSheehy PMJ et al: The effect of calcium-regulating hormones and prostaglandins on bone resorption by osteoclasts disaggregated from neonatal rabbit bones, *Endocrinology* 60:234-239, 1985.
13. Christiansen C: Consensus development conference: prophylaxis and treatment of osteoporosis, *Am J Med* 90:107-110, 1991.
14. Colditz GA, Stampfer MJ et al: Prospective study of estrogen replacement therapy and risk of breast cancer in postmenopausal women, *J Am Dent Assoc* 264:2648-2653, 1990.
15. Consensus Conference Report on Osteoporosis: *J Am Dent Assoc* 252:799-802, 1984.
16. Cowin SC: *Bone mechanics,* Boca Raton, Fla, 1989, CRC Press.
17. Currey JD: *The mechanical adaptations of bones,* Princeton, 1984, Princeton University Press.
18. Davidovitch Z: Tooth movement, *Crit Rev Oral Biol Med* 2:411-450, 1991.
19. Drinkwater BL, Nilson K, Ott S et al: Bone mineral content of amenorrheic and eumenorrheic athletes, *N Engl J Med* 311:277-281, 1984.
20. Enlow DH: *Principles of bone remodeling,* Springfield, 1963, Charles C Thomas.
21. Eriksen EF, Mosekilde L: Estrogens and bone, *Bone Min Res* 7:273-312, 1990.
22. Frost HM: *Bone remodeling and its relationship to metabolic bone diseases,* Springfield, 1973, Charles C Thomas.
23. Frost HM: The regional acceleratory phenomenon: a review, *Henry Ford Hosp Med J* 31:3-9, 1983.
24. Frost HM: *Intermediary organization of the skeleton,* vol 1, Boca Raton, Fla, 1986, CRC Press.
24a. Frost HM: Skeletal structural adaptations to mechanical usage (SATMU), 2: redefining Wolff's law: The remodeling problem, *Anat Rec* 226:414-422, 1990.
25. Grisso JA, Baum CR, Turner BJ: What do physicians in practice do to prevent osteoporosis? *J Bone Min Res* 5:213-219, 1990.
26. Heaney RP: *Calcium, bone health and osteoporosis.* In Peck WA, editor: *Bone and mineral research,* Amsterdam, 1986, Elsevier Science, pp 255-301.
27. Heaney RP: Estrogen-calcium interactions in the postmenopause: a quantitative description, *Bone Min* 11:67-84, 1990.
28. Helm FR, Poon LC et al: Bone remodeling response to loading of rigid endosseous implants, *J Dent Res* 66:186, 1987 (abstract).
29. Henrich JB: The postmenopausal estrogen/breast cancer controversy, *JAMA* 268:1900-1902, 1992.
30. Holtrop ME, Raisz LG, Simmons HA: The effects of parathyroid hormone, colchicine, and calcitonin of the ultrastructure and the activity of osteoclasts in organ culture, *J Cell Biol* 60:346-355, 1974.
31. Hylander WL: Mandibular function in Galago crassicaudatus and Macaca fasicularis: an in vivo approach to stress analysis, *J Morphol* 159:253-296, 1979.
32. Hylander WL: *Patterns of stress and strain in the Macaque mandible.* In Carlson DS, editor: *Craniofacial biology,* Ann Arbor, Mich, 1981, Center for Human Growth and Development, pp 1-35.
33. Jackson CB, Roberts WE, Morey ER: Growth alterations of the mandibular condyle in Spacelab-3 rats, *ASGSB Bul* 1:33, 1988 (abstract).
34. Jeffcoat MK, Williams RC et al: Nuclear medicine techniques for the detection of active alveolar bone loss, *Adv Dent Res* 1:80-84, 1987.
35. Johnston CC: Osteoporosis—extent and cause of the disease, *PSEBM* 191:258-260, 1989.

36. Johnston CC, Miller JZ, Slemenda C et al: Calcium supplementation and increases in bone mineral density in children, *N Engl J Med* 327:82-1233, 1992.

37. Keeting PE, Scott RE et al: Lack of a direct effect of estrogen on proliferation and differentiation of normal human osteoblast-like cells, *J Bone Min Res* 6:297-304, 1991.

38. King GJ, Thiems S: Chemical mediation of bone resorption induced by tooth movement in the rat, *Archs Oral Biol* 24:811-815, 1979.

39. Lanyon LE: Control of bone architecture by functional load bearing, *J Bone Min Res* 7:S369-S375, 1992.

40. Love RR, Mazess RB, Barden HS et al: Effects of tamoxifen on bone mineral density in postmenopausal women with breast cancer, *N Engl J Med* 326:852-856, 1992.

41. Malluche HH, Faugere MC: Renal bone disease 1990: an unmet challenge for the nephrologist, *Kidney Int* 38:193-211, 1990.

42. Manhartsberger C, Morton JY, Burstone CJ: Space closure in adult patients using the segmented arch technique, *Angle Orthod* 59:205-210, 1989.

43. Martin RB, Burr DB: *Structure, function, and adaptation of compact bone,* New York, 1989, Raven Press.

44. Midgett RJ, Shaye R, Fruge JF: The effect of altered bone metabolism on orthodontic tooth movement, *Am J Orthod* 80:256-262, 1981.

44a. Miura F: *Effect of orthodontic force on blood circulation in periodontal membrane.* In Cook JT, editor: *Transactions of the Third International Orthodontic Congress,* St Louis, 1975, Mosby, pp. 35-41.

45. Morey ER, Baylink DJ: Inhibition of bone formation during space flight, *Science* 201:1138-1141, 1978.

46. Mundy GR, Bonewald LF: *Transforming growth factor beta.* In Gowen M, editor: *Cytokines and bone metabolism,* Boca Raton, Fla, 1992, CRC Press, pp 93-113.

47. Nikolai RJ: *Bioengineering analysis of orthodontic mechanics,* Philadelphia, 1985, Lea & Febiger.

48. Parfitt AM: *The physiological and clinical significance of bone histomorphometric data.* In Recker RR, editor: *Bone histomorphometry: techniques and interpretation,* Boca Raton, Fla, 1983, CRC Press, pp 143-223.

49. Parfitt AM: *Bone remodeling: relationship to the amount and structure of bone, and the pathogenesis and prevention of fractures.* In Riggs BL, editor: *Osteoporosis: etiology, diagnosis, and management,* New York, 1988, Raven Press, pp 45-93.

50. Pead MJ, Lanyon LE: Indomethacin modulation of load-related stimulation of new bone formation in vivo, *Calcif Tissue Int* 45:34-40, 1989.

51. Rapperport DJ, Carter DR, Schurman DJ: Contact finite element stress analysis of porous ingrowth acetabular cup implantation, ingrowth, and loosening, *J Orthop Res* 5:548-561, 1987.

52. Reddy MS, English R et al: Detection of periodontal disease activity with a scintillation camera, *J Dent Res* 70:50-54, 1991.

53. Reitan K: *Biomechanical principles and reactions.* In Graber TM, Swain BF, editors: *Orthodontics, current principles and techniques,* St Louis, 1985, Mosby, pp 111-229.

54. Rhodes R, Pflanzer R: *Human physiology,* Philadelphia, 1989, WB Saunders.

55. Riggs BL: Overview of osteoporosis, *West J Med* 154:63-77, 1991.

56. Rigotti NA, Neer RM et al: The clinical course of osteoporosis in anorexia nervosa, *JAMA* 265:1133-1138, 1991.

57. Roberts WE: Cell kinetic nature and diurnal periodicity of the rat periodontal ligament, *Arch Oral Biol* 20:465-471, 1975.

58. Roberts WE: *Advanced techniques for quantitating bone cell kinetics and cell population dynamics.* In Jarsowski ZRG, editor: *Proceedings of the first workshop on bone morphometry.* San Francisco, 1976, University of Ottawa Press, pp 310-314.

59. Roberts WE: Cell population dynamics of parathyroid hormone stimulated periodontal ligament, *Am J Anat* 143:363-370, 1975.

60. Roberts WE: Rigid endosseous anchorage and tricalcium phosphate (tcp)-coated implants, *Calif Dent Assoc J* 12(7):158-161, 1984.

61. Roberts WE: Bone tissue interface, *J Dent Educ* 52:804-809, 1988.

62. Roberts WE, Katona TR, Paydar NH, Akay HU et al: Stress analysis of bone modeling response to rat molar orthodontics (accepted by *J Biomech*), 1993.

63. Roberts WE, Arbuckle GR, Katona TR: *Bone physiology of orthodontics: metabolic and mechanical control mechanisms.* In Witt E, Tammoscheit U-G, editors: Symposon der Deutschen Gesellschaft für Kieferorthopädie, München, 1992, Urban & Vogel, pp 33-55.

64. Roberts WE, Aubert MM et al: Circadian periodicity of the cell kinetics of rat molar periodontal ligament, *Am J Orthod* 76:316-323, 1979.

65. Roberts WE, Chase DC: Kinetics of cell proliferation and migration association with orthodontically-induced osteogenesis, *J Dent Res* 60(2):174-181, 1981.

66. Roberts WE, Chase DC, Jee WSS: Counts of labelled mitoses in the orthodontically-stimulated periodontal ligament in the rat, *Arch Oral Biol* 19:665-670, 1974.

67. Roberts WE, Ferguson DJ: *Cell kinetics of the periodontal ligament.* In Norton LA, Burstone CJ, editors: *The biology of tooth movement.* Boca Raton, Fla, 1989, CRC Press, pp 55-70.

68. Roberts WE, Garetto LP: Physiology of osseous and fibrous integration, *Alpha Omega* 85:57-60, 1992.

69. Roberts WE, Garetto LP, DeCastro RA: Remodeling of devitalized bone threatens periosteal margin integrity of endosseous titanium implants with threaded or smooth surfaces: indications for provisional loading and axially directed occlusion, *J Indiana Dent Assoc* 68:19-24, 1989.

70. Roberts WE, Garetto LP et al: Bone physiology: evaluation of bone metabolism, *J Am Dent Assoc* 122:59-61, 1991.

71. Roberts WE, Garetto LP, Katona TR: *Principles of orthodontic biomechanics: metabolic and mechanical control mechanisms.* In Carlson DS, Goldstein SA, editors: *Bone biodynamics in orthodontic and orthopedic treatment.* Ann Arbor, 1992, University of Michigan Press, pp 189-255.

72. Roberts WE, Garetto LP, Simmons KE: *Endosseous implants for rigid orthodontic anchorage.* In Bell WH, editor: *Surgical correction of dentofacial deformities,* vol 2, Philadelphia, 1992, WB Saunders, pp. 1231-1263.

73. Roberts WE, Goodwin WC, Heiner SR: Cellular response to orthodontic force, *Dent Clin North Am* 25:3-17, 1981.

74. Roberts WE, Helm FR et al: Rigid endosseous implants for orthodontic and orthopedic anchorage, *Angle Orthod* 59:247-256, 1989.

75. Roberts WE, Jee WSS: Cell kinetics of orthodontically-stimulated and nonstimulated periodontal ligament in the rat, *Arch Oral Biol* 19:17-21, 1974.

76. Roberts WE, Klingler E, Mozsary PG: Circadian rhythm of mechanically mediated differentiation of osteoblasts, *Calcif Tissue Int* 36:S62-S66, 1984.

77. Roberts WE, Marshall KJ, Mozary PG: Rigid endosseous implant utilized as anchorage to protract molars and close an atrophic extraction site, *Angle Orthod* 60:135-152, 1990.

78. Roberts WE, Morey ER: Proliferation and differentiation sequence of osteoblast histogenesis under physiological conditions in rat periodontal ligament, *Am J Anat* 174:105-118, 1985.

79. Roberts WE, Mozsary PG, Klingler E: Nuclear size as a cell-kinetic marker for osteoblast differentiation, *Am J Anat* 165:373-384, 1982.

80. Roberts WE, Mozsary PG, Morey ER: Suppression of osteoblast differentiation during weightlessness, *Physiologist* 24(suppl 6):S75-S76, 1981.

81. Roberts WE, Poon LC, Smith RK: Interface histology of rigid endosseous implants, *J Oral Implantol* 12:406-416, 1986.

82. Roberts WE, Simmons KE et al: Bone physiology and metabolism in dental implantology: risk factors for osteoporosis and other metabolic bone diseases, *Implant Dent* 1:11-21, 1992.

83. Roberts WE, Smith RK, Cohen JA: *Change in electrical potential within periodontal ligament of a tooth subjected to osteogenic loading.* In Dixon A, Sarnat B, editors: *Factors and mechanisms influencing bone growth,* New York, 1982, Alan R. Liss, pp 527-534.

84. Roberts WE, Smith RK et al: Osseous adaptation to continuous loading of rigid endosseous implants, *Am J Orthod* 86:95-111, 1984.

85. Roberts WE, Turley PK et al: Bone physiology and metabolism, *Calif Dent Assoc J* 15(10):54-61, 1987.
86. Roberts WE, Wood HB et al: Vascularly oriented differentiation gradient of osteoblast precursor cells in rat periodontal ligament: implications for osteoblast histogenesis and periodontal bone loss, *J Peridont Res* 22:461-467, 1987.
87. Rodan GA: Perspectives of mechanical loading, estrogen deficiency, and the coupling of bone formation to bone resorption, *J Bone Min Res* 6:527-530, 1991.
88. Rodan GA, Martin TJ: Role of osteoblasts in hormonal control of bone resorption—a hypothesis, *Calcif Tissue Int* 33:349, 1981.
89. Rubin CT, Laynon LE: Regulation of bone mass by mechanical strain magnitude, *Calcif Tiss Res* 37:411-417, 1985.
90. Rubin CT, Lanyon LE: Osteoregulatory nature of mechanical stimuli: function as a determinant for adaptive modeling in bone, *J Orthop Res* 5:300-310, 1987.
91. Rubin CT, McLeod KJ, Bain SD: Functional strains and cortical bone adaptation: epigenetic assurance of skeletal integrity, *J Biomech* 23:43-54, 1990.
92. Rygh P, Moxham BJ, Berkovitz BKB: *The effects of external forces on the periodontal ligament—the response to horizontal loads.* In Berkovitz BKB, Moxham BJ, Newman HN, editors: *The periodontal ligament in health and disease.* Oxford, 1982, Pergamon Press, pp 269-290.
93. Siegele D, Dr-Ing US: Numerical investigations of the influence of implant shape on stress distribution in the jaw bone, *Int J Oral Maxillofac Implants* 4:333-340, 1989.
94. Simmons DJ, Russell JE, Winter F et al: Effect of spaceflight on the non-weight bearing bones of rat skeleton, *Am J Physiol* 244:319-326, 1983.
95. Slemenda CW, Hui SL et al: Predicators of bone mass in premenopausal women, *Ann Int Med* 112:96-101, 1990.
96. Smith RK, Roberts WE: Cell kinetics of the initial response to orthodontically induced osteogenesis in rat molar periodontal ligament, *Calcif Tissue Int* 30:51-56, 1980.
97. Thompson DD, Rodan GA: Indomethacin inhibition of tenotomy-induced bone resorption in rats, *J Bone Min Res* 3:409-414, 1988.
98. Yee JA: Response of periodontal ligament cells to orthodontic force: ultrastructural identification of proliferating fibroblasts, *Anat Rec* 194:603-607, 1979.
99. Yee JA, Kimmel DB, Jee WSS: Periodontal ligament cell kinetics following orthodontic tooth movement, *Cell Tissue Kinet* 9:293-302, 1976.

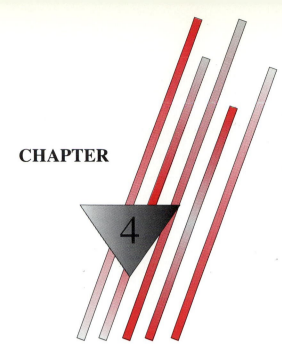

Application of Bioengineering to Clinical Orthodontics

CHAPTER

4

CHARLES J. BURSTONE

Part of the scientific revolution that has been occurring in biology during the last decade has been the broad application of the physical sciences to living tissues. Physics, engineering, and mathematics are disciplines that can be similarly applied with great profit to the field of orthodontics. Of the number of possible applications, this chapter will concern itself with only one, the biophysics of the orthodontic appliance. In a sense we will be asking ourselves whether theoretical mechanics can help us in the design and the clinical manipulation of an orthodontic appliance.

The role of theoretical mechanics has potential possibilities in three areas.

First, basic knowledge from engineering and physics can point the way toward improved design of orthodontic appliances. If the profession is to rely on trial-and-error procedures for the development of new appliances, the developmental horizons, of course, become sharply limited. Empiricism in orthodontic design must give way to a new discipline of orderly appliance development, using concepts from the physical sciences. In a less ambitious way theoretical mechanics may help us in the design of a new appliance by applying knowledge that has been gained from some of our older appliances. For example, if an existing appliance works quite well for a given type of tooth movement, we could use the force system developed by this appliance as a basis for designing a new appliance. Although trial and error has proved valuable in the past history of orthodontics, it is hoped that a more orderly development of orthodontic appliances will be possible with the application of biophysics.

The *second* area of application is the study of the biophysics of tooth movement. If we can quantify the force systems that are applied to teeth, we are in a better position to understand the clinical and histologic responses that take place. To make valid judgments about the response of teeth to orthodontic forces, we must first define fully the force system acting on the tooth. Furthermore, theoretical mechanics can be used to formulate useful concepts of the stress distribution in the periodontal ligament as it relates to bone remodeling.

Third, a knowledge of physics can enable us to produce better treatment results. Every time we make an adjustment in an archwire or any other orthodontic appliance, we are making certain assumptions about the relationship between the appliance and the biology of tooth movement. As our assumptions about the relationship between forces and tooth movement come closer to reality, the quality of orthodontic treatment can improve. For instance, many of the undesirable side effects produced during the course of orthodontic treatment can be directly attributed to a lack of understanding of the physics involved in a given adjustment. There are many variables in orthodontic treatment that we cannot fully control, including growth and the tissue responses to our appliances. However, one variable that we are in a position to control is the force we place on a tooth. In a sense it is almost our duty to understand the physics of these forces so we can better control the one variable that we are in a position to influence so strongly.[13]

Sign conventions. It is important to adopt a universal sign convention for forces and moments that will be applicable to dentistry and orthodontics. The convention is as follows:

Anterior forces are positive (+), and posterior forces are negative (−); lateral forces are positive (+), and medial forces are negative (−) (Fig. 4-1, *A*). Forces acting in a mesial direction are positive (+); forces acting in a distal direction are negative (−). Buccal forces are positive (+); lingual forces are negative (−) (Fig. 4-2, *A*).

Moments (couples) tending to produce mesial, labial, or buccal crown movements are positive (+), and moments tending to produce distal or lingual crown movements are negative (−) (Figs. 4-2, *B* and *C*).

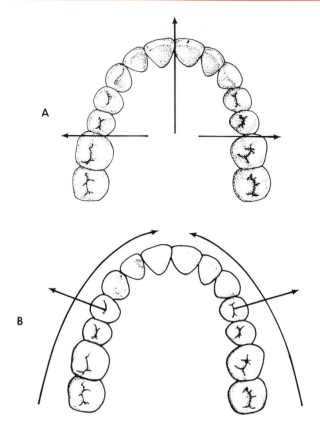

Fig. 4-1   Sign conventions. **A,** Lateral and anterior forces are positive. **B,** Buccal, labial, and mesial forces are positive. (From Burstone CJ, Koenig HA: *Am J Orthod* 65:270, 1974.)

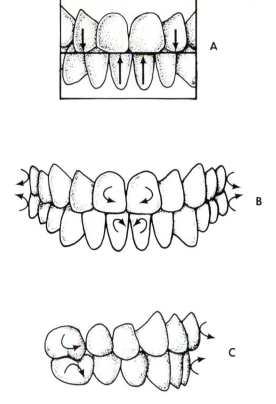

Fig. 4-2   Sign conventions. **A,** Extrusive forces are positive. **B** and **C,** Moments (couples) tending to move crowns to the mesial, buccal, and labial are positive. (From Burstone CJ, Koenig HA: *Am J Orthod* 65:270, 1974.)

The same convention is used for groups of teeth (a segment or an entire arch) and for establishing signs for orthopedic effects on the maxilla or mandible.

BIOMECHANICS OF TOOTH MOVEMENT

From a clinical viewpoint two major problems related to tooth movement can be considered: (1) the type of force system that is required to produce a given center of rotation; and, (2) the force magnitudes that are optimal for tooth movement. Solving these problems requires a thorough understanding of the forces and moments that may act on the teeth as well as a detailed documentation of the tooth movement and the response within the periodontal ligament.

The forces delivered from an orthodontic appliance can be determined by direct measurement with suitable instruments or, in part, by mathematical calculation.[24, 33, 51, 57] The load deflection rates of orthodontic springs or wires may be measured with either electronic strain gauges or mechanical gauges (Fig. 4-3). It should be remembered that most orthodontic appliances deliver a relatively complicated set of forces and moments. In clinical studies, therefore, it is useful to employ appliances of simple construction in which forces are more easily and accurately determined. For the same reason a clinical study in which force variables are controlled is likely to supply more information than are data taken from patients in a routine orthodontic practice.

The problems inherent in studying the response of a tooth subjected to a force system are much more complex and difficult to solve than is the simple measurement of the forces themselves. Three levels of observation can be used to describe the response of a tooth to forces: *clinical, cellular* and *biochemical,* and *stress-strain*. At the clinical level, phenomena such as rates of tooth movement, pain response, tooth mobility, alveolar bone loss, and root resorption can be studied. The cellular and biochemical level gives insight into the dynamics of bone and connective tissue changes in the periodontal ligament. Perhaps the most important and least understood is the stress-strain level of activity in the periodontal ligament. If the stress (force per unit area) level could be accurately determined in different areas of this tissue, it might well offer the best opportunity for correlating force application on a tooth with tooth response. Since at this time it is not possible to place strain gauges in the periodontal ligament to measure stress distributions, our

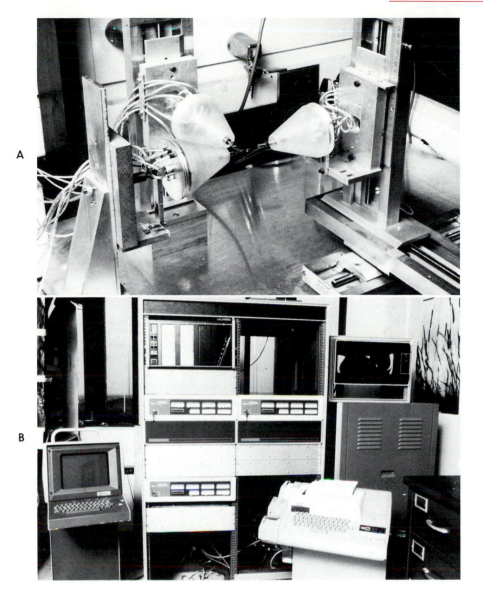

Fig. 4-3 **A,** Strain gauge apparatus used to measure force and moments at a bracket in three planes. **B,** The computer interface allows instantaneous determination and printout of the force system. Simple force or torque gauges do not give sufficient information to determine the force system from an appliance.

knowledge of stress phenomena must depend on another approach. A mathematical model of the tooth and surrounding structures can be constructed based on certain assumptions. From these mathematical models, theoretical stress levels can be calculated if the forces applied to the teeth are known. Unfortunately, however, these mathematical models are no better than the assumptions. Therefore, all such calculation, whenever possible, should be verified by clinical or animal experimentation.

Centers of rotation

Tooth movement is often described in general terms—tipping, bodily movement, and root movement. A more specific method of description can be evolved by locating a center of rotation relative to three mutually perpendicular planes. The three planes are (1) a *buccolingual* or *labiolingual* plane oriented through the long axis of a tooth, (2) a *mesiodistal* plane also oriented through the long axis of a

tooth, and (3) a *transverse* plane that intersects the buccolingual or labiolingual and mesiodistal planes at right angles. To define fully changes in position of a tooth, it is necessary to employ all three planes of reference. For purposes of simplification, the following discussion will consider two-dimensional representations of teeth and thereby only one plane of space will be described. If certain simple assumptions are made about stress distributions (i.e., a uniformly varying distribution for pure rotation and a uniform distribution for pure translation), if a linear stress-strain relationship is postulated and if axial loading is ignored, it is then possible to predict mathematically the force system required for various centers of rotation. These calculations will err as the realities of tooth and periodontal ligament differ from the idealized assumptions just described. A typical central incisor is employed as representative of the application of this theory to centers of rotation. For purposes of presentation the use of actual force values is avoided.

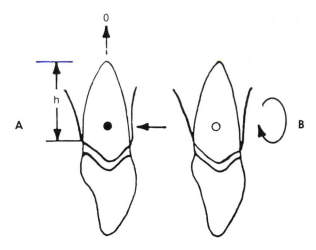

Fig. 4-4 Basic tooth movements. **A,** A force acting through the center of resistance of a tooth produces translation—center of rotation at infinity. **B,** A couple acting on the tooth produces a center of rotation at the center of resistance.

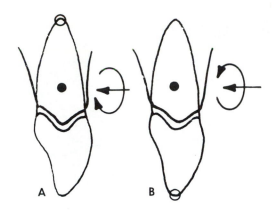

Fig. 4-5 A couple and a force acting through the center of resistance. **A,** A negative couple produces lingual tipping of the incisor crown. **B,** A positive couple produces incisor lingual root movement.

As a tooth translates (bodily movement), a relatively uniform stress distribution along the root is found. In terms of a center of rotation, the center of rotation for translation is at infinity (Fig. 4-4, A). It can be shown that a single force acting through the center of resistance of a root effects pure translation of a tooth. The center of resistance in a single rooted tooth with a parabolic shape is at a point 0.33 multiplied times the distance from the alveolar crest to the apex. The center of resistance coincides with the centroid, which in this case is the geometric center of the part of the root that is between the alveolar crest and the apex. A force placed near the center of the root therefore should be expected to produce pure translation.[20,21]

If a pure moment (a couple) is placed anywhere on a tooth, a center of rotation occurs near the center of resistance of the tooth. In Fig. 4-4, B, the clockwise moment will tend to displace the crown to the lingual and the root to the labial, with a center of rotation near the middle of the root. Unlike pure translation, pure rotation does not produce a uniform stress distribution in the periodontal ligament, but instead a uniformly varying distribution with the highest stresses at the apex and the next highest at the alveolar crest. Zero stress is found at the center of resistance. It can be seen that the center of rotation is located at the level of the root where the stress is zero.

Pure translation (center of rotation at infinity) and pure rotation (center of rotation near the center of resistance) can be considered the two basic types of tooth displacement. Other centers are a combination of pure rotation and pure translation, that is, any center of rotation can be produced by combining a single force through the center of resistance of a root and a pure moment if the proper force/couple ratio is used.[36]

In Fig. 4-5, A, a lingual force is acting through the center of resistance of the root. If a couple is added in a clockwise direction, the center of rotation will move from infinity toward the center of resistance. If the magnitude of the couple is small (relative to the force at the center of resistance), the center of rotation lies at the apex of the root. As the magnitude of the couple is increased, the center of rotation will shift from the apex toward the center of resistance; finally, with increased values of the couple, the center will approach the center of resistance of the root. It can be seen that the relative magnitude of the couple and force acting through the center of resistance determines the specific type of lingual tipping of the tooth if the direction of the moment is clockwise.

On the other hand, a counterclockwise moment plus a force acting through the center of resistance will place the center of rotation somewhere between the center of resistance and infinity (Fig. 4-5, B). More specifically, as the couple force ratio increases, the center of rotation will move from the incisal edge to the level of the bracket and then, finally, will approach the center of resistance. The basis, then, for controlling the center of rotation during tooth movement is the placing of a single force through the center of resistance of the root and a couple of proper direction and magnitude.[49]

In most instances, however, it is not practical to place a force through the center of resistance because of anatomic limitations in the oral cavity. Because of these limitations, a force system must be placed on the crown of the tooth (at a bracket or tube) that is equivalent to the required couple and force acting through the center of resistance. The two force systems are equivalent if the sums of their individual forces are equal (F_x, F_y, and F_z) and if the sums of their moments around any axis of rotation are equal.

The following equivalent force systems acting on a bracket of an incisor are typical effects of altering the couple/force ratio:

A lingually directed single force placed on the crown of a tooth produces a center of rotation somewhere

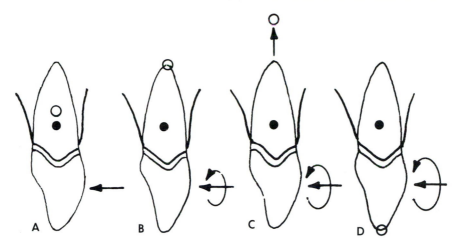

Fig. 4-6   A single force acting on the crown of a tooth produces a center of rotation *(open circle)* slightly below the center of resistance. **A,** If increasingly larger couples are added to the force in the direction shown in **B** through **D,** the center of rotation will be found at the apex **(B),** infinity **(C),** or incisal edge **(D).**

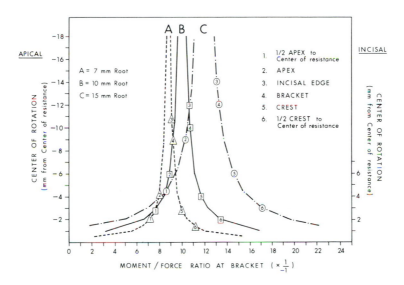

Fig. 4-7   Moment-to-force ratio (M/F) plotted against the center of rotation for three incisor root lengths. Note that identical M/F values produce different centers of rotation if the root length varies.

between the center of resistance and the apex (Fig. 4-6, *A*).

If a counterclockwise moment (lingual root torque) of sufficient magnitude is added, the center of rotation moves to the apex (Fig. 4-6, *B*).

If an additional moment in the same direction is placed on the tooth, the center of rotation moves toward infinity and at this instance the tooth is translating or moving bodily (Fig. 4-6, *C*).

Further increases in the magnitude of the couple will place the center of rotation incisal to the crown of the tooth (Fig. 4-6, *D*), then at the incisal edge, and finally at the bracket.

Any further increase in the moment tends to move the center of rotation toward the center of resistance.

In Fig. 4-7 the M/F ratio is plotted against the center of rotation for three incisor roots: 7 mm, 10 mm, and 15 mm in length. The moment and force are applied at the bracket. The distance of the bracket in all cases is 6 mm from the alveolar crest. The direction of the force applied to the incisor is lingual $(-)$ and the sense of the moment is lingual root torque $(+)$. In the three examples it should be noticed that as the M/F ratio approaches zero, the center of rotation approaches the center of resistance. As the ratio increases, the center of rotation will be found at the apex of the root, infinity, the incisal edge, the bracket, and the alveolar crest.

As the ratio becomes infinitely large, the center of rotation approaches the center of resistance. Small variation in the M/F ratio can make a large difference in the positioning of the center of rotation, with the exception of ratios that produce centers of rotation near the center of resistance. Furthermore, the same M/F ratio will produce different centers of rotation, depending on the length of the root.

Nägerl et al. have developed a general theory of tooth movement based on three-dimensional linear elastic assumptions. The general theory states that in any given plane the distance from the applied force to the center of resistance (a) times the distance from the center of resistance to the center of rotation (b) equals a constant. This constant is sigma squared, which represents the distribution of the restraining forces in the periodontal ligament. As shown in Fig. 4-8, regardless of the point of force application of the force in a given plane, sigma squared remains the same. The experimental determination of sigma squared offers the possibility of determining centers of rotation for given teeth with similar morphology minimizing the number of recordings required experimentally.[41-43]

A number of clinical implications are suggested by the preceding analyses.

First, the center of rotation is dependent on the ratio between the moment and the force applied to the tooth (M/F ratio) and not on the absolute values of each. For example, if a single force were placed on the crown of the tooth, the center of rotation should be the same, irrespective of the magnitude of the force. A *light* or *heavy* force would tend equally to move the crown in one direction and the root in the other. This is in sharp contradiction to the often repeated idea that lighter forces will not displace root apices as much as heavy forces. This statement would be accurate only if a properly directed moment as well as a force were applied to the tooth in question. It is possible that if the moments were identical the tooth with the lower force would have a minimal root displacement.[23]

Recent research suggests that if identical moment/force ratios are delivered to a tooth, the center of rotation may not be exactly identical. Heavier single forces on the crown tend to move the center of rotation slightly apically rather than occlusally.

Second, the moment/force ratio is quite critical in the establishment of any given center of rotation. Small miscalculations in this ratio can change the type of tooth movement that is observed. Since stress distributions in the periodontal ligament are altered as well, a change in the ease of tooth movement also may be produced.

Third, in many instances the load-deflection rate of the force acting on the crown and the torque-deflection (angular) rate of the moment may be quite different. If, for example, a lingual force dissipates faster than the moment (torque), the center of rotation will be modified. The center of rotation in this instance is not constant but shifts because of a changing force/moment ratio.

Laser holography is a new noninvasive technique for accurately studying tooth movement.[14,20,21,45] In Fig. 4-9 the location of the center of rotation is plotted against the M/F ratio for a typical maxillary central incisor. The experimental curves are similar to the curves derived from previously discussed theory.

In addition to analytical methodology and laser holography, numerical techniques have been used to determine centers of rotation of teeth under different loading conditions and to estimate stress in the periodontal ligament. These techniques use a finite element method that is three dimensional. The tooth and the alveolar process are broken down into elements (Fig. 4-10) by accurately determining the shape of the elements and the constitutive mechanical be-

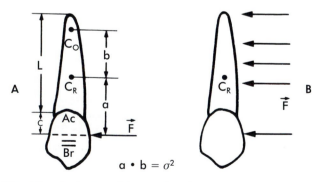

Fig. 4-8   **A,** A general theory of tooth movement states that the product of the distances *a* and *b* equals a constant (α^2). **B,** α^2 is a constant, provided that the single forces are parallel and act in the same plane. Any of the individual forces shown in **B** produces the same α^2. (From Nägerl H, Burstone CJ et al: Centers of rotation with transverse forces: an experimental study, *Am J Orthod Dentofac Orthop* 99(4):337-345, 1991.)

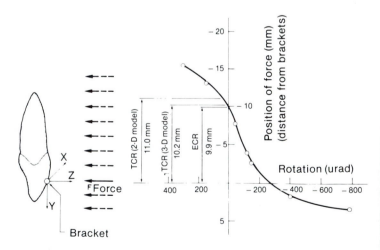

Fig. 4-9   Center of rotation measured from the centroid of the paraboloid of revolution (h/3) as a function of the M/F ratio at the bracket. The center of rotation approaches infinity as the line of action of the applied force approaches the centroid. *TCR,* Theoretical center of resistance; *ECR,* experimental center of resistance.

havior of each of the elements. Centers of rotation are determined using assumed forces on the teeth.[53-56]

As more knowledge becomes available, refinements in mathematical models will enable the clinician to have good estimates of the M/F ratios needed to produce required centers of rotation for teeth with varying geometries and different periodontal supports and for groups of teeth or segments.

Our lack of knowledge of the variation in tooth morphology and support should not deter the clinician from making the best estimates concerning the relationship between the forces from the appliance and the centers of rotation produced. The understanding of theory at its basic minimum will guide the clinician in adjusting the appliances when undesirable centers of rotation are produced.

Nägerl has developed a new concept for describing tooth motion that is not as limiting in three-dimensional space as is the center of rotation concept. Tooth movement is envisioned as a screw that is oriented in a coordinate system. The screw forms an axis around which the tooth rotates; in addition, translation may occur either in or out along that axis.[41,42]

Force magnitude and the rate of tooth movement

Considerable debate in orthodontics has centered on the relationship of force magnitude and the rate of tooth movement.[25,26,50,52,58] Attempts at correlations of this type are more likely to be successful if rates of tooth displacement rather than total displacement (absolute displacement) values are used. Rate of tooth movement is defined as the displacement of a tooth per unit time and is usually measured in millimeters per hour, day, or week. As the increments of time become shorter, it is possible to become more aware of the dynamics of tooth movement and, hence, daily rather than weekly or monthly recordings are preferred.

Average daily rates can be established by dividing the absolute displacement by the number of days when mea

surements are made at less frequent intervals than daily. The tendency of such methods is to smooth out rate curves and eliminate much of the fluctuation in rate that can be observed each day. For practical purposes, if it is not possible to measure daily increments of movements (which is the case in many clinical studies), average rates of tooth movement must be used. Whenever average rates are used, their limitations should always be kept in mind.

Two possible force-rate relationships can be studied. One approach relates force magnitude and tooth displacement. The second approach, which is perhaps more logical, attempts to relate stress-strain phenomena (force per unit area and displacement per unit length) in the periodontal ligament with tooth displacement. Until better experimental methods are devised, the latter method is limited by the fact that the stress-strain values must be calculated from mathematical models rather than obtained by experimentation in the living.

The difficulty of correlating forces and tooth movement is compounded by the great number of variables that can influence the recorded rate of tooth displacement. Connective tissue forces operating through gingival and transseptal fibers or forces from the tongue, perioral musculature, and muscles of mastication may alter the force system acting on the tooth. For these reasons, it is not yet possible to make definitive statements about the relationship between force and tooth displacement. A more complete discussion of the problem must await renewed experimentation in this area.

If a relatively constant force is placed on the tooth, a typical type of graph is obtained when rate of tooth movement is plotted against time (Fig. 4-11). Three phases of tooth movement can be differentiated: *an initial phase, a lag phase,* and *a post-lag phase.* The *initial phase* is char-

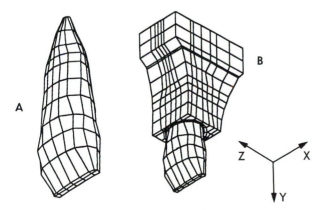

Fig. 4-10   A three-dimensional model for tooth **(A)** and tooth-PDL-alveolar bone system **(B).** (From Tanne K, Koenig HA, Burstone CJ: Moment to force ratios and the center of rotation, *Am J Orthod Dentofac Orthop* 94(5):426-431, 1988.)

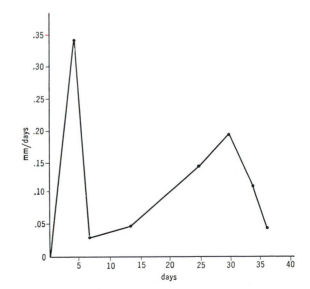

Fig. 4-11   Typical tooth movement graph in which rate is plotted against the number of days after the application of a continuous force (125 g). Rates are given for the reciprocal closure of a diastema between two central incisors.

acterized by a period of rapid tooth movement and normally lasts a few days. The rapidity of displacement and its onset immediately after the application of a force to a tooth suggest that the tooth movement in the initial phase represents, to a large degree, displacement of a tooth in the periodontal space. Immediately after the initial phase *a lag phase* is observed during which the tooth does not move or has a relatively low rate of displacement. A number of explanations could be postulated to explain the presence of a lag period. It has been suggested that the lag is produced by nonvitalization (hyalinization) of the periodontal ligament in areas of maximum stress and that no tooth movement will occur until the area of nonvitalization is removed by cellular processes.[46,48,50] Another explanation is that the lag period may represent the time required for the thicker compact bone of the lamina dura to be absorbed, and hence the rate of tooth movement is reduced. The third phase of tooth movement, the *post-lag phase*, occurs when the rate of tooth movement gradually or suddenly increases. It follows the lag period. (See Chapters 2 and 3.)

During study of the rates of tooth movement the great variation of response to relatively identical force systems is impressive. This is not surprising since the force applied on a tooth is but one of the many variables that determine its displacement. If constant force were placed on a tooth, it might be expected that the tooth would move at a constant rate through the alveolar process. Clinical measurements, however, display a lack of constancy in rate not only during the initial and lag phases but also during subsequent movement of a tooth.

The critical issue in orthodontic therapy is the relationship between force magnitude and rate of tooth movement. The most obvious and appealing relationship is a linear one, in which more force implies greater tooth movement. Appealing as the simplicity of this assumption might be, it does not correspond to the facts as they are observed histologically and clinically in all phases of tooth movement.

During the first part of the initial stage, when the tooth is deflected through the periodontal space, something approaching a linear relationship may exist. As the stress levels in the periodontal ligament further increase, an increased rate of tooth movement is expected. Thus a light force may take days to move a tooth through the width of the periodontal ligament, whereas a heavy force, such as a dental separator, can accomplish the same result momentarily. Response between light and heavy forces show no gross differences if the absolute displacement is measured after 2 or 3 days or if the average rate is calculated for a like period. In Fig. 4-12 average rates of tooth movement are plotted against the number of days after insertion of a continuous force appliance. In comparing the application of 10 g as opposed to 200 g on a central incisor, a similar initial response is observed. It appears that fairly light forces are capable of moving a tooth through a greater part of the width of the periodontal ligament. Once this has been accomplished, it might be expected that higher forces would

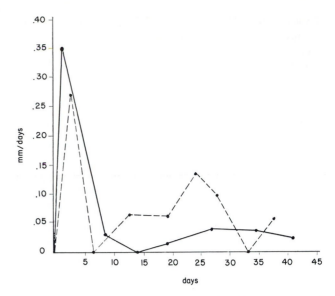

Fig. 4-12 Rates of tooth movement with different force applications. *Dotted line,* 200 g; *solid line,* 10 g. Rates are given for the reciprocal closure of a diastema between two central incisors.

produce additional compression of the ligament. The magnitude of this additional compression is small compared to the initial tooth movement and therefore is not evident on gross measurements of tooth movement. Such variables as the width of the periodontal ligament are of much greater importance than force magnitude in determining the initial absolute displacement of a tooth (Chapter 3).

During the second stage of tooth movement, two processes can be observed in the areas of pressure. Direct resorption may occur on the bone surface facing the root or indirect (undermining) resorption may start in the medullary spaces and work toward the tooth.[46,48] The best that can be hoped for at this time is the development of a working hypothesis to explain and relate these bony changes to stress levels in the periodontal ligament. Until data are available that correlate measured or calculated stress levels with histologically observed bony resorption, assumptions of this type must be considered tentative. Theoretically, if a low stress level is introduced into the periodontal ligament no bony transformation will occur. If this stress level is increased, a point will be reached at which bone resorption can begin (i.e., a threshold stress level). Nothing is known about the magnitude of stress that is capable of initiating bone resorption and apposition. Clinically, however, it is known that relatively small force magnitudes are capable of tipping teeth (10 g or less on the maxillary incisors).[31] Provided it even exists, a threshold force (the lowest possible force that will move a tooth) has a very low magnitude, at least for *simple* tipping movements. Additional stress in the periodontal ligament beyond the threshold stress level can be expected to increase the amount of frontal resorption on the alveolar process. As the stress values increase a reduction in cellular activity can be anticipated because areas of maximum stress produce further compression of blood vessels and cellular elements. Histologically these areas appear hyalinized and may at least in part be described as nonvital. A reduction in bone resorption logically follows, since vital connective tissue is a requisite for direct bone resorption. On the other hand, undermining resorption is associated with high stresses on the periodontal ligament and is a response to a compressed nonvital area of connective tissue.

At low stress levels little indirect resorption occurs. In fact, bone apposition can occur in the medullary spaces. As the stress increases, the magnitude of cellular response also increases; however, once again, a limiting factor is present. A force can be only great enough to displace a tooth against the alveolar process; when this occurs the stress level is limited, and for that given interval of time, no greater stimulus for indirect resorption might be expected.

Under most clinical conditions tooth displacement after the lag phase is produced by a combination of direct and indirect resorptive processes. Concomitant bony and connective tissue changes in the areas of tension are most likely secondary to resorption of bone in the existing pressure regions.

What, then, is the relationship between force magnitude and the rate of tooth movement? At lower force magnitudes, most increases in force enhance the rate of tooth movement. At higher magnitudes, increases in force are responsible in part for hyalinization of the periodontal ligament and result in an increased lag period. Eventually undermining resorption will remove the area of hyalinization and the tooth will move rapidly into the newly created space. For these reasons a wide range of forces, from light to heavy (provided they are continuous), are capable of rapidly moving teeth.

Lighter forces are more likely to move teeth gradually, whereas heavy forces demonstrate a marked lag followed by a period of rapid movement. Over a long time interval the average rate of movement for heavy continuous forces may be greater than those observed for lighter continuous forces. The complexity of the tissue changes, as well as the presence of a great number of variables, suggests that there are inherent difficulties in postulating any simple relationship between force magnitude and the rate of tooth movement.

One of the variables to be considered in evaluating force magnitude and rate of movement is the type of tooth movement (center of rotation). It is possible with the application of identical forces on the crown of a tooth to produce different centers of rotation by altering the applied couple. Although the force remains the same, as the moment is changed the stress distribution is modified in the periodontal ligament. Imagine a simple model of the tooth in its alveolus (a linear stress-strain relationship in the periodontal ligament will be assumed). For simplicity the model has a uniformly thick periodontal ligament and smooth alveolar walls. To be sure, this oversimplifies the nature of the tooth and its surrounding structures. The periodontal ligament is not uni-

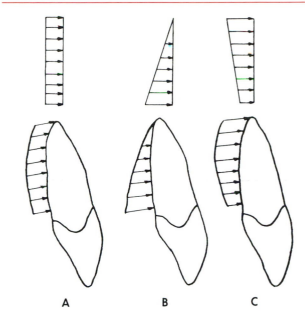

Fig. 4-13 Theoretical stress distributions in the periodontal ligament. **A,** Translation. **B,** Center of rotation at the apex. **C,** Center of rotation at the incisal edge. The force magnitude is identical in the three situations.

formly thick, and the lamina dura is an irregular cribriform plate pierced by numerous holes; yet the tooth model with all its difficulties may prove most useful in comparing stress distribution for different types of tooth movement.

In pure translation or bodily tooth movement a relatively uniform stress distribution is found in the periodontal ligament (actually variations in periodontal ligament thickness alter the stress distribution). Fig. 4-13 shows an imaginary stress distribution for a force system producing translation of a central incisor in a lingual direction. If the movement of the crown is reduced, the center of rotation will shift from infinity toward the apex of the root. Although the lingual force is identical with that used for bodily movement, the stress distribution is markedly altered (Fig. 4-13). In tipping with a center of rotation at the apex, the maximum stress is to be found at the alveolar crest and its magnitude is considerably greater than that seen in translation. If the moment is increased beyond the amount required for translation, the center of rotation shifts from infinity toward the incisal edge. With the center of rotation at the incisal edge, once again a nonuniform stress distribution is observed (Fig. 4-13). In this case the maximum stress is at the apex and its magnitude is greater than the stress found in translation. It should be emphasized that in the three instances (translation, tipping at the apex, and rotation around the incisal edge) the lingual force is identical. To develop the same maximum stress level of bodily tooth movement as in rotation around the apex and the incisal edge, it would be necessary to increase the lingual force and the moment applied to the crown of the tooth. The center of rotation is an important factor that determines stress distribution in the periodontal ligament and hence the degree and type of cellular reaction. Therefore the force system should be well defined in any attempt to relate force magnitude and rate of tooth movement. This includes an awareness of not only the magnitude of all forces and the moments acting as a crown but also their constancy.

Fig. 4-14 shows a tooth in which stresses were studied using the finite element method. If a force is placed to produce translation, as shown in Fig. 4-15, it is apparent that the stresses are not as uniform as described in the simplistic explanations given above.[56] The simplistic explanations may aid in understanding how stress distributions vary with the same magnitude of force. It should be remembered, however, that a tooth is a three-dimensional, irregular body that has a most complicated stress distribution, even during translation.

Not all variables that influence rates of movement involve stress levels in the periodontal ligament. Some involve the structure of the supporting bone of the alveolar process. Clinical observation also suggests a great variation in the response of connective tissues to the stresses of orthodontic

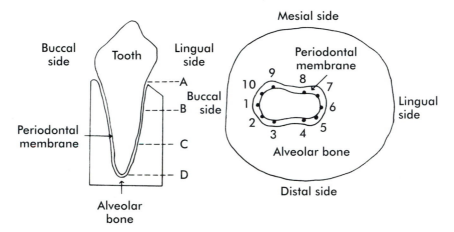

Fig. 4-14   Occlusogingival levels (*A* through *D*) and horizontal points (*1* through *10*) where the principal stresses were determined. (From Tanne K, Sakuda M, Burstone CJ: Three-dimensional finite element analysis for stress in the periodontal tissue by orthodontic forces, *Am J Orthod Dentofac Orthop* 92(6):499-505, 1987.)

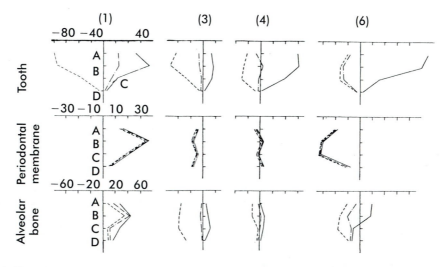

Fig. 4-15   Stress distribution (g/cm²) in loading condition for a lingual force of 100 g and a buccal crown couple of 858.5 g-mm (L₂). Three principal stresses, maximum (——), intermediate (—●—), and minimum (- - - -), are shown for four significant points (*1, 3, 4,* and *6*) at various occlusogingival levels (*A* through *D*). (From Tanne K, Sakuda M, Burstone CJ: Three-dimensional finite element analysis for stress in the periodontal tissue by orthodontic forces, *Am J Orthod Dentofac Orthop* 92(6):499-505, 1987.)

tooth movement. The response of tissues to mechanical stress is as yet obscure. However, biochemical mechanisms in which stress and strain produce bone resorption and apposition are beginning to be better understood. Strain, working through biochemical mediators such as prostaglandins or piezoelectric effects, could be responsible for the biologic response to orthodontic forces.

Relationship of force magnitude to pain and tooth mobility

After an active orthodontic appliance has been inserted, symptoms of pain or discomfort may develop. Objective evaluation of pain is most difficult, since the pain response is determined by the central nervous system and by local tissue changes. It is not too surprising, however, to find a wide range of pain reactions among individuals in whom similar forces have been placed on the teeth.

To evaluate the relationship of force to pain, a classification of pain response is helpful. Three degrees of pain response may be described. *First-degree* pain is produced only by heavy pressure placed on the tooth with an instrument like a band pusher or a force gauge. A first-degree response usually is elicited most easily by placing a force in the same direction as the force produced by the appliance. The patient is not aware of first-degree pain unless the teeth that are being moved with an orthodontic appliance happen to be manipulated. A *second-degree* pain response is characterized by pain or discomfort during clenching of the teeth or heavy biting. The patient maintains the ability to masticate a normal diet without difficulty. If spontaneous pain is present or if the patient is unable to masticate food of normal consistency, a *third-degree* response exists. The proper interpretation of pain data requires the testing of the patient's response to heavy forces placed on the teeth before orthodontic treatment has begun. In this way the patient influences, even controls, future pain and discomfort.

Two types of pain based on time of onset are found: *immediate* and *delayed*. Immediate pain responses are associated with the sudden placement of heavy forces on a tooth. For example, a *hard* figure-eight tie between spaced incisors usually produces an acute pain reaction that gradually subsides. Some hours after an orthodontic adjustment, a delayed response may become evident. Delayed pain responses are produced by a variety of force values from light to heavy and represent hyperalgesia of the periodontal ligament. Usually with the passage of time, the degree of response becomes less. A decreasing gradient is observed when, for instance, the pain reaction passes from a third-degree to a second-degree response and finally to a first-degree or zero-degree response. Although a gradient of this type is generally observed, situations arise where, for no apparent reason, the pain reaction suddenly increases many days after the application of a continuous force.

In general, the magnitude of force applied to a tooth has a definite relation to the pain experienced by the patient. It

has been demonstrated in clinical studies that the incidence of second- and third-degree pain is higher with application of heavier forces to the teeth. Not only is a higher degree of pain evident with a heavy force, but the total number of days in which an abnormal pain response can be elicited is increased. This is not to imply, however, that a linear relationship exists.

The generalization that greater forces produce higher degrees of pain for longer periods is an oversimplification. As in the discussion of rates of tooth movement, once again it is found that force magnitude is only one of the factors that determine the final response of the patient.

An understanding of pain during orthodontic treatment is further obscured by a lack of knowledge about why pain is produced. This difficulty is aggravated because no pain fibers are to be found in the periodontal ligament. If or when the mechanisms of pain production during tooth movement are known, the orthodontist will have better insight into the relationship of force and pain response.

Optimal force and stress

The effect of the couple/force ratio on the center of rotation of a moving tooth has been considered. Another question of great clinical significance is the proper magnitude of force and couple that should be used for the most desirable response. In other words, what force magnitudes are optimal for tooth movement?

From a clinical point of view, an optimal force is one that produces a rapid rate of tooth movement without discomfort to the patient or ensuing tissue damage (alveolar bone loss and root resorption, in particular). From a histologic point of view, an optimal force is one that produces a stress level in the periodontal ligament that (1) basically maintains the vitality of the tissue throughout its length and that (2) initiates a maximum cellular response (apposition and resorption). Optimal forces therefore produce direct resorption of the alveolar process. Since optimal forces require no period of time for repair, it appears that such forces can be made to act continuously.

Histologic studies that correlate factors on the crown or stresses in the periodontal ligament with tissue responses could be most helpful in establishing levels of optimal force for different situations. Unfortunately, the difficulty of obtaining human material is a limiting factor in this type of investigation. At the clinical level, wherein a greater wealth of material is available, the orthodontist is limited to the supply of gross tooth and bone changes or patient symptoms. This is not to imply that careful clinical observation will not prove helpful in determining optimal forces. Lack of pain, minimal mobility, and lack of a marked lag period immediately after an appliance adjustment are examples of clinical responses that suggest desirable stress levels in the periodontal ligament. It is dangerous, however, to use rate of tooth movement by itself as an indicator of optimal force. Rate is deceptive, since both heavy and light continuous forces have the ability to move teeth rapidly. It is a non sequitur to state: "The teeth moved rapidly; therefore, the forces used were optimum."

Long-term histologic and clinical studies are needed to define further the nature of optimal force.

Although investigations into the biomechanics of tooth movement have great promise, it is risky to employ mathematical formulations to describe biologic phenomena because mathematical oversimplification of highly dynamic and variable vital structures and reactions can mislead as well as inform. It is therefore necessary to check biomechanical assumptions with observations on both clinical and histologic levels. A multidisciplinary approach of this type offers the best hope for solving orthodontic problems relating force systems and tooth movement.

THE ORTHODONTIC APPLIANCE

The starting place for the design of any orthodontic appliance is certain assumptions about the nature of an optimal force system to move teeth. The author believes that an optimal force system is one that accurately controls the center of rotation of a tooth during tooth movement, produces optimal stress levels in the periodontal ligaments, and maintains a relatively constant stress level as the tooth moves from one position to the next. For the sake of argument, let us assume that these objectives for the orthodontic appliance are correct; it must then be decided what is needed to design an appliance that will deliver this type of force system.

Active and reactive members

An orthodontic appliance can be considered to have *active* and *reactive* members. The active member of the appliance is the part that is concerned with tooth movement; the reactive member functions for purposes of anchorage and involves the teeth that are not to be displaced. In certain instances a member may function as both an active and reactive member at the same time. This is clearly the case when reciprocal anchorage is used.

On a subclinical level it has been said that our objectives are (1) to control the center of rotation of the tooth, (2) to maintain desirable stress levels in the periodontal ligament, and (3) to maintain a relatively constant stress level. Moving from the subclinical to the clinical level of observation, we find that we are interested in the forces and moments produced by an orthodontic appliance. Specifically, we are interested in three important characteristics that involve active and reactive members. They are (1) the moment/force ratio, (2) the load-deflection rate, and (3) the maximal force or moment of any component of an appliance.

Moment/force ratio. To produce different types of tooth movement, it is necessary for the ratio between the applied moment and force on the crown to be altered. As the moment/force ratio is altered, so the center of rotation will be changed. Crown tipping, translation, and root movement are examples of different types of tooth movement that can be produced with the proper moment/force ratio. The im-

portant consideration is that instances are few in which desirable types of tooth movement can be produced by single forces applied to the crown alone, where crown and root will move in opposite directions. An active member therefore must be capable of producing the desired moment and force if a modern orthodontic appliance is being considered. The moment/force ratio is not only important in the active member of the appliance but is also equally significant in the reactive member. For instance, if preservation of anchorage of the posterior segments in an extraction case is being considered, it is desirable to introduce a moment that tends to move roots forward and crowns back so, in combination with the mesial forces acting on the posterior segments, a more uniform distribution of stresses will be produced in the periodontal ligament. With a more uniform distribution of stress in the posterior segment, forward displacement is minimized. An example of the addition of a moment of this type to the posterior segment to enhance anchorage is the tip-back bend. In short, the moment/force ratio determines the control that the orthodontic appliance will have over both the active and reactive units. Specifically, the moment/force ratio controls the center of rotation of a tooth or a group of teeth.

Load-deflection rate. The second characteristic of an orthodontic appliance, the load-deflection or torque-twist rate, is involved with the delivery of a relatively constant force.[5] By definition, the load-deflection rate gives the force produced per unit activation. As the load-deflection rate becomes lower for a tooth that is moving under a continuous force, the change in force value is reduced. With regard to active members, a low load-deflection rate is desirable for two important reasons: A mechanism with a low load-deflection rate will maintain a more desirable stress level in the periodontal ligament, since the force on a tooth will not radically change magnitude every time the tooth has been displaced. Also a low load-deflection rate member offers greater accuracy in control over force magnitude. For example, if a high load-deflection spring is used, such as an edgewise vertical loop, it is possible that the load-deflection rate might be 1000 g per millimeter. This would mean that an error in adjustment of 1 mm could produce an error in force value of approximately 1000 g. On the other hand, if a low load-deflection spring were used, such as one with a rate of 10 g per millimeter, an error of 1 mm in activation would affect the force value by only 10 g. Flexible members that have low load-deflection rates require long ranges of activation to build up to optimal force values, and hence they give the orthodontist greater control in the magnitude of force employed.

If a low load-deflection rate is desirable for an active member of the appliance, the opposite is true for the reactive member. The reactive member should be relatively rigid; that is, it should have a high load-deflection rate. The anchorage potential of a group of teeth can be enhanced if the teeth displace as a unit. If individual teeth in the reactive unit tend to rotate around separate centers of rotation, then higher stress distributions will be produced in the periodontal ligament and therefore the teeth can be more easily displaced. Another factor to consider is that the equal and opposite forces produced by the active members are usually distributed to localized areas, with just one or a few teeth involved. Localized tooth changes in these areas can be minimized if the reactive members of the appliance have sufficient rigidity. In short, load-deflection rate is an indicator of the force required per unit deflection. In the reactive part of the appliance a high load-deflection rate is needed: when the orthodontist is dealing with a relatively rigid member.

Maximal elastic moment. The last characteristic of an orthodontic appliance that must be evaluated is the maximal elastic load or the maximal elastic moment. The maximal elastic load or moment is the greatest force or moment that can be applied to a member without producing permanent deformation. Active and reactive members must be designed so that they will not deform if activations are made that will allow optimal force levels to be reached. In designing an appliance, it is a good idea to go beyond the required force needs and create a factor of safety. Thus permanent deformation or breakage will not occur by accidental overloading, which can be produced by abnormal activation of an appliance or by abnormal forces during mastication.

All three of these important characteristics are found within the elastic range of an orthodontic wire and hence may be termed *spring characteristics*. Beyond this range are the plastic changes that can occur in a wire up to the point of fracture. Although plastic changes are important in the design of an orthodontic appliance, little reference will be made to them in this discussion.

A number of variables are under the control of the designer and influence spring characteristics. These variables will be considered individually in the sections to follow. The reader should keep in mind at all times the relationship between the variables and three important characteristics that have just been discussed.

Manner of loading

If an active member is to deliver continuous force for tooth movement, it must have the ability to absorb and release energy. Energy absorption in a flexible member is produced as a result of elastic deformations that occur during the application of a force or a load. Elastic deformations are changes in form or configuration that are reversible when the load is removed.

To understand the different types of loading and their significance, it is necessary to visualize a structural axis centrally positioned along a round wire (Fig. 4-16). A force acting along this structural axis of the wire may act to produce either *compression* or *tension*, shortening or elongating the wire. Thus in tension and compression the axial load may increase or decrease the length of the structural axis. This change is produced by force acting along the structural axis and hence is termed an axial load. If a moment operates around the structural axis, that is, at right angles to the lines of the structural axis, *torsion* is produced (Fig. 4-17, A). In torsion the wire rotates around the structural axis, with the greatest elastic deformation occurring at the periphery of the wire. *Bending* or *flexure* is produced when the structural axis changes its configuration transversely or at right angles to its original structural axis. Bending can be produced by either moments acting at right angles to the cross section of the wire (Fig. 4-16, B) or a transverse force acting on the wire (Fig. 4-17, C).

The typical member of an orthodontic appliance is usually not loaded in a simple manner. Tension, compression, torsion, and bending are commonly combined into a more complicated type of loading pattern referred to as compound loading. Fig. 4-18, A, shows two vertical loops in a round wire that can be used clinically to move a tooth buccally or lingually by displacing the central section at right angles to the surface of the paper. In reality a compound deformation takes place, with bending occurring at point B and torsion or twisting at A. During activation of this particular member, both bending or torsion occur. Fig. 4-18, B, shows a vertical loop that can be used as a retraction spring. In a loop of this type, if the horizontal arms are kept parallel during activation, the loading pattern is fairly complicated. Not only are horizontal forces required, but two equal and opposite couples must be used to keep the horizontal arms parallel. Even though the loading pattern is somewhat more complicated in this example, the vertical loop is undergoing only bending.

Certain types of loads, be they forces or moments, are capable of producing certain changes in the structural axis of a wire. Compression, tension, torsion, and flexure refer

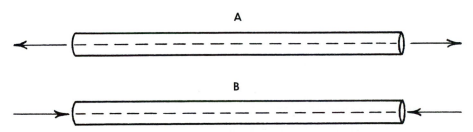

Fig. 4-16 Axial loading. **A,** Tension. **B,** Compression. The force acts along the structural axis (*dotted line*).

to such changes. A more sophisticated way of describing changes in a wire is in terms of the stress distribution throughout the length of the wire. This approach has been avoided, since a knowledge of stress-strain phenomena would be required of the reader. It should be remembered, however, that there are resisting forces acting throughout the wire during loading, resulting in certain internal stresses and strains. Reference will be made to stress and strain only when absolutely necessary to develop a point.

Axial loads producing compression or tension are not useful for spring design, since the load-deflection rate is high. It is commonly observed that an axial pull on a wire will not produce much elastic deformation, even with a heavy force—the reason being that the force is uniformly distributed as stress over each cross section of the wire. On the other hand, when nonuniform stress is distributed over various cross sections of wire (as in torsion and bending) load-deflection rates may be low. For this reason loading that leads to torsion and flexure is useful in the design of the active or flexible members of an appliance.

If the maximal load or maximal torque were maintained as a constant, load-deflection rates would be the lowest in two particular types of loading: (1) torsion; and (2) bending produced by moments alone. The reason such a low load-deflection rate might exist for a given maximal load would be that each cross section of the wire from one end to the other was undergoing the same amount of torsion or bend-

ing. Loading of this type is ideal for spring design, but unfortunately in most instances it is necessary to deliver more than a moment to a tooth. Transverse loads therefore must be introduced, and these do not produce uniform changes along a wire unless the diameter of the wire is not the same at all points along its length: a tapering wire.

In designing an orthodontic appliance, when should we take advantage of tension, compression, torsion, or bending? A number of factors determine the manner of loading that should be used on a given member. First of all, one configuration might be superior to another on the basis of simplicity of design, general space available for it, or comfort in the mouth. Second, the moment/force ratio that would be needed for control of teeth would partly determine the configuration to be used. For example, if equal and opposite moments are required, pure torsion or bending in a wire may be used. On the other hand, if moments and forces are required, most likely bending properties will be used primarily. In considering a reactive member, whenever possible the forces should be distributed as axial loads. For example, a transpalatal lingual arch can better preserve widths of the posterior segments than can a horseshoe lingual, since a horseshoe lingual can bend more easily in this plane of space. Thus one of the early steps in the design of an orthodontic member is to decide on its basic configuration, keeping in mind the objectives listed.

Of the variables that influence the spring characteristics

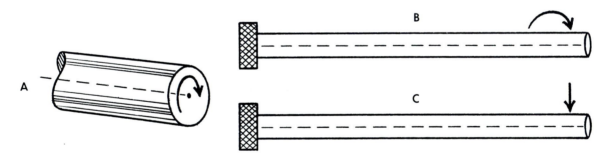

Fig. 4-17   Torsion and bending. **A,** Torsion is produced by a couple acting around the structural axis. **B,** Pure bending is produced by the application of a couple. **C,** Bending is produced by a transverse force.

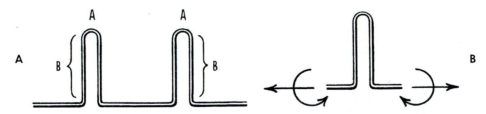

Fig. 4-18   **A,** Displacement of the central portion of the loop at right angles to the page requires a force and a moment. Bending occurs at *B* and torsion at *A*. **B,** Opening of a vertical loop requires both a force and a moment to keep the horizontal arms parallel.

of *load-deflection rate* or *torque-twist rate*, *maximal elastic load* or *maximal elastic torque*, and *moment/force ratio*, only bending will be considered in the sections that follow. Since most orthodontic configurations take advantage of bending as a major type of elastic deformation, many of the concepts (if not the exact formulations) are also applicable to the areas of torsion and axial loading.

Mechanical properties of metals

In describing the mechanical properties of an alloy used in an orthodontic wire, a number of levels are employed. The most superficial is the observational level, on which the clinician operates. On the observational level, forces and deflection can be detected and measured. In other words, a certain amount of force in grams can be applied and the wire will deflect by a certain number of millimeters. On the observational level, the orthodontist is limited as to how much he or she can understand and predict about the nature of appliances.

The second level is the stress-strain level. On this level the orthodontist is dealing with quantities of pounds per square inch and inches per inch: deflection per unit length. These are not values that can be directly measured, but they can be calculated from measurements made on the observational level. Most of the engineering formulations that can be used to predict changes in bodies subject to loads are based on stress-strain phenomena. Finally, at a still more basic level of description is the atomic and molecular level. An understanding of this level further enhances our abilities to predict responses and therefore to design new structures.

Basic behavior of alloys. Fig. 4-19 is a theoretical diagram plotting load against deflection. It might represent, for instance, the load-deflection characteristics of an open coil spring. It can be observed that from *0* to P_{max} (maximal elastic load) on the graph there is a linear relationship between load and deflection. As the force increases, the deflection also increases proportionately. The proportionality is referred to as Hooke's law. Load divided by deflection is a constant through this range and has already been defined as the load-deflection rate. At P_{max} a point is reached where load and deflection are no longer proportionate. Near P_{max}, permanent deformation is being produced in the spring, and the spring will not return to its original shape. P_{max} represents the highest load that can be placed on the spring without permanent deformation—the maximal elastic load. All the behavior found to the left of P_{max} on the graph lies in the elastic range, and behavior to the right lies in the plastic range. Elastic behavior is the ability of a configuration to return to its original shape after unloading; plastic behavior is the occurrence of permanent deformation in a configuration during loading. Finally, at the extreme right of the graph the ultimate load (P_{ult}) is reached, at which point the spring will break. The diagram is a schematic one, and loads and deflections may not be so regular in commonly used orthodontic springs.

Load-deflection diagrams of the type illustrated are limited in application, since a separate diagram would be required for every orthodontic member. However, if the stress-strain level is studied, generalizations can be made about orthodontic alloys that would be applicable for any given alloy, no matter what the configuration might be. Fig. 4-20 is a diagram that plots stress against strain.* A diagram of this type corrects for the dimensions of the wire. The form of the diagram is identical to that of the load-deflection rate diagram, except that the units are different. From *0* to *EL* (elastic limit) a straight line is seen, denoting a linear relationship between stress and strain. This relationship is

---

*Stress in a wire is force per unit area applied to a cross section. Strain is deflection per unit length of the wire.

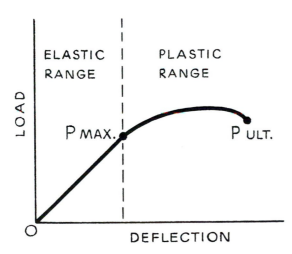

Fig. 4-19   Load deflection. P_{max}, Maximal elastic load; P_{ult}, maximal load before fracture. Note the linear relationship between load and deflection in the elastic range.

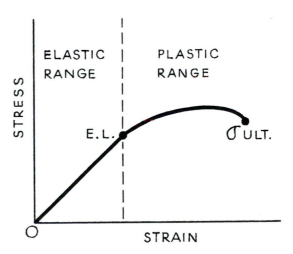

Fig. 4-20   Stress-strain relationship. *EL*, Elastic limit; σ_{ult}, tensile strength. Note the linear relationship between load and deflection in the elastic range.

comparable to the relationship seen on the observational level between load and deflection. The ratio of stress to strain is referred to as the modulus of elasticity (E). As might be expected, it is this mechanical property that determines the load-deflection rate of a spring.[30] The elastic limit (EL) represents the greatest stress that can be applied to the alloy without permanent deformation. It is analogous to the maximal elastic load and is therefore the mechanical property that determines the ability of a member to withstand permanent deformation. A number of other terms describe this general part of the curve, such as yield point, yield strength, and proportional limit; they are close to the elastic limit, although each of them differs by definition. Finally, at the ultimate stress (tensile strength) the wire will fracture. Once again most actual alloys do not present such a regular and definitive type of diagram.

An explanation of elastic and plastic behavior would not be complete without a brief mention of the atomic and molecular events. Fundamentally, elastic behavior involves interatomic bonding. Since atoms are being pulled apart, little wonder that a fairly definite relationship exists between stress and strain. On the other hand, plastic behavior involves displacement along slip planes, which are not atomic in nature but rather are molecular. Plastic behavior therefore is not as linear as elastic behavior.

Elastic limit. The elastic limit (EL) determines the maximal elastic load of a configuration. With respect to only the mechanical properties of the wire, the maximal elastic load varies directly and linearly with the elastic limit. Manufacturers' data will usually include either the yield point or the tensile strength. The yield point is close to the elastic limit, but the tensile strength is higher.

In a given alloy (such as 18-8 stainless steel) a number of factors determine the EL. The amount of work hardening produced during cold drawing of the wire will sharply influence the EL.* Wires that have been considerably cold worked have a hard temper and therefore a high elastic limit. Small round wires may have particularly high elastic limits, since the percentage of reduction by cold working is high. Second, the cold worked outer core becomes proportionately greater in a wire of smaller cross section. Too much work hardening, however, produces a structurally undesirable wire that becomes highly brittle and may fracture during normal use in the mouth. It is far better to have a slightly lower EL, so that an orthodontic member can permanently deform rather than break under accidental loading. Since the work hardening needed to reduce the diameter of a wire increases the EL, the procedure of anodic reduction is a poor method of reducing the size of the wire. Anodic reduction does not cold work a metal, hence a wire is produced that has a lower EL than a work hardened one, which could lead to permanent deformation.

Many orthodontic alloys—Elgiloy and gold—can be

heat treated to raise the EL. This is not true of the most commonly used alloy, 18-8 stainless steel. A stress relief, however, at 850° for 3 or more minutes will raise the apparent EL of 18-8 stainless steel. The mechanism of stress relief is to remove undesirable residual stresses that have been introduced during manufacturing and during fabrication by the orthodontist. The optimal time to relieve stresses in a configuration is after all required bends and twists have been placed in the wire if a single stress relief is used.

Modulus of elasticity. The mechanical property that determines the load-deflection rate of an orthodontic member is the modulus of elasticity (E). Load-deflection varies directly and linearly with E (in torsion, linearly and directly as the modulus of rigidity). Steel has an E approximately 1.8 times as great as that of gold. A reactive member made of stainless steel would be 1.8 times as resistant to deflection as one made of gold. With edgewise brackets and a 0.022 × 0.028 inch archwire, for instance, it is apparent that a steel wire would give greater control over the anchorage unit. On the other hand, activations made in a steel wire for tooth movement, if they were identical to the same ones made in a gold wire of similar configuration, would produce a load-deflection rate almost twice as great. For this reason steel and gold are not directly interchangeable in the design of an orthodontic appliance.[29,30]

The most commonly used alloys for orthodontic wires are of steel. The moduli of elasticity of most steel alloys are almost identical. Unlike the EL, the E is constant for a given alloy. It is not influenced by work hardening or heat treatment.* Thus hard-temper wires do not have higher load-deflection rates than soft-temper wires. When altering the E of a piece of stainless steel, a new alloy must be chosen, for nothing can be done to a steel alloy that will markedly alter its modulus.

Within recent years, two new alloys have been introduced in orthodontics: nickel-titanium and beta-titanium (TMA).

Nitinol was developed by William F. Buehler in the early 1960s. The original alloy contained 55% nickel and 45% titanium, which resulted in a one-to-one stoichiometric ratio of these elements. The most unique feature of this bimetallic (NiTi) compound is its *memory*, which is a result of temperature-induced crystallographic transformations. Andreasen and Hilleman[1] and Andreasen and Morrow[2] have suggested that these shape changes might be used by the orthodontist to apply forces. The shape memory principle is not used clinically. Instead, Nitinol is used for its low force and high springback. Its low modulus of elasticity, only 0.26 that of stainless steel, means that an 0.018 inch Nitinol wire has the approximate stiffness of a 0.013 inch stainless steel wire. The most dramatic characteristic of Nitinol, however, is its resistance to permanent deformation. NiTi wires can be activated over twice the distance that stainless steel can, with minimum permanent deformation;

---

*Orthodontic wires during their manufacture are reduced in size by being drawn through dies in a cold state.

*However, residual stresses or other mechanisms can give an E that is slightly lower after work hardening.[23]

but since permanent deformation is time dependent, additional small deformation will occur between adjustments. After the placement of bends or twists, if the wire is activated in a direction opposite that used in forming the configuration, it will easily deform permanently.[37] Nitinol therefore has its most useful application where low forces and large deflections are needed in relatively straight wires. It is more brittle than stainless steel and cannot be joined by soldering or welding.[1]

A new generation of shape memory alloys has been introduced into orthodontics and is referred to as superelastic.[22,39,40] Unlike Nitinol, these alloys have a much lower transition temperature—either slightly below or slightly higher than mouth temperature. Generally speaking, the austenitic form of these alloys has a slightly higher springback than Nitinol and may be less brittle. Figure 4-21 shows a loading and unloading curve for a superelastic NiTi wire at various activations. At the larger activations, part of the unloading curve is relatively flat. The clinical significance of this finding is that during the deactivation more constant forces are delivered to the teeth. Another interesting finding is that for small activations the stiffness is greater than for large activations. The typical orthodontic wire, however, is different because of a relatively constant load-deflection rate and because it delivers more and more force depending upon the amount of activation. The superelastic NiTi wires are now available in different stiffnesses. A true comparison of stiffness should be made at mouth temperature, since some wires may appear to have lower forces because they are partly martensitic at room temperature. Forces will increase as a phase transformation occurs with mouth temperature.

The superelastic NiTi wires and Nitinol are limited in that they are not easily formed and will lose, by permanent

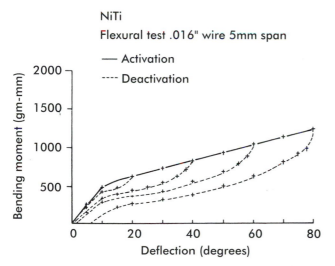

NiTi

Flexural test .016" wire 5mm span

— Activation
---- Deactivation

Fig. 4-21 Activation and deactivation curves for NiTi wire. Unlike the stainless steel and nitinol wires, unloading curves change at different activations. (From Burstone CJ, Qin B, Morton JY: Chinese NiTi wire—a new orthodontic alloy, *Am J Orthod* 87(6):445-452, 1985.)

deformation, bends that are placed, unless a heat treatment process is carried out. The NiTi wires are also reasonably brittle, and are usually applied in procedures that call for relatively straight wires where large deflections without permanent deformation are required.

TMA has a modulus of elasticity intermediate between that of steel and that of Nitinol (approximately 0.4 that of stainless steel).[16,27] It can be deflected up to two times as much as steel without permanent deformation. Unlike Nitinol, TMA is not significantly altered by the placement of bends and twists and has good ductility, equivalent to or slightly better than that of stainless steel. It can be welded without significant reduction in yield strength. Direct welding of finger springs and hooks can be accomplished without solder reinforcement (Fig. 4-22).[11,44]

Ideal orthodontic alloys. The ideal orthodontic wire for an active member is one that gives a high maximal elastic load and a low load-deflection rate. The mechanical properties that determine these characteristics are elastic limit and modulus of elasticity. The ratio between the elastic limit and modulus of elasticity (EL/E) determines the desirability of the alloy. The higher the ratio, the better will be the spring properties of the wire. In the commercial development of new wires the orthodontist should look for alloys that have high ELs and low Es. Small differences in the EL or E will not appreciably alter the ratio. For an alloy to be markedly superior in spring properties, it must possess a significantly higher ratio.

By contrast, in the reactive member of an appliance not only is a sufficiently high elastic limit required but a high modulus of elasticity is also desirable. Since it is common practice to use the same size of slot or tube opening throughout a hookup, it is possible to use different alloys combined in the same appliance so that the needs of both the active and the reactive members can be served.

Four other properties of wire should be mentioned in evaluating an orthodontic wire. (1) The alloy must have a reasonable resistance to corrosion caused by the fluids of the mouth. (2) It should have sufficient ductility so that it will not fracture under accidental loading in the mouth or during fabrication of an appliance. (3) It is desirable to have a wire that can be fabricated in a soft state and later heat-treated to a hard temper. (4) A desirable alloy is one to which attachments can easily be soldered.

A thorough knowledge of the mechanical and physical properties of an alloy is important in the design of an orthodontic appliance. Yet it is but one of the many variables that determine the final form of an orthodontic mechanism.

Wire cross section

A most critical factor in the design of an orthodontic appliance is the cross section of the wire to be used. Small changes in cross section can dramatically influence both the maximal elastic load and the load-deflection rate.[5,9]

The maximal elastic load varies directly as the third power of the diameter of round wire, and the load-deflection rate

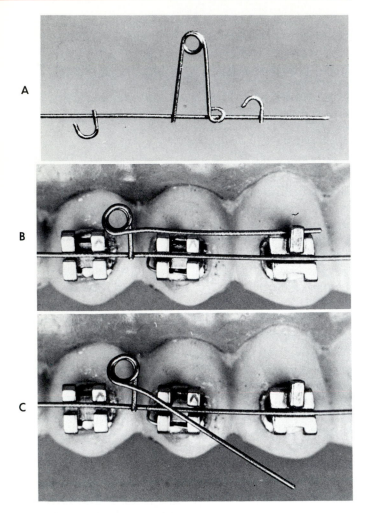

Fig. 4-22 TMA can be directly welded without significant reduction in properties. **A,** Intermaxillary hook, retraction spring, and tieback hook—0.018 inch round on 0.017 × 0.025 inch arch. **B** and **C,** Welded helical spring to erupt a high canine. The canine is now erupted and engaged on the archwire.

varies directly as the fourth power of the diameter. It may seem that the most obvious method of reducing the load-deflection rate of an active member is to cut down the size of the wire. The fallacy in reducing the size of the cross section, however, is that the maximal elastic load is also reduced at an alarmingly high rate (as d^3). In the design of the active member it is good policy to use as small a cross section as possible consistent with a safety factor, so that undue permanent deformation will not occur. Beyond this, any attempt to reduce the size of the cross section to improve spring properties may well lead to undesirable permanent deformation.

The fact that the load-deflection rate varies as the fourth power of the diameter in round wire suggests the critical nature of the selection of a proper cross section. A piece of 0.018 inch wire is not interchangeable with 0.020 inch wire, for with a similar activation (forgetting about play in the bracket) the 0.020 inch wire will deliver almost twice as much force. The dramatic difference between wire sizes can be further demonstrated by comparing two similar activations in a 0.020 inch and a 0.010 inch round wire. The 0.020 inch does not deliver twice as much force but rather 16 times as much force, load-deflection rate varying as the fourth power of the diameter.

In the selection of a proper cross section for the rigid reactive members of an appliance, load-deflection rate rather than maximal elastic load is the prime consideration. Under normal circumstances it is necessary to select a large enough wire cross section beyond the needed maximal elastic load to have sufficient rigidity, so that a sufficiently high load-deflection rate exists.

What is the optimal cross section for a flexible member? Generally for multidirectional activations in which the structural axis is bent in more than one plane, a circular cross section is the one of choice. Furthermore, because of the large amount of round wire that is available for commercial purposes, the mechanical properties of the wire and the cross sectional tolerances are far superior to those of other cross sections. One of the problems of round wire is that, unless it is properly oriented, activations may not operate in the intended plane. Moreover, round wire may rotate in the bracket; and if certain loops are incorporated into the configuration, these can then roll into either the gingiva or the cheek.

Many orthodontic wire configurations, however, undergo unidirectional bending. An edgewise vertical loop used for anterior retraction, for instance, has a structural axis that bends in only one plane. For unidirectional bending, flat wire is the cross section of choice; more energy can be absorbed into a spring made of flat wire than of any other cross section. This principle has been used for years in watch springs and other commercial designs. Hence, flat or ribbon wire can deliver lower load-deflection rates without permanent deformation than can any other type of cross section. Another advantage of flat wire is that the problem of orientation of the wire can be more simply solved than with a round cross section. Flat wire can be definitely anchored into a tube or a bracket so that it will not spin during the deactivation of a given spring. Flat wire can also be used in certain situations when considerable tooth movement is required in one plane, while limited tooth movement is needed in the other. For instance, if continuous ribbon wires were used (long axis oriented occlusogingivally), positive leveling could be produced occlusogingivally over a limited range while buccolingual and labiolingual tooth alignment could be achieved over a long range of action (Fig. 4-23). A configuration of this type is useful when most of the problems are in the horizontal rather than the vertical plane.

With respect to the reactive member, a square or rectangular wire would appear superior to a round one because of the ease of orientation and the greater multidirectional rigidity. This leads to more definite control of the anchorage units. In the edgewise mechanism the assumption may be

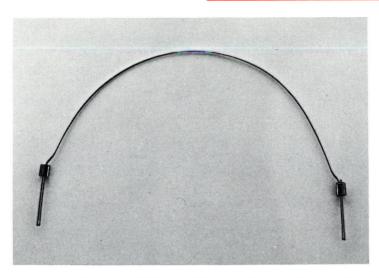

Fig. 4-23   Continuous ribbon arch (0.010 × 0.020 inch). Greater deflections are possible in the horizontal than in the vertical plane.

made that greater rigidity is needed buccolingually or labiolingually than occlusogingivally, since an edgewise wire is employed. This may or may not be the case, depending on how the edgewise mechanism is to be used.

Selection of the proper wire (alloy and cross section)

The selection of proper wire size should be based primarily on the load-deflection rate required in the appliance. Secondarily, of course, it is dependent on the magnitude of the forces and moments required. Many orthodontists will select a cross section of wire on the basis of two other factors, which, although valid, are not as significant. (1) It may be believed that increasingly heavier wires are needed in a replacement technique to eliminate the play between wire and bracket. In an edgewise appliance, however, the ligature wire minimizes a great amount of the play in a first-order direction, since it can fully seat within the brackets. Therefore the clinician does not select an 0.018 inch over a 0.016 inch wire primarily because of the difference in play. (2) A wire also may be selected because it is believed that the smaller the wire the greater will be the amount of maximum elastic deflection possible; in other words, the smaller the wire the more it can be deflected without permanent deformation. This is true, but maximum elastic deflection varies inversely with the diameter of the wire. A 0.016 inch wire would have only 1.15 times as much maximum elastic deflection as an 0.018 inch wire. Therefore the differences would be negligible from a clinical point of view. If the differences were 2:1, as in 0.010 versus 0.020 inch, then, of course, this factor would become clinically significant.

The major reason why the orthodontist should select a particular wire size is the stiffness of the wire or its load-deflection rate. In a replacement technique, for instance, the orthodontist might begin with a 0.014 inch wire that,

deflected over 2 mm, would give the desired force. After the tooth had moved 1 mm, the wire could be replaced with an 0.018 inch, which would give almost the same force with 1 mm of activation.

Small differences in cross section produce large changes in load-deflection rates, since in round wires the load-deflection rate varies as the fourth power of the diameter (Table 4-1). In bending, the stiffness or load-deflection rate is determined by the moment of inertia of the cross section of the wire with respect to the neutral axis. Clinicians are interested in the relative stiffnesses of the wire that they use, but they have neither the time nor the inclination to use engineering formulas to determine these stiffnesses. Therefore a simple numbering system has been developed, based on engineering theory, that gives the relative stiffnesses of wires of different cross sections if the material composition of the wire is the same.[9] The cross-sectional stiffness number (C_s) uses 0.1 mm (0.004 inch) round wire as a base of 1.

A 0.006 inch wire has a C_s of 5.0, which means that for the same activation five times as much force is delivered. Tables 4-2 and 4-3 list, under the C_s column, stiffness numbers based on nominal cross sections. Manufacturing variation in wires or mislabeling of wires obviously can significantly alter the actual C_s number. Two C_s numbers are given for rectangular wires—one for the first-order and one for the second-order direction.

Wire with a cross section of 0.016 inch has a number of 256, which means that for an identical activation it will deliver 256 times as much force as a 0.004 inch round wire. The cross section number of 0.018 × 0.025 inch wire in a first-order direction is 1865. Since 0.016 has a number of 256, an 0.018 × 0.025 inch wire in a first-order direction will deliver 7.3 times as much force for the same activation. We are assuming, for purposes of comparison, that both the

TABLE 4-1

Factors Influencing Load-Deflection Rate, Maximum Load, and Maximum Deflection

Design factor	Load-deflection rate	Maximum load	Maximum deflection
Addition of wire without changing length	Decreases	No change	Increases
Activation in direction of original bending		Increases	Increases
Alteration of cross section to rectangular form	If rate is maintained as constant	Increases as $\dfrac{1}{h}$	Increases as $\dfrac{1}{h}$

Mechanical properties of wire	Varies as E (modulus of elasticity)	Varies as Sp (proportional limit)	Varies as $\dfrac{Sp}{E}$ ↓
Cross section (d)*(round)	d^4	d^3	$\dfrac{1}{d}$
Cross section (b, h)† (rectangular)	bh^3	bh^2	$\dfrac{1}{h}$
Length (L) (cantilever)	$\dfrac{1}{L^3}$	$\dfrac{1}{L}$	L^2

*d, Diameter.
†h, Dimension in the direction of bending; b, direction at right angle to h.

wire configuration and the alloy are identical and that only the cross section varies. To compare any two sections of wire for stiffness involves merely dividing the cross-section stiffness number of one into the other.

Fig. 4-24 shows the cross-section numbers graphically for 0.014-0.018 × 0.025 inch wires. Although the full spectrum of available wire cross sections is not shown, it is apparent that load-deflection rates can vary by factors of 10 or more if different-sized wires of a constant material (e.g., stainless steel) are used.

In the past, wire cross section has been varied to produce different stiffnesses. The overall stiffness of an appliance (S) is determined by two factors; one relates to the wire itself (W_S), and one is the design of the appliance (A_S):

$$S = W_S \times A_S$$

where S is the appliance load-deflection rate, W_S the wire stiffness, and A_S the design stiffness factor.

In general terms

Appliance stiffness = Wire stiffness × Design stiffness

As the appliance design is changed by increasing wire between the brackets or adding loops, the stiffness can be reduced as the design stiffness factor changes; however, the orthodontist is not concerned only with ways by which wire stiffness can be altered. Wire stiffness is determined by two factors—the cross section and the material of the wires:

$$W_s = M_s \times C_s$$

where W_s is the wire stiffness number, M_s the material stiffness number, and C_s the cross sectional stiffness number.

TABLE 4-2

Cross-Sectional Stiffness Numbers (C_s) of Round Wires

Cross section		C_s
(in)	**(mm)**	
0.004	0.102	1.00
0.010	0.254	39.06
0.014	0.356	150.06
0.016	0.406	256.00
0.018	0.457	410.06
0.020	0.508	625.00
0.022	0.559	915.06
0.030	0.762	3164.06
0.036	0.914	6561.00

From Burstone CJ: *Am J Orthod* 80:1, 1981.

In general terms

Wire stiffness = Material stiffness × Cross-sectional stiffness

Wire stiffness is determined by a cross-sectional property (e.g., moment of inertia) and a materials property (the modulus of elasticity).

Previously, since most orthodontists used only stainless steel with almost identical moduli of elasticity, only the size of the wire was varied and no concern was given to the material property, which determines wire stiffness. With the availability of new materials, it is now possible to maintain the same cross section of wire but use different materials with different stiffnesses to produce a wide range of forces and load-deflection rates required for comprehensive orthodontics.

TABLE 4-3
Cross-Sectional Stiffness Numbers (C_s) of Rectangular and Square Wires

| Shape | Cross section | | C_s | |
	(in)	(mm)	1st order	2nd order
Rectangular	0.010 × 0.020	0.254 × 0.508	530.52	132.63
Rectangular	0.016 × 0.022	0.406 × 0.559	1129.79	597.57
Rectangular	0.018 × 0.025	0.457 × 0.635	1865.10	966.87
Rectangular	0.021 × 0.025	0.533 × 0.635	2175.95	1535.35
Rectangular	0.0215 × 0.028	0.546 × 0.711	3129.83	1845.37

| Shape | Cross section | | C_s |
	(in)	(mm)	
Square	0.016 × 0.016	0.406 × 0.406	434.60
Square	0.018 × 0.018	0.457 × 0.457	696.14
Square	0.021 × 0.021	0.533 × 0.533	1289.69

From Burstone CJ: *Am J Orthod* 80:1, 1981.

TABLE 4-4
Material-Stiffness Numbers (M_s) of Orthodontic Alloys and Braided Steel Wires*

	M_s
ALLOYS	
Stainless steel (ss)	1.00
TMA	0.42
Nitinol	0.26
Elgiloy blue	1.19
Elgiloy blue (heat-treated)	1.22
BRAIDS	
Twist-flex	0.18 to 0.20
Force-9	0.14 to 0.16
D-rect	0.04 to 0.08
Respond	0.07 to 0.08

*Based on $E = 25 \times 10^6$ psi.
From Burstone CJ: *Am J Orthod* 80:1, 1981.

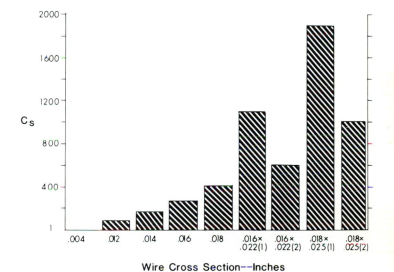

Fig. 4-24 Cross section stiffness numbers (C_s) of orthodontic wires. Forces for any given activation are proportionate to the number. With varying cross sections, stiffnesses can vary as much as 10 or more between wires. (From Burstone CJ: *Am J Orthod* 80:1, 1981.)

Just as it was useful to develop a simple numbering system to describe the relative stiffness of wires based on cross section, so a similar numbering system can be used to compare relative stiffness based on the material. The material stiffness number (M_s) is based on the modulus of the elasticity of the material. Since steel is currently the most commonly used alloy in orthodontics, its M_s number has been arbitrarily set at 1.0. Typical stiffness numbers for other alloys are given in Table 4-4. Although the modulus of elasticity is considered a constant, the history of the wire (particularly that of the drawing process) may have some influence on the modulus. Furthermore, differences in chemistry may make small alterations in the recorded modulus. For practical clinical purposes, however, the material stiffness number (M_s) can be used to determine the relative amount of force that a wire will give per unit activation.

Note that TMA has an M_s number of 0.042, which means that for the same appliance and wire cross section a given activation delivers approximately 0.4 as much force as steel. Elgiloy wires deliver slightly more force than comparable wires of stainless steel, but for all practical purposes this increase is negligible.

In addition to new alloys, braided wires have been introduced in orthodontics. Braids take advantage of smaller cross sections, which have higher maximum elastic deflections, and in the process produce wires that have relatively low stiffnesses. If the reader were to pretend that a braid was a solid wire and if the nominal cross section were used,

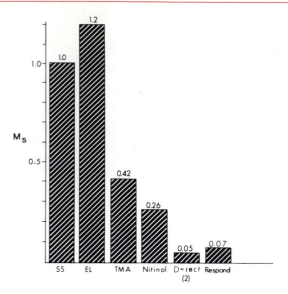

Fig. 4-25 Material stiffness numbers *(M_s)*. Stainless steel has a base number of 1. The numbers for the other alloys and braids denote their stiffness in comparison to stainless steel. With variations in material, a range of stiffness is available equivalent to that with varying cross sections. (From Burstone CJ: *Am J Orthod* 80:1, 1981.)

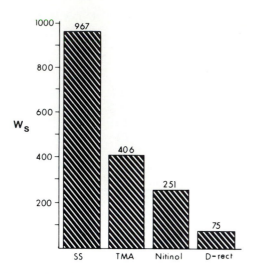

Fig. 4-26 Wire stiffness numbers *(W_s)* of 0.018 × 0.025 inch wires in second-order direction. Forces for the same activations are proportionate to the *(W_s)* numbers. A full range of forces is obtained by using a constant cross section (e.g., 0.018 × 0.025 inch) in different materials. (From Burstone CJ: *Am J Orthod* 80:1, 1981.)

it would be possible to establish an apparent modulus of elasticity. Based on an apparent modulus the material stiffness numbers are given for representative braided wires in Table 4-4. For instance, an 0.018 inch Respond wire braid has an M_S of 0.07 and delivers only 0.07 the force of an 0.018 inch steel wire. The variation in M_S numbers is shown graphically in Fig. 4-25.

The load-deflection rate can be changed by maintaining wire size and varying the load-deflection rate as significantly as by altering the cross section. Maintaining a cross section of 0.018 × 0.025 wire, the wire stiffness (W_S) can be changed by using different materials. To obtain the W_S number it would be necessary to multiply the M_S by the C_S number. For example, in a second-order direction for TMA:

$$W_S = M_S \times C_S$$
$$W_S = 0.42 \times 967$$
$$W_S = 406.1$$

TMA wire with dimensions of 0.018 × 0.025 inch has a stiffness number of 406.1, which is equivalent to an 0.018 round steel wire. Nitinol wire has a stiffness number of 251.4, which is similar to that of 0.016 steel wire. Braided wire with dimensions of 0.018 × 0.025 inch (W_S = 75.4) is similar to 0.012 inch steel wire. A full range of forces can be obtained by varying the material of the wire and keeping the cross section the same (Fig. 4-26). The W_S numbers for 0.018 inch round wires of different materials are shown in Fig. 4-27.

Using the principle of variable cross-section orthodontics, the amount of play between the attachments and the wire

can be varied, depending on the stiffness required. With small low-stiffness wires, excessive play may lead to lack of control over tooth movement. On the other hand, if the principle of variable-modulus orthodontics is employed, the clinician determines the amount of play required before selecting the wire. In some instances more play is needed to allow freedom of movement of brackets along the archwire. In other situations little play is required to allow good orientation and effective third-order movements. Once the desired amount of play has been established, the stiffness of the wire can be produced by using a material with a proper material stiffness. In this way the play between the wire and the attachment is not dictated by the stiffness required but is under the full control of the operator.

The variable-modulus principle allows the orthodontist to use oriented rectangular wires or square wires in light force, as well as heavy force applications and stabilization. A rectangular wire orients in the bracket and hence offers greater control in delivering the desired force system; it is easier to bend, since the orientation of the wire can be carefully checked. More important, when placed in the brackets, the wire will not turn or twist to allow the forces to be dissipated in improper directions.

Wire length

The length of a member may influence the maximal elastic load and the load-deflection in a number of ways, depending on the configuration and loading of the spring. The cantilever has been chosen to demonstrate the effect of length, since the cantilever principle is widely used in orthodontic mech-

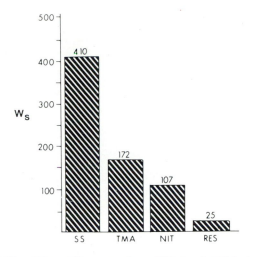

Fig. 4-27 Wire stiffness numbers (W_s) for 0.018 inch round wires. Figs. 4-26 and 4-27 show wide stiffness ranges when the occlusogingival wire dimension is kept constant at 0.018 inch. (From Burstone CJ: *Am J Orthod* 80:1, 1981.)

anisms. A finger spring may be visualized for the following discussion.

Fig. 4-28 shows a cantilever attached at *B* with a vertical force applied at *A*. The distance *L* represents the length of the cantilever measured parallel to its structural axis. In this type of loading the load-deflection rate will vary inversely as the third power of the length; in other words, the longer the cantilever the lower the load-deflection rate. The maximal elastic load varies inversely as the length of the cantilever. Once again, the longer the cantilever the lower the maximal elastic load.

Increasing the length of the cantilever is a better way to reduce the load-deflection rate than is reducing the cross section. Increasing the length of the cantilever markedly reduces the load-deflection rate; yet the maximal elastic load is not radically altered, since it varies linearly with the length. Adding length within the practical confines of the oral cavity is an excellent way of improving spring properties.

Another way of loading the cantilever is shown in Fig. 4-28, this time by means of a couple or moment applied to the free end. Loading of this type is shown in Fig. 4-29. With a couple applied at the free end, the moment-deflection rate varies inversely as the second power of the length. Quite interestingly, the maximal elastic moment is not affected by changes in length at all. If the length is doubled or tripled, the maximal elastic moment is still the same. This is a most desirable type of loading, since additional length can reduce the moment-deflection rate and since there is no reduction in the maximal elastic moment. However, the principle can be applied only if moments alone are required for a given tooth movement.

Increasing the length of a wire with vertical loops is one of the more effective means of reducing load-deflection rates for flexible members and, at the same time, only minimally altering their maximal elastic loads. However, there are limitations in how much the length can be increased. The distance between brackets in a continuous arch is predetermined by tooth and bracket width. Vertical segments in the wire are limited by occlusion and the extension of the mucobuccal fold. An application demonstrating how added length in a wire achieves more constant force delivery without radically sacrificing maximal elastic load is seen in the use of a 0.021 × 0.025 inch depressive base arch (Fig. 4-30). The base arch is used to depress maxillary anterior teeth and erupt posterior teeth in the correction of deep overbite.[6,7,8] The long distance from an auxiliary tube on the buccal stabilizing segment to the midline of the incisor is responsible for a more constantly delivered depressive force on the anterior teeth.

Amount of wire

Additional length of wire may be incorporated in the form of loops or helices or some other configuration. This tends

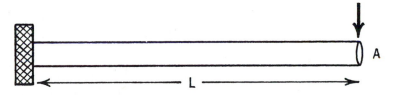

Fig. 4-28   Cantilever with load applied at the free end, *A*.

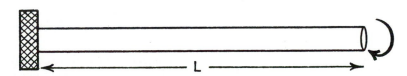

Fig. 4-29   Cantilever with an applied couple. The effect is uniform bending along the wire.

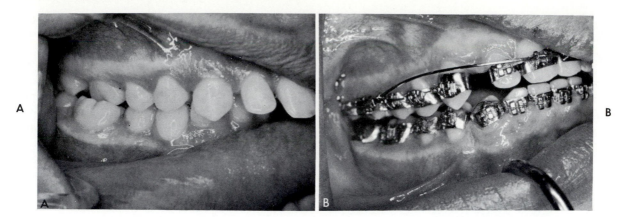

Fig. 4-30 Base arch used for depression. **A,** Before treatment. **B,** After depression of the incisors. The long arm delivers a relatively constant force.

to lower the load-deflection rate and increase the range of action of the flexible member. The maximal elastic load may or may not be affected.

When a member is designed that incorporates additional wire, it is necessary to locate properly the parts of the configuration where additional wire should be placed and to determine the form that the additional wire should take. If location and formation are properly done, it should be possible to lower the load-deflection rate without altering the maximal elastic load merely by adding the least amount of wire that will achieve these ends.

Let us consider the problem of the cantilever as related to the placement of the additional wire. In Fig. 4-31 a cantilever is shown with a vertical force of 100 g at the free end. Along the length of the wire, imaginary vertical sections can be cut and at each of these sections a bending moment can be calculated. The bending moment is found by multiplying the load at the end of the cantilever by the perpendicular distance to the section in question. Thus it is that the bending moment at the point of force application at the free end of the wire is zero. One millimeter closer to the point of support, it is 100 gram-millimeters (g·mm). Two millimeters closer, it is 200 g·mm. Finally at the point of support the bending moment is 1000 g·mm. The bending moment represents an internal moment resisting the 100 g force applied at the free end of the cantilever. The significance of the bending moment is that the amount of bending at each cross section of the wire is directly proportionate to the magnitude of the bending moment; in other words, the greater the bending moment at any particular cross section the more the wire is going to bend at that point along the wire.

The optimal place for additional wire is at cross sections where the bending moment is the largest. In the case of the cantilever the position for additional wire would be at the point of support, since here the bending moment is the greatest: 1000 g·mm. Helical coils can be used to reduce

the load-deflection rate. Fig. 4-32 illustrates the proper positioning of a helical coil for this purpose. The load-deflection rate is maximally lowered for the given amount of wire used if the helix is placed at the point of support rather than anywhere else along the wire.

The placement of additional coils at the point of support in a cantilever does not alter the maximal elastic load. A straight wire of a given length and a wire with numerous coils at the point of support have identical maximal elastic loads, provided they have the same lengths measured from the force to the point of support. This should not be surprising since the maximal elastic load is a function of this length of the configuration rather than the amount of wire incorporated in it. It is also true of many other configurations: load-deflection rate can be lowered without altering the maximal elastic load if additional wire is properly incorporated. From the point of view of design, this is important because, for the first time, we have discussed a method of lowering the load-deflection rate without subsequently reducing the maximal elastic load.

To achieve this objective with the minimal amount of wire, the optimal placement of additional wire is at cross sections where the bending moment is the greatest. A practical way of deciding where these parts of a wire might be is to activate a configuration and see where most of the bending or torsion occurs. These are the sections where the bending moments or torsional moments are the greatest: the cross sections of the wire that have the greatest stress. The configuration of the additional wire should be such that maximal advantage can be taken of the bending and torsional properties of the wire. In short it is not the amount of wire used that is important in achieving a desirably flexible member, but rather it is the placement of the additional wire and its form.

Although additional wire is quite helpful in the design of flexible members for an orthodontic appliance, it should be avoided in the reactive or rigid members. Loops and other

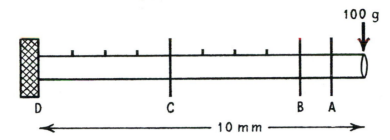

Fig. 4-31   Cantilever with load applied at the free end. *A, B,* and *C,* Imaginary perpendicular sections; *D,* point of support.

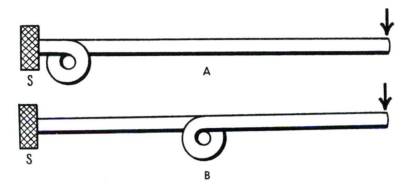

Fig. 4-32   Placement of a helical coil in a cantilever. **A,** Correct. **B,** Incorrect. *S,* Point of support.

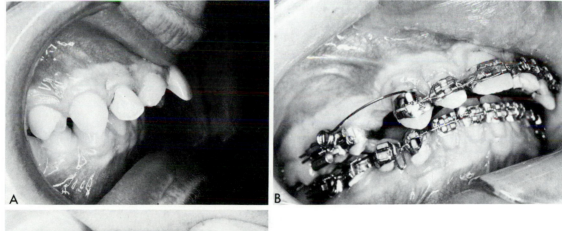

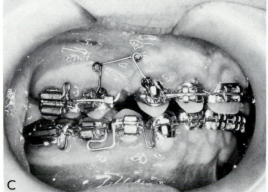

Fig. 4-33   Class II, division 1, therapy. **A,** Before treatment. **B,** During deep overbite correction. Note the helices, which lower the load-deflection rate on an 0.018 × 0.022 inch intrusive arch. **C,** During en masse anterior retraction. Forces and moments are delivered so that the anterior segments will be tipped around a center of rotation at the incisor apices.

types of configurations decrease the rigidity of the wire and hence may be responsible for some loss of control over the anchor units.

An anterior retraction spring is seen in Fig. 4-33. It should be noticed that additional wire has been placed in the four corners, where the stresses are high during bending.

Stress raisers

From a theoretical point of view, the force or stress required to permanently deform a given wire can be calculated; however, in many instances the wire will deform at values much lower than the predicted ones because the presence of certain local stress raisers increase the stress values in a wire far beyond what might be predictable by commonly used engineering formulas.

Two common stress raisers are sudden changes in cross section and sharp bends.

Any *nick* in a wire will tend to raise the stress at that cross section and hence may be responsible for permanent deformation or fracture at this point. It is therefore desirable to mark wires by other means than a file, particularly the wires of small cross section used in the flexible member of an appliance.

A *sharp bend* in a wire also may result in higher stresses than those that might be predicted for a given cross section of wire. A sudden sharp bend will far more easily deform than a more rounded or gradual bend. Unfortunately, with a continuous archwire, the orthodontist is somewhat limited in space between brackets and many times is required to make sharp bends because of this limitation. Flexible members should be designed with gradual bends so that they will be more free from permanent deformation than comparable ones with sharp or sudden bends.

For example, three vertical loops might be compared: a squashed one, a plain one, and one with a helical coil (Fig. 4-34). In terms of permanent deformation, the poorest design would be loop *A*, which, because of its squashed state, has a very sharp bend at its apex. The plain vertical loop *(B)* would be slightly superior, since the bending is more gradual. Nevertheless, a fairly sharp bend occurs at its apex. The configuration with the most gradual bending is the loop with a helical coil *(C)*. Not only would the helical coil enhance the flexible properties of the spring because of its

additional wire, but the lack of sharp bends would further increase its range of action without permanent deformation. Proper direction of activation will be discussed later.

Sections of maximal stress

There are certain sections along a wire where stresses are maximal. These may be called critical sections. It has already been seen that in sections where the bending moments are the largest, areas of high stress exist. These critical sections are important from the point of view of design, for it is here that permanent deformation is most likely to occur.

A number of precautions should be observed at a critical section. *First,* stress raisers should be avoided in these sections at all costs. A nick in a wire, for instance, might not be so disastrous where the stresses are low but might well lead to deformation or fracture where the stress level is high. *Second,* the elastic limit of the wire should be carefully watched at a critical section. Operations such as soldering might overheat the wire and thus reduce its elastic limit. Lowering the elastic limit at another place in the wire where the stresses are low might not be too undesirable but could be responsible for failure at a critical section. Therefore, in high stress areas it is desirable to use other means of attaching an auxiliary than soldering, or if soldering is to be used as the method of attachment it should be done with considerable care.

An example of permanent deformation or fracture produced by a sudden change in cross section and by a lowering of the elastic limit can be seen in the facebow in Fig. 4-35.[4,32] A stress point is found at the juncture of the solder and the outer bow *(A)* and secondarily at the juncture of the solder and the inner bow *(B)*. At *A* the wire may be structurally weak for two reasons: the existence of a stress point associated with the sudden change of cross section, and a lowering of the elastic limit because of the soldering operation. *A* also happens to be a critical section where the stresses are quite high, and for that reason it is a predictable area of fracture in a facebow of this design.

If the orthodontist is in doubt about which parts of an appliance will have critical sections, the appliance can be activated in a typical manner and the parts that exhibit the most bending or torsion noted. These will be found to have high stresses along their cross sections. There are three rules

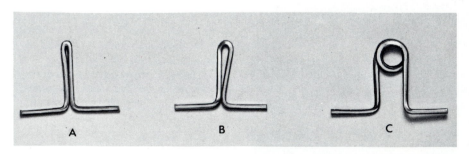

Fig. 4-34 Vertical loops. **A,** Squashed loop. **B,** Plain loop. **C,** Loop with a helical coil.

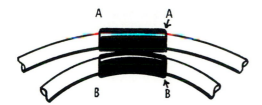

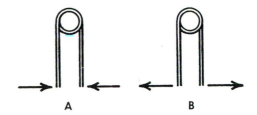

Fig. 4-35 Facebow: the anterior portion of an inner and an outer bow. *A,* There is a stress point at the juncture of the solder and the outer bow. *B,* Another stress point is found at the juncture of the solder and the inner bow.

Fig. 4-36 Activation of a loop with a helical coil. **A,** Correct. **B,** Incorrect.

to be kept in mind as far as design of critical sections: (1) all stress raisers should be eliminated as completely as possible; (2) a larger cross section can be used to strengthen this part of the appliance; and (3) the appliance may be so designed that it will elastically rather than permanently deform under normal loading. Many times a highly flexible member will be more serviceable than a rigid one, because the flexible member can deflect out of the way of the oncoming load. A light flexible spring can withstand occlusal trauma far better than can a more rigidly constructed spring, since it has the ability to displace elastically away from an occlusal force. Because the wings of airplanes are flexible, they are less apt to fracture under normal flying conditions. In a similar manner, increasing the flexibility of a member may be a way of preserving the integrity of the appliance.

Direction of loading

Not only is the manner of loading important, but the direction in which a member is loaded can markedly influence its elastic properties. If a straight piece of wire is bent so that permanent deformation occurs and an attempt is made to increase the magnitude of the bend, bending in the same direction as had originally been done, the wire is more resistant to permanent deformation than if an attempt had been made to bend in the opposite direction. The wire is more resistant to permanent deformation because certain residual stresses remain in it after the placement of the first bend. A flexible member will not deform as easily if it is activated in the same direction as the original bends were made to form the configuration. If a bend is made in an orthodontic appliance, the maximal elastic load will not be the same in all directions. It will be greatest in the direction that is identical to the original direction of bending or twisting. The phenomenon responsible for this differnce is referred to as the Bauschinger effect.

Fig. 4-36 demonstrates a vertical loop with a coil at the apex and a number of turns in the coil under different directions of loading. The loading in *A* tends to wind the coil, increasing the number of turns in the helix and shortening the length. The type of loading seen in *B* tends to unwind the helix, reducing the number of coils and lengthening the

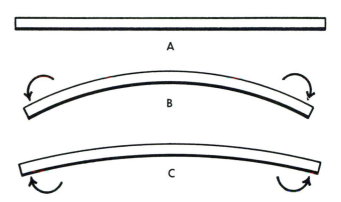

Fig. 4-37 Placing a reverse curve of Spee in a lower arch. **A,** Original straight wire. **B,** Wire overbent. **C,** Final configuration. Note that the last bends are in the same direction as the activation in the mouth.

spring. The loading in Fig. 4-36, *A,* tends to activate the spring in the same direction as it was originally wound and hence is the correct method of activation. In many configurations in which residual stresses are high: a vertical loop employing a number of coils at the apex, the range of action can vary 100% or more between correct and incorrect loading. Obviously this is a much more significant factor in design than are small differences in the mechanical properties of the wire.

The same principles can be applied to less complicated configurations such as in a continuous archwire. The operator should be sure that the last bend made in an archwire is in the same direction as the bending produced during its activation. For example, if a reverse curve of Spee is to be placed in an archwire, the curve should be first overbent and then partly removed. Only then will the activation of the archwire be in the same direction as the last bend (Fig. 4-37). The same is true of a series of tip-back bends. The tip-back bend should be increased beyond the amount required and then some of it removed. The bending that occurs during the activation of the tip-back bend when it is placed in the brackets will then be in the same direction as the last bend.

Attachment

If forces and moments are to be delivered to a tooth, it is necessary to have some means of attachment. If forces alone were sufficient without the use of moments, the attachment could be relatively simple; however, this is not usually the case. Most orthodontic movements require both moments and forces. Moments and forces can be produced if a noncircular wire is oriented in a noncircular bracket. The edgewise bracket and tube are excellent examples of the use of a noncircular cross section for both wire and attachment. It is possible, however, by means of loops to obtain such orientation of round wire, that moments and forces can be delivered.

What are the optimal dimensions for a bracket or a tube? No definitive answer to this question is available, unless the objectives and design of an orthodontic appliance are fully specified. However, some of the factors in making this decision can be discussed.

The starting point in the design of a bracket is to determine bracket width (mesiodistal dimension). From a theoretical viewpoint, a system of forces and moments could be produced regardless of what the mesiodistal width of the brackets might be. Width, however, does become important for two reasons. *First,* wider brackets minimize the amount of play between the archwire and the attachments. A certain amount of leeway must exist between the archwire and the bracket; otherwise it would be impossible to get easy bracket engagement. However, if a bracket is too narrow, considerable play can occur in all planes between wire and bracket. If the bracket is wider, the archwire has a much more positive purchase. *Second,* the greater the distance between the brackets, the lower will be the load-deflection rate. Since at least part of the movement required to treat a patient is produced by adjustments between brackets, it would seem desirable that the distance between attachments be as large as possible. One of the problems of the continuous arch is the sharp limitation of space between brackets, no matter how narrow they might be made. The decision as to proper bracket width lies between two extremes. At one end a bracket might be as wide as the tooth. In this instance, however, the interbracket distance would not be enough to produce sufficient flexibility for adjustment. A knife edge bracket might be at the other end, which would offer the greatest interbracket distance and hence the most desirable load-deflection rates. With a knife edge bracket, however, it would be impossible to deliver the necessary moments, as well as forces, to give full control over tooth movement.[3] Generally speaking, the ideal bracket width is one that is as narrow as possible and is still capable of obtaining positive purchase on an archwire so that moments can be delivered to teeth.

Optimal occlusogingival slot dimensions are determined by the maximal elastic loads required from the active members and the reactive members. A safe rule would be to design on the basis of the reactive members, assuring that the bracket and tube slots were sufficiently large for rigid control of anchor units. It would be a mistake to design primarily on the basis of the active members, which may lead to using slots that were relatively too small to control the anchor teeth or to withstand the forces of mastication.

A vexing problem in orthodontic treatment is that the appliance requirements change between stages of treatment. Teeth that at one time are actively being moved may later become reactive units. For convenience the same dimensions are used in all slots throughout the arch in the typical strap-up. Yet the active and reactive requirements are not the same throughout the arch. One objective in the design of an appliance is the assuring of a positive fit between different cross sections of wire, depending on the needs of the case. An edgewise bracket can become adjustable in a buccolingual or labiolingual direction by means of a ligature tie but is not adjustable occlusogingivally. Thus no definite answer is evident to the question of optimal occlusogingival slot dimension. The decision rests on many factors, including the general concept of treatment and the basic design of an orthodontic appliance.

Forces from a continuous arch

A multibanded appliance, such as that used in edgewise mechanics, produces a complicated set of forces and moments. For instance, a straight or ideal arch placed between irregular brackets on malaligned teeth may deliver both desirable and undesirable forces. An analysis of two-tooth segments (two teeth connected by a straight wire) can demonstrate some of the problems encountered when adjacent brackets are connected by a continuous wire or arch.*

The force system produced in a two-tooth segment is determined by the angle of the bracket (Θ_A and Θ_B) with respect to the straight wire and the interbracket distance (Fig. 4-38). Based on the ratio Θ_A / Θ_B, six classes of force systems can be described (Fig. 4-39). The force system for each class is given in Table 4-5. Note that the ratio of the moments at bracket *A* with respect to bracket *B* is constant for each class. Lines *2* and *3* of Table 4-5 give the force systems acting on the wire; line *4* reverses the direction, showing the forces acting on the teeth. It is apparent that forces and moments as well as their ratios may not be correct

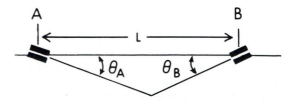

Fig. 4-38 The geometry of the wire to an edgewise bracket is defined by the interbracket distance. *L,* from the angles of the brackets with respect to the interbracket axis. (From Burstone CJ, Koenig HA: *Am J Orthod* 65:270, 1974.)

*References 12, 17, 19, 33, 34, 47, 57.

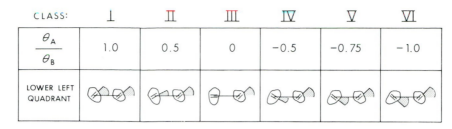

Fig. 4-39 The six basic geometries based on the ratio Θ_A/Θ_B. Classes are independent of interbracket distance. Position *A* is the canine; position *B*, the premolar.

TABLE 4-5

Force Systems by Class

Class	I	II	III	IV	V	VI
$\dfrac{\theta_A}{\theta_B}$	1.0	0.5	0	−0.5	−0.75	−1.0
$\dfrac{M_A}{M_B}$	1.0	0.8	0.5	0	−0.4	−1.0
Force system on wire at yield	531.4 ↑↓ 531.4	477.4 ↑↓ 477.4	398.0 ↑↓ 398.0	265.7 ↑↓ 265.7	160.0 ↑↓ 160.0	
L = 7 mm	1860 ⊆⊆ 1860	1488 ⊆⊆ 1860	930 ⊆⊆ 1860	⊆ 1860	740 ⊇⊆ 1860	1860 ⊇⊆ 1860
Force system on wire at yield	177.0 ↑↓ 177.0	160.0 ↑↓ 160.0	133.0 ↑↓ 133.0	88.6 ↑↓ 88.6	53.3 ↑↓ 53.3	
L = 21 mm	1860 ⊆⊆ 1860	1488 ⊆⊆ 1860	930 ⊆⊆ 1860	⊆ 1860	740 ⊇⊆ 1860	1860 ⊇⊆ 1860
Force system on teeth at yield	531.4 ↑↓ 531.4	477.4 ↑↓ 477.4	398.0 ↑↓ 398.0	265.7 ↑↓ 265.7	160.0 ↑↓ 160.0	
L = 7 mm	1860 ⊇⊇ 1860	1488 ⊇⊇ 1860	930 ⊇⊇ 1860	⊇ 1860	740 ⊆⊇ 1860	1860 ⊆⊇ 1860

From Burstone CJ, Koenig HA: *Am J Orthod* 65:270, 1974.

to produce the desired changes in a malocclusion without side effects.

For example, a Class I geometry is seen in Fig. 4-40, *A*, in which the second premolar is supererupted in relation to the first molar. A straight wire placed on the premolar produces a desirable intrusive force; unfortunately, the moment produced is undesirable, displacing the root mesially. This can be avoided by using a noncontinuous configuration, the rectangular loop. Fig. 4-40, *B*, shows the force system from the rectangular loop, which can be designed to give a single force only on the canine. The equilibrium theory dictates that the moment acting on the buccal segments will be greater than with the continuous arch; therefore greater care is needed with the control of anchorage of the posterior teeth. Fig. 4-41 shows a rectangular loop that is being used to rotate and extrude a premolar. Rectangular loops and other loop designs offer the potential of delivering desired

force systems with minimum side effects, a capability not usually possible with the continuous arch.[6,7] Loops are not used only to lower forces; they change the entire force system.

Principles of spring design

An understanding of the relationships between bioengineering parameters and force systems can offer a rational basis for the design of orthodontic appliances. To achieve an optimum force system, not only must the force magnitude be correct, but the force must be delivered constantly and the required moment/force ratio must be produced to control the center of rotation. In this section all of these factors together will be considered, using the example of an anterior or canine retraction spring.[6,7,10,18]

A canine that requires a translation or bodily movement needs a force applied through its center of resistance (Fig.

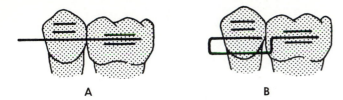

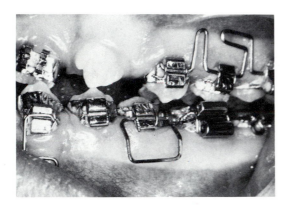

Fig. 4-40 **A,** A straight wire (ideal arch) between the first molar and the premolar produces an undesirable positive movement, displacing the root mesially. **B,** A rectangular loop used for the same bracket malalignment shown in *A* produces no side effects on the bicuspid since only an intrusive force is delivered.

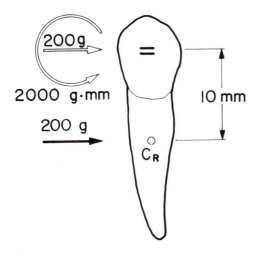

Fig. 4-41 A rectangular loop used to rotate and extrude a premolar. No side effects are produced on the premolar.

Fig. 4-42 A force acting at the center of resistance *(C_R)* of a tooth will translate the tooth. A couple (moment) and a force *(white arrows)* acting at the bracket can produce the same effect. Note that the magnitude of the moment is equal to the force multiplied by the distance from bracket to center of resistance. (From Burstone CJ, Koenig HA: *Am J Orthod* 70:1, 1976.)

4-42). If the force is 200 g, 200 g must be delivered at the bracket and a moment of 2000 g·mm (provided the distance between the bracket and the center of resistance is 10 mm). In other words, a 10:1 moment/force ratio (M/F) would be produced. If a simple vertical loop is used for space closure, a moment encouraging the root to move distally will be produced during activation. For a loop 6 mm long, typically the M/F is low, approximately 2.2:1.[18] This M/F is too low to control the root and prevent it from being displaced mesially. To increase the M/F during activation, a number of strategies can be employed. The loop can be made as long as possible in an apical direction. By increasing the length of the loop to 11 mm, the M/F will be approximately doubled. However, limitations exist as to how far apically a loop can be placed before irritation is produced in the mucobuccal fold. Another strategy is to increase the amount of wire found gingivally at the top of the loop. Fig. 4-43 shows that by increasing the gingival amount of wire (dimension *G*) the M/F is increased and the load-deflection rate is reduced. One of the advantages of the T-loop design over a simple vertical loop is that there is a much higher M/F controlling the root and a low load-deflection rate, thereby giving greater force constancy.[10,38]

The moment produced by a retraction spring during activation is called the *activation moment* and is dependent on the change in angle that the horizontal arms of the spring make with the bracket when a loop is pulled apart. Even if the design is improved by the use of a configuration like a T-loop, the M/F may not be high enough for translation. To effect a higher moment/force ratio, it is necessary to put an angulation or a gable-type bend in the spring. The moment produced by gabling is referred to as the *residual moment*. Ideally a retraction spring should deliver a relatively constant M/F. If the ratio is changing every time the tooth moves, the tooth will not have a constant center of rotation. Three principles to remember in obtaining a constant M/F are (1) to use as high an activation moment and as low a residual moment as possible; (2) to place the spring off center toward the tooth that requires the greatest M/F constancy; and (3) to lower the force-deflection and moment-deflection rates.

Fig. 4-44 shows a retraction mechanism that is used to retract all six anterior teeth en masse.[11] The anterior segment is undergoing controlled tipping, with a center of rotation approaching the apices of the incisors; the posterior teeth, if they come forward at all, will translate or have roots displaced forward ahead of the crowns. The spring is a composite using an 0.018 inch round TMA wire welded to a 0.017 × 0.025 inch base arch (Fig. 4-45).

The load-deflection rate of the spring is relatively low, averaging under 35 g/mm (Fig. 4-46). This load-deflection rate assures a relatively constant force: as the tooth moves 1 mm, there is a dropoff of only 35 g or so in the force magnitude. Typically the spring would be activated 6 mm, producing 201 g of force (Fig. 4-47). Of particular interest is the change in moment/force ratio between the anterior

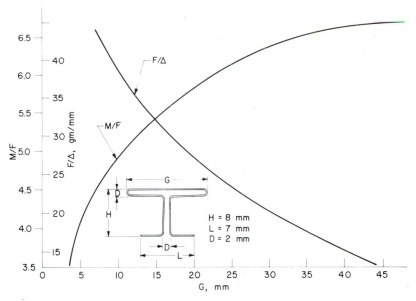

Fig. 4-43   As the gingival horizontal length increases, the M/F increases and the F/δ continues to decrease. (From Burstone CJ, Koenig HA: *Am J Orthod* 70:1, 1976.)

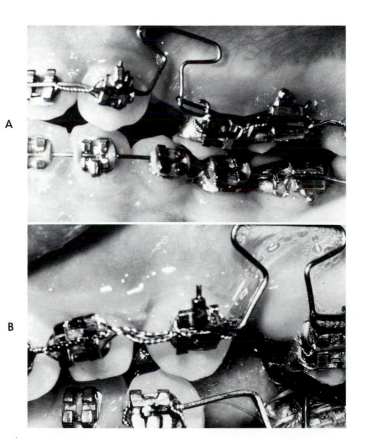

Fig. 4-44   En masse retraction. **A**, *A*, 0.021 × 0.025 inch anterior segment is in place for true segmental space closure with a 0.017 × 0.025 inch TMA attraction spring. **B**, Low-stiffness multistrand wire in the anterior segment allowed the canine to be retracted so additional space could be gained for anterior alignment. After alignment a rigid anterior segment was placed.

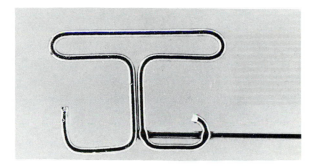

Fig. 4-45   The composite TMA 0.018-0.017 × 0.025 inch retraction spring. An 0.018 inch round T spring is welded directly to a 0.017 × 0.025 inch base arch. (From Burstone CJ: *Am J Orthod* 82:361, 1982.)

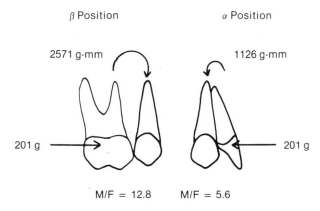

Fig. 4-46   Force systems produced at 6 mm by activation of an 0.018-0.017 × 0.025 inch anterior retraction spring. Note the differential M/F between the anterior segment (α position) and the posterior segment (β position). A large moment at the β position is instrumental in anchorage control. (From Burstone CJ: *Am J Orthod* 82:361, 1982).

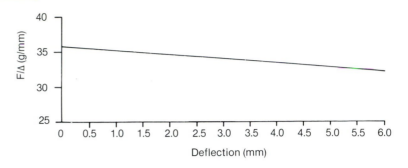

Fig. 4-47 The load-deflection rate for an 0.018-0.017 × 0.025 inch composite retraction spring is low and relatively constant. At full activation it is lowest. (From Burstone CJ: *Am J Orthod* 82:361, 1982.)

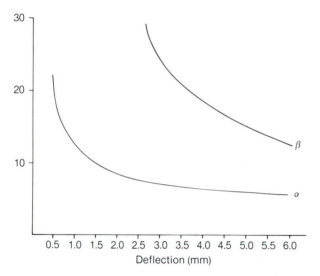

Fig. 4-48 Differential M/F ratios in an 0.018-0.017 × 0.025 inch retraction spring between the α and β positions. As the spring is deactivated, a tip-back effect is placed on the posterior teeth. (From Burstone CJ: *Am J Orthod* 82:361, 1982.)

and posterior teeth (Fig. 4-48). At 6 mm of activation the M/F on the anterior segment (α moment) is 5.6. Over a range of 3.5 mm, the ratio does change a little, which implies a relatively constant center of rotation for the anterior segment. On the other hand, the M/F in the posterior segment (β moment) starts at 12.8 mm and rapidly increases during space closure. This rapid increase has the effect of tipping back the posterior segments during space closure to enhance anchorage further.

A spring of this type is relatively forgiving of mistakes in shape and activation as used by the orthodontist. It should be remembered that an error of 1 mm in activation is an error of only 35 g. Since the residual moment is small, and is produced by a large angular activation, a small error in the angulation or gabling is also relatively insignificant.

Discussion

The design of an orthodontic appliance depends on thorough understanding of both biological and physical variables. It is an area wherein concepts of both biology and physics can be wedded into a true biomechanical discipline.

Although it is not our purpose to attempt a cookbook recipe for appliance design, the merit is in pointing out the steps that may go into the design of an orthodontic appliance.

1. The designer must make certain assumptions about the nature of forces and tooth movement. Objectives relative to tooth movement must be biologically sound, recognizing not only the tissue changes around the tooth but also the generalized growth changes in the face. The biologic objectives of treatment must come first, for without them there is no basis for appliance design.

2. A basic configuration must be selected, depending on the limitations of space in the oral cavity. In part, it will be determined by patient hygiene and comfort. Most important, it must be capable of delivering the required force system. It should possess a desirable maximal elastic load and load-deflection rate, and it must deliver the needed moment/force ratio. The members should be analyzed so stress distribution at critical sections will not result in failure.

3. Once the general configuration has been established, its dimensions may be determined. Length is established consistent with patient comfort and oral hygiene.

4. When the dimensions of a member are known, it is possible to choose the type of material out of which it is to be made. At this time the choice is made as to the alloy.[35]

5. Finally, the cross section of the wire is determined.

This is not to suggest that appliances can always be designed by following the same logical sequence. The many variables in appliance design are related and cannot be separated. Furthermore, it is not suggested that all that is needed in designing an appliance is a group of engineering formulas. Background in the physical sciences can help in the design of appliances, but appliance development still takes a certain amount of intuition, as well as clinical and laboratory experimentation. Basic science, rather than trial and error, offers the greatest possibilities in the development of the orthodontic appliance of the future.

REFERENCES

1. Andreasen GF, Hilleman TB: An evaluation of 55 cobalt substituted Nitinol wire for use in orthodontics, *J Am Dent Assoc* 82:1373, 1971.
2. Andreasen GF, Morrow RE: Laboratory and clinical analyses of Nitinol wire, *Am J Orthod* 73:142, 1978.
3. Andreasen GF, Quevedo FR: Evaluation of friction forces in the 0.022 × 0.028 edgewise bracket in vitro, *J Biomech* 3:151, 1970.
4. Baldini JC, Haack DC, Weinstein S: The manipulation of lateral forces produced by extraoral appliances, *Angle Orthod* 51:301, 1981.
5. Burstone CJ: The application of continuous forces to orthodontics, *Angle Orthod* 31:1, 1961.
6. Burstone CJ: The rationale of the segmented arch, *Am J Orthod* 11:805, 1962.
7. Burstone CJ: Mechanics of the segmented arch technique, *Angle Orthod* 36:99, 1966.
8. Burstone CJ: Deep overbite correction by intrusion, *Am J Orthod* 72:1, 1977.
9. Burstone CJ: Variable-modulus orthodontics, *Am J Orthod* 80:1, 1981.
10. Burstone CJ: The segmented arch approach to space closure, *Am J Orthod* 82:361, 1982.
11. Burstone CJ: Welding of TMA wire clinical applications, *J Clin Orthod* 21(9):609-615, 1987.
12. Burstone CJ: Precision lingual arches-active applications. *J Clin Orthod* 23(2):101-109, 1989.
13. Burstone CJ: *Biomechanical rationale for orthodontic therapy.* In Melsen B, editor: *Controversies in orthodontics,* 1991, Quintessence, pp 131-146.
14. Burstone CJ, Every TW, Pryputniewicz RJ: Holographic measurement of incisor extrusion, *Am J Orthod* 82:1, 1982.
15. Burstone CJ, Goldberg AJ: Maximum forces and deflections from orthodontic appliances, *Amer J Orthod* 84(2):95-103, 1983.
16. Burstone CJ, Goldberg J: Beta titanium: a new orthodontic alloy, *Am J Orthod* 7:2, 1980.
17. Burstone CJ, Koenig HA: Force systems from an ideal arch, *Am J Orthod* 65:270, 1974.
18. Burstone CJ, Koenig HA: Optimizing anterior and canine retraction, *Am J Orthod* 70:1, 1976.
19. Burstone CJ, Koenig HA: Creative wire bending—the force system from step and V bends, *Am J Orthod Dentofac Orthop* 93:59-67, 1988.
20. Burstone CJ, Pryputniewicz RJ: Holographic determination of centers of rotation produced by orthodontic forces, *Am J Orthod* 77:396, 1980.
21. Burstone CJ, Pryputniewicz RJ, Bowley WW: Holographic measurement of tooth mobility in three dimensions, *J Periodont Res* 13:283, 1978.
22. Burstone CJ, Qin B, Morton JY: Chinese NiTi wire—a new orthodontic alloy, *Am J Orthod* 87(6):445-453, 1985.
23. Christiansen R, Burstone CJ: Centers of rotation within the periodontal space, *Am J Orthod* 55:353, 1969.
24. DeFranco JC, Koenig HA, Burstone CJ: Three dimensional large displacement analysis of orthodontic appliances, *J Biomech* 9:793, 1976.
25. Dellinger EL: Histologic and cephalometric investigation of premolar intrusion in the Macaca speciosa monkey, *Am J Orthod* 53:325, 1967.
26. Fortin JM: Translation of premolars in the dog by controlling the moment-to-force ratio in the crown, *Am J Orthod* 59:541, 1971.
27. Goldberg AJ, Burstone CJ: An evaluation of beta titanium alloys for use in orthodontic appliances, *J Dent Res* 58:593, 1979.
28. Goldberg AJ, Burstone CJ, Koenig HA: Plastic deformation of orthodontic wires, *J Dent Res* 62(9):1016-1020, 1983.
29. Goldberg AJ, Morton J, Burstone CJ: The flexure modulus of elasticity of orthodontic wires, *J Dent Res* 62(7):856-858, 1983.
30. Goldberg AJ, Vanderby R Jr, Burstone CJ: Reduction in the modulus of elasticity in orthodontic wires, *J Dent Res* 56:1227, 1977.
31. Groves MH Jr: "Threshold force values for anterior retraction." Thesis, Indiana University School of Dentistry, 1959.
32. Hershey GH, Houghton CW, Burstone CH: Unilateral facebows: a theoretical and laboratory analysis, *Am J Orthod* 79:229, 1981.
33. Koenig HA, Burstone CJ: Analysis of generalized curved beams for orthodontic applications, *J Biomech* 7:429, 1974.
34. Koenig HA, Burstone CJ: Force systems from an ideal arch—large deflection considerations, *Angle Orthod* 59(1):11-16, 1989.
35. Kusy RP, Greenberg AR: Effects of composition and cross section on the elastic properties of orthodontic arch wire, *Angle Orthod* 51:325, 1981.
36. Kusy RP, Tulloch JFC: Moment/force ratios in mechanics of tooth movement, *Am J Orthod Dentofac Orthop* 90:127-131, 1986.
37. Lopez I, Goldberg J, Burstone CJ: Bending characteristics of Nitinol wire, *Am J Orthod* 75:569, 1979.
38. Manhartsberger C, Morton J, Burstone CJ: Space closure in adult patients using the segmented arch technique, *Angle Orthod* 59:205-210, 1989.
39. Miura F, Mogi M, et al: The super-elastic properties of the Japanese NiTi alloy wire of use in orthodontics, *Am J Orthod Dentofac Orthop* 90:1-10, 1986.
40. Miura F, Mogi M, et al: The super-elastic Japanese NiTi alloy wire of use in orthodontics, part III: studies on the Japanese NiTi alloy coil springs, *Am J Orthod Dentofac Orthop* 94:89-96, 1988.
41. Nägerl H, Burstone CJ et al: Centers of rotation with transverse forces: an experimental study, *Am J Orthod* 99:337-345, 1991.
42. Nägerl H, Kubein-Meesenberg et al: *Basic biomechanical principles of tooth movement.* In Hosl E, Baldauf A, editors: *Mechanical and biological basics in orthodontic therapy,* Heidelberg, Germany, 1991, Huthig Buch Verlag Heidelberg, pp 31-49.
43. Nägerl H, Kubein-Meesenberg et al: Theoretische und experimentelle aspekte zur initialen Zahnbewegung, *Orthodontie und Kieferorthopadie Quintessence,* 43-61, 1991.
44. Nelson K, Burstone CJ, Goldberg AJ: Optimal welding of beta titanium orthodontic wires, *Am J Orthod* 92:213-219, 1987.
45. Pryputniewicz RJ, Burstone CJ: The effects of time and force magnitude on orthodontic tooth movement, *J Dent Res* 58:1154, 1979.
46. Reitan K: The initial tissue reaction incident to orthodontic tooth movement as related to the influence of function, *Acta Odontol Scand Suppl* 6, 1951.
47. Ronay F, Kleinert MW et al: Force system developed by V bends in an elastic orthodontic wire, *Am J Orthod Dentofac Orthop* 94(4):295-301, 1989.
48. Sandstedt GW: Einige Beiträge zur Theorie der Zahnregulierung, *Nord Tand Tidskr* 5:236, 1904; 6:1, 1906.
49. Smith RJ, Burstone CJ: Mechanics of tooth movement, *Am J Orthod* 85(4):294-307, 1984.
50. Smith R, Storey E: The importance of force in orthodontics, *Aust Dent J* 56:291, 1952.
51. Solonche DJ, Burstone CJ, Yeamans E: *An automated device for determining load-deflection characteristics of orthodontic appliances.* In *Proceedings,* 25th Annual Conference of Engineering in Medicine and Biology, 359, 1972.
52. Storey E, Smith R: Force in orthodontics and its relation to tooth movement, *Aust Dent J* 56:11, 1952.
53. Tanne K, Burstone CJ, Sakuda M: Biomechanical responses of tooth associated with different root lengths and alveolar bone heights: changes of stress distributions in the PDL, *J Osaka Univ Dent School* 29:17-24, 1989.
54. Tanne K, Koenig HA et al: Effect of moment to force ratios on stress patterns and levels in the PDL, *J Osaka Univ Dent School* 29:9-16, 1989.
55. Tanne K, Nagataki T et al: Patterns of initial tooth displacements associated with various root lengths and alveolar bone heights, *Am J Orthod Dentofac Orthop* 100(1):66-71, 1991.
56. Tanne K, Sakuda M, Burstone CJ: Three-dimensional finite element analysis for stress in the periodontal tissue by orthodontic forces, *Am J Orthod Dentofac Orthop* 92:499-505, 1987.
57. Timoshenko S, Goddier JN: *Theory of elasticity,* ed 2, New York, 1951, McGraw-Hill.
58. Wainwright WM: Faciolingual tooth movement: its influence on the root and cortical plate, *Am J Orthod* 64:278, 1973.

Computer Applications in Orthodontics

CHAPTER

RICHARD P. WALKER

Computers are ubiquitous tools in modern society. Advances in computer hardware technology continue at a remarkable rate; breakthroughs in computing power, speed, graphics capabilities, and storage capacity accelerate, while the ratio of hardware cost to performance declines, often precipitously. Great efforts are being made to make computers easier to use.

The torrid cycle of hardware evolution shows no signs of abatement. Engineering methods for the design and manufacture of microprocessors and memory chips are well established. The hardware design process is somewhat like a cascading waterfall; each team of engineers uses robust tools for design, testing, and manufacture, and pours its work into the next team's pool. Furthermore, abundant capital is available for funding of research and development that is aimed at the next generation of microprocessors and architectures. It is therefore not unreasonable to expect that the current acceleration of hardware advancement will continue for some time to come.

Despite the magnificent progress made in placing ever more powerful and inexpensive computers at our fingertips, it is the computer software that breathes life into hardware. Without software, computers are simply inanimate lumps of silicon. Regrettably, software engineering methods are comparatively poorly established, and the pace of software development lags significantly behind that of hardware. Computer programs continue to be literally handcrafted, line by line, by small teams of developers working in an arcane, abstract world. Programmers use software development tools that are constantly changing and evolving, often several times within the development cycle of one program.

The following description of the construction of a building is a suitable metaphor for the software development process.

Plans for the building are meticulously drawn up before construction begins. During construction, however, many changes are made in the architectural designs and engineering specifications, forcing large portions of the building to be torn down and meticulously rebuilt. At the same time, many of the tools used in construction are replaced with newer and apparently more refined tools. Some of these new tools are robust, reliable, and dependable; others are not. The construction process takes much longer than originally planned and costs considerably more than expected, and the building looks and functions differently than originally envisioned.

The sands which underlie the software developers' feet are continually shifting. Yet great hope and promise lie in the future of software engineering. New programming methods, languages, and environments are emerging that purport to facilitate and shorten the software development process. Despite trailing hardware by a few years, software by any other measure is evolving at a rapid pace. Its rate of advancement pales in comparison to hardware simply because hardware is evolving at a truly frantic pace.

Computers are becoming increasingly easy to use. The term *user interface* refers to the manner in which a user interacts with a computer and its software. A graphical user interface (GUI) is one in which information is displayed or represented as icons or in contextual windows and tasks are accomplished with a pointing device such as a mouse or trackball. All current GUIs are based on original creative work performed by researchers at Xerox's Palo Alto Research Centre (PARC) in the 1970s. This pioneering work led to the development of the mouse, icons, pull-down menus, and windowing environments. Both the Macintosh and Microsoft Windows are examples of graphical-user interfaces and are direct descendants of work at PARC.

268

Currently, over 100 million personal computers are in use around the world. Computers based on Intel's family of microprocessors, generally termed IBM-compatible machines, maintain an overwhelming world market share. The Intel microprocessors, which lie at the hearts of these machines, include the 8086 and 8088, 286, 386, 486, and Pentium. Intel-based machines typically use a combination of DOS and Microsoft Windows as operating system and graphical operating environment. These may be supplanted by Windows NT, a 32-bit multitasking operating system.

Apple computers are based on Motorola's family of microprocessors, including the 68000, 68020, 68030, and 68040. The Macintosh operating system is a 32-bit multitasking operating system that is tightly linked to the underlying hardware and provides a graphical operating environment. Apple and IBM are cooperating in the new technology ventures, Taligent and Kaleida, to develop their collective vision of the next generation of hardware and software environments and multimedia applications.

Computer Applications in Orthodontics

Computers are widely used for a number of tasks in the modern orthodontic practice, including word processing, practice management, diagnosis and treatment planning, and practice marketing. This chapter will explore three current and emerging areas in which computer hardware and software can be applied to orthodontics:

1. Cephalometrics
2. Facial imaging
3. Volume visualization

This chapter is not intended to be an exhaustive survey of computer applications in orthodontics. It is rather intended to serve as an overview of major areas of interest and as an introduction to many of the issues associated with hardware and software development. The references to computer hardware made in this chapter will most certainly be obsolete before this text is published. The software examples provided will likely also be soon outdated. Nevertheless, the concepts which underlie our progression from two- to three-dimensional computer-aided morphometrics will likely remain valid and intact for many years.

Computer Display Fundamentals

Before discussing specific computer applications in orthodontics, a brief discussion of some computer graphics display fundamentals may assist the reader.

Computer applications that convey information pictorially are termed *graphics applications*. Information is graphically displayed on a computer monitor or cathode-ray tube (CRT). The image space on a CRT is made up of tiny rectangular or square picture elements termed *pixels*. Pixels are arranged in a series of horizontal lines on the CRT called *raster lines*. Display *resolution* refers to the total number of pixels displayed on the CRT and is commonly reported as the display width in pixels by the display height in pixels. Common display resolutions include 640 by 480, 800 by 600, 1024 by 768, and 1280 by 1024. The higher the resolution, the more refined the displayed images appear. The entire displayed matrix of pixels is termed a *bitmap*.

Images displayed on a CRT may consist of many different intensities or colors. The number of different intensities or colors that each pixel can assume is termed *color depth* and is measured in bits per pixel. Each pixel in a display of n bits per pixel is capable of 2^n different colors or intensities. Monochrome displays need only 2 (2^1) colors (black or white) and are hence 1-bit bitmaps; each pixel is either on or off. Line drawings, such as cephalometric tracings and superimpositions, are managed adequately with 4-bit (16 color) displays. Grey-scale images may need 256 (2^8) different intensities to be perceived as having continuous shades of grey. Color images may also be displayed on an 8-bit display if the 256 colors are appropriately selected to match the tones of the image.

Pixels in systems with 24-bit displays may assume up to 16,777,216 different colors. Here, 8 bits of data are assigned to each of red, green, and blue. Many color imaging applications do not need 2^{24} different colors in order to adequately display a single image. Recent advances in video controller technology have resulted in inexpensive 15-bit (32,768 colors) and 16-bit (65,536 colors) displays.

The video controller is responsible for the refresh of the CRT display. There are two types of refresh: *interlaced* and *noninterlaced*. With interlaced refresh, half of the raster lines are redrawn during each cycle (typically 1/60 second). The odd-numbered raster lines are refreshed in the first cycle; the even-numbered raster lines are refreshed in the second. The entire display is refreshed every 1/30 second, which represents a rate of 30 Hz (cycles per second). Interlaced displays have a noticeable flicker, inducing eye strain. Video controllers producing noninterlaced signals refresh the entire display at least every 1/60 second. The display is rock solid and comfortable to view. Modern controllers have noninterlaced refresh rates of up to 76 Hz.

CEPHALOMETRIC APPLICATIONS

Clinical cephalometrics is a routine part of the diagnosis and treatment planning process in modern orthodontics. Traditionally, acetate tracings are made and analyzed according to one or more of the many cephalometric analyses that have gained common clinical acceptance. The cephalometric tracing is also used as the starting point during the formulation of so-called visualized treatment objectives (VTO) or surgical treatment objectives (STO). Cephalometric treatment planning manipulations may include estimates of growth, contemplated orthopedic intervention, orthodontic tooth movements, and orthognathic surgery. Actual growth and treatment response are measured by longitudinal superimposition of serial tracings on stable cranial base or regional contours.

Cephalograms are two-dimensional representations of three-dimensional anatomy. Our ability to derive meaningful information from headfilms depends on the reliability with which information can be gathered from them. Fortunately, a reasonably high degree of standardization exists in the methods used to acquire cephalograms. Head position and orientation, source-object distance, and radiographic enlargement have been standardized to a degree that permits a common descriptive language of dentofacial morphology and the development of consistent methods of anthropometric landmark identification. The relative reliability of our ability to locate many commonly used cephalometric landmarks has been well documented.[1]

Computers are useful tools for clinical cephalometrics. If cephalograms are converted into a digital form of representation, computers and software can be used to derive a great deal of clinically useful information, often in a short period of time. Some of this derived information is not necessarily immediately obvious to the casual observer. Many cephalometric tasks are well suited to computer implementation; however, some cephalometric tasks are rather less well suited to computerization.

Clinical cephalometrics can be broadly divided into static functions and dynamic functions. Static functions are those in which information is derived from the radiographic contours that currently exist on a film or collection of films and include cephalometric analysis and superimposition. Dynamic functions are those in which elements of the cephalometric representation are arbitrarily transformed or manipulated and include growth estimation, orthodontic treatment planning, and surgical treatment planning. Later we shall examine the role that computers and software can play in both the static and dynamic cephalometric functions.

Hardware Requirements for Cephalometric Applications

Cephalometric applications have relatively modest computer hardware requirements. Typical systems use a digitizing tablet for landmark coordinate input; a computer with graphics capabilities for display, analysis, and manipulation; and a graphics plotter for hardcopy generation (Fig. 5-1).

A video controller and CRT display capable of displaying 16 colors (4 bits per pixel) is adequate for graphical cephalometric display. This includes elements of the user interface and display of one or more cephalometric tracings and analyses. The display resolution should be a minimum of 640 by 480 pixels. A higher resolution CRT display is desirable; tracings appear smoother and more refined at resolutions of 800 by 600 or 1024 by 768. Noninterlaced display is essential to avoid eye strain and fatigue (Fig. 5-2).

The data structures required to store digitized cephalograms are not particularly large. The digitized coordinates of 100 landmarks take up less than 1 megabyte (MB) of memory. As discussed below, the mode of digitization has

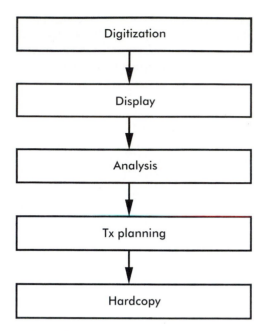

Fig. 5-1 The cephalometric application pipeline.

an influence on storage requirements. Cephalometric applications generally run on machines with 640 kilobytes (KB) to 1 MB of random access memory (RAM). A hard disk with a capacity as low as 40 MB is sufficient to store the digitized coordinates of thousands of cephalograms. Hundreds of digitized films can be archived to a single 1.2 MB or 1.44 MB floppy diskette.

Digitization is a process by which analog information is converted into digital form. An enormous amount of raw information is incorporated in the anatomic contours contained in a cephalogram. A small subset of this information is of interest—precisely that which is needed to assist in making a diagnosis and treatment plan. The task is to reduce the radiographic data to a meaningful, manageable size and is accomplished through the process of digitization. The orthodontist can use a digitizing tablet, a video camera and frame grabber, or a scanner to digitize cephalograms.

Digitizing Tablets

A digitizing tablet, or digitizer, is a device that records the x-y coordinates of points in a Cartesian coordinate system. A digitizing cursor, usually with fine cross hairs, is used to locate radiographic landmarks or contours. Coordinate pairs are transmitted from the digitizer to the computer—typically via serial asynchronous communication—and are recorded and later used for various cephalometric determinations.

Digitizers may be opaque, translucent, or transparent. Translucent or transparent digitizers may be backlit (Fig. 5-3)—an advantage that allows digitization to proceed directly from a radiograph without making an intermediate

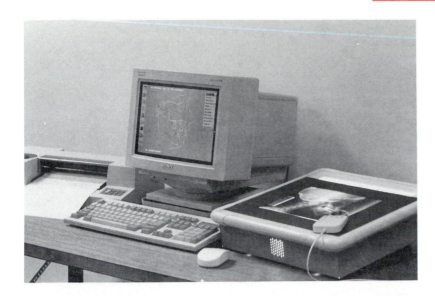

Fig. 5-2 Cephalometric applications generally require a computer, an input device, and an output device.

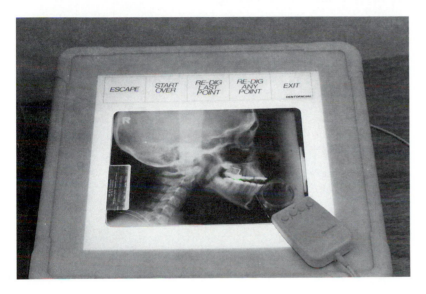

Fig. 5-3 A translucent backlit digitizer allows digitization directly from cephalograms.

acetate tracing and therefore without adding tracing error to the overall process. Two parameters generally used to measure digitizer performance are resolution and accuracy. Resolution refers to the smallest distance that can be resolved by the digitizer and is of the order of 1000 lines per inch or 40 lines per millimeter in current tablets. Accuracy refers to the precision with which a digitizer can record spatial measurements over various regions of its surface and should be of the order of ± 0.25 mm for cephalometric applications.

Early cephalometric applications used off-line digitizers; coordinate pairs were generated on punched cards that were subsequently fed to a computer in batch mode. The competitive hardware pressures concurrent with the advent of computer-aided design (CAD) applications led to the development of inexpensive, accurate digitizing tablets. A digitizer connected directly to a computer (on-line digitization) permits immediate display and analysis of digitized landmarks. Digitizing tablets remain an inexpensive, reli-

able, and accurate means of acquiring cephalometric information.

Two modes of digitization may be used to record information from cephalograms. *Point mode digitization* refers to the discrete location of individual landmarks. The user sequentially locates individual landmarks in a predetermined order, pressing a cursor button when the cursor is accurately positioned over the landmark. One coordinate pair is transmitted for each landmark. A visual representation of a cephalogram is generated by connecting discretely digitized landmarks with lines or curves. If the digitized landmarks are suitably selected and in reasonable proximity, the resulting vector tracing is an effective representation of the original radiographic contours.

Stream mode digitization refers to a process whereby a stream of coordinate pairs is transmitted by the digitizer when a cursor button is pressed. The stream of points is controlled by programmable options. Points may be transmitted at a specified number of coordinate pairs per second or may be transmitted after the cursor has moved a minimum distance. Stream mode is used to manually trace radiographic contours. A large number of adjacent points are transmitted, which, when joined together in a simple point-to-point fashion, provide a representation of radiographic contours.

Each digitizing method has advantages and disadvantages. Point mode digitization is more time consuming than stream mode but provides accurate landmark locations and high quality contours when joined through the use of appropriate curve-fitting algorithms. Stream mode digitization is more technique-sensitive than point mode. Tracing contours in stream mode is rather like drawing with a brick; the operator must possess considerable skill to record accurate contours.

The mode of digitization has a profound influence on computer-aided cephalometric treatment planning. Soft tissue changes associated with orthodontic tooth movements and orthognathic surgery have been documented in a large and growing body of retrospective investigation. Virtually without exception, soft tissue profile response is characterized by changes in location of a common group of specific soft tissue landmarks relative to treatment-induced changes in underlying hard tissue structures.

Computer-aided cephalometric profile prediction should be based on a digitizing model that allows the results of retrospective studies to be easily incorporated into software. It is therefore essential that the locations of key-hard and soft-tissue landmarks be provided to predictive software. Key landmark locations can only be reliably acquired through point mode digitization (Fig. 5-4); stream mode digitization does not inherently provide the location of key landmarks (Fig. 5-5). If the soft tissue profile is digitized in stream mode, a coordinate pair may or may not be transmitted as the cursor passes over a key landmark. It becomes the software engineer's task to attempt to deduce the location of the point which is closest to the key landmark from a stream of points. To date, exceedingly little work has been

published regarding the reliability of automated cephalometric landmark location. For these reasons, point mode is the preferred method of digitization for predictive treatment planning purposes.

An additional advantage of point mode digitization over stream mode is found in cephalometric research applications. If the orthodontist should wish to measure the change in a landmark's location over time, it is essential that he or she know the precise location of the landmark relative to an origin. For example, the practitioner might want to design a research project to study the upper lip changes that occur as a result of Le Fort 1 surgery with V-Y incision closure and would want to track the positional change in soft tissue landmarks, such as subnasale, labrale superius, and stomion superius, relative to hard tissue landmarks, such as A point and the upper incisor tip. Only point mode digitization of pre- and post-surgical cephalograms can accurately deliver this information (Fig. 5-6).

A final difference between point and stream modes of digitization is efficiency in data storage. Cephalometric contours are efficiently stored when represented in point mode, whereas stream mode digitization can easily produce hundreds or thousands of coordinate pairs in the generation of a single tracing.

Video Camera and Frame Grabber

The human eye is sensitive to ratios of intensity levels rather than to absolute values of intensity.[13] The difference in intensity between pixels of value 10 and 11 is perceived as the same as the difference between pixels of value 100 and 110. Grey-scale images are images that are made up of pixels that vary in intensity between black and white. Humans have difficulty discerning more than 256 different shades of grey. This is a fortuitous fact when it comes to acquiring images of cephalograms. Images acquired in 8-bit (256 shades) grey-scale are probably sufficient to discern clinical cephalometric needs. The use of 12 bits of intensity

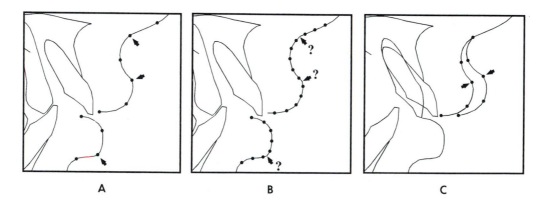

A   B   C

Fig. 5-4 **A,** Point mode digitization allows precise location of essential landmarks for soft tissue profile prediction. **B,** Stream mode digitization may or may not record key profile landmarks. **C,** Point mode digitization allows simple retrospective analysis of changes in landmark location with treatment.

(4096 shades) is more appropriate for research purposes. Grey-scale images can be acquired through the use of a video camera and frame grabber or with a transparency scanner.

Radiographic images can be acquired with the aid of a video camera. The video image is converted to a digital representation using a device called a frame grabber. The digital radiographic image is displayed on a CRT from which landmarks and contours are identified with a pointing device, such as a mouse.

Image quality depends greatly on the type of video signal generated by the video camera. The three common types of signal are composite, S-video, and RGB. Each of these signals manages the color and brightness information in a video signal in a different manner. Composite video combines luminance (brightness) and chrominance (color) information into one signal. S-video, also known as Y-C, uses separate signals for luminance (Y) and chrominance (C) resulting in higher quality images but at greater expense. RGB component video separates the red, green, and blue information into separate signals and produces the highest quality images but at the greatest expense. S-video or RGB video signals are preferred for clinical video imaging, whether it is used in the acquisition of images of cephalograms or in facial imaging.

A frame grabber is a device that provides an interface between a video signal and a computer. The analog video signal from a video camera is converted into a digital image that is subsequently displayed on a CRT. The frame grabber literally grabs an image frame from a continuous video signal. The combination of video camera and frame grabber can be used to acquire a digital image of a cephalogram.

It is essential that digitized cephalograms be accurate representations of the original anatomy. The reliability of images acquired through the use of a video camera and frame grabber is limited by several constraining technical elements of the process.

Video cameras employ at least one charged couple device (CCD) to detect the light that enters the camera through its lens. The resolution of the video image is limited by the pixel count in the CCD and by the resolution inherent in video signals. In North America, video signals comply with the NTSC video standard, which has 525 horizontal scan lines. Only 480 lines of the NTSC video signal are visible. European video signals comply with the PAL or SECAM standards, each of which have 625 scan lines.

If it is assumed that a typical lateral cephalogram is 250 mm by 200 mm, then a video digitized image of a cephalogram is at best represented by an image that has a resolution of approximately 0.5 mm per pixel. Each pixel in the image represents a region of the film that is 0.5 mm by 0.5 mm in size. This resolution is considerably lower than that which is possible with conventional digitizing tablets or with transparency scanning (discussed below). An additional limitation associated with video acquisition of radiographs is related to image distortion. A video camera

uses a lens to focus the image onto the CCD. A measurable amount of image distortion is introduced by the optics associated with any lens, especially in the peripheral regions of the image.[4] The use of a flat-field lens may reduce this distortion but at considerable additional expense.

A video camera and frame grabber may be used, in acknowledgment of their limitations, for the first step in digitization—namely generating a grey-scale digital image on a computer monitor. The second step is cephalometric landmark location, which can be performed in point or stream mode, much as discussed above. A pointing device, generally a mouse, is used to locate individual landmarks or to trace contours on the displayed image.

Clinicians who elect to use a video camera and frame grabber to acquire images of cephalograms should be aware of the weaknesses of the process. Additional research should be directed at more fully quantifying the errors associated with this method. Emerging high-definition television standards will most certainly provide higher resolution video signals in the next decade. Until such time, however, the combination of video camera and frame grabber remains the least accurate means of cephalometric digitization.

Scanners

A most promising method of acquiring images of cephalograms is through transparency scanning. Two types of scanners are prevalent: drum and flat-bed. In a drum scanner the transparency is mounted on a rotating drum, and a finely collimated light beam is directed at it. The amount of transmitted light is measured by a photocell inside the drum. With a flatbed scanner the transparency is placed on a flat transparent surface and a light source is passed over it. The amount of transmitted light is detected by a photocell and is converted into a digital representation of position and intensity.

Scanners are capable of acquiring images at high resolutions and ranges of intensity. Rotating drum scanners can acquire images at resolutions approaching 2000 lines per inch and 24 bits per pixel. Less expensive flatbed transparency scanners are capable of resolutions of up to 300 dots per inch or 12 dots per millimeter (also at 24 bits per pixel). These resolutions and depth exceed our cephalometric requirements by a comfortable margin. A scanned image is displayed on a CRT, from which landmarks and contours are recorded with a mouse, as described above.

Scanned images acquire a large amount of digital data, hence the files necessary for their storage are also extensive. Image compression techniques are emerging that will undoubtedly assist in reducing image file storage requirements. The Joint Photographics Experts Group (JPEG) has developed a public domain image compression standard which is becoming widely adopted. It is a *lossy method,* which means that data is discarded during the compression process. Great care must be exercised in applying a lossy compression method to radiographic images. As yet no scientific

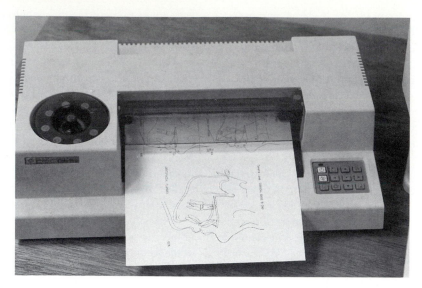

Fig. 5-5 A graphics plotter generates high-resolution cephalometric tracings. Colored pens are used to differentiate superimposed tracings.

study has been initiated to determine the compression ratio at which featural loss is detectable on cephalograms. Alternate lossless methods of compression are preferred for radiographic images.

Transparency scanners are not yet in wide clinical use, but such scanners hold great promise as the future preferred method of cephalometric image acquisition.

Hardcopy Generation

Cephalometric hardcopy is generated using a graphics plotter or a laser printer. A plotter is a device that draws vector tracings, using pens of various colors on paper or acetate, and generates high-quality renderings of cephalometric tracings, analyses, and superimpositions (Fig. 5-7). Laser printers are raster devices; vector tracings must be converted into a raster representation before being sent to a laser printer. Laser printers also require internal memory that is sufficient to produce a full page of bitmapped graphics.

Static Cephalometric Functions

Computers and software are well suited for the task of performing cephalometric analysis. It is, therefore, not surprising that the use of computers for digitization, analysis, and serial superimposition has been widely reported over the past three decades. Walker[47-50] uses a 177-point lateral digitizing regimen and a 133-point posteroanterior regimen to perform cephalometric analyses, serial superimposition, and growth simulation. Bergin[2] et al. use a digitizing model to study errors associated with computer-aided cephalometric analysis and report that digitizer inaccuracy makes a negligible contribution to the method error when compared to errors associated with landmark location. Baumrind and

Miller[1] advocate the use of extra-cranial corner fiducial reference points for precise repeated headfilm digitization.

Computer-aided cephalometric systems use the digitized coordinates of a sequence of cephalometric landmarks as a mathematical model for the anatomic structures they represent (Fig. 5-8). Vector mathematics is used to compute a variety of commonly used cephalometric measurements, including the linear distance between two landmarks, the angle between two lines, and the perpendicular distance from a point to a line. Measurements derived from a patient's digitized cephalogram are compared to a database of age- and sex-specific comparison values. Cephalometric enlargement is accommodated for by scaling the coordinates of all digitized landmarks by a factor that reduces the dimensions of the overall representation to a corrected size.

Digitized cranial base or regionally stable landmarks are used for superimposition of serially digitized cephalograms. The landmarks that represent a second or third film are translated and rotated so that they overlie those of the base film at a target landmark and along a desired line. Spatial changes in landmark location are reported as vectors incorporating magnitude and direction of change. Analyses are calculated for all superimposed coordinate sets.

Most cephalometric analyses lend themselves well to software implementation. However, computer-aided superimposition of digitized cephalograms is rigid and potentially prone to error. During manual superimposition, stable anatomic structures are carefully traced. The best fit of these contours is for cranial base, maxillary, and mandibular superimpositions. It is difficult to implement best-fit vector contour matching in software. Superimposition is generally performed at a specific landmark and along a specific line defined by two terminal landmarks. A small error in the location of either or both of the terminal landmarks (espe-

Steiner analysis

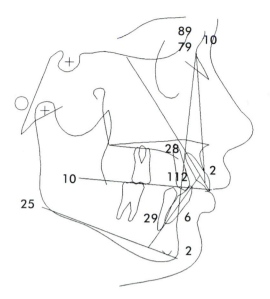

McNamara analysis

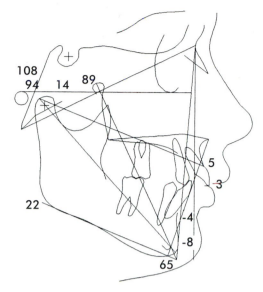

Ricketts analysis

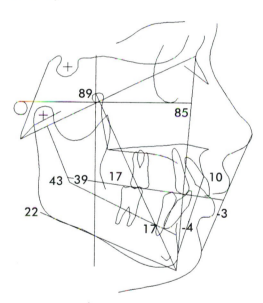

Jarabak analysis

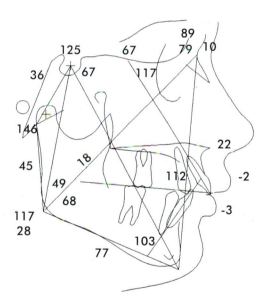

Fig. 5-6 Cephalometric applications are well suited for performing analyses.

cially if they are in close proximity) can profoundly distort the overall superimposition and the conclusions that are drawn from it.

Dynamic Cephalometric Functions

Many of the dynamic cephalometric manipulations which contribute to the formulation of visualized treatment objectives (VTO) or surgical treatment objectives (STO) can be implemented in software. Faber[12] describes an early treatment planning system in which growth prediction and ortho-

dontic tooth movements are interactively performed, including manipulation of some elements of the soft tissue profile. The user controls much of the treatment planning process; decisions are made by the user and immediately evaluated through feedback of graphical images displayed on a CRT. Similar systems* of VTO generation perform growth prediction, orthopedic and orthodontic planning, and

*References 3, 20, 33, 34, 39.

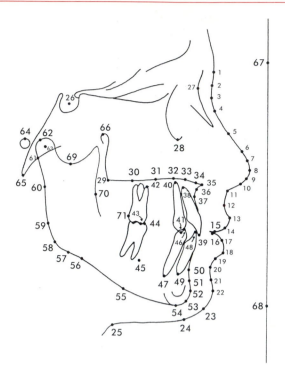

Fig. 5-7 Lateral digitizing regimen which incorporates landmarks required for static and dynamic cephalometric determinations.

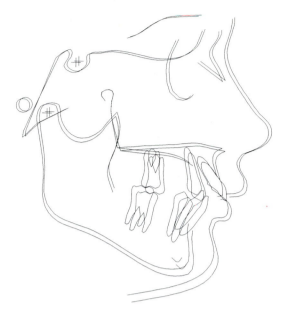

Fig. 5-8 Computer-generated 2-year growth estimate.

orthognathic surgical planning at various levels of refinement and user facility.

In order to perform the skeletal, dental, and soft tissue region transformations that form a VTO, landmarks sufficient to render an adequate depiction of the structures involved must be digitized. For example, to plan upper incisor retraction and estimate its effects on the profile, the upper incisor landmarks and a series of soft tissue profile landmarks must be included in the digitizing regimen. A digitization model that is general enough to permit the vast majority of treatment planning procedures and that can be routinely employed in virtually every case is therefore highly desirable. Such a regimen employs approximately 70 landmarks (Fig. 5-9).

Considerable controversy exists over the reliability of cephalometric growth forecasting techniques. The present discussion is not intended to confirm or deny the accuracy of growth prediction methods; although the term *growth estimation* is perhaps a more representative description of the process. It is sufficient to state here that growth estimation methods can be implemented in software (Fig. 5-10). Ricketts' method[33] is widely used and is easily implemented in software. It assigns mean increments of growth to a series of landmarks along key reference lines determined by the subject's existing anatomy. It can be refined by the use of growth increments that are sensitive to the subject's skeletal age. Ricketts' method regrettably makes no attempt

to predict the post-growth position of many important landmarks, such as sella.

Modern computer user interfaces use a pointing device, such as a mouse, to accomplish tasks. The user points and clicks the mouse to achieve desired effects. This interface can be adapted in an elegant manner to the problem of easing the user's task during complex treatment planning manipulations, wherein position and inclination of skeletal or dental structures are changed on the fly. Target zones are displayed in context-sensitive regions of the displayed cephalometric tracing. Each target zone has a prescribed meaning that is related to the movements that are effected by its use. For example, to interactively simulate the effects of a Le Fort 1 osteotomy in which the maxilla is differentially impacted and advanced, the user clicks the mouse cursor in target zones representing translation and rotation of the maxilla and drags the maxilla to a new location.

As skeletal and dental structures are interactively transformed, the soft tissue profile is modified accordingly. Systematic methods of estimating the soft tissue response to treatment planning movements of the teeth and jaws are applied after every change the user makes.

Soft tissue profile changes in growing individuals may occur as a result of growth, orthopedic changes in the maxilla or mandible, orthodontic movement of the anterior teeth, and postural changes in the soft tissues of the lower face. It is difficult to design a cephalometric research project that effectively studies the isolated profile changes that occur purely as a result of orthopedic movements or purely as a result of retraction or advancement of anterior teeth. That is why our journals are not replete with studies documenting the soft tissue profile changes that accompany, for example, purely orthopedic intervention. Hence it is difficult to write

Superimposed orthodontic plan   Orthodontic plan

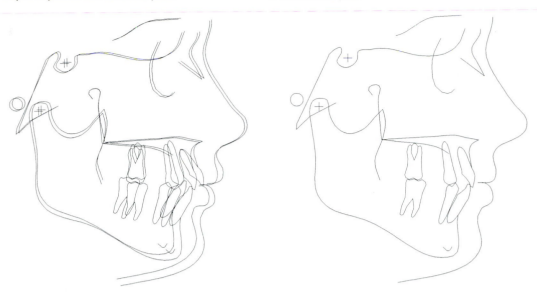

Fig. 5-9 Computer-generated orthodontic treatment plan incorporating growth, orthopedics, and orthodontic tooth movements.

software which incorporates data derived from such a study, and it is difficult to study the predictive accuracy of software models in treated growing individuals (Fig. 5-11).

Profile changes in adult, nongrowing individuals result from orthodontic movement of the anterior teeth, surgical movement of the jaws or portions thereof, and (depending on duration of treatment) aging effects. Here we have a much better chance of designing a cephalometric project to study the isolated effects of orthodontics or orthognathic surgery. The prevalence of rigid internal fixation in orthognathic surgery has improved our lot because many cases require little postsurgical modification in the position and inclination of anterior teeth. If the clinician selects a sample of subjects treated in such a way, he or she can compare cephalograms taken immediately presurgery and again subsequent to treatment and be confident that the greatest part of the change in profile is as a result of surgical intervention. This isolative ability enables the development of better predictive methods for implementation in software.

This very path has been followed by a number of investigators and has produced some excellent data upon which to base our estimates of soft tissue change, whether the data have been gathered manually or in software. An ideal test of the predictive accuracy of software models is to further compare both software predictions and manual predictions to actual treatment results. Regrettably, few have seen fit to test the abilities of skilled clinicians against a software model. Jacobson,[20] in a study of manual and computer predictive accuracy, found that from the few studies that have been performed in this manner, it can be said with some confidence that software predictive models are at least as accurate as manual predictions.

Planning orthodontic treatment through the formulation of a VTO is a valuable pretreatment exercise. Currently no evidence supports the claim that computer-assisted VTOs are any more reliable than those objectives arrived at through exceedingly careful manual methods. The value of using computer-assisted methods to automate some aspects of the manipulations embodied in the VTO process lies in the speed with which these determinations are performed. A modern personal computer can execute in a few moments a multitude of cephalometric tasks that would otherwise require laborious and time-consuming manual efforts. This affords a clinician the luxury of quickly exploring many possible courses of treatment, carefully weighing the growth and patient cooperation required to improve the likelihood of a given plan's success. The anticipated profile changes associated with extractions can be easily compared to a nonextraction approach. Orthognathic surgery can be explored in all of its wondrous and ever growing variety, and the anticipated results can be compared to purely orthodontic treatment. Orthodontists and surgeons can collaborate in front of the computer, finding common and mutually agreeable ground for their combined efforts.

Future Directions for Cephalometric Applications

It has been suggested[40] that human error associated with cephalometric landmark location might eventually be eliminated with the fully automated digitization of cephalograms. This scenario involves a scanner or frame grabber for image acquisition and software that performs automatic contour detection and landmark location. Mostafa[30] uses a video camera and frame grabber to acquire images of ceph-

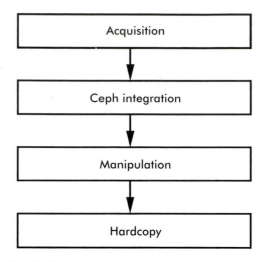

Fig. 5-10   The facial imaging application pipeline.

alograms and describes software for automated detection of soft tissue profile contours and automatic hard and soft tissue landmark location, claiming that the process is reliable.

Predictive algorithms for cephalometric treatment planning can most certainly be enhanced by future study that seeks to isolate more fully the soft tissue profile response to treatment in acknowledgment of the procedures contemplated and the patient's age, sex, and race. It is conceivable that standardized digitizing regimens, which include landmarks universally applicable to a wide range of projects, might facilitate the acquisition of large, multi-institutional samples of digitized cephalograms for further, more robust study of profile response to treatment.

FACIAL IMAGING APPLICATIONS

Orthodontists wield enormous clinical influence over facial esthetics. Orthodontic treatment, either in isolation or in combination with orthognathic surgery, routinely produces profound positive change in facial appearance. Patients are asked to put their faith in the clinicians' clinical judgment, yet many patients have great difficulty visualizing the facial changes that are likely to occur as a result of orthodontics or surgery. It is therefore not surprising that our less conservative treatment plans are occasionally faced with a high level of patient resistance based, not on educated awareness of risks and benefits, but on the fear of unknown and potentially adverse facial changes that might occur. Visualization tools can aid in the process of explaining to patients the rationale behind complex treatment plans and of estimating the nature and extent of facial change that may result from treatment.

Cephalometric tracings provide a wealth of information to trained clinicians. We mentally extrapolate our cephalometric estimation of planned profile relationships into three dimensions, aided by clinical evaluation of facial esthetics and based on the experience gained through countless completed cases, successful or otherwise. Despite the fact that a great deal of effort has gone into improving predictive algorithms for orthodontic and surgical cephalometric planning, prediction tracings are unquestionably of limited value to patients. The profile contours of a cephalometric prediction do not necessarily enable patients to clearly visualize the facial changes that are contemplated. Yet patients and parents remain the ultimate arbiters about whether we may proceed with an ideal plan or if we must compromise the plan to a degree that we know will be esthetically unfavorable.

The concept of linking facial images with cephalograms to visualize in concert surface contours and underlying skeletal structures is not new. Margolis[26] described an early method of photographic manipulation. Hohl et al.[19] describe a method of superimposing clinical photographs over cephalograms in which four radio-opaque markers are affixed to various locations of a subject's face. Lateral and frontal photographs are taken with a 35 mm camera that is mounted on a cephalometric x-ray machine and aligned with the central ray. Positive photographic transparencies are made at the enlargement factor required to precisely superimpose the visible metallic markers over their radiographic equivalents. The resulting photocephalometric montages are used to make soft tissue measurements and to gauge orthognathic soft tissue changes.

Computers and software can be used to carry out a similar process. Several recent technical advances in multimedia hardware have made high-quality desktop imaging significantly more affordable and clinically useful. Great strides have been made in video controller and CRT display technology, image acquisition methods, mass storage devices, and image compression methods. As a result of these developments, computer-aided facial image manipulation systems have emerged as powerful treatment simulation and patient education tools (Fig. 5-12). A facial image is acquired, typically with a video camera and frame grabber. Current systems[36-38] allow interactive manipulation of regions of the image in a cut-and-paste fashion in order to simulate the effects of orthodontic tooth movement, orthopedic appliances, or orthognathic surgery. The image may be linked to a cephalometric tracing through profile superimposition for combined manipulation of cephalometric and image regions. Hardcopy of images representing estimated posttreatment results is generated on a color image printer.

Despite great technical progress and accelerating clinical interest in facial imaging systems, little reliability can be claimed for image prediction. The differences in enlargement and distortion found between digitized video images and cephalograms make it difficult to precisely link these two records. Little scientific study has been directed towards quantifying treatment-induced facial contour changes that occur in regions other than the mid-sagittal plane. Imaging systems are capable of producing dramatic facial images that may or may not represent the changes that can or will be achieved through treatment.

Hardware Requirements for Imaging Applications

A computer intended for use with facial imaging software must possess abundant random access memory (RAM), a high-capacity mass storage device, and a video controller and CRT capable of displaying images at reasonably high resolution and color depth.

The minimum resolution and color depth at which facial images can be photo-realistically displayed is 640 × 480 resolution and 8 bits of color depth per pixel. Video controllers that are 8-bit permit selection of the 256 colors for image display from a palette that typically offers up to 256,000 possible colors. The 256 colors are selected from all of the available colors in the palette to most appropriately represent the colors present in the image. The 256 colors selected for a facial image of a Caucasian patient is dramatically different from those offered for a black patient.

The quality of 8-bit images rendered with such an adaptive approach is remarkably good. However, since each image uses a unique collection of 256 colors, only one image may be displayed on an 8-bit display at a given time. Video controllers capable of generating 15, 16, or 24 bits of color per pixel are termed *high-color* or *true-color* controllers and usually have a fixed palette. The colors available for image display are predetermined, and all colors are available for each image. Hence multiple images may be simultaneously displayed because they all use the same palette. Noninterlaced display is greatly preferred because of the steady nature of the displayed image.

High-resolution, true-color images are large and require considerable RAM and a high capacity permanent storage device. An 8-bit image with 640 × 480 resolution requires over 300 kilobytes (KB) of RAM. A 24-bit image with 1024 × 768 resolution requires over 2 megabytes (MB) of memory. Facial image manipulation software typically maintains more than one image in memory at any given time. Hence 4 MB of RAM is a minimum computer system requirement, and 16 MB is a reasonable system configuration; it is conceivable that imaging systems may require 32 MB or more in the near future.

It is likely that many images may be acquired for a single patient. Lateral, frontal, intra-oral, and radiographic images may be acquired at several stages of treatment. An imaging system therefore requires a large permanent storage device. A hard disk with a capacity of 200 MB is a reasonable minimum requirement, and hard disks with a capacity of up to 1 gigabyte are currently a reliable, cost-effective option for mass storage. Rewritable optical disks are undoubtedly the preferred future method of image archival, albeit with data access and transfer rates somewhat slower than conventional hard disks.

Image files can be compressed in order to reduce storage requirements. The judicious use of JPEG image compression can safely reduce the size of facial image files without noticeably sacrificing image quality. The fact that JPEG is a lossy method is less important with nonradiographic images; ratios of image file compression up to 15:1 or 20:1 are claimed to be clinically acceptable.

Image Acquisition

The simplest method of facial image acquisition is through the use of a video camera and a frame grabber. Frame grabbers and accompanying software allow real-time image preview along with the ability to capture (grab) an image frame in the form of a video snapshot. The requirements for patient positioning and lighting are not dissimilar from those required for clinical photography.

An alternate means of image acquisition is the use of a scanner to scan routine clinical facial photographs. Scanning of photographs may be an appropriate solution in situations where the imaging system is remote from the clinical setting. Inexpensive color flatbed scanners are capable of acquiring 24-bit, 300 dot-per-inch (dpi) images.

Image Manipulation

Once acquired, facial images can be manipulated to simulate changes in facial surface morphology that result from orthodontic tooth movement, the orthopedic effects of extra-oral or functional appliances, and orthognathic surgery. Recall that an image displayed on a CRT is a large two-dimensional array of pixels called a bitmap. Image-manipulation software lets the user identify a source rectangular region of pixels on the bitmap, which is first copied from the visible bitmap to an area of memory and then is copied from memory into another user-specified region on the bitmap. This two-step process creates a cut-and-paste image transformation effect. Rectangular regions may be stretched in a horizontal or vertical direction or be proportionately enlarged or reduced. These basic image transformation capabilities, when performed in various combinations, are used to simulate treatment-induced facial changes.

Regrettably (from the standpoint of image transformation), the human face is rarely well represented as a collection of rectangles. Nevertheless, the clinician can occasionally design a single, relatively large rectangular region of pixels to reasonably match a facial region that changes with treatment. The lower portion of the face, inferior to stomion, may be thus delineated and transformed in simulation of a simple mandibular advancement or setback or in simulation of the insertion of a functional appliance with an anterior bite registration.

A bitmap of the face must more frequently be cut up into smaller patches of pixels in an attempt to simulate treatment-induced facial changes. The simulated posttreatment position and shape of these small regions may not blend contiguously one into another, creating a disjointed, blocky image. Software image retouching tools must then be employed to refine the image to a more acceptable level. These tools consist of a collection of freehand paint capabilities which allow the user to blend and smooth adjacent groups of pixels, much as an artist refines paint on a canvas.

Cephalometric Predictions Can Guide Image Manipulations

A sizeable body of work has been performed in the study of pretreatment and posttreatment cephalograms in order to quantify the soft tissue profile changes that accompany orthodontic and surgical treatment. Retrospective study allows us to prospectively apply our best estimates of profile change to cases that lie before us.

Despite the fact that prediction of the posttreatment profile remains an imperfect art, cephalometric prediction may be used as a guide for facial image manipulations. Before this process can be implemented, bridges must be built between the two forms of record so that changes in one can be made to cause changes in the other. In order to use a cephalometric prediction as a guide for image manipulation, the pretreatment cephalogram must first be linked in a meaningful way to the facial image. The cephalometric profile tracing is superimposed over the image profile and is manually interactively scaled, translated, and rotated so that it matches the image as closely as possible. A precise record is kept of the scaling, rotation, and translation factors required to make the tracing fit the image. These two-dimensional transformations are subsequently applied to a predicted cephalometric profile so that it can be mapped onto the image. The differences between pretreatment and planned cephalometric profiles, when superimposed on the image, guide the manipulation of regions of the bitmap to automatically generate a facial image prediction.

A cephalometric prediction and image transformation can be performed in a manner that appears to be virtually simultaneous (Fig. 5-13). The cephalometric prediction is displayed in one window on the CRT and the image pre-

diction in another, each responding promptly to the user's commands. The tracing may conversely be superimposed on the image even during manipulation of cephalometric target zones, creating an integrated effect. Treatment simulation through the use of linked ceph-image pairs presupposes a reliable cephalometric prediction scheme. The issues previously raised regarding mode of digitization and critical retrospective scrutiny of predictive accuracy come to the fore once more.

Another method of treatment simulation through linking of tracings and images is visually impressive but less reliable. Just as active manipulation of a cephalometric tracing can be applied to a passive facial image, so can active image manipulation be applied to a passive cephalometric tracing. This process attempts to estimate the underlying cephalometric changes that are likely to accompany a facial change of a particular magnitude and direction. Direct manipulations of facial image regions are applied to a linked cephalometric tracing using the reverse of the process described above.

All of our cephalometric research (Figs. 5-14 through 5-18) has been performed using a predictive model in which the soft tissue profile is the dependent variable and underlying hard tissue is the independent variable. The chin might advance during treatment for many reasons. The mandible can grow, the mandible can be encouraged to grow with functional appliances, the mandible can be repositioned anteriorly through a change in occlusal and temporomandibular dynamics, the mandible can be surgically advanced, or the chin itself can be surgically advanced. Each of these eventualities produces a change in the position and appearance of the chin. If that region of a bitmap that corresponds to the chin advances, the orthodontist cannot with certainty divine the underlying skeletal cause as represented cephalo-

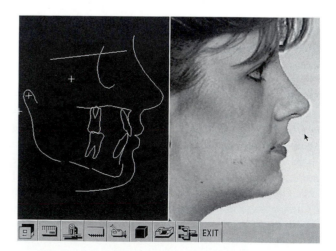

Fig. 5-12 An integrated surgical treatment simulation incorporating LF1 maxillary surgery, mandibular autorotation, mandibular advancement, and genioplasty. Predicted cephalometric profile changes are mapped onto the facial image, guiding image manipulations.

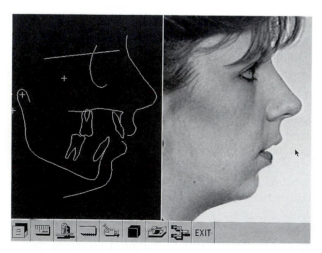

Fig. 5-11 A lateral tracing may be linked to a lateral facial image and simultaneously displayed.

metrically. Hence transformations that begin with a facial image region and end with a cephalometric tracing remain gross visual aids only.

Hardcopy Generation

High quality hardcopy generation of facial image predictions remains a contentious and potentially expensive proposition. The indiscriminate use of printed color image predictions may lead to unnecessary liability in the event that actual treatment results do not approach original targets. Clinicians who routinely give patients hardcopy of treatment simulation images should exercise great caution in regard to claims of predictive accuracy and should counsel patients about the limitations of computer imaging systems.

Four major printer technologies are currently used to produce image hardcopy: laser, ink-jet, thermal wax-transfer, and dye sublimation. Conventional laser printers generate tiny black dots, generally at resolutions of 300 dots per inch. Various combinations of dots (called a dither matrix) are printed that create the appearance of a continuous-tone, grey-scale image. The printer must possess sufficient memory to print a full page of graphics, typically 1.5 to 2 MB. Grey-scale dithered images printed on a laser printer are an inexpensive and creditable method of printing facial images.

Color ink-jet printers combine cyan (C), yellow (Y), magenta (M), and black (K) ink in a print head that heats the ink and causes it to boil, spraying the ink through a nozzle onto the paper. Most ink-jet printers require specially coated paper. Image details are not particularly sharp, and the colors do not blend well, hence image quality suffers. However, these printers are an inexpensive color printing option.

Thermal wax-transfer systems produce glossy color prints of moderate quality. The print head melts dots of cyan, yellow, magenta, and black wax from page-size regions of wax under which the paper passes. The paper is drawn into the printer separately for each color, hence page registration

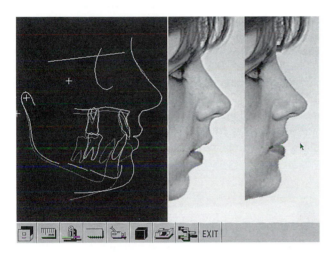

Fig. 5-13 Simultaneous review of cephalometric treatment plan and image treatment simulation.

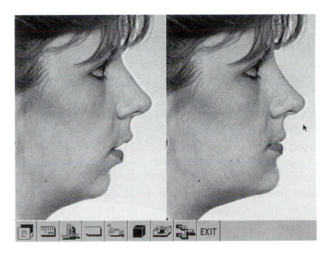

Fig. 5-14 Review of pretreatment image and treatment simulation.

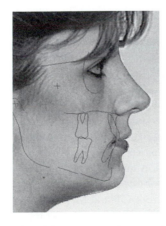

Fig. 5-15 Cephalometric treatment plan superimposed over image treatment simulation.

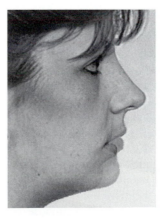

Fig. 5-16 Image transparency may be used to superimpose pretreatment image over treatment simulation.

is exceedingly important for image quality. Image quality is higher than that of ink-jet printers but is not truly photographic in quality.

Dye sublimation printers are related to wax-transfer systems. Plastic film coated with cyan, magenta, yellow, and black ink is passed over a print head with over 2,000 heating elements. When it is heated, the dye becomes gaseous and is transferred to coated paper that absorbs the dye on contact. The paper must pass across the film four times; once for each color. The print head is capable of 255 different temperatures for each element; the hotter the element, the more dye is transferred. This process produces a continuous tone color-printed image that is of spectacular and virtually photographic quality.

Limitations of Imaging Applications

Phillips et al.[32] measure the errors inherent in photocephalometric superimposition, seeking to determine whether lateral and frontal facial photographs can be accurately superimposed over lateral and frontal cephalograms in the manner described by Hohl.[19] A 35 mm camera is mounted in an aluminum bracket on the head of a cephalometric x-ray unit. Stainless steel wires are embedded in a sheet of Plexiglas to form a grid that is used to compare and quantify the enlargement and distortion of both photographic and radiographic contours. The grid is mounted on the cephalostat on a sliding bracket, which allows the distance from the x-ray anode or camera to the grid to be varied at 1 centimeter intervals.

Radiographs and photographs are taken of the grid at 1 cm intervals designed to encompass all possible frontal and lateral features of a subject's head in a cephalostat. A centimeter ruler is mounted in the same plane as the grid to allow precise photographic enlargement. The authors report that photographic images and radiographic images cannot be accurately superimposed at any depth, and therefore the photocephalometric technique described by Hohl and associates cannot therefore be accurately implemented.

The ramifications of this work extend to our attempts to integrate cephalometric prediction with facial images. The cephalometric method is well established; the distance from the anode to the subject's mid-sagittal plane is standardized and cephalometric enlargement is quantifiable and generally ranges between 8% and 12%. The orthodontist can be confident of the ability to locate many cephalometric landmarks and to understand the regions in which it is difficult to reliably locate landmarks. Facial image acquisition methods are much less well established. Variables such as camera resolution, focal length of the lens, distance from the camera to the patient, lighting conditions, patient head positioning, lip position, and mandibular postural position can and do vary greatly. It is therefore not surprising that cephalometric tracings do not accurately superimpose on facial images, regardless of whether facial images are acquired by scanning clinical photographs or through video digitization with a frame grabber. Herein lies the greatest single weakness of image prediction methods.

In order to use cephalometric profile prediction algorithms, the cephalometric soft tissue profile must be linked to the image profile. Predicted changes in the cephalometric profile are mapped onto the image and used as a guide for image region manipulation. The linkage between cephalometric and image profiles is currently performed by distorting the cephalometric profile (contours in which the clinician can have some confidence) to match the image profile (contours in which the clinician has much less confidence). This is not the wisest path to confidence in image predictions.

Cephalometric studies by definition record soft tissue changes in sagittal soft tissue contours only. Of course many three-dimensional changes in facial surface morphology are associated with orthodontic and surgical treatment. Image manipulations attempt to simulate changes in nonsagittal structures, yet virtually no data exists to support the nature and extent of these types of changes.

Three potential solutions to these current inherent weaknesses in facial image prediction are evident. (1) Facial image acquisition methods must be standardized to minimize image distortion and reduce the differences between cephalometric and image profile contours. (2) Independent study must be made of treatment-induced changes in three-dimensional facial surface morphology in a manner that allows the results to be easily applied to bitmapped image manipulation. (3) Methods that have been used to study cephalometric predictive accuracy must be extended to the study of image predictive accuracy.

THREE DIMENSIONAL APPLICATIONS

The anatomy of the craniofacial region can be visualized in three dimensions with the aid of powerful computer graphics workstations and cleverly designed software. The area of computer graphics concerned with representation and manipulation of volumetric data is known as *volume visualization*.

Computed tomography (CT) measures x-ray attenuation coefficients as they spatially vary across a section of anatomy. Osseous structures attenuate x-rays more greatly than do soft tissues, hence CT is often used to visualize hard tissue anatomy although some soft tissue structure is generally apparent.

Magnetic resonance imaging (MRI) records the density or distribution of mobile hydrogen nuclei in tissues. Abundant mobile hydrogen nuclei are found in soft tissues, whereas few or none are found in bone. Hence MR provides excellent resolution and contrast between soft tissues but generates little information about bone.

Data derived from CT and MRI scans generally consists of a series of slices corresponding to the sections of tissue that have been sequentially scanned. Depending on the CT machine used to acquire images, one CT slice is generally represented as 256 by 256 pixels with 12 bits of data per pixel (4096 shades of grey). The intensity value of a pixel is termed its Hounsfield number. These slices of data can be stacked upon one another and used to form a three-dimensional representation of the anatomy contained therein.

Early volume visualization systems (Fig. 5-19) run directly on CT machine consoles, using the CT machine's internal processor to perform the time-consuming calculations necessary for 3D reconstruction of the data. These systems disadvantageously commandeer the resources of the CT machine for 3D reconstructions, when it might otherwise be used for performing CT scans. Later volume visualization systems use stand-alone desktop computer graphics workstations for 3D reconstruction, display, and manipulation. Considerable processing power, graphics capabilities, and mass storage are required to manipulate and view the vast amounts of data that are contained in three-dimensional datasets.

Volume visualization applications are used for visualization of craniofacial anatomy, fabrication of 3D models or graft templates, surgical planning of osteotomies, and intraoperative anatomical visualization. Because of the predominance of CT data, osseous structures are visualized more commonly than soft tissues.

This section explores emerging methods of 3D data representation and visualization and discusses the potential clinical application of these methods to help the reader understand some of the problems associated with deriving meaningful morphometric information from three-dimensional images.

Volume Visualization Methods

Several methods are used for computer-aided reconstruction of 3D datasets. *Surface rendering* is an indirect technique whereby the volume data is first converted into an intermediate surface representation, which is then shaded and displayed on the CRT. *Volume rendering* is a direct technique whereby the volume data is directly visualized without making any such intermediate surface representation.

Surface Rendering

Surface rendering methods are concerned only with the representation of anatomical surfaces. The boundary between one tissue and another, as represented by CT or MR data, is detected and used to form a surface representation, which is in effect a thin veneer. No internal anatomical structure is retained.

An early technique[7,14,42] manually identifies contours that represent tissue boundaries on CT slices. Triangles are constructed between contour lines found on adjacent CT sections and are shaded to impart a three-dimensional appearance. Graphics hardware and software are used to view the reconstruction from any perspective.

Lorensen and Cline[25] describe a 3D surface visualization algorithm called *marching cubes*. This method divides a CT or MR data set into a series of cubes formed by eight pixels from adjacent sections—four from each section. The value of each cube vertex is appraised to determine whether it is above or below or is a threshold value selected to represent the tissue of interest. Bone exhibits a characteristic range

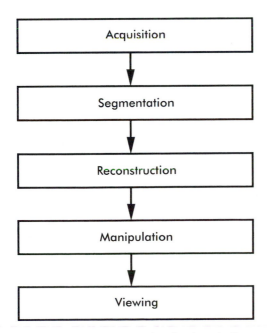

Fig. 5-17   The volume visualization pipeline.

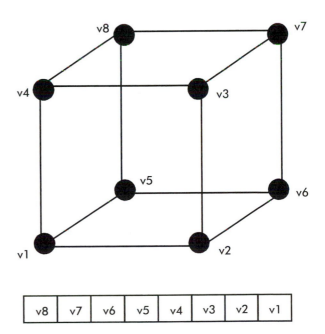

Fig. 5-18   The marching cubes method of surface rendering. Four pixels from each of two adjacent CT or MR slices form the vertices of a cube.

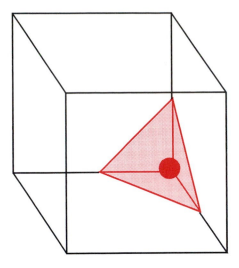

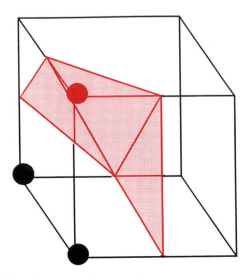

Fig. 5-19   The tissue surface transects the cube edges surrounding a vertex which lies within a threshold tissue range.

Fig. 5-20   Several vertices may lie within the threshold range, producing more intricate surfaces within the cube.

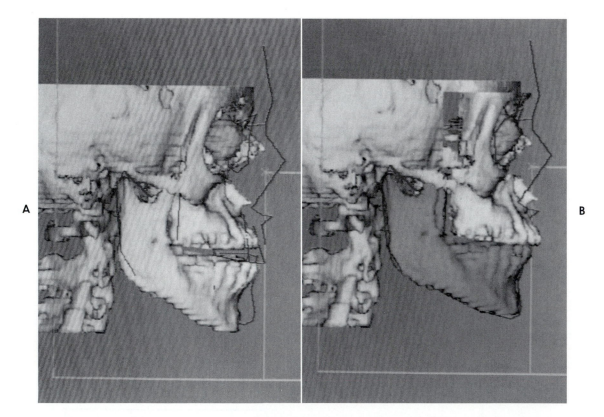

Fig. 5-21   Volume visualization integrated with 3D representation of Bolton cephalometric templates. **A,** Preoperative images. **B,** Planned orbital osteotomies, LF3 advancement, mandibular autorotation. (Courtesy of Dr. D. Altobelli.)

of CT values, as do soft tissue structures. The surface intersects the cube edges between vertices that are above and below the threshold value. Triangles are formed using the surface-cube intersections as vertices. All such cubes in the dataset are evaluated in a similar manner to establish the overall surface anatomy. The triangles formed by this method are rendered and shaded, using conventional graphics methods. A modification of this approach[8] termed *dividing cubes* can be more computationally efficient and produce high-quality surface renderings. Motoyoshi et al[31] project points of light onto the face in known patterns, then integrate multiple facial photographic views to produce surface contours. (See Figs. 5-20 through 5-23.)

Voxel Volume Rendering

Pixels from a CT or MRI image can be extruded to form a parallelepiped shape, which is termed a volume element or *voxel*. Each voxel represents the tiny volume of tissue from which a pixel intensity is derived. Voxel volume rendering techniques construct three-dimensional images by representing the dataset as thousands of such tiny blocks. The collection of voxel cubes derived from a three-dimensional dataset form a structure termed a *cuberille*.[17] If the voxels are small enough and are shaded appropriately, anatomy is depicted in a relatively smooth and contiguous manner.[18,24] (See Fig. 5-24.)

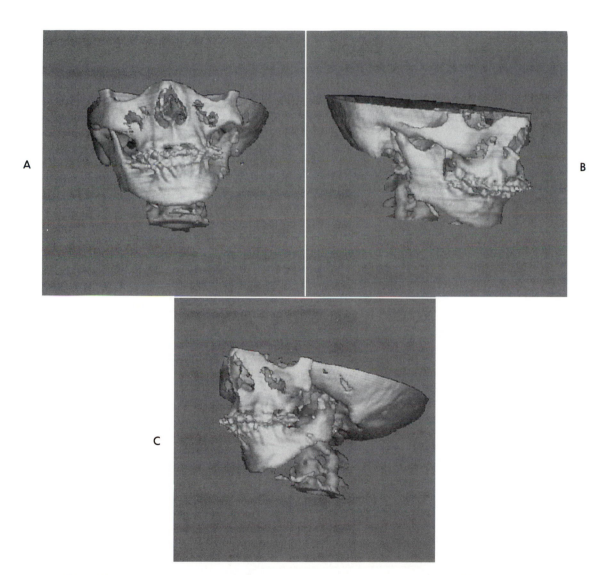

Fig. 5-22 A CT dataset of a case of hemifacial microsomia (Courtesy of Dr. D. J. Vincelli), visualized with a voxel volume technique. **A,** Anterior view of facial asymmetry. Note the bilateral artifactual pseudofenestration in the anterior surface of the maxilla. Radial artifacts emanating from the dentition result from CT scatter from orthodontic appliances. **B,** Right antero-lateral view of unaffected side. **(C)** Left antero-lateral view of affected side. Note the lack of external auditory meatus and zygomatic arch and deformed ramus, condyle, and coronoid process.

Volume Rendering with Ray Casting

Each voxel in a 3D CT or MRI dataset can be described in terms of the tissue or tissues that it represents. Indices representing properties such as color, opacity, and index of refraction may be assigned to each voxel based on the proportion of bone, muscle, or fat contained in the voxel. Ray casting[11,23] is a volume visualization method wherein rays are cast from each pixel on the CRT into the voxel volume. The ray accumulates color and opacity values as it traverses the volume and stops when it registers complete opacity or has made its way entirely through the volume. By changing the vantage point of the two-dimensional pixel plane from which the rays are cast, the volume is viewed from any perspective.

Rays can be cast from front to back, or conversely from back to front through the volume. Voxel opacity values can also be assigned on the basis of boundary detection through gradient evaluation. If a ray encounters voxels in a region of high intensity gradient, color and opacity is added. Voxels in regions of low gradient, despite representing tissues of high opacity, do not add to the color or opacity accumulated by the ray. In this way tissue surfaces are represented by the ultimately displayed image (Fig. 5-25).

Clinical Reliability of Volume Visualization

Hemmy and Tessier[16] critically evaluate the accuracy of voxel reconstructions of CT series of dry skulls. They vary CT section thickness (1.5 mm to 5 mm), surrounding medium (air or normal saline), section orientation (axial or coronal), and scanner model (GE 8800 vs GE 9800). Dry skulls of individuals with Crouzon's syndrome and orbital neurofibromatosis are evaluated under varying sets of conditions. As the section thickness increases, a stair-step effect, known as aliasing artifact, becomes more prominent. Thin regions of bone show artifacts termed pseudoforamina: holes through the 3D reconstruction that are not present in the dry skull.

Christiansen et al.[6] measure errors associated with deriving angular and linear measurements from CT images. An intra- and inter-operator error study compares measurements derived from CT images to those made directly on dry skull and fresh-frozen cadaveric specimens. Errors found in linear CT measurements are of the same order as the pixel size at the chosen CT target factor. Measurements made of mandibular condyles in which pathologic degenerative bony changes are apparent are more variable and less accurate.

Craniofacial and Temporomandibular Visualization

Hemmy et al.[15] advocate volume visualization methods for precise definition of congenital anomalies, complex fractures, and unusual bony defects. Volume visualization performs the three-dimensional reconstruction that radiologists perform mentally when assessing a series of 2D CT or MRI images. Accurate 3D representation permits precise surgical planning and reduces operating time and morbidity by revealing unusual anatomy to a surgeon preoperatively. Totty and Vannier[44] similarly describe the clinical implementation

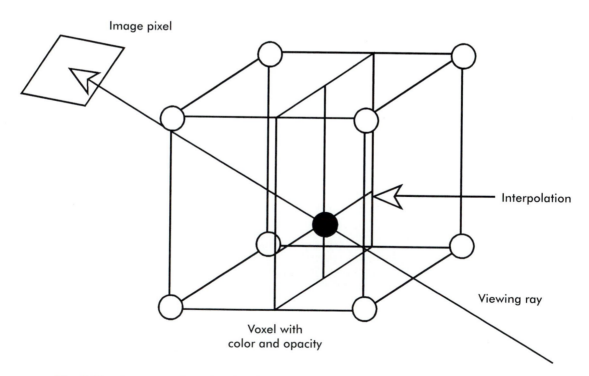

Fig. 5-23   A ray cast through a 3D dataset accumulates color and opacity from the tissues represented by the adjacent voxels.

of a simple voxel volume rendering technique for determining the relative positions and spatial orientation of bone fractures, bone fragments, calcific masses, and tumors.

The target factor used during CT acquisition influences the resolution and cross-sectional surface area of the pixels that comprise each CT slice. High target factors are used to generate high-resolution CT images of the temporomandibular joints. Volume visualization methods are used to investigate TMJ abnormalities.[22,28,35,45] Coronal or subcoronal sections are recommended for visualization of osseous joint structures and have the advantage of imaging both joints in each section. Sagittal CT sections may provide more detail with respect to meniscus position. Current volume visualization methods are capable neither of accurately determining the presence or absence of subtle pathology, such as disk perforations, nor of resolving soft tissue structures, such as the pterygoid musculature.

Treatment Planning

Volume data can be manipulated in order to aid craniofacial surgical planning.* In cases of facial or orbital asymmetry, the volume data representing the normal or unaffected side is reflected into the volume occupied by the affected side. The differences between the reflected volume and the underlying abnormal anatomy are used to plan reconstruction.

Computer-controlled milling machines are used to create 3D models of craniofacial anatomy that can be used for mock surgery, fabrication of implants, templates for autogenous bone grafts, or prostheses. Dental models may be mounted into plastic models to duplicate the patient's occlusion. Osteotomies are planned and performed on the plastic models, guiding the size and shape of bone plates and screws for rigid fixation. Materials such as hydroxyapatite may be directly milled for the creation of precise grafts or implants.

A more challenging volume manipulation task is that of planning treatment through interactive manipulation of portions of volume data. It is not a trivial task to represent volume data in a manner that permits segments or regions of the maxillofacial skeleton to be interactively repositioned in simulation of orthodontic treatment, maxillofacial surgery, or craniofacial surgery. Cutting et al.[9] describe a method of integrating cephalometric data with 3D CT for planning orthognathic surgery. A 3D cephalometric wireframe representation is generated from landmarks which are visible on both lateral and posteroanterior (PA) films. A patient's 3D tracing is compared to a similarly generated *ideal* 3D tracing derived from lateral and PA Bolton standards. The magnitude and direction of surgical skeletal movements required to transform the patient's skeletal pattern to the Bolton *ideal* are calculated, then the cephalometric treatment planning manipulations are transferred to

---

*References 5, 10, 21, 27, 41, 43, 46.

a 3D CT reconstruction for closer visualization of the planned anatomic changes. Le Fort 1, mandibular ramus osteotomies, and genioplasties are simulated in exclusion of the soft tissues.

Moss et al.[29] describe the integration of voxel volume and surface modeling for planning maxillofacial surgery. Laser range-finding devices are used to scan facial surface contours and record three-dimensional surface anatomy as a series of profiles in close proximity. Skeletal volumetric data is derived from CT voxel volume data. The two forms of 3D representation are linked in an attempt to simulate osteotomies through dynamic manipulation of surgical segments. Soft tissue changes are estimated in the midline based on retrospective cephalometric studies of surgical soft tissue change. These are attenuated in regions beyond the influence of the simulated osteotomy in order to render a smooth soft tissue surface.

Orthodontic Applications and Volume Visualization

Refining cephalometric methods to current levels of sophistication has taken over half a century. A vast and growing body of work exists which describes two-dimensional cephalometric analysis and dynamic cephalometric treatment planning manipulations. No such morphometric foundation exists for volume visualization. The vast majority of work to date has been directed at simply displaying volume data in a realistic manner. This is clearly of value in cases of serious dentofacial deformity or TMJ pathology but has limited utility in routine clinical orthodontic diagnosis. Sound tools for systematic three-dimensional analysis of volume data have yet to be developed. In this respect three-dimensional morphometrics remains in its infancy.

The realm of volume visualization needs core studies that address many questions that have largely been answered or continue to be answered with respect to cephalometrics. How reliably can anthropometric landmarks be identified and located in a 3D dataset? What are the effects of landmark location error on the reliability of 3D angular and linear measurements? How can volumetric data be represented so that it can easily be manipulated for treatment simulation? What 3D soft tissue changes accompany growth, orthodontics, and orthognathic surgery? Longitudinal samples of radiographic records took decades to accumulate and to provide us with large bodies of growth data and average values for purposes of cephalometric comparison. Scarcely any 3D facial data exist upon which to base volumetric clinical comparisons for diagnostic purposes.

Computed tomography is an invasive means of imaging in that ionizing radiation is used for image acquisition. It is unrealistic to expect that CT images might be acquired for routine orthodontic diagnosis. It is conceivable that CT images might be acquired for cases involving major maxillofacial surgery or evidence of TMJ pathology. Magnetic resonance imaging is noninvasive; no deleterious effects have yet been demonstrated in subjects exposed to the high magnetic fields required for acquisition of MR images. The cost of MRI unfortunately remains prohibitively high for routine orthodontic use, even if a comprehensive means of morphometric analysis is available.

The computing power required to perform volume visualization and future methods of three-dimensional treatment simulation is significantly greater than that afforded by current personal computer technology. It is anticipated, however, that emerging processors, computer architectures, and graphics technologies will put exceedingly powerful machines at our fingertips and within our budgets in the near future.

Summary

The emergence and refinement of computer applications in orthodontics has paralleled the migration of computing to the desktop. Processing power was embodied in expensive mainframe computers during the 1960s, and orthodontic applications were limited to those institutions that could afford such a computer and the programmers to write software for it. The minicomputer brought computing capabilities to a wider group of orthodontic researchers during the 1970s, although possession of these machines was still largely restricted to institutions. The advent of inexpensive personal computers in the late 1970s and 1980s served to distribute computing power to a much wider group of software developers and users, resulting in a proliferation of applications. More powerful and graphically capable machines will inevitably be developed at concomitantly declining costs. It is highly likely that demand will continue to grow among clinicians, researchers, and training programs for advanced diagnostic, treatment planning, and patient education software applications.

The tendency is to become greatly enamored with computer technology. Computers are wonderful devices for generating numbers and can easily produce more purely analytic information for a given case than is ever likely to be acquired through manual methods. Rather than increasing our reliance on numerical interpretation of dentofacial characteristics, cephalometric software applications should serve simply as tools to facilitate the radiographic portion of diagnosis and treatment planning for the wide variety of cases that are routinely faced. The clinician might wish to evaluate an adult or surgical case in a manner that differs greatly from that of a growing adolescent. Cephalometric applications diminish the time required to perform cephalometric determinations and as a result increase the time available for careful reflection on all essential elements of the diagnostic and treatment planning process, especially patient concerns and clinical examination.

Diagnostic and treatment planning applications should in no way replace or supplant the professional opinion of qualified practitioners. A computer program is a set of instructions dutifully carried out by obedient silicon. Software tools for developing applications incorporating artificial intelligence have fallen far short of the expectations of a decade ago. Computer generation of rigidly interpreted *cookbook* treatment plans are in the author's opinion a disservice to practitioners and patients alike and serve to diminish much of what is espoused through graduate-level orthodontic training.

However, interesting possibilities are plentiful for the embodiment of orthodontic knowledge in software applications. A great deal of orthodontic wisdom is accumulated through years of clinical experience, tempered by the results of thousands of treated cases. A young clinician, faced with a difficult, ambiguous, borderline treatment planning dilemma might ask, "How would Don Woodside treat this case?" or "How would Bill Proffit manage this?" Talented, experienced clinicians are rarely available for a chairside consultative chat, but it is conceivable that portions of a clinician's collective knowledge and experience might be incorporated into software knowledge modules that could subsequently be selectively queried through the supply of appropriate data. The development of such a system would not, however, be a trivial task.

The purpose of this chapter is to explore three areas of current and emerging computer applications that pertain to orthodontics. The past twenty years have seen a steady evolution of cephalometric applications, culminating in widespread clinical acceptance of computer-aided cephalometrics. These applications are well suited for performing cephalometric analyses but must be used carefully when superimposing serial tracings. Digitization in point mode has advantages over stream mode, especially for soft tissue profile prediction associated with treatment planning manipulations. It is more feasible to implement predictive algorithms for profile changes resulting from orthognathic surgery than from growth, orthopedics, or orthodontic tooth movements.

The issues associated with facial imaging applications are currently being addressed with varying degrees of success and clinical efficacy. Computer-aided facial imaging systems are excellent visualization tools for case presentations and serve a useful purpose in educating patients about possible facial changes. Cephalometric tracings and video images cannot currently be reliably superimposed; hence imaging applications are not refined to a degree that permits detailed treatment planning. Clinicians should exercise great caution when providing image hardcopy of treatment simulations to patients and should counsel patients about the limitations of imaging systems.

The future of diagnostic and treatment planning software lies in applications that represent the face and the dentition in a truly three-dimensional manner. Current methods of representing volume data include surface modeling, voxel volume rendering, and ray casting techniques. Voxel volume rendering methods may introduce spurious features such as pseudoforamina and aliasing into 3D images. Volume rendering is used for visualization of anatomy and pathology, fabrication of surgical models and templates, and simulation of maxillofacial surgery. Volume visualization methods do not yet permit three-dimensional morphometric analysis at a level of usefulness demanded by clinical orthodontics.

The next decade will be one in which the practitioner will see great changes in the methods by which clinicians routinely evaluate and plan treatment for their patients and communicate their ideas to patients, parents, and colleagues. The emergence of more robust software development tools coupled with the onrush of powerful new hardware will stimulate the design and implementation of a new generation of useful orthodontic applications.

REFERENCES

1. Baumrind S, Miller DM: Computer-aided headfilm analysis: the University of California San Francisco method, *Am J Orthod* 78(1):41-65, 1980.

2. Bergin R, Hallenberg J, Malmgren O: Computerized cephalometrics, *Acta Odontol Scand* 36:349-357, 1978.

3. Bhatia SN: A computer-aided design for orthognathic surgery, *Br J Oral Maxillofac Surg* 22(4):237-253, 1984.

4. Bochacki V, Queveda J, Walker R: Comparative analysis of various system configurations for computer-aided cephalometric analysis, *JADR* 71:142, 1992.

5. Brewster LJ, Trivedi SS et al: Interactive surgical planning, *IEEE Comput Graphics Appl* 4(3):31-40, 1984.

6. Christiansen EL, Thompson JR, Kopp S: Intra- and inter-observer variability and accuracy in the determination of linear and angular measurements in computed tomography, *Acta Odont Scand* 44:221-229, 1986.

7. Christiansen HN, Sederberg TW: Conversion of complex contour line definitions into polygonal element meshes, *Comput Graphics* 12(3):187-192, 1978.

8. Cline HE, Lorensen WE et al: Three-dimensional segmentation of MR images of the head using probability and connectivity, *J Comput Assist Tomogr* 14:1037-1045, 1990.

9. Cutting C, Bookstein FL et al: Three-dimensional computer-assisted design of craniofacial surgical procedures: optimization and interaction with cephalometric and CT-based models, *Plast Reconstr Surg* 77(6):877-885, 1986.

10. Donlon WC, Young P, Vassiliadis A: Three-dimensional computed tomography for maxillofacial surgery: report of cases, *J Oral Maxillofac Surg* 46:142-147, 1988.

11. Drebin RA, Carpenter L, Hanrahan P: Volume rendering, *Comput Graphics* 22(4):65-74, 1988.

12. Faber RD, Burstone CJ, Solonche DJ: Computerized interactive orthodontic treatment planning, *Am J Orthod* 73(1):36-46, 1978.

13. Foley JD, van Dam A, Feiner SK, Hughes JF: *Computer graphics principle pract*, 1990, Addison-Wesley, p. 565.

14. Fuchs H, Kedem ZM, Uselton SP: Optimal surface reconstructions from planar contours, *Comm ACM* 20(10):693-702, 1977.

15. Hemmy DC, David DJ, Herman GT: Three-dimensional reconstruction of craniofacial deformity using computed tomography, *Neurosurgery* 13(5):534-541, 1983.

16. Hemmy DC, Tessier PL: CT of dry skulls with craniofacial deformities: accuracy of three-dimensional reconstruction, *Radiology* 157:113-116, 1985.

17. Herman GT, Liu HK: Three-dimensional display of human organs from computed tomograms, *Comput Graphics Image Process* 9:1-21, 1979.

18. Herman GT, Udupa JK: Display of 3-D digital images: computational foundations and medical applications, *IEEE Comput Graphics Appl* 3(5):39-45, 1983.

19. Hohl TH, Wolford LM: Craniofacial osteotomies: a photocephalometric technique for the prediction and evaluation of tissue changes, *Angle Orthod* 48:114-125, 1978.

20. Jacobson RS: "The reliability of soft tissue profile prediction in orthognathic surgery." Thesis, Northwestern University, 1989.

21. Kaplan EN: 3-D CT images for facial implant design and manufacture, *Clin Plast Surg* 14(4):663-676, 1987.

22. Kursunoglu S, Kaplan P et al: Three-dimensional computed tomographic analysis of the normal temporomandibular joint, *J Oral Maxillofac Surg* 44:257-259, 1986.

23. Levoy M: Display of surfaces from volume data, *IEEE Comput Graphics Appl* 8(3):29-37, 1988.

24. Liu HK: Two- and three-dimensional boundary detection, *Comput Graphics Image Process* 6:123-134, 1977.

25. Lorensen WE, Cline HE: Marching cubes: a high resolution 3D surface construction algorithm, *Comput Graphics* 21(4):163-169, 1987.

26. Margolis HI: A basic facial pattern and its application to clinical orthodontics II. Craniofacial skeletal analysis and dento-craniofacial orientation, *Am J Orthod* 39:425-443, 1993.

27. Marsh JL, Vannier MW et al: Computerized imaging for soft tissue and osseous reconstruction in the head and neck, *Clin Plast Surg* 12(2):279-291, 1985.

28. Moaddab MB, Dumas AL et al: Temporomandibular joint: computed tomographic three-dimensional reconstruction, *Am J Orthod* 88(4):342-352, 1985.

29. Moss JP, Grindrod SR et al: A computer system for the interactive planning and prediction of maxillofacial surgery, *Am J Orthod Dentofac Orthop* 94(6):469-475, 1988.

30. Mostafa YA, El-Mangoury NH et al: Automated cephalographic soft-tissue analysis, *J Clin Orthod* 24(9):539-543, 1990.

31. Motoyoshi M, Namura S, Arai H: A three-dimensional measuring system for the human face using three-directional photography, *Am J Orthod Dentofac Orthoped* 101:431-440, 1992.

32. Phillips C, Greer J et al: Photocephalometry: errors of projection and landmark location, *Am J Orthod* 86(3):233-243, 1984.

33. Ricketts RM et al: *Orthodontic diagnosis and planning: their roles in preventive and rehabilitative dentistry,* 2 vol, Denver, 1982, Rocky Mountain Data Systems.

34. Ricketts RM, Bench RW et al: An overview of computerized cephalometrics, *Am J Orthod* 61:1-28, 1972.

35. Roberts DR, Pettigrew J et al: Three-dimensional imaging and display of the temporomandibular joint, *Oral Surg* 58:461-474, 1984.

36. Sarver DM, Johnston MW: Video imaging in treatment planning and counseling in orthognathic surgery, *J Oral Maxillofac Surg* 46:935-945, 1988.

37. Sarver DM, Johnston MW: Video imaging: techniques for superimposition of cephalometric radiography and profile changes, *Int J Adult Orthod Orthognath Surg* 5:241-248, 1990.

38. Sarver DM, Matukas VJ, Weissman SM: Incorporation of facial plastic surgery in the planning and treatment of orthognathic surgical cases, *Int J Adult Orthod Orthognath Surg* 6:227-239, 1991.

39. Slavicek R: Clinical and instrumental functional analysis for diagnosis and treatment planning. Part 6. Computer-aided diagnosis and treatment planning, *J Clin Orthod* 22(11):718-729, 1988.

40. Solow B: Computers in cephalometric research, *Comput Biol Med* 1:41-49, 1970.

41. Stoker NG, Mankovich NJ, Valentino D: Stereolithographic models for surgical planning: preliminary report, *J Oral Maxillofac Surg* 50:466-471, 1992.

42. Sunguroff A, Greenberg D: Computer generated images for medical applications, *Computer Graphics* 12:196-202, 1978.

43. Toth BA, Ellis DS, Stewart WB: Computer-designed prosthesis for orbitocranial reconstruction, *Plast Reconst Surg* 81(3):315-322, 1988.

44. Totty WG, Vannier MW: Complex musculoskeletal anatomy: analysis using three dimensional surface reconstruction, *Radiology* 150(1):173-177, 1984.

45. Tyndall DA, Renner JB et al: Positional changes of the mandibular

condyle assessed by three-dimensional computed tomography, *J Oral Maxillofac Surg* 50:1164-1172, 1992.

46. Vannier MW, Marsh JL, Warren JO: Three-dimensional CT reconstruction images for craniofacial surgical planning and evaluation, *Radiology* 150(1):179-184, 1984.

47. Walker GF: Cephalometrics and the computer, *J Dent Res* 46:1211, 1967.

48. Walker GF: Summary of a research project on the analysis of craniofacial growth, *NZ Dent J* 63:31-38, 1967.

49. Walker GF: A new approach to the analysis of craniofacial morphology and growth, *Am J Orthod* 61(3):221-230, 1972.

50. Walker GF, Kowalski CJ: Computer morphometrics in craniofacial biology, *Comput Biol Med* 2:235-249, 1972.

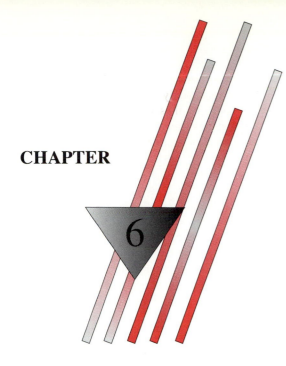

CHAPTER 6

Interceptive Guidance of Occlusion with Emphasis on Diagnosis

JACK G. DALE

As we learn more about growth and its potentials, more about the influences of function on the developing denture, and more about the normal mesiodistal position of the denture in its relation to basal jawbones and head structures, we will acquire a better understanding of when and how to intervene in the guidance of growth processes so that Nature may better approximate her growth plan for the individual patient. In other words, knowledge will gradually replace harsh mechanics, and in the not-too-distant future the vast majority of orthodontic treatment will be carried out during the mixed-dentition period of growth and development and prior to the difficult age of adolescence.[64]

Charles H. Tweed

The term *serial extraction* was first introduced by Kjellgren[34] in 1929. Unfortunately, the phrase that emphasizes extraction has resulted in the indiscriminate removal of a myriad of teeth by individuals who have not appreciated the need for the special knowledge that is required to carry out the procedure successfully. The misconception exists that the procedure is easy because it simply implies the removal of teeth in a serial manner.

Hotz,[30] on the other hand, referred to the procedure as *guidance of eruption*. This is a superior title because it implies that a knowledge of growth and development is necessary to direct the teeth as they erupt into occlusion.

The term *guidance of occlusion* is even more appropriate because clinicians are interested in the final destination of eruption: the occlusion. It is necessary to have a thorough understanding of growth and development with all its ramifications, and it is also essential to be aware of occlusion of the dentition, with its relationship to the craniofacial structures and with function.

Thus this chapter will discuss the serial extraction of the primary teeth in an effort to guide the eruption of the permanent teeth into a favorable occlusion to intercept, in part, the occurrence of a major malocclusion.

When the practitioner is contemplating the correction of an orthodontic problem, the most critical decision to make is whether teeth should be extracted. Even more demanding is adding the dimension of time, complicating that with the

growth and development of the dentition and the craniofacial complex, and carrying out the procedure in a serial manner.

Serial extraction is not easy—as so many mistakenly believe, and it should never be initiated without a comprehensive diagnosis. Teeth may be extracted with the greatest of ease during so-called serial extraction procedures; however, if the basic principles of diagnosis are ignored, the results will be failure and disappointment. Not only will it be injurious to the patient, but subsequently it will be injurious to the reputation of the practitioner and ultimately to the profession.

Unfortunately, since the time that serial extraction was introduced to the profession by Bunon,[14] exactly 250 years ago, it has been grossly misunderstood. Lack of understanding and knowledge has created disastrous results, including a deterioration of the dentition and facial balance. It has been criticized and maligned—unfairly—by individuals who have never used the procedure in practice nor acquired the necessary knowledge that is required to perform it well.

If it is based on a thorough diagnosis and carried out carefully and properly on a select group of patients, the procedure can be an excellent and valuable treatment. It can reduce appliance treatment time, the cost of treatment, discomfort to the patient, potential iatrogenic sequelae and time lost by the patient and the parents.

It is logical to intercept a malocclusion as early as possible and to reduce or, in rare instances, to avoid multibanded mechanotherapy at the sensitive teenage period. Why allow an unfavorable dental, skeletal, or soft tissue relationship to exist for a number of years if it can be corrected, or practically corrected, early, with a minimum of appliance treatment time?

Before attempting the treatment of an orthodontic patient using *guidance of occlusion,* the practitioner must be prepared to meet the challenge of *diagnosis.* Without question, the secret of success in orthodontic treatment is a thorough understanding of diagnosis. The orthodontist can have the most comprehensive and sophisticated treatment plan at work in the patient's mouth; however, if the plan is implemented in the wrong patient, treatment will fail. This chapter will discuss guidance of occlusion with a special emphasis on diagnosis.

The quotation by Charles Tweed at the beginning of this chapter is an interesting statement by a man who devoted over 40 years of his life to the treatment of the permanent dentition and to the development of precision edgewise mechanotherapy, sometimes referred to as "harsh mechanics." However, during the last 13 years of his life he was vitally interested in treatment during the mixed dentition period, including preorthodontic guidance, guidance of occlusion, and serial extraction.

He found, as many others have found, that serial extraction, especially in Class I tooth-size jaw-size discrepancy malocclusions, improves the alignment of the teeth when they emerge into the oral cavity. As a result it creates a better environment "so that Nature may better approximate her growth plan." Tweed also discovered that the interception of dentofacial deformities using "growth and its potentials" and biologic principles rather than "harsh mechanics" was an exhilarating and rewarding experience.

Although mixed dentition treatment has made significant advances in recent years, it will be some time before the "vast majority of orthodontic treatment will be carried out during the mixed dentition period"—completely, that is. Class II, Class III, and the majority of Class I malocclusions, even subsequent to serial extraction, still require a period, albeit a shorter period, of "harsh mechanics" or, at least, precision mechanotherapy to produce a successful and stable treatment result characterized by a high standard of excellence. It must be stressed most emphatically that serial extraction does not replace mechanotherapy. Nevertheless, in a rewarding number of instances it reduces it significantly at the "difficult age of adolescence."

Early consideration of the corrective measures necessary to remedy any type of malocclusion should be the prime concern of modern orthodontics. Whatever method is chosen, a minimum of treatment time should be the goal.[68]

In this day when so much emphasis is being placed on avoiding bands and on *invisible braces,* serial extraction becomes even more important. The best way to hide appliances is not to use them or at least diminish their use. By using the benefits of serial extraction in Class I mal-

occlusions, orthodontists can more fully concentrate on the time-consuming and technically demanding Class II and Class III malocclusions and thus increase their usefulness to their profession and to society.

At the present time malocclusions are being treated in ever increasing numbers by other members of the dental profession; the practice of dentistry is changing and the delivery of orthodontic care is experiencing a transformation. Advances in dental science and preventive procedures have markedly reduced the incidence of caries and the loss of teeth, while the rapid increase in education and the use of auxiliaries has relieved the dentist of traditional duties. As a result dentists are now undertaking a much greater variety of services. When this enlargement of scope and interest goes hand in hand with professional competence, everyone can benefit. If not, the risks to the public may be unfortunate.[10] It is not so important who provides the treatment, but it is important that the orthodontist make a concerted effort to prepare for the responsibility being undertaken. A thorough knowledge of the basic principles of diagnosis and treatment is essential.

Serial extraction has often been criticized as being a *bad* procedure, and it certainly can be more harmful than beneficial if not done properly (Fig. 6-1). The two girls in Figs. 6-2 and 6-3 are both 13 years of age, just at the beginning of adolescence. The girl in Fig. 6-2 has a severe Class I tooth-size jaw-size discrepancy. Her treatment required the extraction of four premolar teeth and 30 months of multibanded mechanotherapy beginning at 13 years of age. The retention period was prolonged because the teeth had been allowed to remain in a crowded irregular relationship for several years. The girl in Fig. 6-3 had a similar malocclusion, but her treatment was completed by 13 years of age. Serial extraction was begun at 8 years, and the multibanded appliance was inserted at 12 years. The retention period was minimal. Thus two girls with similar malocclusions were

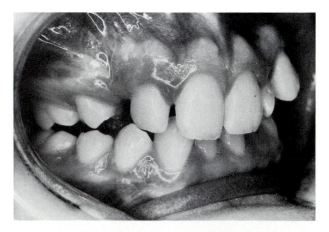

Fig. 6-1   Class II, division 2, malocclusion with an impacted permanent maxillary right canine. During a *bad* serial extraction procedure one mandibular incisor and the maxillary right first premolar were extracted.

treated quite differently. Whereas one was just beginning 30 months of treatment at 13 years of age, the other was already finished and with a more stable result.

The recommended, routine-basis office procedure done before serial extraction treatment is discussed in the following pages.

EXAMINATION AND CONSULTATION

During the course of the first appointment the orthodontist determines whether or not a malocclusion exists. If so, the parents must be familiarized with orthodontic treatment. An explanation (in general terms) of the tentative diagnosis must be given, possible treatment that will be required, time that will be involved, the total cost, and the need for diagnostic records and a case presentation. The appointment should be conducted in a relaxed atmosphere and in privacy. Preferably it takes place in the operatory, with the parents present and the patient seated in the chair.

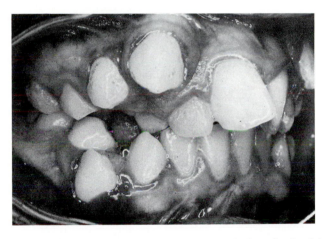

Fig. 6-2   A 13-year-old girl who did not have the benefit of serial extraction and early treatment.

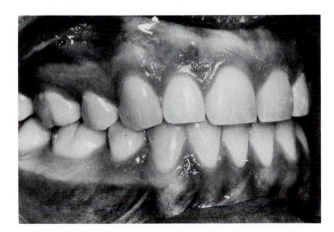

Fig. 6-3   A 13-year-old girl who did have the benefit of serial extraction and early treatment.

DIAGNOSTIC RECORDS

During the second appointment, a complete set of diagnostic records is acquired, including intraoral radiographs, cephalometric radiographs, facial photographs, study models, and intraoral slides of the dentition. Adequate time should be scheduled for doing this, with meticulous care and with as little discomfort and anxiety to the patient as possible. These records are then studied and analyzed in preparation for the case presentation. The objective of taking quality records is to secure clinical accuracy for the purpose of establishing a sound diagnosis.

Intra-oral radiographs

One record that must be obtained before the initiation of serial extraction is the complete series of periapical radiographs or a panoramic radiograph. Can you imagine extracting four first premolar teeth and then discovering that the second premolars are congenitally absent? Dental radiographs must be taken for the

1. Protection of the patient and the orthodontist
2. Detection of congenital absences of teeth
3. Detection of supernumerary teeth
4. Evaluation of the dental health of the permanent teeth, especially the first molars (Fig. 6-4)
5. Detection of pathologic conditions in the early stages
6. Assessment of trauma to the teeth after an injury (Fig. 6-5)
7. Detection of evidence of a true hereditary tooth-size jaw-size discrepancy, such as the resorptive pattern on the mesial of the roots of the primary canines (Fig. 6-6)
8. Determination of the size, shape, and relative position of unerupted permanent teeth
9. Evaluation of the eruptive patterns of unerupted permanent teeth (Fig. 6-7)
10. Determination of dental age of the patient by assessing the length of the roots of permanent un-

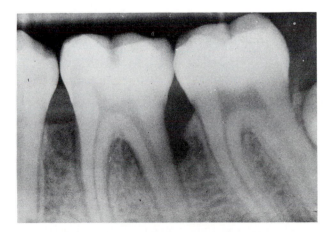

Fig. 6-4   Bone loss surrounding the permanent first molar as a result of periodontal disease.

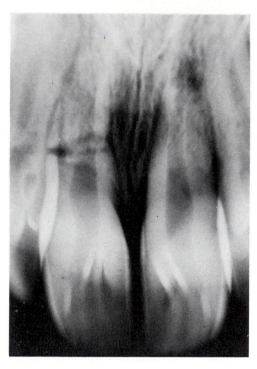

Fig. 6-5   Fractured maxillary left central incisor immediately after an accident. (From Dale JG: *Dent Clin North Am* 26:565, 1982.)

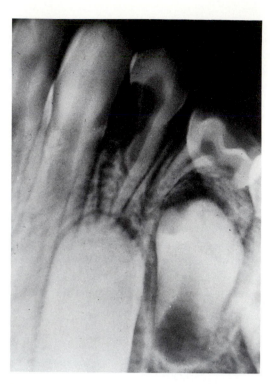

Fig. 6-6   Root resorption of the primary canine as a result of crowded permanent incisors.

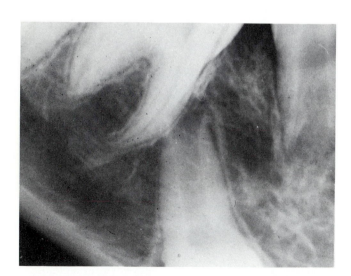

Fig. 6-7   Grotesque eruption pattern of the mandibular second premolar. (From Dale JG: *Dent Clin North Am* 26:565, 1982.)

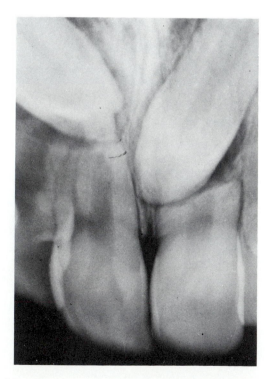

Fig. 6-8   Root resorption of the maxillary central incisors by impacted canines. (From Dale JG: *Dent Clin North Am* 26:565, 1982.)

erupted teeth and the amount of resorption of primary tooth, as in dental age analysis (p. 339) (Figs. 6-89 through 6-96)

11. Calculation of the total space analysis (p. 331) (Figs. 6-75 through 6-88)
12. Detection of root resorption before, during, and after treatment (Fig. 6-8)
13. Evaluation of third molars before, during, and after treatment
14. Final appraisal of the dental health after orthodontic treatment

Cephalometric radiographs

Sound orthodontic treatment, including serial extraction, is based on the intelligent use of cephalometric radiographs and analyses—including the evaluation of numbers. There is absolutely nothing wrong with attempting to assess craniofaciodental discrepancies with the aid of linear and angular measurements. This is a valuable diagnostic technique that demands precision and discipline. To avoid its use because of its weaknesses, in the face of its manifest and manifold virtues, is either to ignore unlimited opportunity for the best service or to shirk supinely an insistent and moral responsibility.

Cephalometric radiographs are used for the following:

1. Evaluation of craniofaciodental relationships before treatment
2. Assessment of the soft tissue matrix
3. Classification of facial patterns (as in the proportional facial analysis) (Figs. 6-14 through 6-27)
4. Calculation of tooth-size jaw-size discrepancies (as in the total space analysis)
5. Determination of mandibular rest position (as in the occlusal curves analysis)
6. Prediction of growth and development
7. Monitoring of skeletodental relationships during treatment
8. Detection of pathologic conditions before, during, and after treatment
9. Assessment of trauma after facial injuries
10. Study of relationships before, immediately following, and several years after treatment for the purpose of long-range improvement in treatment planning

Facial photographs

Fig. 6-9 illustrates the American Board of Orthodontics' requirements for facial photographs.[1]

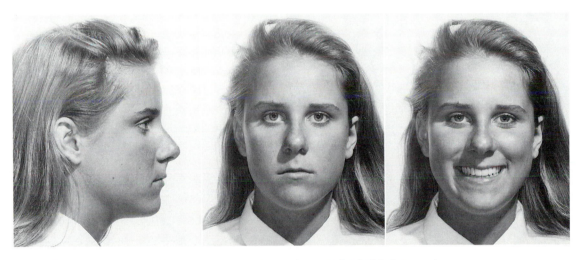

Fig. 6-9   American Board of Orthodontics requirements for facial photographs.

Requirements:

Quality, standardized facial photographic prints either in black and white or color
Patient's head oriented accurately in all three planes of space and in the Frankfort horizontal plane
One lateral view; facing to the right; serious expression; lips closed lightly to reveal muscle imbalance and disharmony
One anterior view; serious expression
Optional: One lateral view and/or one anterior view with lips apart
Optional: One anterior view, smiling
Background free of distractions
Quality lighting revealing facial contours, with no shadows in the background
Ears exposed for purpose of orientation
Eyes open and looking straight ahead; glasses removed

(From American Board of Orthodontics: Specific instructions for candidates, St Louis, 1993.)

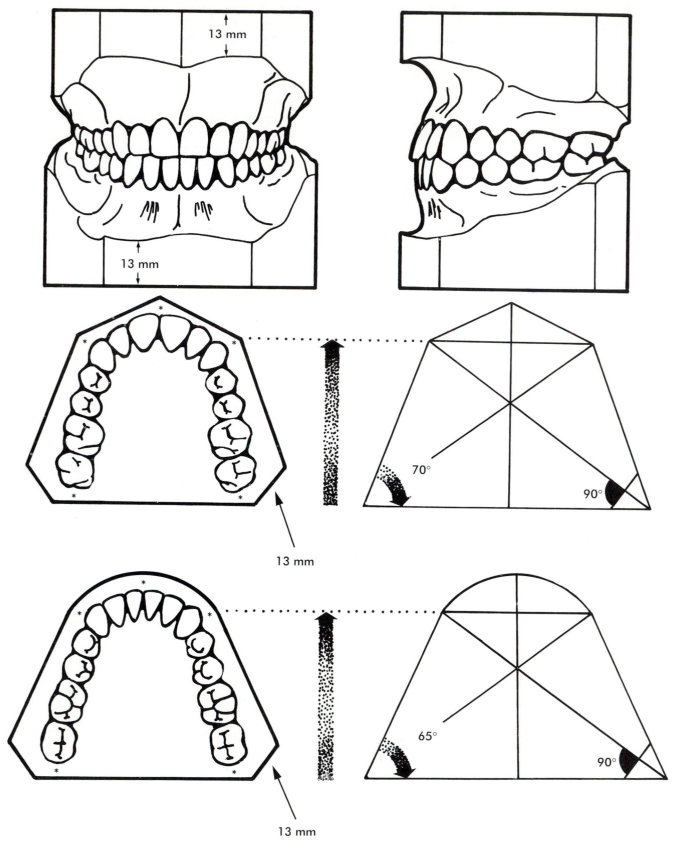

Fig. 6-10 American Board of Orthodontics requirements for study models. (From American Board of Orthodontics: Specific instructions for candidates, St Louis, 1993.)

Facial patterns play an extremely important role in serial extraction. Like cephalometric radiographs they are invaluable in the

1. Evaluation of craniofacial (and dental) relationships and proportions before treatment
2. Assessment of soft tissue profile
3. Proportional facial analysis
4. Total space analysis
5. Occlusal curves analysis
6. Monitoring of treatment progress
7. Study of relationships before, immediately following, and several years after treatment to improve treatment planning

In addition, they are useful for (1) detecting and recording muscle imbalance and balance, (2) detecting and recording facial asymmetry, and (3) identifying patients.

During the case presentation the orthodontist should be careful to point out to parents that treatment is *not* being made to produce a *normal* face. (What does a normal face look like?) Also care should be taken *not* to suggest that treatment is being made to produce an *esthetic* face. Esthetic appreciation is personal and subjective. Most parents will not admit that a need exists for improvement in esthetics, even if they believe the contrary. The prime objective of treatment in relation to the face should be the creation of harmony and balance: a favorable, proportionate relationship between the teeth, skeletal pattern, and soft tissue matrix, including the profile.

Study models

Fig. 6-10 illustrates the American Board of Orthodontics' requirements for study models.[1]

Study models provide a three-dimensional record of the dentition and are essential for many reasons. They are used to

1. Calculate total space analysis (If for no other reason they should be taken for this invaluable diagnostic procedure.)
2. Assess and record the dental anatomy
3. Assess and record the intercuspation
4. Assess and record arch form
5. Assess and record the curves of occlusion (occlusal curves analysis)
6. Evaluate occlusion, with the aid of articulators
7. Measure progress during treatment
8. Detect abnormalities (e.g., localized enlargements, distortion of arch form)
9. Provide a record before, immediately after, and several years following treatment for the purpose of studying treatment procedures

Intra-oral photographs

Fig. 6-11 illustrates the American Board of Orthodontics requirements for intraoral photographs.[1]

Treatment could be performed without the use of color transparencies of the dentition. However, they are extremely valuable for one reason: to record for future reference the structure of the enamel. This is particularly important when bands or brackets are removed. It is quite possible that the orthodontist could be accused of producing decalcification, or an imperfection in the enamel, that was already present before treatment was begun. Intraoral photographs add the dimension of color to the records, which aids in assessing and recording the health or disease of the teeth and soft tissue structures.

With regard to serial extraction, photographs allow the clinician to record the steps in the technique, frequently without making study models. This is important for self-evaluation and for discussion with students and colleagues.

Finally, photographs complete the records that may be taken before, immediately following, and several years after treatment for the purpose of assessing treatment methods.

CASE PRESENTATION

The case presentation includes a detailed description of all aspects of treatment with the aid of the patient's own diagnostic records. Both the parents and the child are present, again in a relaxed atmosphere and in the privacy of the office. This appointment affords the orthodontist an opportunity to explain certain basic principles associated with treatment.

The cause or causes, diagnosis, treatment plan, and prognosis are outlined. For example, serial extraction may be explained as a procedure that has been in existence for 250 years[14] and is based on the fact that arch length does not increase. Growth and development do not provide for an increase in the existing arch length but provide space for the unerupted second and third molars to the posterior of the visible dentition. If crowding exists at 8 years of age, it will increase with time.

The case presentation can be one of the most valuable, most rewarding, and most enjoyable appointments that are scheduled throughout treatment. The orthodontist is obliged to sit down and study the malocclusion, set objectives, and discuss all aspects of treatment with the parents and the patient. It constitutes the only opportunity in many instances to meet with the parents, especially the father, and to stress that the treatment must be a group effort. It creates a better understanding, reduces misconception, ensures greater cooperation, and in general provides for smoother more enjoyable treatment. It is one of the most important, positive, and effective office procedures that an orthodontist can employ in promoting good public relations and a favorable image of the specialty.

DIAGNOSIS

To differentiate, categorize, and treat specifically and successfully on a routine basis requires an understanding of the fundamental principles of diagnosis. Several analyses related to the face and teeth will be discussed. These examples

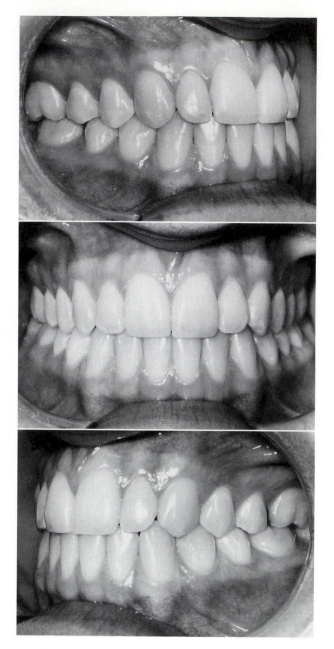

Fig. 6-11   American Board of Orthodontics requirements for intra-oral photographs.

Requirements:

Quality, standardized intraoral prints in color
Patient's dentition oriented accurately in all three planes of space
One frontal view in maximum intercuspation
Two lateral views—right and left
Optional: Two occlusal views—maxillary and mandibular
Free of distractions—check retractors, labels, and fingers
Quality lighting revealing anatomical contours and free of shadows
Tongue retracted
Free of saliva and/or bubbles
Dentition clean

(From American Board of Orthodontics: *Specific instructions for candidates*, St Louis, 1993, The Board.)

of the procedures should be done if treatment is to be successful and serial extraction effective.

The face

Duncan says in *Macbeth**
There's no art to find the mind's construction in the face.

However, several arts and sciences are concerned with the construction of the face, and one of these is orthodontics.

The human face is a living mirror held out to the world. Natural, marked, painted, or adorned, it has the power to attract, charm, captivate, brighten, or seduce. Individuals of the past and present—including natives, warriors, athletes, and performers—in their efforts to be noticed or to conform to caste systems, religious rituals, tribal ceremonies, and social functions, have all adorned or mutilated the face.[67]

To help the reader identify characters, novelists often build word pictures of the face. For instance, Irving Stone[61] in his book *The Origin,* a biographical novel of Charles Darwin, describes the character John Henslow in this manner:

He was . . . the most handsome, pleasure-giving face in all Cambridge. He had a big head, a mop of soft, richly textured black hair, long and full sideburns down to the jawbone. The heroic forehead was high, broad, strong, and bold features toned down by the personal modesty of the man: wide-spaced, general but all consuming eyes, arching eyebrows, ample but non-assertive mouth and mildly dimpled chin with the clean, finely textured sun-bronzed skin of the outdoors man.

You undoubtedly have heard the expression "I may forget a name but I never forget a face." Probably nothing fascinates a person more than the sight of another human face. One of the first images recognized by an infant is its mother's face, and throughout life the brain's memory center identifies individuals by their particular facial features more than by the features of any other part of the body.

According to Angle[2]
The study of orthodontia is indissolubly connected with that of art as related to the human face. The mouth is a most potent factor in making or marring the beauty and character of the face and the form and beauty of the mouth largely depend on the occlusal relationship of the teeth. Our duties as orthodontists force upon us great responsibilities and there is nothing in which the student of orthodontia can be more keenly interested in than art generally, and especially in its relation to the human face, for each of his efforts, whether he realizes it or not, makes for beauty or ugliness, for harmony or disharmony, or for the perfection or deformity of the face. Hence, it should be one of his life's studies.

According to a chapter entitled "Childhood Facial Growth and Development," written by Donald Enlow and me in the textbook *Oral Histology: Development, Structure, and Function,*[63] facial patterns have changed throughout evolution, just as they can drastically change throughout the development of the individual. The human face is unusual compared to most other mammalian faces. It lacks an elongated graceful snout and muzzle flowing back onto a streamlined neurocranium. Instead, humans possess a large rounded head with rather bizarre combinations of facial features. Extraordinarily wide, flat, and vertical, the human face has a forehead above a small razor-thin fleshy proboscis and a chin below. Owl-like orbits point nearly straight forward, and a tiny mouth rests between muzzle-less jaws. No one knows for certain what factors initiated the evolutionary chain leading to the face of modern humans, although a number of hypotheses have been set forth. Brachiation and the development of a huge brain have been suggested as possible factors leading to changes and adaptations. Although the precise evolutionary sequence of the face is speculative, the anatomic consequences and the functional and developmental relationships involved are fairly well understood. This knowledge is important; it helps to explain inherent tendencies toward malocclusion and provides an insight into the causes of developmental abnormalities, including crowding of the dentition.

The human body has made many adaptations to its upright stance, some of which are reflected in the skull and face. Together with the awesome enlargement of the human cerebral hemispheres, marked flexure of the cranial floor has occurred; this contrasts sharply with the flat basal cranium of other mammals. Rather than projecting horizontally, the spinal cord has become vertically disposed and the brain and foramen magnum are positioned at the ventral rather than the posterior aspect of the skull. The orbits, however, still point in the horizontal direction of body movement because of the cranial base flexure. The bipedal posture has freed the arms and led to the development of hands with dexterous fingers. Stereoscopic vision and the lack of an elongated muzzle allow humans to see and manipulate close objects. The defensive, offensive, and vocational functions of the jaws have been taken over by the hands. The decreased relative size of the human jaws has thereby not presented a threat to survival. The mammal's sizable snout with its thermoregulatory function has been replaced by a nearly hairless integument containing many sweat glands and an elaborate vasomotor control system for heat loss and retention capabilities.

Several interrelated factors have contributed to the vertical disposition of the human face. These involve increases or decreases in the relative sizes of facial regions and, also, a series of anatomic rotations of the facial and cranial parts. The sizable enlargement of the frontal lobes of the cerebrum accommodates the addition of a bulging vertical forehead above the face. The supraorbital rims have rotated to an upright position overlying the anterior orbital rims. At the

---

*Act I, Scene 4, Lines 12 and 13.

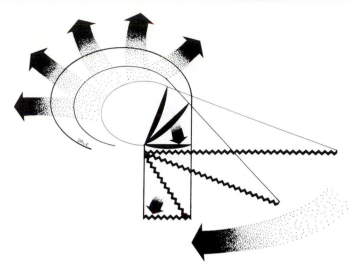

Fig. 6-12 Progression from the mammalian to the human cranium. As the cerebral hemispheres enlarge (outwardly directed arrows), the olfactory bulbs (black saucer shapes) rotate from the obliquely vertical position of the typical mammal to the horizontal position of the human. In almost all mammals (including humans) the nasomaxillary complex (triangle formed by solid and zigzag lines) projects in a perpendicular direction from the olfactory bulbs. Thus as the bulbs become displaced horizontally, the human face becomes upright in alignment. To provide a horizontal occlusal plane, a new compartment (the suborbital region), occupied by the maxillary sinus, was added to the human maxilla, thus lowering the occlusion into a functional position. (From Dale JG: In Ten Cate AR et al: *Oral histology: development, structure, and function,* St Louis, 1980, Mosby.)

same time a forward rotation of the lateral orbital rims has occurred ahead of the greatly enlarged frontal and temporal lobes of the cerebrum. The composite result is a vertically aligned set of orbits pointed nearly straight forward. The massive enlargement of the cerebrum also relates to another key rotation: the olfactory bulbs and the floor of the anterior cranial fossa have been displaced from their typical obliquely upright position to a distinctively horizontal one (Fig. 6-12). This change has had a major rotational effect on the whole nasomaxillary complex, because the nasomaxilla in humans is directly continuous with the anterior cranial fossa and is articulated to it by sutures. As a functional generalization, the snout of a mammal points in a direction essentially perpendicular to the olfactory bulbs. With the downward rotational displacement of the olfactory bulbs from a nearly vertical to a horizontal plane, and the olfactory nerves from horizontal to vertical, the fleshy proboscis of the human face with its downward-directed nares ushers air inflow toward the ceiling of the nasal chambers. Because of the rotation of the olfactory bulbs and sensory nerves, the nerve endings are located in the roof of the nasal chamber rather than in its posterior wall, as in other mammals. The nasomaxillary complex has correspondingly become rotated downward and backward into an upright rather

than a horizontal position. Significantly, dental arch length has been reduced. Because of the orbital rotation toward the midline, often referred to as biorbital convergence, the anatomic region between the eyes has undergone a reduction in size. This region houses the root of the nose, which is markedly thinner. A nose with a more narrow base must be less prominent. As the snout becomes reduced, jaw prominence and the maxillary dental arch length also are reduced since the nasal and oral regions share a common bony palate. The composite of all these various rotations, brain enlargements, facial reductions, and realignment adaptations has produced a wide, flat, and vertically disposed face and has contributed to the anatomic basis for the various malocclusions that can occur in the human face, including tooth-size jaw-size discrepancies.

The infant's face is not simply a miniature of the adult's face (Fig. 6-13). The linkage of the terms *growth* and *development* indicates that the enlargement of the face involves more than the progressive increases in size. Growth is a differential process, in which some parts enlarge more or less than others and in a multitude of directions. It is a gradual maturational process taking many years and requiring a succession of changes in regional proportions and the relationships of various parts. Many localized alterations occur that are associated with a continuous process of soft and hard tissue remodeling. An understanding of the mechanisms of growth and development of the face is essential to the practice of dentistry. To achieve this understanding, it is necessary to have some knowledge of faces.

Three essential processes bring about the growth and development of the various cranial and facial bones: size increase, remodeling, and displacement. The first two are closely related and are produced simultaneously by a combination of bony resorption and deposition. The third process, displacement, is a movement of all the bones away from one another in their articular junctions as each undergoes a size increase. It must be understood that these various growth processes occur more or less simultaneously. Normal growth is imbalanced and therefore progressive and, quite noticeably, alterations in facial form and pattern take place. These differential growth processes not only produce a wide range of topographic facial variations but also constitute the developmental basis for malocclusions and congenital facial abnormalities. To control and use the complex processes of growth in clinical procedures, it is essential that dentists understand the various concepts.

Proportional Facial Analysis

The proportional facial analysis is basically a classification of facial patterns based on the Steiner,[60] the Merrifield and Tweed cephalometric analyses,[43,65] and especially on the counterpart analysis of Enlow.[20] It includes an evaluation of the following relationships (Fig. 6-14, *A*):

Anterior cranial base *(1, 2)*
Posterior cranial base *(2, 3)*

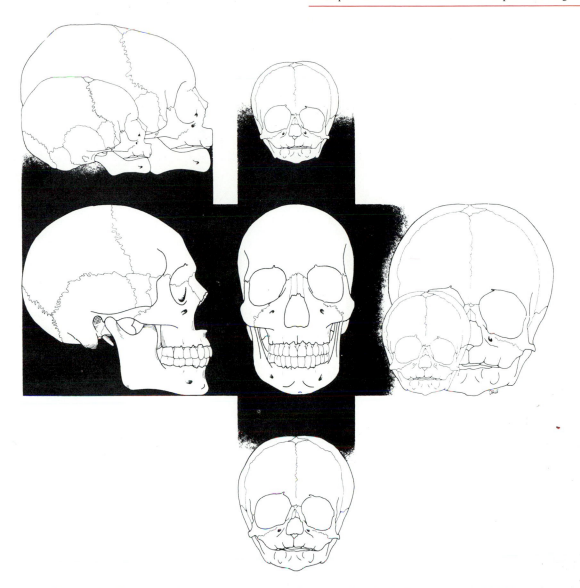

Fig. 6-13 Changes in facial proportions throughout growth and development from infancy to maturity. To show the regional differences in height, depth, and breadth, the newborn skull has been enlarged to the same size as the adult skull. (From Dale JG: In Ten Cate AR et al: *Oral histology: development, structure, and function*, St Louis, 1980, Mosby.)

Cranial base angle *(1, 2, 3)*
Ramus of the mandible *(3, 4)*
Corpus of the mandible *(4, 5)*
Gonial angle *(3, 4, 5)*
Nasomaxillary complex *(6, 7, 8, 9)*
Maxillary dentition *(10, 11)*
Mandibular dentition *(12, 13)*

PM (posterior maxillary plane) is possibly the most significant plane in the craniofacial complex. It delineates, naturally, the various anatomic counterparts and is a developmental interface between the series of counterparts in front of and behind it. It thus retains a number of basic relationships throughout the growth process.

Anterior to *PM* are the following:
a, Frontal lobe of the brain
b, Anterior cranial fossa
c, Anterior cranial base
d, Nasomaxillary complex
e, Maxillary dentition
f, Mandibular dentition
g, Corpus of the mandible
Posterior to *PM* are the following:
h, Temporal lobe of the brain
i, Middle cranial fossa
j, Posterior cranial base
k, Posterior oropharyngeal space
l, Ramus of the mandible

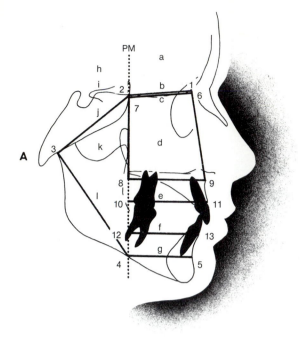

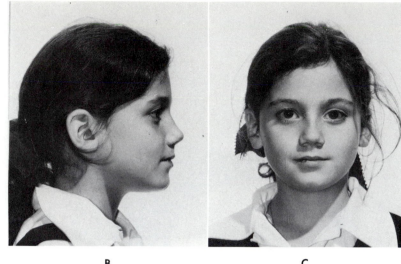

Fig. 6-14 Standard or orthognathic facial pattern. **A,** The basic units associated with the proportional facial analysis. **B** and **C,** The patient.

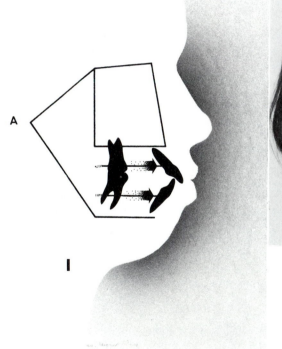

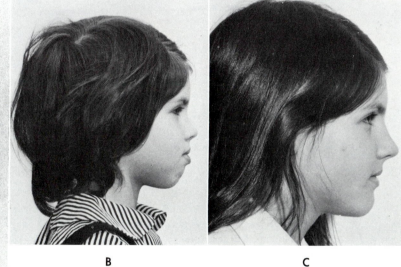

Fig. 6-15 **A,** Class I, maxillary mandibular alveolodental protrusion. **B,** Before treatment. **C,** After treatment. Note the improvement in facial harmony, balance, and proportion.

The standard. The standard or orthognathic face, as seen in Fig. 6-14, *B* and *C,* exhibits a harmonious relationship between the facial structures and the cranium, between the maxilla and the mandible, between the maxilla and the maxillary dentition, between the mandible and the mandibular dentition, between the maxillary dentition and the mandibular dentition, and between the soft tissue profile and the underlying hard tissue structures ("the mesiodistal position of the denture in its relation to the basal jawbones and head structures").[64]

Alveolodental protrusion

Class I: maxillary mandibular alveolodental protrusion (Fig. 6-15). Both the maxillary and the mandibular dentitions are relatively forward and the teeth are in a Class I relationship. This facial pattern, in general, responds well to extraction and, when caution is exercised, to serial extraction.

Class II: maxillary alveolodental protrusion (Fig. 6-16). The maxillary dentition is relatively forward and the teeth are in a Class II relationship, but everything else is favor-

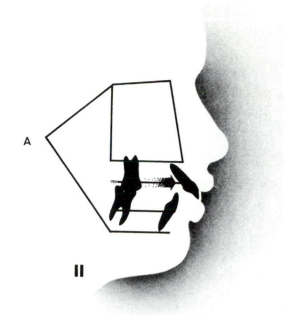

able. Routinely this malocclusion can be treated by the extraction of two maxillary first premolars and by serial extraction in the maxilla only.

Class III. In the interest of brevity and relevance the Class III category of this analysis will not be included in the discussion. Class III malocclusions are not suitable for serial extraction procedures. Mixed dentition Class III treatment is a complicated undertaking. It is often extensive and prolonged and may have to be repeated. Concerning this type of malocclusion, Tweed[65] has said:

> *The size of the orthodontist's heart and his inherent decency have much to do with the success or failure of such treatment.*

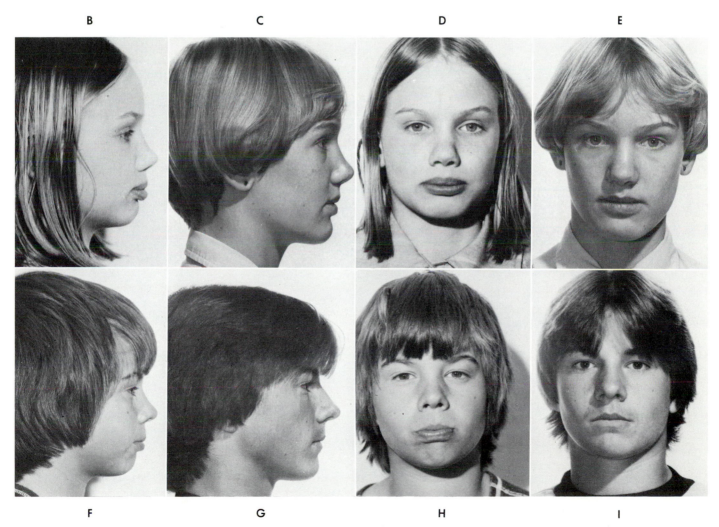

Fig. 6-16 **A,** Class II, maxillary alveolodental protrusion. Note the improvement in muscle balance in both instances. **B** and **D,** Before treatment. **C** and **E,** After treatment. **F** and **H,** Before treatment. **G** and **I,** After treatment.

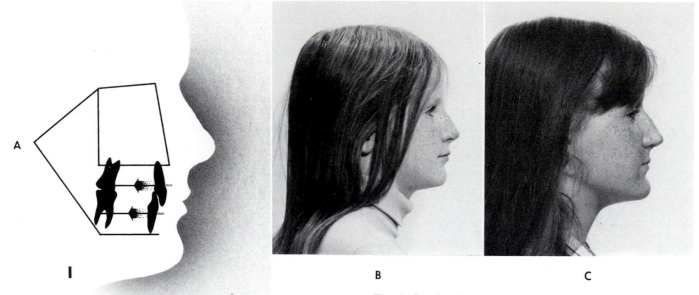

Fig. 6-17   **A,** Class I, maxillary mandibular alveolodental retrusion. **B,** Before treatment. **C,** After treatment. Note the concave nature of the profile in spite of nonextraction treatment.

Fig. 6-18   **A,** Class II, mandibular alveolodental retrusion. **B** and **D,** Before treatment. **C** and **E,** After treatment. Note the subtle improvement in the lower lip area as a result of uprighting the mandibular incisors.

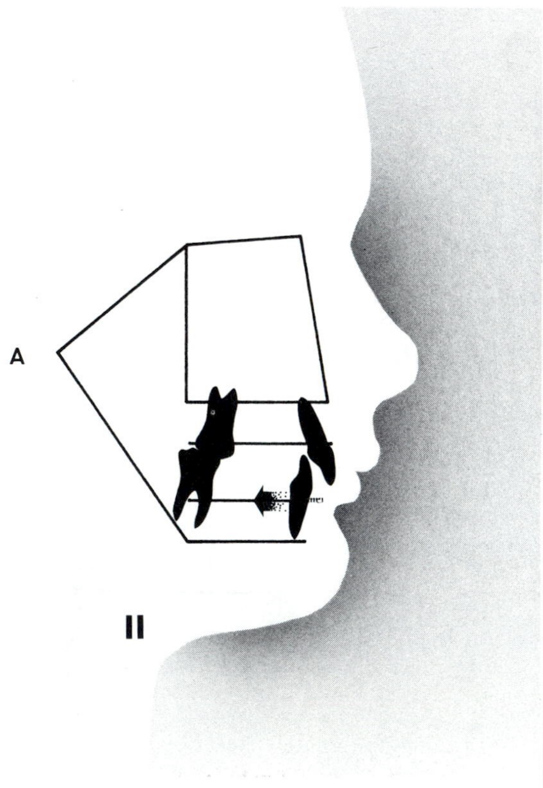

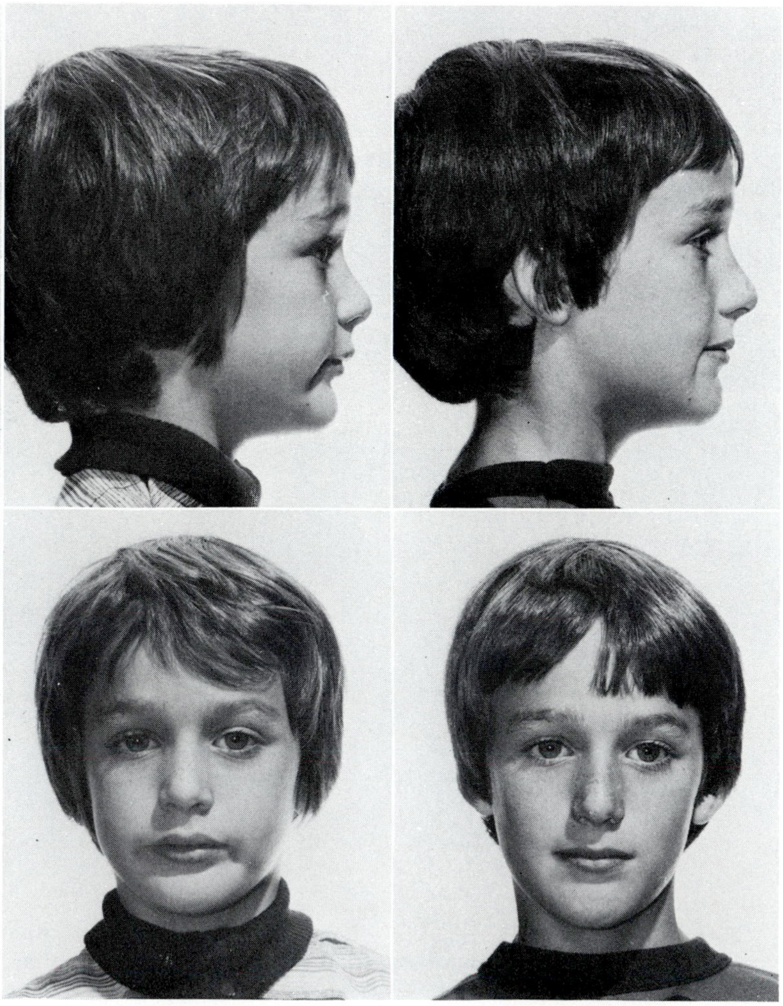

Alveolodental retrusion

Class I: maxillary mandibular alveolodental retrusion
(Fig. 6-17). Both the maxillary and the mandibular dentitions are relatively back and the teeth are in a Class I relationship. The orthodontist must be particularly careful in
the treatment of this type of facial pattern. If possible, treatment should be done without the extraction of teeth. This
appearance can be seen in individuals who have had no
orthodontic treatment and in patients who have had treatment with extractions and without. A *dished-in face* cannot
always be avoided, regardless of the treatment. This patient
was treated without extractions.

Class II: mandibular alveolodental retrusion (Fig. 6-
18). The mandibular dentition is relatively back and the
teeth are in a Class II relationship. Again, the practitioner
must be careful about extracting teeth in this type of facial
pattern. This patient was treated by a functional appliance
followed by Tweed edgewise mechanotherapy without the
extraction of teeth.

Prognathism

Class I: maxillary mandibular prognathism (Fig. 6-19).
In maxillary mandibular prognathism both jaws are relatively forward and the teeth are in a Class I relationship.
Quite often this is a most esthetic facial pattern. Many
motion picture stars exhibit this type of profile. If the teeth
are severely crowded, serial extraction should be performed.
However, because of the increase in the size of the jaws,
extractions are not always indicated.

Class II: maxillary prognathism (Figs. 6-20 and 6-21).
In maxillary prognathism the maxilla is relatively forward
and the teeth are in a Class II relationship. This relationship
may be because the maxilla itself is forward (Fig. 6-20) or
it may be due to a long anterior cranial base. Also the cranial
base angle may be relatively flat, creating a downward and
forward position of the nasomaxillary complex (Fig. 6-21).
This, in turn, may rotate the mandible down and back. These
are difficult Class II malocclusions to treat and certainly
demand more than serial extraction. They are complicated

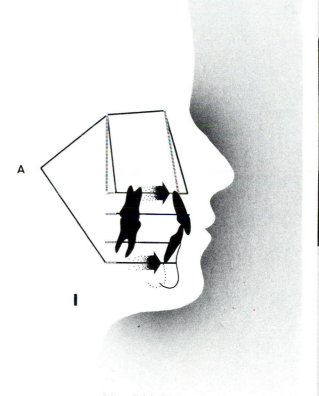
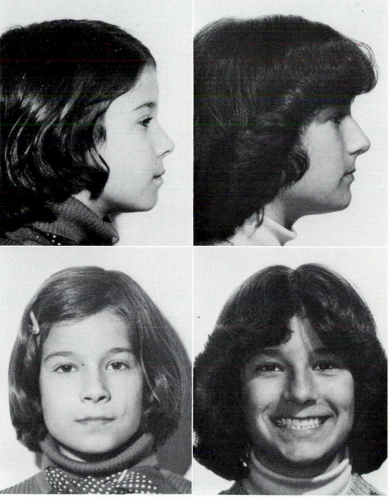

Fig. 6-19 **A,** Class I, maxillary mandibular prognathism. **B** and **D,** Patient before treatment, **C** and **E,** After
treatment.

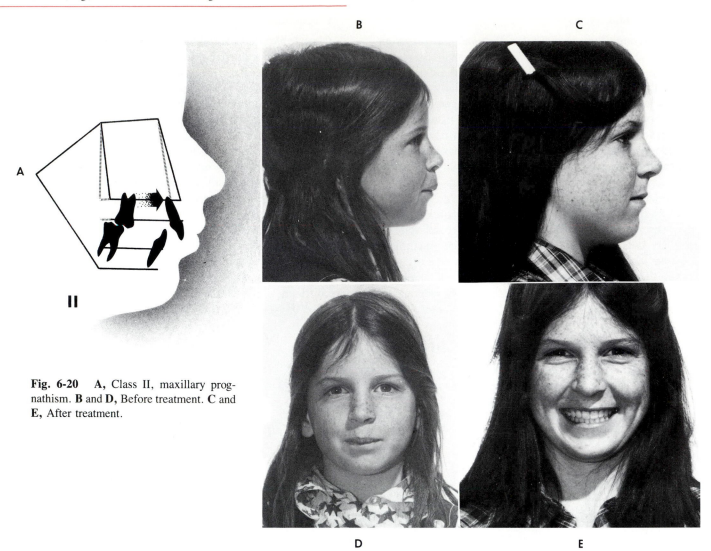

Fig. 6-20   **A,** Class II, maxillary prognathism. **B** and **D,** Before treatment. **C** and **E,** After treatment.

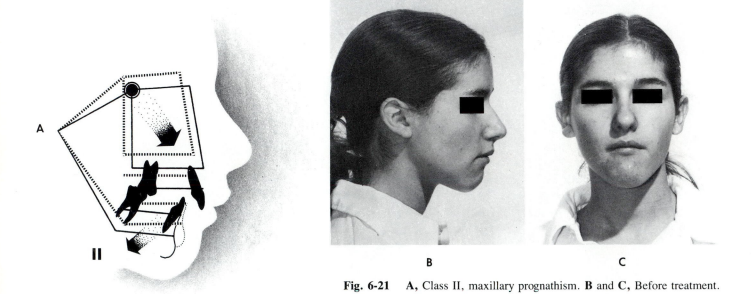

Fig. 6-21   **A,** Class II, maxillary prognathism. **B** and **C,** Before treatment.

skeletal discrepancies that may require not only comprehensive multibanded mechanotherapy but also surgical intervention. *Midface protrusions,* as they are sometimes called, are difficult profiles to correct satisfactorily by orthodontic treatment alone. The nose, at the end of treatment, often is relatively prominent.

Retrognathism

Class I: maxillary mandibular retrognathism (Fig. 6-22). In Class I malocclusions of this type both the maxilla and the mandible are relatively back in relation to the other craniofacial structures. It is difficult to produce a favorable profile in these patients because of the lack of horizontal growth and the recessive nature of their profiles. Every effort should be made to encourage a forward development of the jaws. However, this is difficult because the dentition is in a Class I relationship. Over a long time such a profile can become relatively more recessive and, if serial extraction is being done, the orthodontist could be saddled with the blame. It is extremely important to explain to the parents

during the case presentation that this patient appears to have an unfavorable growth pattern that may get worse regardless of treatment.

Class II: mandibular retrognathism (Figs. 6-23 through 6-25). In Class II malocclusions of this type the mandible is relatively back. It may be that the corpus of the mandible is relatively small (Fig. 6-23) or that the ramus is relatively narrow. The gonial angle may be proportionately acute (Fig. 6-24). There may be excessive vertical development in the nasomaxillary complex (Fig. 6-25). This, in turn, rotates the mandible down and back, producing a retrognathic mandible and a tendency to open bite. If this is the cause of the retrognathic mandible, the treatment of preference may be surgery or, if less extreme, extraction of the permanent molars. Regardless, a patient with this facial pattern is not a good candidate for serial extraction. McNamara[40] found the most common characteristic of Class II malocclusions to be a retrognathic mandible with excessive vertical development.

According to the proportional facial analysis, a Class I

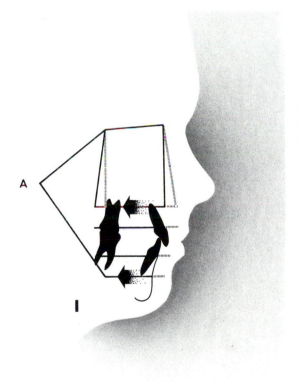

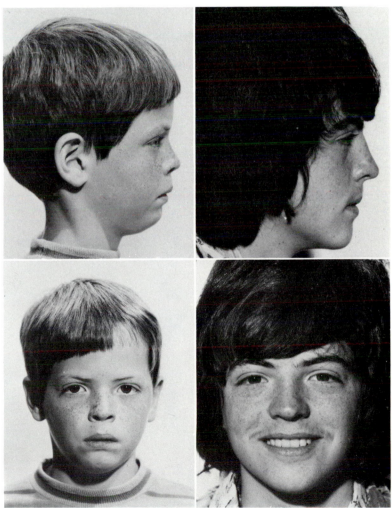

Fig. 6-22   A, Class I, maxillary mandibular retrognathism. **B** and **D,** Before treatment, **C** and **E,** After treatment.

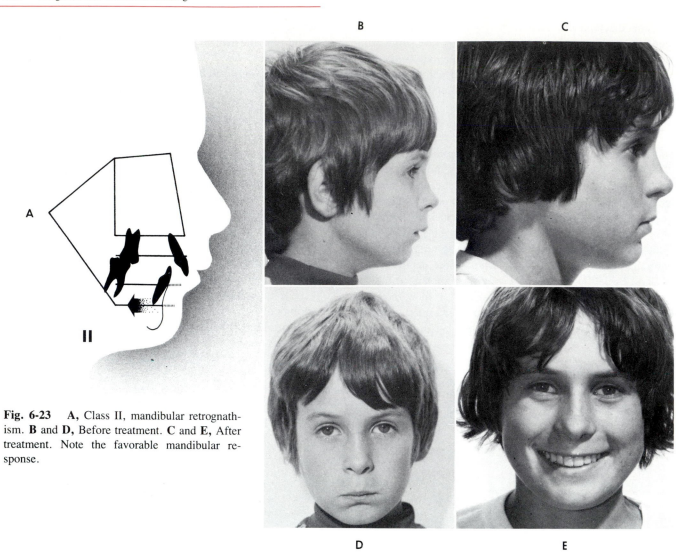

Fig. 6-23   **A,** Class II, mandibular retrognathism. **B** and **D,** Before treatment. **C** and **E,** After treatment. Note the favorable mandibular response.

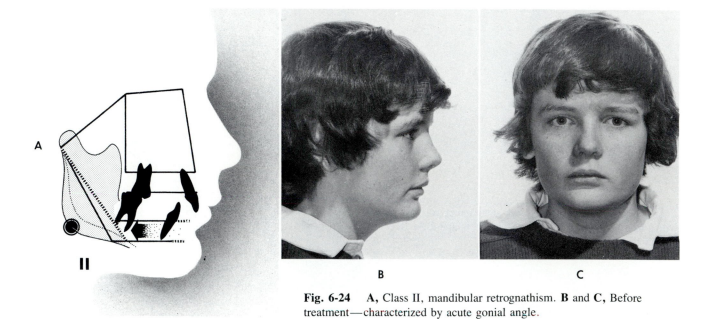

Fig. 6-24   **A,** Class II, mandibular retrognathism. **B** and **C,** Before treatment—characterized by acute gonial angle.

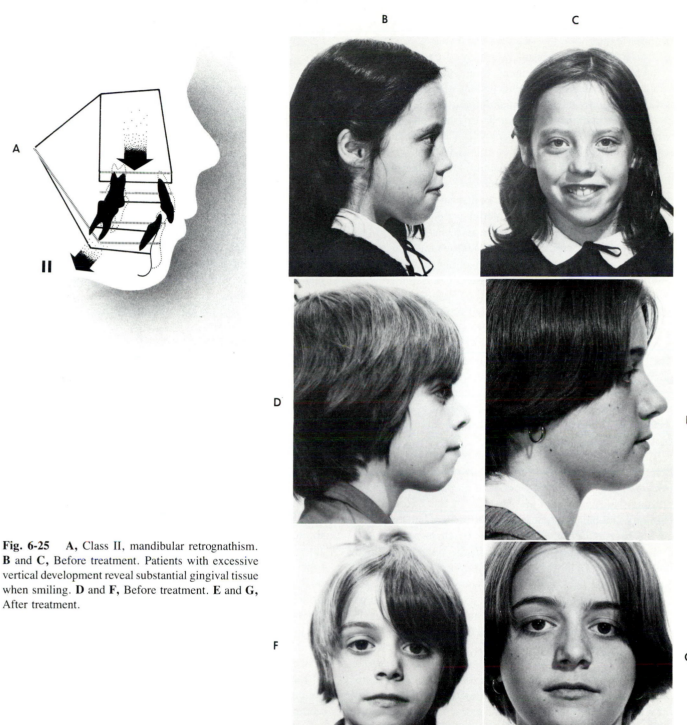

Fig. 6-25   A, Class II, mandibular retrognathism. **B** and **C,** Before treatment. Patients with excessive vertical development reveal substantial gingival tissue when smiling. **D** and **F,** Before treatment. **E** and **G,** After treatment.

malocclusion could be associated with a facial pattern that is characterized by a maxillary mandibular alveolodental protrusion, a maxillary mandibular alveolodental retrusion, a maxillary mandibular prognathism, a maxillary mandibular retrognathism (even orthognathism), or a combination of these features.

It is evident from this analysis that to treat all Class I malocclusions in the same manner would not be using sound clinical judgment. Class I malocclusions with excessive vertical development of the nasomaxillary area might be better treated by extraction of the four first molars rather than by serial extraction followed by removal of the four first premolars (Fig. 6-136).

Similarly a Class II malocclusion could be the result of a maxillary alveolodental protrusion; a mandibular alveolodental retrusion; a prognathic maxilla caused by a forward nasomaxillary complex, long anterior cranial base, or relatively flat cranial base angle; a retrognathic mandible caused by a short corpus, narrow ramus, acute gonial angle, and excessive vertical development of the nasomaxillary complex; or a combination of these features.

It is even more evident that serious thought should be given serial extraction in Class II malocclusions. It aids in the correction of tooth-size jaw-size discrepancy but not necessarily in the correction of a Class II relationship. Therefore the orthodontist must be prepared to place appliances for an extended time. The diagnosis is particularly important because permanent teeth other than the four first premolars may be extracted in the treatment of these malocclusions, referred to later in the discussion of total space analysis (pp. 328 to 339).

The proportional facial analysis describes clearly the multifactorial basis for malocclusion. It also explains how *compensation* may occur to prevent or minimize a discrepancy. A patient's facial pattern may include a Class I profile with harmony and balance that is the result of a relatively small cranial base angle (which is a Class III characteristic) and a short corpus (which is a Class II characteristic). Since both the maxilla and the mandible tend toward retrognathism, the profile that results is in balance. Similarly, a *combination* of factors could result in a more severe malocclusion. A patient might have a Class I malocclusion as a result of excessive vertical development (a Class II characteristic) and a large gonial angle (a Class III characteristic). However, in this instance the two factors would not balance one another but would combine to make the malocclusion more severe. This Class I dentition would not be a good candidate for premolar extraction or for serial extraction (Fig. 6-136).

High angle (hyperdivergent[58]) (Fig. 6-26). This facial pattern includes a steep mandibular plane and is usually associated with a prognathic maxilla, a retrognathic mandible, a maxillary mandibular alveolodental protrusion, an open bite relationship of the incisor teeth, an incompetent lip relationship, a long sloping forehead with a heavy glabella and supraorbital rims, an aquiline or Roman nose that is long and thin, and a flattened recessive chin exhibiting mus-

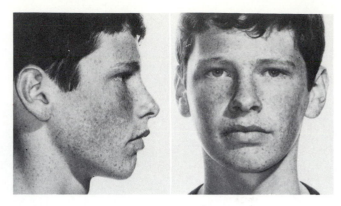

Fig. 6-26 High angle facial pattern.

cle tension. Cephalometrically the mandibular plane to S-N angle is greater than 32° in the Steiner analysis. The FMA is greater than 25° in Tweed analysis. Additional features include dolichocephalic head form, leptoprosopic facial form, large gonial angle, short ramus, small coronoid process, antegonial notching, long anterior face height, short posterior face height, long lower face height relative to upper face height, large cranial base angle (which is responsible for a downward and forward position of the nasomaxillary complex), and a downward and backward position of the mandible. This, in turn, contributes to a steep occlusal plane and frequently to an exaggerated curve of occlusion. The following are characteristic: microgenia, narrow and long symphysis, high and narrow palate, tooth-size jaw-size discrepancy caused by relatively large teeth, impacted third molars, small interincisal angle, overerupted incisors in spite of an open bite tendency, convex soft tissue profile, weak masseter muscles situated posterior to the buccal teeth and producing an anterior component of force, weak temporal muscles, restricted pharyngeal space with the tongue forward, mouth breathing, narrow nasal apertures, vertical mandibular growth, and ectomorphic body type with relatively slow skeletal development and poor posture. The extraction of teeth is routinely part of the orthodontic treatment plan in these facial patterns. It is necessary to relieve crowding, to assist in the correction of the openbite tendency, and to upright mandibular incisors. Depending on the severity, serial extraction may be permissible.

Low angle (hypodivergent[58]) (Fig. 6-27). This facial pattern routinely exhibits a low mandibular plane angle accompanied by a favorable horizontal skeletal relationship or an orthognathic facial pattern, a maxillary mandibular alveolodental retrusion, a deep overbite relationship of the incisor teeth, a prominent chin, a straight or dished-in, soft tissue profile, and a shorter or *pug* nose. Cephalometrically the mandibular plane to S-N is less than 32° in the Steiner analysis. The FMA is less than 25° in the Tweed analysis. Additional features include a broad brachycephalic head form, a euryprosopic facial form, wide-set eyes, prominent

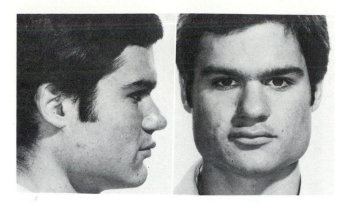

Fig. 6-27   Low angle facial pattern.

cheek bones, bulbous forehead, less prominent glabella and supraorbital ridges, small gonial angle, broad and long ramis, large coronoid processes, and no antegonial notching on the lower border of the mandible. The anterior face height equals the posterior face height. Compared to the upper face height, the lower face height is relatively small. There is a small cranial base angle, which is responsible for an upward and backward position of the nasomaxillary complex and an upward and forward position of the mandible. Macrogenia is common. The palatal vault is flat with a wide dental arch and relatively small teeth. The mandibular incisors may be crowded as a result of a deep overbite, or there may be a spaced dentition. A high percentage of congenital absence of teeth is characteristic. There is more abrasion of teeth along with early formation and eruption of teeth; thin lips; deep mentalis sulcus; heavy masseter muscles, with vertical pull; strong temporal muscles; large pharyngeal space, with a relatively posterior tongue position. There is less tongue thrusting. The nasal apertures are large. The mandibular growth is horizontal. The body is endomorphic with advanced skeletal age and upright posture. In these patients there is less need for extraction. Every effort is made to avoid the extraction of teeth. Arch length can be gained by correcting the deep overbite and uprighting mandibular teeth. Serial extraction, in most instances, is contraindicated.

The Teeth

According to the Burlington Growth Study,[15] 34% of 3-year-old children enjoy a *normal* occlusion. By the time they reach 12 years of age, only 11% have a normal intercuspation—a reduction of 23%. This is attributed to local environmental factors. For example, crowded dentitions result from a loss of arch length caused by the premature loss of primary teeth.

With regard to the 66% of 3-year-old children destined to suffer the ravages of malocclusion, 41% are in a Class I dental relationship, 23% are in a Class II, and only 2%

are in a Class III. By the time these children reach 12 years of age, 55% have Class I malocclusions, 32% have Class II, and 2% still have Class III—a total increase of 23%. To repeat, this increase is due primarily to local environmental factors.

Serial extraction is an interceptive procedure designed to assist in the correction of hereditary tooth-size jaw-size discrepancies. Since the malocclusions of the 66% of 3-year-old children are hereditary in nature (with a significant number of tooth-size jaw-size discrepancies), serial extraction is an invaluable adjunct to interceptive treatment. This is especially true in the 41% Class I malocclusions and, to a lesser extent, the 23% Class II malocclusions.

Class I malocclusions are more ideal for serial extraction because the dentition is basically in a favorable relationship and successful treatment is possible with a minimum of mechanotherapy. The ideal conditions for serial extraction are (1) a true, relatively severe hereditary tooth-size jaw-size discrepancy; (2) a mesial step mixed dentition developing into a Class I permanent relationship; (3) a minimal overjet relationship of the incisor teeth; (4) minimal overbite; and (5) a facial pattern that is orthognathic, or with a slight alveolodental protrusion.

Clinical analysis

Hereditary crowding. The signs of a true hereditary tooth-size jaw-size discrepancy may be outlined as follows:
1. Maxillary mandibular alveolodental protrusion without interproximal spacing (Fig. 6-28)
2. Crowded mandibular incisor teeth
3. A midline displacement of the permanent mandibular incisors, resulting in the premature exfoliation of the primary canine on the crowded side (Fig. 6-29)
4. A midline displacement of the permanent mandibular incisors with the lateral incisors on the crowded side blocked out, usually lingually (Fig. 6-30) but occasionally labially (Fig. 6-31)
5. A crescent area of external resorption on the mesial aspect of the roots of the primary canines, caused by crowded permanent lateral incisors (Fig. 6-6)
6. Bilateral primary mandibular canine exfoliation, resulting in an uprighting of the permanent mandibular incisors; this, in turn, increases the overjet (Fig. 6-32) and/or the overbite (Fig. 6-33)
7. A splaying out of the permanent maxillary or mandibular incisor teeth caused by the crowded position of the unerupted canines (Fig. 6-34)
8. Gingival recession on the labial surface of the prominent mandibular incisor (Fig. 6-35)
9. A prominent bulging in the maxilla or mandible caused by the crowding of the canines in the unerupted position (Fig. 6-36)
10. A discrepancy in the size of the primary and permanent teeth, reducing the leeway space
11. Ectopic eruption of the permanent maxillary first molars, resulting in the premature exfoliation of the

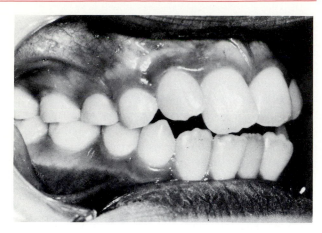

Fig. 6-28   Maxillary mandibular alveolodental protrusion.

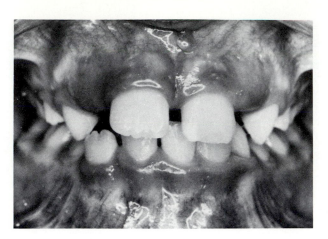

Fig. 6-29   Premature exfoliation of one primary mandibular canine with a resulting midline discrepancy.

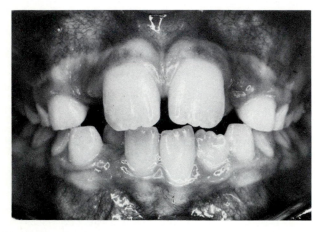

Fig. 6-30   One permanent mandibular lateral incisor blocked out lingually with a midline discrepancy.

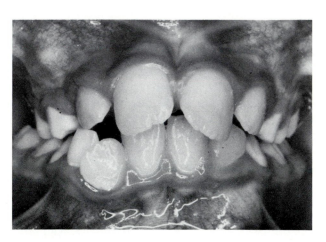

Fig. 6-31   One permanent mandibular lateral incisor blocked out labially with a midline discrepancy. (From Dale JG: *Dent Clin North Am* 26:565, 1982.)

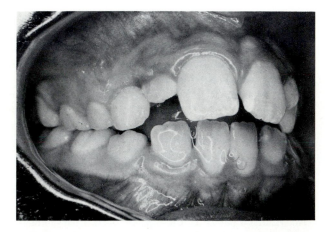

Fig. 6-32   Bilateral exfoliation of primary mandibular canines resulting in an increase in overjet.

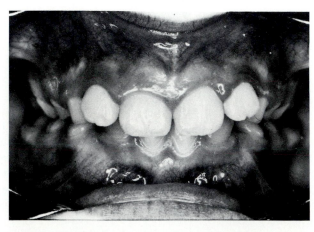

Fig. 6-33   Bilateral exfoliation of primary mandibular canines resulting in an increase in overbite. (From Dale JG: *Dent Clin North Am* 26:565, 1982.)

primary second molars; this indicates a lack of development in the tuberosity area (Fig. 6-59)

12. A vertical palisading of the permanent maxillary first, second, and third molars in the tuberosity area, again indicating a lack of jaw development (Fig. 6-37)

13. Impaction of the permanent mandibular second molars in the absence of treatment

True hereditary tooth-size jaw-size discrepancies must be differentiated from crowded dentitions resulting from factors that are more environmental in nature. It is quite likely that true hereditary crowding will be treated with the aid of extractions and, if discovered early, with serial extraction. On the other hand, crowding resulting from environmental factors may be treated without extractions.

Environmental crowding. Environmental crowding may result under the following conditions:

1. Trauma (Fig. 6-38)
2. Iatrogenic treatment (Fig. 6-39)

3. A discrepancy in the size of individual teeth (Fig. 6-40)
4. A discrepancy between mandibular tooth size and maxillary tooth size
5. An aberration in the shape of teeth (Fig. 6-41)
6. An aberration in the eruptive pattern of the permanent teeth (Fig. 6-42)
7. Transposition of teeth (Fig. 6-42)
8. Uneven resorption of primary teeth (Fig. 6-43)
9. Rotation of teeth (Fig. 6-44)
10. Suppression of primary teeth (Fig. 6-45)
11. Premature loss of primary teeth resulting in the reduction of arch length due to subsequent drifting of permanent teeth (Figs. 6-57, 6-58, 6-60, and 6-61)
12. A reduction of arch length caused by interproximal caries in the primary teeth (Fig. 6-56)
13. Altered emergence sequence (Fig. 6-69)
14. Exfoliation sequence of primary teeth (Fig. 6-60)

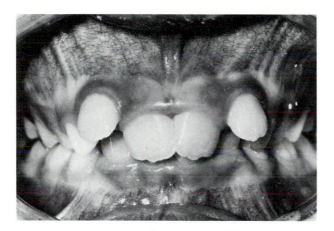

Fig. 6-34 Splayed maxillary lateral incisors.

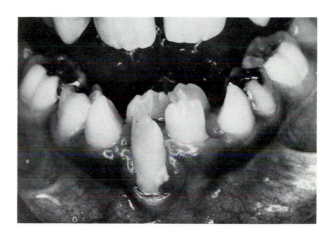

Fig. 6-35 Gingival recession. (From Dale JG: *Dent Clin North Am* 26:565, 1982.)

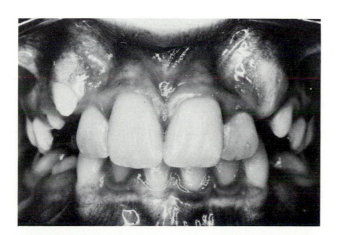

Fig. 6-36 Canine bulging in the maxilla. (From Dale JG: *Dent Clin North Am* 26:565, 1982.)

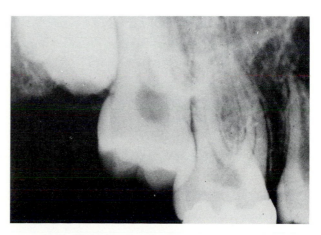

Fig. 6-37 Palisading of the maxillary molars.

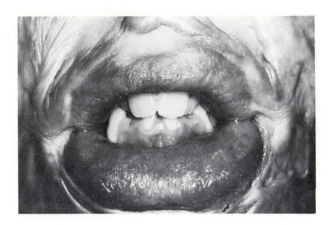

Fig. 6-38   Crowded dentition as a result of severe facial burns.

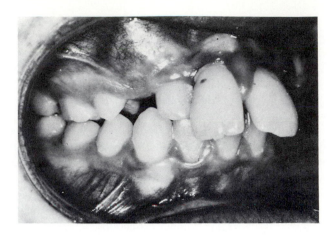

Fig. 6-39   Irregularity and extrusion caused by an elastic placed around the maxillary central incisors.

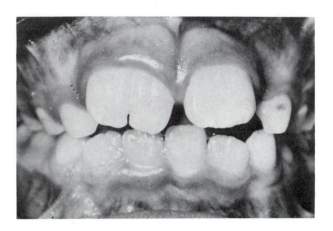

Fig. 6-40   Discrepancy in the size of individual teeth.

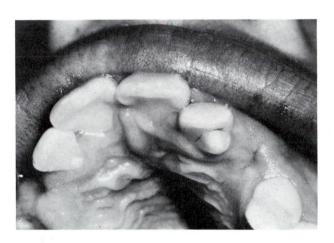

Fig. 6-41   Rotated maxillary incisor with an enlarged cingulum.

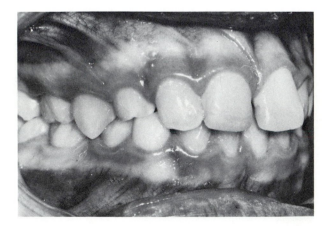

Fig. 6-42   Maxillary canine erupted in the premolar position.

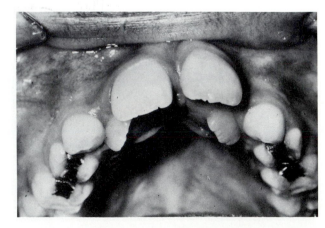

Fig. 6-43   Irregularity caused by uneven resorption of the primary maxillary canines.

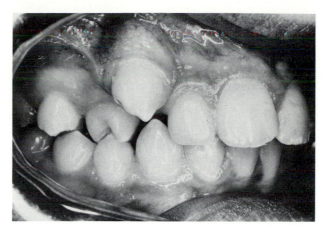

Fig. 6-44 Rotated maxillary premolar consuming more space than it would in its normal position.

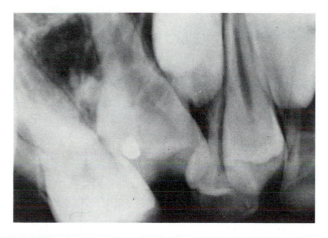

Fig. 6-45 Irregularity caused by a suppressed primary maxillary second molar. Note the restoration in spite of the fact that the tooth is covered by gingival tissue.

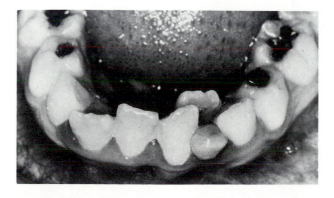

Fig. 6-46 Irregularity caused by prolonged retention of the primary teeth.

15. Prolonged retention of primary teeth (Fig. 6-46)

Since serial extraction is performed during the mixed dentition period, it is of utmost importance that the transformation from the primary to the permanent dentition be examined carefully.

Dental development

Primary dentition. The first paper ever published on the primary dentition was by Jacobi[33] in 1860. Meredith,[41] in the *Journal of Dental Research,* reviewed extensively all the papers on the primary teeth prior to 1946. He found that only one sixth of the studies on the primary dentition were published in the dental literature; the balance appeared in journals associated with anthropology, biology, child development, etc. Lundt and Law,[38] writing in the *Journal of the American Dental Association,* have completed the review subsequent to 1946.

The oldest age at which a patient has been recorded as having no primary teeth visible is 13 months, and the youngest age with all primary teeth visible is 13 months. The range for the emergence of all twenty teeth is between 18 and 30 months.

According to Robinow et al.[57] late eruption is a more common variable and second molars are the most variable in eruption.

Baume,[5-9] in his classic articles in the 1950s, showed that the relationships of the primary teeth could be divided into three categories: (1) straight terminal plane—76%; (2) mesial step—14%; and (3) distal step—10% (Fig. 6-47). The mesial step is an ideal relationship that routinely guides the permanent first molars into a favorable Class I intercuspation. The straight terminal plane, which is by far the most frequently occurring relationship, is the one that must be observed the most critically. Depending on a number of factors, it can guide the permanent molars into a normal Class I or an abnormal Class II. The transformation reduces arch length in either the maxillary dentition or the mandibular depending on the situation. This is critical in the evaluation of the amount and type of crowding prior to treatment. The distal step, as a rule, guides the permanent first molars into an abnormal Class II malocclusion.

Delabarre in 1918[18] was the first to describe interproximal spacing in the primary dentition. Baume concluded in 1950 that there is no physiologic spacing after the eruption of primary teeth and emphasized that one has either a *spaced* or a *closed* dentition (Fig. 6-48). *Primary spacing* occurs in the maxilla in 70% of the patients and in the mandible in 63%. There are no spaces in the maxillary dentition in 30% of the patients and none in the mandibular in 37%. The intercanine distance in the maxilla is 1.7 mm more in *spaced* dentitions than in *closed* dentitions. In the mandible it is 1.5 mm more. According to Baume, a primary dentition without spacing is followed by crowding in the permanent dentition 40% of the time. Contrary to a widely held misconception, arch length is reduced after the premature loss of a primary incisor (Fig. 6-49). This is particularly true if

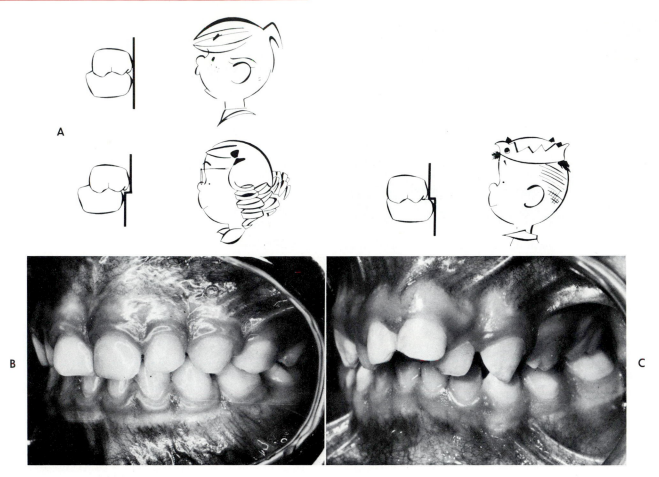

Fig. 6-47 Baume's classification. **A,** Straight terminal plane. **B,** Ideal mesial step. **C,** Abnormal distal step.

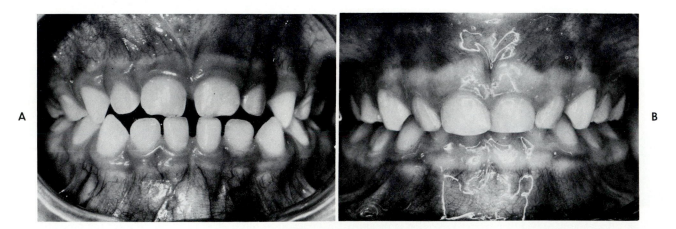

Fig. 6-48 **A,** *Spaced* and, **B,** *closed* dentitions.

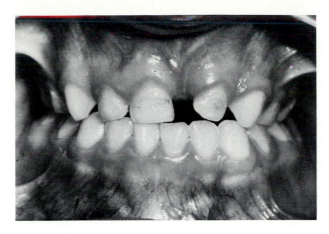

Fig. 6-49   Space reduction after the premature loss of a primary maxillary central incisor.

the incisor is lost early. It is also true if the primary dentition is a *closed* dentition, if there is a tendency to a Class II relationship of the molars, and if there is a deep overbite relationship of the incisors.

Overbite is related to the growth of the jaws and to the rate of eruption of the incisor teeth. It decreases from the primary dentition to the permanent 10% of the time; it remains constant 43% of the time; and it increases 47% of the time. According to Baume 40% of primary dentitions have a slight overbite. By the time the permanent dentition erupts this has been reduced to 19%, a drop of 21%. Twenty-nine percent have a medium overbite, which drops by two to 27%, and 31% have a severe overbite, which rises to 54% in the permanent dentition, an increase of 23%. Thus overbite increases from the primary dentition to the permanent.

Zsigmundy in 1890[69] was the first to measure arch dimensions in the primary dentition. Again, according to Baume arch dimension does not change during the primary dentition period: arch length does not change in the maxilla in 89% of the cases, and in the mandible in 83%; arch width does not change in the maxilla in 82% of the cases, and in the mandible in 83%.

Franke in 1922[24] was the first to describe the reduction of arch length with the natural loss of the primary teeth. Since then many investigators have confirmed these findings.

Mixed dentition. At present there is overwhelming scientific evidence to indicate that the posterior teeth move forward throughout life. This would tend to reduce arch length. Moorrees[50] has established that arch length decreases 2 to 3 mm between 10 and 14 years of age, when the primary molars are being replaced by the permanent premolars (Fig. 6-50). He has also demonstrated that the arch circumference is reduced approximately 3.5 mm in the mandible of boys and 4.5 mm in girls during the mixed dentition period. De Kock[17] has measured a 10% decrease in arch length for males and 9% for females over a period of 10 years beyond the period of the mixed dentition, from 12 years of age to 26 (Fig. 6-51). Brodie[13] has observed that in newborn infants the tongue tends to fill the oral cavity and often encroaches on the alveolar ridge area. As a consequence of the more rapid anterior growth of the jaws in the postnatal period, the tongue lags behind and comes to occupy a relatively more posterior position in the oral cavity. This is consistent with the uprighting of the incisors that occurs in many adolescents as noted by Enlow[19] (Fig. 6-52), Björk[11] (Fig. 6-53), Tweed,[65] and others. These findings suggest that as facial growth continues in an anterior direction into adulthood it thrusts the mandible into the facial musculature, which produces a posterior force vector on the crowns of the incisors. Thus arch length decreases from the anterior as well as the posterior. To repeat, serial extraction is based on the fact that arch length does not increase. If crowding is evident at 8 years of age, it will not improve with further growth and development.

First molars. Several situations can exist for the permanent first molars:

In patients with a *spaced* primary dentition and a straight terminal plane relationship of the primary molars, the permanent mandibular first molars emerge at approximately 6 years of age, move the primary molars mesially, close the space distal to the primary canines, convert the straight terminal plane to a mesial step relationship, reduce arch

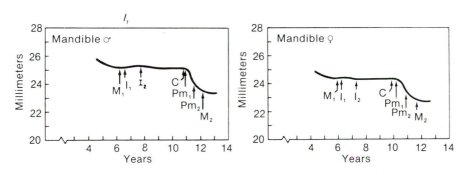

Fig. 6-50   Reduction in arch length as a result of the moving forward of posterior teeth. (From Moorrees CFA, Reed RB: *J Dent Res* 44:129, 1965.)

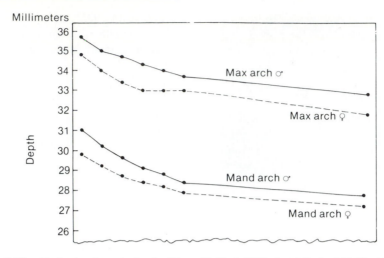

Millimeters

Fig. 6-51   Reduction in arch depth. (From DeKock WH: *Am J Orthod* 62:56, 1972.)

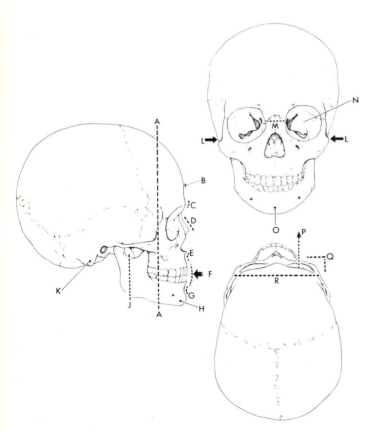

Fig. 6-52   Reduction in arch length because of evolutionary changes, resulting in the uprighting of incisors. (From Enlow DH: *The human face,* New York, 1968, Hoeber Medical Division, Harper & Row.)

length in the mandibular dentition, and allow the permanent maxillary molars to emerge into a Class I relationship. This has been referred to as *the early mesial shift* (Fig. 6-54).

In patients with a *closed* primary dentition and a straight terminal plane the permanent maxillary and mandibular first molars emerge into a cusp-to-cusp relationship simply because there are no spaces to close. At approximately 11 years of age the primary mandibular second molars are exfoliated and the permanent mandibular first molars migrate mesially into the excess leeway space provided by the differences in mesiodistal dimensions of the primary second molars and the permanent second premolar teeth. Again, this reduces arch length, converts the straight terminal plane to a mesial step, and provides for a Class I relationship of the permanent first molars. It has been referred to as *the late mesial shift* (Fig. 6-55) and is substantiated by the investigations of Moorrees[50] (Fig. 6-50).

If the permanent maxillary first molars emerge before the mandibulars, just the reverse of the early mesial shift—an abnormal Class II relationship—will occur and a reduction in the maxillary arch length will result.

If extensive interproximal caries is allowed to develop in the maxilla, a similar situation will occur—a reduction of arch length causing crowding (Fig. 6-56).

If the caries is so extensive that extraction of the primary maxillary second molars is necessary, again crowding will result (Fig. 6-57).

Similarly, and this is contrary to popular belief, premature loss of the primary maxillary first molars will cause crowding (Fig. 6-58).

Ectopic eruption of the permanent maxillary first molars, resulting in premature exfoliation of the primary second molars and loss of arch length, is indicative of a lack of development of the tuberosity. This results in not only crowding but also a Class II molar relationship (Fig. 6-59).

If the exfoliation sequence of the primary second molars

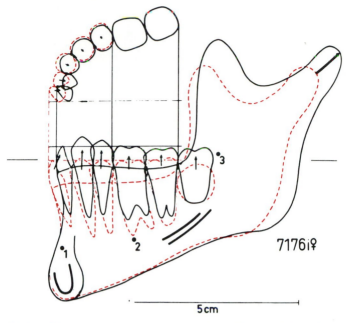

Fig. 6-53   Uprighting of incisors with forward growth. (From Björk A: *J Dent Res* 42:400, 1963.)

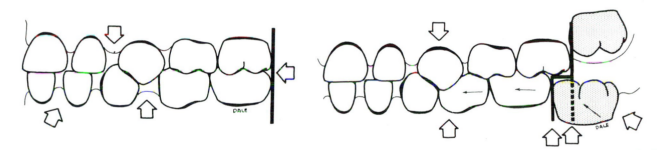

Fig. 6-54   Early mesial shift. (From Baume LJ: *J Dent Res* 29:331, 1950.)

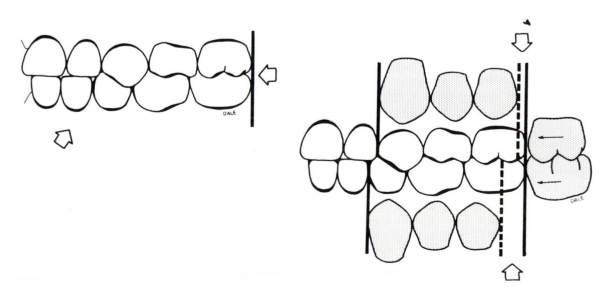

Fig. 6-55   Late mesial shift. (From Baume LJ: *J Dent Res* 29:331, 1950.)

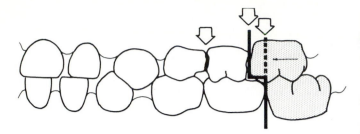

Fig. 6-56   Reduction in arch length as a result of caries.

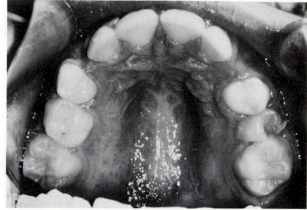

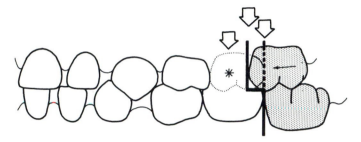

Fig. 6-57   Reduction in arch length as a result of premature loss of primary maxillary second molars.

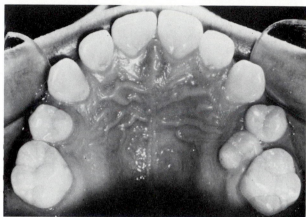

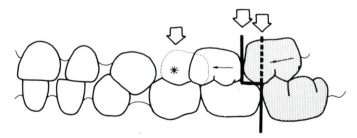

Fig. 6-58   Reduction in arch length as a result of premature loss of the primary maxillary first molars.

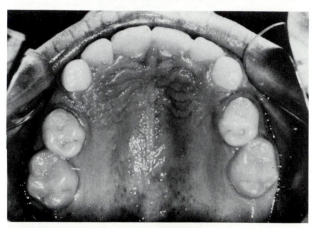

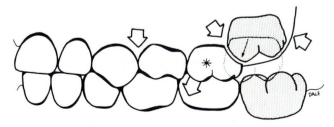

Fig. 6-59   Reduction in arch length as a result of ectopic eruption of the permanent maxillary first molars.

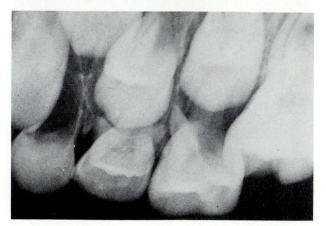

is reversed and the maxillary molar is lost before the mandibular, a Class II relationship of the permanent first molars will result. Again, arch length will be reduced and crowding will occur in the maxilla (Fig. 6-60).

On the other hand, if the primary mandibular second molar is lost far too early, the mandibular arch length will be reduced to such an extent that the normal leeway will be exceeded and crowding will occur (Fig. 6-61).

The normal leeway, according to Moyers, is 2.6 mm (1.3 mm on each side) in the maxilla and 6.2 mm (3.1 mm on each side) in the mandible. However, this leeway varies considerably and should be measured on each patient. It is possible that a discrepancy exists between the size of the primary teeth and the size of the permanent to such an extent that there is no positive leeway available. There may even be a negative leeway. According to Horowitz and Hixon,[29] correlations in size between a single primary tooth and its successor range from r = 0.2 to r = 0.6. This means that anywhere from 4% to 36% of the time there is a favorable correlation. In other words, if the primary tooth is small its successor will be small. According to Arita and Iwagaki,[3] Hixon and Oldfather,[28] Lewis and Lehman,[36] Moorrees and Chadha,[52] and Moorrees et al.,[56] the size correlation between all the primary teeth and their successors is approximately r = 0.5. Therefore 25% of the time there is a positive relationship. That is not too good.

Incisors. Several situations can exist also for the incisors:

Ideally the *primary spacing* of the spaced primary dentition will be sufficient, together with other factors, to allow for the accommodation and favorable alignment of the succedaneous permanent incisors (Fig. 6-62).

In closed primary dentitions the permanent mandibular lateral incisors emerge and the primary mandibular canines are moved laterally. Thus a space is created that enables the permanent maxillary lateral incisors to emerge into a favorable alignment. This is referred to as *secondary spacing* and was first described by Baume in 1950 (Fig. 6-63). Secondary spacing also occurs when the permanent mandibular central incisors are emerging (Fig. 6-64).

Both these observations have been substantiated by the findings of Moorrees[50] that show an increase in intercanine width during the period of incisor emergence (Fig. 6-65). Moorrees[48] has also demonstrated an increase in arch circumference in the maxilla of boys of 1.5 mm and of girls of 0.5 mm during this period of development.

If the primary canines are reduced in size (Fig. 6-66) or extracted when this natural phenomenon is occurring, an increase in intercanine distance and *secondary spacing* may not occur. Thus borderline discrepancies may be converted from a nonextraction treatment to extraction.

Research conducted by Moorrees and Chadha[53] has revealed that there is an increase in the crowding of both

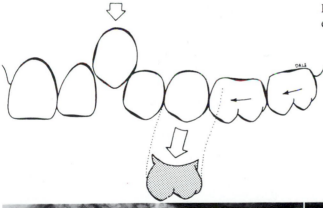

Fig. 6-60 Reduction in arch length as a result of premature exfoliation of the primary maxillary second molar.

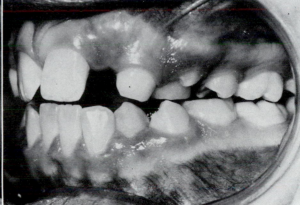

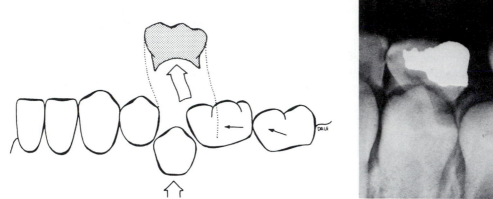

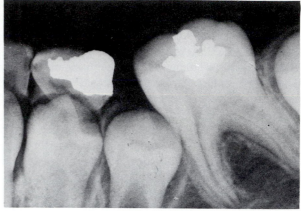

Fig. 6-61   Reduction in arch length as a result of premature loss of the primary mandibular second molar.

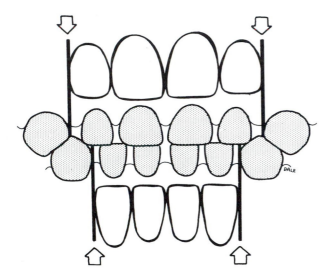

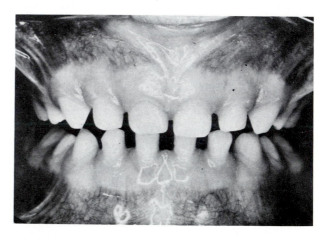

Fig. 6-62   *Primary spacing.*

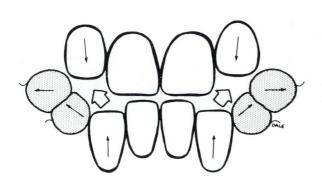

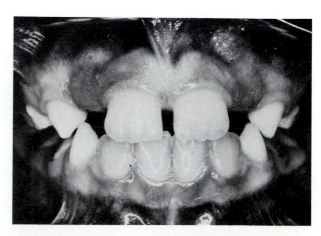

Fig. 6-63   *Secondary spacing* occurring when the permanent mandibular lateral incisors are emerging.

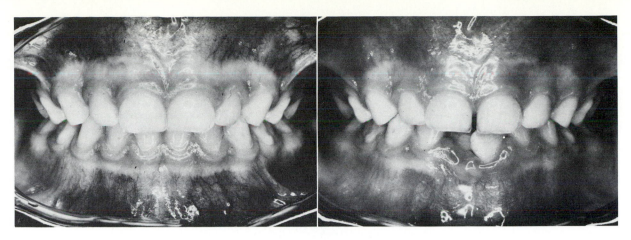

Fig. 6-64 *Secondary spacing* occurring when the central incisors are emerging.

Millimeters   + 4   + 2   0   _ 2   _ 4

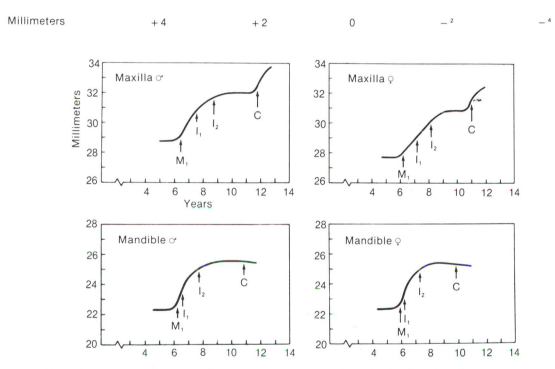

Fig. 6-65 Average intercanine distance. (From Moorrees CFA, Reed RB: *J Dent Res* 44:129, 1965.)

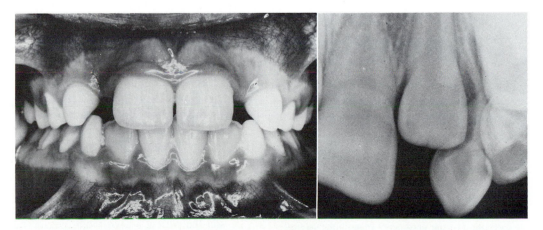

Fig. 6-66 Effect of interproximal reduction of the primary canines on secondary spacing.

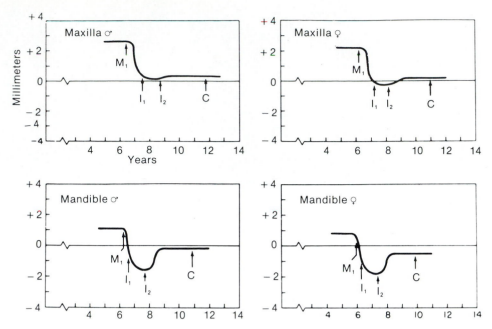

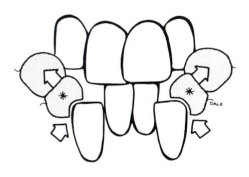

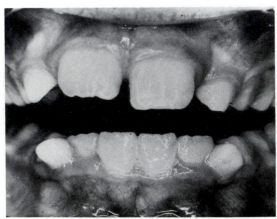

Fig. 6-67   Available space in the incisor segment. (From Moorrees CFA, Chadha IM: *Angle Orthod* 35:12, 1965.)

Fig. 6-68   Ectopic eruption of the permanent mandibular lateral incisors and its effect on secondary spacing.

maxillary and mandibular incisors when they are emerging into the oral cavity. However, 2 mm of crowding in the incisor segment in the mandible of boys will recover to 0 crowding by 8 years of age on the average. Girls recover to approximately 1 mm of crowding. In the maxillary dentition of both boys and girls there is not the same tendency to crowding. However, during the eruption of the incisors, 2 to 3 mm of spacing is reduced to 0 (Fig. 6-67). This is a significant finding because it tells the clinician not to be alarmed with a slight amount of crowding in the early stages of emergence of the permanent incisors. The reduction in size, or extraction, of the primary canines should be deferred. In fact, it may not be an extraction case at all.

Intercanine distance increases more in the maxilla and in closed dentitions. A true hereditary tooth-size jaw-size discrepancy is characterized by an ectopic eruption of the permanent mandibular lateral incisors and a premature exfoliation of the primary canines (Fig. 6-68).

Warren Mayne,[39] in writing this chapter for this textbook in 1969, described a concept he termed *incisor liability*. In his discussion he outlined how it could be used clinically in the determination of anterior crowding.

He described the following four principal variables:
1. *Incisor liability.* According to Black[12] the four permanent maxillary incisor teeth are, on the average, 7.6 mm larger than the primary incisors. The four permanent mandibular incisors are 6.0 mm larger. This size differential is the *incisor liability*. It varies greatly from individual to individual, and for this reason the patient's own tooth measurements should be used in the analysis.

A favorable incisor liability exists when the primary spacing of the spaced dentition is sufficient to allow for the eruption of the permanent incisors without any crowding (Fig. 6-62).

A more precarious incisor liability situation exists when there is no *primary spacing* in a closed primary dentition. Then the individual must rely on the development of *secondary spacing* to create sufficient space for the permanent incisors to emerge without crowding (Figs. 6-63 and 6-64).

An impossible situation exists when the incisor liability is of such magnitude that growth and development will never be able to meet the space demands required by the permanent incisors. Such patients are doomed to severe crowding and irregularity from the outset (Fig. 6-68).

2. *Interdental spacing.* In the primary dentition the interdental spacing may range between 0 and 10 mm in the maxilla, with an average of 4 mm, and between 0 to 6 mm in the mandible, with a range of 3 mm.

3. *Intercanine arch width.* During the period of permanent incisor eruption notable amounts of intercanine arch width development occur in both the maxillary and the mandibular dentition. In the mandible the increase occurs between 6 and 9 years of age for boys and between 6 and 8 years for girls. In the maxilla it increases longer, to 16 years in boys and 12 years in girls (Fig. 6-65). After 10 years of age there is little intercanine arch width change to be expected in the mandible of either boys or girls. According to Moorrees[50] the average increase in the mandibular dentition of boys and girls is approximately 3 mm; in the maxilla it is approximately 4.5 mm (Fig. 6-65).

4. *Incisor position.* According to Mayne[39] the permanent incisor teeth erupt slightly labial to the arch position of the primary incisors and, for a time at least, are more procumbent. Baume has estimated that the permanent incisors, after full eruption, are 2.2 mm forward of the primary incisors in the maxilla and 1.3 mm in the mandible. This particular calculation may be questionable, since several investigators have established that arch length decreases after eruption and several have established that the uprighting of incisors contributes to this decrease. Nevertheless, incisor position is important and will be discussed further under "Total space analysis" (p. 328).

Incisor crowding may be assessed by using the four variables just described.

First, the *favorable* situation, described earlier, exists when sufficient *primary spacing* is present in the spaced primary dentition to allow for the eruption of the permanent incisors without crowding (Fig. 6-62) (Table 6-1).

Second, the *precarious* situation exists when there is a closed primary dentition and it is necessary to have a substantial increase in intercanine width to provide *secondary spacing* so that the permanent incisors erupt without appre-

TABLE 6-1

Incisor Liability

Situation	Maxilla (mm)	Mandible (mm)
Favorable—Primary Spacing		
Incisor liability	− 6.2	− 4.3
Interdental spacing	+ 4.0	+ 3.0
Incisor position	+ 2.2	+ 1.3
	6.2	4.3
Amount of crowding	—	—
Precarious—Secondary Spacing		
Incisor liability	− 9.2	− 7.3
Interdental spacing	+ 4.0	+ 3.0
Intercanine arch width	+ 3.0	+ 3.0
Incisor position	+ 2.2	+ 1.3
	9.2	7.3
Amount of crowding	—	—
Impossible—Ectopic Eruption		
Incisor liability	− 14.2	− 12.3
Interdental spacing	+ 4.0	+ 3.0
Intercanine arch width	+ 3.0	+ 3.0
Incisor position	+ 2.2	+ 1.3
	9.2	7.3
Amount of crowding	5.0	5.0

ciable crowding (Fig. 6-63) (Table 6-1). It is in these patients that the practitioner avoids the interproximal reduction or the extraction of primary canines (Fig. 6-66).

Finally, the *impossible* situation exists when there is a true hereditary tooth-size jaw-size discrepancy and an incisor liability that cannot be compensated by interdental spacing, an increase in intercanine arch width, or the labial positioning of the permanent incisors (Fig. 6-68) (Table 6-1). It is in these individuals that serial extraction can be beneficial.

Canines, premolars, and second molars. The most frequently occurring sequence of eruption in the maxilla is as follows: permanent first molar, central incisor, lateral incisor, first premolar, second premolar, canine, second molar. The most frequently occurring sequence in the mandible is permanent first molar, central incisor, lateral incisor, canine, first premolar, second premolar, second molar. According to Lo and Moyers[37] this combination produces the highest incidence of favorable occlusion and more girls than boys have a favorable combination.

An unfavorable sequence can produce crowding. For instance, if the second molars erupt relatively early, they may impact the canines in the maxilla and the second premolars in the mandible (Fig. 6-69). Maxillary second molars erupt ahead of mandibular molars in 89.11% of Class II patients whereas in only 56.5% do maxillary first molars erupt ahead of their mandibular counterparts.[37] Therefore second molars

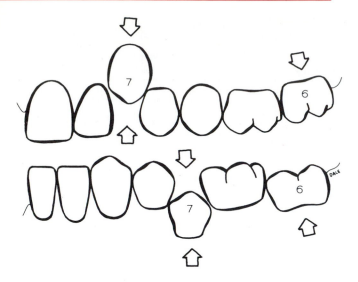

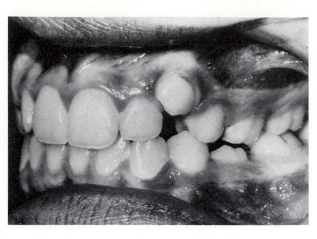

Fig. 6-70 Prolonged retention of the primary maxillary second molar causing crowding of the permanent canine.

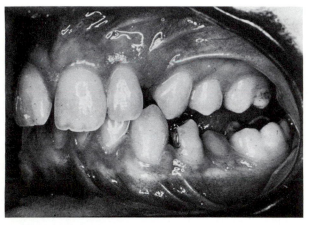

Fig. 6-69 Unfavorable emergence sequence. The permanent second molars are emerging relatively early blocking the maxillary canines and mandibular second premolars.

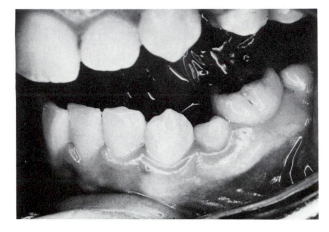

Fig. 6-71 Prolonged retention of the mandibular second molar causing crowding of the first premolar.

are more important than first molars in the development of a Class II relationship.

Early exfoliation of primary teeth can disrupt the alignment of the dentition, reducing arch length in the maxilla (Figs. 6-57, 6-58, and 6-60) and in the mandible (Fig. 6-61).

Prolonged retention of primary teeth can cause crowding of the permanent teeth in either the maxilla (Fig. 6-70) or the mandible (Fig. 6-71).

Clinically it appears that primary second molars resist mesial migration to some extent. Rarely does the orthodontist observe primary mandibular second molars tipped mesially after the premature loss of primary first molars. On the other hand, the permanent mandibular first molars are observed to have an exaggerated mesial inclination after the premature loss of the primary second molars. The relative position of the unerupted premolars is critical in this situation. When the primary mandibular second molars are lost prematurely, the permanent second premolars are quite

often deep in the alveolar bone. This may encourage the permanent first molar to tip forward. When the primary mandibular first molar is lost prematurely, the permanent first premolar (which is scheduled to emerge before the second premolar) is not so deeply embedded in bone. Therefore the tendency for tipping of the primary second molar is not as great. The unerupted first premolar tends to support the primary second molar.

Contrary to popular belief, arch length can be reduced and space can be lost after premature exfoliation or extraction of the primary first molar (Fig. 6-58). This is especially true in the mandible, where one observes the formation of a knife-edge ridge of alveolar bone obstructing and retarding the emergence of the underlying first premolar (Fig. 6-106).

The premature loss of primary molars immediately leads one to consider space maintenance. However, using space maintainers is dependent on a thorough diagnosis, and it may be modified with subsequent treatment planning. If a patient has a normal dentition, or the treatment plan does

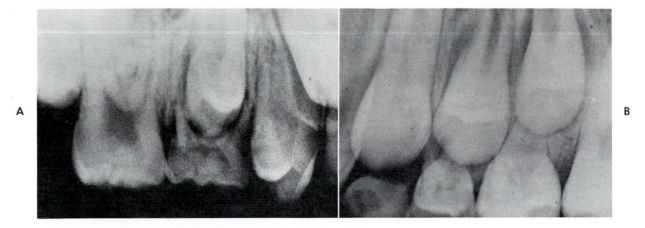

Fig. 6-72 **A,** Sequence of eruption in the maxilla that is favorable for extraction. **B,** Unfavorable sequence.

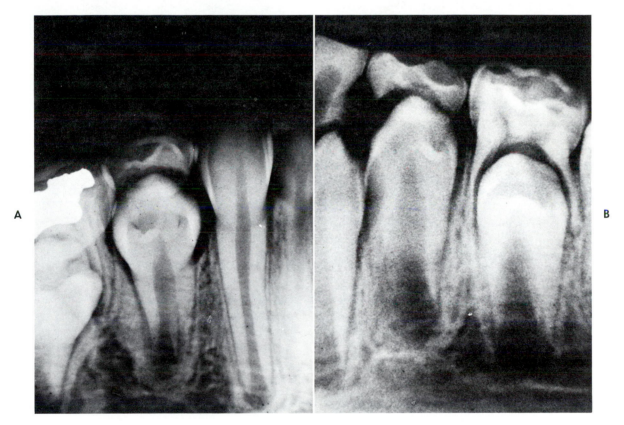

Fig. 6-73 **A,** Sequence of eruption in the mandible that is unfavorable for serial extraction. **B,** Favorable sequence.

not include the extraction of permanent teeth, a space maintainer may be placed.

In the maxilla approximately 90% of the time the first premolar emerges ahead of the canine (Fig. 6-72) (Table 6-2). This is favorable for serial extraction and for maintenance of the overbite because the maxillary incisors are not held forward. Approximately 10% of the time the se-

quence is unfavorable for both serial extraction and the overbite.

In the mandible approximately 80% of the time the canine emerges ahead of the first premolar[37] (Fig. 6-73) (Table 6-2). This, according to Baker,[4] decreases overbite because it maintains the mandibular incisors in a forward position. However, it is not favorable for serial extraction. Approx-

TABLE 6-2
Sequences of Eruption in the Maxilla and Mandible

		Cases	Percentage
Maxilla			
1	6 1 2 4 5 3 7	115	48.72
2	6 1 2 4 3 5 7	38	16.01
3	6 1 2 4 5 7 3	28	11.87
4	6 1 2 3 4 5 7	14	5.93
5	6 1 2 4 3 7 5	13	5.51
6	6 1 2 5 4 3 7	6	2.54
7	6 1 2 4 7 5 3	5	2.12
8	6 1 2 4 7 3 5	4	1.69
9	6 1 2 5 3 4 7	2	0.84
10	6 1 2 3 4 7 5	2	0.84
11	1 6 2 4 5 3 7*	2	0.84
12	6 1 2 3 5 4 7	1	0.42
13	6 1 2 5 4 7 3	1	0.42
14	6 1 2 3 7 4 5	1	0.42
15	6 1 2 7 4 5 3	1	0.42
16	6 4 1 2 5 3 7*	1	0.42
17	6 1 5 2 4 3 7*	1	0.42
18	1 2 6 4 3 5 7*	1	0.42
		236	100.00
Mandible			
1	6 1 2 3 4 5 7	108	45.77
2	6 1 2 3 4 7 5	44	18.64
3	6 1 2 4 3 5 7	20	8.47
4	6 1 2 3 7 4 5	14	5.93
5	6 1 2 4 5 3 7	14	5.93
6	6 1 2 5 3 4 7	6	2.54
7	6 1 2 3 5 4 7	6	2.54
8	6 1 2 4 3 7 5	5	2.12
9	6 1 2 5 4 3 7	4	1.69
10	6 1 2 4 5 7 3	3	1.27
11	6 1 2 3 5 7 4	3	1.27
12	1 6 2 3 4 5 7*	3	1.27
13	1 2 6 3 4 5 7*	2	0.84
14	6 1 2 5 7 3 4	1	0.42
15	6 1 2 7 4 5 3	1	0.42
16	1 6 2 4 5 3 7*	1	0.42
17	1 2 6 4 5 3 7*	1	0.42
		236	100.00

From Lo RT, Moyers RE: *Am J Orthod* 39:460, 1953.
*All cases marked with an asterisk in this table are taken from the files of the Faculty of Dentistry, University of Toronto. They show an abnormal sequence of eruption of the first three teeth. This enabled us to follow them over a longer time than the Red Cross data allowed. They are inserted into subsequent tables to avoid prejudicing the final sequence percentages.

imately 20% of the time the sequence is favorable for serial extraction but not for maintenance of the overbite; that is, the first premolars are ahead of the canines.

Serial extraction is beneficial in the prevention of resorption of the roots of the maxillary lateral incisors by impacted canines. When the maxillary canine is extracted in serial extraction, the space between the lateral incisor and the primary first molar is substantially reduced. However, when

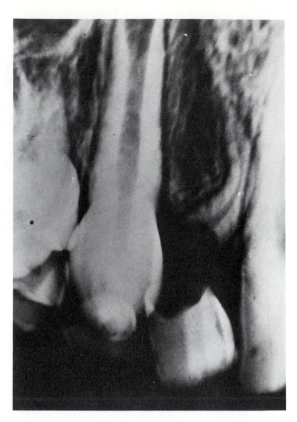

Fig. 6-74 Impacted permanent maxillary canine causing unfavorable resorption of the root of the lateral incisor.

the primary first molar is extracted at the proper time, the first premolar will erupt and this allows the unerupted permanent canine to move away from the root of the lateral incisor. Upon extraction of the first premolar, the canine then erupts into place without difficulty and without danger to the lateral incisor. There are times, which will be discussed later, when primary first molars are extracted before the primary canines to allow the premolars to erupt. This may even be done, if there is concern, in nonextraction malocclusions. To inject a personal comment at this time, I have never had a lateral incisor root resorbed by an impacted canine in 33 years of practice using serial extraction procedures. The example in Fig. 6-74 was contributed by a dental colleague.

Total Space Analysis

The mixed dentition analyses that I learned as a dental student were dentally oriented. Unfortunately, even today, tooth-size jaw-size discrepancies diagnosed in the mixed dentition period are still evaluated by dental-oriented analyses. These will be referred to as conventional methods. Their aim is to evaluate, as accurately as possible, future crowding in the permanent dentition using a prediction of the mesiodistal width of the permanent mandibular canines and premolars. The value obtained is added to the already known measurement of the permanent mandibular incisors. This represents *space required*. The resulting calculation is subtracted from the arch circumference of *space available*. If the result is significantly negative, future crowding can be predicted.

Tweed,[66] studying the relationship between the mandibular incisors and the mandibular plane, found that if the teeth are not in a stable relationship with the basal bone after treatment, the result may relapse. In view of this the dental-oriented mixed dentition analysis, alone, is not adequate. A facial-oriented analysis, incorporating the relations of the incisor teeth to the basal bone, is preferable. This will be described as the *Tweed method*.

Furthermore, the various mixed dentition analyses demonstrate the discrepancy only and do not indicate the exact area where the discrepancy occurs. In many instances, the problem is confined to one specific area. Since it is possible to direct treatment specifically to one area, it is desirable to know the area affected. The total space analysis provides this precise information.

The total space analysis was developed by Levern Merrifield,[44] of The Charles H. Tweed International Foundation for Orthodontic Research, and is currently being evaluated and tested by him and his associates at the Foundation.

Javier Garcia-Hernandez, while a postgraduate student at the Faculty of Dentistry, University of Toronto, and I[25] completed a study of 60 patients in my practice. One objective was to compare the conventional method, the Tweed method and the total space analysis method in the diagnosis of tooth-size jaw-size discrepancies before serial extraction.

Sixty individuals (30 boys and 30 girls) with a mean chronologic age of 8 years 4 months (range 7 years 7 months to 11 years 3 months) were selected from the records of the practice.

All subjects had a Class I mixed dentition malocclusion. Study models, periapical radiographs, cephalographs, facial photographs, and intraoral color transparencies were available for all subjects. Several mixed dentition analyses were performed for each individual.

Conventional method. The calculations were done as follows:

For *space required* the four mandibular incisors were measured at their greatest mesiodistal crown diameter by means of a sliding Boley gauge with pointed beaks. All measurements were made with the gauge parallel to the incisal edges of the teeth, and all readings were to the nearest 0.1 mm (Fig. 6-75). The values for unerupted canines and premolars were obtained by measuring their greatest mesiodistal crown diameter or their images on the periapical radiograph (Fig. 6-76).

To reduce the radiographic enlargement, the formula recommended by Huckaba[31] was used in all radiographic measurements:

$$x = \frac{(y)(x^1)}{y^1}$$

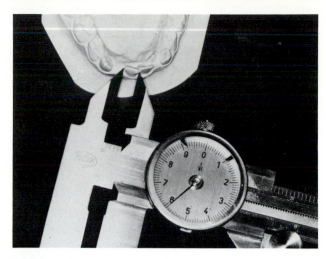

Fig. 6-75   Measurement of space required on study models with a Boley gauge.

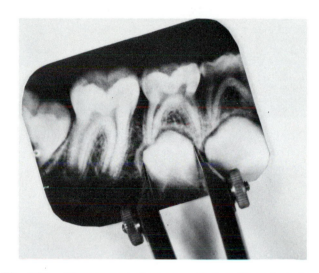

Fig. 6-76   Measurement of space required on the periapical radiograph with a Boley gauge.

where x is the estimated size of the permanent tooth; x^1, the radiographic size of the permanent teeth; y, the size of the primary mandibular second molar on the cast (Fig. 6-77); and y^1, the radiographic size of the primary molar.

The values obtained for the mandibular incisors on the cast and those for the canines and premolars on the radiograph were added to provide the space required.

The *space available* was obtained by extending a brass wire (0.033 inch) from the mesiobuccal of the first permanent molar on one side to the mesiobuccal of the molar on the opposite side, passing through the buccal cusps and incisal edges of the remaining teeth (Fig. 6-78). The wire was carefully straightened and measured with a pointed Boley gauge to the nearest 0.1 mm.

The difference in the values obtained for space required and space available was the amount of the discrepancy.

Tweed method. The values for space required and space available were obtained as described for the conventional method (Figs. 6-75 through 6-78).

An assessment of the relations between the axial inclination of the mandibular incisors and the basal bone was made on a tracing of the lateral cephalogram. The amount of alveolodental protrusion or retrusion was assessed and incorporated into the mixed dentition analysis (Fig. 6-79).

Tweed Foundation research has established the following relationships:

> When the FMA is between 21° and 29°, the FMIA should be 68°.
> When the FMA is 30° or greater, the FMIA should be 65°.
> When the FMA is 20° or less, the IMPA should not exceed 92°.

If for a specific FMA (30°) the FMIA (49°) did not correspond, an objective line was traced to form the required FMIA (65°). Then the distance between this objective line

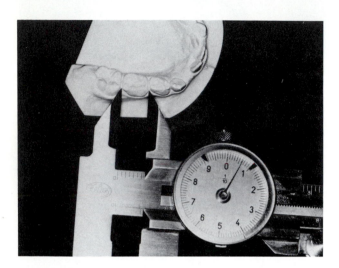

Fig. 6-77 Measurement of the primary second molar on the study model with a Boley gauge to aid in establishing a radiographic enlargement.

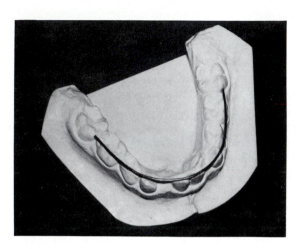

Fig. 6-78 Measurement of space available on the study model with a brass ligature wire.

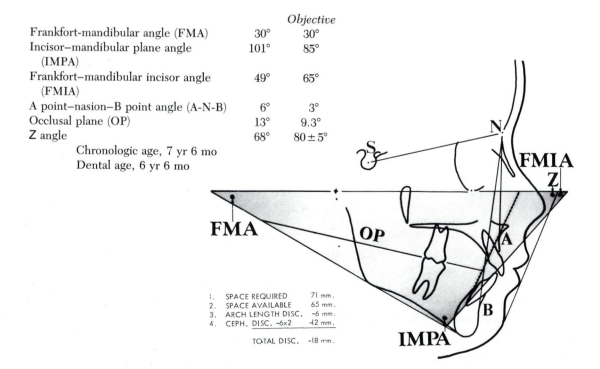

		Objective
Frankfort–mandibular angle (FMA)	30°	30°
Incisor–mandibular plane angle (IMPA)	101°	85°
Frankfort–mandibular incisor angle (FMIA)	49°	65°
A point–nasion–B point angle (A-N-B)	6°	3°
Occlusal plane (OP)	13°	9.3°
Z angle	68°	80 ± 5°

Chronologic age, 7 yr 6 mo
Dental age, 6 yr 6 mo

1.	SPACE REQUIRED	71 mm.
2.	SPACE AVAILABLE	65 mm.
3.	ARCH LENGTH DISC.	-6 mm.
4.	CEPH. DISC. -6×2	-12 mm.
	TOTAL DISC.	-18 mm.

Fig. 6-79 Tweed method. Cephalometric correction.

and the line that passed through the actual axial inclination of the mandibular incisors was measured on the occlusal plane with pointed calipers to the nearest 0.1 mm (6 mm). This figure was multiplied by 2 to include right and left sides (12 mm). The total was the cephalometric correction, which was then added to the difference between space required and space available to yield the total discrepancy (Fig. 6-79).

Total space analysis. This method was divided into three areas—anterior, middle, and posterior—and the resulting values for each area were added together to yield the final deficit (Table 6-3).

Anterior area. For this area the calculation of the difference between space required and space available was done as before. However, the *space required* included, in addition to tooth measurement and cephalometric correction, soft tissue modification.

Tooth measurement. Measurements of mandibular incisor widths on the cast were added to the values obtained from the radiographic measurements of the canines. Both measurements were made according to a previously described technique (Figs. 6-75 through 6-77).

Cephalometric correction. The cephalometric correction was calculated as for the Tweed method. However, instead of measurements being made of the distance (in millimeters) on the occlusal plane between the objective line and the line indicating the true axial inclination of the mandibular incisors, the actual FMIA (in degrees) was subtracted from the proposed angle and the difference (in degrees) was multiplied by a constant (0.8) to give the difference in millimeters (Fig. 6-80) (Table 6-3).

Soft tissue modification. Whereas the Tweed method added the anterior skeletal dental relationships to the dental-oriented mixed dentition analysis, this method adds a consideration of the soft tissue profile. Thus the teeth, jaws, and soft tissue all are involved in the assessment.

The soft tissue modification was derived by measuring the Z angle of Merrifield[43,44] and adding the cephalometric

TABLE 6-3

Total Space Analysis

	Deficit	Surplus
Anterior		
Required space		
Tooth width $\overline{3\ 2\ 1\ \vert\ 1\ 2\ 3}$	39.0	
Cephalometric correction ($68 - 50 = 18 \times 0.8 = 14.4$)	14.4	
Soft tissue modification ($58° + 18° = 76°$)	—	
Available space		36.0 (brass wire)
	17.4	
Middle		
Required space	58.0	
Tooth width $\overline{6\ 5\ 4\ \vert\ 4\ 5\ 6}$		
Curve of occlusion $\left(\dfrac{1.5 + 1.5}{2} = 1.5 + 0.5 = 2.0\right)$	2.0	
Available space		60.0 (brass wire)
	0.0	
Posterior		
Required space	42.0	
Tooth width $\overline{8\ 7\ \vert\ 7\ 8}$		
Available space		
Presently available		4.0
Estimated increase $\left(\begin{array}{l}14\ \text{yr} - 8.3\ \text{yr} = 5.7\ \text{yr}\\ 5.7\ \text{yr} \times 3 = 17.1\ \text{mm}\end{array}\right)$		17.1
	20.9	
Total	38.3	

Total deficit: 38.3 mm (anterior 17.4, posterior 20.9).
Extraction of first premolars: 16 mm (correct anterior deficit).
New deficit: 38.3 − 16.0 = 22.3 mm.
Extraction of third molars: 20 mm (correct posterior deficit).
Final deficit: 22.3 − 20.0 = 2.3 mm.

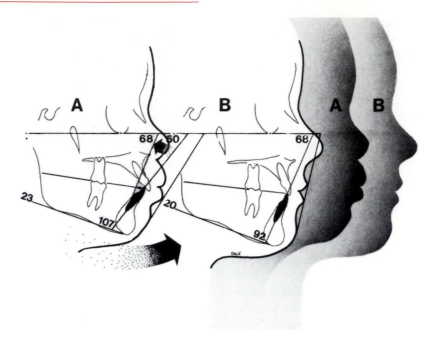

Fig. 6-80 Total space analysis. Anterior arch cephalometric correction.

correction (in degrees) to it. If the corrected Z angle was greater than 80°, the mandibular incisor inclination was modified as necessary (up to an IMPA of approximately 92°). If the corrected angle was less than 75°, additional uprighting of the mandibular incisors was necessary. Upper lip thickness was measured from the vermilion border of the lip to the greatest curvature of the labial surface of the central incisor. Total chin thickness was measured from the soft tissue chin to the N-B line.

If lip thickness was greater than chin thickness, the difference (in millimeters) was determined, multiplied by 2, and added to the space required. If it was less than or equal to chin thickness, no soft tissue modification was necessary.

Fig. 6-81 portrays *patient M.L.,* described in Fig. 6-80 and Table 6-3, who had a typical Class I malocclusion with an alveolodental protrusion and an incompetent lip relationship (Fig. 6-81, *A* and *B*). Note the improvement in muscle balance and facial harmony after serial extraction and active treatment (Fig. 6-81, *C* and *D*).

The *space available* was obtained by placing a brass wire (0.033 inch) from the mesiobuccal of the primary first mandibular molar to the mesiobuccal of the opposite molar (Fig. 6-82). The wire was then straightened and measured with a pointed caliper to the nearest 0.1 mm. This value was subtracted from the total space required to yield the deficit (Table 6-3).

Middle area. For this area calculations were made of the difference between *space required* and *space available*. In this instance, however, the mandibular curve of occlusion was considered.

Tooth measurement. The crown widths of the permanent mandibular first molars were measured at their greatest me-

siodistal diameter on the cast. These values were added to the measurements of the premolars obtained from the radiographs (Figs. 6-75 to 6-77).

Curve of occlusion. The calculations for the curve of occlusion were done as follows:

The *space required* to level the mandibular curve of occlusion was determined (Fig. 6-83). A flat object was placed on the occlusal surfaces of the mandibular teeth contacting the permanent first molars and the incisors. The deepest point between this flat surface and the occlusal surfaces of the primary molars was measured on both sides. The curve of occlusion formula was applied and the space required for leveling was determined. This was added to the tooth measurements to complete the space required (Table 6-3). The curve of occlusion formula used the greatest depth of each side:

$$\frac{\text{Right side depth} + \text{Left side depth}}{2} + 0.5 \text{ mm}$$

The *space available* was determined by placing two brass wires (0.033 inch) from the mesiobuccal of the primary first molars to the distobuccal of the permanent first molars (Fig. 6-84). These were measured as before, added together, and subtracted from the space required (Table 6-3).

Posterior area. For this area determinations were made of the space required and space available (including that presently available and that predicted).

The *space required* consisted of the sum of the mesiodistal widths of the two second and third molars, which were unerupted in these patients (Fig. 6-85). Because they were unerupted, radiographic enlargements had to be calculated. However, the formula used for the conventional method was

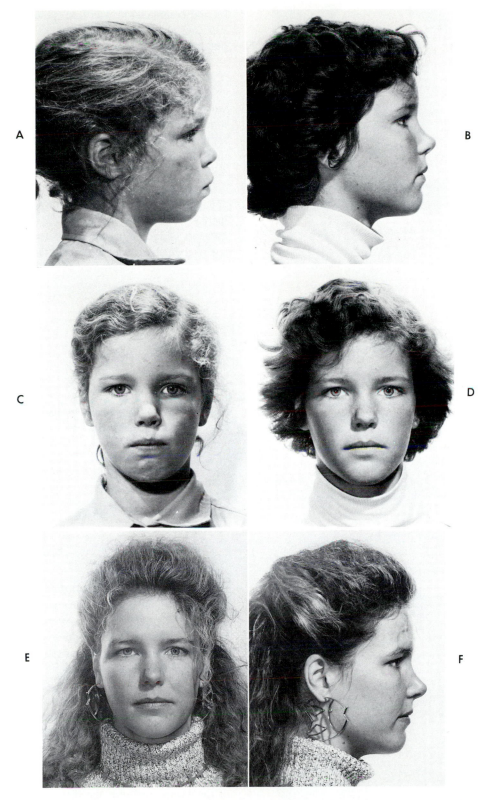

Fig. 6-81   Patient M.L. **A** and **C,** Before treatment. **B** and **D,** After treatment. **E** and **F,** Balance and harmony persist as an adult, fifteen years later.

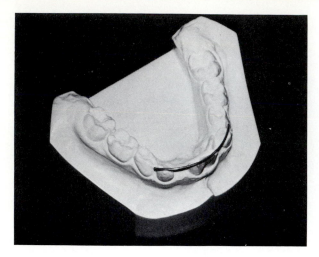

Fig. 6-82   Total space analysis. Measurement of space available in the anterior area.

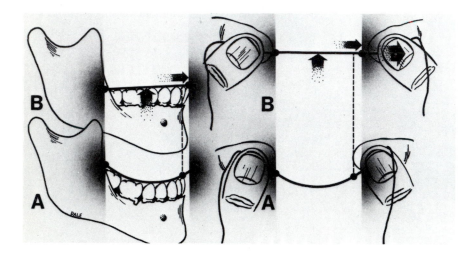

Fig. 6-83   Total space analysis. Curve of occlusion.

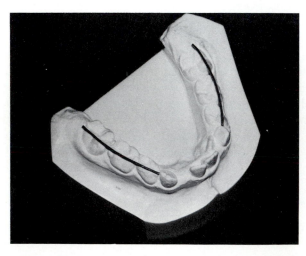

Fig. 6-84   Total space analysis. Measurement of space available in the middle area.

modified. In this instance the permanent mandibular first molars were substituted for the primary second molars. A second complication was that quite often the third molars were not visible on the radiographs. In this case Wheeler's measurements were used and the calculation was as follows:

$$x = \frac{y - x^1}{y^1}$$

where x is the estimated value of the permanent mandibular third molar in the individual patient; x^1 is Wheeler's value for third molars; y is the actual size of permanent mandibular first molar on the cast; and y^1 is Wheeler's value for first molars.

The *space available* consisted of the space presently available plus the estimated increase or prediction. The estimated increase was 3 mm per year (1.5 mm for each side) until 14 years of age in girls and 16 years in boys. Therefore the age of the patient was subtracted from either 14 or 16. The result was multiplied by 3 to obtain the estimated increase for the individual patient. The space presently available was obtained by measuring the distance on the occlusal plane between a perpendicular line drawn from the occlusal plane tangent to the distal surface of the permanent first molar to the anterior border of the ramus on the lateral cephalometric tracing (Fig. 6-85). After the presently available space and the predicted space were totaled to give the space available, the space required was subtracted (Table 6-3).

Discussion.   Since the total space analysis involves the permanent molars, it was not possible to compare its results with those of the other two procedures. However, when the results of the conventional method are compared with those of the Tweed method, the differences become highly significant.

The assessment of axial inclination of the mandibular anterior teeth with respect to the basal bone must be included in the analysis of mixed dentition malocclusions so there

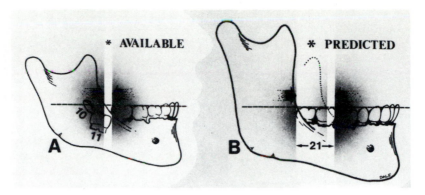

Fig. 6-85   Total space analysis. Measurement of the available and predicted space in the posterior area.

will be harmony in the facial profile and stability in the dentition. The cephalometric correction in the Tweed method accounts for 9.8% of the space required, a considerable amount.

Table 6-4 illustrates the differences between the conventional method and the Tweed method in one of the subjects of the investigation. When the techniques are compared, it is evident that completely different treatment plans will result.

According to the conventional method *patient L.S.* would have been treated without extraction, even if the profile had presented the unfavorable appearance portrayed by *patient M.L.* (Fig. 6-81, *A* and *B*). Certainly the beautiful balance and harmony evident in Fig. 6-81, *C* and *D*, and *E* and *F*, would not have been possible without consideration of the alveolodental protrusion and without extraction of the premolar teeth. The Tweed method indicated that extractions were necessary to produce a successful treatment result even though it did not indicate specifically which teeth.

The total space analysis enables the clinician to identify the specific area of the dental arch where crowding or spacing exists, and results indicate that extraction of teeth will vary considerably depending on the location and extent of the discrepancy. When two patients have a tooth-size jaw-

size discrepancy, the treatment plans may be different depending on the amount of crowding and the location. For example, in Table 6-5 *patient M.M.* will require extraction of the first premolars to alleviate crowding in the anterior area followed by the extraction of third molars to alleviate crowding in the posterior. However, *patient L.D.* will be treated by extraction of the second premolars only. Anterior teeth will be moved distally to relieve the discrepancy in the anterior area, and the molars will be moved mesially to relieve the discrepancy in the posterior. The malocclusion of *M.M.* will be more suitable for serial extraction than that of *L.D.* since the ultimate teeth extracted will be the first premolars. Both patients had a Class I malocclusion.

Patient M.L. (Figs. 6-80 and 6-81, Table 6-3) exemplifies an ideal serial extraction situation: a Class I mixed dentition malocclusion with an anterior discrepancy in the form of an alveolodental protrusion and a posterior discrepancy with a medium angle facial pattern. The first premolars were extracted to correct the anterior discrepancy, and the third molars were extracted to correct the posterior discrepancy.

Patient M.R. (Fig. 6-133, Table 6-6) also is a good example of a favorable serial extraction situation: a Class I mixed dentition malocclusion with an anterior discrepancy in the form of a moderate alveolodental protrusion and a posterior discrepancy with a relatively high angle facial pattern. The same teeth were extracted as in *M.L.* for somewhat different reasons. The anterior discrepancy is more related to the alveolodental protrusion in *M.L.* than in *M.R.* The posterior discrepancy is more related to the high angle facial pattern in *M.R.* than in *M.L.*

Patient J.L. (Fig. 6-136, Table 6-6) would not have been a good candidate for serial extraction when he was younger, even if there had been a Class I tooth-size jaw-size discrepancy. He had a severe high angle facial pattern that was contributing to the posterior middle discrepancy and the open bite. The first molars were extracted to correct the posterior discrepancy and to rotate the mandible favorably in an upward and forward direction, which, in turn, contributed to the reduction of the severe open bite. Serial

TABLE 6-4

Mixed Dentition Analysis—Comparison of the Conventional and Tweed Methods

L.S.	Conventional method (mm)	Tweed method (mm)
Space required	− 69.3	− 69.3
Space available	+ 69.1	+ 69.1
Discrepancy	− 0.2	− 0.2
Cephalometric correction	—	− 8.0
Total discrepancy	− 0.2	− 8.2
Difference between two methods		− 8.0

TABLE 6-5
Total Space Analyses—Comparison of Patients M.M. and L.D.

	M.M. (mm)		L.D. (mm)	
Anterior				
Required space		−44.9		−39.6
Tooth widths $\overline{3\ 2\ 1\ |\ 1\ 2\ 3}$	−35.9		−37.6	
Cephalometric correction*	− 9.0		− 2.0	
Available space		+32.9		+33.5
Deficit		−12.0		− 6.1
Middle				
Required space		−50.3		−55.9
Tooth widths $\overline{6\ 5\ 4\ |\ 4\ 5\ 6}$	−48.6		−54.2	
Curve of occlusion*	− 1.7		− 1.7	
Available space		+54.1		+59.6
Surplus		+ 3.8		− 2.4
Posterior				
Required space		−40.0		−41.0
Tooth widths $\overline{8\ 7\ |\ 7\ 8}$	−40.0		−41.0	
Available space		+19.9		+36.0
Presently available	+ 4.0		+ 9.0	
Estimated increase*	+15.0		+27.0	
Deficit		−20.1		− 5.0
TOTAL DISCREPANCY		−28.3		−13.5

M.M.
Total deficit: 28.3 mm (anterior 12.0, middle +3.8, posterior 20.1)
Extraction of first premolars: 16.0 mm
New deficit: 28.3 − 16.0 = 12.3 mm
Extraction of third molars: 20.0 mm
Final surplus: 20.0 − 12.3 = 7.7 mm

L.D.
Total deficit: 13.5 mm (anterior −6.1, middle −2.4, posterior −5.0)
Extraction of second premolars: 16.0 mm
Final surplus: 2.5 mm
Move anterior teeth back into middle surplus
Move posterior teeth forward into middle surplus

*Soft tissue and Class II factors have been eliminated from this specific description of the analysis.

TABLE 6-6
Total Space Analysis, Mandibular Dentition, for Four Patients (Millimeters) Included in this Chapter

M.R. (Fig. 6-133)		J.L. (Fig. 6-136)		J.O. (Fig. 6-137)		G.L. (Fig. 6-98)	
Anterior deficit	16.6	Anterior deficit	0.0	Anterior deficit	15.4	Anterior deficit	18.0
Middle deficit	0.0	Middle deficit	16.0	Middle surplus	1.5	Middle deficit	5.0
Posterior deficit	12.0	Posterior deficit	9.0	Posterior deficit	15.0	Posterior deficit	11.0
Total deficit	28.6	Total deficit	25.0	Total deficit	28.9	Total deficit	34.0
Extraction $\frac{4\ |\ 4}{4\ |\ 4}$	16.0	Extraction $\frac{6\ |\ 6}{6\ |\ 6}$	23.0	Extraction $\frac{4\ |\ 4}{4\ |\ 4}$	16.0	Extraction $\frac{4\ |\ 4}{4\ |\ 4}$	16.0
New deficit	12.6			New deficit	12.9	New deficit	18.0
Extraction $\frac{8\ |\ 8}{8\ |\ 8}$	20.0			Extraction $\frac{8\ |\ 8}{8\ |\ 8}$	20.0	Extraction $\frac{8\ |\ 8}{8\ |\ 8}$	20.0
FINAL SURPLUS	7.4	**FINAL DEFICIT**	2.0	**FINAL SURPLUS**	7.1	**FINAL SURPLUS**	2.0

extraction does not culminate in the extraction of four first molars, nor is it advisable in severe high angle posterior discrepancy patients.

Patient J.O. (Fig. 6-137, Table 6-6) has a moderately high angle facial pattern with a posterior discrepancy, a Class II malocclusion, and an open bite with an anterior discrepancy. The four first premolars were extracted to correct the anterior discrepancy, and the four third molars were extracted to correct the posterior discrepancy. All responses were favorable.

Patient G.L. (Fig. 6-98, Table 6-6) is somewhat similar to *patient J.O.* Both have Class II malocclusions, both have anterior and posterior discrepancies, and both had the same teeth extracted. *G.L.,* however, did not benefit from serial extraction.

Thus each of these individuals was treated differently depending on the results of the various diagnostic procedures, including total space analysis.

Harris[45] has developed a graphic format that enables the clinician to visualize, in an easily understood and simple manner, the results of the total space analysis. It is possible to calculate from the graph the efficiency of treatment on a monthly basis and on an office visit basis; it is also possible to determine if treatment objectives have been accomplished.

Fig. 6-86 illustrates the Harris graph. The *anterior discrepancy* (AD) is plotted in the vertical direction, on the Y axis in millimeters, and the *middle discrepancy* (MD) is plotted in the horizontal direction along the X axis. Diagonal lines are drawn at 5 mm intervals from the X to Y axes.

If a patient has an AD of 15 mm and an MD of 5 mm a dot is placed on the graph to correspond to these measurements. The dot rests on the 20 mm diagonal line, which indicates that 20 mm of treatment is required to complete the correction of the malocclusion. When the treatment goal is achieved, the dot should come to rest on the *XY* intersect.

Treatment efficiency ratio. TER is the treatment delivered in millimeters divided by the number of months of active treatment: TER = TD divided by months. In this patient, 20 mm of treatment were required to correct the malocclusion, and the objective was achieved. Therefore 1.0 mm of progress was noted each month: 20 mm divided by 20 months = 1.0. If 10 mm were corrected in 20 months, the TER would have been 0.5, indicating ½ mm of progress per month. If 20 mm were corrected in 10 months, the TER would have been 2.0, indicating 2 mm of

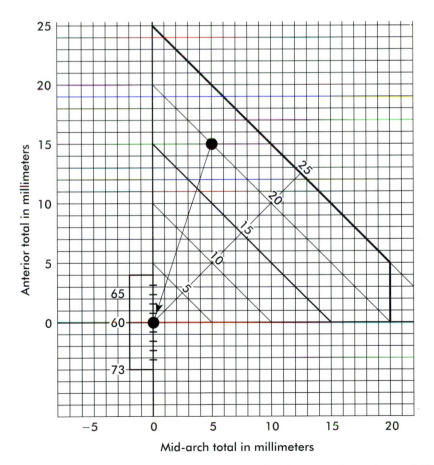

Fig. 6-86   Graphic display of total space analysis. (Harris GS: *J Tweed Foundation* 13:28-52, 1985.)

progress each month. Harris reported that a range of 0.5 mm to 1.2 mm of progress per month is common when measuring typical cases treated by members of the Tweed Foundation.

Treatment delivered per office visit. TD/OV is the treatment delivered divided by the number of the office visits during active treatment. In this patient, 15 office visits were required to complete treatment. Thus 1.33 mm of progress were achieved between each visit: 20 mm divided by 15 visits = 1.33. If 20 visits were required, 1 mm of progress would have been achieved between each appointment. If only ten visits were required, two millimeters of progress would have been recorded.

Treatment delivered divided by treatment required. TD/TR is a useful measurement of orthodontic expertise and is expressed as a percentage value. It is a measurement of the orthodontist's skill in the management of the patient's malocclusion. If 20 mm of treatment are delivered (as with this patient) where 20 mm are required, the orthodontist is 100% successful. If only 10 mm are delivered, the orthodontist is only 50% successful.

Fig. 6-87 illustrates how the graph indicates the extraction decision based on AD and MD measurements. If the dot is placed within the triangle representing 0-8 AD and 0-8 MD based on this analysis, the patient should be treated without the extraction of teeth, third molar notwithstanding. If the AD ranges from 8 to 15 and the MD ranges approximately from 0 to 8, four first premolars should be extracted. The anterior discrepancy is greater. Thus the first premolars are closest to the problem, and the orthodontist should extract as close to the problem as possible to reduce treatment time. If the dot is placed in the area measured by the MD 8 to 15 and AD 0 to 8, maxillary first and mandibular second premolar extraction are indicated. Mandibular incisors are in a relative upright and favorable position. Care must be taken to prevent further uprighting, which could create a concave profile. The further out the dot is placed in graph, the more involved the treatment becomes, including the extraction of molars and orthognathic surgery.

Serial extraction was plotted on the graph in Fig. 6-88 for two of Harris' patients: 27 and 11. *Patient 27's* dot, AD 9 to MD 6, fell within the AD 8 to 15, MD 0 to 8 area; therefore, four first premolars were ultimately extracted. Two millimeters of MD remained untreated following *serial extraction.* This would have been corrected during the active treatment period. *Patient 11's* dot, 8 AD to 9 MD, fell within the AD 0 to 8, MD 8 to 15, indicating that the maxillary first and the mandibular second premolars were

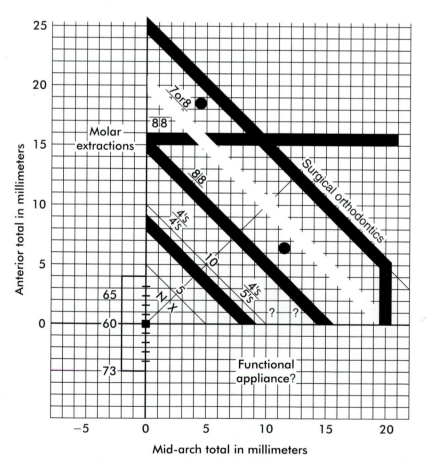

Fig. 6-87 Harris graph illustrating extraction alternatives.

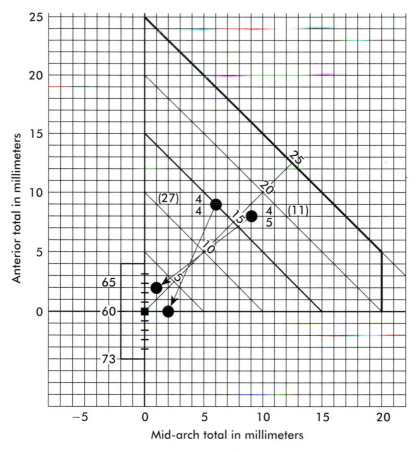

Fig. 6-88 Harris graph illustrating serial extraction progress.

extracted following *serial extraction*. Two millimeters of AD and 1 mm of MD remained to be treated during appliance therapy.

Dental Age Analysis

In orthodontics the practitioner is interested in predicting the ultimate size, the rate of maturation of the jaws, the emergence of teeth into the oral cavity, and the ultimate treatment result. The adolescent growth spurt of the body and its relation to the accelerated growth in the craniofacial complex is also of interest, as well as the relationship between chronologic age, skeletal age, and dental age.

Using information derived from longitudinal studies, the clinician who is attempting to guide the teeth into a favorable occlusion can more accurately predict important events in the development of the dentition. For instance, the unerupted permanent tooth is literally standing still until half its root is formed. With this knowledge the orthodontist would hesitate to extract the primary first molar if its permanent successor had less than one half root formation. This would delay rather than accelerate the eruption of the premolar. The practitioner also knows that (1) teeth emerge into the oral cavity when three quarters of their roots are formed

(Fig. 6-89); (2) it requires 2½ years for the canine root to go from one quarter to one half root length and 1½ years to go from a half to three quarters (Fig. 6-90); (3) it requires 1¾ years for the first premolar root to go from one quarter to one half root length and 1½ years to go from a half to three quarters (Fig. 6-90). Armed with this information the clinician, on inspecting the periapical radiograph, can predict the emergence of these teeth and can time their extraction more precisely. For instance, if a periapical radiograph shows that the canine has one quarter of its root formed, then it is obvious that 4 years will be needed for the canine to develop three quarters of its root length and emerge into the oral cavity. Also, if it is observed that the first premolar has one quarter of its root formed, then obviously 3¼ years must elapse for the root to reach three quarters of its length and the tooth to emerge into the oral cavity. Similar information associated with the maxillary incisors can be used to guide the timing of partial multibanded treatment and interceptive procedures. Information associated with the second premolars and second molars can also be used in the initiation of multibonded mechanotherapy and permanent dentition treatment. Multibonded appliances are inserted when the maxillary permanent canines and mandibular second premolars have erupted sufficiently. In deep

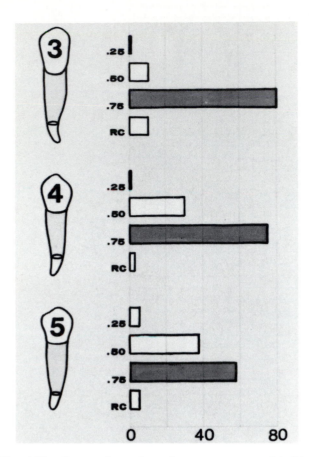

Fig. 6-89 Extent of root formation at emergence. (Modified from Moorrees CFA, Fanning EA, Grøn AM: *Angle Orthod* 33:44, 1963.)

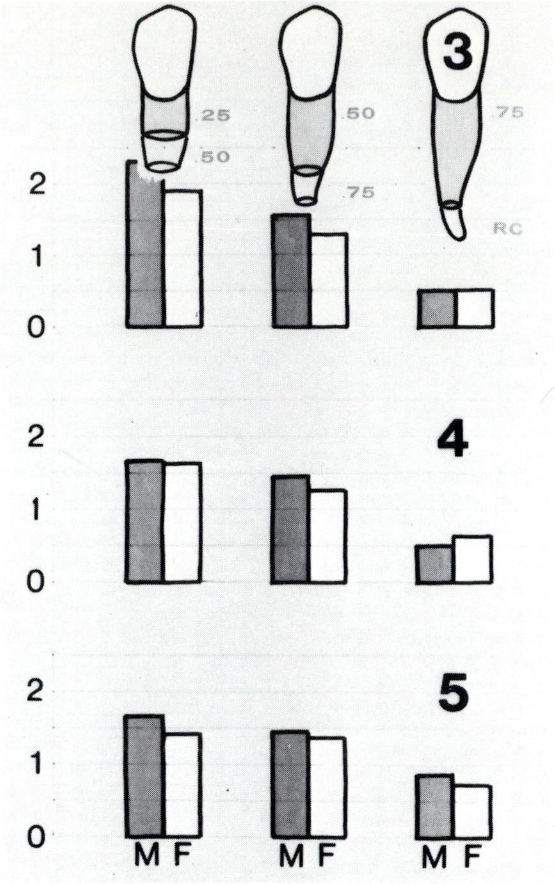

Fig. 6-90 Average time for the development of quarter stages of root length. (Modified from Moorrees CFA, Fanning EA, Grøn AM: *Angle Orthod* 33:44, 1963.)

overbite malocclusions the placement of appliances is delayed until the permanent second molars have emerged.

Before the case presentation and when the diagnostic records are being studied and evaluated, the dental age is determined according to the method outlined by Moorrees* and his associates, Fanning,[21,23] Grøn,[27] and Lebret.[35] This enables the orthodontist to predict precisely when the canines, premolars, and second molars will emerge into the oral cavity. As a result it is possible to outline the treatment plan more specifically and with more confidence during the case presentation.

The longitudinal growth and development studies conducted by Moorrees, Meredith,[42] Sillman,[59] and others have provided a scientific basis for prediction in relation to (1) the development of the dentition, (2) the guidance of occlusion, including serial extraction, and (3) the timing of treatment.

The dentition counts as a separate tissue system in the growth process, and the timing of its growth changes is dependent on the formation of the teeth. An absolute prerequisite for the prediction of events in the development of the dentition therefore is the establishment of the patient's dental age.

Tooth emergence is a convenient method for age assessment, but its value is limited. Emergence is a single fleeting occurrence in the continuous process of tooth eruption, and the chance that the time of inspection will coincide with the actual moment of emergence is small. Moreover, eruption may be influenced by exogenous factors, such as infection, injury, obstruction, crowding, and extraction of teeth. The rate of eruption may be decreased by deficiency of vitamin A or D, hypothyroidism, and sickness; it may be increased by prolonged intrauterine development, prolonged sleep, semistarvation, hyperthyroidism, cortisone administration, and increased activity (to mention only a few).

Tooth formation is preferable to tooth emergence for assessing dental age. It is not influenced as markedly by exogenous factors, and a rating is possible at all times from birth to the completion of the third molars.

Root resorption of the primary dentition is also used for

---

*References 47, 49, 51, 54, 55.

determining dental age from 4 to 12 years; however, it is subject to considerable variation. Combined with formation and emergence it completes the developmental history of the dentition.

In 1949, Hurme,[32] working at the Forsyth Infirmary, published an extensive study on the emergence of teeth based on 93,000 children throughout the world. It was an extensive undertaking that involved 100 years of publications in eight different countries. As a result of this study a chart was produced that has become a classic in the field. For the first time an emergence chart indicated variability and sex differences. According to Hurme, girls erupt their teeth 5 months earlier than boys; the mandibular canines show the most sex difference, with 11 months between girls and boys, and the maxillary first molars show the least difference, with 2 months between the sexes. As regards variability, the mandibular second premolars show the most, with a difference of 3 years 5 months, and the mandibular central incisors show the least, with 1 year 4 months difference. Hurme's chart presented the emergence data for girls and boys in both the maxillary and the mandibular permanent dentition. It also indicated the mean, together with one standard deviation (SD) early and late, for 68.35% of the population. The emergence times range from that of the mandibular central incisors (which are the least variable) through those of the maxillary first molars, mandibular first molars, maxillary central incisors, mandibular lateral incisors, maxillary lateral incisors, mandibular canines, mandibular second molars, maxillary second molars, maxillary canines, mandibular first premolars, maxillary first premolars, and maxillary second premolars to, finally, that of the mandibular second premolars (which are the most variable). In regards to sex difference, the maxillary first molars have the least. They are followed by the maxillary central incisors, mandibular first molars, mandibular central incisors, maxillary second premolars, mandibular lateral incisors, maxillary first premolars, maxillary second molars, mandibular second molars, maxillary lateral incisors, mandibular second premolars, mandibular first premolars, maxillary canines, and finally mandibular canines (which have the most sex difference) (Fig. 6-91).

In 1978 Moorrees published, with Kent, Jr.,[54] a new set

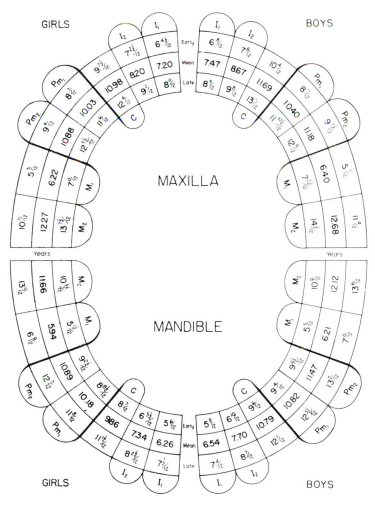

Fig. 6-91 Assessment of dental age by mean age of tooth emergence (± 1 SD). (From Hurme VO: *J Dent Child* 16:11, 1949.)

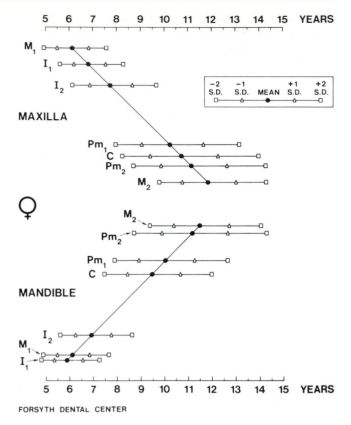

Fig. 6-92 Assessment of dental age by tooth emergence. (From Moorrees CFA, Kent RL, Jr: In McNamara JA, Jr, editor: *Monograph 6: craniofacial growth series,* Ann Arbor, 1978, Center for Human Development, University of Michigan.)

of norms for tooth emergence (Fig. 6-92). Median ages for emergence of the permanent maxillary and mandibular teeth were given on horizontal lines together with ± 1 and 2 SD limits. Oblique lines conveyed the median time interval between emergence of successive teeth and also indicated the order in which maxillary and mandibular teeth emerge. By drawing a vertical line representing the chronologic age from the top scale to the bottom the dental age can be calculated. This combined with the clinical observation of the precise moment of emergence enabled comparison of the dental age with the chronologic age for a determination of whether emergence was late or early, and by how much.

Note that on the emergence charts the teeth appear to fall into two groups: early and late. In other words, a time gap exists between emergence of the incisors and first molars and that of the canines, premolars, and second molars. This situation was used by Moorrees and his group to establish another set of charts that aided in the assessment of dental age. These charts, based on the number of teeth visible in the oral cavity at a given time, removed the frustration of not being present when a specific tooth emerged through the gingival tissue. The method was referred to as a *step function* (Fig. 6-93). By this method the median ages of attainment for number of teeth present, determined separately for 12 early-emerging teeth (incisors, first molars) and 16 late-emerging teeth (canines, premolars, second molars), could be shown for boys and for girls as functions on a log scale.

Essentially, if the early teeth have emerged early, a fairly accurate prediction can be made that the late teeth will emerge early as well. Correlation coefficients of 0.72 in

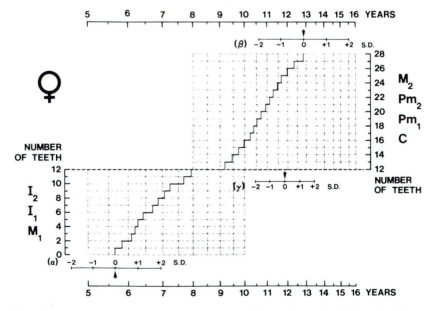

Fig. 6-93 Assessment of dental age by emergence. (From Moorrees CFA, Kent RL, Jr: *Ann Hum Biol* 5:1, 1978.)

boys and 0.78 in girls indicate that a consistency in dental emergence is evident. For instance, on the chart for girls (Fig. 6-93) eight teeth in the oral cavity at 7 years of age can be observed. If only five are apparent, then the patient's dental age is approximately 6½ years. In other words, the patient is 1 SD late according to *goodness of fit* with the norm. If this has been a consistent observation from 5 to 9 years, the orthodontist can predict with reasonable accuracy that the late teeth will emerge 1 SD late as well. (Refer to the article by Moorrees and Kent[54] for a more detailed description of this fascinating technique.)

In 1962 Moorrees, Fanning, Grøn, and Lebret published charts for the assessment of dental age by tooth formation. One of these charts, associated with the eruption of the canines and premolars for girls, is seen in Fig. 6-94. To understand its use, refer to Fig. 6-95. *A* is a radiograph of a girl chronologically 8 years of age. The second premolar is just initiating its root formation. *B* also is a radiograph of a girl chronologically 8 years of age. However, the second premolar has half its root formed. *C* is a close-up view of the second premolar area on the tooth formation chart for girls (Fig. 6-94). Since both girls are chronologically 8 years of age, a vertical line is drawn from 8 on the top scale to 8 on the bottom scale. According to the chart the mean for root initiation (R_i) is 7 years of age; therefore the girl in Fig. 6-95, *A*, has a dental age of 7 years. Again, according to the chart the mean for half root formation is 9 years of age; thus the girl in Fig. 6-95, *B*, has a dental age of 9.

Multibonded treatment will begin when the second premolars emerge into the oral cavity. The Moorrees data instructs that the second premolars emerge at three quarters root development. According to the chart the mean for root three quarters is 10 years of age. Therefore treatment will begin for the girl in Fig. 6-95, *A*, at 11 years of age chronologically and for the girl in Fig. 6-95, *C*, at 9 years chronologically, a difference of 2 years.

A set of charts (Fig. 6-96) has been produced at the Forsyth Dental Center that are an improvement on the orig-

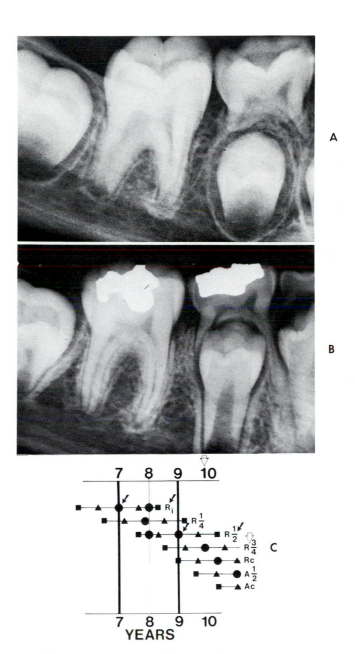

Fig. 6-95 Chronologic age, 8 years. The second premolar, **A,** is just initiating its root formation and, **B,** has half its root formed. **C,** Detail of chart (Fig. 6-94) in the second premolar area.

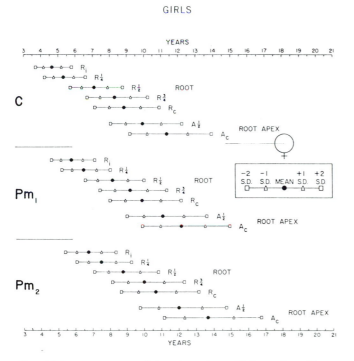

Fig. 6-94 Assessment of dental age by tooth formation. (From Moorrees CFA, Fanning EA, Grøn AM, Lebret J: *Eur Orthod Soc Trans* 38:87, 1962.)

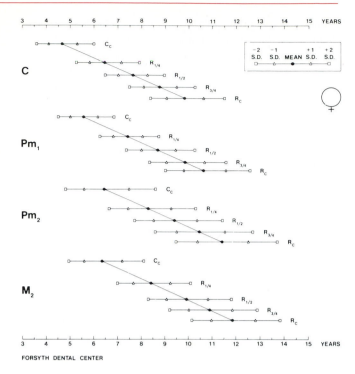

Fig. 6-96 Formation stages for permanent mandibular teeth. (From Moorrees CFA, Kent RL, Jr, Lebret L: Unpublished material, 1982.)

inal because they include the second molars. Nevertheless, they are used in precisely the same manner. The charts are based on an extensive and comprehensive longitudinal twin study conducted under the supervision of Dr. Moorrees, but they have not been published previously. However, Dr. Lebret, the investigator in this instance, has very kindly given her permission to include them in this discussion. There are similar charts available for assessing dental age according to (1) primary tooth formation, (2) primary tooth resorption, (3) permanent incisor tooth formation, and (4) third molar tooth formation.

Does planned removal of the primary teeth exercise some control over the eruptive sequence of the permanent teeth? The answer is yes. In the January 1962 issue of *The Angle Orthodontist*,[21] Fanning describes the effects of primary tooth extraction on the rate of root formation, eruption, and the underlying permanent tooth. No change in the rate of root formation of the premolar was observed after extraction of the primary molar. However, an immediate spurt occurred in the eruption of the premolar regardless of the stage of development and the age at which the primary molar was extracted. Early clinical emergence occurred if extraction of the primary molar coincided with the later development of the premolar. Three factors may be applied by the clinician in deciding the optimum time for the removal of teeth in the guidance of occlusion: (1) the effect of extraction of the primary tooth on the eruption of its permanent successor;

(2) the amount of root formation at the time of emergence; and (3) the length of time for the attainment of various stages of root development.

Serial extraction, if carried out too early in the primary dentition, can delay the eruption of permanent successors. In the case of early extraction of the primary molar, Fanning[21] reported an initial spurt in eruption of the premolar. This leveled off and the tooth then remained stationary, erupting later than its antimere with a normally shedding primary precursor. If serial extraction is initiated with the extraction of the primary canines, the length of the roots of the premolars is not an important consideration. If, however, the orthodontist is contemplating initiating serial extraction by the removal of the primary first molars, then the length of the root of the premolar is an important consideration and guide for the commencement of the procedure.

The relative eruptive rates of the permanent canines and first premolars influence the decision about which primary teeth should be extracted. When an examination of the periapical radiographs is made and the permanent mandibular first premolar crown is observed ahead of the permanent canine crown, the premolar has less than half its root formed, and the mandibular incisors are crowded, then the primary canine should be extracted to relieve the crowding. The primary first molar should be left until the first premolar has attained half its root length. If, on examining the radiographs, the orthodontist observes the premolar crown even with the canine crown, the premolar with half its root formed, and an alveolodental protrusion, then the primary first molar should be extracted to encourage the emergence of its successor.

Dental age, assessed particularly by root length, is an essential requirement in the decision of a serial extraction program and in the initiation of interceptive and definitive multibonded treatment. A knowledge of root development, relative eruptive rates, and the emergence of permanent teeth, together with root resorption of the primary teeth and the factors that influence these processes, is mandatory in the timing of serial extraction.

TREATMENT

Throughout my career I have adhered primarily to the principles and objectives of the Tweed philosophy,[16] defined as

The search for the truth and the quest for excellence in diagnosis and treatment. It is characterized by honesty with ourselves, with our colleagues and above all with our patients. It is sincerity of purpose and action, with the belief that the service rendered is infinitely more important than the reward received. It assumes that the orthodontist will limit his practice to the number of patients who can properly be cared for, and that he will conduct himself in such a manner as to reflect credit upon his profession.

Clinically Dr. Tweed advocated maximum facial harmony and balance. To achieve this goal, he recognized that mandibular incisor teeth must be placed upright over basal bone. This, in turn, routinely requires anchorage preparation and the extraction of teeth.

The primary objective of The Charles H. Tweed International Foundation for Orthodontic Research today is the spatial positioning of the dentition within the oral environment to obtain maximum health, esthetics, function, and stability. Specifically it is excellence in tooth alignment, arch form, and axial inclination of the teeth, with optimal occlusal intercuspation of the maxillary and mandibular dentitions through the use of one of the most precise instruments for the correction of malocclusions that exist in the world today.

Tweed[16] once said

The world should be a beautiful place for a child to live. If he is handicapped by facial deformity that is marring his happiness, we should make every effort to restore that happiness. To say that there is no use trying to help a patient because he has a certain facial type, or he has a facial pattern with serious abnormal deviations, is not courageous. We must strive for maximum harmony and balance as near to normal as conditions will allow.

With the Tweed philosophy as it exists at present—including such modern developments as (1) differential diagnosis, (2) total space analysis, (3) proportional facial analysis, (4) dimensions of the dentition, (5) directional force systems including 10-2 concepts, (6) action, reaction, and interaction of forces, (7) precision wire manipulation, (8) prescription arches, (9) *readout* procedures to monitor tooth position, and (10) performance standards evaluation—the clinician is in an ideal position to establish "maximum harmony and balance as near to normal as conditions will allow."

Objectives of treatment include the following:

1. Decrease in the FMA, indicating a favorable rotation of the mandible
2. Decrease in the IMPA, indicating the reduction of the alveolodental protrusion
3. Increase in the FMIA, also indicating an uprighting of the mandibular incisor teeth
4. Decrease in the occlusal plane angle throughout treatment, indicating that one is not extruding the posterior teeth or *dumping* the anterior teeth forward
5. Decrease in the A-N-B angle, indicating a correction of the skeletal discrepancy
6. Increase in Merrifield's Z *angle,* indicating improvement in facial harmony and balance

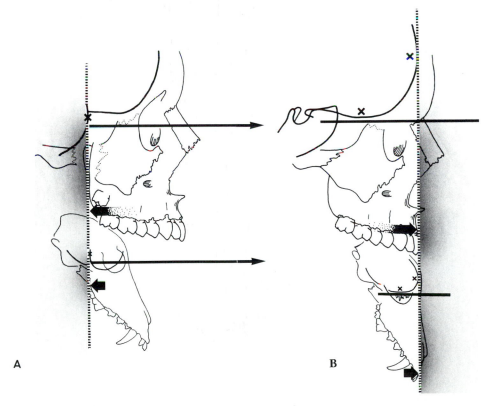

Fig. 6-97   **A,** Posterior limits of the nasomaxillary area: a line perpendicular to the line of sight passing through the junction of the anterior and middle cranial fossae. **B,** Anterior limit of the nasomaxillary complex: a line extending from the internal surface of the frontal bone and running perpendicular to the ethmoid. (Modified from Enlow DH: *Handbook of facial growth,* Philadelphia, 1982, WB Saunders.)

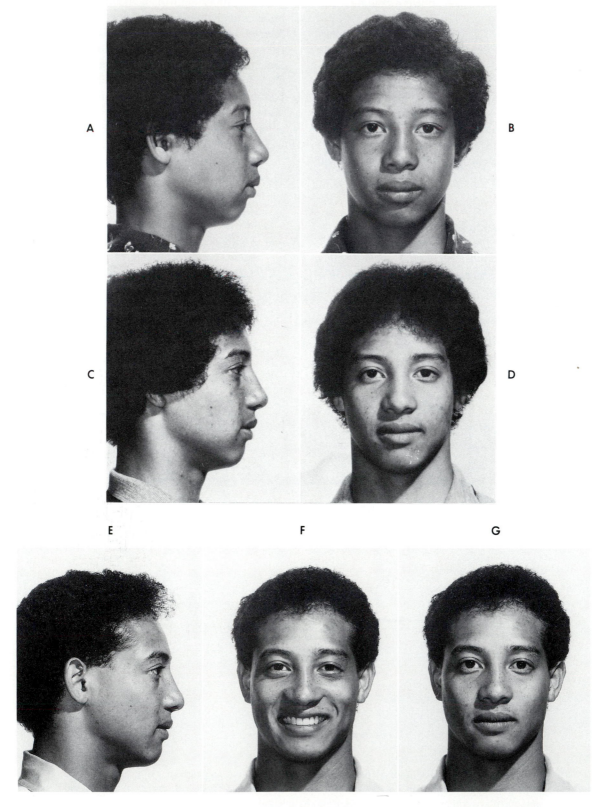

Fig. 6-98   Patient G.L. Facial configuration. **A** and **B,** Before treatment. **C** and **D,** After treatment. **E, F,** and **G,** Ten years after treatment.   *Continued.*

In addition, Tweed orthodontists feel uncomfortable when there is an expansion of the dentition laterally, anteriorly, or posteriorly. This is substantiated by the scientific investigations of Enlow,[19] who describes, quite specifically, the boundaries of the nasomaxillary complex (Fig. 6-97).

The treatment record of *patient G.L.* (Fig. 6-98, Table 6-6) graphically illustrates these objectives. Gregory has a typical Class II, division 1, malocclusion with an alveolodental protrusion. Before treatment his cephalometric analysis showed an FMA of 30°. Throughout the course of treatment this was reduced to 25°, a favorable response. His

IMPA before treatment was 107°, indicating an alveolodental protrusion. After treatment it was 89°, again a favorable response. This reduction was also reflected in an increased FMIA (from 43° to 66°). The OP angle was reduced from 6° to 0°, indicating good control in the dentition throughout treatment. The Z angle increased from 55° to 72°, again a favorable response to treatment. The S-N-A remained at 80°, indicating that the maxilla had not been changed. The S-N-B increased from 71° to 76°, denoting a good response in mandibular position. The A-N-B decreased from 9° to 4°, which signified improvement in the skeletal discrepancy (Fig. 6-98, *N* to *P*). The Steiner analysis showed that the

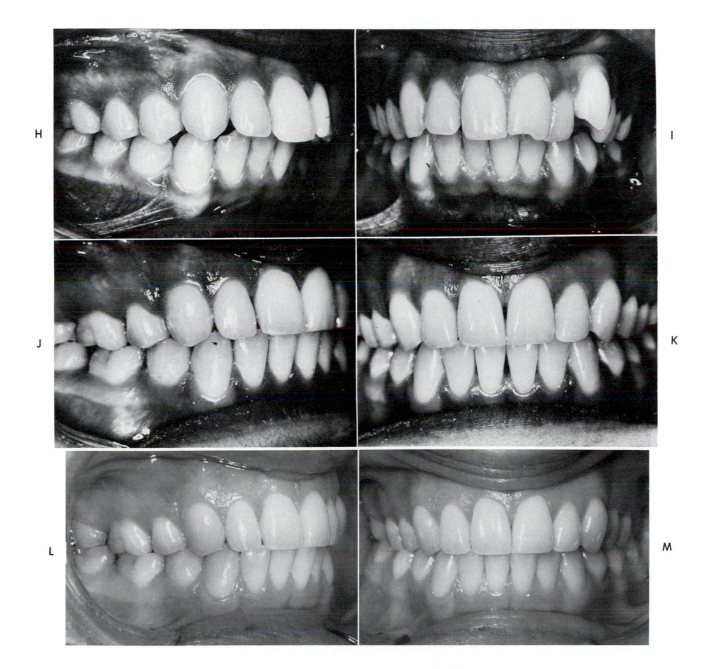

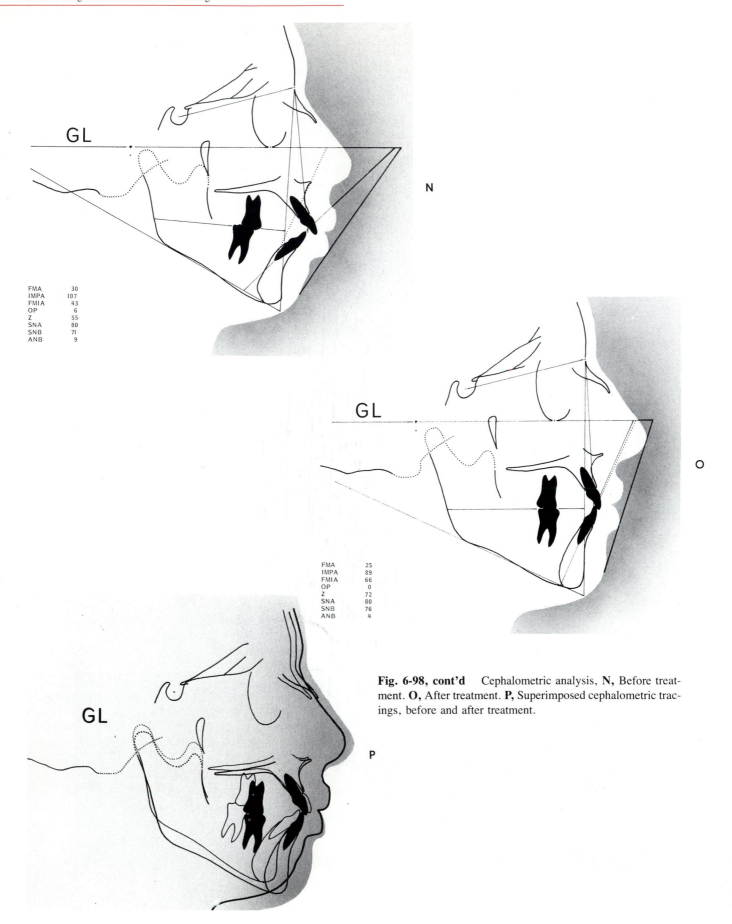

FMA	30
IMPA	107
FMIA	43
OP	6
Z	55
SNA	80
SNB	71
ANB	9

FMA	25
IMPA	89
FMIA	66
OP	0
Z	72
SNA	80
SNB	76
ANB	4

Fig. 6-98, cont'd Cephalometric analysis, **N,** Before treatment. **O,** After treatment. **P,** Superimposed cephalometric tracings, before and after treatment.

maxillary incisors had gone from 6 to 4 mm and from an angle of 30° to 20°, while the mandibular incisors had gone from 12 to 7 mm and from 43° to 23°. The total space analysis showed an anterior discrepancy characterized by an alveolodental protrusion and a posterior discrepancy with a relatively high angle facial pattern. Extraction of the first premolars aided in the correction of the anterior discrepancy, and extraction of the third molars benefited correction of the posterior discrepancy. All changes showed a favorable response to the mechanotherapy according to the Tweed philosophy (see Chapter 11).

Many orthodontists have found from bitter experience that they cannot extend arch length posteriorly, anteriorly, or laterally unless the position of the teeth is due to environmental factors, such as premature loss of the primary teeth. Most of the problems during treatment and retention have been associated with creating space and maintaining alignment where teeth have not been extracted. If retainers are required for a prolonged time, the teeth have not been placed in the correct position relative to the skeletal pattern and soft tissue matrix. The ideal conditions for stability are achieved when teeth are placed in a harmonious relationship early. If prolonged retention is required, either the occlusion is not satisfactory or the dentition is not in harmony with associated structures. There are exceptions, however. Mandibular fixed retainers should be maintained in patients for a prolonged time to preserve the incisor alignment when there is horizontal growth of the mandible. This is done between the ages of 13 and 17, when the mandible is still growing after the maxilla has stopped (see Chapter 2).

Serial extraction allows teeth to become aligned when they emerge into the oral cavity, rather than to stay in a crowded unfavorable condition for several years. In the case of alveolodental protrusion the procedure allows the mandibular incisors to be uprighted lingually into a position of balance. This alone will reduce multibonded mechanotherapy by 6 months and will contribute to the stability of the treatment result. In many of these patients the need for retention is minimal. However, the orthodontist must remember that under ideal serial extraction conditions he or she is not dealing with severe skeletal discrepancies or severe overjet and overbite problems. As a result the need for retention should be less.

Two questions that may be asked are (1) "If the roots of the permanent incisor teeth complete their formation in a more favorable position, is their stability enhanced?" It seems logical that if a tooth completes its formation in a site where it will remain when treatment is completed, it will be more stable. Conversely, if a tooth is left in a crowded, tipped, and rotated position for several years and then is moved to a new position relatively rapidly, it will be less stable for a time and will require a longer retention period (see Chapter 2 and 16).

(2) "Does the initiation of serial extraction with the removal of primary teeth always mean that the permanent teeth will be removed?" Once initiated, serial extraction more often than not will culminate in the extraction of four premolar teeth because arch length, which is deficient to begin with, is reduced even more. In spite of a thorough diagnosis, the treatment plan will occasionally need to be changed to nonextraction. The practitioner should always be prepared to treat with nonextraction if it appears that this can be done successfully with stability. If not, then patients should not be required to wear a retainer for a prolonged time nor should they be subjected to an additional period of unscheduled treatment.

At the beginning of treatment the parents should be informed that extractions may be necessary to produce a successful and stable treatment result. Later they will be relieved and happy if extractions are not necessary. It is best to prepare the parents during the case presentation, when they are a captive audience and when all phases of the treatment for their child are being discussed.

An important objective in using the serial extraction technique is to make treatment easier and mechanotherapy less complicated, less extensive, and shorter (especially during the teenage period). Treatment can be divided into four categories:

1. *A period of interceptive guidance,* extending approximately 5 years, from age 7½ to 12½. This consists entirely of the guidance of occlusion, including serial extraction, and is the most ideal service that can be provided. Unfortunately, it is possible also to produce excellent occlusion in only a few patients with serial extraction alone. When it is accomplished, it is most rewarding and satisfying because the results are achieved without mechanotherapy.

2. An initial *period of interceptive guidance,* extending approximately 4 years, from age 7½ to 11½, plus a second *period of multibonded treatment* extending approximately 1 year (from 11½ to 12½). Class I and specific types of dental Class II fall into this category.

3. An initial *period of interceptive treatment,* extending approximately 1 year, from 8½ to 9½, plus a *period of interceptive guidance* extending approximately 2 years, from 9½ to 11½, and a second *period of mechanotherapy* extending approximately 1½ years, from 11½ to 13. Class II malocclusions fall primarily into this category.

4. A *period of multibonded treatment,* extending for 1½ to 3 years, from age 11½ to 14½. Serial extraction is not involved in this treatment. Wherever possible, the orthodontist should try to avoid extensive treatment in the teenage period.

Of course, this is a general classification. It may vary considerably depending on the individual patient, the malocclusion, and the dental age.

CLASS I TREATMENT

The classic procedure of serial extraction has been the elimination of the primary canines, primary first molars, and permanent first premolars. This has been the most popular and widely used procedure since Bunon.[14] With scientific investigation and clinical experience it has become increasingly sophisticated and precise. Results will be more rewarding if the orthodontist does not cling to a particular sequence but varies it according to the diagnosis. The sequence that he or she believes is indicated for each patient should be selected. The sequences described next are applicable to Class I malocclusions.

Treatment Procedure A—Interceptive Guidance, Active Treatment

Serial Extraction in Class I Treatment

Group A—anterior discrepancy: crowding

Step 1. Extraction of the primary canines (Fig. 6-99). This is a typical serial extraction problem—severe crowding, a developing Class I malocclusion, a favorable overjet-overbite relation of the incisor teeth, and an ideal orthognathic facial pattern. On examining the radiographs you will often note a crescent pattern of resorption on the mesial of the primary canine roots (Fig. 6-6). This is an indication of a true hereditary tooth-size jaw-size discrepancy. It signifies that the first premolars are emerging favorably, ahead of the permanent canines. None of the unerupted permanent teeth have reached one half root length. Because of this the primary first molars would not be extracted. The primary canines should be extracted to relieve the incisor crowding.

Step 2. Extraction of the primary first molars (Fig. 6-100). The incisor crowding has improved; the overbite has increased, and the extraction site is reduced in size. The radiographs reveal that the first premolars have reached one half root length. It is now time to extract the primary first molars to encourage the eruption of the first premolar teeth.

Step 3. Extraction of the first premolars (Fig. 6-101). These teeth are emerging into the oral cavity. Since the permanent canines have developed beyond one half root length, indicating that they are prepared to accelerate their eruption, the premolars are extracted.

Step 4. Multibonded treatment (Fig. 6-102). This is the typical result of serial extraction, a relatively deep overbite with a distoaxial inclination of the canines, a mesioaxial inclination of the second premolars, a Class I molar relationship, an improved alignment of the incisors, and residual spaces at the extraction sites.

Step 5. Retention (Fig. 6-103). When mechanotherapy is completed, an ideal occlusion should be observed, with minimal overjet overbite relationship of the anterior teeth, parallel canine and premolar roots, ideal arch form, and no spaces. In addition, the dentition should be aligned in harmony with the craniofacial skeleton and soft tissue matrix.

Step 6. Postretention (Fig. 6-104). Again, you should observe an ideal occlusion with stability. Initiating the serial extraction procedure with elimination of the primary mandibular canines tends to deepen the overbite. The primary first molars should be extracted when the

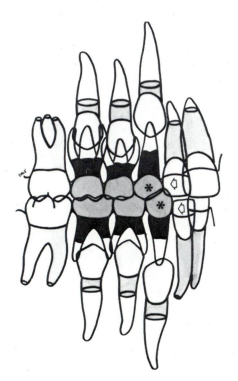

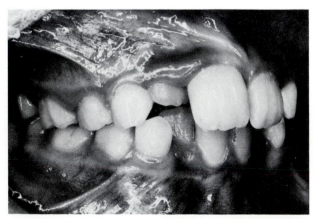

Fig. 6-99

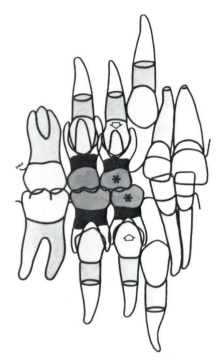

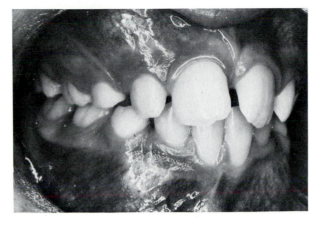

Fig. 6-100

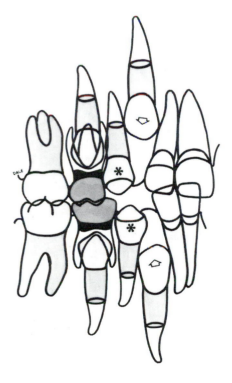

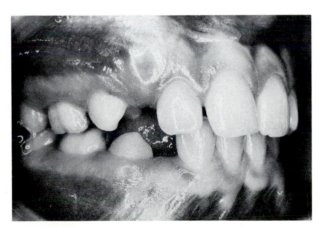

Fig. 6-101

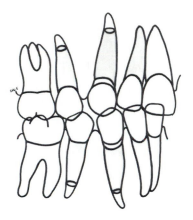

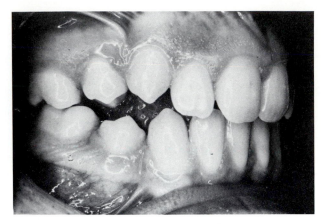

Fig. 6-102

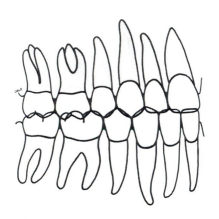

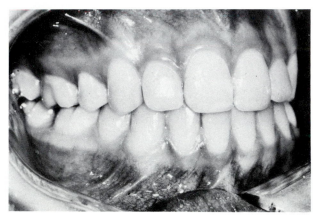

Fig. 6-103

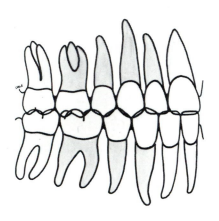

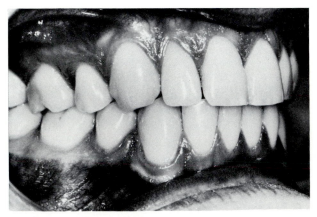

Fig. 6-104

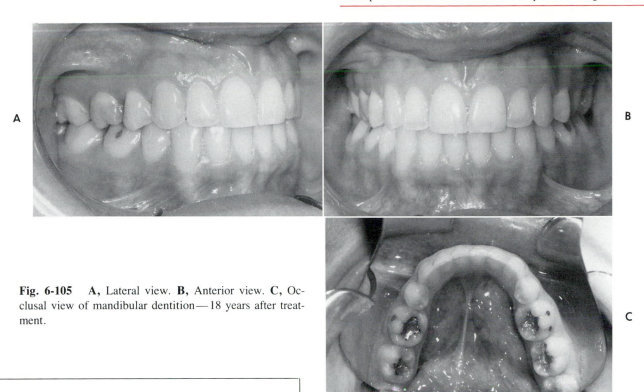

Fig. 6-105   **A,** Lateral view. **B,** Anterior view. **C,** Occlusal view of mandibular dentition—18 years after treatment.

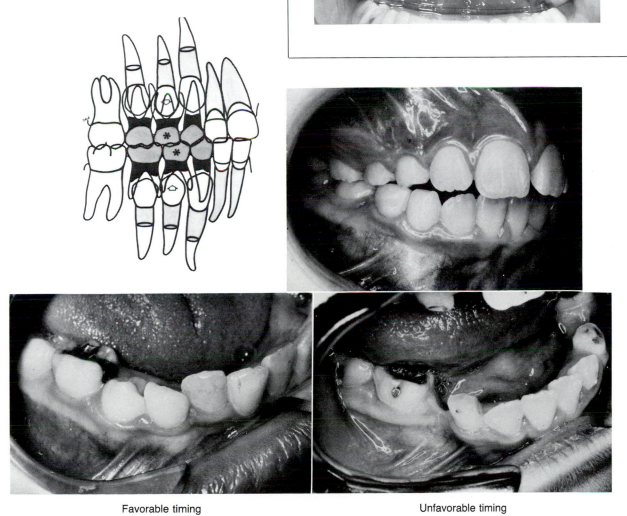

Favorable timing   Unfavorable timing

Fig. 6-106

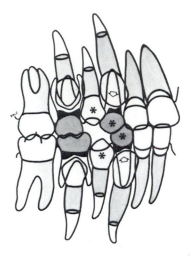

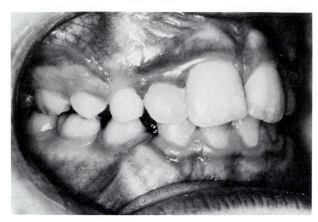

Fig. 6-107

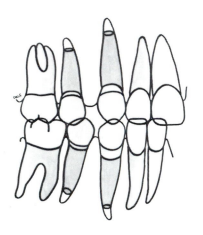

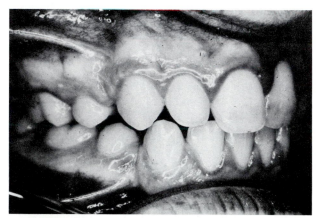

Fig. 6-108

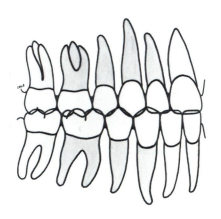

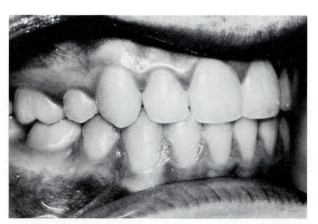

Fig. 6-109

underlying first premolars have reached half their root length. If this is done, risk of collapse will be minimal. If the mandibular incisors are crowded, the primary canines should be extracted first, in preference to the primary first molars. The orthodontist will rarely be satisfied with the improved alignment of the incisors when the primary molars are extracted first. Again, the decision is based on the relative position and length of the roots of the first premolars and canines. Fig. 6-104 illustrates the occlusion 18 years after treatment. Fig. 6-105 illustrates another patient 18 years after treatment.

Group B—anterior discrepancy: alveolodental protrusion

Step 1. Extraction of the primary first molars (Fig. 6-106). There is a minor irregularity of the incisor teeth. Instead of crowding, the patient has an alveolodental protrusion. The crowns of the first premolars and canines are at the same level. However, the canines are beyond one half root length and are erupting faster than the premolars. Since the first premolars have one half their root length developed, the primary first molars should be extracted to accelerate eruption of the first premolars. This will ensure that the premolars emerge into the oral cavity ahead of the canines. Timing is most important to prevent the formation of a knife-edge ridge (Fig. 6-106, *lower*).

Step 2. Extraction of the primary canines and first premolars (Fig. 6-107). When the first premolars have emerged sufficiently, they are extracted along with whatever primary canines remain. No effort is made to prevent lingual tipping of the incisor teeth since the objective is to reduce the alveolodental protrusion.

Step 3. Multibonded treatment (Fig. 6-108). Note how beautifully the dentition is aligning itself. Little mechanical treatment will be required.

Step 4. Retention (Fig. 6-109). Retention in the mandible is less crucial, since there was minimal irregularity before treatment.

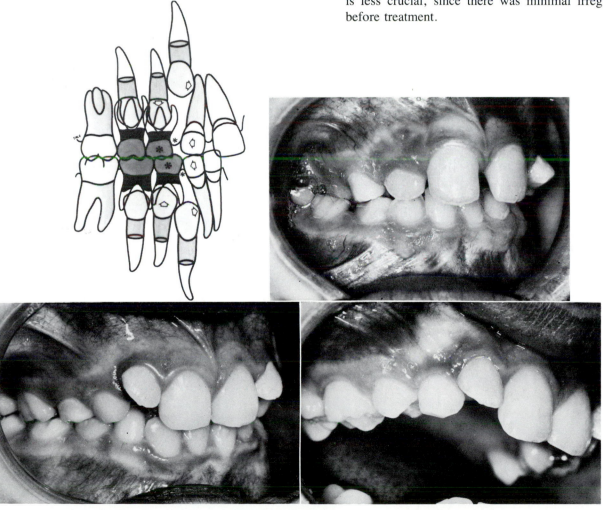

Splayed incisors, space
distal to primary canines

Favorable premolar
emergence

Fig. 6-110

Group C—middle discrepancy: impacted canines

Step 1. Extraction of the primary first molars (Fig. 6-110). The tooth-size jaw-size discrepancy is severe, causing premature exfoliation of the primary canines. Note the splaying of the incisors because of crowding in the apical area. Quite often parents will interpret this spacing as evidence for nonextraction treatment. It must be explained that this is a sign of severe crowding. The radiograph will reveal that the first premolars are ahead of the canines in eruption and have attained one half their root length. Here you must begin with the extraction of the primary first molars.

The impacted permanent maxillary canines may cause severe splaying of the maxillary incisors to such an extent that the lateral incisors do not contact the primary canines (Fig. 6-110, *lower*). In this situation it does little good to extract the primary canines first. Better advice is to extract the primary first molars to encourage the first premolars to emerge as early as possible. The canines will then have space to migrate away from the apices of the incisors and begin their eruption into the oral cavity. In this instance the practitioner should be concerned more with correcting canine crowding than with incisor irregularity. Every effort should be made to avoid correcting the incisors with multibonded appliances for fear of causing the incisor roots to resorb (Fig. 6-74).

Step 2. Extraction of the first premolars (Fig. 6-111). For reasons explained in Group A, *Step 3*, the first premolars are now due for extraction.

Step 3. Multibanded treatment (Fig. 6-112). Note the typical result of serial extraction.

Step 4. Retention (Fig. 6-113). Again, note the desired result of mechanotherapy.

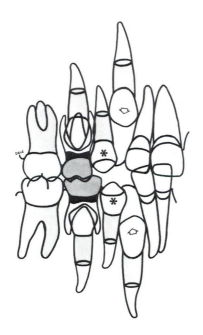

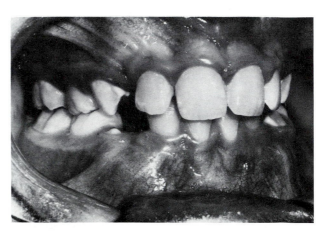

Fig. 6-111

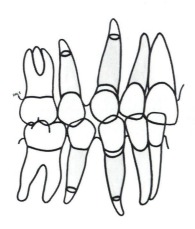

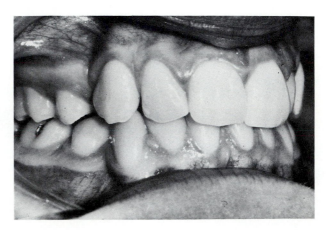

Fig. 6-112

Group D—enucleation in the mandible

Step 1. Extraction of the primary first molars and enucleation of the mandibular first premolars (Fig. 6-114). If it is evident that the canines will emerge into the oral cavity ahead of the first premolars, the primary first molars can be extracted and the first premolars, enucleated. This will encourage distal migration of the canines as they erupt.

Step 2. Extraction of the primary maxillary canines and maxillary first premolars (Fig. 6-115). In the maxilla the first premolars usually emerge before the canines. Therefore enucleation is less likely to be indicated. At this point the mandibular canines can be observed emerging favorably into the oral cavity.

Step 3. Mechanotherapy (Fig. 6-116).

Step 4. Retention (Fig. 6-117).

Group E—enucleation in the maxilla and mandible

Step 1. Extraction of primary canines and primary first molars and enucleation of the first premolars (Fig. 6-118). On occasion the canines in both the maxilla and the mandible will erupt before the first premolars. If this is the case, the orthodontist might elect to extract the primary canines and first molars and enucleate the first premolars. This would be more acceptable if there were absolutely no opportunity to place multibanded appliances at the completion of serial extraction. Otherwise, there is an alternative to enucleation that is preferable.

Step 2. Mechanotherapy (Fig. 6-119).

Step 3. Retention (Fig. 6-120).

Group F—alternative to enucleation

Step 1. Extraction of the primary first molars (Fig. 6-121). When the permanent canines are erupting ahead of the first premolars and if there is an opportunity to place multibonded appliances at the completion of serial extraction, enucleation of the premolars should be avoided. When the first premolars have attained one half their root length, the primary first molars should be extracted.

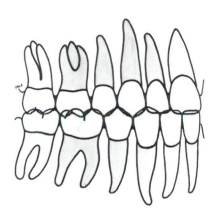

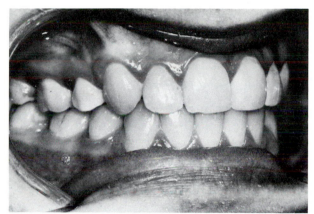

Fig. 6-113

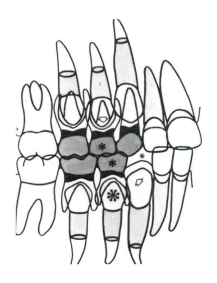

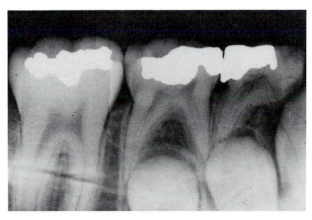

Fig. 6-114

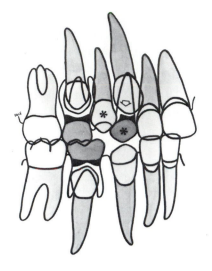

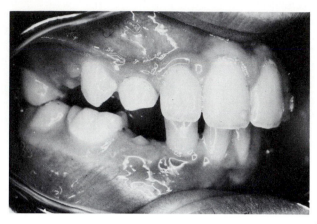

Fig. 6-115

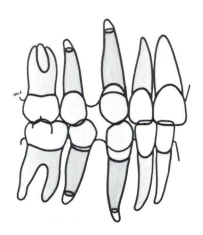

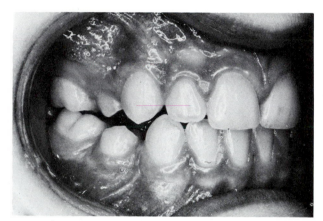

Fig. 6-116

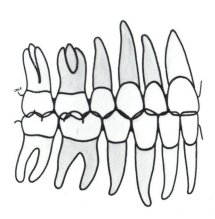

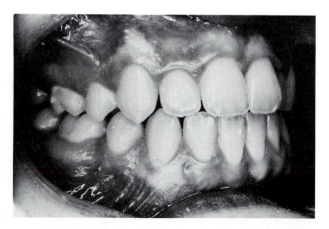

Fig. 6-117

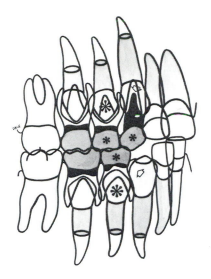

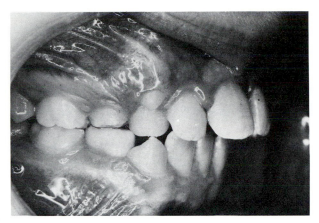

Fig. 6-118

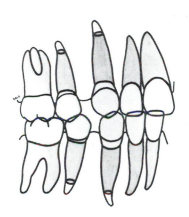

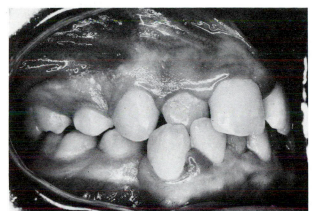

Fig. 6-119

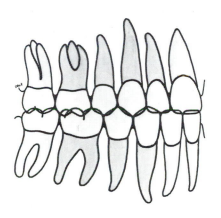

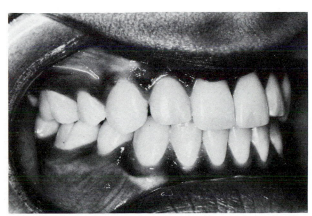

Fig. 6-120

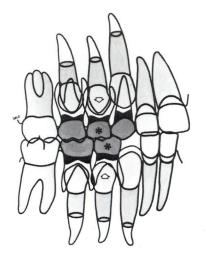

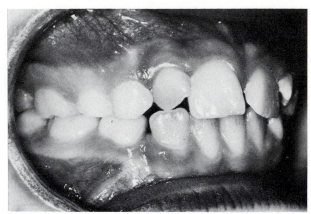

Fig. 6-121

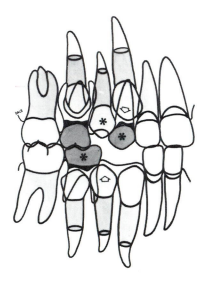

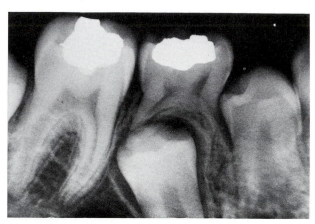

Fig. 6-122

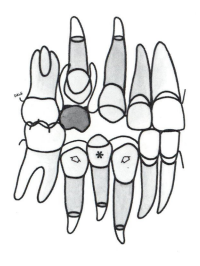

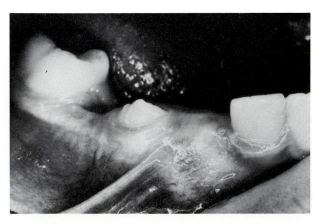

Fig. 6-123

Step 2. Extraction of the primary maxillary canines, maxillary first premolars, and primary mandibular second molars (Fig. 6-122). Some 6 to 9 months later, when the emerging mandibular first premolar appears to be obstructed by the mesial contour of the primary second molar, the orthodontist should extract the offending tooth. However, this sequence is usually not necessary in the maxillary dentition.

Step 3. Extraction of the mandibular first premolars (Fig. 6-123). When these teeth emerge sufficiently, they are extracted.

Step 4. Mechanotherapy (Fig. 6-124). With this particular sequence the least desirable extraction result is achieved. However, it does not prolong the multibonded treatment significantly.

Step 5. Retention (Fig. 6-125).

Group G—interproximal reduction. Rarely should the mesial surfaces of the primary canines be reduced. However, this can be accomplished when the practitioner does not intend to extract the permanent teeth and where there is a localized interference resulting in the rotation of the lateral incisor.

Occasionally in nonextraction malocclusions the primary second molars will be retained for an unusually long time. Since these teeth are wider mesiodistally than the underlying second premolars, they force the first premolars into a forward position in the dental arch and thus impact the permanent canines (Fig. 6-126, *A*). The long retention of these primary second molars may also interfere with the eruption of the first premolars after the permanent canines have emerged (Fig. 6-126, *B*). In each instance the mesial surface of the primary second molars should be reduced the amount of the leeway space (Fig. 6-126). This usually results in a favorable alignment of the permanent teeth (Fig. 6-127).

It may at times be necessary to reduce the distal surfaces of the primary second molars (Fig. 6-128) to ensure conversion of a straight terminal plane into a mesial step in preparation for a Class I relationship of the permanent first molars. This is accomplished when the primary maxillary second molars are exfoliated before those in the mandible and when there is space to allow the molars to move mesially. Ideally the mandibular molars should be lost first. (For more detailed discussion of interproximal reduction of primary teeth, read the excellent article by Hotz.[30])

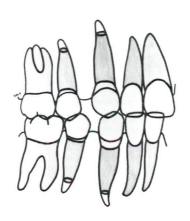

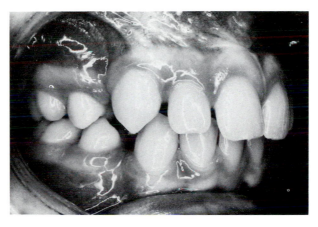

Fig. 6-124

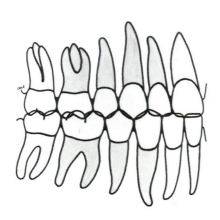

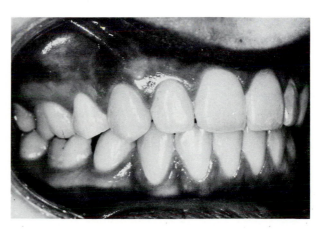

Fig. 6-125

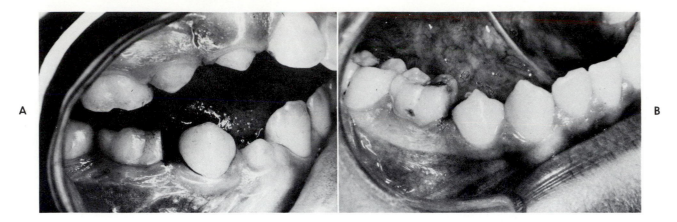

Fig. 6-126   Interproximal reduction of the primary second molar to allow for emergence of, **A,** the permanent canine and, **B,** the first premolar.

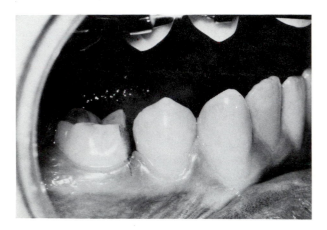

Fig. 6-127   Favorable alignment after reduction of the primary second molar.

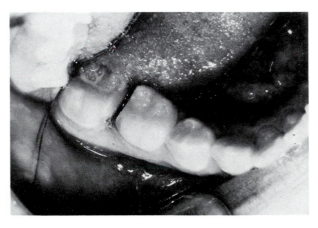

Fig. 6-128   Reduction of the distal surface of the primary second molar to convert a straight terminal plane into a mesial step.

Group H—congenital absence. It is of utmost importance in these patients to proceed with the conventional orthodontic diagnosis and treatment planning *as if the teeth were present.* Having done this you can then alter the treatment to cope with the missing tooth or teeth. It matters little whether the teeth are missing as a result of injury, disease, or developmental aberration; which teeth are missing and what is left to work with are the important factors in total correction of the malocclusion.

Maxillary incisors. The maxillary lateral incisors are frequently missing or malformed. The percentage varies depending on the study consulted, but in most practices it is approximately 5% of the patients treated.

If a maxillary lateral incisor is congenitally absent, the dentition should be allowed to emerge completely before initiating multibonded treatment. Examine the crown of the canine carefully after emergence before deciding to place it in the lateral incisor position or in its usual position. Do not rely on periapical radiographs to evaluate the shape of unerupted teeth. Often it is wiser to place restorations rather than to use canines as lateral incisors. When they are used as laterals, the orthodontist seems to be constantly fighting interproximal spaces during the retention period; and in most instances it is just not esthetic.

Depending on the basic orthodontic diagnosis and the anatomy of the maxillary canines, the decision may be to replace the incisors with canines. The two patients in Fig. 6-129 have also had mandibular first premolars extracted. This has resulted in a Class I molar relationship. Quite frequently only one incisor will be missing. In this instance the patient would have a Class I molar relationship on one side and a Class II molar relationship on the other if no mandibular teeth were extracted.

Mandibular incisors. Fig. 6-130 illustrates a treated patient, two of whose permanent mandibular incisors were missing. The treatment plan was altered from extraction of

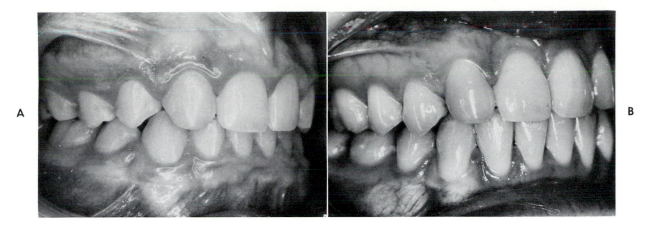

Fig. 6-129   **A,** During the developmental period the permanent canines were guided into the lateral incisor positions in the maxilla and serial extraction was conducted in the mandible. Here the canines have replaced the lateral incisors satisfactorily and the molars are in a Class I relationship. **B,** Same treatment, different patient, several years after retention. Esthetic and stable result.

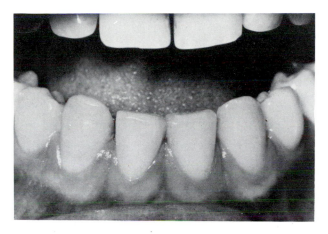

Fig. 6-130   Alignment of the mandibular dentition after treatment in a patient with congenital absence of two incisors. The first premolars were extracted in the maxilla.

the four premolar teeth to extraction of the two maxillary premolars. The incisor space was closed, and a satisfactory occlusion resulted.

The patient in Fig. 6-35 was treated by extraction of the mandibular central incisors. This is disturbing. Patients who have severe recession and malposition of the centrals can be treated by routine serial extraction. The extraction of mandibular incisors, especially during development, is definitely not recommended; it complicates the total treatment plan and necessitates a compromise result. Every effort should be made to maintain the mandibular incisors, especially in unilateral situations.

There have been times when the canine was moved into the incisor position. Again, it depends on the basic diagnosis. To repeat, every effort should be made to maintain the mandibular incisors, especially in the unilateral situation

and during development. If one of the mandibular incisors is missing, it may be advisable to avoid extracting a premolar in that quadrant and use the canine as an incisor. If it is an extraction case, the molars on the affected side will be in a Class I relationship; if it is not, they will be in a Class III relationship.

Premolars. Fig. 6-42 illustrates a patient who had two maxillary first premolars missing. The clinical appearance that resulted was unusual. The canines erupted into the premolar locations, and the primary canines were retained. The treatment plan was altered to include extraction of the primary canines and movement of the permanent canines forward into their proper position. The remaining maxillary teeth were moved forward into a Class II molar relationship.

Mandibular second premolars are frequently missing. Depending on the basic orthodontic diagnosis, you may treat by moving the molars forward or by having the missing teeth replaced by bridges. Class II malocclusions that involve extractions may be treated by moving the maxillary protruding incisors into the space provided by the extraction of the maxillary first premolars, and the Class II molar relationship may be corrected by moving the mandibular molars forward into the second premolar area where the teeth are congenitally absent.

Mandibular second premolars are constantly presenting difficulties in orthodontic treatment. They frequently are missing or erupting in the wrong direction (Fig. 6-7). Often they are badly shaped (Fig. 6-131). This particular serial extraction patient's treatment plan should have been altered to include extraction of the second premolars rather than the first.

When one mandibular second premolar is congenitally missing, the clinician should proceed with serial extraction as normally done, extracting all four primary canines, or primary first molars, depending on the development. When the four first premolars have emerged, three of them are

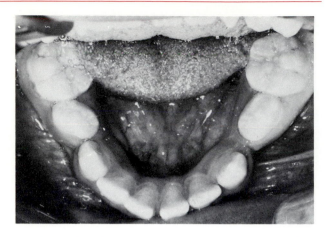

Fig. 6-131 Serial extraction in a patient in whom the mandibular second premolars should have been extracted rather than the first premolars.

extracted. In the quadrant where the second premolar is missing, the primary second molar is extracted. The first premolar is then moved into the second premolar site. This allows space for the canine to emerge. Occasionally, the primary second molar must be extracted earlier to allow the first premolar to emerge into a more distal position.

Garn[26] has shown that when there is a congenital absence more often than not the treatment will not require extraction. In other words, congenital absence of teeth is related to small teeth; thus serial extraction is not indicated.

If the diagnosis indicates the extraction of four second premolars or if the four teeth are congenitally missing, serial extraction is not indicated. Second premolar extractions are prescribed for a borderline tooth-size jaw-size discrepancy where the incisors are upright over basal bone. With extraction of the second premolars the minimal crowding in the anterior area is corrected by using a fraction of the extraction space and without producing an alveolodental retrusion. The space that remains will be closed by moving the posterior teeth forward. Primary canines are extracted to relieve severe incisor crowding, and primary molars are extracted to reduce an alveolodental protrusion. Since neither condition exists in these patients, the extraction of primary canines or first molars is not indicated. Also primary first molars are extracted to encourage the eruption of first premolars. Since first premolars are not going to be extracted in these cases, the extraction of primary first molars is not indicated. It is difficult to encourage the emergence of second premolars ahead of the first premolars by extraction of the primary second molars early. Second premolars are notoriously slow in their eruption. Furthermore, if the primary second molars are extracted early the permanent first molars may move mesially too rapidly. Second premolars are extracted when they have partially emerged into the oral cavity.

Quite often the question is asked about creating a *dished-in face* as the ultimate result of serial extraction when the four first premolar teeth are extracted. All orthodontists should be concerned about creating dished-in faces. That is why serial extraction should be done only on a specific group of patients and only after a comprehensive diagnosis. Because of this concern the clinician should constantly monitor the position of the mandibular incisors. These should be allowed to tip lingually to the desired position and then held. Some patients will have a dished-in profile whether treated by extraction or nonextraction or left untreated. They exhibit a maxillary mandibular alveolodental retrusion, a low mandibular plane angle, a deep overbite of the incisor teeth, a relatively short anterior facial height, a prominent chin, a relatively prominent nose, and a tense perioral musculature. If a severe tooth-size jaw-size discrepancy is superimposed, extraction may be called for to produce a stable result. It is often advisable to defer extractions until all the permanent teeth have emerged rather than perform serial extraction. If serial extraction is performed, it must be done with extreme caution and in conjunction with holding appliances.

A word of caution is necessary at this point regarding holding appliances, the labial uprighting of permanent mandibular incisors, and the distal movement of permanent mandibular first molars by the use of a multibonded appliance, lingual arch, or lip bumper. The reaction could impact the permanent mandibular second molars (Fig. 6-132).

Typical Patient for Class I Serial Extraction

A typical Class I malocclusion with an anterior discrepancy manifested by an alveolodental protrusion and a posterior discrepancy manifested by a relatively high angle configuration is illustrated by *patient M.R.* (Fig. 6-133). The dentition when the patient came for examination and consultation is presented in *A*. The primary canines had already been extracted. In these patients the clinician prefers to extract the primary first molars first to encourage emergence of the first premolars so they can, in turn, be extracted as early as possible. This facilitates correction of the alveolodental protrusion by uprighting of the incisor teeth. With relatively straight alignment of the incisor teeth it is not necessary to extract primary canines early. In *B* the primary first molars have been extracted. Note the early eruption of the maxillary first premolar. It is possible that a large restoration and a periapical infection of the primary molar were factors in this situation. The orthodontist should wait until the other premolars have emerged into the oral cavity before advising extraction of these teeth (*C*). Note in *D* that the four premolars have been extracted and the incisor teeth are beginning to upright over basal bone. In *E* the permanent mandibular canines are beginning to emerge into the oral cavity. Note that the maxillary right primary second molar has been lost early. The premolar has emerged and the first molar has drifted somewhat mesially. In *F* all the primary second molars have now been lost and the second premolars are emerging. Note the further uprighting

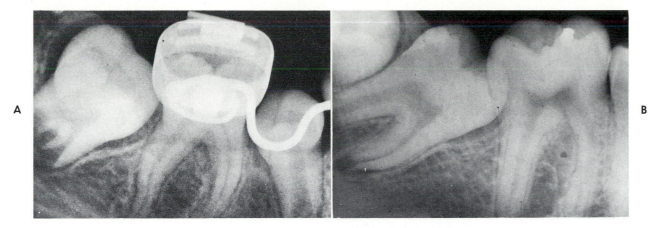

Fig. 6-132 **A,** Impending problem caused by the improper use of a mandibular lingual arch. **B,** Result of the lingual arch maltreatment.

of the incisor teeth. With the emergence of the permanent maxillary canines and second molars, this patient is now ready for multibonded treatment *(G)*. Fig. 6-133, *H*, illustrates the end result, *I* the occlusion 2 years after retention appliances were removed, and *J*, 15 years after retention. Cephalometric radiographs were taken of *patient M.R.*

1. Before treatment
2. After the extraction of the primary canines
3. After the extraction of the primary first molars
4. After the extraction of the permanent first premolars
5. After the edgewise treatment

It is interesting to observe that the response to serial extraction during interceptive guidance—superimpositions of cephalometric tracings number *1* and *4* (Fig. 6-133, *K*)—is significantly greater than the response during the edgewise treatment—superimposition of cephalometric tracings *4* and *5* (Fig. 6-133, *L*).

Fig. 6-133, *M,* illustrates the response during the total treatment—interceptive guidance and edgewise appliance. The mandibular incisors gradually move upright, reducing the alveolar dental protrusion; the mandibular molars move upward and forward, accounting for an upward and forward rotation of the mandible.

The Tweed objectives are:

1. An upward and forward rotation of the mandible-decreasing FMA and ANB angles
2. Correcting the alveolar dental protrusion by uprighting the mandibular incisors; decreasing the IMPA angle and increasing the FMIA angle
3. Flattening the occlusal plane; reducing the occlusal plane angle
4. Decreasing the jaw discrepancy; reducing the ANB angle
5. Averting the expansion of the dentition
6. Creating balance and harmony in the soft tissue profile; increasing the Z angle; all occur during interceptive guidance, without any appliance in place. The same

response continues to a lesser degree during the Tweed edgewise treatment.

Fig. 6-134 presents the facial appearance before and following serial extraction and after multibonded treatment. Note that this patient before treatment has a moderate high angle facial pattern and alveolodental protrusion. After treatment the facial configuration exhibits harmony and balance. The smile has improved following serial extraction and again following multibanded treatment. Balance and harmony persist fifteen years after treatment.

Before treatment the cephalometric analysis of *M.R.* showed an FMA of 31°. This represents a relatively high angle face. Throughout the course of serial extraction the FMA was reduced to 27°, and throughout the course of multibonded treatment to 25°. The 6° reduction indicated a favorable upward and forward rotation of the mandible. The patient's IMPA before treatment was 91°, suggesting a moderate alveolodental protrusion for a high angle facial pattern. During serial extraction the mandibular incisors were uprighted to 88° and during active treatment to 86°. This reduction of 5° in the IMPA resulted in a slightly more balanced and harmonious soft tissue profile. The overall increase in the FMIA of 11° (from 58° to 69°) reflected a reduction in both the FMA and the IMPA, as well as a favorable rotation of the mandible and correction of the alveolodental protrusion. The reduction of the occlusal plane angle from 13° to 8° during serial extraction indicated a mesial migration of the posterior teeth and an uprighting of the mandibular incisor teeth, both favorable responses in the treatment of this particular facial pattern. The reduction of the OP angle from 8° to 7° during active treatment indicated good control. The overall increase in the Z angle of 18° (from 57° to 75°) reflected a favorable rotation of the mandible and correction of the alveolodental protrusion. The maxilla grew slightly during the serial extraction period, from 78° to 80°, and remained relatively constant during active treatment. Mandibular growth and rotation accounted

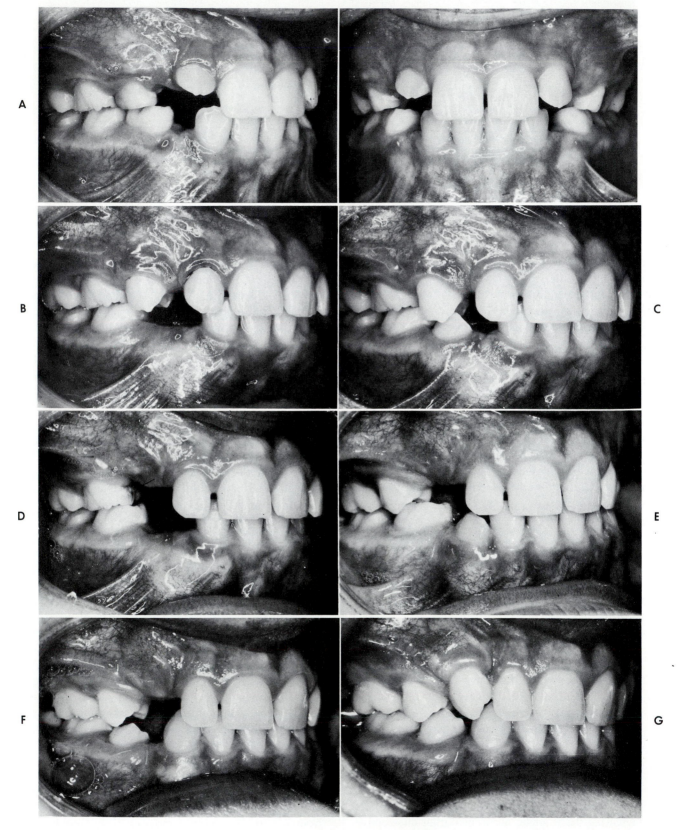

Fig. 6-133 For legend see opposite page.

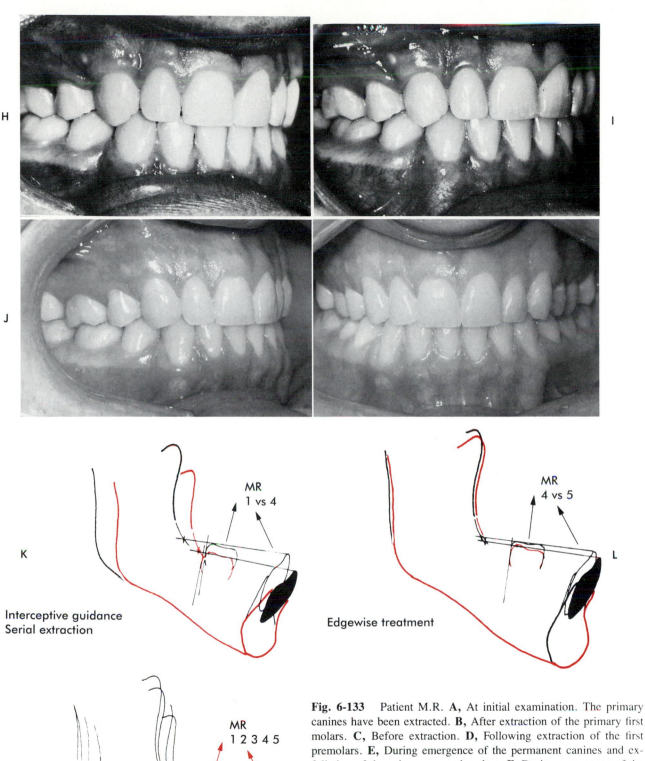

Fig. 6-133   Patient M.R. **A,** At initial examination. The primary canines have been extracted. **B,** After extraction of the primary first molars. **C,** Before extraction. **D,** Following extraction of the first premolars. **E,** During emergence of the permanent canines and exfoliation of the primary second molars. **F,** During emergence of the seconds premolars. **G,** Before, and **H,** Following multibanded treatment. **I,** Two years after retention. **J,** Fifteen years after treatment (lateral and anterior view). **K,** Response during interceptive guidance. **L,** Considerably less of response during edgewise treatment. **M,** Response as indicated by the five cephalometric tracings *(1, 2, 3, 4, 5)* that were taken at each step in the treatment: *(1)* Before treatment; *(2)* After the extraction of the primary canine; *(3)* After the extraction of the primary first molars; *(4)* After the extraction of the first premolars; and *(5)* After the edgewise treatment.

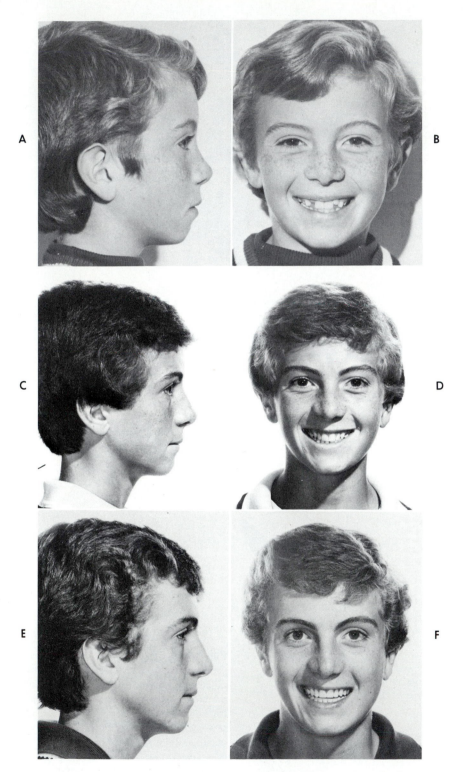

Fig. 6-134 Facial appearance of patient M.R. **A** and **B,** Before, and **C** and **D,** following serial extraction. **E** and **F,** After the multibanded treatment. *Continued.*

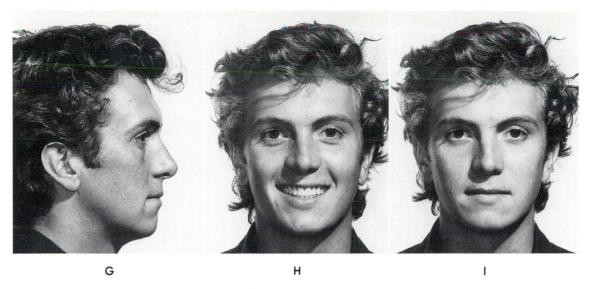

G   H   I

Fig. 6-134, cont'd   G, H, and **I,** Fifteen years after treatment.

for 3° during the serial extraction period and for one more degree during the active period of treatment. Throughout total treatment the A-N-B was reduced from 3° to 1°, indicating a modest improvement in the jaw relationship (Fig. 6-135).

It was important in *M.R.'s* case that the tooth-size jaw-size discrepancy not be corrected by extension of the teeth posteriorly, anteriorly, laterally, or vertically. If this had been done in such a relatively high angle facial pattern, the molar extrusion would have resulted in an unfavorable downward and backward rotation of the mandible. With extrusion of the molars and the *dumping* forward of the incisors, the occlusal plane would have been tipped unfavorably and the alveolodental protrusion worsened. With the mandibular rotation and the tipped occlusal plane the maxillary incisor would have been rabbited downward and backward, revealing more gingival tissue. Concomitantly the posterior molars would have been impacted; the dental arches would have been expanded; the mandibular incisors would have been tipped off basal bone, creating an unstable situation that required prolonged retention; and the harmony and balance of the facial profile would have been worsened considerably.

The total space analysis indicated an anterior and posterior space discrepancy (Table 6-6). The anterior discrepancy was corrected by serial extraction and extraction of the permanent first premolars. The posterior discrepancy was corrected by extraction of the permanent third molars.

Often high angle facial patterns are associated with an open bite relationship of the anterior teeth. To preface the discussion of this type of Class I malocclusion, the characteristic features of a true hereditary open bite malocclusion as described by Subtelny[62] will now be outlined:

1. An excessively steep mandibular plane angle or a high angle facial configuration

2. A retrognathic mandible relative to cranial base
3. A significantly greater anterior vertical dimension of the skeletal face, especially in the lower portion
4. A maxillary mandibular alveolodental protrusion
5. A relatively short ramus height
6. A relatively large gonial angle
7. A relative overeruption of the maxillary molars and incisor teeth (this is an extremely important observation and must be considered when planning treatment)
8. A relatively shorter posterior cranial base
9. A relatively obtuse angle between the posterior and anterior cranial bases
10. A relatively distal maxillary alveolar process in relation to the anterior cranial base

A word of caution is important relative to Subtelny's remarks with regard to the overeruption of the maxillary molars, which contributes to the open bite relationship. It is quite possible that extraction of the permanent molars would be preferable to extraction of the premolars in an attempt to correct this malocclusion. Molar extraction has the same effect as molar intrusion: it encourages the mandible to rotate up and forward, which, in turn, reduces the steep mandibular plane angle, the long lower anterior face height, the retrognathism of the mandible, and the anterior open bite.

A typical example of the treatment plan preferred for the severe high angle Class I discrepancy malocclusion is illustrated in the case of *patient J.L.* (Fig. 6-136). Before treatment the patient's cephalometric analysis indicated that he had an FMA of a whopping 47°. Throughout the course of multibonded treatment, which followed extraction of the permanent first molars, this angle was reduced to 43°—indicating a favorable upward and forward rotation of the mandible. His IMPA before treatment was 68° and his FMIA

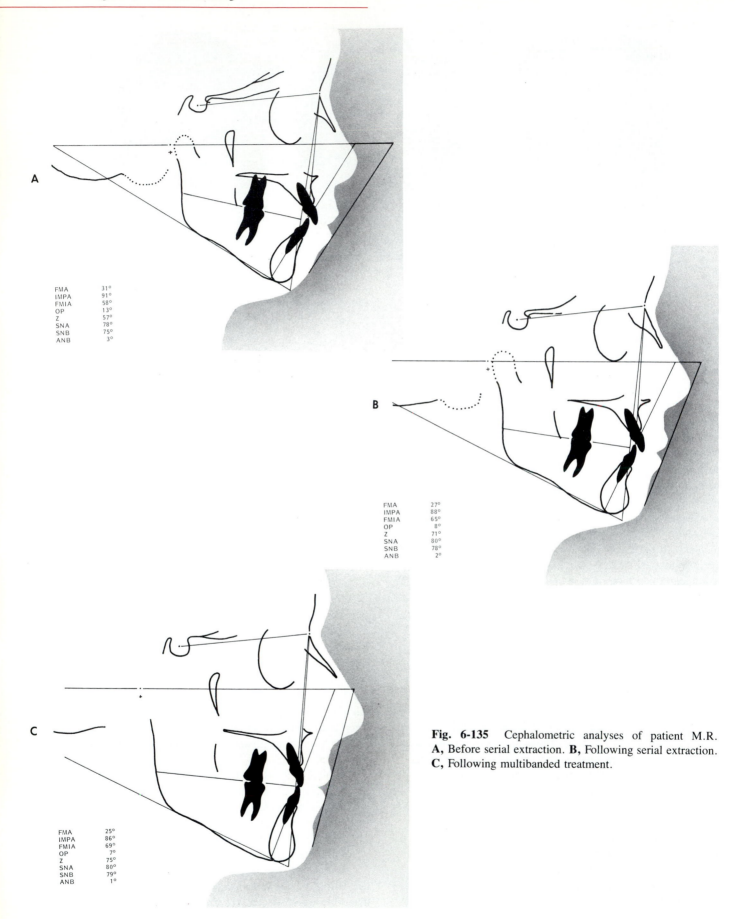

FMA	31°
IMPA	91°
FMIA	58°
OP	13°
Z	57°
SNA	78°
SNB	75°
ANB	3°

FMA	27°
IMPA	88°
FMIA	65°
OP	8°
Z	71°
SNA	80°
SNB	78°
ANB	2°

FMA	25°
IMPA	86°
FMIA	69°
OP	7°
Z	75°
SNA	80°
SNB	79°
ANB	1°

Fig. 6-135 Cephalometric analyses of patient M.R. **A,** Before serial extraction. **B,** Following serial extraction. **C,** Following multibanded treatment.

65°. Both these figures denote that the mandibular incisors had a favorable axial inclination. In addition, the alignment of these teeth was favorable as indicated by the study models. The S-N-A was 75°, the S-N-B, 73°, and the A-N-B, 2°. This implies that the maxilla was well related to the mandible but that both were in a retrognathic position. The OP angle was steep, and the Z angle was small. Throughout treatment the mandibular incisors were maintained in a favorable relationship as indicated by the IMPA. The S-N-A remained constant but the S-N-B increased by 2°, suggesting a favorable forward rotation of the mandible. It has

been said that an extremely high angle facial pattern is a potential Class III malocclusion. This statement is substantiated by the reduction of the A-N-B from 2° to 0° during treatment.

Throughout the first year of mechanotherapy, no attachments were placed on the mandibular dentition. The mandibular molars were allowed to drift mesially. As a result the mandible rotated favorably, and the occlusal plane angle was reduced from 17° to 13°. This further improved the Z angle and the soft tissue profile.

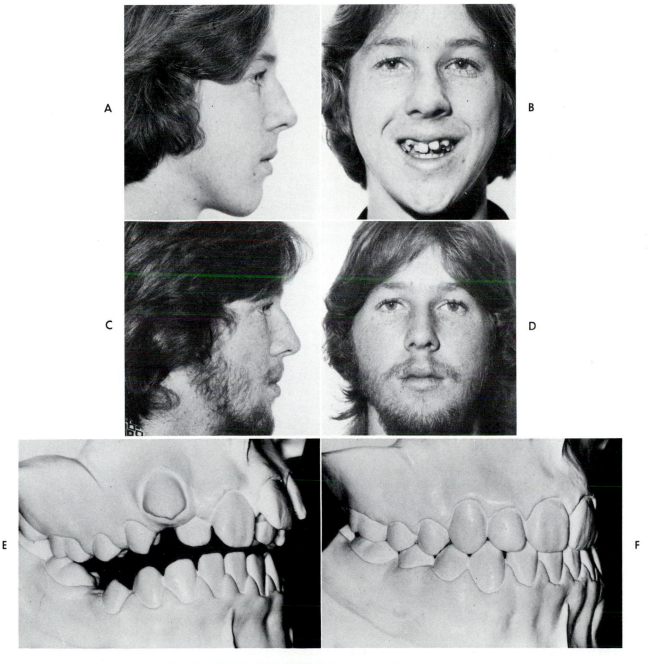

Fig. 6-136   Patient J.L. Facial configuration before, **A** and **B,** and after, **C** and **D,** treatment. Study models of the dentition before, **E,** and after, **F,** treatment.   *Continued.*

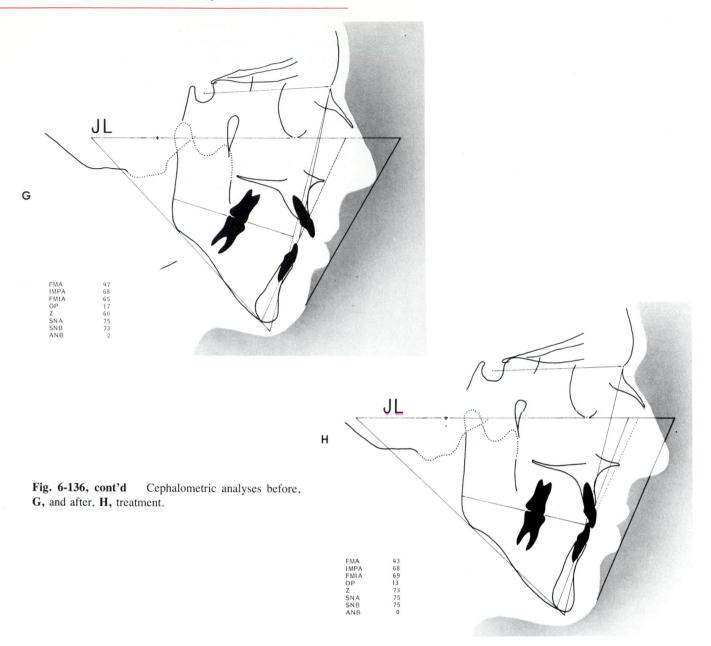

FMA	47
IMPA	68
FMIA	65
OP	17
Z	60
SNA	75
SNB	73
ANB	2

FMA	43
IMPA	68
FMIA	69
OP	13
Z	73
SNA	75
SNB	75
ANB	0

Fig. 6-136, cont'd Cephalometric analyses before, **G,** and after, **H,** treatment.

The favorable axial inclination and alignment of the mandibular incisors was reflected in a 0 mm deficit in the anterior arch area of the total space analysis. The 16 mm deficit in the middle area reflected a mesial migration of the mandibular molars, causing a crowded condition of the premolar teeth. The deficit of 9 mm in the posterior arch area reflected a severe high angle configuration. The total deficit of 25 mm, which was primarily toward the posterior area, was relieved by extraction of the permanent first molars. To bring about a more favorable relationship, the mandibular curve of occlusion was not completely leveled (Table 6-6).

CLASS II TREATMENT

Serial extraction can be an important part of Class II treatment; however, if extreme caution is not exercised, the malocclusion can be aggravated. The orthodontist should always inform the parents that appliances will be required to treat the Class II discrepancy when all the permanent teeth have emerged. Again, it must be stressed, that serial extraction does not replace mechanotherapy, particularly in Class II malocclusions. Nevertheless, in a rewarding number of instances, it does reduce it significantly at the *difficult* age of adolescence.

Treatment procedure B—interceptive treatment, interceptive guidance, active treatment

Initial period of interceptive treatment. During this period, which may extend 1 to 1½ years, the primary first molars and maxillary first premolars are extracted as early as possible. This provides space for retraction of the permanent maxillary anterior teeth. Appliances are placed on the four permanent maxillary incisors and first molars and on the primary second molars. With a maxillary edgewise arch and an anterior high pull headgear, the maxillary incisors are retracted, intruded, and torqued. This reduces the overjet and overbite.

The primary objective of the initial period of interceptive treatment is to decrease the vulnerability of and possible injury to the maxillary incisors. In the mandible the primary canines are extracted to relieve the permanent incisor crowding. Later the primary first molars and the premolars are extracted. To prevent collapse of the mandibular incisors and accentuation of the curve of occlusion, appliances are placed on the permanent incisors and first molars and on the primary second molars. Progress is made from round leveling arches to ideal edgewise arches.

In the interceptive phase, the method of treatment used to correct a Class II malocclusion is determined by the type of Class II. It can be seen from the proportional facial analysis that there are several types. With this analysis and with the total space analysis, the treatment of Class II malocclusions may involve nonextraction or one of the following series of extractions: (1) maxillary first premolars, (2) four first premolars, (3) maxillary first premolars and mandibular second premolars, (4) permanent maxillary first molars and mandibular third molars, (5) permanent maxillary second molars and mandibular third molars, (6) third molars, (7) four premolars plus permanent maxillary first molars and mandibular third molars, (8) four premolars plus permanent maxillary second molars and mandibular third molars, or (9) four first premolars and four third molars. Or jaw surgery may be performed. Since serial extraction usually culminates in the extraction of the first premolars, it is obvious from this list that it is not indicated in the treatment of all Class II malocclusions.

Period of interceptive guidance. During this period retention appliances are worn and serial extraction is continued. The parents are informed that appointments will be required every 3 months for assessment of growth and development with the aid of diagnostic records and that teeth will be extracted periodically as indicated.

Second period of active treatment. When all the permanent teeth have emerged, a multibonded appliance is placed and the Class II is corrected, adhering to the principles of Tweed edgewise mechanotherapy.

Patient J.O. (Figs. 6-137 through 6-139) is a good example of a Class II malocclusion treated by serial extraction and edgewise mechanotherapy.

A relatively high angle facial pattern, a prognathic maxilla and retrognathic mandible, a skeletal discrepancy, and a maxillary mandibular alveolodental protrusion with open bite relationship of the anterior teeth are present.

Fig. 6-137, *A,* illustrates the malocclusion before serial extraction. Note the Class II intercuspation of the molars and the open bite relationship of the anterior teeth. *B* shows the dental relationship after serial extraction and before multibonded appliance therapy. Significant improvement has been made in both the incisor and the molar relationships. To this point no mechanotherapy has been used. *C* shows the complete multibonded appliance with edgewise arches during final space closure. *D* shows the final occlusion after treatment, and *E* and *F,* the 2-year appearance.

The soft tissue profile and facial appearance before and after serial extraction, and after treatment, are illustrated in Fig. 6-138. Note the prognathic maxilla, retrognathic mandible, and moderately high angle facial pattern before serial extraction. Improvement may be seen as treatment progresses, particularly in the mandible and in the smile.

Before serial extraction the FMA was 32°, indicating a relatively high angle facial pattern; this improved to 30° during serial extraction and to 29° during active treatment. Reduction in the FMA suggests a favorable upward and forward rotation of the mandible. During serial extraction the IMPA was reduced 5° (from 96° to 91°) and the FMIA increased 6° (from 53° to 59°), both signifying a reduction in the alveolodental protrusion and an uprighting of the mandibular incisors. Further improvement took place during active treatment, with the IMPA decreasing to 89° and the FMIA to 62°. Throughout treatment the skeletal discrepancy improved: A-N-B was reduced from 9° to 3°; the maxilla became less prognathic (from 86° to 82°); and the mandible became less retrognathic (from 77° to 79°). The occlusal plane remained fairly constant, indicating good control throughout treatment. The Z angle increased from 64° to 76°, denoting improvement in the facial harmony and balance (Fig. 6-139).

In the total space analysis the anterior arch area had a deficit of 15.4 mm. Two thirds of this was cephalometric correction, indicating an alveolodental protrusion. The middle arch area had a surplus of 1.5 mm, and the posterior arch area a deficit of 15.0 mm. The anterior deficit was corrected by extraction of four first premolars, and the posterior deficit was corrected by extraction of the four third molars (Table 6-6).

Mechanotherapy

The treatment objectives after the serial extraction phase are (1) closure of residual extraction spaces, (2) improvement of the axial inclination of individual teeth, (3) correction of rotations, (4) correction of midline discrepancy, (5) correction of a residual overbite, (6) correction of a residual overjet, (7) correction of crossbites, (8) refinement of the intercuspation of individual teeth, (9) improvement and coordination of arch form, and (10) correction of the Class II relationship in some Class II patients.

When the serial extraction phase has been completed, the

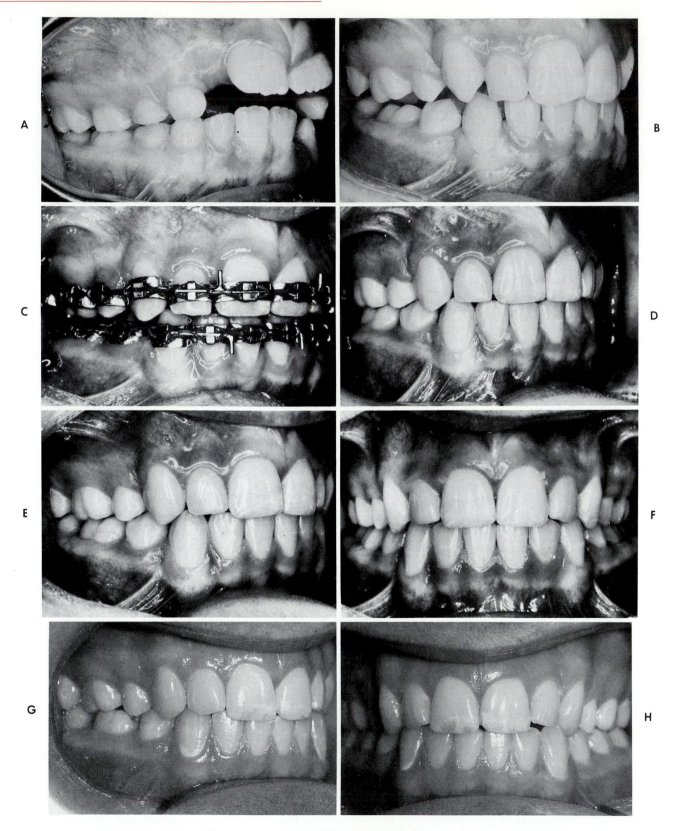

Fig. 6-137   Patient J.O. **A,** Before, and **B,** following serial extraction. **C,** Final stage of over-treatment. **D,** End of treatment. **E** and **F,** Two years after retention. **G** and **H,** Seven years after retention. Note chipped enamel on the maxillary incisors, caused by a blow while playing football without a mouth guard.

A, B, C

D, E, F

G   H

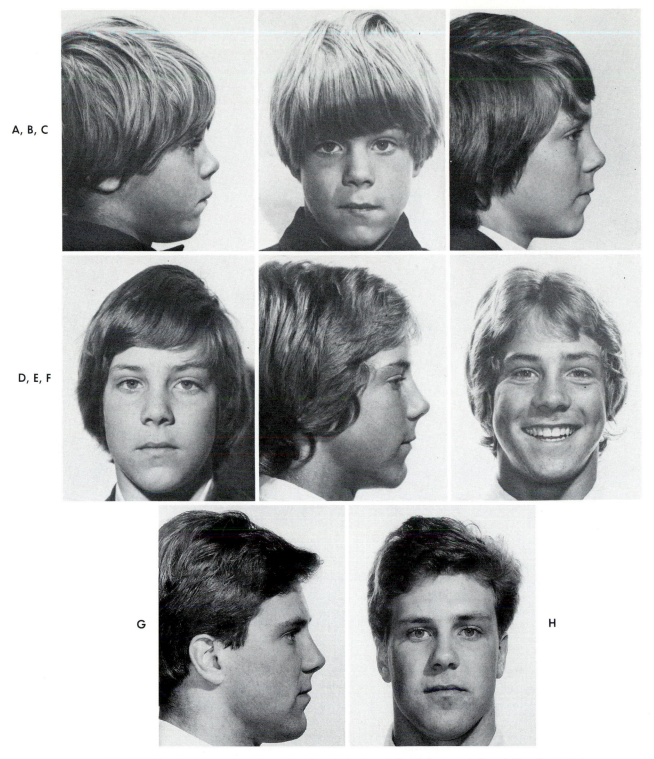

Fig. 6-138   Facial configuration of patient J.O. **A** and **B,** Before, and **C** and **D,** after serial extraction. **E** and **F,** Following active treatment. **G** and **H,** Seven years after treatment.

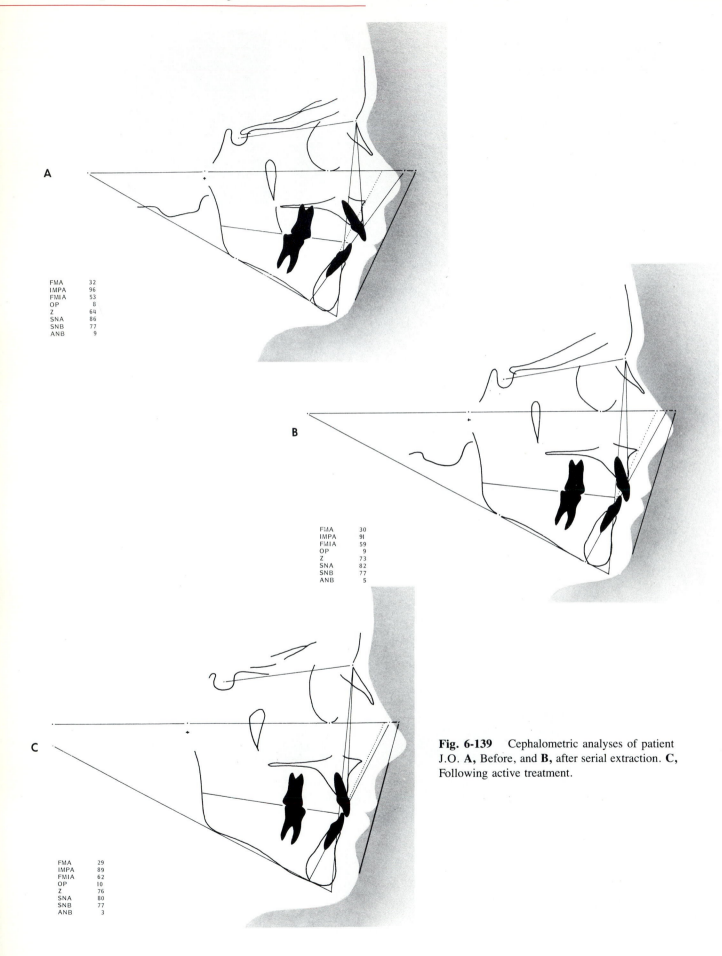

FMA	32
IMPA	96
FMIA	53
OP	8
Z	64
SNA	86
SNB	77
ANB	9

FMA	30
IMPA	9l
FMIA	59
OP	9
Z	73
SNA	82
SNB	77
ANB	5

FMA	29
IMPA	89
FMIA	62
OP	l0
Z	76
SNA	80
SNB	77
ANB	3

Fig. 6-139 Cephalometric analyses of patient J.O. **A,** Before, and **B,** after serial extraction. **C,** Following active treatment.

multibonded appliance is placed and treatment is initiated using the traditional concepts of the Tweed philosophy. The modern concepts of The Charles H. Tweed International Foundation for Orthodontic Research can be summarized as follows[44,46] (see Chapter 11):

Directional force systems

10-2 Anchorage

Readout

Prescription arches

Performance testing

Dr. Tweed's primary objectives in treatment included a healthy dentition, stability, optimal function, healthy supporting tissues and optimal facial esthetics. These are excellent treatment goals; nevertheless, they are too general:

The *directional force* technique is a group of force systems using directional control to position the teeth precisely in both the maxilla and the mandible so they will be in optimum harmony with their environment.

The *10-2* concept is a sequential anchorage system wherein the archwire stabilizes 10 teeth while 2 teeth receive the active force. Instead of 12 teeth being involved in the anchorage preparation at one time, only 2 are receiving active force. The sequence begins with the second molars and is completed with the second premolars. When this type of improved anchorage preparation is used, there is less risk that the dentition will move unfavorably downward and forward and patient cooperation is not as crucial.

With *readout* the objectives of orthodontic treatment can be defined by accurate measurement. Tooth movements can be predetermined, monitored during treatment, and checked for accuracy of final placement.

Prescription arches include the tabulation of second-order angulation associated with *10-2 anchorage* and *readout*. They also permit the precise measurement and tabulation of buccolinguoaxial inclinations of teeth so third-order bends can be incorporated in the archwire. Finally, they include the horizontal first-order bends. These prescription arches are designed specifically for individual malocclusions.

Performance testing is a relatively recent development that involves the serial measurement of tooth movement and dental relationships so treatment progress can be evaluated. This particular edgewise appliance, originally designed by Tweed and modified by Merrifield and his associates, is the precision instrument used in achieving treatment goals. It is characterized by simplicity, efficiency, and comfort; it is hygienic and esthetic; and, above all, it has a wide range of versatility.

When the appliance is removed and retainers are placed—a critical stage in the correction of the malocclusion occurs. This is referred to as the *period of recovery*. If the corrective procedures barely achieve the normal relationship of teeth, there will be an inevitable relapse. Any change that occurs will be away from ideal occlusion. However, if treatment is completed by overcorrection, all changes that take place

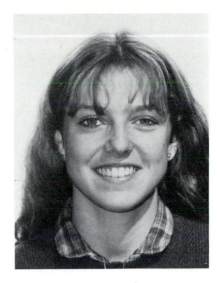

Fig. 6-140   The smile that makes it all worthwhile.

during the recovery period will be toward the ideal relationship. This provides the ideal circumstances for obtaining the original objectives: health of the dentition and the supporting structures, optimal function, stability, and beautiful facial esthetics (Fig. 6-140).

When facial deformity has been corrected and mental anguish eliminated, a dull and unhappy facial expression becomes bright and happy. What greater reward could any orthodontist want or expect.

Charles H. Tweed

I would add . . . the earlier this occurs the better.

REFERENCES

1. American Board of Orthodontics: *Specific instructions for candidates,* St Louis, 1993, American Board of Orthodontics.
2. Angle EH: *Malocclusion of the teeth,* ed 7, Philadelphia, 1907, SS White Dental.
3. Arita M, Iwagaki H: *Studies on the serial observations of dento-facial region in the Japanese children,* Tokyo, 1963, Nihon University School of Dentistry.
4. Baker C: Development of the occlusion of the teeth, *J Am Dent Assoc* 31:1470, 1944.
5. Baume LJ: Physiological tooth migration and its significance for the development of occlusion. I. The biogenetic course of the deciduous teeth, *J Dent Res* 29:123, 1950.
6. Baume LJ: Physiological tooth migration and its significance for the development of occlusion. II. The biogenesis of accessional dentition, *J Dent Res* 29:331, 1950.
7. Baume LJ: Physiological tooth migration and its significance for the development of occlusion. III. The biogenesis of the successional dentition, *J Dent Res* 29:338, 1950.
8. Baume LJ: Physiological tooth migration and its significance for the development of occlusion. IV. The biogenesis of overbite, *J Dent Res* 29:440, 1950.
9. Baume LJ: Developmental and diagnostic aspects of the primary dentition. *Int Dent J* 9:349, 1959.
10. Bilkey ER: Is there writing on the wall? [Editorial.] *Oral Health* 71:4, 1981.

11. Björk A: Variations in the growth pattern of the human mandible; longitudinal radiographic study by the implant method, *J Dent Res* 42:400, 1963.
12. Black GV: *Descriptive anatomy of the human teeth*, ed 5, Philadelphia, 1902, SS White Dental.
13. Brodie A: Late growth changes in the human face, *Angle Orthod* 23:146, 1953.
14. Bunon R: *Essay sur les maladies des dents; ou l'on propose les moyens de leur procurer une bonne confirmation dès la plus tendre enfance, et d'en assurer la conservation pendant tout le cours de la vie*, Paris, 1743.
15. Burlington Orthodontic Research Project, University of Toronto, Faculty of Dentistry, Report no 3, 1957.
16. Dale JG, Rushton JS et al: *A half century of care, a future of caring*, Tucson, Ariz, 1982, The Charles H. Tweed International Foundation.
17. DeKock WJ: Dental arch depth and width studies longitudinally from 12 years of age to adulthood, *Am J Orthod* 62:56, 1972.
18. Delabarre CF: *Traité de la second dentition et méthode naturelle de la diriger suivis d'un apercu de séméiotique buccale*, Paris, 1918.
19. Enlow DH: *The human face; an account of the postnatal growth and development of the craniofacial skeleton*, New York, 1968, Paul B Hoeber.
20. Enlow DH: *Handbook of facial growth*, ed 2, Philadelphia, 1982, WB Saunders.
21. Fanning EA: Effect of extraction of deciduous molars on the formation and eruption of their successors, *Angle Orthod* 32:44, 1962.
22. Fanning EA: Longitudinal study of tooth formation and root resorption, *NZ Dent J* 57:202, 1961.
23. Fanning EA, Hunt EE: Linear increments of growth in the roots of permanent mandibular teeth, *J Dent Res* 43(suppl):981, 1964.
24. Franke G: *Ueber Wachstum und Verbildungen des Kiefers und der Nasenscheidewand auf grund vergleichender Kiefer-messungen und experimenteller Untersuchungen über Knochenwachstum*, Leipzig, 1921, Curt Kabitzsch.
25. Garcia-Hernandez J, Dale JG: "Facial considerations in mixed-dentition analysis in preparation for guidance of occlusion." Postgraduate Thesis, Department of Paedodontics, University of Toronto, Faculty of Dentistry, 1979.
26. Garn SM, Lewis AB: The gradient and the pattern of crown-size reduction in simple hypodontia, *Angle Orthod* 40:51, 1970.
27. Grøn AM: Prediction of tooth emergence, *J Dent Res* 41:573, 1962.
28. Hixon EH, Oldfather RE: Estimation of the sizes of unerupted cuspid and bicuspid teeth, *Angle Orthod* 28:236, 1958.
29. Horowitz SL, Hixon EH: *The nature of orthodontic diagnosis*, St Louis, 1966, Mosby, Chapter 16.
30. Hotz R: Guidance of eruption versus serial extraction, *Am J Orthod* 58:1, 1970.
31. Huckaba GW: Arch size analysis and tooth size prediction, *Dent Clin North Am* p 431, 1964.
32. Hurme VO: Ranges in normalcy in eruption of permanent teeth, *J Dent Child* 16:11, 1949.
33. Jacobi A: Course of lectures on dentition and its derangements, *Am Med Times* 1:416, 1860.
34. Kjellgren B: Serial extraction as a corrective procedure in dental orthopedic therapy, *Eur Orthod Soc Trans* p. 134, 1947-1948.
35. Lebret L: Personal communications.
36. Lewis SM, Lehman IA: A quantitative study of the relation between certain factors in the development of the dental arch and the occlusion of the teeth, *Int J Orthod* 18:1015, 1932.
37. Lo RT, Moyers RE: Studies in the etiology and prevention of malocclusion. I. The sequence of eruption of the permanent dentition, *Am J Orthod* 39:460, 1953.
38. Lundt RC, Law DB: A review of the chronology of calcification of deciduous teeth, *J Am Dent Assoc* 89:599, 1974.
39. Mayne WR: *Serial extraction*. In Graber TM, editor: *Current orthodontic concepts and techniques*, Philadelphia, 1969, WB Saunders, Chapter 4.
40. McNamara J: Components of Class II malocclusion in children 8-10 years of age, *Angle Orthod* 51:177, 1981.
41. Meredith HV: Order and age of eruption for the deciduous dentition, *J Dent Res* 25:43, 1946.
42. Meredith HV, Knott V: *Childhood changes of head, face, and dentition—a collection of research reports*, Iowa City, 1973, Iowa Orthodontic Society.
43. Merrifield LL: The profile line as an aid in critically evaluating facial esthetics, *Am J Orthod* 52:804, 1966.
44. Merrifield LL: Differential diagnosis with total space analysis, *J Charles H Tweed Int Found* 6:10, 1978.
45. Harris GS: Graphic display of total space analysis, *J Tweed Foundation* 13:128-152, 1985.
46. Merrifield LL: The systems of directional force, *J Charles H Tweed Int Found* 10:15, 1982.
47. Moorrees CFA: Growth changes of the dental arches—a longitudinal study, *J Can Dent Assoc* 24:449, 1958.
48. Moorrees CFA: *The dentition of the growing child; a longitudinal study of dental development between 3 and 18 years of age*, Cambridge, Mass, 1959, Harvard University Press.
49. Moorrees CFA: Dental development—a growth study based on tooth eruption as a measure of physiologic age, *Eur Orthod Soc Trans* 40:92, 1964.
50. Moorrees CFA: Changes in dental arch dimensions expressed on the basis of tooth eruption as a measure of biologic age, *J Dent Res* 44:129, 1965.
51. Moorrees CFA: Normal variation in dental development determined with reference to tooth eruption statistics, *J Dent Res* 44:161, 1965.
52. Moorrees CFA, Chadha JM: Crown diameters of corresponding tooth groups in deciduous and permanent dentition, *J Dent Res* 41:466, 1962.
53. Moorrees CFA, Chadha JM: Available space for the incisors during dental development; a growth study based on physiological age, *Angle Orthod* 35:12, 1965.
54. Moorrees CFA, Kent RL Jr: *Patterns of dental maturation*. In McNamara JA editor: *The biology of occlusal development, Monograph 6, Craniofacial growth series*, Ann Arbor, 1978, Center for Human Growth and Development, University of Michigan.
55. Moorrees CFA, Kent RL Jr: A step function model using tooth counts to assess the developmental timing of the dentition, *Ann Hum Biol* 5:55, 1978.
56. Moorrees CFA, Thomsen S et al: Mesiodistal crown diameters of the deciduous and permanent teeth in individuals, *J Dent Res* 36:39, 1957.
57. Robinow M, Richards TW, Anderson M: The eruption of deciduous teeth, *Growth* 6:127, 1942.
58. Schudy FF: The rotation of the mandible resulting from growth; its implications in orthodontic treatment, *Angle Orthod* 35:36, 1965.
59. Sillman JH: Dimensional changes of the dental arches; longitudinal study from birth to 24 years, *Am J Orthod* 50:824, 1964.
60. Steiner C: Cephalometrics in clinical practice, *Angle Orthod* 29:8, 1959.
61. Stone I: *The origin*, Garden City, NY, 1980, Doubleday.
62. Subtelny JD, Sakuda M: Openbite, diagnosis and treatment, *Am J Orthod* 50:337, 1964.
63. Ten Cate AR, et al: *Oral histology: development, structure, and function*, St Louis, 1980, Mosby.
64. Tweed CH: Treatment planning and therapy in the mixed-dentition, *Am J Orthod* 49:900, 1963.
65. Tweed CH: *Clinical orthodontics*, St Louis, 1966, Mosby.
66. Tweed CH: The diagnostic facial triangle in the control of treatment objectives, *Am J Orthod* 55:651, 1969.
67. Virel A: *Decorated man*, New York, 1980, Harry N. Abrams.
68. Wagers LE: Preorthodontic guidance and the corrective mixed-dentition treatment concept, *Am J Orthod* 69:1, 1976.
69. Zsigmundy O: Ueber die Veränderungen des Zahnbogens bei der zweiten Dentition, *Arch Anat* p 367, 1890.

ADDITIONAL READINGS

Bolton WA: The clinical application of a tooth size analysis, *Am J Orthod* 48:504, 1962.

Clifton OW: Lower first premolar extraction: a viable alternative? *Am J Orthod Dentofac Orthop* 90(2):158-163, 1986.

Dale J: J.C.O. interviews: Dr. Jack G. Dale on serial extraction, *J Clin Orthod* 10:44, 116, 196, 1976.

Dewel BF: Serial extractions in orthodontics; indications, objections, and treatment procedures, *Int J Orthod* 40:906, 1954.

Dewel BF: A critical analysis of serial extraction in orthodontic treatment, *Am J Orthod* 45:424, 1959.

Dewel BF: Serial extraction, its limitations and contraindications in orthodontic treatment, *Am J Orthod* 53:904, 1967.

Dibbets JM et al: Long-term effects of orthodontic treatment, including extraction, on signs and symptoms attributed to CMD, *Eur J Orthod* 14(1):16-20, 1992.

Garfinkle RL, Artese A et al: Effect of extraction in the late mixed-dentition on the eruption of the first premolar in Macaca nemestrina, *Angle Orthod* 50:23, 1980.

Gianelly AA et al: Condylar position and extraction treatment, *Am J Orthod Dentofac Orthop* 93(3):201-205, 1988.

Gianelly AA et al: Longitudinal evaluation of condylar position in extraction and nonextraction treatment, *Am J Orthod Dentofac Orthop* 100(5):416-420, 1991.

Gilmore CA et al: Mandibular incisor dimensions and crowding, *Am J Orthod* 86(6):493-502, 1984.

Greer GW, Artese A et al: Effect of extraction in the early mixed-dentition on the eruption of the first premolar in Macaca pemestrina, *Angle Orthod* 50:34, 1980.

Hägg U, Taranger J: Maturation indicators and the pubertal growth spurt, *Am J Orthod* 82:299, 1982.

Heath J: The interception of malocclusion by planned serial extraction, *N Z Dent J* 49:77, 1953.

Heath J: Dangers and pitfalls of serial extraction, *Eur Orthod Soc Trans* 37:60, 1961.

Hotz R: Active supervision of the eruption of teeth by extraction, *Eur Orthod Soc Trans* p. 34, 1947-1948.

Jacobs SG: A re-assessment of serial extraction, *Aust Orthod J* 10(2):90-97 (15 ref), 1987.

Jegou I: Indication and limits on the choice of extraction of 14-24 and 35-45 in treating Angle class-II malocclusion by a Tweed-Merrifield analysis of the total space, *Orthod Fr* 55(2):485-494, 1984.

Jones O et al: Orthodontic management of a patient with Class I malocclusion and severe crowding, *Am J Orthod Dentofac Orthop* 98(3):189-196, 1990.

Klapper L et al: The influence of extraction and nonextraction orthodontic treatment on brachyfacial and dolichofacial growth patterns, *Am J Orthod Dentofac Orthop* 101(5):425-430, 1992.

Krogman WM: Biological timing and dento-facial complex, *J Dent Child* 35:175, 328, 377, 1968.

Leighton BC, Hunter WS: Relationship between lower arch spacing/crowding and facial height and depth, *Angle Orthod* 82:418, 1982.

Little, R.M.: The effects of eruption guidance and serial extraction on developing dentition, *Pediatr Dent* 9(1):65-70, 1987.

Little RM, Riedel RA, Årtun J: An evaluation of changes in mandibular anterior alignment from 10-20 years post retention, *Am J Orthod Dentofac Orthop* 93:423-428, 1988.

Little RM, Waller TR, Riedel RA: Stability and relapse of mandibular anterior alignment—first premolar extraction cases treated by traditional edgewise orthodontics, *Am J Orthod* 80:349-365, 1981.

Little RM et al: Serial extraction of first premolars—postretention evaluation of stability and relapse, *Angle Orthod* 60(4):255-262, 1990.

Lloyd ZB: Serial extraction as a treatment procedure, *Am J Orthod* 42:728, 1956.

McNamara JA, Brudon WL: *Orthodontic and orthopedic treatment in the mixed dentition,* ed 1, Ann Arbor, 1993, Needham Press.

McReynolds DC et al: Mandibular second premolar extraction—postretention evaluation of stability and relapse, *Angle Orthod* 6(2):133-144, 1991.

Moorrees CFA: Variability of dental and facial development, *Ann NY Acad Sci* 134:846, 1966.

Moorrees CFA, Fanning EA, Grøn AM: Consideration of dental development in serial extraction, *Angle Orthod* 33:44, 1963.

Moorrees CFA, Fanning EA, Grøn AM, Lebret J: Timing of orthodontic treatment in relation to tooth formation, *Eur Orthod Soc Trans* 38:87, 1962.

Moorrees CFA, Fanning EA, Hunt EE Jr: Age variation of formation stages for ten permanent teeth, *J Dent Res* 42:1490, 1963.

Moorrees CFA, Fanning EA, Hunt EE Jr: Formation and resorption of three deciduous teeth in children, *Am J Phys Anthropol* 21:99, 1963.

Moorrees CFA, Reed RB: Biometrics of crowding and spacing of the teeth in the mandible, *Am J Phys Anthropol* 12:77, 1954.

Moorrees CFA, Reed RB: Correlations among crown diameters of human teeth, *Arch Oral Biol* 9:685, 1964.

Moorrees CFA, Reed RB, Chadha JM: Growth changes of the dentition defined in terms of chronologic and biologic age, *Am J Orthod* 50:789, 1964.

Ortial JP: The Tweed technic. Choice of extraction and treatment strategy. I. *Actual Dent* 3(16):10-1, 13-5, 17-21 *passim,* 1987.

Renfoe EW: The philosophy of extraction in orthodontics: 1966 (classified article), *Int J Orthod* 27(1-2):3-8, 1989.

Richardson ME: Late lower arch crowding in relation to primary crowding, *Angle Orthod* 52:300, 1982.

Richardson ME: The effect of mandibular first premolar extraction on third molar space, *Angle Orthod* 59(4):291-294, 1989.

Sanin C, Savara B, Sekiguchi T: Longitudinal dentofacial changes in untreated persons, *Am J Orthod* 55:135, 1969.

Tanner JM: *Growth at adolescence,* ed 2, Cambridge, Mass, 1962, Blackwell Scientific Publications.

Toshniwal NG: A review of serial extraction, *J Indian Dent Assoc* 61(12):291-293, 1990.

Tweed CH: The Frankfort-mandibular plane angle in orthodontic diagnosis, classification, treatment planning, and prognosis, *Am J Orthod Oral Surg* 32:175, 1946.

Tweed CH: The Frankfort-mandibular incisor angle in orthodontic diagnosis treatment planning and prognosis, *Angle Orthod* 24:121, 1954.

Tweed CH: *Pre-orthodontic guidance procedure, classification of facial growth trends, treatment timing.* In Kraus BS, Reidel RA, editors: *Vistas in orthodontics,* Philadelphia, 1962, Lea & Febiger, Chapter 8.

Yamaguchi K et al: The effects of extraction and nonextraction treatment on the mandibular position, *Am J Orthod Dentofac Orthop* 100(5):443-452, 1991.

Techniques and Treatment

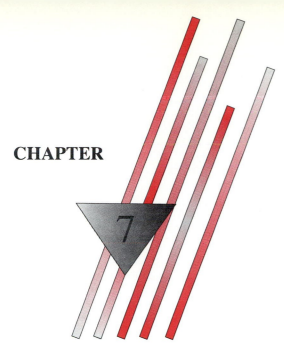

CHAPTER 7

Functional Appliances

THOMAS M. GRABER

THE ANDRESEN ACTIVATOR

Origin. Theories on bone plasticity may be traced back to Roux[165] and Wolff,[213] who believed that form was intimately related to function. Changes in functional stresses produced changes in internal bone architecture and external shape. Although Robin[164] introduced a *monobloc* early in the twentieth century, which effectively postured the mandible forward, it was not intended to effect structural change or guide jaw growth. Rather, it was used as a passive positioning device in neonates with micromandible and cleft lip and palate (later referred to as the Pierre Robin syndrome) to prevent glossoptosis, or literally swallowing of the tongue. For Viggo Andresen,[7] however, who was unaware of the Robin appliance, the possible effect of function on bone shape, size, and position offered hope in correcting sagittal malrelationships, primarily Class II, division 1 malocclusions, in the growing child, by changing the functional pattern of the stomatognathic system. The working hypothesis was tested on his daughter, who went away to camp during the summer. Andresen removed the fixed labiolingual appliances and placed a modified Hawley-type retainer on the maxillary arch, but he added a lower lingual horseshoe flange that guided the mandible forward some 3 to 4 mm when the teeth were brought into maximum interarch contact (Fig. 7-1). This was done to prevent any relapse over the 3-month vacation period.[7] On his daughter's return from camp, Andresen was pleasantly surprised to see that the nighttime wearing of the appliance had produced a complete sagittal correction and a significantly improved facial profile. The result was stable. Trying this on numerous other

patients who were going away for the summer and then on patients under routine care, Andresen observed a significant sagittal basal bone and neuromuscular improvement that he could not produce with conventional fixed appliances.[8,9]

Rationale. The explanation behind the sagittal changes is that the appliance activated or increased the activity of the

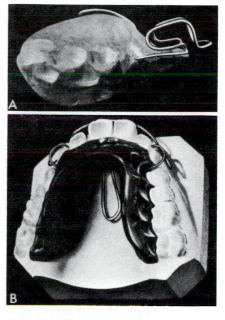

Fig. 7-1 Andresen-Häupl activator. No tooth-moving parts. The original appliances were made of Vulcanite. In this appliance, being used to treat a Class II, division 1, malocclusion, the palatal acrylic has been cut out and a heavy Coffin spring laid across the palate for stability. The loops at the canine region stand away from the teeth, allowing maxillary intercanine development. These loops are the forerunner of the Balters Bionator loops, which extended to the distal of the deciduous second molars, holding off cheek pressure—also a forerunner of the Fränkel buccal shields. (From Andresen V, Häupl K: *Funktionskieferorthopädie. Die Grundlagen des "norwegischen Systems,"* ed 2, Leipzig, 1939, H. Meusser.)

Special credit is given to the late Professor Olav Slagsvold and to WB Saunders Company for permission to use some of the illustrations and factual material from *Activator development and philosophy*, in Graber TM, and Neumann B: *Removable orthodontic appliances*, ed 1, Philadelphia, 1977, WB Saunders.

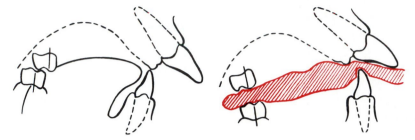

Fig. 7-2 Construction bite. Correcting the buccal segment relationship from Class II to Class I, or approximately a 6 mm advancement. Note that the overjet is still excessive in this case, probably because of labial malposition of the upper incisor segment. This would be corrected after the sagittal relationship was normalized. There is a 3 to 4 mm vertical opening to allow the mandible to come forward sufficiently to correct the anteroposterior buccal intercuspation. (From Andresen V, Häupl K: *Funktionskieferorthopädie. Die Grundlagen des "norwegischen Systems,"* ed 2, Leipzig, 1939, H. Meusser.)

protractor and elevator muscles, with concomitant relaxation and stretching of the retractors. Eliminating the abnormal perioral muscle function by mandibular protraction prevented deforming and restrictive action by the lower lip trap and hyperactivity of the mentalis and the submandibular muscle groups (Figs. 7-2 and 7-3). The change in muscle pattern thus would produce not only a new and more favorable muscle pattern but also a change in bony structures as they adapted to the new functional stresses[8] (Fig. 7-4). The intermittent forces produced by the loose appliance were thought to create favorable tooth position changes, even though the appliance was worn only at night. Like Robin's monobloc, the appliance used by Andresen was passive, with no intrinsic force systems.[8-10] The extrinsic force came from the loose appliance's stimulating the elevators and protractors to contract as the patient bit into the appliance. It was hypothesized that growth increments were greater at night, providing optimal tissue response.

The original name used by Andresen for this type of treatment was biomechanical orthodontics, and only later after further work on the concepts and technique refinements with Karl Häupl was it changed to *functional jaw orthopedics,* which was more descriptive.[11-13] The concepts were broadened to include the potential of altering skeletal relationships, depending on the amount and direction of jaw growth. The forward posturing of the construction bite activated the muscles, which in turn enhanced a sagittal skeletal change, harnessing the growth potential—hence the functional orthopedic connotation. To much of the orthodontic world, however, it became known as *the Norwegian system,* despite the fact that Andresen was a Dane and Häupl a German (both were teaching at the dental school in Oslo, Norway).

THE BITE-OPENING CONTROVERSY

Whereas the sagittal construction bite advancement concept was generally accepted by most clinicians in Europe (it varied from 3 to 6 mm, depending on the severity of the anteroposterior malrelationship and resultant abnormal buc-

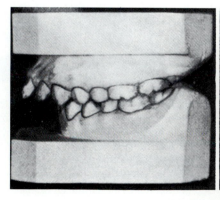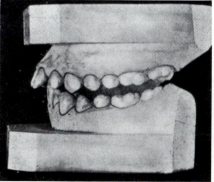

Fig. 7-3 Lateral view of study models of severe Class II, division 1, malocclusion (Fig. 7-2) shown in habitual occlusion and in a proper construction bite. In this case the lingual inclination of the lower incisor segment is a favorable characteristic, as is the deeper than normal overbite, improving the treatment prognosis. (From Andresen V, Häupl K: *Funktionskieferorthopädie. Die Grundlagen des "norwegischen Systems,"* Leipzig, 1942, J.A. Barth.)

cal segment interdigitation), the functional jaw orthopedic concepts elicited considerable controversy, even among Norwegian orthodontists, over the amount of vertical opening and the effect produced by the appliance on the muscles. Selmer-Olsen,[176] who became professor of orthodontics at the University of Oslo after World War II, felt that muscles could not actually be stimulated or activated during sleep, since Nature had designed them to rest at night and swallowing took place only 4 to 8 times an hour. He interpreted the activator action as a stretching of the muscles, fascial sheets, and ligaments when the mandible was opened beyond postural resting position. The activator was, in truth, a foreign body and the tooth-moving force produced was due not to the kinetic energy of muscle function but to the potential energy of stretched tissues. Woodside[214,215] and Woodside et al.[216] were to refer to this later as the *viscoelastic* properties of the tissue. Current debate on the exact nature of the activator effect still reflects this dichotomy of opinion. Condylar unloading seems to be a factor.

Andresen's interpretation presupposed freedom for the mandible to assume rest position. Slagsvold[179] noted that it did not appear from the literature and his own observations that Andresen considered the degree of mandibular displacement in relation to this position. Nevertheless, it would mean a violation of his principles to displace the mandible beyond it. Andresen had only a 2 mm interocclusal clearance between the upper and lower jaw, or the thickness of a match. Even later when changed to 2 to 4 mm, it would still be within the freeway space limits of most patients, particularly for sleeping individuals.[14] Too wide an opening made compliance more difficult and could introduce potentially depressing action on the posterior teeth.

The Selmer-Olsen, Harvold,[81,82] and Woodside interpretations are based on the fact that in most activators, as modified from the original appliance, the interocclusal separation did, indeed, exceed the postural rest position if for no other reason than to keep the appliance in place at night

during sleep to maintain a sagittal corrective stimulus.[158] The cognitive interpretations of Selmer-Olsen were subsequently corroborated by Ahlgren,[1-5] Thompson,[188] Witt,[209,210] Witt and Komposch,[211] and Witt and Meyer.[212]

Rolf Grude,[74,75] an associate and disciple of Andresen, believed that the appliance worked best only if the vertical dimension established did not exceed postural resting position. If it was increased beyond that, the action became fundamentally changed. Fränkel[56] and Fränkel and Reiss[59] concurred in this assessment.

The concepts and explanations of Paul Herren[93,94] had a significant impact on activator use and philosophy. He stated that the traditional nighttime loose-fitting appliance did not work as claimed. (Reitan[161] had already questioned the Roux *shaking of the bone* theory espoused by Andresen and Häupl with his monumental doctoral dissertation on tissue reactions in 1951.) Herren came to the conclusion that the activator did not increase the frequency of closing movements, even if the freeway space was not exceeded. Tooth movement forces thus were not created by nocturnal functional movements stimulated by the activator. The Herren interpretation was as follows:

Various forces acting on the mandible are in equilibrium by virtue of constant adjustments between them. Gravity and air pressure are dominant independent variables, and muscle tonus and tension are dominant dependent variables. When there is a gravity component change or an intraoral air pressure change, the mandible is moved or pulled to a new position wherein the initial changes are compensated for by reactive changes in muscle tension and tonus. Also changes in muscle tonus are compensated for by a change in muscle tension as the mandible tends to relocate. The mandibular position determined by the activator is the desired postural position rather than a momentary rest position that is free of appliance guidance. The activator limits mandibular movement in all planes of space except an opening or vertical movement. When the mandible would normally have a number of rest positions during sleep (depending on body position), the activator tends to prevent it from moving to these positions, splinting the lower jaw

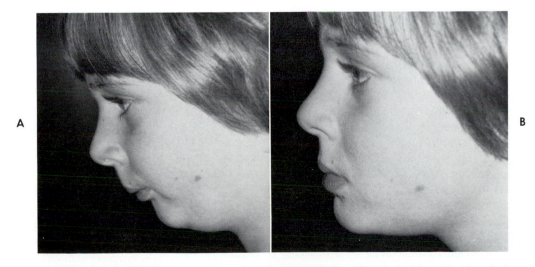

Fig. 7-4   Profile with the jaw in habitual Class II occlusion, **A,** and protracted into Class I sagittal relationship, **B,** A good clinical test for demonstrating the dramatic change possible in the profile.

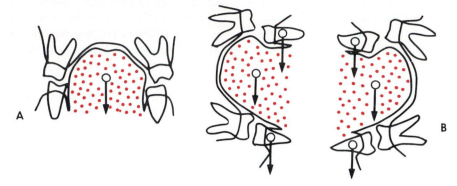

Fig. 7-5 Various forces acting on the upper and lower arches. In this instance the influence of gravity is quite different when the head is erect, **A,** from what it is when the patient is sleeping with the head turned to one side or the other, **B,** The activator then tends to prevent the normal change or adaptation to varying postural and gravitational forces, which elicits a positive reaction from the buccinator mechanism and the protractor and retractor muscles. Since a patient swallows only four to eight times an hour during sleep, this action would more likely be responsible for the changes produced by the activator. (From Herren P: *Am J Orthod* 45:512, 1959.)

in the desired centric relationship regardless of sleeping posture (Fig. 7-5). The muscle forces that would normally be acting at night to maintain mandibular postural equilibrium with changing body positions are thus transmitted to the appliance, which in turn exerts force on the teeth and alveolar bone, causing the resultant movement. Any mandibular movements that occur are of minor importance.

Head posture during sleep. Since head position changes many times during sleep, the direction of the resultant force on the activator also changes. At any particular moment the rest position depends on head and body posture, so the restriction of muscle movement that would create the desired mandibular position change without the activator in place varies constantly, involving different muscle groups and creating different force vectors on the activator. The plane of sleep (light or deep), the intraoral air pressure, the dream cycle, and the state of mind are additional conditioning factors, all uncontrolled by the orthodontist. Only the mandibular position held by the appliance is determined by the clinician; however, this splinting effect on the mandible is such that it can help predetermine the net effect of the variable forces. If the activator is designed properly and worn as prescribed, the resultant of all the controlled and uncontrolled forces is usually to enhance adaptation to the position created by the appliance (Figs. 7-6 and 7-7).

Herren[93] attempted to assess the magnitude of the resultant forces acting on the mandible, as well as the interaction between them. He pointed out that the weight of the mandible, tongue, and appliance are constant, averaging about 250 g. Muscle tonus and tensions vary, depending on the degree of stretching, the control from the central nervous system, the relation with the bed or pillow, whether the head is prone or supine, etc. If the patient is dorsally recumbent while sleeping and the head is upright, then the muscle forces must balance the weight of the lower jaw, associated soft tissue structures, and appliance. It is clear that the forces

active are entirely different in multiple prone, supine, rotated combinations from what they are in an alert, awakened, upright head posture. Over a prolonged period the duration that a particular position is held and the resultant forces would be factors to consider. The forces created are basically intermittent, however, even though some teeth or groups of teeth may be subject to pressure for a protracted time. The loose appliance is responsible for some of the intermittent action. Removal of the appliance during the day also produces a net intermittent action, calling up a new muscle engram to establish the neuromuscular engram consistent with diurnal postural changes and activities. Hence the same conclusion was reached by Herren as by Selmer-Olsen but with a different basis for reasoning.

Working hypotheses. Thus for the conventional nighttime wear of the passive Andresen activator, there are two working hypotheses as far as the effect on the teeth themselves is concerned:

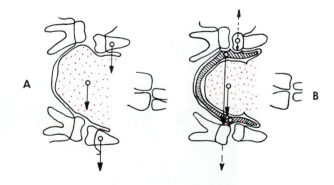

Fig. 7-6 Instead of the postural alterations evoked by changes in body position, **A,** as shown in Fig. 7-5, the activator splints the jaws in a more normal transverse, sagittal, and vertical relationship when it is worn, **B,** (From Herren P: *Schweiz Monatsschr Zahnheilkd* 63:829, 1953.)

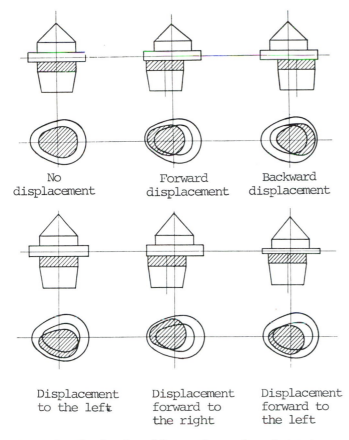

No
displacement

Forward
displacement

Backward
displacement

Displacement
to the left

Displacement
forward to
the right

Displacement
forward to
the left

Fig. 7-7 The direction of force acting on the activator at any particular moment depends on the spatial relationships between the posture induced by the activator and the momentary rest position. The view is from the top of the head with the face to the left of the ovoid outline. (From Herren P: *Schweiz Monatsschr Zahnheilkd* 63:829, 1953.)

1. The original Andresen-Häupl theory[14] attributed tooth movement to a loose-fitting functionally generated mobility providing intermittent forces created by the elevator and protractor muscles, as well as by elements of the buccinator mechanism, that jolted or shook the teeth, pushing the appliance back into position on the maxillary teeth when it dropped away. A prerequisite was that the bite opening could not exceed the normal interocclusal clearance or freeway space.[14] This approach, using nocturnal wear of a loosely fitting appliance, is espoused by Ahlgren.[1-5]

2. The second hypothesis,[178] as described previously and closely following the Herren analysis, denied the nocturnal functional activity during sleep. Rather, it suggested that the activator at rest moves the teeth and creates the desired changes. The appliance is squeezed between the jaws most of the time, splinting them in the *ought to be* sagittal relationship and preventing compensatory postural changes that would normally occur without the activator in place. The resultant forces created vary from time to time and change in magnitude. They are intermittent, but the net result is that they are transmitted to the activator, which distributes them to the teeth and alveolar bone, enhancing the adaptive process. The action is still considered to be primarily interrupted or intermittent in nature. The forces produce a strain in the tissues and are a mechanical phenomenon, whether the strain is due to muscles directly or whether it acts indirectly through the appliance* (Fig. 7-8).

---

*References, 2, 13, 48, 72, 81-83, 98-101, 168-173, 187, 211, 215, 216.

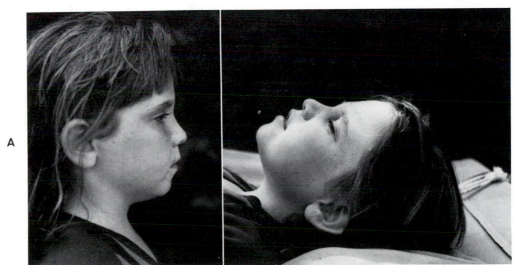

A   B

Fig. 7-8 When the patient is awake and upright, **A,** muscle tonus, muscle tension, and atmospheric pressure balance the weight of the mandible and associated tissues plus the activator. If the mouth is open, then the weight and gravitational effect are balanced by the muscles alone. If the patient sleeps reclined while wearing the activator, **B,** then muscle tension, muscle tonus, and gravity all act in the same direction. When the patient is asleep, the lips drop open; then *function,* as far as any appliance is concerned, is minimal.

Sagittal change. The desired sagittal change needed to correct the anteroposterior malrelationship is produced by the forward posturing of the mandible in the construction bite. This was recognized as dependent on growth guidance to achieve the skeletal alteration required, as well as favorable dentoalveolar adjustment. Controversy still surrounds this working hypothesis, despite definitive research by Petrovic et al.[151-157] on rats and the primate studies by Elgoyhen et al.,[45] Graber,[64] Graber,[68] McDougall et al.,[123] McNamara,[127-130] McNamara et al.,[131,132] and Stutzmann et al.[186,187]

Their studies indicate that mandibular growth enhancement occurs as well as redirection of condylar growth and maxillary horizontal growth with forward posturing appliances, worn during a growing period (a headgear effect). A number of studies on treated patients* also indicate that when treated Class II patients are compared with nontreated controls, mandibular length is enhanced by functional appliances. The results are variable, as Graber[64] has shown in a study of 58 completed Fränkel appliance patients, but the potential for change seems to be there. The *unloading* of the condyle is considered a potentially significant factor by Johnston.[111]

The same philosophy is applicable for the Herbst appliance. The working hypothesis is that all growth restrictions are removed (Fig. 7-9). This is in spite of articles by Creekmore and Radney,[38] Gianelly et al.,[63] and Ricketts[162] that

do not find enhanced mandibular growth specifically attributable to functional appliances. But then these clinicians have had limited experience with functionals.

The net effect is that patients attain the *achievable optimum,* with the most favorable functional environment, freed of any restrictive neuromuscular aberrations resulting from compensatory, adaptive, or homeostatic activity. The correct comparison should be with similar malocclusions, not so-called normals. This means controls matched for sex, age, pattern of growth direction, or morphology.

Vertical opening variations. A number of modifications of the original Andresen activator have been introduced. This is because of the ongoing controversy over the amount of vertical opening and degree of forward posturing created by the activator, as well as the differing views regarding nocturnal wear versus full-time wear (which would provide potentially active functional stimulus and predictable forces from relatively constant head posture), and the arguments for loose appliances versus functional appliances *anchored* to the maxilla.

Whereas Andresen and his disciples recommended an opening of no more than 4 mm within the confines of the freeway space, as do Fränkel, Fleischer, and others, many clinicians* have turned to varying degrees of mandibular advancement and larger vertical openings of the construction bite (ranging from 4 to 15 mm). Some[14,51,187,211] recommend a specific intermolar clearance, varying from the Andresen

---

*References 21, 22, 39, 40, 55, 60, 71, 84-88, 115, 122, 128, 131, 140-142, 149-151, 154-158.

*References 2, 14, 48, 72, 81-83, 98-101, 133, 170-172, 174, 187, 211, 215-217.

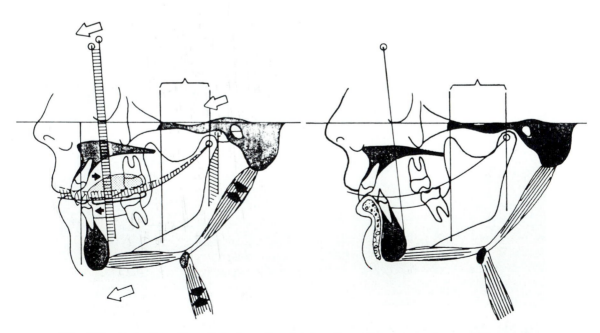

Fig. 7-9   Immediate effect of placing a functional appliance that postures the mandible forward. The condyle is brought forward in the fossa, which removes the usual functional stresses and constraints. The retractor muscles of the mandible are activated, and the resultant force is directed against the maxillary arch. (From Bimler P: In Graber TM, Neumann B: *Removable orthodontic appliances,* ed 2, Philadelphia, 1984, WB Saunders.)

recommendation by different amounts. Others* prefer to open the construction bite a specific amount beyond the postural rest position (Fig. 7-10).

A definite problem exists in rest position determination. Day and night rest positions are usually significantly different, mainly because of change in body and head posture and spatial relationships. Experience has shown that postural resting position varies from morning to night in the same individual depending on posture, mental anxiety, and fatigue.[67] The variability is greater at night, and the variation is great among individuals, even with normal occlusions. Thus any formula that recommends a specific distance for all patients is arbitrary and unrealistic. Even the most precise orthodontic interocclusal measurements in the dental chair are hardly likely to be replicated at night when the activator is worn. With malocclusions, vertical intermolar distance determinations must depend on relative infraclusion or supraclusion of buccal segment teeth. Differential eruption may be needed in some cases but should be avoided in others. As long as the original 2 to 4 mm opening recommended by Andresen and Häupl[13] was observed, it was probable that the activator construction bite would be within the limits of the freeway space and would not impinge on rest position, except in anterior open bite malocclusions, with overeruption of buccal segments. However, most appliance modifications subsequently introduced have had larger vertical openings and displace the mandible beyond the muscularly determined daytime postural resting position part of the time or all of the time they are worn.[172] It is

---

*References 2, 3, 77-80, 84, 85, 98-101, 160-162, 214-216.

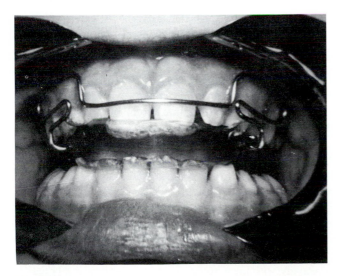

Fig. 7-10 A number of activators require a larger vertical opening. The Herren, Harvold, Hamilton, Woodside, and L.S.U. activators all exceed the freeway space or postural rest position, eliciting the viscoelastic properties of the associated tissues. In this illustration there is an 8 mm opening between the first molars. The lower incisors are capped by the acrylic to provide more stability and reduce the tendency to procline these teeth.

emphasized again that nocturnal rest position is usually different, with a greater interocclusal clearance, and is modifiable by various head positions during sleep.

As Slagsvold and Kolstad[180] ask, can such appliances logically be called activators in the true sense? What do they activate if they call on stretch reflex or viscoelastic properties of the tissues?

This is not to question that many so-called activator modifications work, regardless of the vertical opening or variations in the amount of horizontal mandibular advancement. Part of this is a testimony to the great adaptability of the human organism. Normal is a range and seldom a point. The success of these modifications may be due to different combinations of muscle force, elastic tissue reaction, horizontal versus vertical displacement, age at time of use, length of wear, sleeping posture, and choice of cases to be treated based on growth intensity, direction, and amount left. The justification of each approach by the various proponents of different construction bites makes interesting reading. One unanswered question is, "What is the role of nocturnal parafunctional activity (bruxing and clenching)?"

Egil Harvold,[81-83] one of the foremost proponents of a high construction bite, feels that the wider jaw opening enlists the elastic properties in the elevator and retractor muscles (the "viscoelastic force of the associated soft tissues," as Woodside[214] terms it). This force is transmitted to the teeth; and the appliance, which is worn at night, is more likely to stay in place, producing the desired changes.

As previously noted Paul Herren[93,94] subscribes to this philosophy; and Robert Shaye[178] does the same.

Herren based his observations on patients who wore activators that displaced the mandible 2 or 3 mm below intercuspal position. Even with this relatively small interocclusal distance, he felt that the activator was literally squeezed between the jaws most of the time that it was worn. Since he believed that the same status existed for activators that opened the bite much beyond rest position, he concluded that the action was the same for all activators, regardless of the amount of vertical displacement. However, the forces are more continuous in action and constant in direction when the bite is opened more widely. In addition, their magnitude is greater, with one exception. When the mouth is open, the rest vertical dimension is modified to a more caudal position and the pressure of the closing muscles thus decreases with adaptation to the appliance being worn.

Ahlgren[1] concurred with Herren, basing his conclusions on considerable electromyographic and neurophysiologic research. As long as the appliance is in place, with a vertical opening exceeding the postural rest vertical dimension, the muscles are subject to stretch. Being elastically extensible, they respond similarly to a rubber band, with the tension increasing exponentially as the amount of vertical opening increases. The action also elicits a phenomenon referred to by Sherrington as stretch reflex—either the tonic or the phasic type. A maintained stretch incites a long-lasting tonic stretch reflex contraction whereas a momentary stretch elicits a transient phasic stretch reflex response. Hence the activator produces a tonic stretch reflex in most instances. The tonic reflex response varies inversely with each level of sleep. It is greatest during the wakeful state, active but less intense during the rapid eye light plane of sleep, and nonexistent in the deep phase of sleep.

When the activator is worn during the day, the frequency of deglutition is enhanced while the activator is in place and there is increased phasic muscle activity; but during sleep, even in the deep plane of sleep, phasic muscle contractions can be discerned in the tongue and contiguous jaw musculature. During the deep sleep phase, when the muscles are atonic, myoclonic twitches of the tongue and associated musculature push the activator into place against the teeth, creating intermittent forces. This is in contradistinction to the effect during daytime wear, when the passive tension and tonus of the stretched muscles exert a more continuous force on the teeth and investing tissues.

Schwarz,[174] in his wider open activator studies, noted that the force created varied with the changing magnitude of the blood pressure and the tetanic oscillations of the muscle contractions. He did not observe an increase in the frequency of mandibular movements when the appliance was worn. Again, the vertical opening was beyond postural resting position, eliciting a stretch reflex and viscoelastic tissue response (in contradistinction to the small vertical opening recommended by Andresen, to stay within the confines of the interocclusal clearance and permit optimal forward posturing for the needed sagittal correction).

Eschler[48,52] became quite prominent in the functional orthopedic field and wielded considerable influence with his research and deductions. He developed a working hypothesis, based on his own electromyographic studies, that varied from those previously cited. To him the response was primarily a stretch reflex. When the appliance is in the mouth, it elicits isotonic contractions in the elevator muscles. These are replaced by tonic (isometric) proprioceptively oriented contractions after the mandibular teeth are fully seated in the appliance. Since the mandible is prevented by the appliance from achieving a normal postural rest position, the muscles remain stretched. They fatigue in due course, relax, and allow the mandible to drop. The cycle is repeated when the muscles recover. Eschler saw no evidence of direct activation of the protractor muscles. The therapeutic effect was attributed to the stretch reflex. Hence the effect was proportionate to the opening, with a recommendation of 4 to 6 mm for optimum patient tolerance and cooperation. His research indicated increased frequency of mandibular movements with activator wear, confirming Andresen's observations. Thilander and Filipsson[187] also conducted electromyographic studies on patients wearing activators, but conducted the studies during waking hours. They found only insignificant muscle activity when the activator was at rest. During mandibular movements, however, an increased activity was seen, especially in the retracting muscles. There was also an increased swallowing activity, probably caused by increased saliva flow.

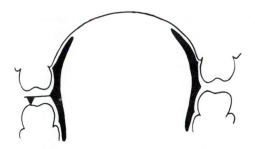

Fig. 7-11 Transducer placement in the interproximal space of an activator worn at night. Note the contact with the lower left molar. Long periods of transducer activity were observed during sleep. (From Witt E, Komposch G: *Fortschr Kieferorthop* 32:345, 1971.)

Clearly although there is essential agreement between Ahlgren,[3] Harvold,[81] Herren,[93] Selmer-Olsen,[176] and Thilander and Filipsson,[187] differences of opinion by Eschler[48] and Schwarz[174] could be a matter more of interpretation than of actual findings. Eschler is actually in partial agreement with both broad hypotheses.

Nocturnal activity. Elucidating the arguments on the exact effect of the vertical opening of the activator construction bite are studies by Komposch and Hockenjos,[114] Schmuth,[170-172] and Witt and Komposch.[211] These authors used transducers at night to assess the type and amount of force generated by activators opened beyond postural resting position (Fig. 7-11). They found long periods of continuous pressure from the mandibular teeth against the activator when the intermolar distance exceeded 4 to 6 mm (Figs. 7-12 and 7-13). This pressure consisted of three components[114,209-212]:

1. A basic pressure varying with the amount of mandibular displacement, head position, and plane of sleep
2. Oscillations synchronized with breathing rhythm
3. Oscillations synchronized with blood pulse

When the vertical displacement was 4 to 6 mm and the horizontal forward posturing half the width of a premolar (3 to 5 mm), the mean sagittal forces ranged from 315 to 395 g for a group of sleeping adults (Fig. 7-13). With the same amount of vertical opening but with no forward posturing the means were much less: between 145 and 270 g. The mean vertical forces ranged from 70 to 175 g. In most subjects the forces were greater when the mandible was displaced downward and forward than when displaced downward only, but this tendency was not statistically significant. However, Ahlgren[1] has observed that the stretch reflex activity of temporal and masseter muscles correlates positively with the amount of mandibular opening (Figs. 7-14 and 7-15).

Witt and Komposch[211] also confirmed that forces exerted on the teeth and supporting structures varied with the plane of sleep and head position (Fig. 7-16). Relatively small depressing forces were found in patients sleeping on their back, while sagittal forces were relatively strong. During the initial stages of sleep the forces were varied but stronger.

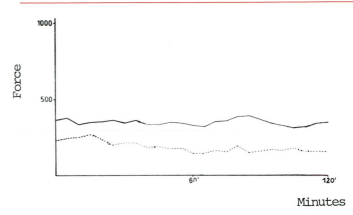

Fig. 7-13   Charting of force increments in grams for downward *(dotted line)* and downward and forward *(solid line)* displacement in 30 adult activator patients. Based on means of individual registrations every 5 minutes. (From Witt E, Komposch G: *Fortschr Kieferorthop* 32:345, 1971.)

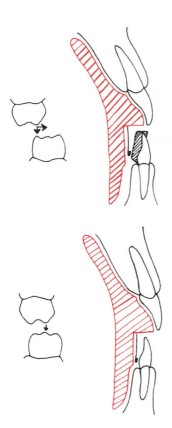

Fig. 7-12   Transducer placement for registration of posterior forces against the activator and anterior forces against the lower incisors and activator during activator therapy. The forward posturing of the mandible was increased by addition of a splint on the linguo-incisal aspect of the lower incisors. (From Witt E, Komposch G: *Fortschr Kieferorthop* 32:345, 1971.)

As the plane of sleep became deeper, the variability was less but the magnitude was significantly reduced.

Recent experiments by Sander[167,168] have shed additional light on functional appliance action. Schmuth[170,172] and Sander separately measured the forces produced between the upper and lower jaws with different construction bites and found that the amount of force was dependent on the vertical height and sagittal position of the lower jaw. Sander[167] also measured the interocclusal clearance in patients with and without activators worn during sleep, since it is important in determining the vertical construction bite, as previously indicated. He showed that in patients who have large horizontal displacements, there was a tendency to disclude the lower jaw from the appliance to avoid the large forces produced. With vertical opening there was less of an effect.

However, a study of mandibular activity patterns in controls not wearing an activator showed a broad range of activity. At the beginning of the night, frequent mandibular movements, including wide-open movements, could be seen. These frequently occurred with tooth contact. After the first sleep phase the lower jaw slowly opened, probably under the influence of gravity, although some closing movements could still be seen. In one control there was an open-

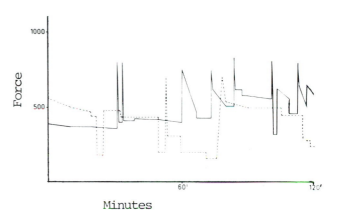

Fig. 7-14   Variation of posterior forces exerted against the activator over a 2-hour period for both downward and downward and forward displacement. (From Witt E, Komposch G: *Fortschr Kieferorthop* 32:345, 1971.)

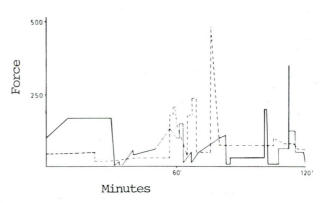

Fig. 7-15   Variation in vertical forces exerted against the activator during a 2-hour period. (From Witt E, Komposch G: *Forstchr Kieferorthop* 32:345, 1971.)

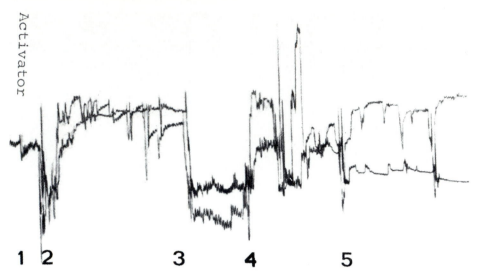

Activator

1 2 3 4 5

Fig. 7-16 Variations in the amount of force exerted by an activator over a 15-minute period of restless sleep with changes in body posture: *1*, Body and head on the right side; *2*, sleeping on the back; *3*, head turned to rest on the right side; *4*, head turned to rest on the left side; *5*, body and head both turned to rest on the left side. (From Witt E, Komposch G; *Fortschr Kieferorthop* 32:345, 1971.)

ing movement that preceded the closing movement. As time passed, the interocclusal clearance increased. Long periods of muscle inactivity were interrupted by active periods during the night. Closing movements reached maximum intercuspation only briefly. The lower jaw would then open, sometimes actively and sometimes passively, because of gravity. Experimental results confirmed that a nocturnal rest position exists that does not mimic the diurnal registration. Near maximum or maximum occlusal contact was recorded less than 0.8% of the total sleep time.[167,168] The implications again stress the time-linked variability of mandibular position and function, making it difficult to assess the exact role of the activator when it is worn.

The mode of action of activators that have a vertical opening of 4 to 6 mm below intercuspal position is well documented. The teeth are subject to almost continuous force when the activator is in place, although the force magnitude varies considerably from patient to patient, as well as within the same patient, depending on the factors just listed. The inescapable conclusion is that these are not functional jaw orthopedic appliances in the truest sense. Perhaps the term suggested by Slagsvold[179] would be more appropriate. He calls them tools for *the muscle stretch method.* Thus the term *monobloc* originally used by Robin and preferred by Hotz is semantically more correct[98]; however, usage has made *activator* the preferred term.

REACTION TO ACTIVATOR THERAPY

As with the range of recommendations on the amount of vertical and sagittal opening for the activator, so there are variations on the theme of tissue response. Since activators are used primarily on Class II, division 1 and Class II,

division 2 problems, most of the literature and case reports are directed to treatment results in these categories. Remarkable results are shown in some cases; in others, poor or partial correction; and in still others, actual detrimental exacerbation of the malocclusion. Conditioning factors are the morphogenetic pattern, severity of the malocclusion, growth increments, growth direction, growth timing, patient cooperation, design of the appliance, amount of vertical or sagittal displacement, and original inclination of the teeth. A correct diagnosis is clearly a prerequisite for successful activator therapy, no less than for fixed appliances.

Expansion. Expansion of the maxillary arch with activator therapy has been demonstrated routinely.[74] Slagsvold and Kolstad[180] found increased molar width in all cases studied (Fig. 7-17).

Overbite. Reduction of excessive overbite is to be expected in most patients properly chosen and treated (Fig. 7-18). One prerequisite for case selection is a deep bite condition. The vertical change must be documented by careful studies.[3,160] Cephalometric analyses[83,107,181] have shown that with eruption may also come a posterior mandibular rotation, as the bite is opened. A significant part of this change is due to differential eruption of the lower molar teeth; however, elimination of a functional retrusion may offset this potentially deleterious effect. In addition, some withholding of maxillary incisor eruption is likely with activator wear, although actual depression is not to be expected, except with wide construction bites. Clark actually allows free eruption of lower molars with twin block therapy.

Sagittal change. Sagittal changes have been the primary objective and have been studied extensively. Variation is perhaps greatest in the accomplishment of this vector of change, whose conditioning factors have already been

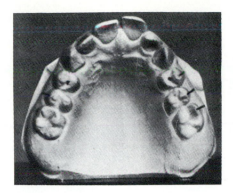
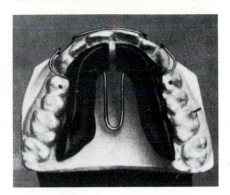

Fig. 7-17   Because most Class II, division 1, malocclusions have a narrow maxillary arch, particularly in the canine region, expansion has been an accepted procedure in activator therapy. This can be done ahead of time (as with the Clark twin block and Hamilton Expansion-Activator approach) or afterward. Use of buccal shielding wires, as with the Bionator, or buccal shields of the Fränkel appliance permits significant expansion without *pushing out from within*. However, many activators have been designed with jackscrews or Coffin springs in midpalate to expand the buccal segments, allowing retraction of the maxillary incisors with the labial wire. Note the expansion achieved by a common type of activator. (From Slagsvold O: In Graber TM, Neumann B: *Removable orthodontic appliances,* Philadelphia, 1977, WB Saunders.)

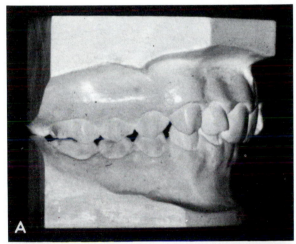

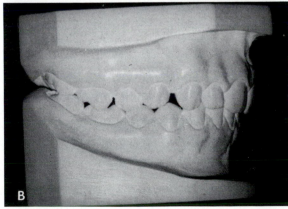

Fig. 7-18   Treatment of a Class II, division 2, malocclusion with an activator. The elimination of the deep overbite, with correction of the sagittal malrelationship was accomplished in less than 2 years. (From Slagsvold O: In Graber TM, Neumann B: *Removable orthodontic appliances,* Philadelphia, 1977, WB Saunders.)

listed. However, successful apical base change can be achieved, as documented in the literature;* retardation of anterior maxillary growth or an actual lingual tipping of the maxillary anterior teeth may contribute part of this.† Of course there are many‡ who believe that mandibular growth is stimulated by the activator. The research of McNamara,[124,125,127-130] McNamara et al.,[126,131,132] Petrovic,[151-153] Petrovic et al.,[154-157] and Stutzmann et al.[185,186] has clearly shown the potential for this effect on experimental animals. Enhanced condylar growth, selective areas of change (usually the posterosuperior condylar aspect), and change in trabecular alignment all are documented. Changed orofacial muscle activity also occurs, with an increase in lateral pterygoid contractions (Fig. 7-19). A skeletal adaptation to the new position and a gradual disappearance of the modified neuromuscular pattern have been observed.

Condylar response.   The unique nature of the phylogenetically and ontogenetically secondary cartilage status of the condyle makes it physiologically different from primary cartilage seen in epiphyses and diaphyses, cranial base cartilages, and the nasal septum. It grows by division of undifferentiated cells, the prechondroblasts, and its growth is regulated to a greater extent by local factors than by growth hormones[152] (Fig. 7-20). Petrovic et al.[157] have concluded from their extensive studies that condylar growth is an expression of locally structured homeostasis for the establishment and maintenance of a functionally coordinated stomatognathic system. The growth depends on continuous information from the teeth (periodontal mechanoreceptors),

---

*References 39, 42, 55, 60, 64, 65, 88, 89, 130, 140, 181, 189.
†References 39, 42, 79, 88, 89, 107, 140, 181, 189, 214-216.
‡References 21, 22, 45, 53-59, 87, 95, 123-132, 151-157, 184, 186.

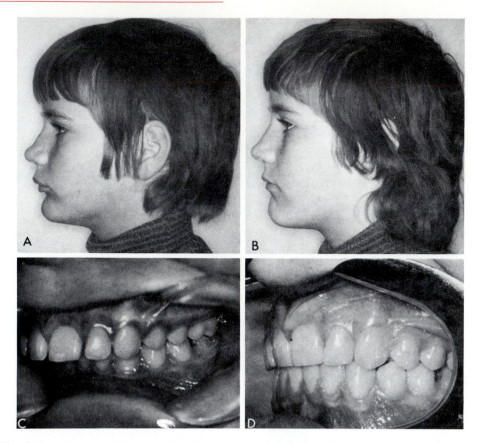

Fig. 7-19   Example of the sagittal and vertical change possible with activator treatment. Before, **A** and **C,** and after, **B** and **D,** facial and intra-oral views show a significant improvement in facial balance, with elimination of the excessive overjet and overbite and establishment of normal perioral muscle function. The treatment was aided for a short time with a cervical extra-oral appliance. Treatment time was 16 months. (From Slagsvold O: In Graber TM, Neumann B: *Removable orthodontic appliances,* Philadelphia, 1977, WB Saunders.)

as well as from the muscles and TMJ itself. A strong role for lateral pterygoid activity is described.[154] In experiments in which the lateral pterygoid was excised, significantly reduced condylar growth was observed. According to Petrovic,[151] activation of the muscles is the key to condylar growth enhancement. Appliances that merely splint the mandible in an anterior position do not activate these muscles and therefore do not stimulate condylar growth. Thus muscle tonus and monosynaptic and polysynaptic reflexes must be maintained. In the deep plane of sleep the activator has little effect on mitotic activity of the prechondroblasts. Growth hormone, although less effective on the condylar cartilage than local factors, does enhance activator effectiveness. It is suggested that the lateral pterygoids, which supply the functional stimulus and also the blood and nutritional supply, are a major pathway to the cartilage metabolism.[24,157]

The question exists, however, about stimulation of condylar growth by an appliance that is worn only during sleeping hours. Gerber[62] and, as pointed out earlier, Herren[93,94] found no increase in muscle activity when the activator was worn. However, Witt[210] studied the Bionator, a modified

activator worn during the day, and did observe increased activity, with the mandible being moved reflexly forward, substantiating the high mitotic activity in the prechondroblasts seen by Stutzmann et al.[185] when appliances are worn during waking hours. So it is questionable whether there is optimal condylar growth stimulation with activator wear limited to sleeping hours only. Other adjustive factors must be present—dental response, possible maxillary horizontal growth restriction, change in the condylar trabecular orientation (Stutzmann angle), remodeling of the articular fossa itself, and elimination of a posterior condylar displacement so often seen with Class II, division 2 deep overbite problems and less frequently, but still of concern, with many Class II, division 1 malocclusions.

Tooth movement. A number of investigators* have studied activator-related anteroposterior dental arch changes with casts and cephalograms. Björk[28] and Parkhouse[150] observed forward displacement of the lower anterior teeth and alveolar bone. Jacobsson[107] observed bodily movement of the lower incisors. Ascher,[16] Dietrich,[42] and Trayfoot and

---

*References 16, 28, 39, 42, 76, 83, 107.

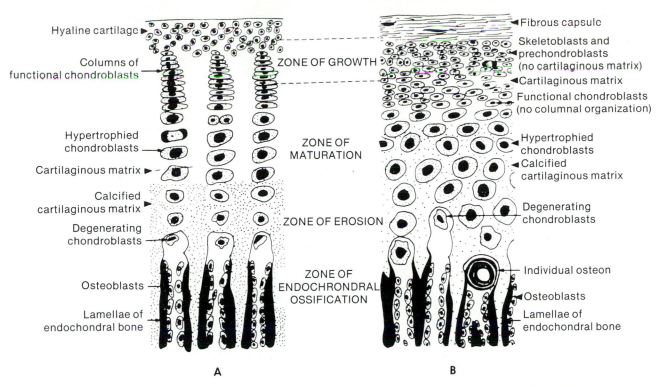

Fig. 7-20   **A,** Primary cartilage growth centers (e.g., in the epiphyses of long bones, in the nasal septum) have a columnar arrangement. **B,** In contrast, the secondary cartilage of the condyle grows by division of the undifferentiated prechondroblast cells. Secondary cartilage is regulated to a lesser extent by hormones and to a greater extent by local factors than is primary cartilage. (From Petrovic A, Stutzmann J, Oudet C: In McNamara JA, Carlson DS, Ribbens KA, editors: *The effect of surgical intervention on craniofacial growth, Monograph 12, Craniofacial growth series,* Ann Arbor, 1982, Center for Human Growth and Development, University of Michigan.)

Richardson[191] reported labial tipping of the lower incisors; yet Moss[140] reported lingual tipping in at least half of his material. Demisch[40] observed accelerated mesial drift of the lower buccal segments whereas Harvold and Vargervik[83] and Softley[181] concluded that the lower dental arch remained stable on its base. Hagerström[76] and Slagsvold and Kolstad[180] saw increased spacing in the lower dental arch.

From the wealth of material studied, it seems likely that the lower dental arch does come forward some during activator treatment. If the lower incisors are already labially inclined initially, or if such reaction is not acceptable, some other form of therapy may be indicated. Conditioning factors also are the direction and amount of growth, length of appliance wear, and (most important) design of the activator—whether there is incisal capping, whether forward posturing involves labial pressure on the teeth and alveolar bone or alveolar bone only, and the degrees of forward advancement and vertical opening that are needed for the construction bite.

Many case reports show that the maxillary anterior teeth can be retracted with activators.* The axial inclination of

these teeth may also be improved. The primary action is lingual tipping, however, and this can be undesirable because overbite is increased with the uprighting of maxillary incisors and premature contact may be created in the incisal region, restricting optimum forward mandibular posturing for basal sagittal correction, as well as eliminating functional retrusion. Torque or bodily movement of incisors is difficult if not impossible to achieve, even with a modified activator.

The question of distalization of maxillary posterior segments by activator treatment is not completely answered. Withholding of the fullest potential of maxillary horizontal growth is accepted by most investigators. Clinically, a space can frequently be seen, particularly in young patients. A distal tipping of buccal segment teeth can also be seen in many cases. Demisch[40] has concluded that the maxillary molars either are stopped in their normal path of eruption or move distally. Woodside[214,215] and Woodside et al.[216] strive to withhold the normal eruption of maxillary molars while allowing the mandibular molars to move mesially and superiorly. Harvold and Vargervik[83] could not confirm distalization. McNamara[129] has reported practically no maxillary change in his Fränkel appliance studies; but Lee Graber[64] has shown a headgear distalization effect in some Fränkel

---

*References 83, 107, 159, 181, 190.

Fig. 7-21 In this untreated Class II, division 2, malocclusion there is a strong upward and forward rotation of the mandibular growth pattern leading to a marked mentolabial sulcus, decreased anterior face height, and enhancement of the original overbite problem. Correction with any type of conventional orthodontic therapy is difficult. Vertical correction is as important as sagittal. Activator therapy here would attempt to stimulate all possible upward and forward eruption of lower posterior segments. (From Björk A: *Nord Klin Odontol* 1:1, 1966.)

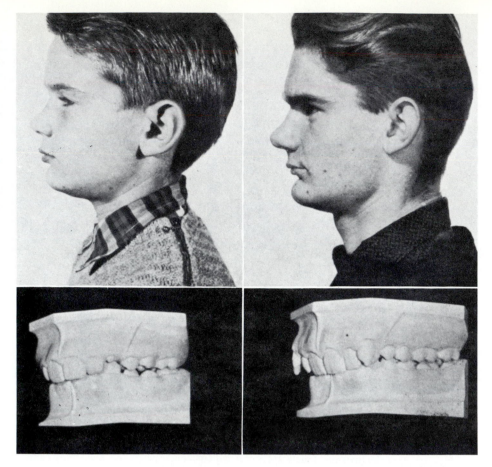

Fig. 7-22 This downward and backward rotational growth pattern does not respond well to activator therapy. Short ramus height, excessive anterior face height, compensatory tongue posture, and function all team up to aggravate the original open bite malocclusion. (From Björk A: *Nord Klin Odontol* 1:1, 1966.)

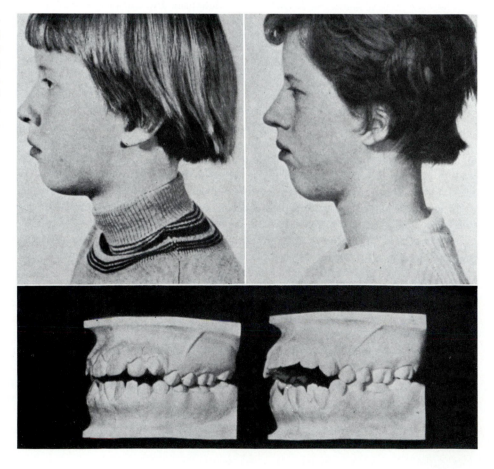

case reports and a wide variation of reaction in patients. Again, growth amounts, growth direction, growth timing, appliance design, appliance wear, selective grinding, and use of the eruptive potential of posterior teeth all can affect the degree of correction (Figs. 7-21 and 7-22). Nocturnal parafunctional activity could also be a consideration. Patient cooperation and full-time wear versus nighttime-only wear obviously will qualify the final result.

APPLIANCE DESIGN

Andresen appliance. The traditional one-piece appliance, involving both dental arches, is passive and has no active parts like springs, jackscrews, or elastics (Fig. 7-23). The maxillary labial arch is passive but can be activated if necessary to tip upper incisors lingually. It is worn only at night and has a vertical opening within the limits of the freeway space, or 2 to 4 mm at most, with an average mandibular advancement of 3 to 5 mm. Generally it is used for less severe Class II malocclusions, with deeper than normal overbite and upright or lingually inclined lower incisors. Lower incisors were not capped with acrylic in the original appliance, although most current use of this appliance incorporates indexing or capping, or a lower labial wire, to reduce the labial tipping tendency of the lower anterior segment. Since the purpose of this chapter is to

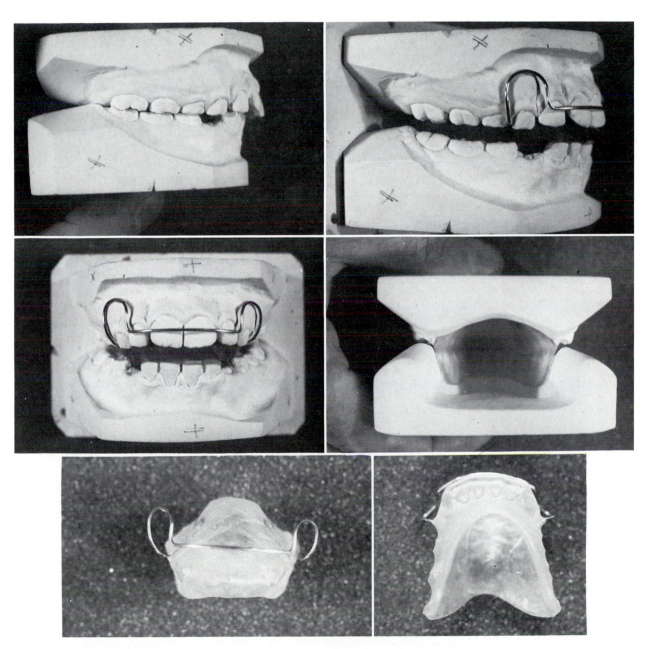

Fig. 7-23 The classical Andresen activator for nighttime wear. It is passive in the sense that there are no tooth-moving parts. (Courtesy Johan Ahlgren.)

present the philosophy and general details and tissue reactions, the appliances mentioned are not discussed in detail. Refer to books by the author[67] together with Bedrich Neumann,[70] Thomas Rakosi,[160] and Alexandre Petrovic[151-157] for construction minutiae.[70,71] Current use by clinicians such as Johan Ahlgren[3-5] carefully documents the response.

Activator modifications. A number of changes have been introduced through the years to attempt to achieve different treatment objectives. The most common is the incorporation of one or more jackscrews to expand the upper, lower, or both dental arches. Modification of the labial archwire to extend posteriorly in the Bionator, opposing the posterior teeth, serves to relieve cheek pressure. Finger springs have been added for limited tooth movement. Acrylic capping of the lower incisors is generally incorporated to increase resistance of the lower incisors to labial tipping. The bulk of the original appliance has been reduced by many clinicians—notably Balters,[18] Bimler,[25-27] Fleischer and Fleischer-Peters,[53] Fränkel,[54-57] Fränkel and Fränkel,[58] Fränkel and Reiss,[59] Klammt,[113] Schmuth,[170,172] and Stockfisch.[182,183] A cross-palatal wire or Coffin spring has been substituted for the acrylic. Of course, the original sagittal and vertical mandibular displacements have been varied, mostly by increasing the vertical bite opening. These will be discussed in more detail in the section on construction bite.

The Bionator, as developed by Balters,[18] is the most frequently used activator modification today (Fig. 7-24). Significant success has been achieved by Fleischer, with his Bio-Modulator modification of the Balters Bionator (Figs. 7-25, 7-26, and 7-30 to 7-35). Reversing the transpalatal loop, replacing the single labial arch with upper and lower labial arches, reducing the acrylic bulk significantly, enhancing maxillary anchorage by the addition of interprox-

imal spurs and C-stops at the mesial of the first permanent molars and canines, and using a thin metal plate between the upper and lower occlusal surfaces to serve as functional occlusal plane permit both horizontal and vertical control[53] (Fig. 7-26). The metal plate is used for selective retardation or guidance of eruption to establish a normal vertical and horizontal relationship. For a fuller discussion of this important modification of the Bionator, in addition to other appliances used by Shaye, Janson, Hamilton, and Schmuth, refer to the second edition of *Removable Orthodontic Appliances* by Graber and Neumann,[70] as well as *Dentofacial Orthopedics with Functional Appliances* by Graber, Rakosi, and Petrovic.[71]

The development of various other skeleton activators has also allowed full-time wear, day and night. The advantages, as far as tissue response is concerned, have already been described.

The Fränkel appliance. A fundamental activator modification is the Fränkel function regulator[54-59] (Fig. 7-27). It resorts to the same basic forward posturing of the mandible for sagittal correction but postures by steps instead of all at once. A critical requirement is that the appliance be fixed to the maxillary arch, anchored by interproximal wires in the molar and canine area to enhance maxillary anchorage, rather than left loose or free-floating, as recommended by Andresen and Häupl. With the exception of a maxillary molar rest to prevent maxillary molar eruption, the remainder of the appliance has minimal tooth contact. As a passive exercise device there are no active parts.

A unique characteristic is the incorporation of buccal shields and anterior lip pads, which serve to relieve cheek and lip pressure and to break up abnormal perioral muscle habits. They are extended into the depths of the vestibule to exert a stretch effect on the vestibular mucosa and underlying periosteal layer, in an attempt to enhance basal

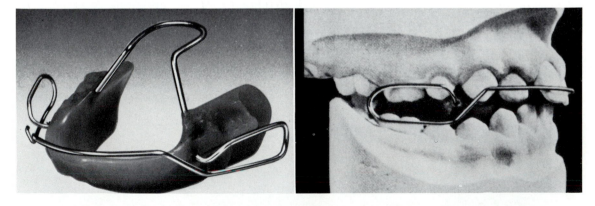

Fig. 7-24 The Bionator, as modified from the original activator by Balters, uses a heavy Coffin-type transpalatal wire instead of an acrylic cover. The labial wire is not a tooth-moving adjunct but a screening wire, holding the lip away from the teeth and extending into the buccal sulcus as far as the distal of the deciduous second molars. To enhance eruption in the desired direction, the acrylic is removed and trimmed in the interdental area. The construction bite is usually taken in an end-to-end incisal relationship if this permits passage of interocclusal wiring. The appliance is an effective adjunct in many TMJ problems requiring forward posturing of the mandible.

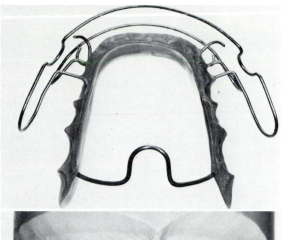

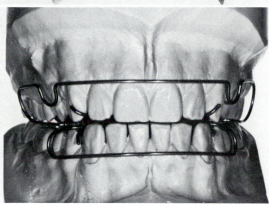

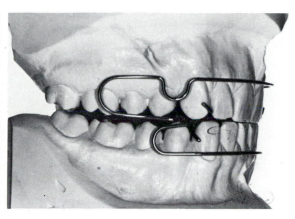

Fig. 7-25   The basic Bio-Modulator of Fleischer. The labial wire is similar to its progenitor, the Bionator; but the lower labial wire (lip bumper), which intercepts the abnormal lower lip trap, screens the lower incisors to allow autonomous improvement with the release of the abnormal perioral muscle deforming action. No acrylic is interposed between the occlusal surfaces so as not to impede eruption. (Courtesy Erich Fleischer.)

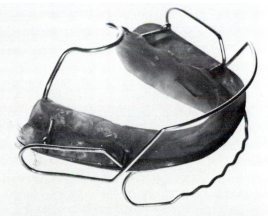

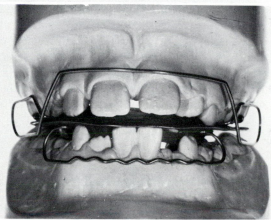

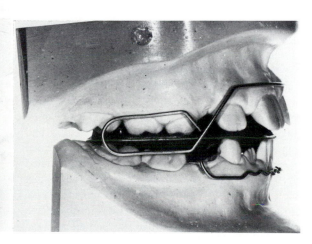

Fig. 7-26   The Fleischer Bio-Modulator, with the stainless metal interocclusal plane. This allows proprioceptive contact of selected teeth that do not need to erupt while stimulating teeth that are in infraclusion and not touching the metal plane. The skeleton appliance is easier to wear than the conventional activator and does not require the precise and sometimes arduous selective trimming of the acrylic for control of guided eruption. (Courtesy Erich Fleischer.)

Fig. 7-27   The Fränkel function regulator makes maximum use of the vestibule as its area of operation, screening away abnormal lip and cheek pressures. **A,** Labial model. *a,* Labial bow; *b,* canine loop; *c,* buccal shield; *d,* lip pads. **B,** Lingual model. *a,* Palatal bow; *b,* protrusion bow; *c,* lower lingual wires; *d,* buccal shield; *e,* lower lip pads; *f,* lower lingual plate. The wire assemblage anchors the FR on the maxillary arch. There is no interocclusal acrylic or interference with eruption of the mandibular teeth with either the FR I or the FR II. The lingual acrylic pad and its passive wires, which lie lingual to the lower anterior teeth, are the only contact in the lower arch since the construction bite maintains the lower jaw in a forward position in the trough formed by the lingual acrylic pad and the labial lip pads. For optimum tissue reaction and patient acceptance and cooperation, the 6 mm sagittal change is usually accomplished in two stages of 3 mm each. The posturing trough is advanced by a simple adjustment with the same appliance. (Courtesy Rolf Fränkel.)

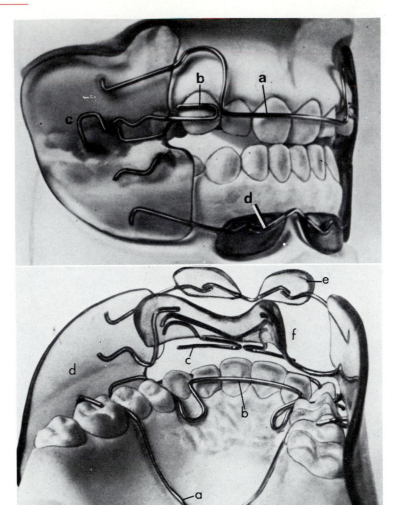

bone development. The concepts are based on well-reasoned and well-researched philosophies. The work of Enlow,[46] Hoyte and Enlow,[102] Moffett,[138] and Moffett and Koskinen-Moffett[139] shows that stimulation of bone growth is possible with periosteal pull. Recent studies by L. W. Graber[64] and T. M. Graber[68] confirm the enhanced transverse maxillary growth induced by the buccal shields, both on primates and in human patients.

Whereas Andresen and Häupl looked for autonomous neuromuscular function and improvement resulting from nocturnal activator wear, Fränkel demands full-time wear and a rigorous program of oral gymnastics. The FR is truly an exercise device and achieves optimum results only if so used. Again, diagnosis, case selection, growth amounts and direction, growth timing, and patient cooperation are qualifying factors in the ultimate treatment result. There can be no denying the dramatic sagittal basal bone, dental, and profile improvement, as well as the restoration of normal perioral muscle function in the properly selected and treated cases (Fig. 7-28). Unlike the activator, however, which can be modified many ways and still produce an acceptable response, the Fränkel appliance demands a rigid discipline of fabrication, fitting, and patient wear for the best possible

correction.[70,71] Some recent reports that attempt to assess the efficacy of the appliance are unfortunately tainted by poor case selection, improper fabrication, improper use, lack of anchoring the appliance on the maxilla (letting it float free in the mouth), and itinerant patient cooperation. Misuse of the appliance negates any conclusions drawn.[38,63,162] Oral exercises are a critical part of the Fränkel regimen but are largely ignored by many American orthodontists. This cannot produce the best results, for a truly functional appliance requires elimination of abnormal perioral function, muscle adaptation to an optimal sagittal jaw relationship, and neuromuscular reinforcement of the new and improved jaw relationship. Of all the so-called functional appliances, the Fränkel is the one that relies most on function. The reader is again referred to books by the author on these appliances for a more extensive discussion of all aspects of use.

THE CONSTRUCTION BITE

One of the most important aspects of activator fabrication is the establishment of proper horizontal and vertical mandibular displacement before construction of the appliance.

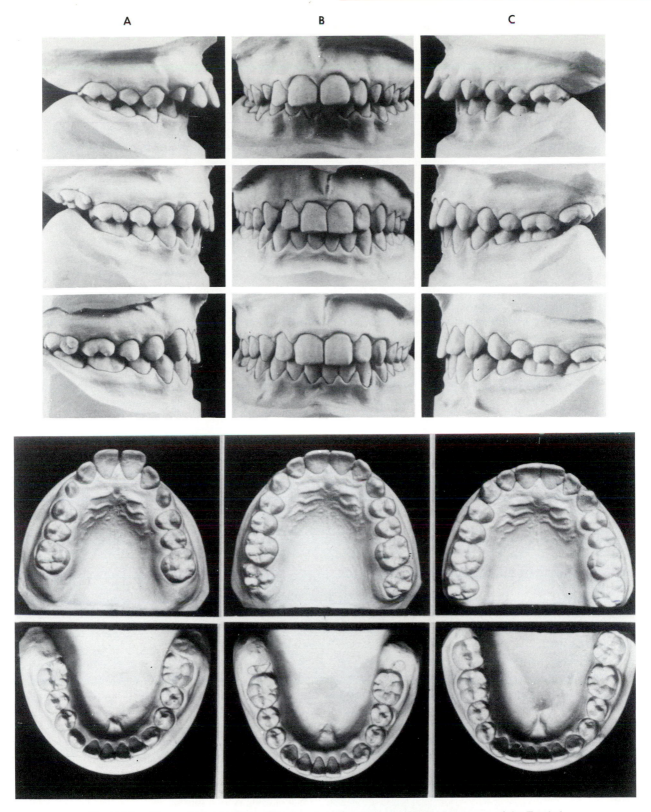

Fig. 7-28   Plaster casts. **A,** Type of treatment result to be expected by correct use of the Fränkel appliance in a properly selected Class II, division 1, malocclusion. **B,** Autonomous expansion caused by screening of aberrant muscle activity by the buccal shields and lip pads, which occupy the vestibule. The expansion is stable in the great majority of cases. **C,** Three and one half years posttreatment with no appliance control. (**A** to **C** courtesy Rolf Fränkel.)

There is no one *cookbook* for determining the relationships. Much depends on the type of activator used, the case selection, the dentofacial morphology, the growth pattern, the desired result, and the need for other therapeutic assists (e.g., fixed appliances, extraoral force, extraction). Since the Bionator, or skeleton activator, and its modifications are currently the most frequently used functional appliances, this section will be devoted to a discussion of the construction bite for that appliance.

A complete diagnostic discipline is essential before selecting a patient for the functional appliance. As Rakosi[160] stresses, it is no less important to do a thorough cephalometric, cast, and functional analysis for the functional orthopedic regimen than it is to do these for a full fixed appliance problem. Facial pattern is important; growth amounts and growth direction are equally important. Only if the case analysis satisfies the demanding criteria for a functional appliance, and *only if patient cooperation is likely to be good,* should such an appliance be used. The operator should always keep in mind that this is primarily an interceptive appliance, seldom capable of achieving full correction and complete dental detailing, and an interceptive appliance should be considered a first-phase effort in the total treatment planning. In this short survey chapter the concern is primarily with the use of functional appliances in Class II mandibular retrusion problems. The reader is referred to *Removable Orthodontic Appliances* by Graber and Neumann[70] and to *Dentofacial Orthopedics with Functional Appliances* by Graber et al.[71] for management of Class III malocclusions with functional appliances.

Anterior Mandibular Posturing

Generally, for the conventional activator and modifications like the Bionator, if the severity of the malocclusion is not too great, the protraction is planned to achieve an end-to-end incisal contact relationship. For practical purposes it should not exceed 4 to 6 mm in most cases (Fig. 7-29). Patient acceptance is likely to be less, and the danger of lower incisor procumbency is greater with larger amounts. As a general rule the anterior positioning should always be 3 mm or more posterior to the most protrusive mandibular position possible. This measurement is checked by having the patient move the jaw forward as much as possible and then drop back 3 to 4 mm. When there is severe lingual inclination of the lower anterior segment, a larger anterior repositioning may be used, with the objective of allowing the lower incisors to tip labially to a better inclination, increasing canine space and reducing the excessive overjet. However, this must still follow the 3 mm drop-back from extreme functional protrusion. Usually in severe problems it is better to bring the mandible forward in two or three steps of 2 to 3 mm each. Research by Petrovic et al.[157]

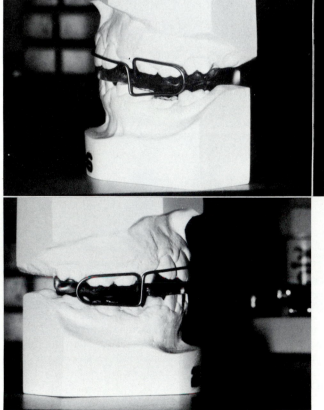

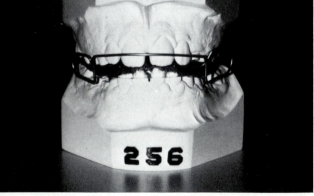

Fig. 7-29 Bionator functional appliance on working models. The mandible is postured forward for correction of the sagittal discrepancy. The lower incisors are capped with acrylic. Minimal bite opening is used for this appliance, which strives for an end-to-end incisal relationship in the construction bite; this is not true of the Woodside, Herren, L.S.U., or Hamilton activators.

and Shaye[178] has shown that tissue response and reactivation are better in the condyle with this procedure. Patient adjustment and cooperation are enhanced. Such a staged mandibular protraction is recommended by Fränkel[56] and his disciples in the use of the function regulator (FR).

Since the maxillary incisors are frequently tipped labially and are often spaced, it may be preferrable to use an active plate (or limited fixed appliances) to retract and rotate the incisors first for a short time and then use the activator; or the construction bite may disclose the need for incisor retraction during functional appliance wear, and a forward position can be established that is 2 or 3 mm less than end-to-end incisal contact.

In most routine cases, however, when adequate growth increments are expected and the growth direction is favorable, an advancement of 4 to 6 mm to establish the supportive, proprioceptively desirable, end-to-end incisal relationship is standard operating procedure and is likely to produce the desired result, with proper patient compliance (Fig. 7-29). Many of these patients have a 1.0 to 1.5 mm posterior condylar displacement associated with mandibular overclosure, so this retruded habitual occlusion position is also eliminated by the forward posturing. The vertical opening is within interocclusal space limits, resulting in a thin construction bite. Both elevator and protractor muscles are activated; and there is a greater hyoid musculature compensation or retractive force, which is distributed against the maxillary arch. This slightly inhibits normal anterior maxillary dentoalveolar relocation. Biting into the appliance and swallowing enhance the neuromuscular and osseous adaptation to the new posture. No effect is expected on the inclination of the maxillary base, and usually it is not necessary to construct more than one appliance in moderate sagittal discrepancy cases.

Vertical mandibular posturing

The opening of the bite varies with the severity of the malocclusion, the amount of anterior displacement, the growth amounts and direction projections, and the type of appliance used. The following general considerations will guide the clinician in most problems, however, recognizing that there is variance in vertical opening used by different authors and clinicians (Fleischer and Fleischer-Peters,[53] Fränkel,[55-57] Fränkel and Fränkel,[58] Fränkel and Reiss,[59] Hamilton,[79] Moss,[140-142] Rakosi,[160] Schmuth,[170-172] Shaye,[178] Woodside,[214,215] and Woodside et al.[216]

1. Mandibular postural displacement is essential to creating the neuromuscular activation required for correction in sagittal or vertical directions, or both.
2. The greater the anterior mandibular displacement for the construction bite, the less the vertical opening should be. For example, in extreme sagittal protraction (6 to 7 mm) the vertical opening should just clear the cusps, or 2 to 3 mm at most. The treatment objective in such cases is to achieve the greatest possible horizontal correction of the anteroposterior discrepancy. Such positioning is

recommended when there is likely to be a more horizontal growth vector. Only enough opening is created to permit interocclusal wires, rests, or the metal plate of the Fleischer Bio-Modulator. This is true for the Fränkel appliance as well. The vertical opening is usually within the limits of the postural resting position, as used by Andresen and his followers. Witt[209] measured the forces produced by such a maneuver and found a range of 315 to 395 g for the horizontal force and a variance from 70 to 175 g for the vertical component. In an attempt to eliminate the need for more than one appliance, the clinician is again cautioned against attempting extreme change in the sagittal mandibular posture. Shaye[178] and others have introduced jackscrew adjustments to allow progressive forward posturing or reactivating, which is better from both tissue reaction and patient cooperation aspects.

3. When there is the probability of a more vertical growth direction for the mandible, the vertical opening can be more extensive, beyond the postural rest position. Such opening elicits both stretch reflex and viscoelastic response from the mandibular elevator muscles and soft tissues. Although less sagittal mandibular response can be expected from this construction bite, the wider vertical opening is more effective in controlling the inclination of the maxillary base, withholding maxillary posterior face height enhancement, and allowing the anterior end of the maxillary plane to tip downward and help compensate for the vertical mandibular growth pattern. Woodside[216] has discussed this changing of palatal and occlusal planes and particularly the desirable therapeutic effects achieved by tipping down of the occlusal plane.

The interocclusal vertical relationship is achieved by having a thicker wax wafer for the construction bite. Too large a vertical opening, however, makes patient acceptance more difficult, as does too large a sagittal correction. In most cases the mandible should not be opened more than 4.0 mm beyond the postural rest position. Fränkel has stressed many times that the vertical opening should not be so great as to prevent the patient from doing lip seal exercises; and if any oral gymnastics are to be prescribed, the same admonition applies to the activator. With the results shown by Fränkel for the FR and his strong reliance on this appliance as an exercise device, it seems logical that lip seal exercises should be beneficial with Bionator wear also. The elimination of lip incompetence and enhancement of nasal breathing are firstline treatment objectives.

In wider open vertical construction bites, dentoalveolar compensation is usually greater. Maxillary incisors are likely to be inclined more to the lingual, and mandibular incisors are more labially tipped.

4. In open bite problems, when little or no sagittal change is desired, the more extreme vertical opening of the bite is essential. The thick interocclusal acrylic wafer elicits both stretch reflex and viscoelastic depressive response

on the posterior teeth, interfering with normal eruption. Woodside et al.[216] have shown dramatic results using the posterior bite block effect, which allows upward and forward rotation of the mandible, closing down the anterior open bite. Repelling magnets in a twin block appliance or Dellinger appliance may enhance posterior tooth depression. The effect is similar to the changes produced by the Milwaukee brace (but of much lesser magnitude, of course). This effect is combined with the downward tipping of the anterior maxillary base and occlusal plane to produce the ultimate correction. The efficacy of the activator in deep overbite cases has been documented in metric studies, but the effect varies from patient to patient in open bite problems.[179] In a study of 30 severe open bite cases treated with a function regulator, Fränkel and Fränkel[58] showed significant improvement in the anterior/posterior height ratio, a change in the direction of mandibular rotation, a closing down of the bite, and a real improvement in the soft tissue profile.

MECHANISMS OF CLASS II CORRECTION WITH FUNCTIONAL ORTHOPEDICS

Thousands of case reports attest to the beneficial changes produced by functional appliances. Dramatic facial changes seldom seen with conventional fixed appliances not only are possible but also are fairly routine (Figs. 7-30 through 7-35). The reasons for these changes, however, are more obscure and they vary from patient to patient. The oversim-

plistic assignment of the change to *condylar growth stimulation* has clouded the picture. We are dealing with a cybernetic process. A number of the conditioning factors have already been discussed. Morphogenetic pattern, growth timing, amounts and direction of sagittal and vertical discrepancies, neuromuscular patterns, functional displacement, dentoalveolar compensation, type of appliance used, and patient compliance are the most important variables; but the list is incomplete.[160] Such nebulous entities as *tissue response* or *rate of fibroblast turnover* may be as important although more difficult to assess. (See Chapters 2, 3.) The controversy over the effect on condylar growth has not been resolved, yet the fact is that sagittal change of major magnitude is achieved. How does this happen? A listing of probable components responsible for the change has been developed by the author. The millimetric values assigned are arbitrary and vary from case to case. The response and interrelationship of the various components are equally variable. (Compensation is the name of the game.) The reader is referred to the discussion of this question by Stöckli and Teuscher in Chapter 8 (p. 446).

Class II correction, the likely scenario*

The amount of sagittal correction needed is 6 to 7 mm. The following anticipated growth increments and other changes are typical:

*The varying amounts of each component depend on growth increments, direction, timing, and length of treatment.

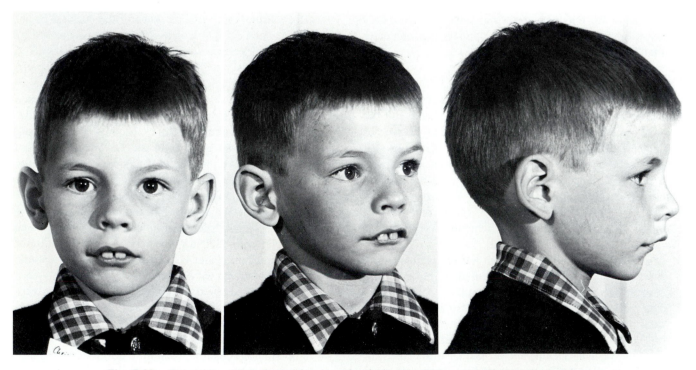

Fig. 7-30 Boy with a Class II, division 1, malocclusion treated by a modified Bionator (Bio-Modulator). Typical hypotonic upper lip, mouth breathing, marked mentolabial sulcus, and hypertonic mentalis activity were in evidence. (Courtesy Erich Fleischer.)

1. Condylar growth amounts, 1.0 to 3.0 mm (mandible outgrows maxilla 1 to 5 mm)
2. Fossa growth and adaptation, 0.5 to 1.0 mm
3. Eliminating functional retrusion, 0.5 to 1.5 mm
4. More favorable growth direction (trabecular angle), 0.5 to 1.0 mm

5. Withholding of downward and forward maxillary arch movement, 1.0 to 2.0 mm
6. Differential upward and forward eruption of lower buccal segments, 1.5 to 2.5 mm
7. Headgear effect, 1.0 to 2.0 mm

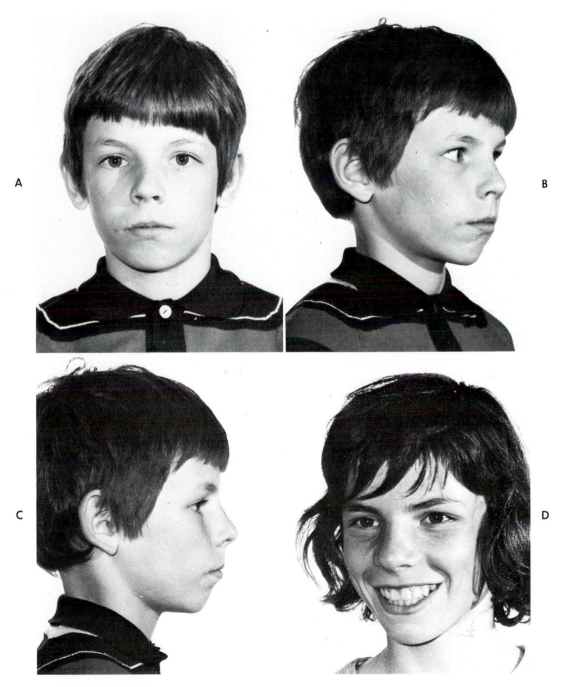

Fig. 7-31 Despite a severe mandibular retrusion, **A** to **C** show a marked facial improvement during treatment. **D** shows eruption of the premolars with the establishment of a normal occlusion, normal muscle activity, and good facial balance. Fleischer often uses a thin stainless steel bite rim interocclusally (like Cervera) for selective guidance of eruption. This obviates the need for selective grinding of acrylic, as is done with most activators. (Courtesy Erich Fleischer.)

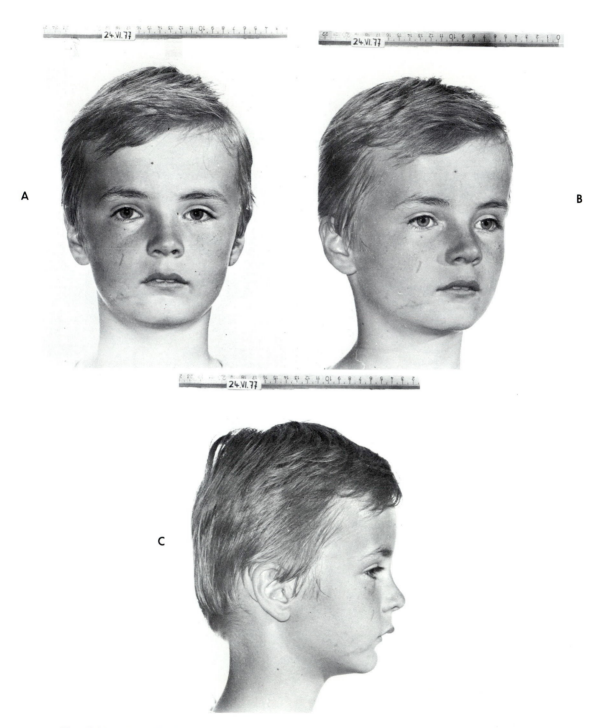

Fig. 7-32   Class II, division 1, malocclusion in a 11-year-old boy with a retained infantile swallowing habit. **A** to **C,** Initial success with the Bionator was limited because of lack of patient cooperation. After 2 years of intermittent success, the patient's attitude changed and cooperation improved and remained at a high level till the end of treatment. (**A** to **F** courtesy Erich Fleischer.)

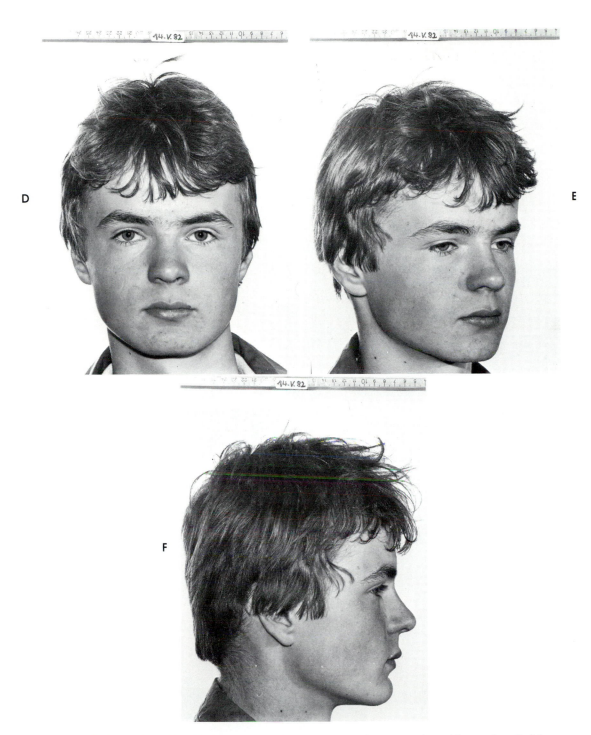

Fig. 7-32, cont'd   D to **F,** After 4 years of treatment. Satisfactory results and harmonious facial relationships are shown in Fig. 7-33 taken before and after treatment. Only the modified Bionator (Bio-Modulator) appliance was used.

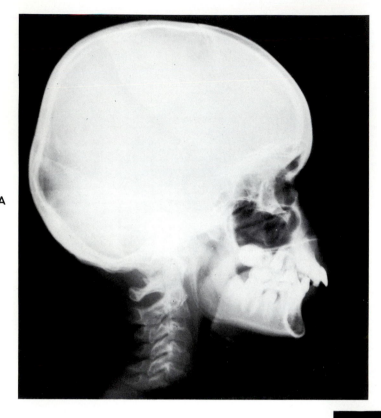

A

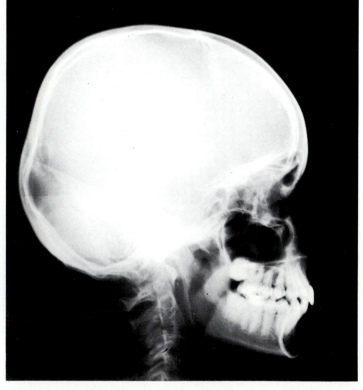

B

Fig. 7-33 Cephalograms of the patient in Fig. 7-32 treated with the Fleischer modified Bionator. The original deep bite and shallow mandibular plane are favorable characteristics for functional appliance treatment. **A,** Before treatment, age 10 years 3 months. **B,** After treatment, age 12 years 9 months. (**A** to **C** courtesy Erich Fleischer.)

	10 yr 3 mo	12 yr 9 mo
S-N-A	84°	83°
S-N-B	76°	78°
A-N-B	8°	5°
A to N (perp)	1 mm	− 1 mm
1 to A	+ 5 mm	+ 2 mm
1̄ to Pog	+ 5 mm	+ 6 mm
Pog to N (perp)	− 10 mm	− 8 mm
Max length	90 mm	91 mm
Mand length	107 mm	114 mm
Skel diff	17 mm	23 mm
Saddle angle	125°	127°
Ar to Ptm	31 mm	31 mm
Mand pl angle	19°	20°
Ant face height	68 mm	69 mm
Post face height	51 mm	56 mm
Ant cranial base length	70 mm	71 mm
1 to S-N	110°	102°
1̄ to Mand pl	104°	108°

C

Fig. 7-33, cont'd   C, Cephalometric summary.

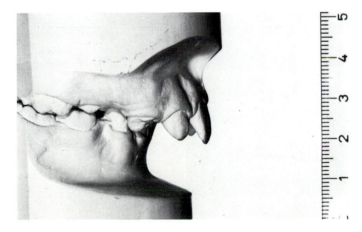

Fig. 7-34   Lateral study cast of a boy 9 years 7 months old with a severe Class II, division 1, malocclusion. (Courtesy Erich Fleischer.)

A

B

C

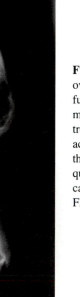

Fig. 7-35   Cephalograms of the patient in Fig. 7-34. **A,** Severe overbite and overjet are exacerbated by abnormal perioral muscle function. **B,** At the end of treatment (13 years 7 months). Normal muscle function. **C,** At 16 years 2 months (about 3 years out of treatment). Result still stable. The modified Bionator was used to achieve this result. Full-time wear during active treatment, rather than nighttime only, is a major requirement, as opposed to requirements of the conventional Andresen activator. The appliance can then be used at night only as a retainer. (**A** to **D** courtesy Erich Fleischer.)

	9 yr 7 mo	13 yr 7 mo	16 yr 2 mo
S-N-A	82°	83°	80°
S-N-B	75°	78°	79°
A-N-B	7°	5°	1°
A to N (perp)	+ 3 mm	+ 4 mm	+ 1 mm
1 to A	+ 7 mm	+ 2 mm	+ 6 mm
1̅ to Pog	0 mm	+ 5 mm	+ 1 mm
Pog to N (perp)	− 3 mm	− 1 mm	+ 4 mm
Max length	89 mm	95 mm	92 mm
Mand length	107 mm	102 mm	126 mm
Skel diff	18 mm	25 mm	34 mm
Saddle angle	130°		128°
Ar to Ptm	34 mm	35 mm	35 mm
Mand pl angle	17°	20°	15°
1 to S-N	115°	95°	98°
1̅ to mand pl	99°	103°	98°
Ant facial height	55 mm	67 mm	70 mm
Post facial height	43 mm	49 mm	55 mm
Ant cranial base length	66 mm	69 mm	72 mm

D

Fig. 7-35, cont'd **D,** Cephalometric summary.

Recognizing that skeletal malocclusions are three-dimensional, with the majority of Class II malocclusions demonstrating a narrow maxillary arch and a sagittal discrepancy, with changed tongue position and function, Hamilton introduced his expansion activator approach. The first generation of appliances was removable and yet achieved fairly stable results. Many activators have incorporated jackscrews for expansion purposes, with development of the dental arches during sagittal correction a valid treatment objective. The latest advance has been his bonded activator, which achieves rapid and dramatic correction with a truly functional appliance. If it is worn all the time, after being bonded to the maxillary arch, there is no compliance problem and the young patients adapt to the forward posturing functional position quickly. As shown some years ago by Melanson and Van Dyken[133] at Michigan in their study on primates, unloading the temporomandibular joint actually stimulated optimal growth and adaptation. The bonded Herbst appliance enlists the same approach (see "Mixed Dentition Treatment," in Chapter 9) with comparable results. With the Hamilton bonded expansion activator, however, forward

guidance of the mandible is achieved primarily by proprioceptive guidance from the lingual flanges of the bonded appliance. There is no actual joining of maxillary and mandibular arches, as there is with the bonded Herbst appliance (Fig. 7-36). That this approach is an excellent adjunct for mixed dentition treatment or even deciduous dentition interception in severe cases, eliminating abnormal, deforming perioral muscle function, has been shown in many cases by Hamilton (Figs. 7-37 through 7-40). Similar results are shown by Joho and colleagues.

Hamilton points out, as does Graber and others, that most of these functional appliance cases ultimately require bonded, bracketed, tooth-borne appliances to complete the detailing, to achieve correct individual tooth positions, and to eliminate rotations. With bonding this phase is relatively easy and usually completed in well under a year.

Controversy continues as to whether the traditional activator or even the bionator or Fränkel function regulator are really what the name implies: functional appliances—if worn only at bedtime (the recommendation made by so many orthodontists). It is more likely that the appliance

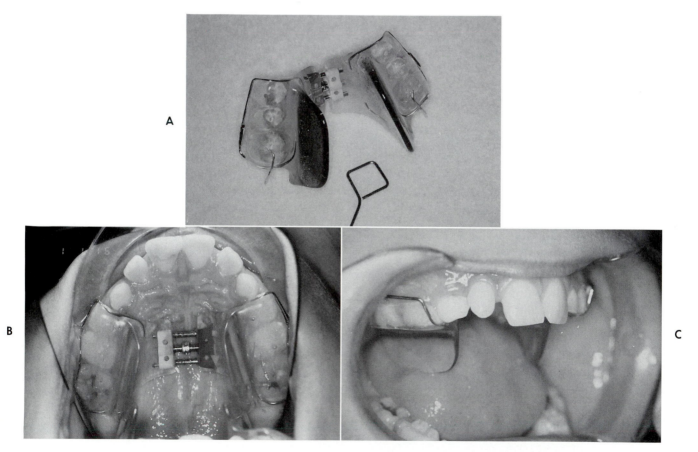

Fig. 7-36 **A,** Hamilton bonded activator from below. Lingual flanges in dark extend toward the viewer. The palatal jackscrew is partly open. The impressions of the lower posterior teeth are imbedded in the occlusal extensions in a forward postured relationship. **B,** Hamilton appliance, bonded to maxillary arch, jackscrew in center of palate. The lingual flanges that guide the mandible forward extend toward the viewer. **C,** Bonded Hamilton expansion-activator on maxillary arch. Lingual guiding flanges extend toward the lower arch and tongue.

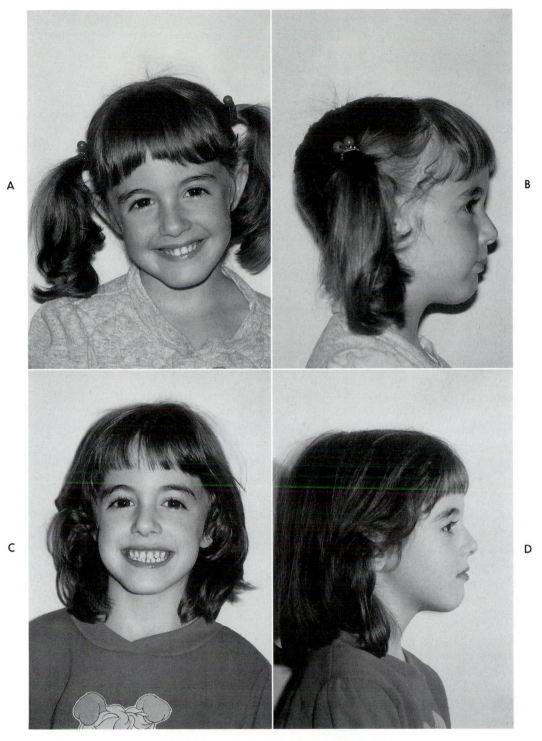

Fig. 7-37   Hamilton bonded expansion activator case. Girl (5 years, 2 months) with severe Class II, division 1 malocclusion with constricted maxilla and retruded mandible. Perioral muscle activity was compensatory and enhancing the malocclusion. The tentative treatment plan was to institute the primary stage of treatment immediately, with defined options of treatment in either/or mixed dentition and permanent dentition. Bonded activator was placed and the malocclusion was over-treated in an 8-month period. Upper and lower removable acrylic retainers were worn for an additional 6 months. The current state at 7 years is a Class I relationship with excellent skeletal and dental relations. No additional therapy is contemplated. **A** and **B,** Beginning facial views. **C** and **D,** Facial photos 2 years later.

serves as a transient posturing splint. Since the average person swallows only 4 to 8 times an hour during sleep and probably only twice that when wearing a functional appliance, this is a small percentage of time for any stimulating or unloading effect to occur from forward posturing. Petrovic and Stutzmann[156] have shown that there is an excitation of the retrodiskal pad (posterior disk attachment) and some lateral pterygoid activity which would enhance metabolism of the temporomandibular joint in a growing child. However, for the appliance to be optimally effective, it would have to provide continual and repeated functional stimuli. To achieve this objective, some proponents require daytime wear. It has always been a major thesis of Rolf Fränkel[57] that function regulators should be worn both day and night. He refers to his appliance as an exercise device. His impressive results seem to achieve maximum stimulation of optimal condylar growth and direction. The problem is that most functional appliances such as activator, monobloc, LSU activator, and Fränkel appliance, are bulky, thereby making it difficult to speak. With allergies and respiratory problems, patients complain about breathing difficulties. Initial adjustment is not easy, and some young patients find the appliances relatively uncomfortable and remove them as soon as the parent is out of the room. Patient compliance is a continuing problem. Thus many clinicians,

who have tried functional appliances because of the demonstrated results and biologic justification, have given up because of a lack of continued patient cooperation, as well as the clinician's inability to determine just how much the patient has worn the appliance (protestations to the contrary notwithstanding).

Martin Schwarz recognized the compliance difficulties when he made his double plate[173]; it consisted of upper and lower removable appliances that were held by suitable retention wires and that had opposing occlusal acrylic guiding ramps that postured the mandible forward on complete closure. With half the bulk of a monobloc, it is easier to wear such appliances; minor tooth movement can actually be accomplished at the same time with wire appurtenances.

William Clark has emulated Schwarz' thinking with his twin blocks, which are modified Schwarz' double plates. His success with occlusal guide planes has been well documented. And now, with the incorporation of rare earth magnets in the attraction mode, the success is enhanced and more rapid (Figs. 7-41 through 7-58). Like Hamilton, Clark recognizes the need to restore normal maxillary width and does this in his arch development stage of treatment, before sagittal correction with the twin-block appliance and using fixed or removable expansion appliances, such as the jackscrew or quad helix fixed appliance (Figs. 7-41 and 7-51).

Text continued on p. 420.

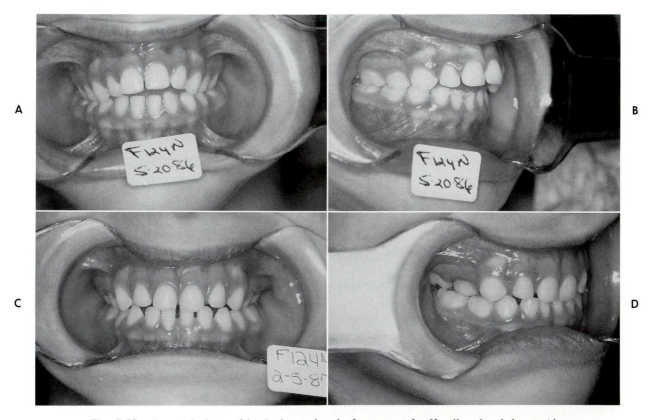

Fig. 7-38 Intraoral views of beginning and end of treatment for Hamilton bonded expansion activator patient in Fig. 7-37. No appliances are being worn now. **A** and **B** at 5 years and 2 months. **C** and **D,** 21 months later.

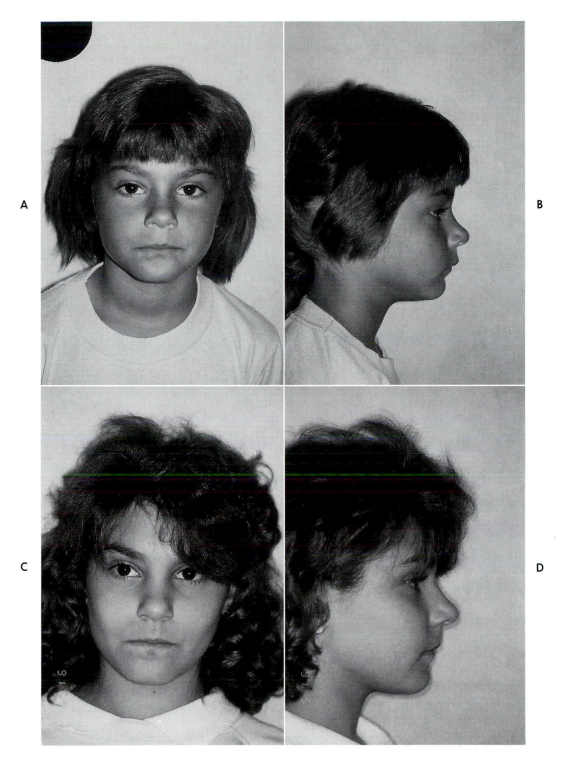

Fig. 7-39   Severe mixed dentition Class II, division 1 (8 year, 1 month girl). Moderate prognathism of restricted maxillary arch. The tentative treatment plan called for a bonded Hamilton expansion activator for 7 months, a rapid palatal expansion appliance for 3 months. Comprehensive treatment and arch length enhancement was to be carried out with partial fixed appliances as needed for detailing. A functional retainer with built-in overtreatment was to be worn as needed. In actuality, the first stage was carried out with highly satisfactory results and no additional care was necessary. **A** and **B,** Facial views at 8 years, 1 month. **C** and **D,** Final facial views at 13 years, 9 months.

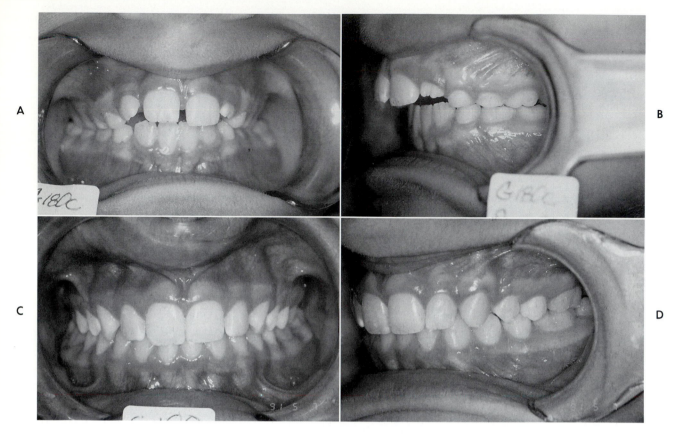

Fig. 7-40   Intra-oral views of patient in Fig. 7-39 at beginning and end of treatment, as well as post-treatment observation period. No appliances have been worn for some time.

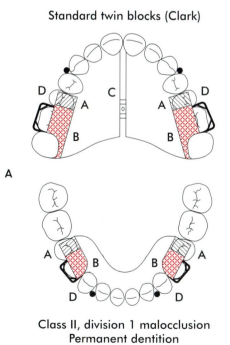

Standard twin blocks (Clark)

Class II, division 1 malocclusion
Permanent dentition

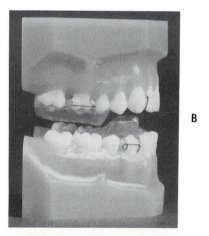

Fig. 7-41   **A,** Drawing of Clark twin block appliances. Attracting rare earth magnets can be embedded in the small 70 degree angulated inclined planes *(hash-marked areas)*, *A*. The occlusal acrylic surfaces, *B*, do not cap the buccal cusps. The lower appliance terminates at the distal of the lower second premolar to allow for upward and forward lower molar eruption. The heavily shaded occlusal cover in the maxillary appliance is trimmed later for controlled eruption. The jackscrew, *C*, in the maxillary appliance can be used as needed for arch width changes. Retention wires and clasps, *D*, provide intra-arch stability. **B,** Twin block on models. Note inclined forward posturing planes, with imbedded attracting rare earth magnets.

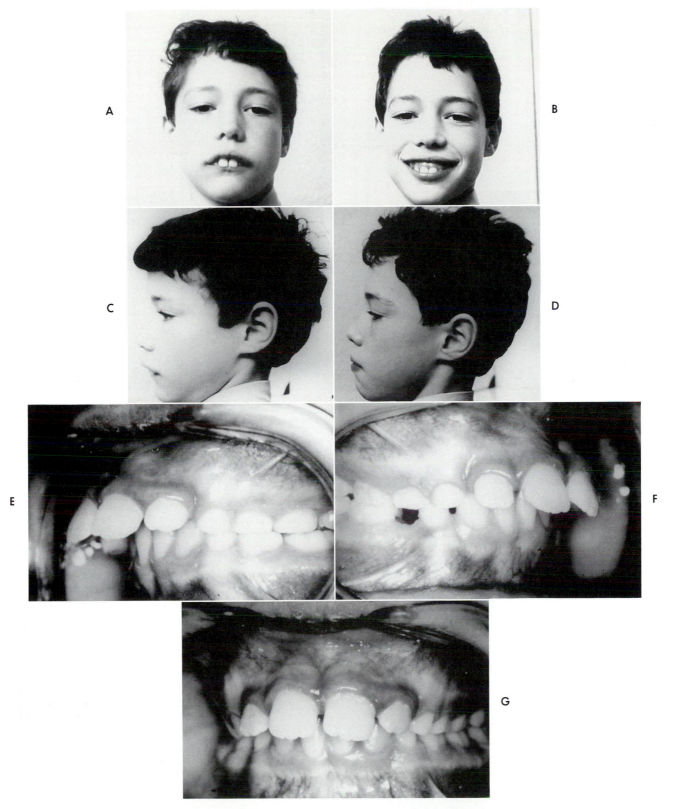

Fig. 7-42 *Case J.C.* **A** and **B,** Boy (8 years, 9 months,) with disfiguring Class II, division 1, malocclusion. Perioral musculature is abnormal, with a lower lip trap that further enhances the overjet. Lower incisors occlude in palatal tissue. Other sequelae are a narrow maxillary arch and a *gummy* smile. **C** and **D,** Profile views taken before and immediately after insertion of forward posturing functional magnetic appliances. **E, F, G,** Intra-oral views before therapy.

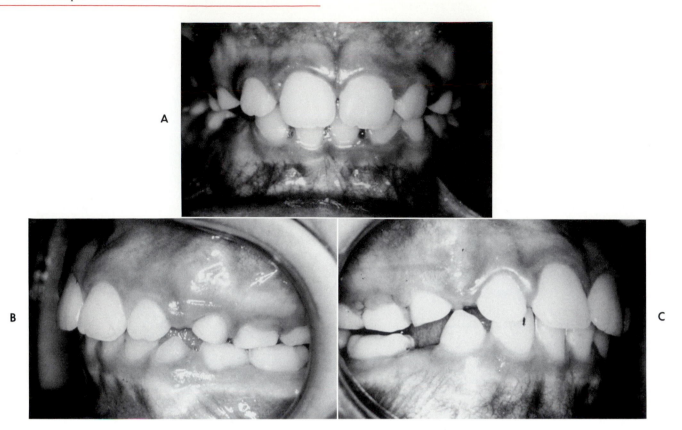

Fig. 7-43 *Case J.C.* Intraoral views, after 8 months of magnetic twin block treatment.

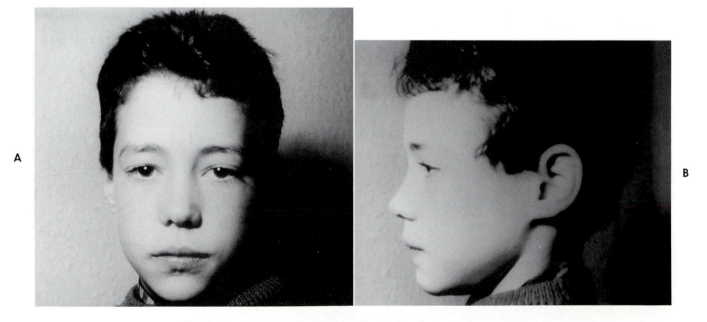

Fig. 7-44 *Case J.C.* Facial views 8 months after start of treatment.

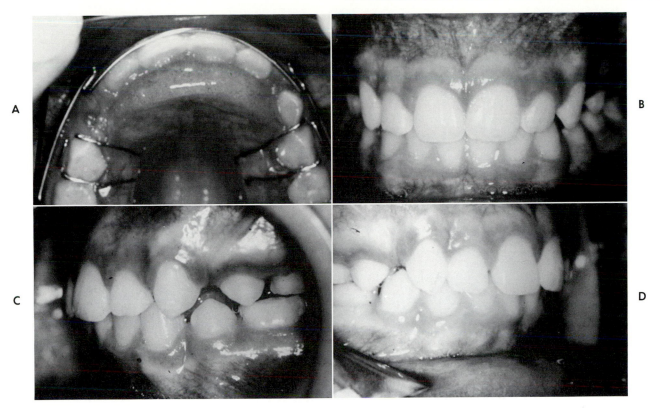

Fig. 7-45 *Case J.C.* **A,** Upper retainer with inclined ramp behind maxillary incisors, worn until fixed appliance phase. **B, C, D,** Intra-orals before second phase fixed appliance detailing.

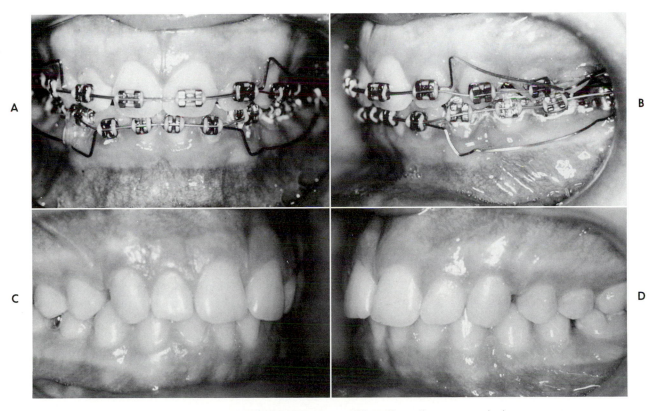

Fig. 7-46 *Case J.C.* **A** and **B,** Bonded brackets and intruding adjustments on incisor segments to eliminate excessive overbite and reduce excessive gingival display. **C** and **D,** Intra-oral views 1 year out of retention.

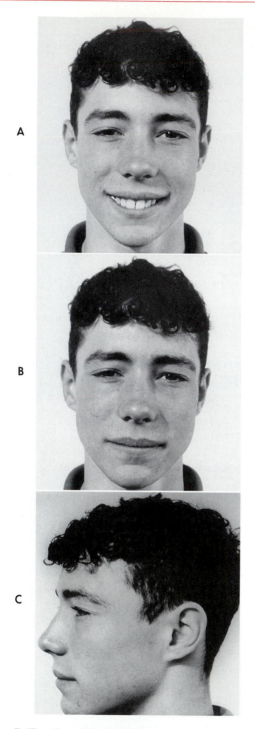

Fig. 7-47   *Case J.C.* Facial views, 1 year out of retention.

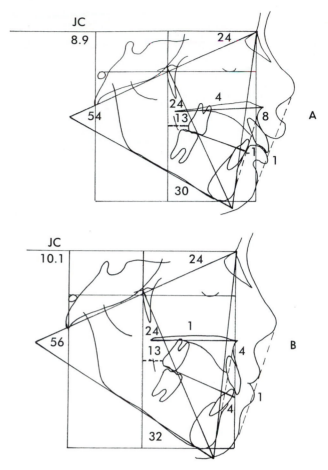

Fig. 7-48   *Case J.C.* Cephalometric tracings before and after twin block therapy (approximately a 14 month interval).

If only mild expansion is needed, it can be accomplished by the palatal jackscrew in the bonded maxillary twin block element and will also improve alignment as needed.

The orthopedic phase with the twin blocks recognizes the need for eruption of lower molars to eliminate excessive overbite. By not covering the mandibular molars they are free to erupt in an upward and forward vector, aiding the Class II correction. The occlusal acrylic does not cover the buccal cusps of both upper and lower posterior teeth (Figs. 7-41 and 7-43). It should be emphasized that functional appliances resort to reciprocal dental Class II correction in a noninvasive manner, avoiding the potential iatrogenic sequelae of periodontal involvement, gingival inflammation, crestal bone loss, root resorption, or dilaceration. This reciprocal upper and lower arch dental adjustment must be controlled, of course. Too often it has not been controlled with conventional functional appliances, because the mandibular incisors are excessively proclined. It is not maltreatment, however, to obtain dental correction with biocompatible measures.

For Phase I of twin block therapy the magnets in attraction mode are embedded in the 70 degree inclines of the upper and lower appliances (Fig. 7-41, *A*) to enhance functional activity and inter-arch contact in the protrusive relationship (Fig. 7-41, *B*). The patient is instructed to wear the appliances all the time, removing them only for cleaning. Note the positions of the inclines differ in the upper and lower appliances (anterior, upper; posterior, lower). Moss and Shaw (1990) have reported using repelling magnets in a different configuration on upper and lower appliances, again

Text continued on p. 428.

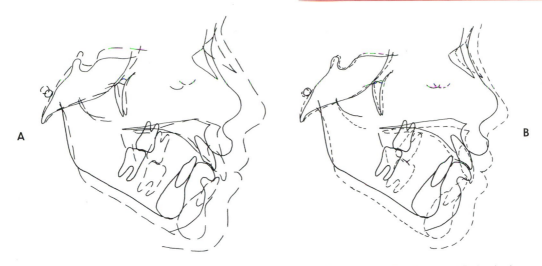

Fig. 7-49   *Case J.C.* Cephalometric superimpositions of **A** tracings in Fig. 7-48, and **B,** beginning treatment and an additional year after previous examination (comparing age 8.9 and 11.1).

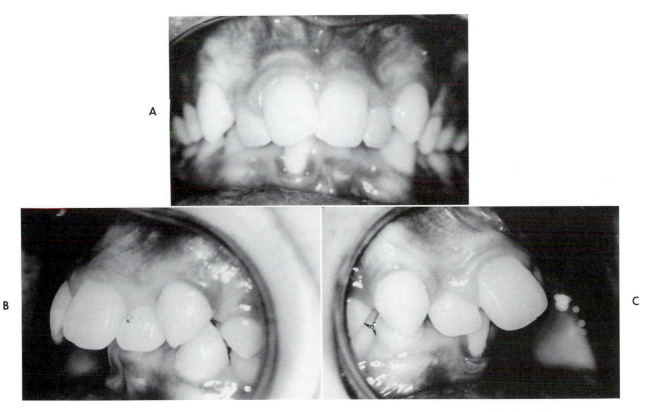

Fig. 7-50   *Case F.H.* **A, B, C,** At initial examination (14 years, 11 months), with a full Class II, division 1, malocclusion, complicated by crowding in both arches. Overjet was 10 mm, with a deep impinging overbite. A chronic labial gingival inflammation existed in the lower right central incisor area. The first phase of arch development treatment was with an upper quad helix and lower fixed lingual appliances for 6 months. The following twin magnetic block phase was for 5 months only because of minimal skeletal involvement. The full fixed bioprogressive phase took 20 months. The labially compromised lower left central incisor was torqued back into the alveolar process, the lower labial frenum resected and the labial gingival infection eliminated. Retention was for 1 year.

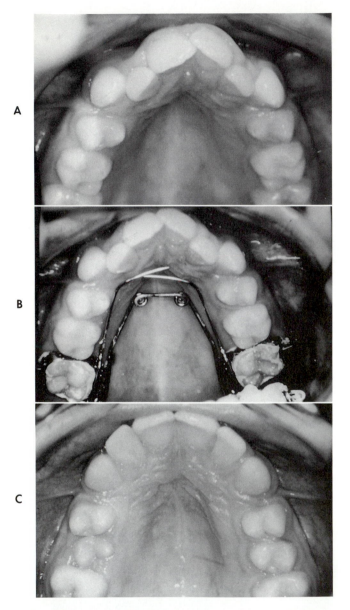

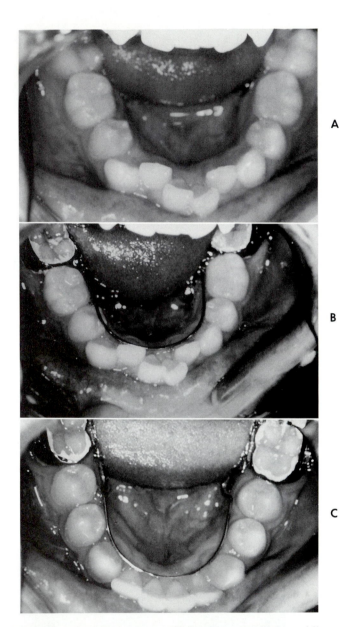

Fig. 7-51 *Case F.H.* Arch development phase, **A, B, C,** using quad helix appliance.

Fig. 7-52 *Case F.H.* Lower arch development with looped lingual arch: **A, B,** and **C.**

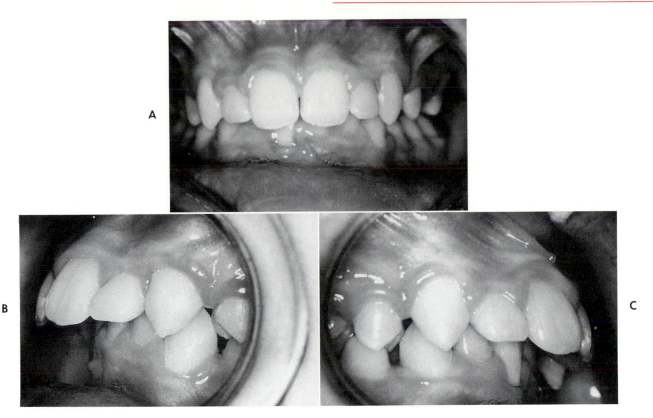

Fig. 7-53   *Case F.H.* Intraorals before twin block magnetic phase.

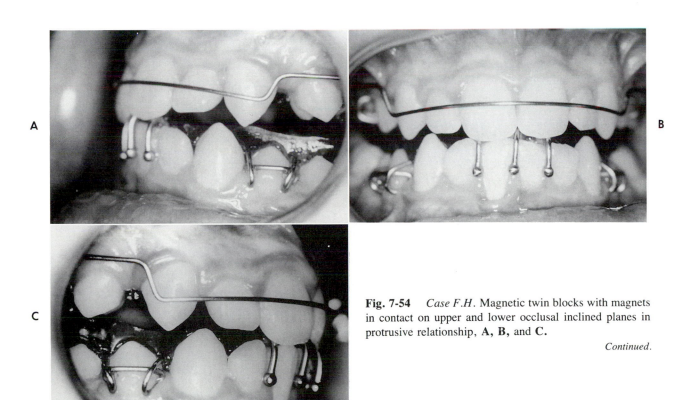

Fig. 7-54   *Case F.H.* Magnetic twin blocks with magnets in contact on upper and lower occlusal inclined planes in protrusive relationship, **A, B,** and **C.**

Continued.

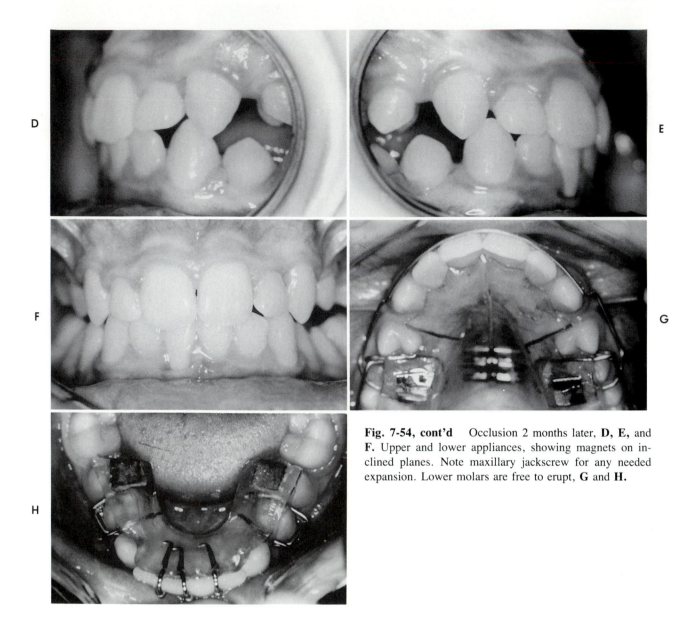

Fig. 7-54, cont'd   Occlusion 2 months later, **D, E,** and **F.** Upper and lower appliances, showing magnets on inclined planes. Note maxillary jackscrew for any needed expansion. Lower molars are free to erupt, **G** and **H.**

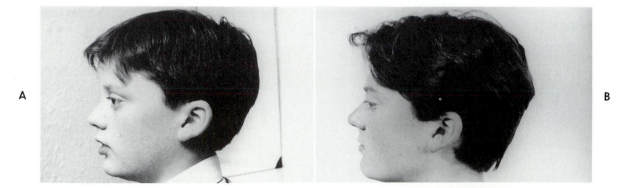

Fig. 7-55   *Case F.H.* **A** and **B,** Profile changes after magnetic twin block therapy (1 year interval).

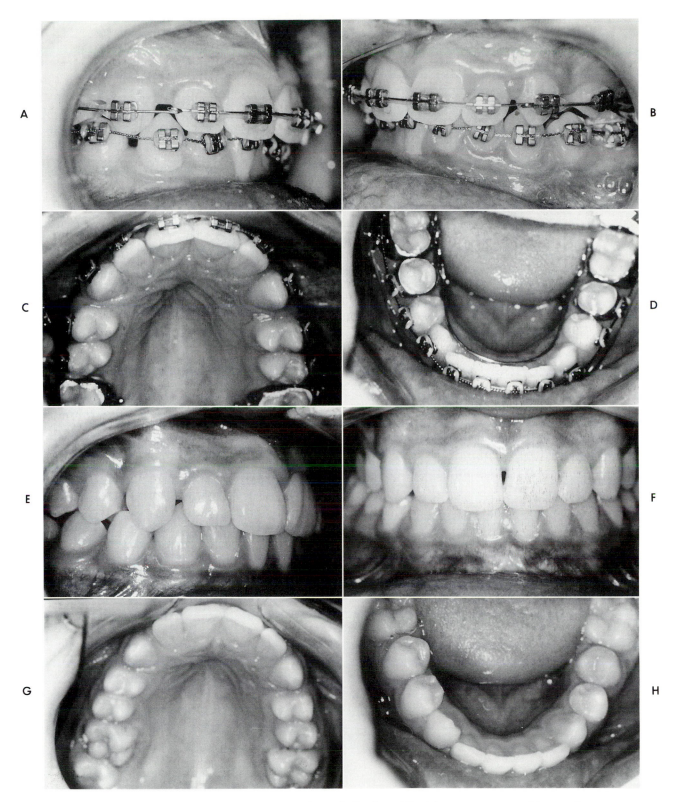

Fig. 7-56   *Case F.H.* Fixed appliance phase, **A, B, C,** and **D.** After treatment, age 17 years, 8 months, **E, F, G,** and **H.**

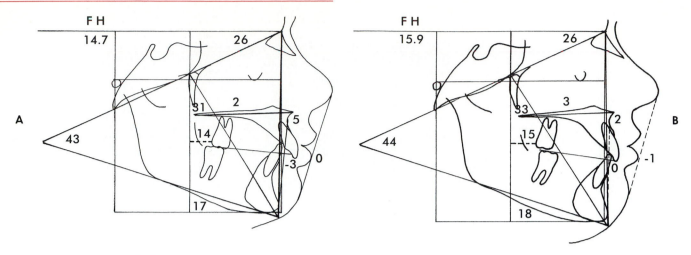

Fig. 7-57 *Case F.H.* Cephalometric tracings, at beginning of treatment and after twin block therapy (1 year interval).

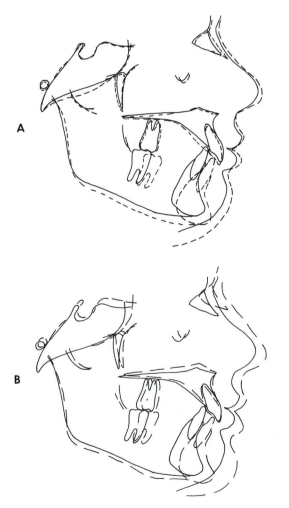

Fig. 7-58 *Case F.H.* Cephalometric superimpositions. **A,** 14′7″ and 15′9″. **B,** 14′7″ and 17′8″, after fixed appliances. Major change occurred in magnetic twin block phase.

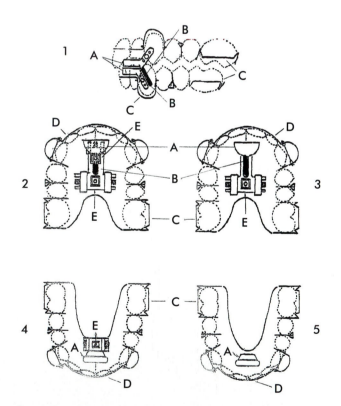

Fig. 7-59 Functional Magnetic Appliance (FMA) **1.** Lateral view with magnets together in protrusive relationship. **2.** Maxillary appliance, with jackscrews for both expansion and incisor segment protraction. **3,** Maxillary appliance, with expansion screw only. Note guidance prongs in maxillary appliances. **4.** Mandibular appliance with expansion jackscrew. **5.** Mandibular appliance with magnet only imbedded in lingual acrylic. *A,* Miniaturized rare earth magnets. *B,* Maxillary forward guidance prong. *C,* Retention clasps. *D,* Labial arch wire, *E,* Jackscrew.

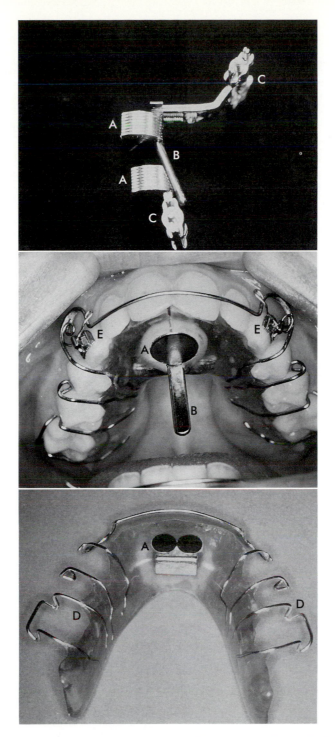

Fig. 7-60 FMA of Vardimon. Upper and lower modified Schwarz plates, similar to the Clark twin block functional approach. Instead of bilateral angled magnetic inclines, lingual midline magnets are imbedded in the acrylic. A maxillary guiding prong which slides on the lingual acrylic of the lower appliance during closure brings the mandible forward into the desired protrusive relationship as the magnets come into contact. This unloads the condyles, much the same as conventional functional appliances—only the functional stimulus of the two-part system is significantly more frequent and apparently greater. Patient compliance is better than with a single *monobloc* appliance. Jackscrews may be incorporated in both appliances as needed for transverse control. In top view, magnets, *A,* approach each other, along lingual guidance prong. *B,* Retention tags, *C,* insert in acrylic of upper and lower appliances. In middle view, note magnet, *A,* and guidance prong, *B,* imbedded in palatal acrylic. Retention clasps, *D,* may be supplemented by small elastics, hooking over bonded brackets, *E.* This increases resistance to dislodgement by magnetic action. Either single or double magnets, *A,* round or oblong, may be used in lower appliance, bottom view.

to aid in forward posturing. Repelling magnets require a different orientation of the inclines.

Following the rapid and desired sagittal correction, the twin blocks are worn for an additional 2 to 3 months to stabilize the occlusion and allow for needed posterior eruption, which occurs more slowly. The acrylic is trimmed away from the maxillary occlusal surfaces of the maxillary molars and premolars gradually to allow for their downward and forward eruption. The lower appliance is discarded and an inclined plane is added to the maxillary appliance, which serves as a short term retainer for Phase II to continue stabilization and allow posterior segment eruption that is needed.

Vardimon and associates,* as well as Joho and Derendelilier,[111a] have been aware of the potential of the use of rare earth magnets in orthodontics and dentofacial orthopedics for some time and have produced a series of research reports on the efficacy and specific applications of rare earth magnets. Blechman[30a,30b] has been a pioneer in the magnetic field, albeit not with functional appliances. Taking advantage of the miniaturization of these powerful and small permanent magnets made of samarium cobalt and neodymium-iron-boron, both upper and lower removable appliances may have strategically placed magnets, delivering attracting or repelling force that is extremely effective and rapid. Considerable experimentation has been done on the size, shape,

*References 194-203.

and placement of the magnet. If the magnets are too strong, they clamp the two appliances together, effecting a monobloc, which defeats the purpose. If they are too strong, they tend to dislodge the removable appliances from their respective jaws. If the magnets are too small, they do not have a stimulating effect on jaw position. The correct size, shape, and angulation of opposing magnets are all-important, as shown by Vardimon (Figs. 7-59 through 7-61).

After continuing experimentation on animals and human patients, a technique has now evolved that satisfies the criteria needed to maintain sufficient stability of the appliance in each arch and the demands for constant functional stimulation of forward and backward movement, yet reasonably retains the facility of speaking and swallowing. These appliances serve as functional, loading and unloading, repetitive mechanisms, not only during swallowing but also innumerable times during the waking hours. Appliances should be removed for eating and cleaning. They are considered effective tools in the functional appliance armamentaria. A good example of mixed dentition, Phase One FMA therapy, is seen in Figs. 7-62 through 7-65. Eight months of functional guidance at the right time greatly reduces sagittal basal discrepancy; eliminates deforming perioral muscle function and speech problems; and makes Phase Two fixed mechanotherapy much shorter, easier, and more likely to be successful without premolar extraction and undue reliance on prolonged extra-oral force.

Current research is exploring the use of light bonded

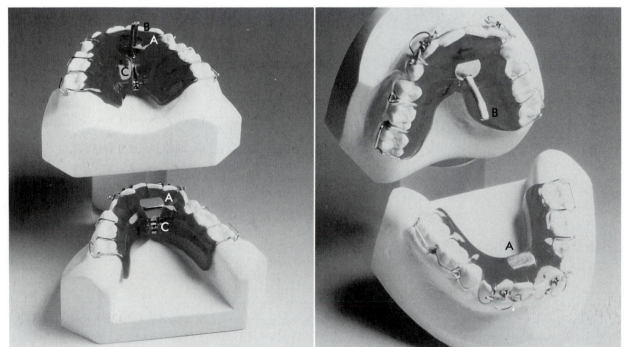

Fig. 7-61 Upper and lower FMA, using jackscrews for expansion. Small double magnets, *A,* are imbedded in palatal acrylic immediately anterior to guidance prong, *B,* and jackscrew, *C.* Lower oblong magnet, *A,* is attached to jackscrew, *C,* so as not to interfere with widening process. Maxillary guidance prong slides down the magnetic surface during closure.

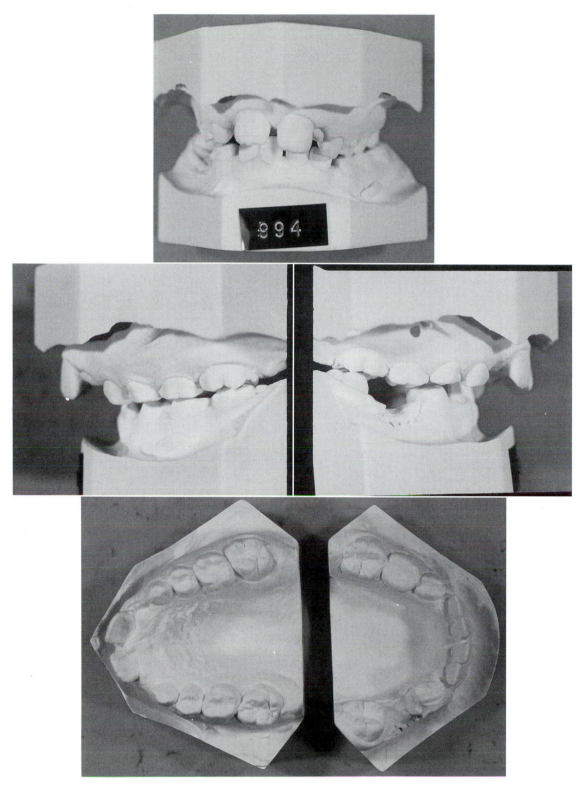

Fig. 7-62 *Patient S.D.* Severe Class II, division 1 (8 year old girl), lip trap compensation, lower incisors forced lingually, with premature deciduous lower canine loss.

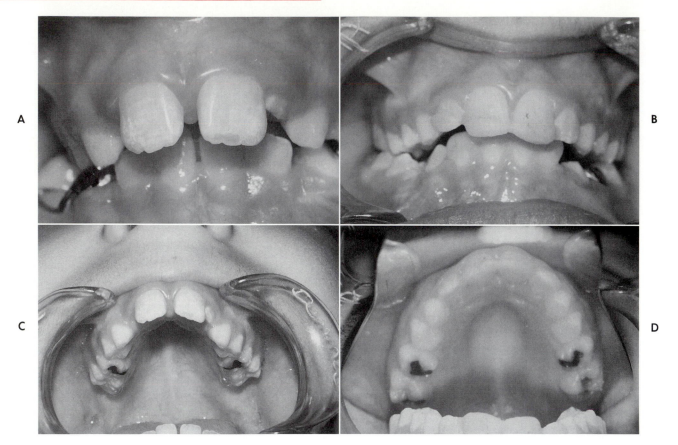

Fig. 7-63 *Patient S.D.* Magnet functional therapy, phase I. **A,** Anterior view at beginning of mixed dentition stage one. **B,** Eight months later with marked reduction of overjet and elimination of abnormal lip habit. **C,** Narrow maxillary arch caused by abnormal lip and tongue function and posture. **D,** Eight months of magnetic functional, combined with jackscrew slow palatal expansion.

acrylic upper and lower appliances, which incorporate angulated attraction magnets to optimize sagittal correction. Magnets may also be used in the palatal midline of the upper appliance at the same time to achieve the desired expansion.[197] Following this phase of treatment, brackets are bonded on individual teeth as needed to complete the detailing.

Blechman has been involved in medical use of electromagnetic fields and has pioneered in orthodontic usage.[30b] He hypothesized that static magnetic fields may have some electric field effect that potentiates tissue response. In vitro orthodontic research on this hypothesis has produced mixed results thus far. Clinically, however, in magnet deimpaction of palatally malposed maxillary canines, the eruption into the mouth is as little as one third of the time required by conventional appliances.[203] However, it is not likely that magnets in functional appliances would have any electric field effect on the condyle. Magnetic functional appliances, of course, cannot be any more effective in a nongrowing child than any other functional appliance. Improperly designed magnetic appliances or improper case selection can result in proclination of the lower incisors, even as it does with other types of activators. At present, the buccal shields

of the Fränkel appliance or the buccal loops of the bionator have not been incorporated in magnetic functionals. Since they seem to relieve pressure from the buccinator mechanism and tend to enhance autonomous expansion, there is no reason why they could not be added in the future without unduly jeopardizing speech and patient cooperation. Today, magnets seem to offer an exciting advance in achieving better functional efficiency and stimulation of optimal growth amounts and direction with minimum bulk. At last, functional appliances can truly live up to their name.

ADVANTAGES OF FUNCTIONAL APPLIANCES

It is pertinent to ask, "Why functional appliances? Do they have any advantages over fixed appliances?" The answer is not absolute and is couched in probabilities, but it is definitive enough to accept for the majority of cases.

The activator allows more effective oral prophylaxis and maintenance of better hard and soft tissue integrity. Of particular concern are the potential for root resorption, sheared alveolar crests, decalcification of enamel surfaces, gingival hypertrophy, chronic inflammation, and the potential fibrotic

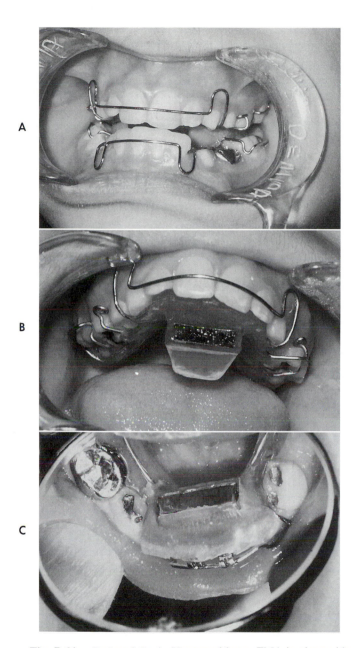

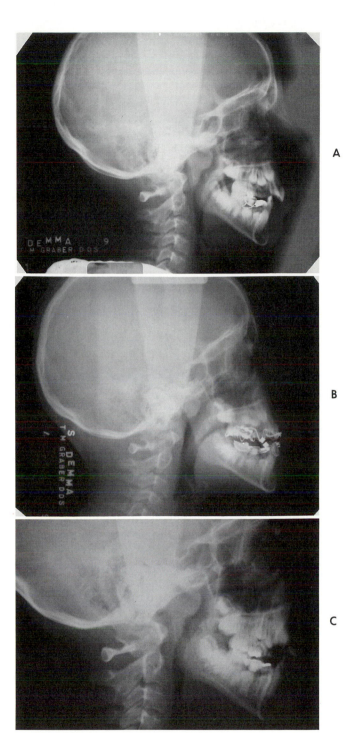

Fig. 7-64 *Patient S.D.* **A,** Upper and lower FMA in place with magnets in contact in attractive mode. This is a transient position, repeated countless times during the day and night, with swallowing breathing, kinetic action. **B,** Angulated oblong magnet in maxillary appliance, with acrylic customized guidance ramp at approximately 70 degrees—similar to Clark twin block. Jackscrew has already been opened. **C,** Mandibular oblong magnet seen in mirror image of lingual surface of lower appliance. Lower brackets may be bonded to labial surfaces of lower incisors, for labial wire to snap below, enhancing retention during continuing functional exercises.

Fig. 7-65 *Patient S.D.* Lateral cephalograms at beginning of treatment. **A,** Note severe overjet and lingually inclined lower incisors. **B,** Upper and lower FMA appliances in place. Arrow shows opposing angulated attractive mode brackets, imbedded in acrylic lingual to incisors. **C,** Lateral cephalogram after 8 months of FMA treatment. Second phase of fixed appliances is planned in permanent dentition, but basal dysplasia and abnormal deforming perioral muscle function have largely been eliminated.

changes too often seen with fixed appliances that have not been taken care of properly by the patient. When there is periodontal disease or a hormonal problem, removable appliances are kinder to the tissue. The problems of decalcification associated with fixed appliances need not be elaborated; they are well known, whether full bands or direct bonded attachments are used. Trapping of acidogenic debris is a real hazard. Too often the question has been, "What price orthodontics?" These are the cases that appear in litigation.

To the question of elimination of abnormal perioral muscle function that is an associated factor in most Class II, division 1 malocclusions, the answer is also in favor of functional appliances. Regardless of where the clinician stands on the question of the relationship of form and function, and the potentially deleterious effects of the hyperactive mentalis and hyoid musculature and the *lip trap,* there is little doubt that elimination of abnormal muscle activity is beneficial (Figs. 7-30 to 7-35). Many fixed appliance regimens now use lip bumpers and shields, emulating functional appliances, in appreciating this aspect.

The answer to the crucial question of whether functional appliances can stimulate condylar growth beyond normal pattern is still open to discussion and needs more clinical research on actual patients to have any air of finality. Animal experiments have produced overwhelming evidence of the possibilities, however, and cephalometric measurements on properly selected and treated patients show a variable response but produce many examples of enhanced mandibular growth during functional appliance wear.[64] Is this *catch-up* growth? Is it due merely to the elimination of restrictive abnormal perioral muscle function and functional retrusion? Or is it merely fortuitous timing with a growth spurt?

The research of Graber[64] and Graber[68] on humans and nonhuman primates and Stutzmann et al.[185] on rats shows that the trabecular angle can be changed by forward advancement of the mandible, producing a change in growth direction that would help reduce the sagittal discrepancy. However, trabecular changes are temporary and actual changes in mandibular morphology caused by them are hard to measure. Until we know more, the best that can be said is that functional appliances do eliminate factors that may stand in the way of accomplishing the most favorable growth pattern and they permit the attainment of the achievable optimum. When we realize the adaptability of the living organism, and recognize the range of normal response, and when we see that the Japanese people are, on the average, 4 inches taller now than they were before World War II largely because of diet (Americans are taller, too, though by not as much), we cannot deny the potential for change.

The question of change in sagittal position is a corollary to condylar response. Firm clinical evidence exists of a large number of Class II, division 1 malocclusions with deep bite that also have a most retruded condylar position in the fossa on habitual occlusion. Functional appliances are capable of eliminating the functional retrusions effectively, particularly in Class II, division 2 malocclusions. As our *most likely scenario* shows, the total sagittal change is the result of multiple factors, no one of which is responsible for the major change. Modified functional appliances are an important tool in TMD cases. They may also prevent development of TMD problems.

Animal experimentation shows significant remodeling of the articular fossa in subjects with mandibular advancement. Although this is one area of lesser potential for significant change, it is a membranous bone region and is adaptable to normal and abnormal function. The changes induced in the articular eminence and condylar path after the eruption of the deciduous incisor teeth show the potential for functional effect on these structures. It is likely that functional appliances are more effective than fixed appliances in producing any such changes.

The potential for slight restriction of horizontal maxillary growth exists for functional appliances. Redirection of maxillary growth or relocation of the maxilla in a more vertical direction is demonstrated in selected cases. However, fixed appliance orthopedic procedures are more effective than functional appliances in this regard—which leads to the obvious conclusion that a combination of fixed and functional appliances could produce the best possible of all orthodontic worlds, using each component of the appliance for the effect it produces best. The following chapter, by Stöckli and Teuscher, as well as Chapter 9 by McNamara, makes this philosophy a practical reality.

REFERENCES

1. Ahlgren J: An electromyographic analysis of the response to activator (Andresen-Häupl) therapy, *Odontol Rev* 11:125, 1960.
2. Ahlgren J: The neurophysiologic principles of the Andresen method of functional jaw orthopedics. A critical analysis and new hypothesis, *Sven Tandlak Tidskr* 63:1, 1970.
3. Ahlgren J: A longitudinal clinical and cephalometric study of 50 malocclusion cases treated with activator appliances, *Trans Eur Orthod Soc* p. 285, 1973.
4. Ahlgren J: Changes in length and torque of the masticatory muscles produced by the activator appliance, *Swed Dent J* (suppl 15), 1982.
5. Ahlgren J: Munskärmaktivator: en modifierad Andresen-plät, *Tandläkartidningen* 75:300, 1983.
6. Altuna G, Niegel S: Bionators in Class II treatment. *J Clin Orthod* 19:185, 1985.
7. Andresen V: Beitrag zur Retention, *Z Zahnaertzl Orthop* 3:121, 1910.
8. Andresen V: Bio-mekanisk ortodonti: et ortodontisk system for privatpraksis og skoletannklinikker, *Nor Tannlaegeforen Tid* 41:71, 161, 442, 1931.
9. Andresen V: Bio-mekanisk ortodonti: et ortodontisk system for privatpraksis og skoletannklinikker, *Nor Tannlaegeforen Tid* 42:131, 215, 295, 1932.
10. Andresen V: Ueber das sogenannte "norwegische System der Funktions-Kiefer-Orthopädie," *Dtsch Zahnaerztl Wochenschr* 39:235, 283, 1936.
11. Andresen V, Häupl K: *Funktionskieferorthopädie. Die Grundlagen des "norwegischen Systems,"* ed 2, Leipzig, 1939, H. Meusser.
12. Andresen V, Häupl K: *Funktionskieferorthopädie. Die Grundlagen des "norwegischen Systems,"* ed 3, Leipzig, 1942, JA Barth Verlag.
13. Andresen V, Häupl K: *Funktionskieferorthopädie. Die Grundlagen des "norwegischen Systems,"* ed 4, Leipzig, 1945, JA Barth Verlag.
14. Andresen V, Häupl K, Petrik L: *Funktionskieferorthopädie,* ed 6, Munich, 1957, JA Barth.

15. Arat M, Iseri H: Orthodontic and orthopaedic approach in the treatment of skeletal open bite, *Eur J Orthod* 14:207, 1992.

16. Ascher F: Kontrollierte Ergebnisse der Rückbissbehandlung mit funktionskieferorthopädischen Geräten, *Fortscher Kieferorthop* 32:149, 1971.

17. Ballard CF: A consideration of the physiological background of mandibular posture and movement. *Dent Pract Dent Rec* 6:80, 1955.

18. Balters W: *Eine Einführung in die Bionatorheilmethode: ausgewählte Schriften und Vorträge,* Heidelberg, 1973, C Herrmann.

19. Barbre RE, Sinclair PM: A cephalometric evaluation of anterior openbite correction with the magnetic active vertical corrector, *Angle Orthod* 6:93, 1991.

20. Battagel JM: The relationship between hard and soft tissue changes following treatment of Class II, division 1 malocclusion using Edgewise and Fränkel appliance techniques, *Eur J Orthod* 12:154, 1990.

21. Baume LJ: Cephalo-facial growth patterns and the functional adaptation of the temporomandibular joint structures, *Eur Orthod Soc Rep Congr,* p 79, 1969.

22. Baume LJ, Derichsweiler H: Is the condylar growth center responsive to orthodontic therapy? An experimental study in *Macaca mulatta, Oral Surg* 14:347, 1961.

23. Bierbaek L, Melsen B, Terp S: A laminagraphic study of the alterations in the temporo-mandibular joint following activator treatment, *Eur J Orthod* 6:157, 1984.

24. Biggerstaff RH: "The condylar plexus." Personal communication, July 1983.

25. Bimler HP: Die elastischen Gebissformer, *Zahnaerztl Welt* 4:499, 1949.

26. Bimler HP: JCO/interviews Dr. H.P. Bimler on functional appliances, *J Clin Orthod* 17:39, 1983.

27. Bimler HP: *The Bimler appliance.* In Graber TM, Neumann B: *Removable orthodontic appliances,* ed 2, Philadelphia, 1984, WB Saunders.

28. Björk A: The principle of the Andresen method of orthodontic treatment, a discussion based on cephalometric x-ray analysis of treated cases, *Am J Orthod* 37:437, 1951.

29. Björk A: Prediction of mandibular growth rotation, *Am J Orthod* 55:585, 1969.

30. Björk A, Palling M: Adolescent age changes in sagittal jaw relation, alveolar prognathy, and incisal inclination, *Acta Odontol Scand* 12:201, 1954-1955.

30a. Blechman AM: Magnetic force systems in orthodontics: clinical results of a pilot study, *Am J Orthod* 87:201-210, 1985.

30b. Blechman AM, Smiley H: Magnetic force in orthodontics, *Am J Orthod* 79:435-443, 1978.

31. Bolmgren GA, Moshiri F: Bionator treatment in Class II, division 1, *Angle Orthod* 56:255, 1986.

32. Bondevik O: How effective is the combined activator-headgear treatment? *Eur J Orthod* 13:482, 1991.

33. Breitner C: Experimentelle Veränderung der mesiodistalen Beziehungen der oberen und unteren Zahnreihen, *Z Stomatol* 28:134, 620, 1930.

34. Brieden CM, Pangrazio-Kulbersh V, Kulbersh R: Maxillary skeletal and dental change with Fränkel appliance therapy—an implant study, *Angle Orthod* 54:226, 1984.

35. Chabre C: Vertical control with a headgear-activator combination, *J Clin Orthod* 24:618, 1990.

36. Chang HF, Wu KM et al: Effects of activator treatment on Class II, division 1 malocclusion, *J Clin Orthod* 23:560, 1989.

37. Charlier JP, Petrovic A, Herrmann-Stutzmann J: Effect of mandibular hyperpropulsion on the prechondroblastic zone of young rat condyle, *Am J Orthod* 55:71, 1969.

38. Creekmore TD, Radney LJ: Fränkel appliance therapy: orthopedic or orthodontic? *Am J Orthod* 83:89, 1983.

39. Demisch A: Effects of activator therapy on the craniofacial skeleton in Class II, Division 1, malocclusion, *Eur Orthod Soc Rep Congr,* p 295, 1972.

40. Demisch A: *Herren's dentofacial orthopedics.* In Graber TM, Neumann B, editors: *Removable orthodontic appliances,* ed 2, Philadelphia, 1984, WB Saunders.

41. Dermaut LR, van den Eynde F, de Pauw G: Skeletal and dentoalveolar changes as a result of headgear activator therapy related to different vertical growth patterns, *Eur J Orthod* 14:140, 1992.

42. Dietrich UC: Aktivator-mandibuläre Reaktion, *Schweiz Monatsschr Zahnheilkd* 83:1092, 1973.

43. Drage KJ, Hunt NP: Overjet relapse following functional appliance therapy, *Br J Orthod* 17:205, 1990.

44. Eirew HL, McDowell F, Phillips JG: The Fraenkel appliance—avoidance of lower incisor proclination, *Br J Orthod* 8:189, 1981.

45. Elgoyhen JC, Moyers RE, et al: Craniofacial adaptation to protrusive function in young rhesus monkeys, *Am J Orthod* 62:469, 1972.

46. Enlow DH: *The dynamics of skeletal growth and remodelling.* In *Scientific foundations of orthopedic surgery,* London, 1981, Heinemann Medical.

47. Enlow DH, DiGangi D, McNamara JA Jr, Mina M: An evaluation of the morphogenic and anatomic effects of the functional regulator utilizing the counterpart analysis, *Eur J Orthod* 10:192, 1988.

48. Eschler J: Wesen und Möglichkeiten der Verwendung von kontinuierlicher und intermittierenden Kräften im Rahmen des Andresen-Häupl'schen Behandlungssystems, *Oesterr Z Stomatol* 47:53, 1950.

49. Eschler J: *Die funktionelle Orthopädie des Kausystems.* Munich, 1952, C Hanser.

50. Eschler J: Die muskuläre Wirkungsweise des Andresen-Häuplschen Apparates, *Oesterr Z Stomatol* 49:79, 1952.

51. Eschler J: Elektrophysiologische und pathologische Untersuchungen des Kausystems. IV. Mitteilung: Elektromyographische Untersuchungen über die Wirksamkeit muskeltonussteigernder Medikamente bei Anwendung des Andresen-Häupl Apparates, *Dtsch Zahnaerztl Z* 10:1421, 1955.

52. Eschler J: Die Kieferdehnung mit funktionskieferorthopädischen Apparaten: der Funktionator, *Zahnaertzl Welt* 63:203, 1962.

53. Fleischer E, Fleischer A: *Bionator modification; the Bio-M-S therapy.* In Graber TM, Neumann B: *Removable orthodontic appliances,* ed 2, Philadelphia, 1984, WB Saunders.

54. Fränkel R: Concerning recent articles on Fränkel appliance therapy (letter), *Am J Orthod* 85:441, 1984.

55. Fränkel R: *Technik und Handhabung der Funktionsregler,* Berlin, 1973, VEB Verlag Volk und Gesundheit.

56. Fränkel R: *Biomechanical aspects of the form/function relationship in craniofacial morphogenesis: a clinician's approach.* In McNamara JA, Ribbens KA, Howe RP, editors: *Clinical alteration of the growing face, Monograph 14, Craniofacial growth series,* Ann Arbor, 1983, Center for Human Growth and Development, University of Michigan.

57. Fränkel R: "The functional strategy in the orofacial area." Presented at the 83rd annual session, American Association of Orthodontists, Boston, May 1983.

58. Fränkel R, Fränkel C: A functional approach to treatment of skeletal open bite, *Am J Orthod* 84:54, 1983.

59. Fränkel R, Reiss W: Problematik der Unterkiefernachentwicklung bei Distalfällen, *Fortschr Kieferorthop* 31:345, 1970.

60. Freunthaller P: Cephalometric observations in Class II, division 1 malocclusions treated with the activator, *Angle Orthod* 37:18, 1967.

61. Gaumond G: Hyperpropulsor activator, *J Clin Orthod* 20:405, 1986.

62. Gerber M: Beobachtungen an schlafenden Aktivatorträgern, *Fortschr Kieferorthop* 18:205, 1957.

63. Gianelly AA, Brosnan P, Martignoni M, Bernstein L: Mandibular growth, condyle position, and Fränkel appliance therapy, *Angle Orthod* 53:131, 1983.

64. Graber LW: "Results of Fränkel appliance therapy on Class II, division 1 malocclusion patients: clinical research with functional appliances." Presented at the 83rd annual session, American Association of Orthodontists, Boston, May 1983.

65. Graber TM: Postmortems in posttreatment adjustment, *Am J Orthod* 52:331, 1966.

66. Graber TM: Maxillary second molar extraction in Class II malocclusion, *Am J Orthod* 56:331, 1969.

67. Graber TM: *Orthodontics; principles and practice,* ed 3, Philadelphia, 1972, WB Saunders.

68. Graber TM: "The effect of buccal shields on the maxillary dental arch width in the squirrel monkey *(Saimiri sciureus)*." Presented at the 83rd annual session, American Association of Orthodontists, Boston, May 1983.

69. Graber TM: *Physiological principles of functional appliances,* St Louis, 1985, Mosby.

70. Graber TM, Neumann B: *Removable orthodontic appliances,* ed 2, Philadelphia, 1984, WB Saunders.

71. Graber TM, Rakosi T, Petrovic A, editors: *Dentofacial orthopedics with functional appliances,* St Louis, 1986, Mosby.

72. Grohs R, Petrik L: Die Funktionskieferorthopädie als Helferin der Prothetik, *Z Stomatol* 42:160-178, 1944.

73. Grossman WJ, Greenfield BE, Timms DJ: Electromyography as an aid in diagnosis and treatment analysis, *Am J Orthod* 47:481, 1961.

74. Grude R: Myofunctional therapy. A review of various cases some years after their treatment by the Norwegian system had been completed, *Nor Tannlaegeforen Tid* 62:1, 1952.

75. Grude R: Ortodontisk terapi med avtagbar apparatur, *Nord Klin Odont* 3/15(6):1, 1966.

76. Hagerström L: Sex fall av distalbett med retruderade överkäksinsisiver behandlade med expansion *Sven Tandlaekarfoerb Tidn* 61:826, 1969.

77. Hale LR, Tonge EA: A long-term follow-up of four cases treated with the Andreasen appliance, *Br J Orthod* 13:195, 1986.

78. Hamano Y, Ahlgren J; A cephalometric study of the construction bite of the activator, *Eur J Orthod* 9:305, 1987.

79. Hamilton, DC: "Integration of functional and fixed appliances. The expansion activator system." Presented at the 83rd annual session, American Association of Orthodontists, Boston, May 1983.

80. Hansen K, Pancherz H: Long-term effects of Herbst treatment in relation to normal growth development: a cephalometric study, *Eur J Orthod* 14:285, 1992.

81. Harvold EP: *Distalokklusjon, Behandlingsmetodik, Tandlaegebladet* 50:146, 1946.

82. Harvold EP: *The activator in interceptive orthodontics,* St Louis, 1974, Mosby.

83. Harvold EP, Vargervik K: Morphogenetic response to activator treatment, *Am J Orthod* 60:478, 1971.

84. Hasund A: The use of activators in a system employing fixed appliances, *Eur Orthod Soc Rep Congr,* p 329, 1969.

85. Häupl K: *Gewebsumbau und Zahnverdrängung in der Funktionskieferorthopädie: eine funktionell-histologische Studie,* Leipzig, 1938, JA Barth.

86. Häupl K: Transformation of the temporomandibular joint during orthodontic treatment, *Am J Orthod* 47:151, 1961 (Abstract).

87. Häupl K, Psansky R: Experimentelle Untersuchungen über Gelenkstransformation bei Verwendung der Methoden der Funktionskieferorthopädie, *Dtsch Zahn Mund Kieferheilkd* 6:439, 1939.

88. Hausser E: Wachstum und Entwicklung unter dem Einfluss funktionskieferorthopädischer Therapie, *Fortschr Kieferorthop* 24:310, 1963.

89. Hausser E: Functional orthodontic treatment with the activator, *Trans Eur Orthod Soc* p. 427, 1973.

90. Hausser E: Funktionskieferorthopädische Behandlung mit dem Aktivator, *Fortschr Kieferorthop* 36:1, 1975.

91. Haynes S: Anterior vertical changes in function regulator therapy, *Eur J Orthod* 5:219, 1983.

92. Haynes S: Profile changes in modified functional regulator therapy, *Angle Orthod* 56:309, 1986.

93. Herren P: Die Wirkungsweise des Aktivators, *Schweiz Monatsschr Zahnheilkd* 63:829, 1953.

94. Herren P: The activator's mode of action, *Am J Orthod* 45:512, 1959.

95. Hoffer O: Les modifications de l'articulation temporomandibulaire par l'action des moyens orthopédiques, *Orthod Fr* 29:97, 1958.

96. Hollender L, Lindahl L: Radiographic study of articular remodeling in the temporomandibular joint after condylar fractures, *Scand J Dent Res* 82:462, 1974.

97. Hopkins JB, Murphy J: Variations in good occlusions, *Angle Orthod* 41:55, 1971.

98. Hotz R: Die funktionelle Beurteilung der Bisslage als Ausgangspunkt für die Prognose und die Begrenzung des Behandlungs, *Fortschr Kieferorthop* 16:255, 1955.

99. Hotz RP: Application and appliance manipulation of functional forces, *Am J Orthod* 58:459, 1970.

100. Hotz R: *Orthodontics in daily practice: possibilities and limitations in the area of children's dentistry,* Bern, 1974, H Huber.

101. Hotz R, Mühlemann H: Die Funktion in der Beurteilung und Therapie von Bissanomalien, *Schweiz Monatsschr Zahnheilkd* 62:592, 1952.

102. Hoyte DAN, Enlow DH: Wolff's law and the problem of muscle attachment on resorptive surface of bone, *Am J Phys Anthropol* 24:205, 1966.

103. Humerfelt A, Slagsvold O: Changes in occlusion and craniofacial pattern between 11 and 25 years of age. A follow-up study of individuals with normal occlusion, *Eur Orthod Soc Rep Congr* p. 113, 1972.

104. Ingervall B: Relation between retruded contact, intercuspal, and rest positions of the mandible in children with Angle Class II, division 2 malocclusions, *Odontol Rev* 19:1, 1968.

105. Ingervall B, Bitsanis E: Function of masticatory muscles during the initial phase of activator treatment, *Eur J Orthod* 8:172, 1986.

106. Isaacson KG, Reed RT, Stephens CD: The Harvold activator: simplified construction and use, *J Clin Orthod* 17:845, 1984.

107. Jacobsson SO: Cephalometric evaluation of treatment effect on Class II, division 1 malocclusions, *Am J Orthod* 53:446, 1967.

108. Jacobsson SO, Paulin G: The influence of activator treatment on skeletal growth in Angle Class II: 1 case: a roentgenocephalometric study, *Eur J Orthod* 12:174, 1990.

109. Johannesen B: "Overjet and labio-lingual position of incisor teeth in treated Class II, division 1 malocclusions." Thesis. University of Oslo, 1972.

110. Johannesen B: A critical evaluation of treatment planning Class II, division 1, malocclusions, *Studieweek* p. 112, 1975.

111. Johnston LE: Seminar at the University of Chicago, November 1979.

111a. Joho JP, Derendeliler MA: Magnetic activator device II (MAD II) for correction of Class II, division 1 malocclusions, *Am J Orthod Dentofac Orthop* 103:223-239, 1993.

112. Kerr WJ, TenHave TR, McNamara JA, Jr: A comparison of skeletal and dental changes produced by function regulators (FR-2 and FR-3), *Eur J Orthod* 11:235, 1989.

113. Klammt G: Der offene Aktivator, *Dtsch Stomatol* 5:322, 1955.

114. Komposch G, Hockenjos C: Die Reaktionsfähigkeit des Temporomandibularen, *Fortschr Kieferorthop* 38:121, 1977.

115. Korkhaus G: Ein kieferorthopädisch interessantes Zwillingpaar, *Fortschr Kieferorthop* 32:257, 1971.

116. Koski K: Cranial growth centers: facts or fallacies? *Am J Orthod* 54:566, 1968.

117. Lehman R, Hulsink JH: Treatment of Class II malocclusion with a headgear-activator combination, *J Clin Orthod* 23:430, 1989.

118. Lehman R, Romuli A, Bakker V: Five-year treatment results with a headgear-activator combination, *Eur J Orthod* 10:309, 1988.

119. Loh MK, Kerr WJ: The function regulator III: effects and indications for use, *Br J Orthod* 12:153, 1985.

120. Lund K: Mandibular growth and remodelling processes after condylar fracture: a longitudinal roentgencephalometric study, *Acta Odontol Scand* 32 (suppl 64), 1974.

121. Madone G, Ingervall B: Stability of results and function of the masticatory system in patients treated with the Herren type of activator, *Eur J Orthod* 6:92, 1984.

122. May FJ: "A laminagraphic and cephalometric evaluation of dental and skeletal changes occurring during activator treatment." Thesis, University of Minnesota. Cited in Hirzel HC, Grewe JM: Activators; a practical approach, *Am J Orthod* 66:557, 1974.

123. McDougall PD, McNamara JA, Dierkes JM: Arch width development in Class II patients with the Fränkel appliance, *Am J Orthod* 82:10, 1982.

124. McNamara JA, Jr: The functional regulator (FR-3) of Fränkel, *Am J Orthod* 88:409,1985.

125. McNamara JA, Jr: Dentofacial adaptations in adult patients following functional regulator therapy, *Am J Orthod* 85:57, 1984.

126. McNamara JA, Jr, Bookstein FL, Shaughnessy TG: Skeletal and dental changes following functional regulator therapy on Class II patients, *Am J Orthod* 88:91, 1985.

127. McNamara JA: Neuromuscular and skeletal adaptations to altered function in the orofacial region, *Am J Orthod* 64:578, 1973.

128. McNamara JA: Functional determinants of craniofacial size and shape, *Eur J Orthod* 2:131, 1980.

129. McNamara JA: Components of Class II malocclusions in children 8-10 years of age, *Angle Orthod* 51:177, 1981.

130. McNamara JA: *A method of cephalometric analysis*. In McNamara JA, Ribbens KA, Howe HP, editors: *Clinical alteration of the growing face, Monograph 14, Craniofacial growth series*, Ann Arbor, 1983, Center for Human Growth and Development, University of Michigan.

131. McNamara JA, Graber LW: Mandibular growth in the rhesus monkey *(Macaca mulatta)*, *Am J Phys Anthropol* 42:15, 1975.

132. McNamara JA, Hinton RJ, Hoffman DL: Histologic analysis of temporomandibular joint adaptation to protrusive function in young adult rhesus monkeys, *Am J Orthod* 82:288, 1982.

133. Melanson E, Van Dyken C: "Studies in condylar growth." Thesis, University of Michigan, Ann Arbor, 1972.

134. Mills JR: The effect of functional appliances on the skeletal pattern, *Br J Orthod* 18:267, 1991.

135. Mills JRE: The stability of the lower labial segment, *Dent Pract Dent Rec* 18:293, 1968.

136. Mills JRE: *Clinical control of craniofacial growth: a skeptic's viewpoint*. In McNamara JA, Ribbens KA, Howe RP, editors: *Clinical alteration of the growing face, Monograph 14, Craniofacial growth series*, Ann Arbor, 1983, Center for Human Growth and Development, University of Michigan.

137. Mills JRE: A clinician looks at facial growth, *Br J Orthod* 10:58, 1983.

138. Moffett BC: *Responses of the craniofacial skeleton to mechanical forces*. In *Symposium on clinical and bioengineering aspects of dentofacial orthopedics*, University of Connecticut, October 1981.

139. Moffett BC, Koskinen-Moffett L: *A biologic look at mandibular growth rotation*. In Carlson DS, editor: *Craniofacial biology, Monograph 10, Craniofacial growth series*, Ann Arbor, 1981, Center for Human Growth and Development, University of Michigan.

140. Moss JP: Cephalometric changes during functional appliance therapy, *Eur Orthod Soc Trans*, p 327, 1962.

141. Moss JP: Function—fact or fiction? *Am J Orthod* 67:625, 1975.

142. Moss JP: An investigation of the muscle activity of patients with a Class II, division 2, malocclusion and the changes during treatment, *Trans Eur Orthod Soc* p. 87, 1975.

143. Neumann B: Funktionskieferorthopädie. Rückblick und Ausblick, *Fortschr Kieferorthop* 36:73, 1975.

144. Nielsen IL: Facial growth during treatment with the function regulator appliance, *Am J Orthod* 85:401, 1985.

145. Orton HS, Noble PM: Fixed-removable approach to presurgical orthodontic treatment, *J Clin Orthod* 24:296, 1990.

146. Owen AH III: Frontal facial changes with the Fränkel appliance, *Angle Orthod* 58:257, 1988.

147. Owen AH III: Clinical management of the Fränkel FR II appliance, *J Clin Orthod* 17:605, 1983.

148. Owen AH III: Clinical application of the Fränkel appliance, case reports, *Angle Orthod* 53:29, 1983.

149. Ozerovic B: Some changes in occlusion and craniofacial pattern obtained during treatment with removable orthodontic appliances, *Eur Orthod Soc Rep Congr* p. 329, 1972.

150. Parkhouse RC: A cephalometric appraisal of cases of Angle's Class II, division 1 malocclusion treated by the Andresen appliance, *Dent Pract Dent Rec* 19:425, 1969.

151. Petrovic A: Recherches sur les mécanismes histophysiologiques de la croissance osseuse cranio-faciale, *Ann Biol* 9:303, 1970.

152. Petrovic AG: Mechanisms and regulation of mandibular condylar growth, *Acta Morphol Neerl Scand* 10:25, 1972.

153. Petrovic AG: "Experimental investigation on the modus operandi of various orthopedic appliances." Continuing education course, American Dental, Association, GV Black Institute and Kenilworth Research Foundation, Chicago, March 1983.

154. Petrovic A, Gasson N, Oudet C: Wirkung der übertriebenen posturalen Vorschubstellung des Unterkiefers auf das Kondylenwachstum der normalen und der mit Wachstumshormon behandelten Ratte, *Fortschr Kieferorthop* 36:86, 1975.

155. Petrovic A, Oudet C, Gasson N: Unterkieferpropulsion durch eine im Oberkiefer fixierte Vorbissfurung mit seitlicher Biss-sperre von unterschiedlicher Höhe. Auswirkungen bei Ratten während der Wachstumsperiode und bei erwachsenen Tieren, *Fortschr Kieferorthop* 43:243, 1982.

156. Petrovic A, Stutzmann J: Le muscle ptérygoïdienne externe et al croissance du condyle mandibulaire. Recherches expérimentales chez le jeune rat, *Orthod Fr* 43:271, 1972.

157. Petrovic A, Stutzmann J, Oudet C: *Defects in mandibular growth resulting from condylectomy and resection of the pterygoid and masseter muscles*. In McNamara JA, Carlson, DS, Ribbens KA, editors: *The effect of surgical intervention on craniofacial growth, Monograph 12, Craniofacial growth series*, Ann Arbor, 1982, Center for Human Growth and Development, University of Michigan.

158. Pfeiffer JP, Grobéty D: Simultaneous use of cervical appliance and activator: an orthopedic approach to fixed appliance therapy, *Am J Orthod* 61:353, 1972.

159. Qwarnström KE, Sarnäs KV: Röntgenkefalometriska studier av förändringar vid funktionskäkortopedisk behandling av distalbett, 7 fall av Angle Klass II:1, *Odontol Rev* 5:118, 1954.

160. Rakosi T: *Biomechanics of functional orthopedic appliances*. In McNamara JA, Ribbins KA, Howe RP, editors: *Clinical alteration of the growing face, Monograph 14, Craniofacial growth series*, Ann Arbor, 1983, Center for Human Growth and Development, University of Michigan.

161. Reitan K: "The initial tissue reaction incident to orthodontic tooth movement as related to the influence of function. An experimental histological study on animal and human material." Thesis, University of Oslo, 1951.

162. Ricketts RM: *Orthopedics in the eyes of the clinician*. In *Symposium on clinical and bioengineering aspects of dentofacial orthopedics*, University of Connecticut, October 1981.

163. Righellis EG: Treatment effects of Fränkel, activator and extraoral traction appliances, *Angle Orthod* 53:107, 1983.

164. Robin P: Observation sur un nouvel appareil de redressement, *Rev Stomatol* 9:423, 1902.

165. Roux W: *Gesammelte Abhandlungen über Entwicklungsmechanik der Organismen*, Leipzig, 1895, W. Engelmann.

166. Sahm G, Bartsch A, Witt E: Micro-electronic monitoring of functional appliance wear, *Eur J Orthod* 12:297, 1990.

167. Sander FG: *Zur Frage der Biomechanik des Aktivators—Entwicklung und Erprobung neuer Unterrrsuchungsmethoden*, Wiesbaden, 1980, Westdeutscher Verlag GmbH.

168. Sander FG: *The effects of functional appliances and Class II elastics on masticatory patterns*. In McNamara JA, Ribbins KA, Howe RP, editors: *Clinical alteration of the growing face, Monograph 14, Craniofacial growth series*, Ann Arbor, 1983, Center for Human Growth and Development, University of Michigan.

169. Schmuth GPF: Milestones in the development and practical application of functional appliances, *Am J Orthod* 84:48, 1983.

170. Schmuth GPF: Untersuchungen über die auf das FKO-Gerät einwirkende Kaumuskeltätigkeit während des Schlafes, *Fortschr Kieferorthop* 16:327, 1955.

171. Schmuth GPF: Muskeltätigkeit und Muskelwirkung im Bahmen der Funktionskieferorthopädie, *Dtsch Zahn Mund Kieferheilkd* 32:4, 1960.

172. Schmuth GPF: Behandlungszeit—Retentionszeit—Rezidive, *Fortschr Kieferorthop* 27:22, 1966.

173. Schwarz AM: Grundsätzliches über die heutigen kieferorthopädischen Behandlungsverfahren, *Oesterr Z Stomatol* 47:400, 448, 1950.

174. Schwarz AM: Die Wirkungsweise des Aktivators, *Fortschr Kieferorthop* 13:117, 1952.

175. Scott JH: The growth of the human face, *Proc R Soc Med* 47:91, 1954.

176. Selmer-Olsen R: En kritisk betraktning over "Det norske system," *Nor Tannlaegefor Tid* 47:85, 134, 176, 1937.

177. Sergl HG: Changes in craniofacial pattern caused by functional adaptation—an experimental study in young rabbits, *Eur Orthod Soc Rep Congr*, p. 197, 1972.

178. Shaye R: J.C.O. interviews: Dr. Robert Shaye on functional appliances, *J Clin Orthod* 17:330, 1983.

179. Slagsvold O: *Activator development and philosophy.* In Graber TM, Neumann B: *Removable orthodontic appliances,* ed 1, Philadelphia, 1977, WB Saunders Co.

180. Slagsvold, O, Kolstad I: "Class II, division 1 malocclusions treated with activators: a study of posttreatment stability." Unpublished.

181. Softley JW: Cephalometric changes in seven "post normal" cases treated by the Andresen method, *Dent Rec* 73:485-494, 1953.

182. Stockfisch H: *Der Kinetor in der Kieferorthopädie. Die Praxis des polyvalenten bimaxillären Apparates und seine rationelle Technik mit Plastik—Fertigteilen,* Heidelberg, 1966, A. Hüthig.

183. Stockfisch H: Possibilities and limitations of the Kinetor, *Trans Eur Orthod Soc* p. 457, 1973.

184. Stöckli PW, Willert HG: Tissue reactions in the temporomandibular joint resulting from anterior displacement of the mandible in the monkey, *Am J Orthod* 60:142, 1971.

185. Stutzmann J, Petrovic A, Graber TM: Auswirkungen seitlicher Vestibularsschilder nach Fränkel auf das maxillare Breitwachstum der Ratte, *Stomatol DDR* 33:753, 1983.

186. Stutzmann J, Petrovic A, Malan A: Seasonal variations of human alveolar bone turnover. A quantitative evaluation in organ culture, *J Interdiscipl Cycle Res* 12:177, 1981.

187. Thilander B, Filipsson R: Muscle activity related to activator and intermaxillary traction in Angle Class II, division 1 malocclusions. An electromyographic study of the temporal, masseter and suprahyoid muscles, *Acta Odontol Scand* 24:241, 1966.

188. Thompson JR: The rest position of the mandible and its significance to dental science, *J Am Dent Assoc* 33:151, 1946.

189. Tonge EA, Heath JK, Meikle M: Anterior mandibular displacement and condylar growth, *Am J Orthod* 82:277, 1982.

190. Trayfoot J, Richardson A: Angle Class II, division 1 malocclusions treated by the Andresen method, *Br Dent J* 124:516, 1968.

191. Trenouth MJ: A functional appliance system for the correction of Class II relationships, *Br J Orthod* 16:169, 1989.

192. Tryti T: "Angle Kl. II, 1 malokklusjoner korrigert med fasialbue og aktivator." Thesis, University of Oslo, 1974.

193. Tulley WJ: The scope and limitations of treatment with the activator, *Am J Orthod* 61:562, 1972.

194. Vardimon AD, Graber TM: Expansion of palatal sutures in diverse force magnitude and application, *J Dent Res* 66:347-348, 1987, (abstract).

195. Vardimon AD, Graber TM, Voss LR: Splitting and remodelling of circum-maxillary sutures with conventional versus magnetic appliances, *Society* p. 78, 1987.

196. Vardimon AD, Graber TM et al: Magnetic versus mechanical expansion with different force thresholds and points of force application, *Am J Orthod Dentofac Orthop* 92:455-466, 1987.

197. Vardimon AD, Mueller HG et al: Effects of Teflon coating on corrosion and magnetic forces in neodymium-iron-boron rare earth magnets, *Br J Dent Res* 69:312, 1988, (abstract).

198. Vardimon AD, Graber TM, Voss LR: Stability of magnetic versus mechanical palatal expansion, *Eur Orthod Jour* 11:107-115, 1989.

199. Vardimon AD, Stutzmann JJ et al: Functional orthopedic magnetic appliance (FOMA)—modus operandi, *Am J Orthod Dentofac Orthop* 97:371-387, 1989.

200. Vardimon AD, Graber TM et al: Functional orthopedic magnetic appliance (FOMA) III—modus operandi, *Am J Orthod Dentofac Orthop* 97:135-148, 1990.

201. Vardimon AD, Graber TM: Determinants controlling iatrogenic external root resorption during and after palatal expansion, *Angle Orthod* 61:113-124, 1991.

202. Vardimon AD, Graber TM, Pitaru S: Ursachen und Reparaturvorgänge der externen Wurzelresorption nach Gaumennahterweiterung mit magnetischen und konventionellen Dehnapparaten, *Festschrift GPF Schmuth Fortschritte f Kieferorthop* 52:193-203, 1991.

203. Vardimon AD, Graber TM et al: Rare earth magnets and impaction, *Am J Orthod* 100:494-512, 1991. (Dewel Award for best clinical article in the *AJO/DO* for 1991. Presented May, 1992, St Louis.)

204. Vardimon AD, Graber TM, Pitaru S: Repair process of external root resorption subsequent to palatal expansion treatment, *AJO/DO* 103, February 1993.

205. Vargervik K, Harvold EP: Response to activator treatment in Class II malocclusions, *Am J Orthod* 88:242, 1988.

206. Watson WG: Functional appliances questioned, *Am J Orthod* 82:519, 1982.

207. Williams S, Melsen B: Condylar development and mandibular rotation and displacement during activator treatment, *Am J Orthod* 81:322, 1982.

208. Williams S, Melsen B: The interplay between sagittal and vertical growth factors—an implant study of activator treatment, *Am J Orthod* 81:327, 1982.

209. Witt E: Investigations into orthodontic forces of different appliances, *Eur Orthod Soc Rep Congr*, p 391, 1966.

210. Witt E: Muscular physiological investigations into the effect of bimaxillary appliances, *Trans Eur Orthod Soc* p. 448, 1973.

211. Witt E, Komposch G: Intermaxilläre Kraftwirkung bimaxillärer Geräte, *Fortschr Kieferorthop* 32:345, 1971.

212. Witt E, Meyer U: Indications for and working action of bimaxillary appliances, *Eur Orthod Soc Rep Congr*, p. 321, 1972.

213. Wolff J: *Das Gesetz der Transformation der Knochen,* Berlin, 1892, Hirschwald.

214. Woodside DG: Some effects of activator treatment on the mandible and the midface, *Trans Eur Orthod Soc* p 443, 1973.

215. Woodside DG: *The activator.* In Graber TM, Neumann B: *Removable orthodontic appliances,* ed 1, Philadelphia, 1977, WB Saunders Co.

216. Woodside DG, Altuna G et al: Primate experiments in malocclusion and bone induction, *Am J Orthod* 83:460, 1983.

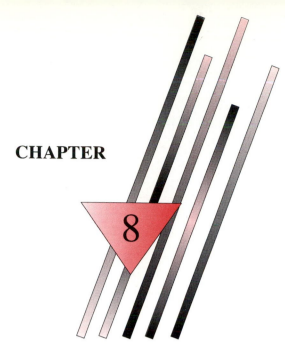

CHAPTER 8

Combined Activator Headgear Orthopedics

PAUL W. STÖCKLI
ULLRICH M. TEUSCHER

BASIC CONSIDERATIONS OF FACIAL GROWTH AND DEVELOPMENT

To be able to adapt treatment to the growth processes in an optimal manner, the clinician must respect the relationships between the displacement trends of the different facial units. The movement of the mandibular symphysis relative to the rest of the face is of paramount importance. The superimposition in Fig. 8-1, representing average growth expression during a 3-year interval, shows that the symphysis moves downward, as well as forward. This is also illustrated by the displacement of gnathion along the Y-axis of Downs or, in a similar manner, along the facial axis of Ricketts. A growth axis of this kind represents nothing more than the result of vertical and sagittal displacement. In average facial growth (Fig. 8-1) the basis for the constancy of pattern must be a balance of displacements among the several components of the facial mosaic.

Vertical factors exert a dominant influence on the anteroposterior displacement of the symphysis.* Pathologic conditions (e.g., the longitudinally documented case of congenital muscular dystrophy published by Kreiborg et al.[68]) exemplify the impact of excessive vertical development with utmost clarity (Fig. 8-2). As a consequence of the missing vertical control—in this case related to the marked atrophy of the mandibular elevator muscles—the symphysis was drastically displaced downward and backward during the 8-year growth period.

Counterpart analysis

In an average growth pattern (Fig. 8-1) with downward and forward displacement of the mandibular symphysis along the Y-axis, the descent of the glenoid fossae and the vertical growth of the condyles balance the vertical down-

ward movement of the maxillary body and upper alveolar process plus the upward movement of the lower alveolar process (Fig. 8-3). If the vertical development of the maxilla and of the upper plus the lower alveolar processes is less than the vertical contribution of fossae and condyles, the symphysis will move predominantly forward. Thus the sagittal greatly surpasses the vertical fraction, as expressed by a closing reaction of the Y-axis (Fig. 8-4). However, if the vertical development of the maxilla and of the alveolar processes is greater than the vertical contribution of fossae and

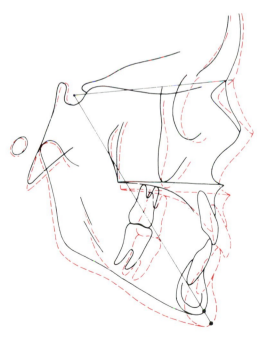

Fig. 8-1 Average displacement of maxillary and mandibular structures during a 3-year period. Superimposition on the anterior cranial base. Point of registration at sella.

---

*References 22, 23, 26, 34, 61, 62, 107-109, 119, 136, 137.

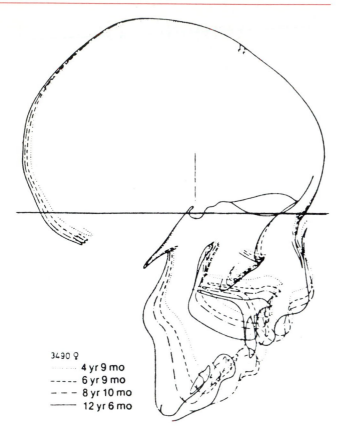

3490 ♀
.... 4 yr 9 mo
----- 6 yr 9 mo
- - - 8 yr 10 mo
——— 12 yr 6 mo

Fig. 8-2   Excessive vertical development of the facial structures with backward rotation of the mandible in a child with congenital muscular dystrophy. (From Kreiborg S et al: *Am J Orthod* 74:207, 1978.)

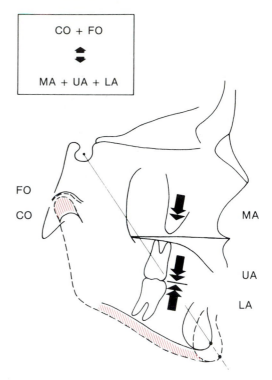

Fig. 8-3   The vertical growth of the mandibular condyles *(CO)* and the descent of the glenoid fossae *(FO)* balance the vertical downward movement of the maxilla *(MA)* and upper alveolar process *(UA)* plus the upward movement of the lower alveolar process *(LA)*. Average growth pattern with downward and forward displacement of the mandibular symphysis (gnathion) along the Y-axis.

condyles, then the symphysis will move almost exclusively downward, thereby opening the Y-axis (Fig. 8-5). In conclusion, if the growth factors of fossae and condyles are maintained at a constant level, the vertical components of maxilla plus upper and lower alveolar processes will strongly influence the inferior displacement of the mandibular symphysis and thereby its anteroposterior position.

The order of magnitude of these natural growth processes is highly relevant in appraising treatment concepts. Approximate calculations, based on the studies of Björk and Skieller,[24,25] Luder,[71] Riolo et al.,[105] Teuscher,[123] and others, indicate a descent of the maxillary complex of about 0.7 mm* per year relative to the cranial base (Fig. 8-6) with a dentoalveolar height gain of almost 1 mm in the upper (Fig. 8-7) and around 0.75 mm in the lower (Fig. 8-8) jaw. Thus vertical development of the maxillary complex measured in the molar region amounts to some 1.5 to 2 mm per year. If the lower dentoalveolar increase is included, an overall vertical development of between 2 and 3 mm can be expected. As a counterpart the movement of the glenoid fossa and the amount of condylar growth must be taken into account. The

*25.4 mm = 1 inch.

vertical downward movement of the fossa is estimated to be only about 0.25 to 0.5 mm per year[14,21,105,123] (Fig. 8-9). By far the greatest annual change in this interplay is in the condylar region, where on the average an addition of more than 2.5 mm can be registered[71,103,123] (Fig. 8-10). Comparing the vertical contribution of the glenoid fossae and the mandibular condyles with the vertical contributions of the maxilla and the upper and lower alveolar processes reveals that the stated equilibrium is also quantitatively apparent within biologic limits. Basically the condylar element must compensate for the vertical development of three facial components, each of which is relatively small. This equilibrium of displacements can be easily disturbed when orthodontic and/or orthopedic treatment is superimposed. In most treatment procedures the tendency is to increase the vertical dimension of the dentoalveolar regions or even of the midfacial structures. The fact that the extrusive mechanical aspect present in most devices does not result in a biologic response in all cases can be attributed to the control effect of the occlusal forces deriving from the adductor muscles. In many instances, however, the efficacy of orthodontic appliances prevails over the antagonistic occlusal forces. In view of the mere 2.5 mm annual growth increase in the

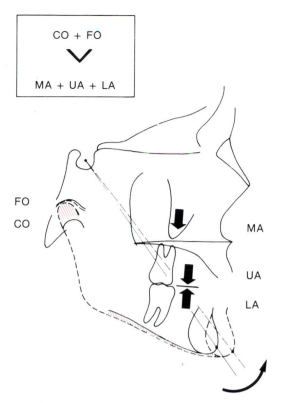

Fig. 8-4 The vertical contributions of the maxilla *(MA)* and the upper *(UA)* and lower *(LA)* alveolar processes are less than those of the glenoid fossae *(FO)* and condyles *(CO)*. Closing rotation of the mandible with predominantly forward displacement of the symphysis.

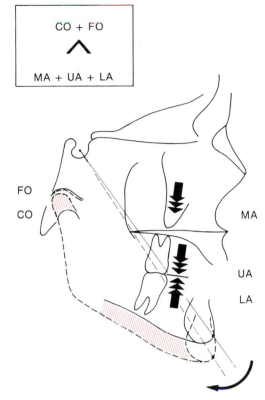

Fig. 8-5 The vertical contributions of the maxilla *(MA)* and the upper *(UA)* and lower *(LA)* alveolar processes are greater than those of the glenoid fossae *(FO)* and condyles *(CO)*. Opening rotation of the mandible with predominantly downward displacement of the symphysis.

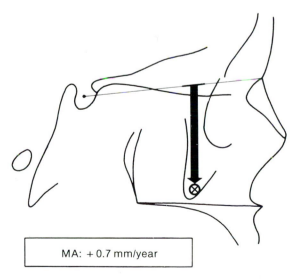

Fig. 8-6 Average vertical displacement of the basal maxillary structures *(MA)*. Approximate annual increase in the distance from the anterior cranial base to the implant in the zygomatic process. (According to Björk A, Skieller V.[24,25])

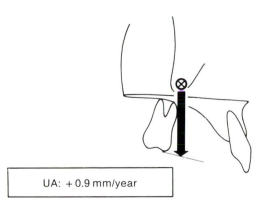

Fig. 8-7 Average vertical growth of the upper alveolar process *(UA)*. Approximate annual increase of the distance from the implant in the zygomatic process to the occlusal plane mesial to the first molar. (According to Björk A, Skieller V.[24,25])

vertical dimension, even a minor additional elongation in the dentoalveolar region of the buccal segments must have a significant effect on mandibular rotation and thereby on the anteroposterior position of the mandibular symphysis. In Fig. 8-11 such an effect is simulated. With extrusion of the upper and lower molars 1 mm each, the geometric consequence in the depicted pattern is an opening of the Y-axis by 2.5° and a decrease in S-N-B of 2.5°. Effects of this kind can indeed be observed as a result of the mechanical impact of orthodontic appliances (Fig. 8-12). In this context

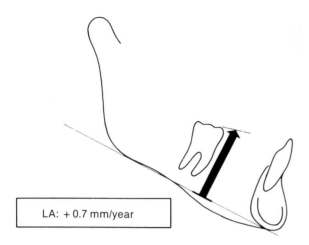

LA: + 0.7 mm/year

Fig. 8-8 Average vertical growth of the lower alveolar process *(LA)*. Approximate annual increase of the distance from the mandibular plane to the mesial cusp of the first molar. (According to Riolo ML et al,[105] Teuscher UM.[123])

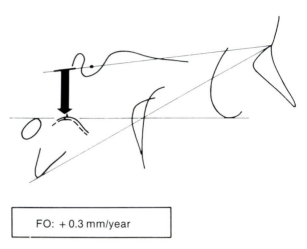

FO: + 0.3 mm/year

Fig. 8-9 Average vertical displacement of the glenoid fossae. Approximate annual increase in the distance from the anterior cranial base to the fossa. (This value is an estimation based on the work of Ricketts RM and the investigations of Baumrind S et al,[13] Björk A,[21] Riolo ML et al,[105] Teuscher UM.[123])

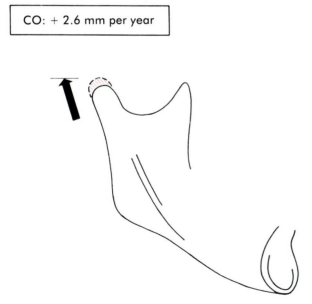

CO: + 2.6 mm per year

Fig. 8-10 Average annual growth increment at the mandibular condyles. (According to Luder HU,[71] Ricketts RM,[103] Teuscher UM.[123])

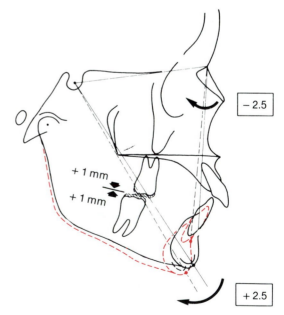

+ 1 mm
+ 1 mm
− 2.5
+ 2.5

Fig. 8-11 The consequence of 1 mm extrusion of the upper and lower molars on the position of the mandibular symphysis. In this facial pattern S-N-B will decrease by 2.5° and the Y-axis will open by 2.5°.

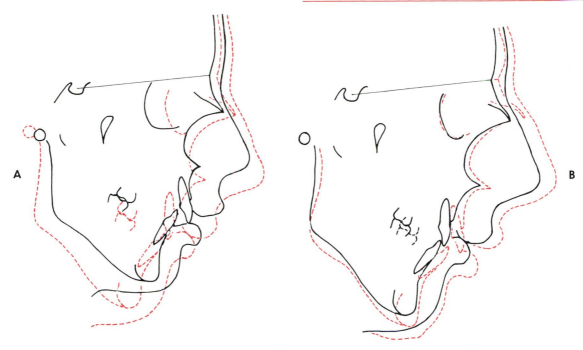

Fig. 8-12 Severe backward rotation of the mandible can occur during orthodontic treatment. The usual claim that a poor facial growth pattern during active treatment was responsible for the reaction observed in **A** must be questioned. More likely it was extrusive mechanics on the molars and excessive posterior rotation of the occlusal plane that caused the excessive downward and backward displacement of the mandibular symphysis. The superimposition of the posttreatment period, **B,** confirms that the basic growth pattern in this case was probably quite normal.

the claim of facing a poor growth pattern must be interpreted, in many instances, as iatrogenic deflection of the natural growth path.

In a concept for skeletal Class II treatment these negative counterproductive side effects should be avoided, even if their probability of becoming manifest appears low.

EVOLUTION OF A GROWTH RELATED CONCEPT FOR SKELETAL CLASS II TREATMENT

One of the key requirements for a solid concept of skeletal Class II treatment must be that natural growth factors contributing to the correction of the sagittal maxillomandibular imbalance should not be disturbed. In fact, they should be enhanced to allow expression of their full potential.

With reference to the superimposition on the anterior cranial base (Fig. 8-1), the average natural displacement pattern of the maxilla and mandible is depicted schematically in Fig. 8-13. The resultant vector of growth expression can be divided into a horizontal and a vertical component of displacement. Normally the forward thrust of the mandible during development is slightly greater than that of the maxilla, leading gradually to a flattening of the face. The difference in anterior displacement is notable at the bottom of Fig. 8-13. In skeletal Class II treatment this difference between mandibular and maxillary anterior displacement

should be increased; otherwise no skeletal correction can be expected. Functional jaw orthopedics aims at stimulating mandibular forward growth. The additional anterior growth vector of the mandible should bring about the so-called jumping of the bite (Fig. 8-14). In all appliances that should produce this reaction—whether the numerous variations of the activator,[50,52,59] the Fränkel,[80] or even the old Herbst appliance—there is one common denominator: the mandible is forced into a forward position by the orthopedic device. The idea is to stimulate condylar growth so that after a certain period this position will be stabilized by compensatory structural adaptation.

The most emphatic statement about this concept has been made by Korkhaus[67]: "We effect the correction of distocclusion exclusively through the mesial development of the entire lower jaw." Nevertheless, the matter remains controversial despite extensive research.[56-58,112,129,130] The basic question has been whether adaptive processes can, in principle, be initiated in the condylar region by mere artificial forward displacement of the mandible. Animal experiments* have proved histologically that an adaptive reaction in the condylar region can be produced by artificial hyperpropulsion of the mandible. Increase and redirection of mandibular growth can be substantiated by quantitative meth-

---

*References 11, 12, 28, 29, 32, 55, 74-76, 78, 79, 93-95, 114-116.

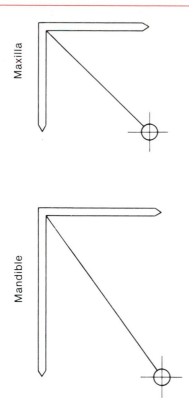

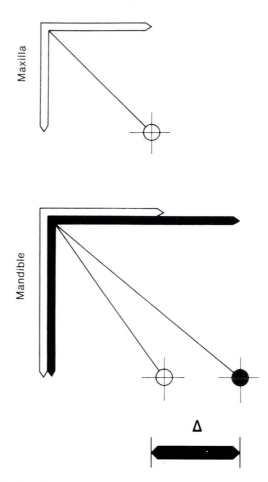

Fig. 8-13 Overall superimposition exhibited in Fig. 8-1. Average natural displacement pattern of the maxilla (point *A*) and mandible (pogonion) relative to the anterior cranial base. The horizontal and vertical components *(white)*, as well as the resultant vector of displacement, are shown. In an average facial growth pattern the forward component of mandibular symphysis displacement is slightly greater than that of the anterior apical base of the maxilla. The difference (Δ) is marked at the bottom.

Fig. 8-14 Concept of stimulating forward mandibular displacement *(black)* to bring about the so-called jumping of the bite in Class II treatment with functional jaw orthopedic appliances. The additional anterior displacement manifestly exceeds the documented amount. Furthermore, concurrent unaffected displacement of maxillary skeletal and/or dentoalveolar structures could not be substantiated by functional jaw orthopedic appliances. This diagram expresses nothing more than an unfulfilled orthodontic dream.

ods.* Remodeling processes at the glenoid fossa indicate a tendency to a reactive forward and downward drift.[114,115] In clinical studies one group of authors† could not find cephalometric indications of a mandibular reaction in either length or improved anterior position after hyperpropulsive treatment. Rather dentoalveolar and maxillary reactions accounted for occlusal and skeletal changes. Another group,‡ however, reported that mandibular reaction in length and position[70] did in effect also contribute to an improvement of the maxillomandibular relationship during Class II treatment when the concept of forced forward positioning of the mandible was employed. The diverging results can be partly attributed to different methods of investigation and also to the fact that different propulsive appliances seem to evoke various types of condylar reaction depending on their designs and uses. Nevertheless, if the results are carefully analyzed, it becomes clear that significant mandibular re-

sponse is found mainly in a limited range of facial patterns and that, in many instances, unfavorable sequelae involving the dentoalveolar and maxillary components are concomitant side effects.

From the standpoint of anchorage and future stability, these untoward implications are not desirable; they may even be counterproductive regarding profile improvement. In none of the reports has condylar adaptation been of such magnitude that it could account for all or even most of the skeletal Class II correction. The scheme in Fig. 8-14 was and still is an unrealistic concept. The additional horizontal displacement of the mandible indicated manifestly exceeds the documented amount. Concurrent unaffected maxillary dentoalveolar and skeletal displacement could not be shown so far, nor could it rationally be expected after the appli-

*References 42, 74, 78, 93-95, 114, 115.
†References 20, 35, 39, 45, 53, 63, 64, 71, 72, 115, 126, 135, 140.
‡References 13-15, 37, 38, 46, 71-73, 81, 91, 92, 110.

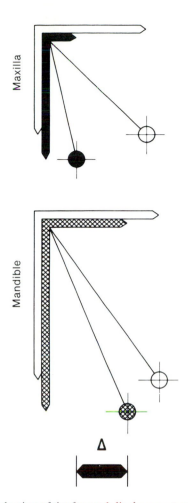

Fig. 8-15 Reduction of the forward displacement component of maxillary skeletal and/or dentoalveolar structures (*black horizontal;* compare with average *white* vector). This is a realistic therapeutic possibility that can be brought about with functional jaw orthopedic appliances, and more effectively with extra-oral forces. In many instances, however, rotational and elongating reactions of the maxilla and upper alveolar structures create additional vertical demands (*black vertical;* compare with *white* vector). Thus the mandible is forced to an opening rotation (*crosshatched*). *The sagittal gain in the maxillary structures thereby dilutes the overall result by promoting a sagittal loss in mandibular position.*

cation of an intermaxillary anchorage system. Fig. 8-14 expresses nothing more than wishful thinking and an unfulfilled orthodontic dream.

A more realistic orthopedic possibility to increase the difference in anterior growth expression between mandible and maxilla is the reduction of the forward vector of maxillary displacement (Fig. 8-15). The efficiency of posteriorly directed maxillary orthopedics has been reported in many animal experiments* and in clinical investigations.† With

*References 27, 40, 41, 47, 83, 113.

†References 1, 5, 7, 13, 15-19, 30, 34, 36, 48, 49, 60, 66, 69, 70, 82, 84-86, 99, 102, 104, 106, 128, 132-134.

activator treatment and, more effectively, with headgear treatment forward maxillary displacement can be influenced significantly. Dramatic S-N-A reductions accomplished through cervical pull on the upper arch can be demonstrated (Figs. 8-16, *A,* and 8-17). A major component of this effect is the posterior rotation* of the maxilla, probably because the sutures are predominantly exposed to shear and tensile forces. The rotational and elongating reactions of the maxilla, especially the anterior alveolar process, however, create additional vertical demands so the mandible on its part is forced to a posterior rotation (Fig. 8-16, *B*). Sagittal gain in the maxillary complex thereby dilutes the overall result by promoting a sagittal loss in mandibular position (Figs. 8-15 and 8-17). The difference in anterior displacement between the maxilla and mandible has nevertheless been increased, thus contributing to a Class II correction (bottom of Fig. 8-15). However, the profile lacks the improvement that natural advancement of the mandibular symphysis would have provided had it not been deflected downward or even backward. The question arises whether the vertical side effects could be so controlled that natural undisturbed mandibular growth would contribute fully to correction of anteroposterior jaw discrepancy. This idea is demonstrated in Fig. 8-18. The vertical component of skeletal and dentoalveolar maxillary displacement is not intensified despite the reduction of the forward component. The mandibular growth vector follows its natural path. Thus the principle of preservation of the contributing growth factors for Class II correction is respected, and therapy is no longer burdened with adverse treatment effects.

This is the basic premise envisioned in the treatment concept to be presented.[118,120] The difference in anterior displacement between the upper and lower jaws (Fig. 8-18, *bottom*) is substantially enlarged in comparison to that shown in Fig. 8-15. Carrying the idea still further, efficacy could be increased if not only the anterior but also the vertical component of maxillary displacement were diminished (Fig. 8-19). Because of autorotation, the mandibular symphysis would then reach a position even further forward than the natural growth path could have accomplished.

If a hyperpropulsive device could indeed produce an additional component of forward mandibular growth displacement, this *plus* might be added to the model just discussed (Fig. 8-20). The sum of these factors—vertical and sagittal

*In the description of rotational influences and effects the following terms are used in this chapter: *posterior rotation* (i.e., clockwise) means downward in front, and *anterior rotation* (i.e., counterclockwise) means upward in front. Clockwise and counterclockwise apply to cephalometric tracings that face to the right. In addition, for the mandibular symphysis, *downward and backward* or *opening* and *upward and forward* or *closing* are used synonymously. We agree entirely with the view that clinical terminology should be based on the subject not the viewer, so succinctly expressed in "Does the Clock on the Other Side of the Tower Run Counterclockwise?" (Thurow R: *Angle Orthod* 52:174, 1982). We are aware that the expressions *posterior rotation* and *anterior rotation* are not perfect either, but since they are universally employed in the orthodontic literature, no new suggestions are made.

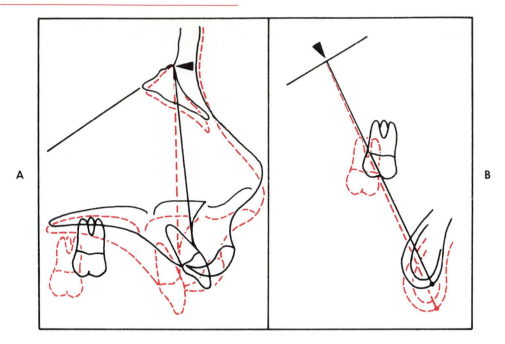

Fig. 8-16 Clinical example related to Fig. 8-15. Note the dramatic change in maxillary position, **A,** after cervical headgear application. However, rotational and elongating components produce a more vertical displacement of the mandibular symphysis, **B.** (From Ricketts RM et al: *Biopro-gressive therapy,* Denver, 1979, Rocky Mountain/Orthodontics.)

reduction of maxillary displacement, autorotation, and increased forward displacement of the mandible—would then culminate in an efficient concept for correcting skeletal Class II discrepancies. Not only would arrangement of teeth and coordination of the upper and lower arches be envisaged but an optimal balance of the bony framework of the face would also result. This balance should not be reached by a rotational orthopedic effect on the maxilla; rather the forward mandibular growth displacement should be enhanced.

BIOMECHANICAL ASPECTS

The prescription in orthodontics is force application. The mechanical influence of the appliances produces a reaction in the biologic system under stress. Local response can be anticipated in the affected tissue areas; and during the growing period, growth dynamics may also be modified. The quantity of force can be controlled rather well. However, exact prediction of the tissue response and the growth behavior in an individual case is highly speculative. It is therefore mandatory to monitor the mechanics according to the reactions observed at each treatment visit—and each time the question must be asked whether the intermediate treatment response is such that the final goal is being approached along the straightest possible line.

Since force is the treatment agent, it is imperative to master the fundamentals of biomechanics.* (See also Chap-

*References 31, 33, 51, 87, 88, 100, 101, 117, 131, 141.

ters 2, 3, and 4.) The design of the force system predetermines the general direction in which a tooth, group of teeth, or skeletal unit responds. The combination of force vectors, couples, and moment/force ratios applied is the means by which the operator strives for the reactions desired in the treatment plan.

The center of resistance of the unit or units to be moved is the basic point of consideration for the arrangement of a force system. Applying a simple force through the center of resistance will lead to a pure translatory movement along the force vector (Fig. 8-21). No rotation will occur because the center of rotation is at infinity. The location of the center of resistance of a biologic entity cannot be exactly determined in advance and furthermore is subject to alteration by tissue and other factors. Only careful observation of the reaction helps the operator modify the force system accordingly. If the force vector runs eccentrically to the center of resistance, a combined translatory and rotational movement will occur. The amount of rotational effect will depend on the distance of the force vector at a right angle from the center of resistance (Fig. 8-22). An inversely proportionate relationship exists; therefore placing the force vector closer to the center of resistance will move the center of rotation, in this example, toward the apex of the tooth and finally to infinity as in the situation depicted in Fig. 8-21. However, if the force vector is placed further away from the center of resistance, the center of rotation will approach and finally become identical with it. Then only rotation will occur, the same as if a pure moment (a couple) were placed anywhere

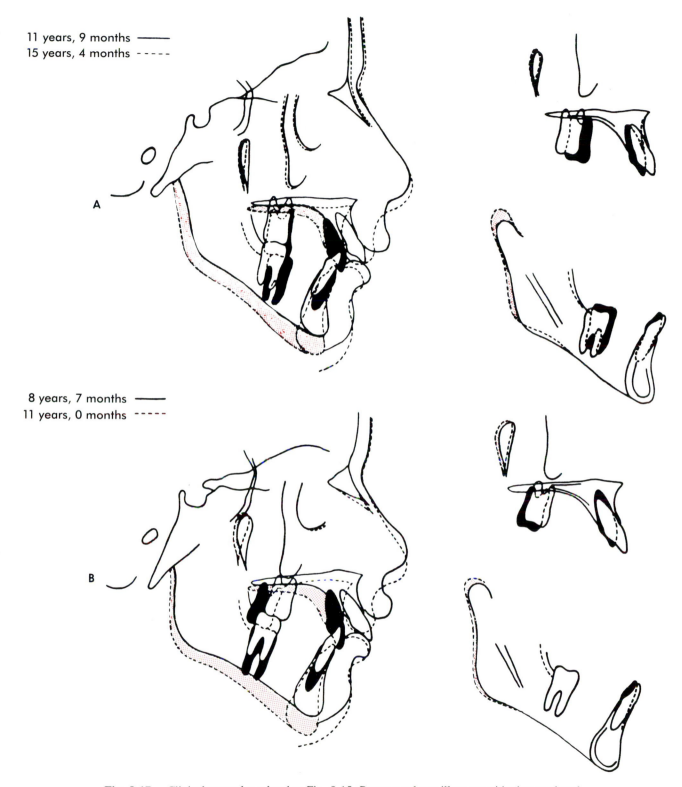

11 years, 9 months ———
15 years, 4 months - - - -

8 years, 7 months ———
11 years, 0 months - - - -

A

B

Fig. 8-17   Clinical examples related to Fig. 8-15. Pronounced maxillary repositioning produced with cervical headgear therapy in an extraction, **A,** and a nonextraction, **B,** case. Note the downward deflection and absent forward component of the mandibular symphysis displacement. (From Meikle MC: *Am J Orthod* 77:184, 1980.)

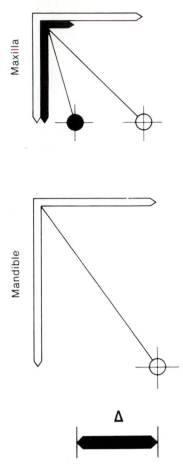

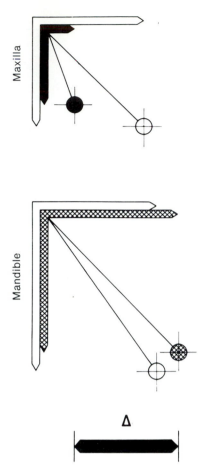

Fig. 8-18 Reduction of the anterior skeletal and/or dentoalveolar displacement of the maxilla without intensifying the vertical displacement vector *(black)*. The undisturbed displacement of the mandibular symphysis follows its natural path *(white)*. The difference (Δ) of forward displacement between the upper and lower jaws is significantly enlarged compared to that in Fig. 8-15. The principle of preservation of the contributing growth factors for Class II correction is respected. This is the basic premise envisioned in the treatment concept to be presented.

Fig. 8-19 The efficacy of skeletal Class II treatment could theoretically be increased if not only the sagittal but also the vertical vector of maxillary displacement could be decreased *(black)*. Mandibular autorotation *(crosshatched)* would, in addition, contribute to improvement of the bony profile.

on the tooth. Since the kind of reaction to an applied force system is so strongly dependent on the site of the center of resistance, it is of paramount importance to estimate where its location will be. This also applies when several dental units are to be influenced in combination. Fig. 8-23 demonstrates the estimated position of the center of resistance derived from clinical experience in a utility arch setup and when all teeth in front of the 6-year molars are included.

It is reasonable to postulate that the nasomaxillary complex, suspended as it is by a sutural system comparable to the desmodontal system of a tooth, possesses a center of resistance.[88,117,118] According to observed clinical reactions the location must be somewhere in the area of the posterosuperior aspect of the zygomaticomaxillary suture (Fig. 8-24). The prognosis of reaction, as far as the direction is concerned, can be made analogously as for a single tooth

(Figs. 8-21 and 8-22). Since the handle for applying force to the maxilla is the teeth, a given force vector must be analyzed relative to the center of resistance of the dental units, as well as to the center of resistance of the skeletal unit. If no rotational effect ensues in either one, then the force vector must be passing through both centers of resistance and therefore is exactly defined in direction (Fig. 8-25).

When planning the direction in which the dental and skeletal units should move to approach a given treatment goal, the operator must consider the effects of growth on the displacement of these structures. The force vector and the growth vector together determine the resultant vector of spatial displacement (Fig. 8-26).

In clinically relevant examples of headgear application, the reactive vectors of the dental and maxillary units, as well as the growth vector, were analyzed[123] (Fig. 8-27). As a first step the relation of the force vector applied to the center of resistance of the stabilized upper arch and the center of resistance of the maxilla was established. Knowl-

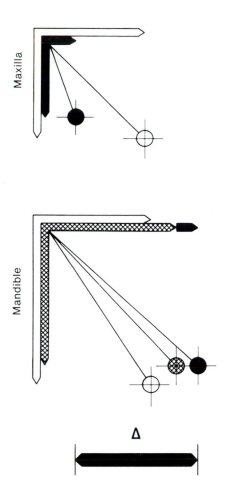

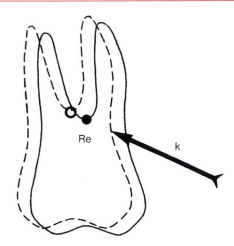

Fig. 8-21 Approximate center of resistance of an upper molar *(Re)*. If a force vector *(k)* passes through the center of resistance, translatory (bodily) movement of the tooth occurs in the direction of the force vector. The center of rotation is at infinity.

Fig. 8-20 If a hyperpropulsive device could indeed produce an additional component of forward mandibular growth displacement, this plus (*black* on the mandibular horizontal component) could be added to the models of Figs. 8-18 or 8-19. (The difference (Δ) of forward displacement would thereby be significantly enlarged despite the fact that the length of the additional component would by far not reach the effect shown in Fig. 8-14.)

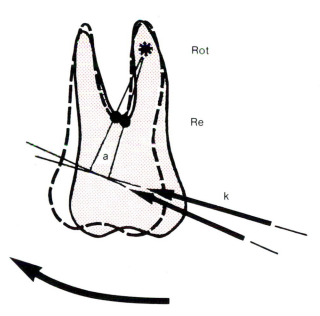

edge of the distances from each of them permitted the approximate location of the centers of rotation to be determined for both the upper arch and the maxilla (Fig. 8-27, *A*). The reactive displacement path of any given point of the dental arch can be determined from the two centers of rotation with a pair of compasses. When the growth vector is included, the resultant displacement vector can be deducted by vector addition (Fig. 8-27, *B*). Of course, localization of the center of resistance, and particularly the center of rotation, for each unit is approximate at best. Also the exact direction and length of the vectors cannot be determined because they vary according to, among other factors, the amount and duration of force application and the tissue response (on the one hand) and the pattern, intensity, and length of the growth period under consideration (on the other).

Although some simplifications are inherent, the models

Fig. 8-22 Eccentric force vector *(k)*. The distance *(a,* at right angle to the vector) from the center of resistance *(Re)* will determine the center of rotation *(Rot)*. An inversely proportionate relationship exists: placing the force vector closer to the center of resistance will move the center of rotation toward infinity (see Fig. 8-21); placing it further away will move the center of rotation closer to the center of resistance; finally, with the force vector at infinity a pure rotation at *Re* will occur as if a couple has been applied. If a force vector does not pass through *Re* (pure translation) or at infinity (pure rotation), a combined translatory and rotational movement will be induced.

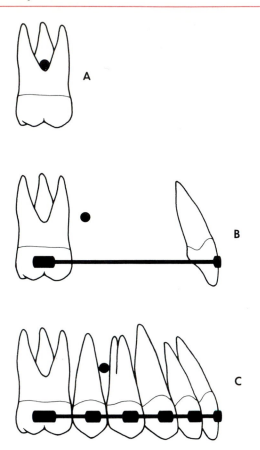

Fig. 8-23 Approximate centers of resistance *(black dots)* of an upper first molar; **A,** a utility arch setup, **B;** and an upper arch with full mixed appliance, **C.**

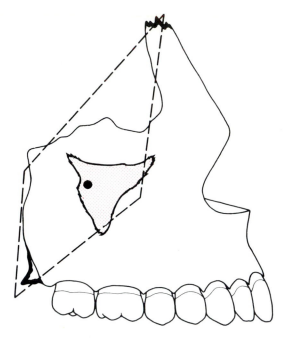

Fig. 8-24 Approximate center of resistance *(black dot)* of the maxilla in the area of the posterosuperior aspect of the zygomaticomaxillary suture.

in Fig. 8-27 nevertheless indicate the overall reaction that can be expected in average clinical application. The tendency toward extrusion or intrusion in the molar and incisal area will be determined by the direction of the force vector and notably by the rotational effects deriving from the relations of the force vector to both centers of resistance. It is, furthermore, demonstrated that the rotation of the maxilla and dental arch can be varied so that, in the setup of Fig. 8-27, *A* and *D,* posterior rotation for both and, in Fig. 8-27, *C* and *E,* posterior rotation for the maxilla but anterior rotation for the upper dental arch will result. In the examples presented, the change of the occlusal plane deriving from the vertical and rotational effects is most relevant. It can readily be seen that the least vertical and rotational change is obtained in an arrangement wherein the applied force vector passes between the centers of resistance of the upper arch and maxilla in an upward and backward direction (Fig. 8-27, *E*). This is therefore the preferred setup for optimal vertical control. It would be desirable to establish an arrangement that placed the applied force vector through the centers of resistance of both the upper arch and the maxilla (Fig. 8-25), but so far it has not been possible to construct a stable yet acceptable headcap for anchoring such a steep

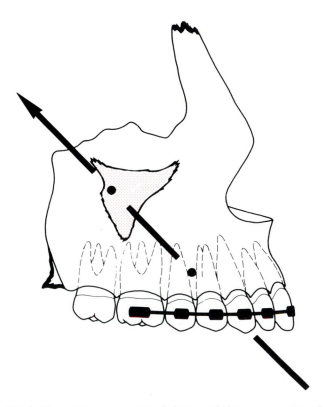

Fig. 8-25 A force vector *(black dots)* would have to pass through the center of resistance of the dentition and through the center of resistance of the maxilla if no rotational effects are to be induced.

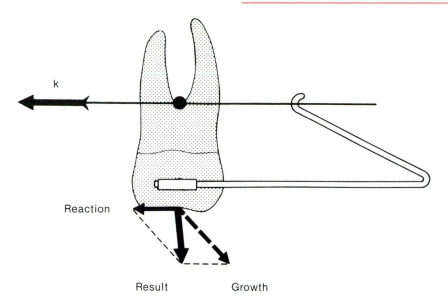

Fig. 8-26   The reaction to the force vector plus the growth vector will determine the resultant vector of spatial displacement. In this example the molar will move downward and even slightly forward despite the distally oriented force vector *(k)*.

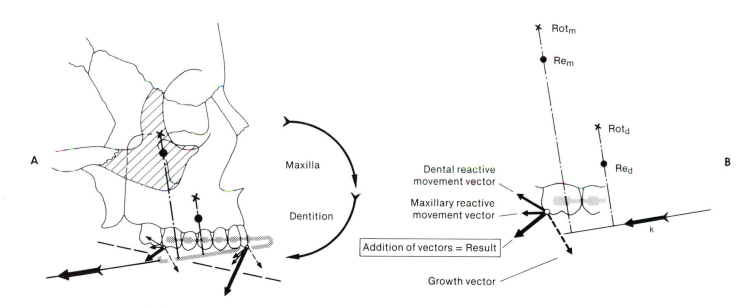

Fig. 8-27   Analysis of the reaction to different applications of extraoral force vectors. In all cases the dentition is stabilized with an edgewise archwire including all dental units mesial to the first permanent molars. **A,** Cervical pull, force vector inferior to both centers of resistance. The distances of the force vector to the centers of resistance of the dentition and maxilla *(black dot)* will determine the corresponding centers of rotation *(X)*. Small arrows indicate the reactive movement vectors of the dentition and maxilla; dashed arrows, the overall growth displacement vectors; and large black arrows, the resultant vectors at the particular points. **B,** Enlargement of the analysis for the distal cusp of an upper molar. Centers of resistance of the maxilla *(Re_m)* and dentition *(Re_d)*; corresponding centers of rotation *(Rot_m, Rot_d)*, depending on the direction and distance of the force vector *(k)* relative to Re_m and Re_d. By adding the derived movement vectors *(small black arrows)* and the growth vector *(dashed arrow)* one can obtain the resultant vector *(large arrow)* by vector addition. In *A* a posterior rotation of the maxilla and dentition must be anticipated. The incisor region will move inferiorly to a greater extent than will the molar region. Accordingly, the occlusal plane will rotate posteriorly *(dashed line)*.   *Continued.*

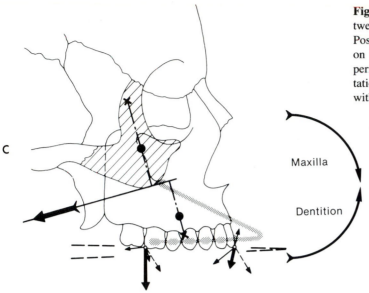

C

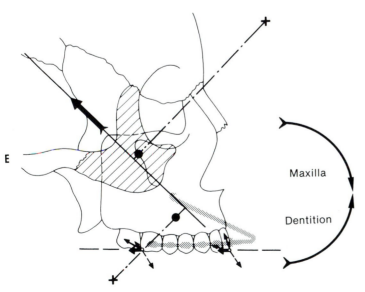

E

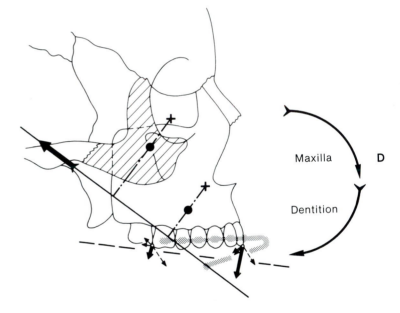

D

Fig. 8-27, cont'd **C,** Cervical pull, force vector passing between the centers of resistance of the maxilla and the dentition. Posterior rotational effect on the maxilla, anterior rotational effect on the dentition. Vector addition reveals that the molars will experience more downward influence than the incisors: anterior rotation of the occlusal plane. Excessive extrusive action is obvious with this setup.

D, Occipital pull, force vector inferior to both centers of resistance. Posterior rotational effect on the maxilla and dentition. The reactive movement vectors for the molars are intrusive but for the incisors are extrusive *(thin arrows)*. Posterior rotation of the occlusal plane.

E, Occipital pull, force vector passing between the centers of resistance of the maxilla and dentition at a very small distance from each. Overall, a small amount of posterior rotation of the maxilla and a slightly greater amount of anterior rotation of the dentition will result. In a particular setup each can neutralize the other. In this case vector addition reveals no extrusion in the incisor or molar region. Vertical control is optimal. The occlusal plane will experience no or only a slight anterior rotational effect.

Curved arrows in **A, C, D,** and **E** indicate the direction (but not the amount) of the rotational effects on the dentition and maxilla to be expected in the setup.

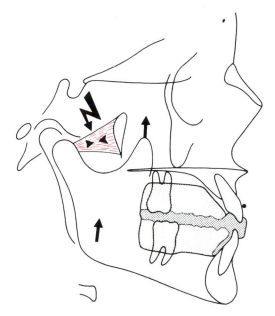

Fig. 8-28 Theory of pure neuromuscular response. Reminder effect of the appliance: the lateral pterygoid muscle by increased activity secures the forward posture of the mandible. No retractive forces would be transmitted to the anchoring structures.

force vector. The shape of the posterosuperior part of the calvarium will, therefore, be a limiting factor governing the maximum slope of the force vector that can be obtained in an individual case.

Another biomechanical consideration deals with the effects that derive from actively dislocating the mandible. Clinical and experimental observations suggest that dislocation of the condyle downward and forward out of the fossa for a prolonged period is necessary if an adaptive condylar response, in direction or even in amount, contributing to Class II correction is to be initiated. The degree of mandibular displacement is determined with a construction

bite and then maintained with a correspondingly fashioned intermaxillary device. This is the common denominator of all functional jaw orthopedic appliances,[50,52,59,80] including the Herbst appliance[90] for Class II correction. The forced forward positioning of the mandible strains the soft tissue and, above all, the muscles involved in anchoring the lower jaw to the head and neck. In a simplified interpretation, two basic patterns of reaction can be identified when the relevant literature* is reviewed: one is a neuromuscular response; the other is related to elastic properties of muscles:

1. The neuromuscular response can lead to an adaptive change in postural activity. According to this view the appliance serves only to remind the muscles to maintain the mandible in the dictated position. After a short period of adaptation the lateral pterygoid muscle, particularly the superior head, secures the forward posture by sustained increased activity (Fig. 8-28). In monkey experiments with a propulsive mandibular appliance it has been demonstrated electromyographically by Mc-Namara[74,76] that indeed lateral pterygoid activity is increased, not only during movement of the lower jaw but also during postural maintenance over a prolonged period of observation (Fig. 8-29). If this pattern of neuromuscular response prevailed, then no or almost no retractive force would be transmitted to the appliance and from there to the anchoring structures.

2. On the other hand, the forward and downward positioning of the mandible affects the length-tension relationship of the musculature involved.[3] Stretching an unstimulated skeletal muscle will increase the tension exponentially because of its elastic properties (passive tension, Fig. 8-30). When, in addition, the muscle is stimulated, the total tension resulting can be measured. A slight decline will be observed if, by further stretching, the resting length of the muscle is exceeded. This effect

*References 2-4, 6, 43, 44, 74, 75, 76, 84, 724, 738, 739, 772.

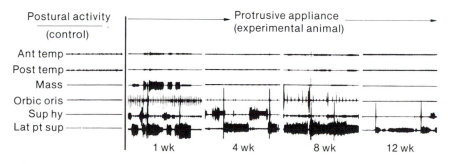

Fig. 8-29 Change in postural muscle activity after insertion of a protrusive appliance in the monkey. Electromyographic recordings of an animal anesthetized with ketamine (which exerts only minor and transitory effects on the neuromusculature). Note the increased activity in the superior head of the lateral pterygoid muscle *(Lat pt sup)* over a prolonged period. No decrease is observed before 12 weeks. (From McNamara JA Jr: *Monograph 1, Craniofacial growth series,* Ann Arbor, 1972, Center for Human Growth and Development, University of Michigan.)

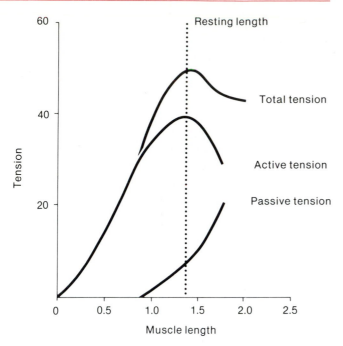

Fig. 8-30 Effect of increased muscle length on tension. Stretching an unstimulated skeletal muscle will increase its tension exponentially because of its elastic properties (passive tension). In a stimulated muscle (tonic reflex contraction) a decline in maximal tension will be observed when the resting length is passed (active tension). The two components will determine the total tension. (From Report to the NRC Committee on Artificial Limbs: *Fundamental studies of human locomotion and other information relating to design of artificial limbs*, University of California, Berkeley, 1947, vol 2; see also Ahlgren J.[3])

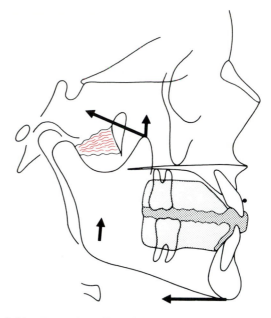

Fig. 8-31 Retracting effect of the posterior part of the temporal and suprahyoid muscles after forced forward positioning of the mandible. The forces are transmitted to the appliance and from there to the anchoring structures.

is caused by the pronounced decrease in active tension—the difference between total and passive tension. The active tension elicits a tonic reflex contraction; however, the increased tonus is dependent on whether the individual is awake or in light sleep or deep sleep. In any case, tension of the muscles, whether elastic only or augmented by tonic reflex contraction, is transmitted to the appliance unless offset by neuromuscular adaptation. The latter can be expected only when the individual is awake.

Clinical results after Class II treatment with jaw orthopedic appliances document a strong anteroposterior influence on the upper and lower dentition and on the upper jaw (decreased S-N-A angle). It is therefore reasonable to assume that the elastic properties of muscles play a dominant role,[142,143] particularly the retracting effects of the posterior part of the temporalis and the suprahyoid (Fig. 8-31). These obviously overpower the possible compensatory postural maintenance activity of the lateral pterygoid in most instances. This is not to say, however, that postural activity does not play a significant role. A broad spectrum of differences in muscular response can be found depending on

the type of appliance, especially between daytime and nighttime wear. In many cases it is obvious that a positional adaptation does indeed take place during Class II treatment with functional jaw orthopedic appliances; however, the tendency to function in a forward mandibular position does not guarantee that structural adaptation will follow spontaneously. Severe centric relation–habitual occlusion discrepancies may be observed in the form of dual bite, succinctly termed *Sunday bites*. They may disappear shortly after appliance removal, or they may persist in some instances. Either aftermath is detrimental.

The biomechanical implications of placing a functional jaw orthopedic appliance for Class II correction, with consequent increased tension in the elevator, and particularly in the retractor muscles, must be taken into account. The resultant force vector will be positioned inferior and posterior to the center of resistance of the upper dentition and maxilla (Fig. 8-32, *A*). A similar relation will result as in the specific headgear arrangement of Fig. 8-27, *D*. Admittedly, the lengths of the muscular vectors are an estimation at best. They certainly vary from individual to individual and may vary in the same individual. However, even by optimistic manipulation of the vectors—lengthening the advantageous and shortening the disadvantageous—the clinician will not improve the resultant force vector substantially if the frame of biologic limitations is respected.

Investigations of dentoalveolar and maxillary reactions after treatment with functional jaw orthopedic appliances generally substantiate the assumption that the estimated resultant force vector in Fig. 8-32, *A*, represents the actual

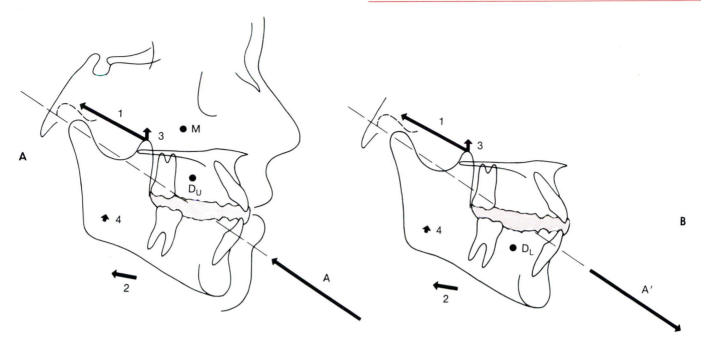

Fig. 8-32   A, Resultant force vector *(A)*, by vector addition of the retracting force vectors (*1* and *2*) (posterior part of the temporal and suprahyoid muscles) and of the force vectors of the adductors (*3* and *4*) (middle part of the temporal and masseter-medial pterygoid muscles). Vector *A* is directed posterosuperiorly and passes inferiorly to the centers of resistance of the upper dentition *(D$_U$)* and maxilla *(M)*. A similar relationship is established as depicted in Fig. 8-27, *D*. **B,** On the mandibular structures force vector *A'*, of the same length as vector *A* but in an opposite direction, will be created. It passes superiorly to the center of resistance of the lower dentition *(D$_L$)*.

situation quite closely. With insertion of a splint-type Class II activator covering all occlusal surfaces, the eccentric force vector will place the greatest stress on the maxillary molars and the lower incisors. According to the relationship of the force vector to the center of resistance of the upper dentition, a backward tipping of the dental units and a posterior rotation of the dentition will result. The rotational effect can be compared to the pattern analyzed in Fig. 8-27, *D*. Lingual tipping and extrusion of the upper incisors are likely to occur. Relative to the center of resistance of the maxilla, the force vector is even more eccentric; thus additional posterior rotation of the palatal plane with an increased downward movement of the anterior nasal spine is observed in many cases of activator-only treatment. The indicated force vector acts in the opposite direction on the mandibular dentition (Fig. 8-32, *B*). The anteriorly oriented component would tip the dental units forward. This does indeed occur if anchorage is not extended to the lingual part of the alveolar process. However, the rotational effect cannot be fully controlled and may result in, among other sequelae, protrusion of the lower incisors.

Examples demonstrating some of the consequences described when Class II treatment with activator only is performed are shown in Fig. 8-33. When adding the reactions to the created force vector, the practitioner can expect correction of the Class II intercuspation and reduction of the

overjet. However, the accompanying posteriorly rotating components demand vertical dimension; thus even if some stimulation in the condylar cartilage has been initiated, the spatial consequence is nevertheless a predominantly downward movement of the symphysis. Increased anterior face height and lack of profile improvement must be anticipated as a possible consequence. Of course, the basic growth pattern will determine whether these untoward influences can be at least partly absorbed or whether they will lead to a severe deterioration. The efficiency of correcting a Class II intercuspation mainly by posterior rotation of the occlusal plane can be intensified by increasing the vertical height of the intermaxillary bite block.[52] As a result the force vector will be placed even more eccentrically (Fig. 8-34). With this concept of raising the bite as much as 8 to 12 mm, however, the accentuated rotational effects of the dentition will intensify downward skeletal deflection (Fig. 8-15). This treatment approach is diametrically opposed to the objectives that should be realized according to the discussion presented in the first part of this chapter.

APPLIANCE DESIGN

In 1968, at our clinic, we started to combine activator treatment with a cervical headgear attached to the upper molars. Hasund[54] reported in 1969 on his results achieved with a similar procedure. Pfeiffer and Grobéty[96] also used this approach and refined the combined orthopedic concept further to better cope with the demands of differential diagnosis.[97,98] Since 1975 we have attached the facebow directly to the activator and applied occipital traction to

achieve better vertical and rotational control during orthopedic Class II treatment.[118,120] At that time Thurow[125] presented his approach with a removable acrylic splint in the upper arch to obtain en masse dental control. A facebow was directly incorporated and occipital pull applied to restrain downward and forward displacement of the maxillary complex. Bass[8-10] also used an upper plate but attached a J-hook headgear to helices of an incisal torque mechanism. Later he extended the appliance to achieve additional forward mandibular displacement.

The appliance to be presented for skeletal Class II treatment consists of an activator with an attached headgear (Fig. 8-35). The mere combination of these two appliances does not in itself warrant a treatment approach respecting the principles outlined up to this point. On the contrary, combination of the two elements increases also the potential for mistreatment. It is imperative to understand the basic growth and displacement dynamics of the facial skeleton and of the dentoalveolar processes, as well as the effects of biomechanical influences on these structures. Appreciation of the neuromuscular and soft tissue involvement is also required, however limited the present understanding in this respect still is.

The prime target of the treatment concept employing the activator headgear combination is to restrict developmental contributions that tend toward a skeletal Class II and to

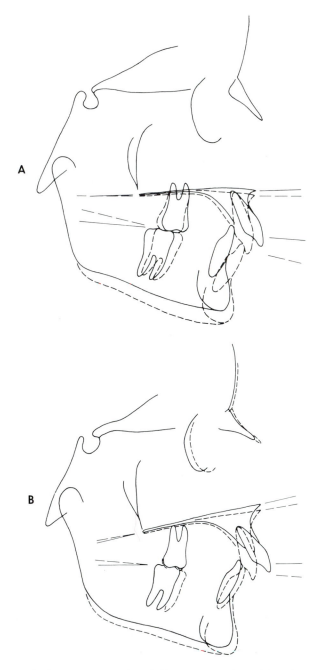

Fig. 8-33 Two examples of Class II correction with activator-only treatment: posterior rotation of the nasal line and occlusal plane, *S-N-A* reduction, retrusion of the upper incisors, protrusion of the lower incisors. In **A** the posterior rotation of the occlusal plane is more pronounced than in **B.** As a consequence the mandibular symphysis is displaced more downward than forward. In **B** ample condylar growth has probably compensated for the untoward vertical effects so the Y-axis was not opened.

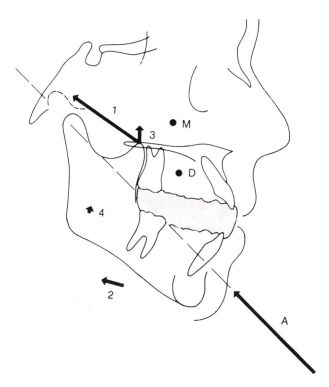

Fig. 8-34 Effect of increasing the vertical dimension of the bite block. Force vector A will pass more eccentrically relative to the centers of resistance of the upper dentition *(D)* and maxilla *(M)* than in the situation shown in Fig. 8-32. The rotational effects and downward skeletal deflection will be intensified.

enhance developmental contributions that tend to harmonize the anteroposterior relations of maxillomandibular structures. It is of paramount concern that no untoward deflections of growth-displacement vectors be introduced (Figs. 8-5 and 8-15) when a treatment device is used to influence facial growth.

Maxillary component

The following influences should be exerted on the maxillary complex (Fig. 8-36):

1. Inhibitory control of the sagittal and vertical growth vectors of the dentoalveolar process and dentition
2. Restraint on the basal structures counter to the line of displacement

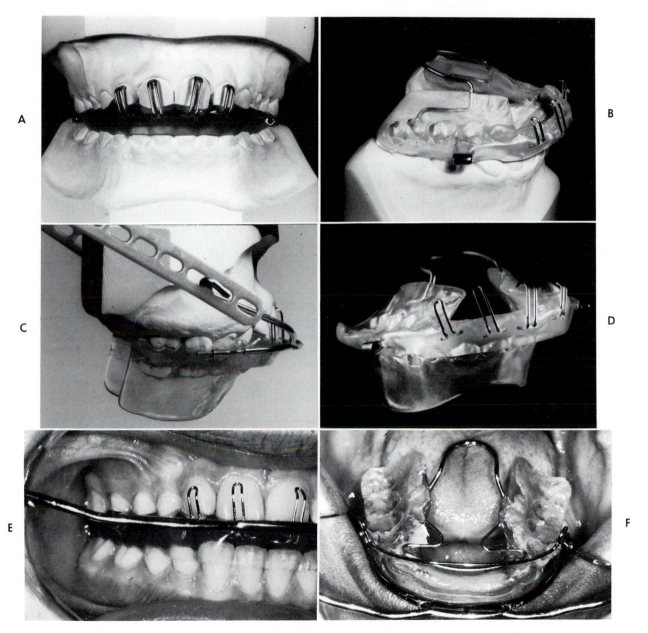

Fig. 8-35 The activator headgear appliance along with extraoral arrangements. **A,** Vestibular extension and torquing springs. **B,** Appliance placed on the lower cast; note the upper front area, with torquing springs, palatal extension of the acrylic, and a transpalatal wire. **C,** Appliance placed on the upper cast and facebow inserted; note the lower lingual extension. **D,** Splint-type activator. **E,** Activator facebow combination in situ. **F,** Activator facebow combination in situ on the lower arch with the mouth opened; note the relationship of the tongue to the transpalatal wire. In this activator the combination of lingual and labial wire for the upper front teeth instead of torquing springs is shown.

Continued.

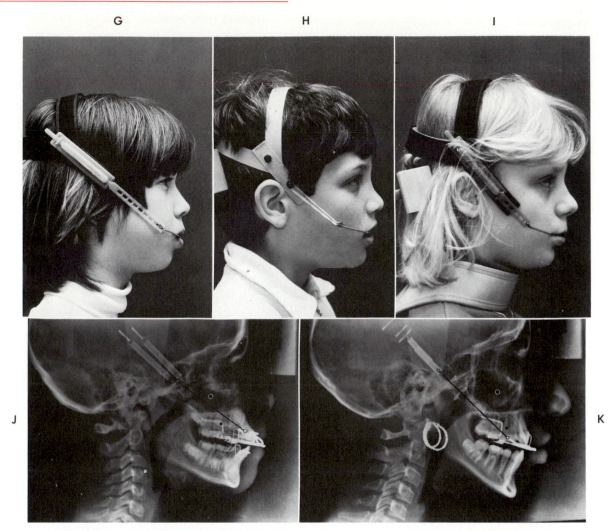

Fig. 8-35, cont'd **G,** Anteriorly placed force vector, estimated in this case to pass just inferior to the center of resistance of the maxilla. Some anterior rotation of the dentition must be anticipated. Requires ample condylar growth for compensation. **H,** Average steepness of the force vector, estimated in this case to pass slightly superior of the center of resistance of the upper dentition. The amount of posterior rotational effect of the maxilla and of anterior rotational effect on the dentition should so neutralize each other that no change in inclination of the occlusal plane is expected. **I,** Posteriorly placed force vector, estimated in this case to pass just inferior to the center of resistance of the dentition. Posterior rotation of the maxilla and dentition must be anticipated. This setup is used in patients with an open bite tendency or if the prognosis for condylar growth is poor. **J** and **K,** Cephalometric check of the relationship of the force vector *(line connecting circle at end of outer arms of facebow and circle at springs of head cap)* to the centers of resistance of the maxilla *(white circle)* and upper dentition *(black dot)*.

The clinical situations: **J** is comparable to the scheme in Fig. 8-27, *E,* and **K** to the scheme in Fig. 8-27, *D.*

Ideally these influences should be exerted with no rotational side effects. A force vector will be required that passes through the centers of resistance of both the upper dentition and the maxilla (Fig. 8-25). Such a steep force vector cannot be realized because of instability of the head cap. The arrangement that approximates the requirement of least rotational effects and still is acceptable in clinical use places the force vector between the two centers of resistance (Figs. 8-27, *E,* and 8-35, *J*). In this way the rotational effects neutralize each other so the cant of the occlusal plane is kept unaltered. The classical time for Class II treatment with the activator headgear assembly is in the period of the mixed dentition when all deciduous teeth in the buccal segment are still firmly anchored. The magnitude of the extra-oral

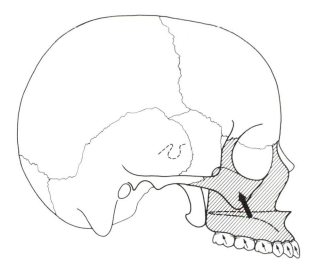

Fig. 8-36   Idealization of the intended influence on maxillary structures.

force should not exceed 300 g* per side. (For variations see pp. 473, 475, and 476.) In some Class II malocclusions, however, tipping of the occlusal plane is part of the treatment plan. The force vector must then be modified accordingly (Figs. 8-27, *D,* and 8-35, *K*). (See under "Biomechanical Aspects," p. 444.)

Anchorage in the maxillary arch is secured by the upper part of the appliance, which embraces with its acrylic replica relief all occlusal and incisal surfaces of the teeth (Figs. 8-35, *B* and *C,* and 8-37, *A* and *B*). The acrylic extends laterally to the buccal cusps. In the canine and incisor region about 2 mm is covered on the vestibular surface of the crowns. On the lingual side about 3.5 mm of acrylic support is provided for the incisor crowns (Figs. 8-35, *B,* 8-37, *A* and *B,* and 8-38, *A*). In the buccal segment from the mesial

---

*Grams are used to indicate amounts of force (31 g = 1 oz). In fact, they are units for measuring mass. The correct units for measuring force would be newtons (1 N = 1 m · kg · s⁻²). However, it has been decided to use the physical terms with which orthodontists are familiar (in spite of the fact that they are incorrect!).

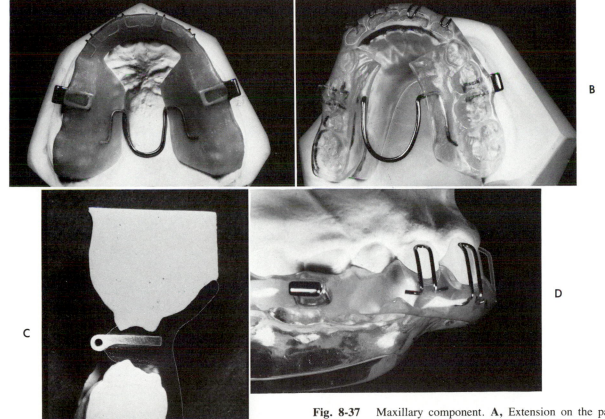

Fig. 8-37   Maxillary component. **A,** Extension on the palatal side. Placement of headgear tubes and palatal wire; retention area of torquing springs. **B,** Occlusal and incisal replica relief of the upper teeth. **C,** Interocclusal placement of the headgear tube. **D,** Design and position of the torquing springs. Only the palatally curved tip should touch the crown immediately coronal to the gingival margin.

of the canine, the acrylic is extended toward the palatal vault. Instead of covering the entire palate across and forward up to the incisors, it is more comfortable for the patient if a transpalatal bar (1.2 mm in diameter) is used and the palate is kept free so as much room as possible remains for the tongue (Figs. 8-35, *F*, and 8-37, *B*). For linking the activator to the inner arch of the facebow a specially constructed tube* is fastened in the acrylic between the upper and lower arches. Vertically, it is placed closer to the upper teeth, since in this region no removal of the acrylic should be performed during treatment (Fig. 8-37, *C* and *D*). About 1 mm of acrylic between the occlusal surface of the upper tooth and the anchoring part of the tube should be provided so that no breakage occurs when the tube is stressed by extraoral forces. It has to be emphasized that the sagittal positioning of the tube is not critical in determination of the force vector that is to be applied to the system. For practical purposes the optimal placement is in the area between the first and second deciduous molars or premolars (Fig. 8-37, *A* and *B*). The dangers of distortion and breakage of the inner arch are thereby minimized. The inner arch of the facebow is closely adapted to the activator, almost touching the acrylic (Figs. 8-35, *C* and *F*, and 8-54, *A*).

With an activator headgear assembly it must be realized

*Microna P, Reinhard AG, Spreitenbach, Switzerland.

that the upper arch is not stabilized in the same manner as with a heavy edgewise archwire. The forces applied are transmitted eccentrically from the acrylic covering the occlusal and incisal portions of the teeth; thus bodily control is lacking. The posteriorly directed component of the recommended force vector (Figs. 8-27, *E*, and 8-35, *J*) therefore tends to tip the crowns backward. Combined with this individual tendency toward backward tipping is an anterior rotational effect exerted on the whole upper dentition, which persists as long as the force vector passes superior to the center of resistance of the upper dentition. The rotational effect is comparable to the situation of an upper arch stabilized with an edgewise archwire as demonstrated in Fig. 8-27, *E;* the rigid control of each tooth, however, is not provided in the activator headgear setup. To counteract this tendency of the crowns to backward tipping and to at least approximate the situation of a stabilized upper arch, a palatal root tipping force should be applied to the upper incisors. For this purpose torquing springs are fabricated of 0.5 or 0.6 mm resilient stainless steel wire. The lower part, with a horizontal leg on each side, is well embedded in the acrylic (Figs. 8-37, *A* and *D*, and 8-38, *A*). The vertical part must stay away from the acrylic so an optimal range of resiliency is obtained. Only the palatally curved tip should touch the crown immediately coronal to the gingival margin. It is essential that the tooth be well secured by the incisal acrylic

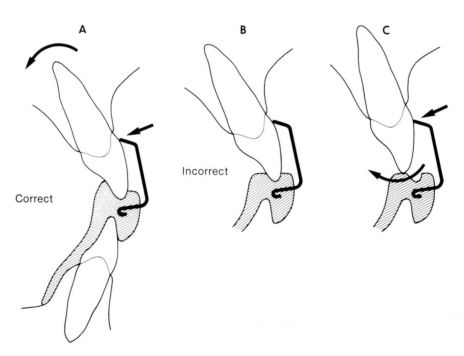

Fig. 8-38 **A,** Correct setup of a torquing spring: curved bend between the horizontal part (embedded in acrylic) and the vertical part (free of acrylic) to provide resiliency. The incisor must be well secured with acrylic on the palatal side. On the labial side about 1.5 to 2 mm of the crown is covered with acrylic. Note, in addition, the extension of the acrylic labial to the lower incisor and lingually along the lower alveolar process down to the floor of the mouth. **B,** Lacking palatal support for the upper incisor can lead to, **C,** lingual tipping of the crown if the torquing spring is activated.

extension, particularly on the palatal side; otherwise, the activated torquing springs can easily cause a palatal tipping of the crown rather than the root (Fig. 8-38). Another design of a torquing mechanism for removable appliances has been suggested by Bass.[8,9]

The torque control auxiliaries are used in the activator headgear combination to prevent lingual crown tipping of the incisors (Fig. 8-56) rather than to move the roots in a palatal direction. They serve therefore mainly to reinforce the anchorage. For this purpose a relatively rigid system is desired rather than a low-load, high-deflection mechanism. The amount of activation required depends on the axial inclination of the incisors at the start of treatment. If they are slightly procumbent, no preactivation is needed, since a force at the tip of the torquing auxiliary will be automatically introduced as soon as the crowns tend to tip lingually. If the axial inclination is correct initially, it is advisable to activate the springs moderately to maintain the ideal relationship. For an active torque mechanism, springs of 0.5 mm diameter are preferable. The upper limit of 1300 to 1500 g · mm* should not be exceeded. The force at the tip

---

*Grams (g) × Millimeters (mm).

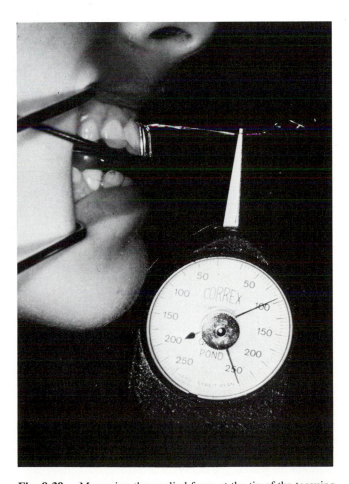

Fig. 8-39 Measuring the applied force at the tip of the torquing spring.

can be easily measured with a Corex instrument (Fig. 8-39). If 100 to 150 g is applied and the arm of the torquing spring is about 6 to 8 mm long, then enough axial control will be secured so long as the heargear force is kept within the limits of 300 to 400 g per side. It would be futile to try to change the axial inclination of initially too uprighted or even retroinclined upper incisors with a rigid type of torquing spring. When protrusion is required, the upper incisor region of the activator must be modified (p. 466). For more complex requirements, preparatory therapy with a utility arch is indicated.

The use of activated torquing springs in an activator-only concept is contraindicated. The force applied with the torquing springs would exert a posterior rotational effect on the activator (Fig. 8-41, *B*), and the inherent tendency of activator-only treatment to induce posterior rotation would be severely aggravated by this effect (Fig. 8-32, *A*), leading to extrusion of the incisors. It is mandatory therefore that activated torquing springs in general be combined with a posterior high pull headgear providing a force vector for vertical control of the upper incisors (Fig. 8-27, *E*). It is advisable to secure the inner arch of the facebow with little bends at the distal of the tubes so that it cannot be removed by the child (Fig. 8-54, *A*). Thus the temptation to wear the activator without headgear is prevented.

The torquing auxiliaries add another advantage to the system. As discussed earlier, the extraoral force vector should usually be placed between the centers of resistance of the maxilla and the upper dentition (Fig. 8-27, *E*). Since the muscular force vector deriving from mandibular advancement is located inferiorly to both centers of resistance (Fig. 8-32, *A*), the extraoral force vector should be placed closer to the center of resistance of the maxilla for compensation (Fig. 8-40). When this is done, however, a position is easily reached where the activator will be destabilized, as is the case if the force vector passes in front of the acrylic covering of the central incisors (Fig. 8-41, *A*). Thus the activator will be disengaged in the buccal segment. Addition of torquing springs can counteract this tendency (Fig. 8-41, *B*). By activation, occlusal pressure on the buccal segments can be exerted.

For checking clinically whether the optimal positioning of the extraoral force vector has been attained without destabilizing the appliance from the maxillary arch, the activator is placed in the mouth and the headgear hooked to the outer arms. Then the mouth is opened (Fig. 8-42). If the posterior part of the activator becomes disengaged, the force vector passes too far in front of the appliance (Fig. 8-43, *A*). Either the direction of the force vector must be adjusted by appropriate bending of the outer arms or, if so desired, the torquing springs must be activated accordingly. If disengagement in the incisor area occurs, the force vector is placed too far posteriorly (Fig. 8-43, *B*). In Fig. 8-43, *C*, a situation is depicted in which the appliance touches all occlusal surfaces. Whether in this instance the vertical pressure is the same in front as in the rear of the arch can be

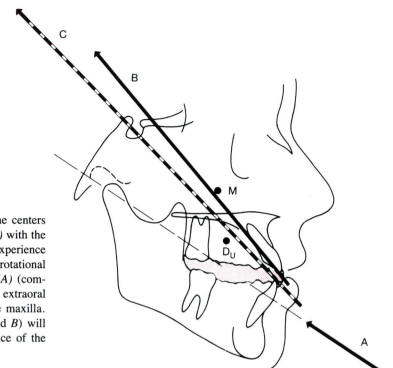

Fig. 8-40   Relationship of force vectors applied to the centers of resistance of the maxilla *(M)* and upper dentition *(D_U)* with the activator headgear appliance if the occlusal plane is to experience no posterior (and preferably no or only slight anterior) rotational effect. The distinctly eccentric muscular force vector *(A)* (compare Fig. 8-32, *A*) is compensated for by placing the extraoral force vector *(B)* close to the center of resistance of the maxilla. The resultant force vector *(C)* (vector addition of *A* and *B*) will thereby still be positioned above the center of resistance of the dentition *(D_U)*.

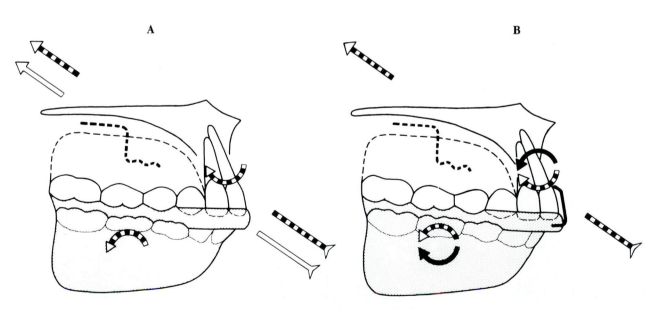

Fig. 8-41   **A,** In an attempt to place the extraoral force vector *(straight white arrow)* closer to the center of resistance of the maxilla *(straight broken arrow)*, the activator may be destabilized. More force will be dissipated on the incisor region the further superiorly the force vector is moved; if it passes above the acrylic edge of the incisor region *(straight broken arrow)*, the buccal area will disengage *(curved broken arrows)*. **B,** With torquing springs added, a countermoment can be exerted *(curved black arrows)* that restabilizes the activator. In general, the degree of activation of the torquing springs and the extraoral force vector will jointly determine the force distribution to the occlusal surfaces of the upper teeth.

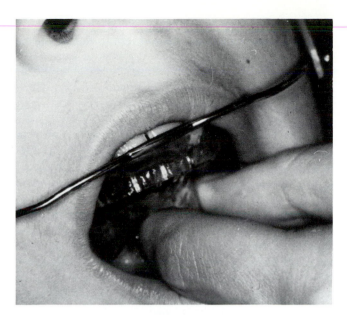

Fig. 8-42 Checking the force distribution to the upper arch clinically. The appliance is inserted, the outer arms adjusted, and the extraoral force applied; then the patient is asked to open. A pronounced disengagement in the frontal or molar region will be discerned immediately (compare Fig. 8-43). By differential pulling at the lower wings the approximate anteroposterior force distribution can be evaluated. A more precise method is to disengage the appliance slightly with a scaler first in the front and then in the molar region to feel the amount of pressure.

checked by slightly disengaging the appliance with a scaler first in the front and then in the molar region or by analogously pulling on the mandibular wings of the activator (Fig. 8-42). Whether a slight rotational component and in which direction—up in the front or up in the molar region—should be introduced depends on the treatment plan. Accordingly, a bite opening or bite closing action can be effected (Fig. 8-35, *J* and *K*). If the uppermost position of the force vector must be established, then the activator should barely touch the molars or even exhibit a slight tendency to disengage posteriorly. The closing muscles of the mandible will still provide a close fit of the appliance in the buccal segment.

Mandibular component

The operator strives to achieve four main objectives with the mandibular part of the appliance (Fig. 8-44):
1. Deblocking the occlusion
2. Selective vertical management of mandibular molar eruption
3. Stimulation and redirection of condylar growth
4. Inducing a less backward and more downward remodeling pattern of the glenoid fossae

The influence on the condyles and glenoid fossae should produce a more forward, structurally stable, mandibular position. The cardinal consideration is that the amount, as

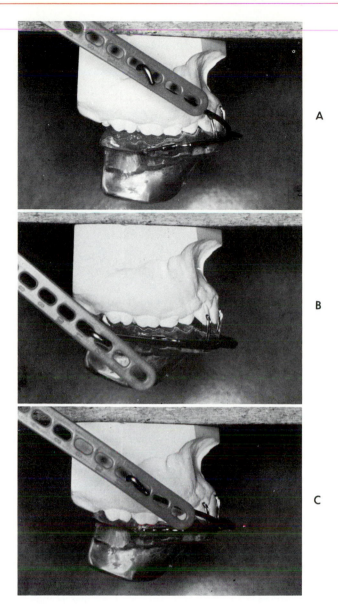

Fig. 8-43 **A,** Force vector applied too far anteriorly. Causes disengagement of the appliance in the buccal area. **B,** Force vector applied too far posteriorly. Causes disengagement in the frontal area. **C,** Force vector passing through the contact point of the lateral incisor and deciduous canine. The anteroposterior force distribution must be checked with a scaler.

well as the direction of mandibular symphysis displacement, contribute to the improvement of the bony profile. It is therefore of paramount importance that vertical development of the maxillary components and the mandibular alveolar structures is controlled at the same time (pp. 437 to 447).

Deblocking the occlusion seems to be an essential factor in Class II treatment. The studies of Tuenge and Elder[127] on monkeys have shown that posteriorly directed headgear forces applied to the upper arch are transmitted from the maxilla to the mandible through occlusal intercuspation,

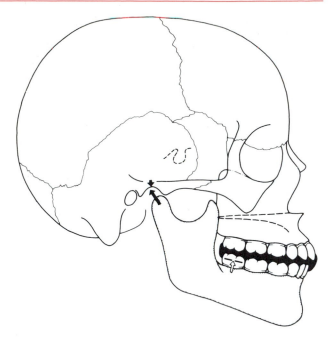

Fig. 8-44 Treatment objectives with a mandibular component of the activator headgear appliance.

causing the condyles to function dorsally to normal position. Resorptive activity in the posterior region of the condyles and mandibular necks and a posterior drift by remodeling of the glenoid fossae were found as adaptive processes. These reactions were comparable to those observed by Joho[65] after the application of a posteriorly directed headgear force to the mandible itself.

The therapeutic positioning of the mandible is determined by the operator with a wax registration bite, which serves to orient the casts for appliance construction (Fig. 8-45, *B*). The amount of sagittal and vertical mandibular displacement recommended in treatment concepts for Class II malocclusion with functional appliances varies widely among different authors.* In our concept we attempt neither an extreme vertical nor an extreme sagittal activation (Fig. 8-45). The bite should be opened slightly wider than the freeway space to obtain enough stretching of the adductor muscles. In most instances the interocclusal distance between the upper and lower permanent first molars should not be greater than 2 to 4 mm. Aside from the fact that too much opening is uncomfortable and, furthermore, a severe handicap to the maintenance of a competent lip seal, it is quite unfavorable from a biomechanical standpoint. As discussed earlier, the muscular force vector should not be placed more eccentrically than necessary (compare Figs. 8-32, *A*, and 8-34). On the other hand, sufficient acrylic resin between the upper and lower buccal segments and between the upper and lower incisors is needed for embedding the headgear tubes and the torquing springs or other auxiliaries.

---

*References 50, 52, 56, 57, 59, 111, 112.

The forward positioning of the mandible should not exceed 5 or 6 mm measured at the lower incisors. A Class I canine relationship is thus reached or approximated (Fig. 8-45, *B* and *D*). The more vertical the activation introduced, the less should be the sagittal. It cannot be argued that excessive sagittal activation elicits significantly more condylar reaction. With an extreme forward positioning only the muscular forces transmitted by the appliance to the upper and lower teeth and jaws are increased (Fig. 8-32). This may hasten Class II correction by rotational effects or tipping of the teeth, but these are not the reactions striven for in this concept (compare Fig. 8-33). Furthermore, the temporomandibular joint structures may be overstressed and the level of cooperation endangered. Prolonged dislocation of the condyle out of the fossa seems to be the main stimulus needed to influence condylar growth. There are indications that even a cervical headgear to the upper molars can force the mandible to assume such a lowered position that some condylar reaction may be initiated.[13-15] Rather than attempt excessive forward activation initially, it is advisable to proceed step by step. In severe cases a reactivation may be indicated after 8 to 12 months. To secure a good fit of the appliance, it is then preferred to construct a new one.

The forward movement of the mandible should be symmetric for registration with the construction bite. The orthodontist should not attempt to correct midline deviations caused by tipping or migration of the incisors in the arches. These malpositions should be treated either before the activator headgear treatment phase or afterward. If it is decided to postpone the solution of these problems, the relationship of the midlines should be marked in centric relation and should be reproduced in the construction bite.

The extension of the appliance in the lower jaw is most critical. With few exceptions no anterior movement of the lower arch relative to the skeletal base is desirable. Anchorage should therefore derive mainly from the lingual cortical plate. Comparable to complete dentures, the extension is carried as far down as the floor of the mouth permits (Figs. 8-35, *C* and *D*, 8-37, *B*, and 8-46). In the deciduous second and permanent first molar region, the pocketlike area offers room to construct wings of considerable length. On the lateral aspect, irritation derives mainly from the region anterior to the deciduous second molar. If the exact relation of the sensitive mucosa to the rim of the activator is not carefully located, the wings are often mistakenly shortened. There are, however, limitations regarding the design of the posterior wings. If pronounced undercuts are present in this region, the inferior part should be partly blocked out with impression plaster before the appliance is constructed (Fig. 8-46) or they can be slightly flattened by grinding the acrylic when the appliance is being adapted. Otherwise, the child has great difficulty closing into the appliance when the upper part is seated; this in spite of the fact that it is routinely advised to move the mandible forward slightly beyond the lower limit of the appliance and then close into the appliance with a slight retracting movement. The patient should be

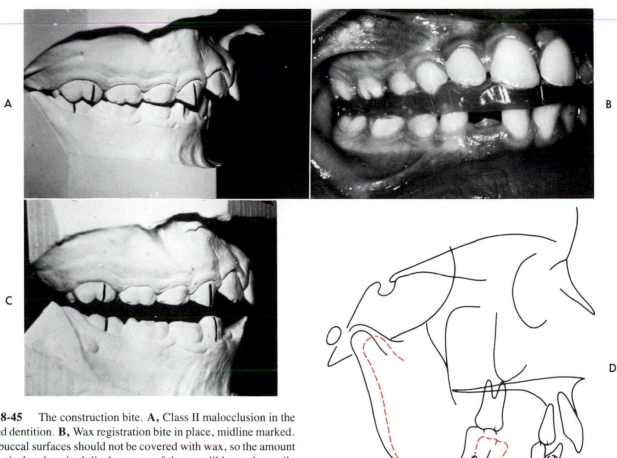

Fig. 8-45   The construction bite. **A,** Class II malocclusion in the mixed dentition. **B,** Wax registration bite in place, midline marked. The buccal surfaces should not be covered with wax, so the amount of vertical and sagittal displacement of the mandible can be easily evaluated. **C,** Mounted casts demonstrating average vertical and sagittal activation in comparison to habitual occlusion. **D,** Cephalometric superimposition: the mandible in habitual occlusion *(solid line)* and the activation determined with the construction bite *(broken line)*. Note the amount of displacement of the condyle despite the only moderate activation recommended.

instructed always to place the appliance first in the upper arch to avoid distorting the torquing springs or the labial wire. There is another important reason for relieving extreme undercuts: during sleep, spontaneous mandibular opening movements may occur. Should vertical movement of the mandible be completely blocked by the undercuts, the appliance may be dislodged from the upper arch.

The lingual region from canine to canine, another area valuable for alveolar anchorage, should be fully used (Figs. 8-35, *D,* 8-37, *B* and *D,* 8-38, *A,* and 8-46). Adequate relief in the acrylic should be provided for the lingual frenum. All teeth should be in touch with the appliance on their lingual and occlusal surfaces. The acrylic is extended to the buccal cusps of the posterior teeth. The canines and incisors are covered also on the vestibular side by about 2 to 3 mm of acrylic to secure good anchorage (Figs. 8-35, *A* and *E,* and 8-38, *A*). Whether and when the occlusal acrylic for the first lower molars should be relieved is discussed on pp. 473 to 475 (Fig. 8-53, *B* and *C*).

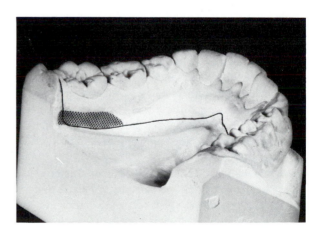

Fig. 8-46   Extension of the appliance on the lingual side of the lower alveolar process. Access should be secured by adequate carving of the cast in the lateral areas of the floor of the mouth. If pronounced undercuts are present in the region of the first molar, they should be blocked out with impression plaster before the appliance is constructed *(screened area).*

Modifications in appliance design and combinations with other appliances

The type of activator that has been discussed is not suited for individual tooth movement. Its characteristic function is to obtain as much overall anchorage as possible for Class II correction. The concept of a simple splint-type construction should not be weakened by introducing all kinds of active parts. Other appliances should be used before or after the activator headgear treatment if intra-arch or coordinative problems must be solved. Within a limited scale, some modifications in activator design, however, may be indicated.

Upper Labial and Lingual Wire (Fig. 8-47)

If torque control of the upper incisors is not critical, a standard labial wire (0.8 mm in diameter) with ∪-loops in the canine region may be used instead of torquing springs (Fig. 8-47, *A* and *F*). The acrylic extensions for the front teeth, however, should be the same. With this setup a two point contact situation is also achieved that can provide some axial control of the upper incisors, although to a much lesser degree than with torquing auxiliaries. This arrangement should be used only in mild Class II cases, requiring a short treatment period.

A labial wire may be indicated for guiding the incisors, if the acrylic must be removed to promote vertical eruption (Fig. 8-59, *F*). It is tempting to use a labial wire to retrude upper incisors. In general, the degree of protrusion of upper incisors is severely overestimated in Class II, division 1, situations. If there is no obvious spacing, then rarely is a pronounced upper incisor protrusion present. The mechanics of Class II treatment tends to tip upper incisors lingually. If a labial wire is used initially to retrude the incisors, they most certainly become too uprighted during treatment. Because of incisal interference, the achievement of a Class I intercuspation will no longer be possible. Moreover, downward and backward rotation of the mandible often results if corrective Class II mechanics are further applied. The labial wire is therefore rarely used for isolated retrusive action on the incisors. Only at the completion of Class II correction can a final light touch with corresponding removal of the acrylic on the lingual be tolerated. Upper protrusion, combined with spacing, should be corrected with a utility arch before activator headgear treatment. The same holds true for other irregularities requiring well-controlled, individual tooth movement.

The combination of a labial and a lingual wire incorporated in the activator may be considered only if minor adjustments are required in upper incisor position (Fig. 8-47, *B* to *D*). The main indications are a slight protrusive movement of all four incisors to the ideal curve of the incisal segment if they are too uprighted initially or a labial movement of the lateral incisors if they are positioned lingually. In both instances, full anteroposterior coordination of the upper and lower arches into a Class I relationship is ob-

structed by incisal interference. Patients with marked retrusion and extrusion upper incisors contacting the lowers must be pretreated with a fixed appliance setup. Those with a tendency to upper incisor retroclination, particularly if correction is initiated in the developmental stage, and those in whom only the lateral incisors are somewhat offset to the lingual may be treated with the combination of a lingual and a labial wire added to the activator. The labial wire is formed according to the ideal incisal curve ultimately intended for that particular case. It does not necessarily touch all the incisors. The lingual wire (0.7 mm in diameter) should also represent the ideal incisal curve and is looped at the distal ends to provide adequate resiliency.

At the start of treatment, as indicated earlier, no wires should be activated and the acrylic should embrace the incisors. When the patient has adapted well to the appliance (usually after 4 to 6 weeks), the acrylic is removed according to the movements planned. If no extrusion is desired, the contact of the incisal edges with the acrylic is maintained. If all incisors are to be moved, the Omega-type spring on the lingual is activated and the labial wire is advanced slightly (Fig. 8-47, *G*). The labial wire serves as a template to which the incisors will be guided. As soon as advancement is completed, the incisal edges are again embedded in cold cure acrylic. If still a great amount of Class II correction lies ahead, it is advisable to replace the wires with torquing springs. When only the lateral incisors must be moved forward, a modification can be considered (Fig. 8-47, *E*). From the beginning of treatment, the central incisors are maintained in their axial inclination with torquing springs. With the lingual wire, or in this situation with two individual lingual springs, the lateral incisors are moved into position and then secured in the activator by means of embedding with cold cure acrylic. They do not need torquing springs because their apices will be lingually positioned.

Lower Labial and Lingual Wires, Lower Lip Bumper (Fig. 8-48)

Slight protrusion in the lower incisor area can easily be corrected with a conventional looped labial wire if some spacing is present. Care must be taken that the acrylic on the lingual is ground away 2 to 3 mm apical to the gingival margin but the anchorage area near the floor of the mouth is maintained (Fig. 8-48, *A*). Depending on the planned incisor movement, an easier and more accurate method is to place a wax relief on the lower cast in the area indicated before the appliance is constructed.

Retroclined lower incisors can be moved labially with a lingual wire. It is somewhat difficult to place an additional wire lingual to the lower incisors, with enough extension for resiliency, without making the appliance rather bulky. Only one loop can be incorporated (Fig. 8-48, *B*). Resiliency can also be gained by extending the wire vertically at its ends. As another alternative, a window in the acrylic where the lingual wire is placed offers room to design ad-

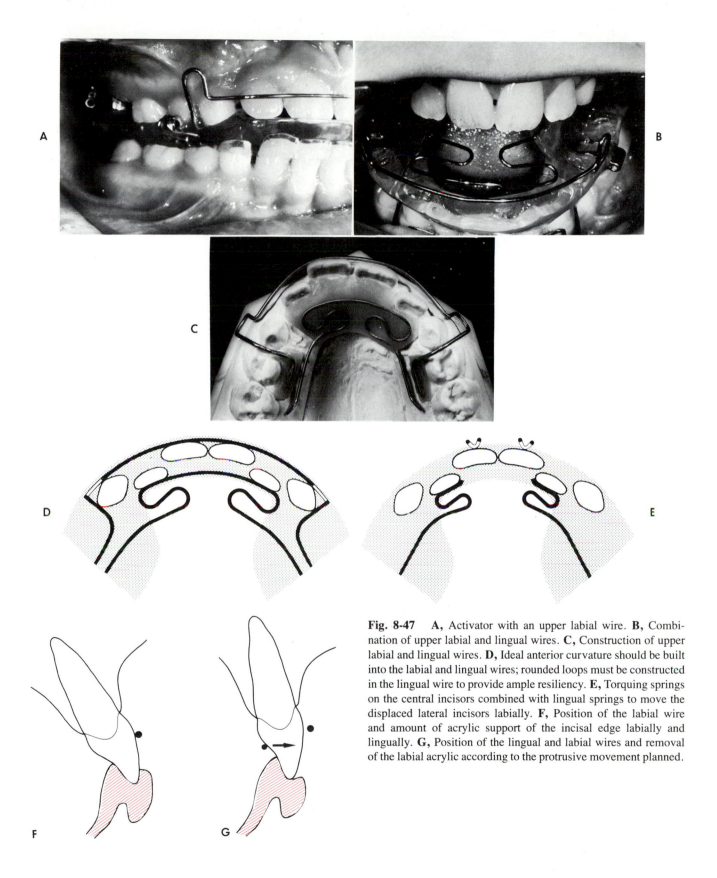

Fig. 8-47 **A,** Activator with an upper labial wire. **B,** Combination of upper labial and lingual wires. **C,** Construction of upper labial and lingual wires. **D,** Ideal anterior curvature should be built into the labial and lingual wires; rounded loops must be constructed in the lingual wire to provide ample resiliency. **E,** Torquing springs on the central incisors combined with lingual springs to move the displaced lateral incisors labially. **F,** Position of the labial wire and amount of acrylic support of the incisal edge labially and lingually. **G,** Position of the lingual and labial wires and removal of the labial acrylic according to the protrusive movement planned.

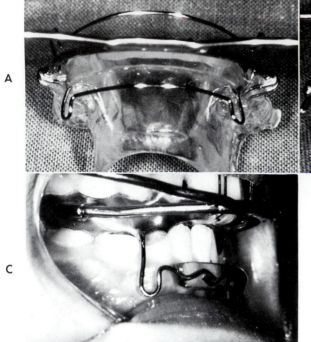

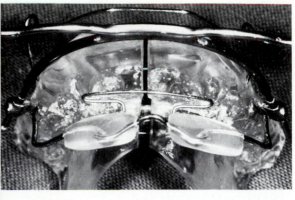

Fig. 8-48 **A,** Lower labial wire. A wax relief was placed on the lingual of the incisors before the appliance was constructed to provide room for uprighting the incisors. Whether this procedure is chosen or the acrylic is ground after appliance construction, the relief should extend about 2 to 3 mm apical to the gingigal margin but the anchorage area near the floor of the mouth should be maintained. **B,** Lingual wire for lower incisor protrusion. Note the screw on the lingual side of the lower incisors for expansion. Labial pads are also added. **C,** Lip bumper added directly to the appliance to assist proclination of the lower incisors. Note the position relative to the lower incisors at about the gingival margin.

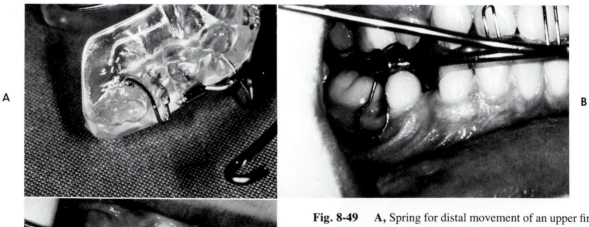

Fig. 8-49 **A,** Spring for distal movement of an upper first molar. Loop for resilience on the buccal side. The acrylic must be ground flat when activation is started, but contact for the cusps should be maintained for vertical control. **B,** Spring for mesial movement of a lower first premolar. **C,** Button bonded eccentrically to the distal of the upper canine. Elastic attached around the tube to move the mesially inclined crown distally.

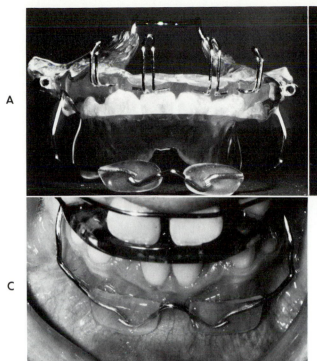

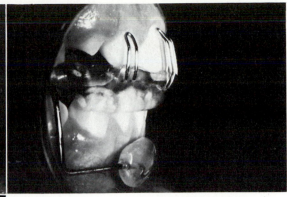

Fig. 8-50 **A,** Activator with added labial pads of the Fränkel type. **B** and **C,** They are positioned deep in the vestibular sulcus to influence mentalis activity and lip seal. The lower labial area must be carved on the working casts before appliance construction.

ditional loops. If desired, a lip bumper, not to be confused with labial pads (Fig. 8-50), can also be added directly to the appliance (Fig. 8-48, *C*).

All tooth moving auxiliaries are exposed to strain whenever the appliance is placed in the mouth. If they are rigidly designed, they will break easily. On the other hand, good, firm stability must be provided. Relatively thick wires should be used, therefore, but adequate extensions should be built in for resiliency. Activations should be performed only in small steps so correct positioning of the wires against the teeth to be moved is achieved every time merely by *closing into the appliance*.

Springs for Individual Tooth Movement (Fig. 8-49)

If an upper first molar has tipped forward somewhat after the loss of the second deciduous molar, it can be guided back to its correct position with a resilient spring as depicted in Fig. 8-49, *A*. The acrylic resin must be ground away to allow distal movement of the crown, but vertical control should be maintained. Once the planned movement has been achieved, the appliance must be locally relined with cold cure acrylic resin so that the crown is once again well seated in the activator. Another application of a spring for moving a tooth to the mesial is shown in Fig. 8-49, *B*. A displaced tooth or an ectopic canine can also be directed with an elastic from a bonded attachment to an appropriately placed hook in the activator (Fig. 8-49, *C*). All these additional tooth moving auxiliaries should, however, be limited to one or two areas and should aim at helping to resolve local de-

velopmental deviations only. Precise resolution of complex irregularities in tooth position does not lie within the domain of the activator.

Lower Labial Pads (Fig. 8-50)

In cases of mentalis hyperactivity, the addition of lower labial pads as proposed by Fränkel has proved helpful for achieving correct lip seal. The contours of the lower labial region must be modified on the working casts to obtain proper extension. The labial pads must be positioned deep in the vestibular fold, parallel to the alveolar process, and should be teardrop shaped (Fig. 8-50). (For details of construction, see McNamara and Huge[80].) A lower lip bumper (Fig. 8-48, *C*) and lower lip pads have different indications and are different in construction and position.

Relining and Expansion Procedures, Expansion Screws (Figs. 8-51 and 8-52)

A great number of Class II, division 1, cases exhibit a constricted upper arch, which needs expansion if coordination in a Class I relationship is to be achieved. In particular, the upper canine region often locks the lower arch in a distal (or posterior) position. If freedom for further forward positioning of the mandible is not present, the transverse problem must be resolved before corrective anteroposterior mechanics. The activator is not an effective appliance for fast expansion. Severe transverse deviations should therefore be resolved first with devices for rapid expansion. After a few weeks of active expansion and about 3 months of re-

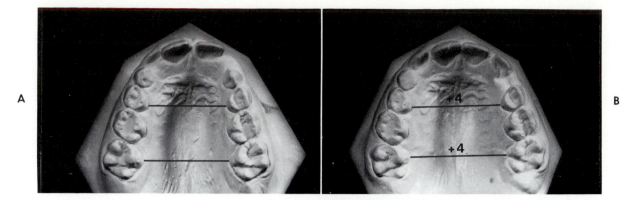

Fig. 8-51   Repetitive relining procedures can bring about considerable expansion of the upper arch. **A,** Initial record. **B,** After 1 year and 4 months of treatment. Six relining procedures had been performed during this period. Initially a transpalatal bar of the Goshgarian type was used for rotation of the first permanent molars.

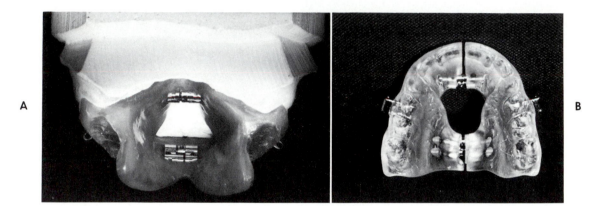

Fig. 8-52   **A,** Placement of two slender jackscrews for expansion, one in the palatal vault and one lingual to the lower incisors. **B,** Sagittally split appliance. Both screws opened by two quarter-turns.

tention, they can usually be removed. Since most cases are overexpanded, relapse to or close to the desired transverse dimension should be allowed before activator headgear treatment for Class II correction is initiated. The time lapse between impressions and insertion of the activator should then not amount to more than 4 days. The activator will be able to maintain the transverse correction provided the upper arch expansion was properly indicated and executed. All cases exhibiting a fully locked lower arch or a transverse deficiency of 3 or 4 mm and more should be expanded before activator headgear treatment.

If the mandible can slide forward freely from the intercuspal position into or close to a Class I relationship without interferences from maxillary transverse deficiencies, Class II treatment with the activator headgear combination can be started without delay. This is permissible despite the fact that in the simulated Class I relationship, complete transverse coordination may be lacking because the upper arch is a bit too narrow. It must be emphasized in this context that the present discussion applies to typical mixed dentition cases. In most instances they exhibit ample freedom in positioning the lower arch forward because of attrition of the deciduous teeth. The transverse deficiency is therefore not an urgent problem since it does not interfere immediately with the anteroposterior correction. Improvement can be accomplished in small steps during the rather long period required for concurrent resolution of the sagittal discrepancy. In our experience 3 to 4 mm of upper arch expansion over a period of 1 year or more is possible with the relining technique only. The procedure can be repeated at intervals of about 8 weeks.

The occlusal reliefs of the upper buccal teeth are ground to shallow grooves without removing acrylic where the cusp tips contact. It is most important to maintain vertical control. Then an ample amount of cold cure acrylic is put in the area of both upper buccal segments, including the extensions to the palate. The acrylic should be of such viscosity that it stays rather well in place but still flows easily. The activator is briefly rinsed in cold water to offset the somewhat unpleasant taste and is then inserted in the patient's mouth. The child is instructed to bit hard for a few minutes. Excess acrylic is removed with a spatula. When the acrylic has started to set but is still somewhat plastic, the activator is carefully disengaged. This stage should not be missed—it is a traumatic experience to attempt removal of the activator when the acrylic has fully set!

After this initial removal the activator is again placed in the patient's mouth to ensure that the fit is perfect. Either an almost full setting is allowed or the activator is placed immediately after this second check in a pressure pot for about 10 minutes. The latter step aids polymerization and imparts a shiny surface, superior from a hygienic standpoint, to the newly added acrylic. The excesses are removed and the areas exposed to the tongue are polished. The whole procedure can be performed by well-trained auxiliary personnel. The close fit accomplished by the relining procedure does indeed cause a slight increase in transverse arch dimension. Considerable changes can be brought about by repetitive relining (Fig. 8-51). It is mandatory, however, that the activator be used in combination with a directly fitted posterior high pull headgear to achieve this result. The close fit in the upper incisor region must be maintained; at least every other time, this area must be included in the relining procedure. Relining should be performed whenever exact fit has been lost and must be done routinely about every 6 months in the upper arch, even if no transverse correction is necessary. Relining is also advisable in the lower arch after about 8 months of treatment.

In rare cases some expansion may be indicated in the lower arch and in the upper arch. Then two jackscrews should be placed: one in the palatal vault and one lingual to the lower incisor segment at the midline (Fig. 8-52). Effectiveness and stability are thereby enhanced. It is then necessary, temporarily, to give up the close fit in the incisor region so that these teeth can drift mesially and prevent diastema formation. The double screw setup also may be used if only relatively efficient upper expansion is desired. In this case the activator is constructed with the two screws opened two quarter-turns and with a midsagittal separation that permits closing of the screws by two quarter-turns (Fig. 8-52, B). After the patient has worn the appliance for about 6 weeks, the screws are closed (decreasing the transverse dimension), relining is performed in the upper arch, and the screws are opened again by two quarter-turns (which equals an activation of almost 0.5 mm). The appliance will fit the lower arch as before, but it will expand the upper arch. This procedure can be repeated about every 5 weeks; but again, it must be emphasized, even with this method the required expansion should be 4 mm at the most. In our clinic only about 6% of the activators used in treatment during the mixed dentition stage are equipped with screws.

Advancement Procedures

Progressive forward activation of mandibular position can be achieved by means of a specially designed screw anchored in the maxillary and as well as the mandibular part of a horizontally split activator.[111] After activation, relining of the mandibular portion is necessary. So far, however, we prefer to replace the appliance after 8 to 12 months of treatment if a severe Class II discrepancy needs to be resolved. At this time the mandible is advanced with the new construction bite into or slightly beyond Class I from the current attained result.

Grinding Procedures

Considerations for the management of lower permanent first molars will be discussed later (pp. 474 to 476). If eruption of the lower permanent molars is to be enhanced, the acrylic is removed occlusally. Removal should extend onto the distal portion of the deciduous second molar (Fig. 8-53, A and B). On the lingual, vertical relief is provided in the gingival area (Fig. 8-53, C). When the exchange process in the buccal segment is about completed, the clinician may need to remove acrylic occlusal to the lower premolars so the curve of Spee can be flattened and settling can take place (Fig. 8-53, E). If lower arch length appears to be critical, it is advisable to secure the first molar mesially with a wire spur from the activator.

Whenever a permanent tooth erupts, some adjustments on the activator should be performed (Fig. 8-53, D). Permanent canines, especially, are larger in the buccolingual, so adequate acrylic must be removed from the lingual extensions of the activator. Appropriate management helps guide the teeth to proper position. A common mistake is to offer too much room for vertical eruption of the upper premolars, particularly if they erupt before the lowers. This will easily establish a curve of Spee that is too pronounced. It is essential to provide freedom for some distal migration of the upper first premolar so that the upper canine can profit from the extra space offered by the deciduous second molar (Fig. 8-49, C). This consideration is also important because it helps guide the first premolars into a Class I relationship. Depending on the developmental situation, concomitant mesial slicing of the deciduous second molar might be indicated (Fig. 8-59, E).

Special attention must be given to the eruption of permanent second molars if activator headgear treatment is performed at this developmental stage. The acrylic should be routinely extended distally from the permanent first molars to prevent vertical overeruption of the permanent second molars (Fig. 8-53, A). As soon as their crowns have reached the desired level of eruption, they are included in the appliance by relining procedures.

Combination with Transpalatal Bar and Lingual Arch (Fig. 8-54)

Often a mesiolingual rotation of the upper first molars is found in Class II cases (Fig. 8-51). For its reciprocal cor-

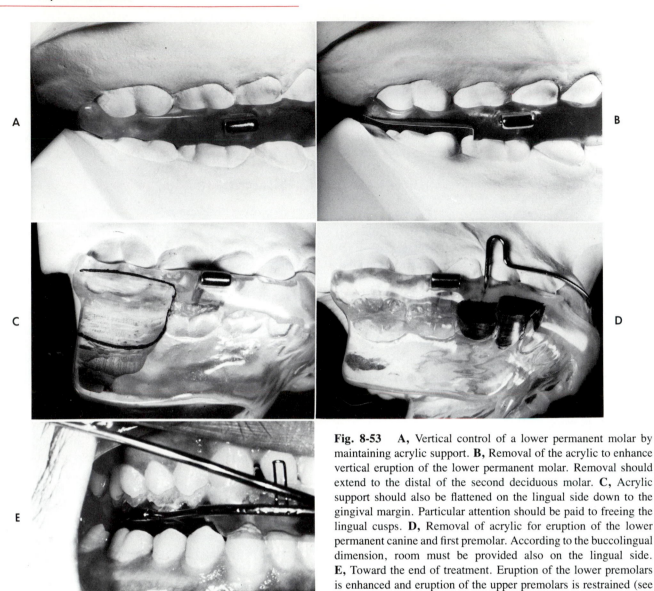

Fig. 8-53 **A,** Vertical control of a lower permanent molar by maintaining acrylic support. **B,** Removal of the acrylic to enhance vertical eruption of the lower permanent molar. Removal should extend to the distal of the second deciduous molar. **C,** Acrylic support should also be flattened on the lingual side down to the gingival margin. Particular attention should be paid to freeing the lingual cusps. **D,** Removal of acrylic for eruption of the lower permanent canine and first premolar. According to the buccolingual dimension, room must be provided also on the lingual side. **E,** Toward the end of treatment. Eruption of the lower premolars is enhanced and eruption of the upper premolars is restrained (see relining) to flatten the curve of Spee and promote settling.

rection a removable transpalatal bar of the so-called Goshgarian type is efficient and revision can be performed within a short time before activator headgear treatment is started. To maintain the molars for a prolonged period in the new position, the transpalatal bar can be kept in place in conjunction with the activator (Figs. 8-54, *A,* and 8-59, *E*). The impression is usually taken with the transpalatal bar in place. On the cast the technician puts some wax around the molar attachments and in the area where the transpalatal bar leaves the tubes and follows the alveolar process. Thus a small groove is created in the acrylic of the activator, providing room for the inserted transpalatal bar. To avoid interfering with the transpalatal bar in the palatal vault, the transpalatal wire of the activator must be modified and positioned further forward. A transpalatal bar is also often placed in high angle cases (p. 474).

Bonded retainers used after correction of upper incisor position and lower 2-2 or 3-3 retainers can be left in place when activator treatment is started. Lower lingual arches can be included if space maintenance is critical or if prolonged retention of a treated lower arch is indicated (Fig. 8-54, *B*). Adequate room in the acrylic of the activator is provided by corresponding wax relief on the working casts.

Combination with Fixed Appliances (Fig. 8-55)

Typically, fixed appliances are used before or after activator headgear therapy. The bonding technique has provided a high degree of flexibility in the application of different appliances during the different phases of overall treatment. In some situations, however, fixed appliances and activator may be used simultaneously. If desired, activator headgear treatment can be initiated immediately; however,

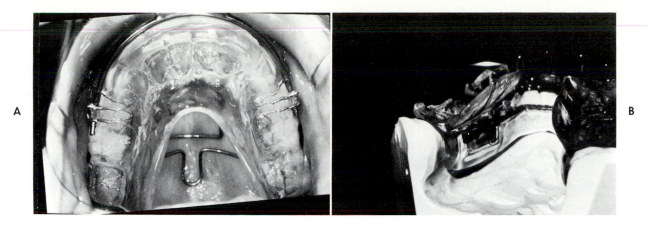

Fig. 8-54   A, Combination with a transpalatal bar and upper molar bands. In the area of the lingual tubes and toward the palatal vault, acrylic relief must be provided in the activator. Modification of the transpalatal wire of the activator is required. **B,** Combination with lower molar bands and lingual arch.

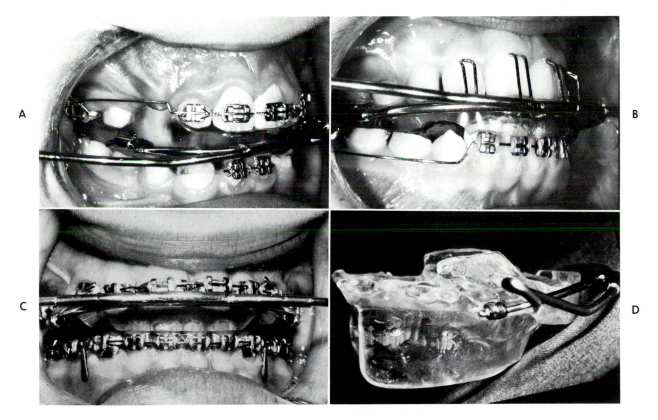

Fig. 8-55   A, Pretreatment with an upper utility arch and sectional in the lower incisor region. Interposed activator headgear treatment for Class II correction without removing the components of the fixed appliance. After eruption of the canines, continuation of fixed appliance therapy is planned for this patient, in whom the upper first premolars were extracted to compensate for agenesis of the lower central incisors. **B,** Lower utility arch used in the pretreatment period and kept in place passively during activator headgear treatment for space maintenance. **C,** Full fixed appliance therapy in an extraction case. Toward the end of treatment. Superimposed activator headgear treatment to complete Class II correction. Space closure in the lower arch is continued. **D,** If used in combination with fixed appliance therapy providing torque and axial control, the activator can be designed as a simple acrylic splint without any auxiliaries.

some arrangement in the upper or lower anterior region may be necessary, whether for coordinative reasons or for providing improved conditions for buccal segment development, particularly for the permanent canines. Bonding of the incisors for closing a diastema or for other small corrections can be performed while the activator is still being worn. Even a simple utility arch setup may be considered whereby the molar area remains secured in the acrylic (Fig. 8-55, *A* and *B*). Such maneuvers should not be initiated before several months of activator headgear combination treatment have elapsed, and they should be delayed until a stage of treatment in which the major part of Class II correction has been attained and maximum anchorage is no longer critical. As soon as the goal of the minor corrections is reached, the teeth are again encased with acrylic (Fig. 8-55, *B*). The attachments may be maintained if a final treatment with full fixed appliances is planned after the activator is discontinued.

More often the simultaneous combination is used whenever complex treatment calls first for extensive fixed appliance therapy. At the stage when the major intra-arch and coordinative problems have been solved an activator headgear assembly is applied rather than extensive use of Class II elastics to correct a residual anteroposterior discrepancy (Fig. 8-55, *C*). The fixed appliances remain inactively in place as an intra-arch retentive device and will be used again for fine tuning of the occlusion after the superimposed activator headgear treatment. For this purpose the activator is constructed as a simple splint with no wires or other auxiliaries (Fig. 8-55, *D*). If lingual attachments will not be needed for final fixed appliance treatment, their removal is advised before impressions are taken. This sequence of events is often practiced in the permanent dentition, whether extraction or nonextraction, and can be extremely efficient if performed during the adolescent growth spurt—which may be a reason to initiate additional activator headgear treatment even before space closure is completed in extraction cases. The latter decision may also be based on the consideration that the practitioner wants first to evaluate the reaction to the activator headgear assembly. During this period slow lower space closure can be performed despite simultaneous activator wear, provided the anterior segment is in correct position. Acrylic is removed without giving up the vertical cuspal contact in the lower buccal segment, to permit mesial movement while the incisors and canines, eventually including first premolars, remain well embedded in the acrylic. If excellent skeletal reaction from activator headgear application ensues, retraction of the upper incisors will no longer be necessary. The upper spaces can also be closed from back to front, which may be preferable with respect to profile esthetics. If the activator headgear phase is not successful, the remaining upper spaces are used to retract the canines and incisors for overjet reduction.

In the permanent dentition, precoordination of the upper and lower arches is critical to arriving at a Class I relationship with the activator headgear treatment. Tooth interferences obstruct successful correction.

INDICATIONS, DIFFERENTIAL MANAGEMENT, AND TIMING

Correction of skeletal Class II discrepancies in growing patients is the operational field of the activator headgear appliance.

Not all Class IIs are alike. Several elaborate diagnostic classifications have been suggested.[77,87] The many dental components can be relatively well controlled by efficient force systems, but from our point of view some therapeutic limitations on skeletal control still need to be accepted. Reduction of the anterior growth vector of the maxillary complex can be produced relatively well. Stimulation of forward mandibular growth to the extent that full skeletal Class II correction could be accomplished is, however, no orthopedic reality. Although with the activator headgear concept all provisions are undertaken to provoke as much mandibular reaction as possible, it must be realized that, in the last analysis, the major contributions derive from maxillary dentoalveolar reactions and normal mandibular growth. Even if the diagnostic baseline calls for exclusive mandibular advancement, orthopedic treatment will always substantially affect the maxillary region (although some proponents of functional jaw orthopedics claim the opposite).

The degree of maxillary contribution to skeletal Class II correction, however, can be modulated with the kind of treatment procedure. At one end, exclusive headgear treatment to the upper arch with heavy forces up to 1000 g per side for 16 or even 24 hours a day can elicit a maximal maxillary contribution; at the other end, headgear forces in the light to moderate range (200 to 400 g) for 12 to 14 hours may result in a minimal contribution. If therefore, with the activator headgear setup, minimal maxillary and maximal mandibular contributions to skeletal Class II correction are to be achieved, only moderate headgear forces should be used; consequently a prolonged treatment time must be accepted. Fast correction of a skeletal Class II always arouses strong suspicion that maxillary reaction has contributed almost exclusively to the change. Substantial mandibular contribution needs time and cannot be expected, on average, in less than 2 years.

The application of an activator headgear setup is therefore indicated if a skeletal Class II deviation is present in which an anterior movement of the chin prominence is desirable and at least some posteriorly directed maxillary dentoalveolar reaction is acceptable. To some degree, the maxillomandibular contributions can be regulated by varying the amount and vector of headgear force, as well as the time allowed for correction, and possibly also reactivating the forward mandibular position in several steps. Dental Class II situations with a skeletal Class I profile should not be treated with this setup; an unpleasant concave profile may be created. The decision concerning the feasibility of striving for anterior movement of the mandibular symphysis is primarily based on clinical judgment. For a rough evaluation the patient is asked to move the mandible forward into a Class I relationship. This can give only an impression of the future situation if the patient can protrude the mandible without encountering interference. In deep bite cases with steep incisal guidance the mandible must be lowered to an excessive degree, exaggerating anterior face height. The diagnostic mandibular advancement simulates basically a surgical result. Orthopedic reality, together with normal growth of a 2-year period, will generally be about halfway. Careful analysis of the lateral head film (not only numbers!) will further aid in determining the desirable changes and, above all, estimating the degree to which they can be attained. It must be made clear that the activator headgear treatment cannot result in miracles.

Deviations in the vertical pattern do not exclude activator headgear treatment. High angle cases are a particular domain of this combination since, unlike the use of activator only treatment, vertical control is optimal. Of course, excessive vertical growth that is due to structural, muscular, or functional disturbances cannot be totally regulated with any appliance. The following recommendations are presented only as general rules, since occlusal aspects may call for modifications:

1. In vertically critical cases the force vector of the headgear is so adjusted that even pressure is distributed between the incisal and molar regions (i.e., through the center of resistance of the upper dentition) (Fig. 8-23, C). The amount of force should not be less than 400 g. No acrylic is removed in the lower molar region.

2. In cases with a hypodivergent trend the force vector of the headgear is positioned above the center of resistance of the dentition so the incisors experience an intrusive influence while the molars remain virtually untouched. A low amount of force is applied, only about 200 to 300 g, and the acrylic around the lower molars is removed to allow additional eruption.

3. Hypodivergent patterns of the deep bite type, with severe vertical deficiencies and pogonion positioned in a skeletal Class III rather than Class II, should not be treated with this appliance. The dental Class II must be corrected, with dental movements and downward displacement of the mandibular symphysis produced by other therapeutic means.

Besides the basic skeletal pattern, the occlusion requires careful consideration. Transverse aspects have already been discussed (pp. 467 to 469). The steepness of the condylar path in protrusive movement, the inclination of the occlusal plane, and the incisal guidance are other key aspects that influence treatment planning. In combination with the skeletal pattern they determine the mode of therapeutic handling. For a general clinical evaluation, the patient is asked to protrude the mandible into a Class I relationship maintaining occlusal contact. In cases with irregularities of sagittal incisor position and/or axial deviations in the incisor segments, with transverse or other interferences, the patient will not be able to attain a Class I relationship without lowering the mandible excessively. This is indicative of intermaxillary discoordination. These situations will be dis-

cussed later (p. 474). If no sagittal obstructions are encountered and the incisor segments either exhibit correct position with correct axial inclination or do not contact at all, a direct classification will be possible. A Class I relationship in the canine and molar region will be achieved under one of the following conditions:

Type 1: Incisal contact at about 2 mm overbite with no or only the slightest vertical clearance in the buccal segment

Type 2: Incisal contact at about 2 mm overbite with moderate or pronounced vertical clearance in the buccal segment

Type 3: No incisal contact, only upper and lower buccal segments touching each other

At the end of treatment the *Type 1* situation, with buccal support, should be achieved in all three types as a result. *Type 2* would not provide stability, and *Type 3* would be unsatisfactory from a functional standpoint. Therefore a decision regarding the vertical management of the incisor and buccal segments must be made. It will depend on the skeletal pattern, growth potential, relationship of the incisors to the lip embrasure, and finally degree of performability of the desirable dentoalveolar changes in vertical position. Intrusion, extrusion, the combination of intrusion and extrusion in the buccal versus the incisor segments, or changing the inclination of the occlusal plane is the maneuver to be selected in the individual case. During facial growth, intrusion and extrusion have not necessarily the strict meaning of absolute tooth movement in one of these directions. Selective restraining and promoting of vertical dentoalveolar development in buccal or incisor segments can be interpreted as relative intrusion and extrusion respectively.

In a *Type 1* situation the splint construction of the activator should be maintained. No removal of acrylic to promote vertical development of the lower buccal segment should therefore be performed during the first phase of treatment. The vertical dimension is not enhanced until sagittal correction has progressed. The decision to remove acrylic in the lower molar region later depends on the vertical contribution of condylar growth. If after substantial sagittal correction the buccal segments are still in contact when a Class III relationship is assumed by protrusive movement of the mandible, additional vertical development of the lower molars should not be promoted therapeutically. On the other hand, obvious disclusion when this check is performed is indicative of excellent potential for vertical contribution from the condylar growth. Some additional eruption of the lower molars (and of the lower buccal segments when the premolars erupt) is required to provide occlusal support. This cautious evaluation, waiting for the kind of reaction and observing the type of growth, is recommended because initially both cannot be foreseen exactly.

In a *Type 2* situation either the incisors are overerupted, the buccal segments are undererupted, or both deviations are combined. The question to be answered is whether and to what degree active intrusion of the incisors or extrusion of the lower buccal segment must be performed before activator headgear treatment or whether restraint of vertical development of the incisors and promotion of vertical development of the lower buccal segment during the activator headgear treatment is the appropriate measure to take. In a hyperdivergent pattern all extrusive manipulations in the buccal segments should be avoided; it is desirable to achieve the vertical coordination by incisor intrusion exclusively. From a biomechanical standpoint active intrusion of the incisors with a utility arch will induce reciprocal extrusion of the buccal segments. This unfavorable reaction in a hyperdivergent pattern must be minimized. In the upper arch, high pull headgear forces and a transpalatal bar will help prevent extrusion. In the lower arch the molars can be controlled vertically to some degree with active buccal root torque and, additionally, with a posterior bite plate. Lower headgear application should be avoided in Class II cases. Some help in vertical control of the buccal segments can be obtained by increasing the occlusal forces through muscle training. An excellent condition is offered if an intrusive utility arch setup can be installed from ankylosed deciduous second molars. In critical Class II cases (i.e., a pronounced hyperdivergent skeletal pattern combined with a dental deep bite) one can even consider ankylosing these teeth artificially. Diagnostic evaluation and prognosis of the condylar growth potential will dictate whether only limited or no countermeasures against extrusion of the lower molars are indicated during the preparatory treatment phase.

When there is a hypodivergent tendency with a good prospective horizontal growth pattern, it may even be desirable to promote molar extrusion by adding Class II elastics. It must be realized, however, that the displacement path of the mandibular symphysis will then be deflected downward unless corresponding vertical growth of the condyles compensates for the increased vertical dentoalveolar development. If in an average skeletal pattern the buccal clearance is only moderate when diagnostic protrusion of the mandible into a Class I relationship is performed, then pretreatment is not indicated from the vertical dental aspect. Additional eruption of the lower molars can be induced during the activator headgear treatment by relieving the acrylic in this area. Intrusion of the upper incisors can also be achieved with the activator headgear setup if the correct extraoral force vector and palatal root torque are applied. With these three components buccal support will be established, in many instances simultaneously, with a proper overjet-overbite relationship at the end of Class II correction. It is always advantageous if vertical development of lower molars can be promoted because their upward and forward eruption path contributes to the dental Class II correction. This factor, however, should not be exploited at the expense of deflecting the mandibular symphysis downward. During Class II correction all precautions must be taken not to extrude upper molars or promote their vertical development. The acrylic support in this area is therefore never removed.

The *Type 1* and *Type 2* background cannot be properly identified with the diagnostic forward mandibular movement into Class I if incisal interferences are due to uprighted or even retroclined upper incisors, to protruded lower incisors, or to irregularities in incisor position, particularly lingually malposed upper lateral incisors. The only information that can be gained in these instances is that proper overjet conditions with correct incisor inclination and coordination of the incisal segments will be necessary for unobstructed protrusive movement of the mandible. Thus vertical problems cannot be evaluated directly. They can be checked only after preliminary clinical adjustment of the incisor segments (a possible alternative would be gnathologic registration, mounting the casts and incisor setup). However, during these adjustments it is helpful to know how the incisor and buccal segments must be handled vertically so incisal guidance and buccal support can be harmonized. In these cases the extrusive and intrusive requirements must be analyzed initially from clinical and cephalometric information. After the obstructing interferences are removed (which usually does not require more than a few months of treatment), the aforementioned dynamic checking procedure can be performed and further vertical manipulations undertaken.

In *Type 3* situations no incisal guidance can be observed. The forward positioning of the mandible into Class I reveals either an anterior open bite or a residual overjet discrepancy. In the latter case the upper and lower incisors, because of an extreme deep bite and discoordinated incisor position, do not contact or just barely contact each other. This condition is frequently a result of upper incisor protrusion or lower incisor retrusion or a combination of these. The vertical interincisal relationship and the clinical and cephalometric evaluation will determine the degree of incisor intrusion and/or buccal extrusion indicated during the correction of the excessive overjet. In anterior open bite caused by undereruption of the anterior segments the therapeutic prognosis is good, provided the skeletal pattern is within normal range. Often crowding, particularly in combination with a narrow upper arch, is the cause of incomplete eruption. Rapid expansion may solve both problems. Interfering habits and tongue and/or lip positions are other typical factors in Class II conditions. They can be controlled in most instances during activator headgear treatment. Lip seal exercises may also be indicated. The incisal area, whether upper alone or upper and lower, is relieved from acrylic so that further eruption can take place. No torquing springs can then be applied. If an upper labial wire is used, it should not contact or should only barely touch the incisors, unless pronounced lingual tipping is indicated. In most instances, however, relief of lip pressure is required, which to some degree can be accomplished by positioning the wire 1 or 2 mm in front of the incisors. The vector of the headgear force must be adjusted to obtain a stable fit of the activator in the upper buccal segments. The amount of force should be minimal so no distal tipping is produced. As soon as eruption of the incisors to the desired level has occurred, relining is performed and, if indicated, the upper labial wire can be replaced with torquing springs. The vector and amount of headgear force are then adapted to the improved anchorage.

A more complex situation is encountered in high angle cases when intrusion of the buccal segment rather than further eruption of the incisors would be the ideal solution. The therapeutic possibilities for dentofacial orthopedics to achieve this goal are extremely meager. The main effort must be to refrain from all manipulations that exert an extrusive influence on the buccal segments. An extraoral force vector as steep as possible should be applied with the activator headgear combination. It should pass through the center of resistance of the upper dentition or even a little posteriorly. Since the acrylic in the incisal region will be removed in many cases to promote further eruption, the center of resistance will move backward. A slightly eccentric vector position to the posterior might be desirable to exert a bit more vertical force on the molars than on the canines. As a consequence a posterior rotation of the dentition and the maxilla must be expected (Fig. 8-27, *D*). It could be argued that the construction bite should be somewhat higher than average to increase the vertical force also on the lower buccal segment. However, an extremely high construction bite may induce additional lengthening of the elevator muscles, which might add to increased vertical growth of the dentoalveolar structures. Furthermore, lip competence is strained. When intrusion of the buccal segment is desirable in these cases, the activator headgear can be combined with a transpalatal bar from banded upper molars (Figs. 8-54, *A,* and 8-59, *E*) (see pp. 471 and 482). In some instances a slight intrusion of the upper molars can be observed. Judicious grinding of the occlusal contact points of the deciduous teeth until contact at the permanent molars is reestablished will contribute to a slight decrease in vertical dimension and a closing rotation of the mandible. Relining from time to time is recommended to maintain close fit of the appliance.

The activator headgear combination can be used for Class II corrections in the deciduous, mixed, or permanent dentition. By far the best developmental period for this kind of treatment is the early mixed dentition, when all incisors have erupted and the deciduous teeth are still firm enough to provide good anchorage. At this stage the reactive potential of the tissues is still pronounced and patient cooperation poses the least problems. If the patient is sleeping 10 to 11 hours at night, he or she can be expected to wear the activator, in total, for 12 to 14 hours each day. An unfavorable period for starting activator headgear treatment is when the deciduous teeth in the buccal segment are loose or most of them are lost. If only upper incisors and first permanent molars are available to provide anchorage, activator headgear treatment can be detrimental, especially if heavy forces are applied during this period (Fig. 8-56). The major effect will be lingual and distal tipping of these teeth. That is not to say that activator headgear treatment should be discarded when the exchange in the buccal segment is taking place. If caries has not caused early loss of deciduous teeth, the transitional exchange permits inclusion of new units while some deciduous teeth, particularly the second molars, are still firm. When treatment is started in the early mixed dentition, the major anteroposterior correction is usually achieved by the time anchorage conditions in the buccal segments begin to deteriorate. The headgear force can then be decreased from 300 to 150 g per side. The activator can help if appropriate adjustments are made to guide the erupting teeth into proper position (p. 469). In this way the appliance may be worn until the permanent dentition is fully established even though the anteroposterior correction is accomplished much earlier. (See Chapter 9.)

When fixed appliances are needed regardless, it is preferable to discontinue the activator headgear after stable sagittal correction has been achieved and wait until treatment in the permanent dentition can be initiated. In this manner, patient cooperation will not be unnecessarily strained.

It has been stressed several times that in a considerable number of patients, pretreatment in the early mixed dentition may be necessary before activator headgear therapy. If started early, the pretreatment appliances can be removed. If started at a later developmental stage, the fixed appliances

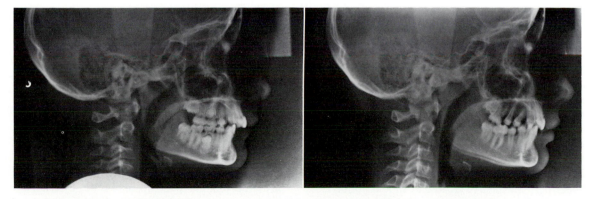

Fig. 8-56 Detrimental sequelae result if excessive extra-oral force is applied. Anchorage is weakened because of tipping in the buccal segments, impaction of second molars and lack of axial control of the upper incisors.

remain, sometimes only partly, and fixed appliance therapy is resumed after an interposed period of activator headgear treatment. (See Chapter 9.)

In another group of patients, referred rather late for treatment and in whom complex problems, mostly combined with extractions of permanent teeth, must be solved, the intra-arch and coordinative problems are first solved with fixed appliance therapy. Then, after removal of the attachments, an activator headgear assembly is used to complete Class II correction. Local bonded retainers can be combined well with this appliance.

It should be emphasized in this context that during the treatment phases with fixed or preparatory appliances the conceptual guidelines of skeletal Class II treatment presented in this chapter must also be respected. The activator headgear treatment phase should not be burdened to resolve untoward side effects of other treatment procedures.

The activator headgear is also well suited for retention of a corrected Class II. The stability of the result will depend on the balance between the growth components of the maxilla plus the dentoalveolar processes and the growth contributions of the condyles and the glenoid fossae (Fig. 8-3). Relapse is imminent if discoordination persists after treatment. With the activator headgear appliance, an intermaxillary and a kind of skeletal retention related to the growth dynamics can be achieved. When used for retention purposes, the construction bite must be modified so that only a minor advancement of the mandible is combined with the opening. Not even a full Class I should be established in the canine region. Mandibular advancement must therefore be much less than the 5 to 6 mm used with the construction bite when Class II correction is being initiated and should not exceed 1.5 to 2 mm.

In summary, a limited number of skeletal Class II patients can be treated exclusively with the activator headgear appliance. The majority, however, require a combination with other appliances. The complexity of the problems to be resolved, the considerations of timing, and the degree of occlusal perfection attempted will dictate a sequence of a combination of approaches deriving from the following basic scheme:

1. Preparatory intramaxillary treatment, quad helix, W-appliance, rapid expansion, utility arches, etc.)
2. *Skeletal Class II correction with activator headgear*
3. Intramaxillary detailing and intermaxillary coordination (full fixed appliances)
4. *Final skeletal Class II correction and/or retention of Class II correction with activator headgear*

The most frequent combinations are either 1 and 2 or 3 and 4. Only in severe discrepancies may the sequences 1, 2, 3 or 2, 3, 4 or even 1, 2, 3, 4 be used. However, an overall 3-year period of active treatment should not be exceeded. In many instances combination with the activator headgear can significantly shorten the duration of fixed appliance therapy, which is advantageous from the aspect of patient cooperation and potential iatrogenic response. The patients are usually happy to complete Class II correction with the activator headgear when removal of the fixed appliances is offered. Most of them also accept the activator headgear easily for a prolonged retention period.

If no further treatment with other means is planned, the activator headgear therapy should not be stopped abruptly. When Class II correction is fully achieved and the attained Class I relationship has corresponded to centric relation for several months, then the wearing time is reduced step by step: first to every other night, and later to twice a week.

CLINICAL HANDLING

Impressions and Construction Bite

Critical areas for appliance construction are the palatal vault and the lower lingual region. Also the occlusal surfaces of the teeth must be perfectly represented in the impressions. Voids in the plaster caused by entrapment of air during the pouring up process should be filled.

Take the construction bite with a horseshoe wafer of medium-hard wax. It should be thin; only the impressions of the occlusal surfaces should be obtained. Contact with the gingiva, the retromolar region, or the palatal tissue should be avoided or cut away; otherwise orientation of the cases may be inaccurate. Taking the construction bite is a critical procedure. In some patients preliminary exercise and one or two trial runs may be necessary.

Mark the midline relationship in centric relation and check it in the position of the construction bite.

Assess the established canine relationship and height of the construction bite, preferably by putting marks on the teeth and measuring.

Cool the wax in the patient's mouth and put it in a cup of ice water after removal.

Recheck in the mouth by evaluating the amount of mandibular advancement from centric relation to the position established. (The technician is not to make any arbitrary adjustments after the working casts have been mounted with the construction bite.)

Appliance Placement

Check the fit first in each arch separately and then both together when the jaws are closed.

Instruct the patient to place the appliance first in the upper arch; otherwise torquing springs or other auxiliaries may be distorted. The patient must get the feeling of how much the mandible needs to be advanced to *close into* the appliance. If difficulties arise, relieve undercuts and carefully shorten the lingual flanges. No wire elements should be activated initially.

Place the junction of outer and inner arms of the headgear in correct relation to the lip embrasure. Check it again during final adjustments for the desired vector and the amount of extraoral force. The outer arms should extend far enough posteriorly that their ends correspond in the frontal plane to the distal cusps of the first permanent molars. Thus the full range for rotational activations is provided.

Place marks on the cheeks where to locate the centers of resistance of the maxilla and the upper dentition. Adjust the outer arms vertically and hook them to the head cap. Check the desired force vector in relation to the approximately located centers of resistance.

Measure the amount of force applied. Head caps with which elastics can be used are preferred because low force levels are better adjustable (Fig. 8-35, *H*). With headgear springs of the heavy type it is often difficult to reliably administer forces below 500 g (Fig. 8-35, *G* and *I*).

Recommended extra-oral force levels per side (in grams) are as follows:

Full mixed dentition	250 to 300
Mixed dentition during exfoliations in upper buccal segments	150 to 250
Full permanent dentition	400 to 500
Retention in full permanent dentition	150 to 400

In cases in which the prognosis is poor and only a pronounced posterior rotation of the occlusal plane may help to arrive quickly at or close to a Class I intercuspation, as much as 800 g with a posteriorly positioned force vector may be applied at the end of treatment for a relatively short time. Otherwise, an additional upper fixed appliance with utmost axial and torque control is mandatory. However, all the undesirable side effects must then be taken into account and stability will be questionable.

With the appliance in place and hooked to the headgear, instruct the patient to open. If the activator is dislodged from the upper arch, check for undercuts and remove them judiciously. Check the force distribution with a scaler in the incisor and molar region. Adjust the force vector to the treatment needs.

Instruct the patient to wear the appliance 2 hours in the daytime only for the first 3 days and from then on also during sleep. In most cases a 14-hour schedule should be attempted initially. According to the treatment reactions and the problems to be solved, 10 to 12 hours may be sufficient later. When the treatment goals have been met and stability seems secured, a reduction to every other night or twice a week may be offered.

First Control (Check-Up) Session

A first check is recommended after 1 or 2 weeks. The patient should present a *report card* stating exactly when the appliance was worn. This should be required during the entire treatment period.

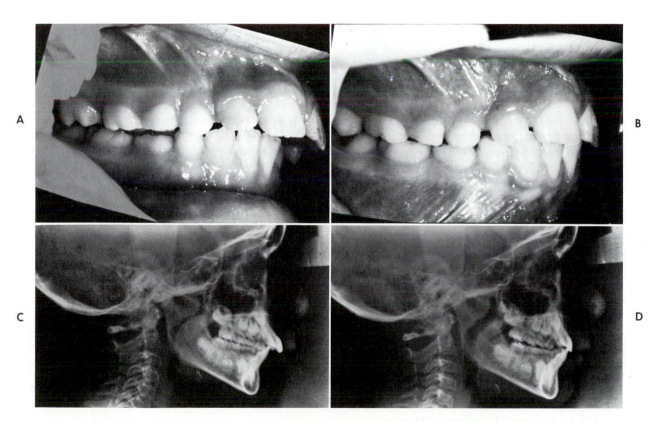

Fig. 8-57 Typical signs of excessive extraoral force application. Distal inclination of the crowns with small steps in the buccal segments as if second-order bends of the anchorage preparation type had been used, **A** and **B.** The corresponding situation is shown on the lateral head films, **C** and **D.**

Take care of all complaints. In the majority of cases, adaptation to the appliance does not pose major problems.

Activation of auxiliaries may now be started. If indicated, light pressure with torquing springs should be initiated and corresponding adjustments of the extraoral force vector made.

Later Adjustment Sessions

During the first phase of treatment, checks are indicated every 3 to 5 weeks. Later, if no activations are necessary, if cooperation is good, and if no critical stages of treatment or development have to be closely supervised, 6-to-8-week intervals may be considered.

At every visit, check the exact fit of the appliance and auxiliaries. Relining must be performed whenever inaccuracies are observed. The torquing springs, extraoral force vector, and force distribution to the upper teeth deserve particular attention.

Assess progress of treatment from centric relation. Advancement of the mandible with occlusal contact into or close to Class I helps to reveal imminent interferences. The reactions must be analyzed in detail and weighed in light of the treatment plan. Appropriate biomechanical modifications must be made. The possible need to promote additional lower molar eruption should also be appraised.

Expect a great variability in cooperation and reaction. The upper arch must be particularly well controlled so any signs of lingual and distal crown tipping will become evident at an early stage. If small steps start to appear in the buccal segment (as if second-order bends for anchorage preparation were made), treatment does not follow the prescription (Fig. 8-57). Either the orthodontist or the patient is overzealously trying to arrive at a dental Class I. Check torque control at the incisors, adjust the force vector, and decrease the amount of force. It should be made clear that the patient must not put two or even three elastics on each side (as some do) to shorten the overall treatment time. Only if, despite these countermeasures, maxillary overreaction persists is the patient asked to decrease the wearing time of the appliance. Fast improvement of the Class II intercuspation must always raise great suspicion that dental reactions prevail.

Repairs

Overall, few problems arise. Simple wires or tubes can easily be replaced or added directly with cold cure acrylic.

Admittedly, the torquing springs are the most delicate parts of the appliance. If constructed with no sharp bends, if embedding of the vertical part and of the inferior curve in acrylic is avoided (during relining, these parts should be covered with wax), and if adjustments are made by hand (not with sharp pliers), they will not break. However, the patient must be careful when seating the appliance.

Should repair be necessary, fit the appliance in the mouth and apply silicone impression material over the vestibular incisor region and the anterior part of the activator. After setting, the activator can be removed with the impression attached to it.

CASE REPORTS

The five cases to be presented in detail were selected to demonstrate the application of the activator headgear concept during different developmental stages, in different sequences of treatment timing, and in different combinations with other appliances.

CASE 1 (Fig. 8-58)

This boy was 9 year 1 month old when he came for clinical evaluation. He was a mouth breather, and his lower lip was interposed between upper and lower incisors most of the time (Fig. 8-58, A and B). At rest the anterior portion of the tongue protruded between the palatal vault and the lower incisors, contacting the lower lip (C). He exhibited a typical Class II profile (B) and a full Class II molar-to-canine relationship on both sides (D). A forward slide of 1 mm from centric relation to habitual occlusion could be detected. The upper incisors exhibited minor spacing, the lower incisors moderate spacing (C). All deciduous teeth were present in the buccal segments, with no obvious root resorption. No sagittal or transverse interferences could be observed on protrusion into a Class I canine relationship, and contact in the buccal segments was maintained. Cephalometric analysis revealed an A-N-B angle of 7° in a slightly prognathic and hypodivergent pattern (G). The upper incisors were protruded only slightly. The lowers, their incisal edges 6 mm in front of N-Pog, were obviously procumbent.

Treatment was started at the age of 9 years 7 months. Initially an upper and lower labial bow was fitted to the activator (Fig. 8-58, E). At the time of treatment (i.e., 6 years before the time of this writing) torquing springs were not used routinely except in critical situations. (Today this boy would be treated with torquing springs applied to the upper incisors.) The extraoral force vector was adjusted to exert slightly more intrusive force on the upper incisors than on the molars. Only 300 g of force was applied to each side. With 12 hours of appliance wear per day, slow uprighting of the lower incisors with the labial bow was begun immediately. After 6 months these teeth were embedded in acrylic and the upper arch was relined. By this time a cusp-to-cusp relationship had been achieved. To promote additional eruption, the acrylic in the lower molar region was removed because diagnostic protrusive movement of the mandible exhibited a small clearance in the buccal segment. After 1 year, Class I in habitual occlusion was achieved. The extra-oral force was decreased to 200 g, and the patient was advised to wear the appliance only during sleeping hours. Treatment was continued in this manner for another 5 months before records were taken at the age of 11 years (F and H to J). A 6-month period without treatment had elapsed after initial records were made, and this was followed by 1 year 5 months of activator headgear treatment. The overall superimposition revealed that sagittal and vertical displacement of the maxilla had been minimal during this period (I). However, forward mandibular displacement was excellent. The local superimposition showed slight changes of incisor and molar position in the upper arch (J). The lower incisors had moved lingually and, as had the molars, become slightly extruded. Condylar growth was favorable in amount and direction.

At this stage (Fig. 8-58, F and H) we could have considered step-by-step slowdown of activator headgear treatment, particularly if fixed appliance therapy had been needed in the permanent dentition. There were, however, no indications for this final treatment. Only the upper permanent canines were still high and mesially inclined. Therefore the upper deciduous canines and first molars were extracted (K). The labial wires were removed from and upper incisor torquing springs added to the appliance. It was decided to use the activator headgear appliance to control the upper buccal segments further until upper permanent canine emergence, to guide the erupting permanent teeth into proper occlusion, and (last but not least) to stabilize the skeletal and dental treatment result achieved thus far. The extraoral force was reduced to 150

g and the wearing time maintained at 9 hours a day for 8 months, after which the appliance was worn only every other night for the following 11 months.

At the age of 12 years 7 months, all permanent posterior teeth had erupted and the permanent canines and second molars were approaching occlusal contact (Fig. 8-58, *L*). Another cephalo-

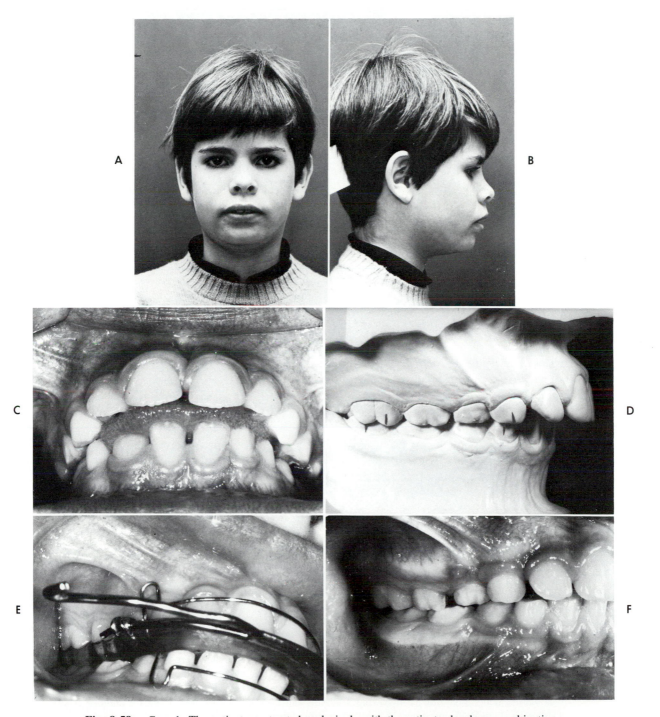

Fig. 8-58   Case 1. The patient was treated exclusively with the activator headgear combination. Initial records, **A** to **D** and **G,** at age 9 years 1 month. A lower labial wire was used to upright the lower incisors during the first 6 months of treatment, **E.** Overall result after 1 year 5 months of activator headgear wear, 12 hours a day, 300 g extraoral force on each side, **F** and **H** to **J.**

Continued.

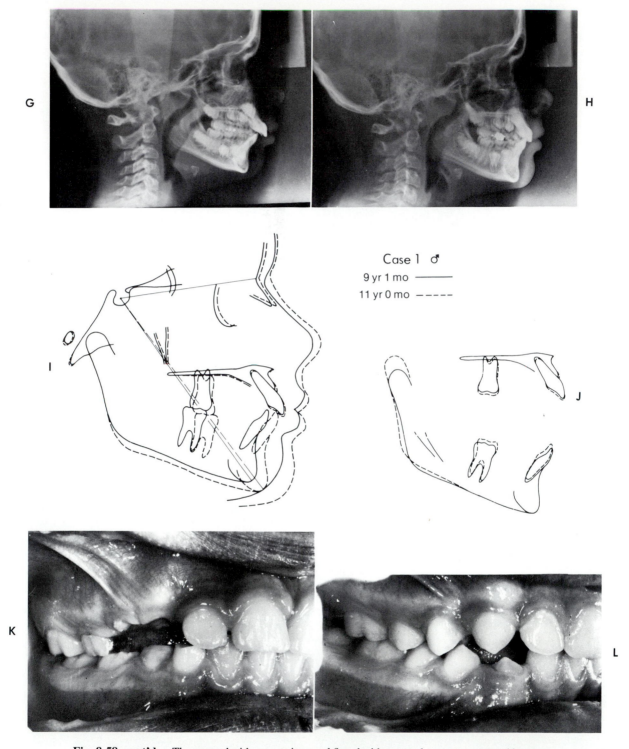

Case 1 ♂
9 yr 1 mo ————
11 yr 0 mo ------

Fig. 8-58, cont'd The upper deciduous canines and first deciduous molars were extracted because the crowns of the upper permanent canines were excessively inclined to the mesial, **K.** Torquing springs to the upper incisors were added, the extraoral force was reduced to 150 g, and the appliance was worn 9 hours a day for the following 8 months and then only every other night for another 11 months. **L** to **P,** Result at age 12 years, 7 months, when treatment was completed. **Q** and **R,** Result 2 years later, without retention.

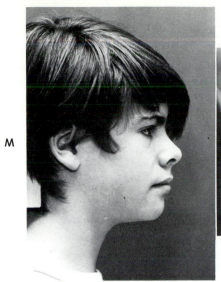

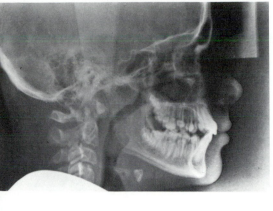

M

N

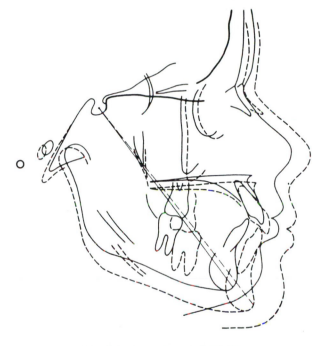

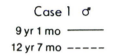

Case 1 ♂

9 yr 1 mo ———

12 yr 7 mo - - - - -

O

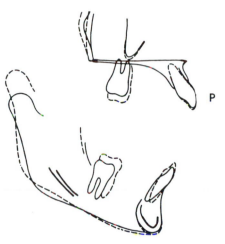

P

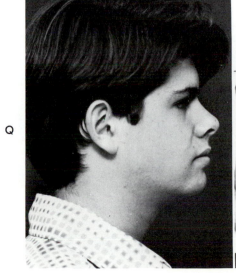

Q

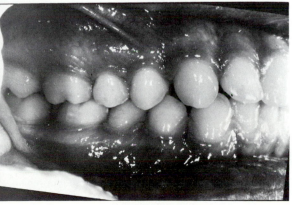

R

metric analysis revealed the overall changes since the age 9 years 1 month (*G* and *N* to *P*). The inclination of the occlusal plane had been well controlled. The local superimposition indicated that almost no vertical or sagittal changes in upper incisor position had occurred relative to the outlines of the basal structures *(P)*. The lower incisors had not been moved labially at all. On the contrary, they had been uprighted during treatment. Condylar growth had predominated slightly over vertical development of the maxilla and

buccal dentoalveolar components (*O* and *P*). The resultant closure of the Y-axis therefore had contributed to the profile improvement *(M)*. No further treatment or retention procedures were performed.

At the age of 14 years 6 months (Fig. 8-58, *Q*), 2 years after completion of treatment, a stable result was exhibited, with the second permanent molars in occlusion *(R)*. An anterior slide of only 0.3 mm could be detected from centric relation to centric (or habitual) occlusion.

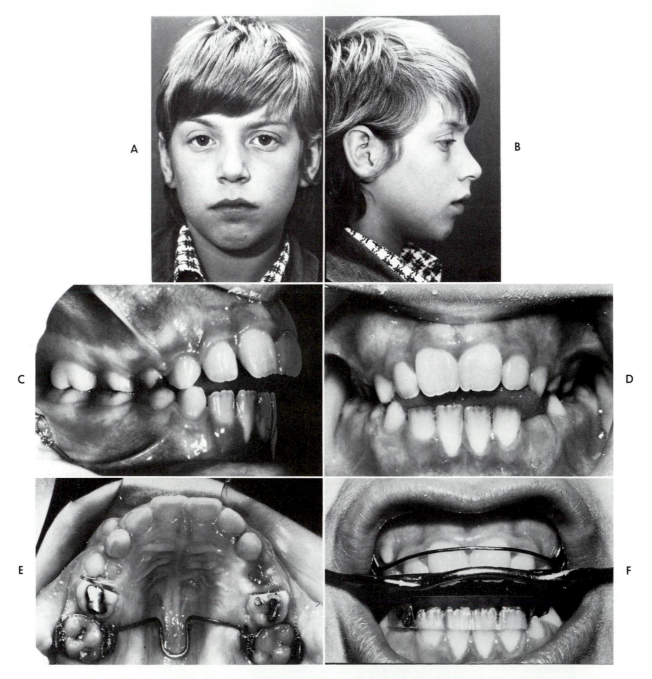

Fig. 8-59 Case 2. Hyperdivergent open bite. The patient was treated with the activator headgear appliance in combination with a transpalatal bar. **A** to **D,** Initial records and, **K,** at 10 years, 11 months. A transpalatal bar was fitted at the start of treatment, **E;** and an activator headgear appliance, **F,** was inserted. The acrylic at the upper incisor region was removed to promote vertical eruption.

This case was selected to demonstrate how the treatment concept is applied beginning in the early mixed dentition and how it can be carried through to the permanent dentition. No preparatory or final treatment with additional appliances was necessary. Only a minority of Class II patients can be treated with the activator headgear combination alone and such a favorable reaction cannot be expected in all cases with so little effort.

CASE 2 (Fig. 8-59)

This patient was clinically examined at the age of 10 years 11 months. His lips were usually apart. For lip closure, mentalis hyperactivity was necessary (Fig. 8-59, *A*). From the initial profile examination a skeletal hyperdivergency combined with an antero-posterior discrepancy was suspected *(B)*. This was corroborated by analysis of the cephalometric head film *(K)*. S-N-A was 81°, S-N-B 74°, and S-N to Me-Go 42°. A dental Class II with an anterior open bite was seen intra-orally *(C and D)*. The tip of the tongue was positioned on the lower incisors. No airway obstruction could be discerned. Protrusion into Class I revealed occlusal contact only at the first permanent molars, thereby increasing the anterior open bite.

A transpalatal bar was fitted to upper molar bands (Fig. 8-59, *E*, shown at a later stage of treatment). An activator headgear assembly, in which the acrylic at the upper incisor region was removed to promote vertical eruption, was also started *(F)*. The labial wire barely touched the central incisors; relative to the laterals it was positioned at a considerable distance, particularly from the right lateral. A lingual wire was used to align the lateral incisors to an ideal incisal curve. With the extraoral force vector more intrusive force was applied to the molars than to the deciduous canines. The amount of extraoral force was 400 g per side. The patient was instructed to wear the appliance every day for 14 hours.

During treatment it was possible to perform some minor occlusal grinding of the deciduous teeth. A particular attempt was made to prevent too much eruption of the permanent teeth in the buccal segments. Of course, at no time was acrylic relieved in the lower molar region. Several relining procedures were performed. The permanent second molars were included in the vertical control as soon as they had reached the occlusal level. The acrylic in the lower incisor region was removed when Class II correction was about to be completed. After 2 years and 2 months of treatment a Class I and normal incisal overbite were achieved (Fig. 8-59, *G* and *H*). The parents requested that treatment be discontinued at this point. Facial appearance had improved, and lip competence

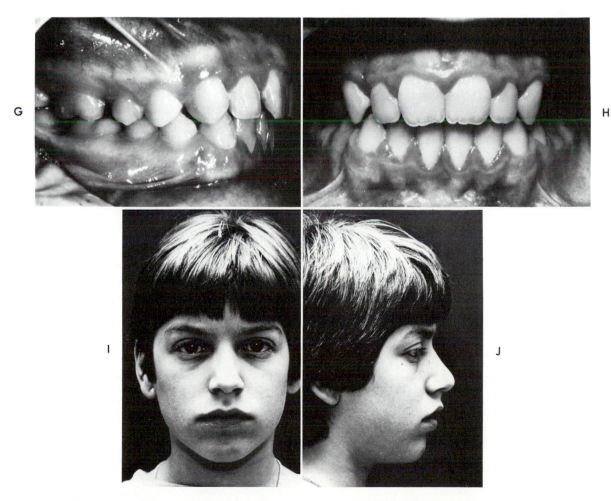

Fig. 8-59, cont'd G to J and L to N, Result after 2 years, 2 months of active treatment. The parents refused further treatment. The patient was checked 5 years later (at age 17 years, 4 months). The result had remained stable. *Continued.*

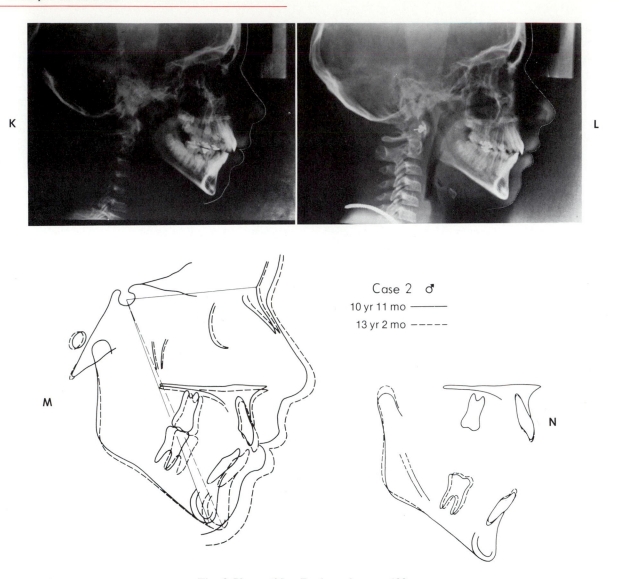

Case 2 ♂
10 yr 11 mo ——————
13 yr 2 mo ————

Fig. 8-59, cont'd For legend see p. 483.

was achieved (*I* and *J*). Comparison of the initial head film at 10 years 11 months of age with the head film at the completion of treatment (at *13* years *2* months) revealed a considerable change of the skeletal pattern (*K* and *L*). The overall superimposition demonstrated a slight posterior rotation of the maxilla and a pronounced closing rotation of the mandible *(M)*. The upper incisors had been extruded slightly when analyzed by local superimposition whereas the upper molars had remained where they were relative to the maxillary contours after treatment *(N)*. The lower incisors had been uprighted and extruded. A slight vertical eruption of the lower molars could be observed. Condylar growth was minimal but, in combination with the vertical control of the dentoalveolar structures, contributed to the vertical and sagittal improvement of the skeletal framework.

The patient was examined 5 years after treatment, and the result had remained stable.

This case demonstrates that hyperdivergency is not at all a contraindication for activator headgear treatment. On the contrary, if adequate appliance manipulation is performed the vertical and sagittal discrepancy can be improved substantially.

CASE 3 (Fig. 8-60)

A receding chin was the most obvious feature of the facial appearance in this 8-year-old boy (Fig. 8-60, *A* and *B*). The cephalometric analysis revealed an A-N-B of 7°, a S-N-A of 81°, and a S-N-B of 74°. Average profile divergency was exhibited, the S-N to Me-Go amounting to 33° *(K)*. Intra-orally a full Class II intercuspation was present on both sides, in combination with a crossbite on the left (*C* and *D*). From centric relation to full occlusion a forward slide of over 1 mm and a lateral slide to the left of 2.5 mm could be discerned. Almost 3 mm of space was lacking for the upper lateral incisors.

Preparatory treatment was indicated in this boy because of the transverse deficiency in the upper arch and the severe functional deviation. Expansion of the upper arch was initiated with a quadhelix appliance (Fig. 8-60, *E* and *F*). During this treatment the

Class II discrepancy was aggravated. One reason was the posterior repositioning of the mandible; the other, the increase in vertical dimension because of contacts on inclined planes as expansion was being achieved *(E)*. After 4 months this appliance was removed and shortly thereafter activator headgear treatment started.

The activator was fitted initially with a lingual and a labial wire to align the upper incisors. These wires were later removed and torquing springs added. The extra-oral force vector was positioned superior to the center of resistance of the dentition, and 400 g was applied as long as all deciduous teeth were present. No acrylic was removed in the region of the lower first permanent molars.

The occlusal result after 1 year and 7 months of activator headgear treatment is shown in Fig. 8-60, *G* and *H*. One month before these pictures were taken the upper deciduous canines and first molars were extracted to allow distal eruption of the permanent canines. Facial appearance had improved substantially during this

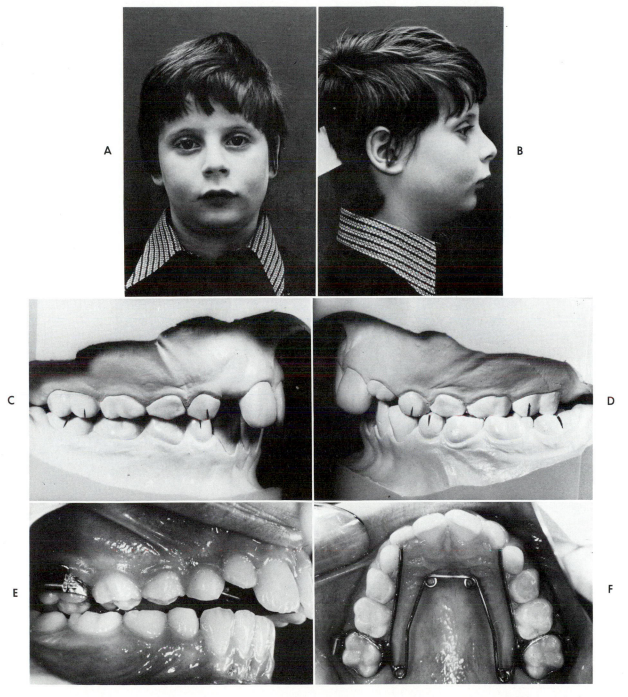

Fig. 8-60   Case 3. Preparatory upper arch expansion with a quad helix before activator headgear treatment. **A** to **D** and **K,** Initial records at 7 years, 11 months. Expansion with the quad helix during 4 months, **E** and **F,** aggravated the Class II discrepancy.   *Continued.*

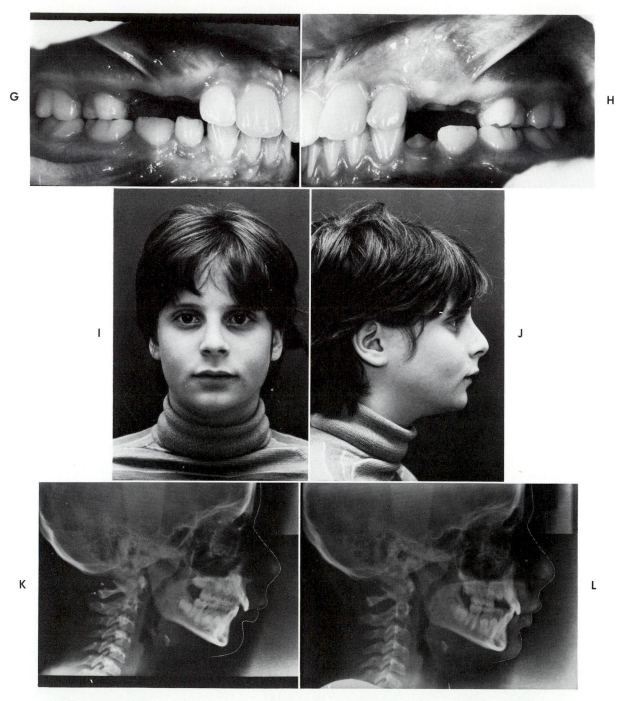

Fig. 8-60, cont'd   **G** and **H** and **L** to **N,** Result at age 10 years after 1 year 7 months of additional activator headgear treatment. At this stage the activator headgear appliance was worn during sleeping hours only until the permanent canines and premolars had emerged; then treatment was discontinued. **O** and **P,** Result after 2 years of posttreatment observation. In cases such as this a decision must be made whether occlusal imperfections like these call for further treatment with fixed appliances.

treatment period (*I* and *J*). The cephalometric comparison between the initial head film at the age of almost 8 years and the progress head film at the age of 10 years revealed the change in the maxillomandibular relationship (*K* and *L*). From the overall superimposition it can be seen that some posterior rotation of the maxilla had occurred *(M)*. The extraoral force vector was probably not managed optimally. Sometimes the shape of the head can be a handicap to achieving as steep an extra-oral force vector as desired. In the case presented it must be remembered, furthermore, that in the 2-year 1-month interval between the two head films, a period of no treatment (2 months) and rapid expansion (4 months) was included. Nevertheless, a favorable mandibular reaction can be observed. The forward displacement of the symphysis surpassed by far the increase in vertical dimension. The Y-axis therefore closed a significant amount *(M)*. The local superimposition demonstrated that minimal molar and incisor movement relative to the outlines of the basal structures had taken place *(N)*.

After this result had been achieved, the activator headgear was worn only during sleep until the upper canines and first premolars started to erupt. Then treatment was discontinued because some cooperation problems were being encountered and the need for final therapy with fixed appliances could not be excluded. The occlusal result after this 2-year observation period is shown in Fig. 8-60, *O* and *P*. A nice Class I intercuspation is present on the right side. On the left, however, the relationship of the canines and first premolars is less than perfect although the permanent first molars are in Class I. A midline deviation of almost 2 mm is present, and from centric relation to habitual occlusion, a lateral shift of 0.5 mm with a minimal sagittal component can be discerned. A decision must be made whether these occlusal discrepancies call for further treatment with fixed appliances or can be tolerated as an esthetically and functionally acceptable result. Treatment of such a problem is delicate.

It should be emphasized that in many patients preparatory treatment is necessary before Class II correction with the activator headgear appliance. Furthermore, the clinician cannot always expect a perfect occlusal relationship after activator headgear treatment, although the basic skeletal discrepancy may have been improved substantially.

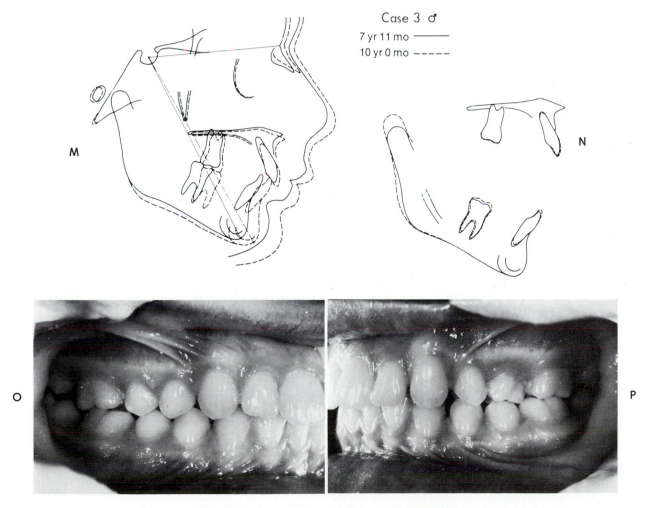

Case 3 ♂

7 yr 11 mo ———
10 yr 0 mo - - - - -

Fig. 8-60, cont'd   For legend see opposite page.

CASE 4 (Fig. 8-61)

This 11-year, 8-month-old girl exhibited an excessive mandibular retrognathia (Fig. 8-61, *A* and *B*). She suffered severely from her facial appearance and told the orthodontist that she did not want "to look like a ghost anymore." A poor skeletal pattern was revealed by the head film *(I)*. The mandibular body (Me-Go) was 11 mm shorter than the anterior cranial base (N-S), and the ramus was also deficient in length. Furthermore, a retroposition of the temporomandibular joint relative to the anterior cranial base could be discerned. S-N-B and S-N-Pog were 70°, the facial angle FH to N-Pog 79°, and the A-N-B 10°. It was anticipated that mandibular surgery would probably be needed later to harmonize the skeletal relationship. Intraorally a Class II intercuspation was observed. The upper central incisor overjet was 8 mm, but the laterals

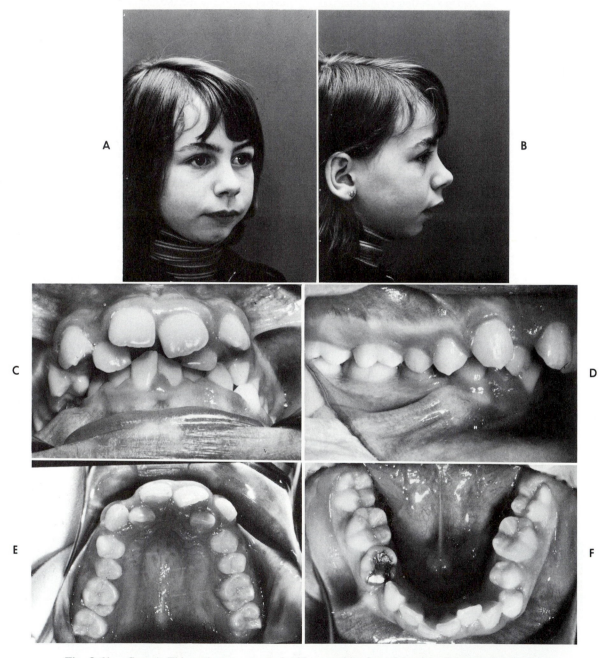

Fig. 8-61   Case 4. This patient was treated with a combination of fixed appliance and activator headgear therapy in four basic treatment phases to resolve severe intraarch, occlusal, and skeletal problems. **A** to **F** and **I,** Initial records at 11 years, 8 months. First phase, 1 year. Extraction of all first premolars, upper edgewise appliance with posterior high pull headgear, and a lower lingual arch, **G** and **H.** Second phase, 1 year, 2 months. Activator headgear treatment without removal of the upper edgewise appliance.

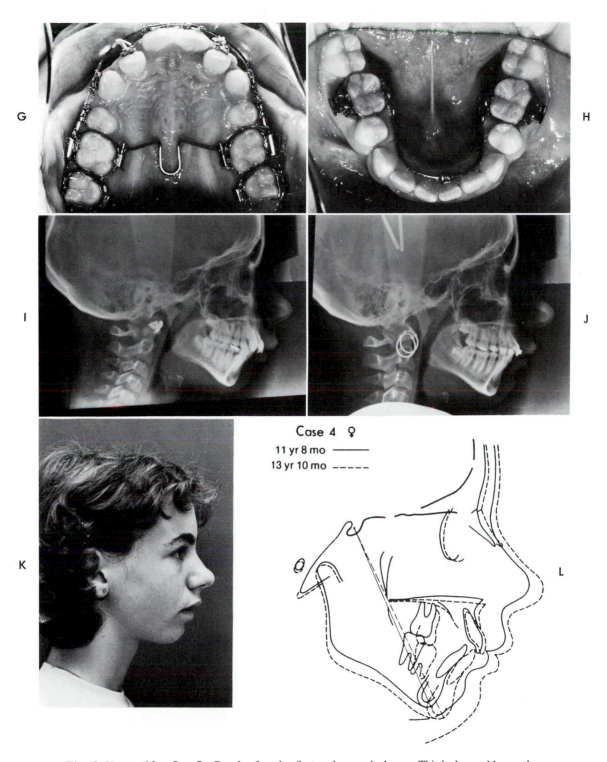

Case 4 ♀
11 yr 8 mo ———
13 yr 10 mo - - - - -

Fig. 8-61, cont'd   J to L, Result after the first and second phases. Third phase, 11 months. Lower arch bonded, fixed appliance therapy to complete occlusal detailing. Fourth phase, 1 year. After removal of the fixed appliances, activator headgear treatment for completion and retention of Class II correction.   *Continued.*

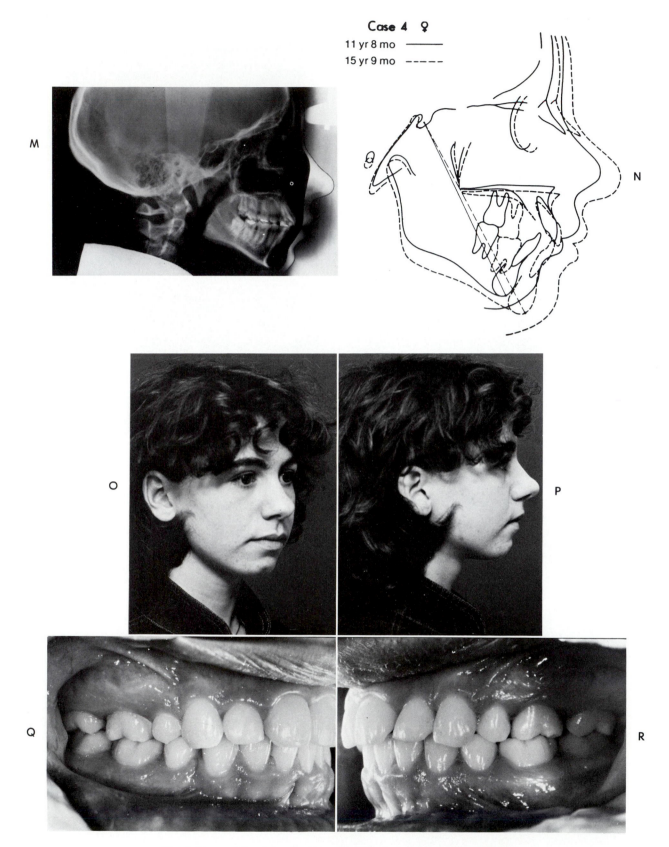

Fig. 8-61, cont'd   M to **R,** Overall result at age 15 years, 9 months.

contacted the lower incisors (*C* and *D*). In the upper arch all permanent teeth except the third molars had erupted. Severe crowding of the incisors was present: both laterals were overlapped labially by the canines (*E*). In the lower arch both permanent second molars had also erupted. Only the lower deciduous second molars persisted, and the emergence of the first and second premolars was obstructed because of crowding (*F*). The overall space deficiency amounted to 10 mm, even with the incisors markedly proclined (*I*). From centric relation to habitual occlusion a sagittal slide of almost 2 mm was detected. Protrusive movement was blocked by the upper lateral incisors.

The goal of the first treatment phase was to correct the irregularities in tooth position and improve the coordination between the two arches. All first premolars were extracted. In the lower arch only the permanent first molars were banded and a lingual wire was placed. In the upper arch all teeth were progressively banded or bonded. A transpalatal bar and posterior high pull headgear were placed. First the canines were retracted to provide room for the alignment of the lateral incisors. Fig. 8-61, *G* and *H*, shows the situation after 9 months of treatment with fixed appliances. Shortly afterward the lateral incisors were aligned and activator headgear treatment was initiated without removing the upper edgewise appliance. According to the treatment plan the activator headgear phase should be started as early as possible to exploit the growth potential during puberty. It was intended as a trial treatment to evaluate whether mandibular surgery after completion of growth could be avoided.

Comparison of the initial head film at the age of 11 years 8 months (Fig. 8-61, *I*) with the head film at age 13 years 10 months (*J*) reveals the progress that was achieved during the overall treatment period of 2 years, 2 months. The superimposition demonstrates a remarkable change in the skeletal relationship, with a predominant mandibular contribution (*L*). Facial esthetics were improved accordingly (*K*).

Following these intermediate records, activator headgear treatment was discontinued and an edgewise appliance fitted to the lower arch. After 11 months of upper and lower fixed appliance therapy, combined with posterior high pull headgear, a second 1-year phase of activator headgear treatment was started for completion and retention of the Class II treatment. Upper and lower incisors and canines were stabilized with lingually bonded retainers. Fig. 8-61, *M*, shows the situation when active treatment at the age of 15 years, 9 months was completed. The overall superimposition reveals the changes accomplished during the 4 years of active treatment (*N*). Facial appearance is documented in *O* and *P*, and the occlusal result in *Q* and *R*.

This case demonstrates that preparatory treatment is imperative if protrusive movement into Class I is obstructed by incisal interference. Furthermore, it illustrates the sequential combination of fixed appliance therapy and activator headgear treatment in the permanent dentition. Because of the severity of the patient's skeletal and dental problems, her developmental conditions, and her skeletal age, treatment proceeded in the following four basic phases:

1. A preparatory phase with fixed appliances after all first premolars had been extracted
2. Activator headgear treatment as soon as the occlusal conditions permitted full advantage to be taken of the pubertal growth activity
3. Completion of intra-arch detailing and improvement of intermaxillary coordination with edgewise appliances
4. Completion of skeletal Class II correction and retention with the activator headgear appliance

It can be argued that almost 4 years of active treatment is too demanding for any patient, regardless of age. Admittedly, the phases with fixed appliances in place could have been managed more efficiently (this patient was treated by graduate students). However, a skeletal improvement of the type and degree demonstrated cannot be completed in a short time.

CASE 5 (Fig. 8-62)

External exposure of the upper incisors, a *gummy* smile, lower lip interposition, and a retrognathic chin were the disfiguring facial features of this 10-year-5-month-old girl (Fig. 8-62, *A* to *C*). Cephalometric analysis revealed a S-N-A of 87° with an A-N-B of 9°, a FH to N-Pog of 85°, and a convexity of 9 mm. In combination with an anterior cranial base of greater than average length, maxillary prognathism (rather than mandibular retrognathism) was the major contributing factor to the skeletal anteroposterior discrepancy (*J*). A 12 mm overjet could be measured in spite of pronounced protrusion of the lower incisors (*D*, *E*, and *J*). The permanent teeth in the buccal segments had erupted or were about to erupt, and a Class II intercuspation with an extremely deep bite was present.

Utility arches and posterior high pull headgear were used first for incisor intrusion. After extraction of all first premolars the incisor segments were retracted and the spaces closed with full edgewise appliances (Fig. 8-62, *F*). The intramaxillary deviations were completely corrected, and the intermaxillary relationships markedly improved. The bands were removed after only 1 year 10 months of treatment, and an activator headgear appliance was inserted to improve the skeletal relations further and provide retention of the treatment result attained thus far (*G*). It should be stressed again in this context that the construction bite must be modified if the occlusal relationship is Class I or close to a Class I (p. 476). The activator was worn for 1 year, 4 months. The occlusal result is shown in *H* and *I*, and the cephalometric result at age 13 years, 11 months in *K*. The overall superimposition demonstrates the extensive dentoalveolar and skeletal reactions after 3 years, 2 months of active treatment in two phases (*L*). Intrusion and uprighting of the upper and lower incisor segments could be achieved without molar extrusion in the upper, and with only minor extrusion of the molars in the lower, jaw (*M*). The superimposition in (*N*), exhibits the fundamental changes accomplished with fixed appliance therapy. During activator headgear treatment the skeletal relationship was substantially improved by advancing the mandibular symphysis 3 mm relative to the forward displacement of the maxillary structures (*O*). The lower incisors were uprighted and the upper incisors protruded slightly to compensate for the difference in forward displacement of the upper and lower jaws. The facial appearance after the two phases of treatment is shown in *P* and *Q*.

In this case the activator headgear appliance was used after occlusal treatment had been completed with fixed appliance therapy. The point should be made that the other phases of treatment should also be performed according to

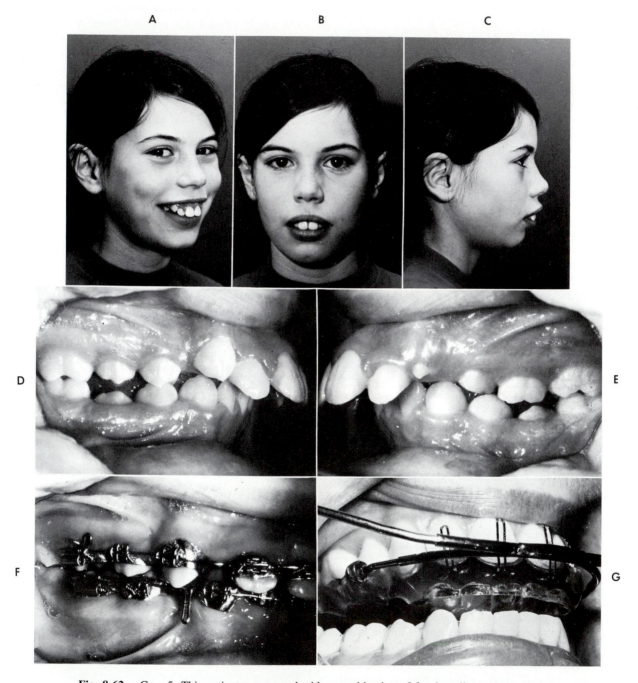

Fig. 8-62   Case 5. This patient was treated with a combination of fixed appliance and activator headgear therapy. **A** to **E** and **J,** Initial records at 10 years, 6 months. Extraction of first premolars, then fixed appliance therapy with posterior high pull headgear. **F,** The fixed appliance was removed after 1 year and 10 months of treatment, and an activator headgear appliance was inserted for 1 year, 4 months to improve the skeletal relationship further and to provide retention of the treatment result attained with fixed appliance therapy, **G.**

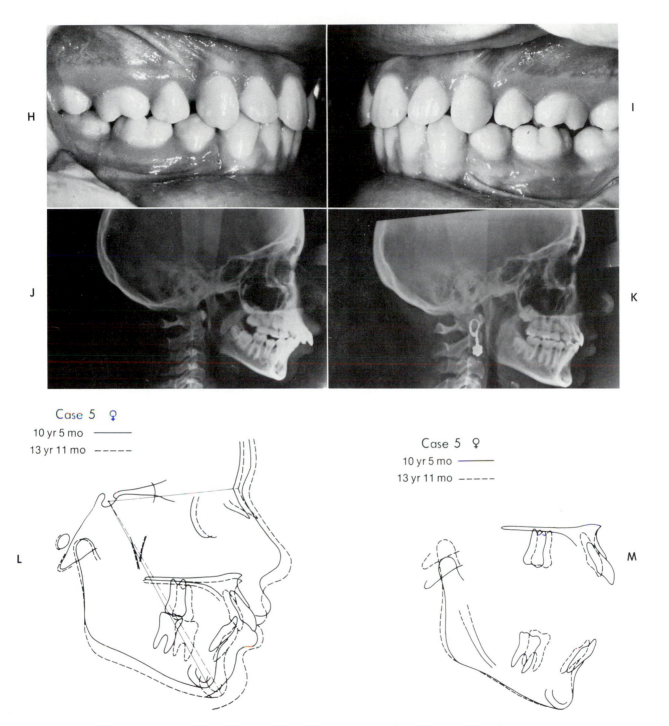

Fig. 8-62, cont'd   Occlusal, **H** and **I,** cephalometric, **J** to **O,** and facial, **P** and **Q,** results after the overall treatment.   *Continued.*

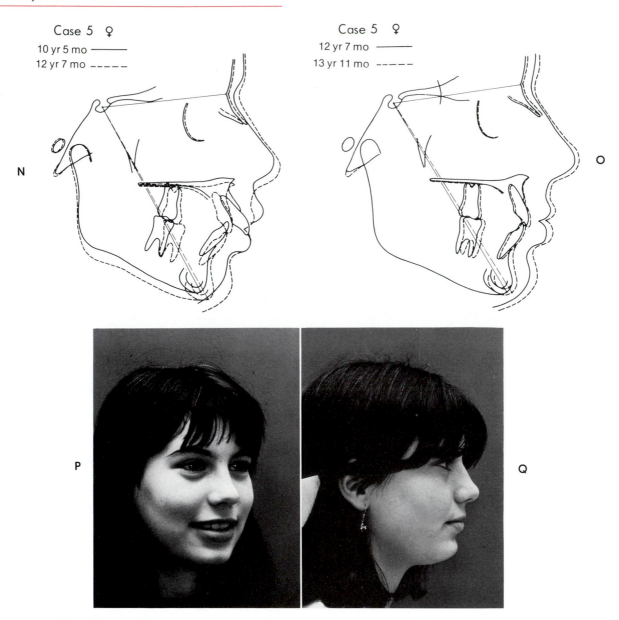

Case 5 ♀
10 yr 5 mo ———
12 yr 7 mo - - - - -

N

Case 5 ♀
12 yr 7 mo ———
13 yr 11 mo - - - - -

O

P

Q

Fig. 8-62, cont'd   The superimposition in **N** exhibits the changes accomplished during the fixed appliance therapy, and in **O** those accomplished during the activator headgear therapy.

the concept outlined in the first sections of this chapter. The activator headgear appliance should not be considered a means for rectifying poorly controlled previous treatment results. This case demonstrates, however, that during retention further improvement of the skeletal relationship can be achieved with the device. Moreover, fixed appliances can be removed at an earlier stage of Class II treatment because, with the activator headgear, occlusal results can be stabilized while basal correction is pursued further.

CASES 6 TO 18 (Figs. 8-63 to 8-75)*

In the following cases only the head films taken before and after activator headgear treatment are presented to provide a general overview of the kind of individual dentoalveolar and skeletal reactions that can be expected when this appliance is used.

In the Cases 6 to 14 the activator headgear was the only therapeutic intervention; neither preparatory nor final treatment with fixed appliances was necessary (Figs. 8-63 to 8-71; *A*, before and, *B*, after treatment).

---

*Figs. 8-63 to 8-71. (Cases 6 to 14.) These patients all were treated exclusively with the activator headgear appliance. In every case, **A** is the age before and **B** the age after treatment; *Iv* is the interval between the head films and *Tt* the active treatment time (years, months).

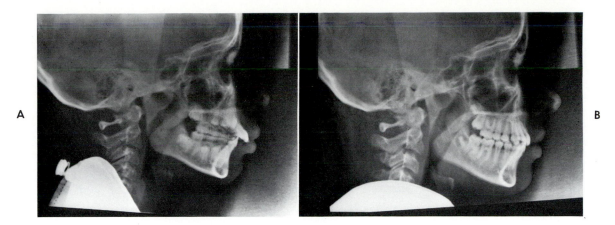

Fig. 8-63   Case 6. **A,** 8.10; **B,** 11.5; *Iv, 2.7; Tt, 2.0.*

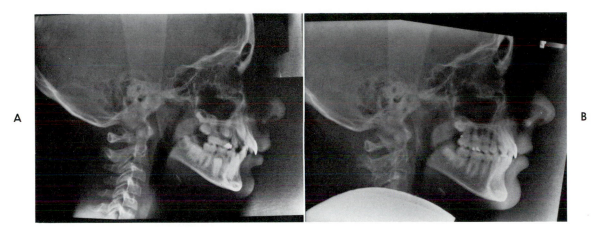

Fig. 8-64   Case 7. **A,** 10.11; **B,** 14.0; *Iv, 3.1; Tt, 2.9.*

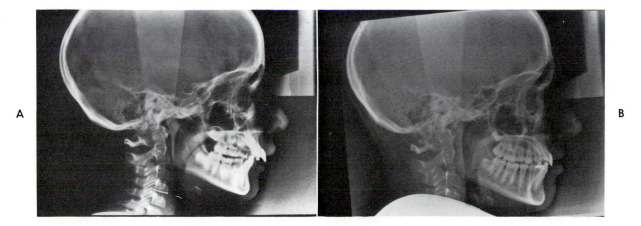

Fig. 8-65   Case 8. **A,** 7.11; **B,** 12.1; *Iv, 4.2; Tt, 3.3.*

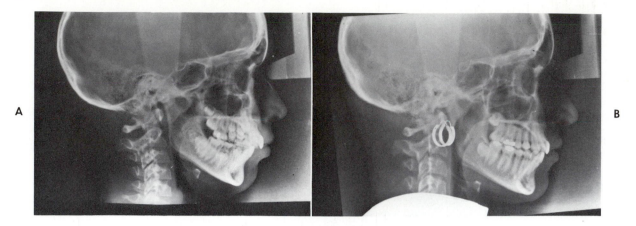

Fig. 8-66 Case 9. **A,** 10.4; **B,** 13.3; *Iv,* 2.11; *Tt,* 2.6.

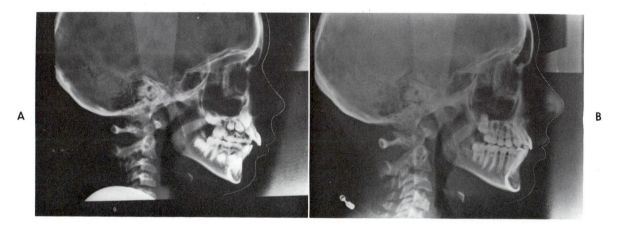

Fig. 8-67 Case 10. **A,** 8.1; **B,** 11.10; *Iv,* 3.9; *Tt,* 3.0.

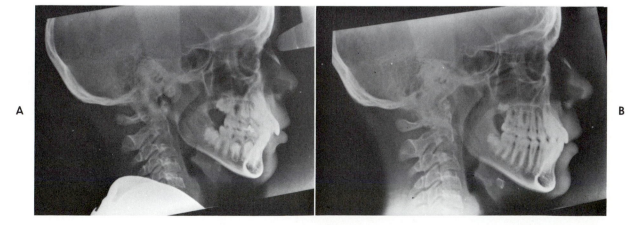

Fig. 8-68 Case 11. **A,** 8.11; **B,** 12.8; *Iv,* 3.9; *Tt,* 2.11.

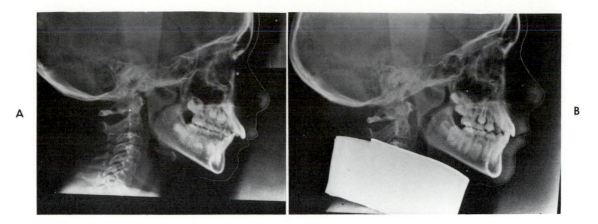

Fig. 8-69   Case 12. **A,** 8.4; **B,** 11.11; *Iv,* 3.7; *Tt,* 3.1.

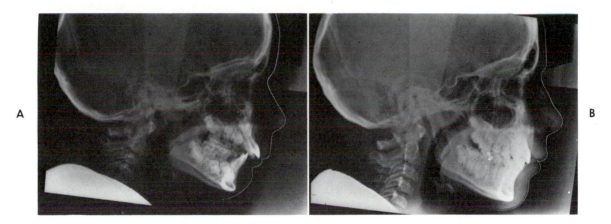

Fig. 8-70   Case 13. **A,** 8.2; **B,** 12.11; *Iv,* 4.9; *Tt,* 3.8.

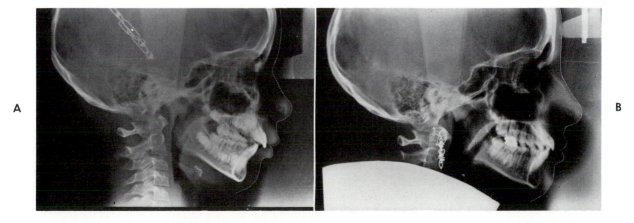

Fig. 8-71   Case 14. **A,** 8.7; **B,** 12.9; *Iv,* 4.2; *Tt,* 3.10.

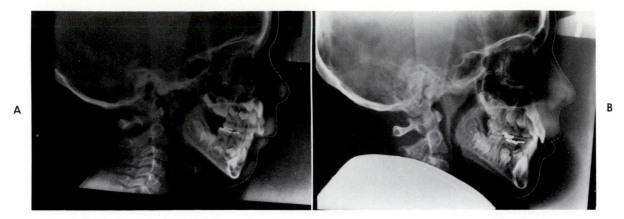

Fig. 8-72   Case 15. Activator headgear treatment started in the deciduous dentition. **A,** 5.11; **B,** 10.7 (1 year after active treatment had been discontinued); *Iv,* 4.8; *Tt,* first appliance 1.10, second appliance 1.6.

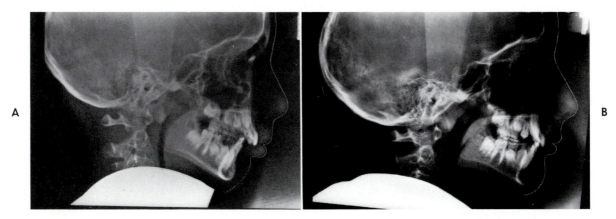

Fig. 8-73   Case 16. Typical start of activator headgear treatment in the mixed dentition. **A,** Second phase of treatment with fixed appliance therapy is planned when the second deciduous molars are about to be lost, a few months after **B. A,** 8.11; **B,** 10.3; *Iv,* 1.4; *Tt,* 1.3.

Case 15 is one of the rare examples in which activator headgear treatment was started in the deciduous dentition (Fig. 8-72, *A*). Two appliances were used consecutively. *B* shows the result in the mixed dentition 1 year after treatment was discontinued. In such cases, during or after eruption of the permanent teeth it must be decided whether a second phase of treatment with fixed appliances will be needed.

The classical approach is exemplified by Case 16. In this patient, with a Class II discrepancy, treatment involved use of the activator headgear during the mixed dentition stage until the exchange in the buccal segments was progressing (Fig. 8-73). Then fixed appliance therapy was initiated for final occlusal adjustments.

Cases 17 and 18 should demonstrate that an aggravation of the skeletal Class II discrepancy often must be expected after preparatory treatment (Figs. 8-74 and 8-75). In Case 17 the parents objected strongly to extraction of permanent teeth (Fig. 8-74, *A*). A transpalatal bar for correction of the transverse problems and a utility arch for incisor arrangement were placed in the upper jaw

and a passive lingual arch for space maintenance in the lower. The cephalometric situation after 8 months of this preparatory treatment is revealed in *B*. An activator headgear appliance was then placed and the result after 1 year is shown in *C*. In Case 18 (Fig. 8-75, *A*) a severe transverse deficiency in the upper jaw had to be resolved with rapid expansion *(B)*. Four months later activator headgear treatment was started, and the result after 2 years is shown in *C*.

INVESTIGATION OF THE AVERAGE EFFECTS OF TREATMENT

A broad investigation was undertaken by one of us[123] to quantitate the average dentoalveolar and skeletal reaction to activator headgear treatment. At our clinic more than 500 patients with Class II discrepancy have been subjected to activator headgear treatment as part of the overall procedure. In the great majority of cases additional fixed appliance

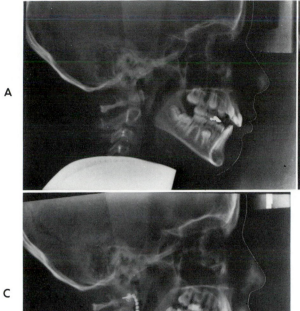

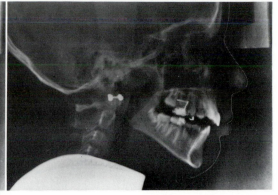

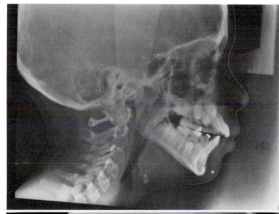

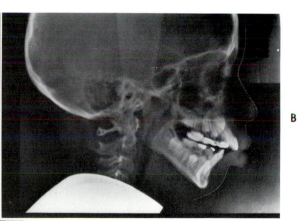

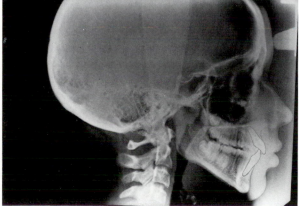

Fig. 8-74   Case 17. **A,** 10.9; **B,** 11.6. After 8 months of preparatory treatment with a transpalatal bar, posterior high pull headgear, and upper utility plus a passive lower lingual arch. The parents (who were dentists!) had refused extraction treatment because no crowding was present. Note the aggravation of the skeletal anteroposterior problem and the vertical discrepancy. **C,** After 1 year of activator headgear treatment following **B** records.

Fig. 8-75   Case 18. **A,** 11.1; **B,** 11.3. Rapid expansion had to be performed because of a severe transverse deficiency in the upper jaw (bilateral crossbite). This procedure caused the skeletal Class II to become more pronounced. After 4 months of retention, activator headgear treatment was started. **C,** 13.7. Result after 2 years of activator headgear treatment.

therapy or combinations with other appliances have been used.

In a pilot study, only the effects of activator headgear treatment were evaluated. A longitudinal control sample of 49 cases (28 boys and 21 girls) was selected at random. These children had had no previous orthodontic treatment, and no skeletal or dentoalveolar criteria were considered. The activator headgear sample consisted of 22 cases (14 boys and 8 girls). The selective criteria were a skeletal and dental Class II, no history of or need for preparatory orthodontic treatment or extractions, no indications for combinations with other appliances, treatment started in the mixed dentition and completed in the permanent dentition, and well-related records of high quality. Neither vertical criteria nor criteria regarding treatment results were applied. Since no cases could be included with intramaxillary or coordinative problems, a large sample size could not be established at the time of evaluation. The size was sufficient, however, to demonstrate the effects of activator headgear treatment.

The mean age at the start of observation of the control group was only 2 months more than the mean at the start of treatment in the activator headgear group, which was 10 years. Mean treatment time was 2 years 5 months. Annual changes were computed. No significant differences could be found between girls and boys in both groups at the age under investigation. True Frankfort horizontal and sella vertical were selected as references from which overall cephalometric changes could be evaluated. This reference system was transferred by structural superimposition of the anterior cranial base from the first to the second head film in each case (Fig. 8-76, A). The maxilla was superimposed on the palatal outline and the nasal floor, the mandible on the structures of the symphysis along the menton-gonion line. The palatal point (P_v) and the landmarks of the symphysis were transferred from the first to the second head film. The system of coordinates for the evaluation of the local changes is shown in Fig. 8-76, B. The landmarks were digitized from pinholes in copies of the cephalograms. The nonparametric Wilcoxon test was applied for statistical analysis. (For details of the investigation, see Teuscher.[123]) Only a small section of the results are presented graphically here to provide an overview of the main effects of activator headgear treatment. For ease of interpretation, a 3-year interval was chosen for illustration.

The pattern of maxillary and upper dentoalveolar displacement is shown in Fig. 8-77, A, for the control and in B for the activator headgear (A-HG) group. The reaction of the basal maxillary structures to activator headgear treatment was minimal over the time interval being considered. Slight inhibition of forward displacement of point A could be discerned, the path of average downward and forward movement being 54° to Frankfort horizontal in the A-HG group versus 46° in the control (Fig. 8-78). However, no significant differences could be found in the vertical and sagittal displacement of any of the maxillary skeletal points investigated. Accordingly, no rotation of the palatal plane was

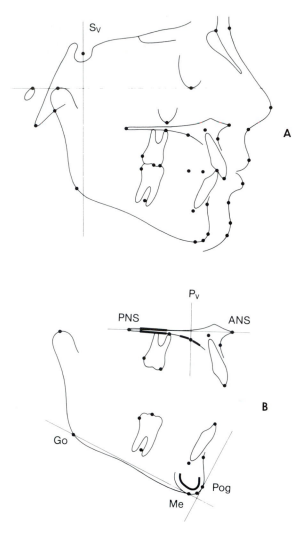

Fig. 8-76 **A,** Reference system, true Frankfort horizontal *(FH)* and sella vertical *(S_v),* to evaluate overall cephalometric changes. The reference system was transferred by structural superimposition on the anterior cranial base from the first to the second head film in each case. **B,** Reference system to evaluate local changes of maxillary structures and of the upper dentition. The maxilla was superimposed along the palatal outline, and the visible parts of the nasal floor. The orientation along the line *ANS-PNS* and the palatal point *(P_v)* were transferred from the first to the second head film in each case. **C,** Reference system to evaluate local changes of mandibular structures and of the lower dentition. The mandible was superimposed along *Me-Go* on the structures of the symphysis. The orientation along the line *Me-Go* and point *Pog* was transferred from the first to the second head film in each case.

observed. Maxillary growth proceeded almost undisturbed. The most important factor is that no untoward deflection was caused by the activator headgear treatment.

The dentoalveolar structures, however, exhibited a pronounced reaction. Forward movement of the molars and incisors was reduced by a highly significant degree in the A-HG group (Figs. 8-77 and 8-79). The axial inclination of the upper incisors was well controlled (Fig. 8-79, B).

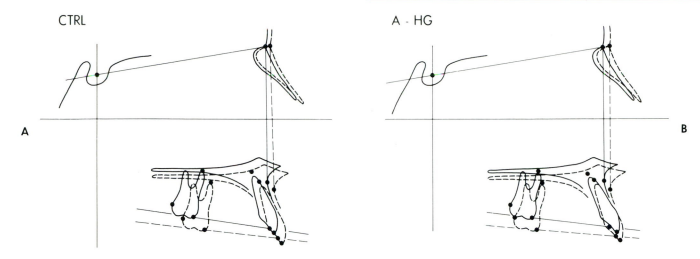

Fig. 8-77 Pattern of maxillary and upper dentoalveolar displacement in the control, **A,** and activator headgear, **B,** groups.

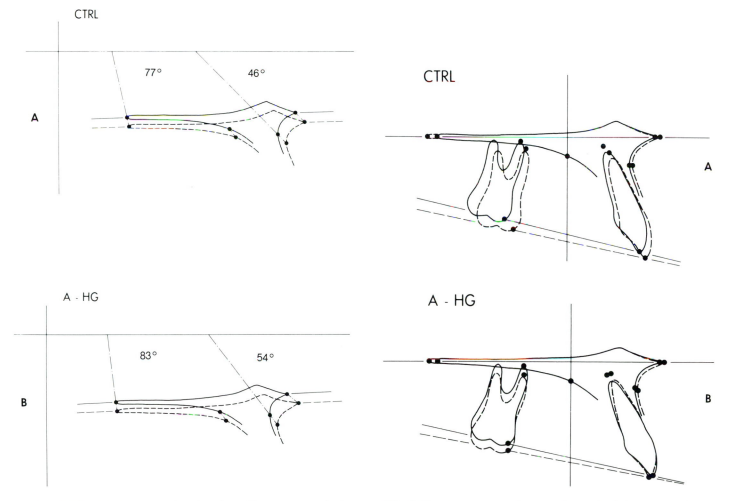

Fig. 8-78 Displacement of the basal maxillary structures in the control, **A,** and activator headgear, **B,** groups.

Fig. 8-79 Amount and direction of growth of the upper molars and central incisors in the control, **A,** and activator headgear, **B,** groups.

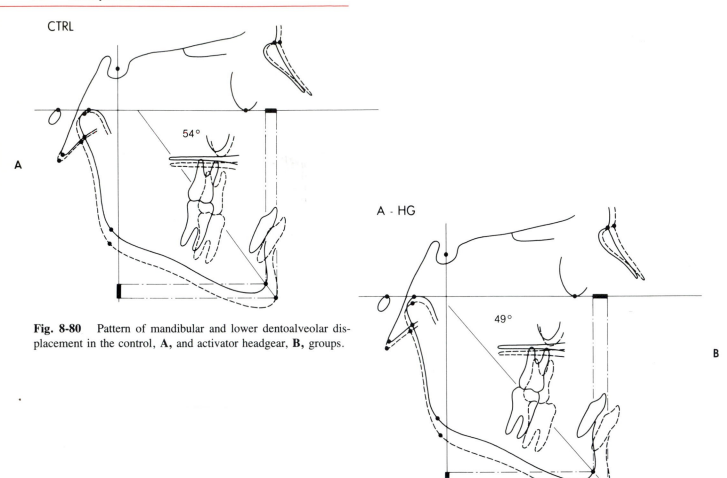

Fig. 8-80   Pattern of mandibular and lower dentoalveolar displacement in the control, **A,** and activator headgear, **B,** groups.

Significant inhibition of the vertical dentoalveolar development could be detected in the incisor region whereas vertical development in the molar region was the same in the control and the A-HG group (Figs. 8-77 and 8-79). The occlusal plane was therefore slightly rotated in an anterior direction. Thus no contribution to Class II correction was provided by rotational effects of maxillary structures. It should be emphasized that the upper dentition was not driven backward. The overall forward displacement was reduced about 40% in comparison to the controls without enhancement of the vertical dimension (Figs. 8-77 and 8-79). This is an extremely important consideration regarding the influence on anterior displacement of the mandibular symphysis.[16,17,19,121]

Relative to the cranial structures, pogonion had advanced significantly further in the A-HG group than in the control (Fig. 8-80). Suprisingly, measurements of annual increases in condylion-pogonion did not reveal any significant differences between the two groups (Fig. 8-81). Only in the angle menton-gonion-condylion could a significant difference be found: it decreased in the control whereas no change was observed in the A-HG group. Accordingly, the direction of condylar growth differed in the two samples (Fig. 8-82). In the A-HG group the condyles grew significantly more in

a posterior direction, exhibiting, however, approximately the same amount of vertical increase as in the control. When the posteriorly directed component of condylar growth is projected on the occlusal plane, the difference in sagittal contribution between the two groups becomes obvious.

The changes of lower incisor position are practically identical in both groups (Fig. 8-82). Uprighting was also observed in the A-HG group,[70,123] confirming that no unfavorable labial tipping need have been feared when the activator headgear combination was used. The same amount of forward drift of the molars was found in both groups. The vertical increase in molar position was slightly greater in the A-HG group but not to a significant degree. The removal of acrylic in the lower molar region in some of the treated patients was probably responsible for this minute difference.

An important finding was the unequal change in condylar position in the two samples (Figs. 8-80 and 8-83). It must be stressed that in the end result centric relation was identical or close to habitual occlusion. In the A-HG group the condyle moved significantly less backward and more downward. The average displacement path of condylion was 46° relative to Frankfort horizontal in the control whereas in the treated sample it was 72° (Fig. 8-83). Moreover, the linear

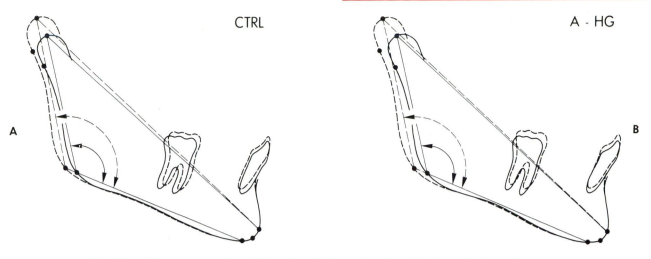

Fig. 8-81 Development of mandibular shape in the control, **A,** and activator headgear, **B,** groups.

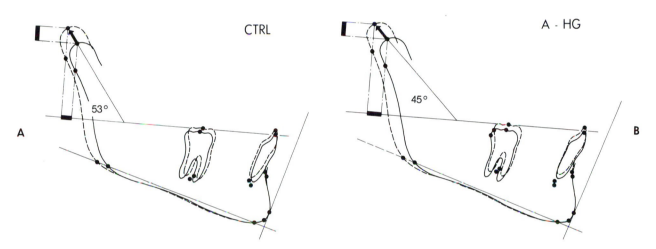

Fig. 8-82 Amount and direction of growth of the mandibular condyles, and of the lower molars and central incisors, in the control, **A,** and activator headgear, **B,** groups.

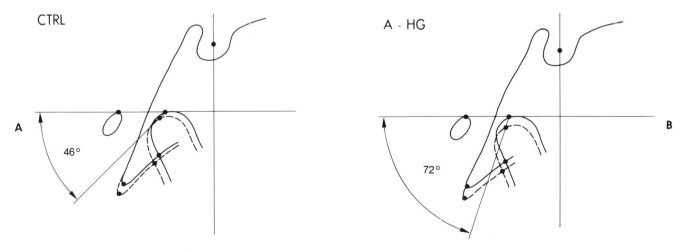

Fig. 8-83 Displacement pattern of condylion and basion in the control, **A,** and activator headgear, **B,** groups.

difference between the initial and final condylar positions was also significantly greater in the A-HG group. All these factors contribute to an anterior rotation of the mandible. Thus the corrective effect on the lower jaw involved a change in mandibular shape and a less backward and more downward remodeling of the glenoid fossae.

In summary, with activator headgear treatment the dentoalveolar reactions in the upper jaw and the exclusively skeletal reactions in the lower jaw contribute about equally to the correction of Class II malocclusions.

The degree of inhibition in anterior displacement of the midfacial structures, together with vertical and rotational management, determines to a large extent the quality of skeletal and profile results in most skeletal Class II cases. The less the need for maxillary inhibition and the more the condylar growth that can contribute to anterior displacement of the symphysis, the better will be the skeletal and profile improvement.

ACKNOWLEDGMENTS

We want to thank Dr. G. Baldini, a former staff member, who contributed with his ideas and drive in many aspects to the realization of the concepts presented. In the struggle to convey our ideas clearly in the English language, Dr. R. Carmichael, a visiting Assistant Professor in Prosthetics from Vancouver, was of great help. Particular thanks are extended to Liselotte Rüegg for her devoted assistance in the preparation of the manuscript, Magdalena Jeannottat for the skillful graphics, and Liselotte Brandenberger for the photographic reproductions.

REFERENCES

1. Abbühl P: Die Wirkung des zervikalen Headgears auf das Fazialskelett—eine klinische Studie, *Inf Orthod Kieferorthop* 8:327, 1976.
2. Ahlgren J: An electromyographic analysis of the response to activator (Andresen-Häupl) therapy, *Odontol Rev* 11:125, 1960.
3. Ahlgren J: The neurophysiologic principles of the Andresen method of functional jaw orthopedics: a critical analysis and new hypothesis, *Sven Tandlak T* 63:1, 1970.
4. Ahlgren J: Early and late electromyographic response to treatment with activators, *Am J Orthod* 74:88, 1978.
5. Armstrong MM: Controlling the magnitude, direction, and duration of extraoral force, *Am J Orthod* 59:217, 1971.
6. Auf der Maur HJ: Electromyographic recordings of the lateral pterygoid muscle in activator treatment of Class II, division 1, malocclusion cases, *Eur J Orthod* 2:161, 1980.
7. Barton JJ: High-pull headgear vs. cervical traction: a cephalometric comparison, *Am J Orthod* 62:517, 1972.
8. Bass NM: Early treatment of skeletal II malocclusion involving preliminary incisor root torquing. *Trans Eur Orthod Soc* p. 191, 1975.
9. Bass NM: Innovation in skeletal Class II treatment including effective incisor root torque in a preliminary removable appliance phase, *Br J Orthod* 3:223, 1976.
10. Bass NM: Dento-facial orthopaedics in the correction of the skeletal II malocclusion, *Br J Orthod* 9:3, 1982.
11. Baume LJ, Derichsweiler H: Is the condylar growth center responsive to orthodontic therapy? An experimental study on *Macaca mulatta*, *Oral Surg* 14:347, 1961.
12. Baume LJ, Häupl K, Stellmach R: Growth and transformation of the temporomandibular joint in an orthopedically treated case of Pierre Robin's syndrome, *Am J Orthod* 45:901, 1959.
13. Baumrind S, Korn EL: Patterns of change in mandibular and facial shape associated with the use of forces to retract the maxilla, *Am J Orthod* 80:31, 1981.
14. Baumrind S, Korn EL, Isaacson RJ et al: Superimpositional assessment of treatment-associated changes in the temporomandibular joint and the mandibular symphysis, *Am J Orthod* 84:443, 1983.
15. Baumrind S, Korn EL et al: Changes in facial dimension associated with the use of forces to retract the maxilla, *Am J Orthod* 80:17, 1981.
16. Baumrind S, Molthen R et al: Mandibular plane changes during maxillary retraction. I. *Am J Orthod* 74:32, 1978.
17. Baumrind S, Molthen R et al: Mandibular plane changes during maxillary retraction. II. *Am J Orthod* 74:603, 1978.
18. Baumrind S, Molthen R et al: Distal displacement of the maxilla and upper first molar, *Am J Orthod* 75:630, 1979.
19. Baumrind S, Molthen R et al: Mandibular plane changes during maxillary retraction. Addendum, *Am J Orthod* 75:86, 1979.
20. Björk A: The principles of the Andresen method of orthodontic treatment: a discussion based on cephalometric x-ray analysis of treated cases, *Am J Orthod* 37:437, 1951.
21. Björk A: Cranial base development, *Am J Orthod* 41:198, 1955.
22. Björk A: Prediction of mandibular growth rotation, *Am J Orthod* 55:585, 1969.
23. Björk A, Skieller V: Facial development and tooth eruption: an implant study at the age of puberty, *Am J Orthod* 52:339, 1972.
24. Björk A, Skieller V: *Postnatal growth and development of the maxillary complex.* In McNamara JA Jr, editor: *Factors affecting the growth of the midface. Monograph 6, Craniofacial growth series,* Ann Arbor, 1976, Center for Human Growth and Development, University of Michigan.
25. Björk A, Skieller V: Growth of the maxilla in three dimensions as revealed radiographically by the implant method, *Br J Orthod* 4:53, 1977.
26. Björk A, Skieller V: Normal and abnormal growth of the mandible. A synthesis of longitudinal cephalometric implant studies over a period of 25 years, *Eur J Orthod* 5:1, 1983.
27. Brandt HC, Shapiro PA, Kokich VG: Experimental and postexperimental effects of posteriorly directed extraoral traction in adult *Macaca fascicularis*, *Am J Orthod* 75:301, 1979.
28. Breitner C: Bone changes resulting from experimental orthodontic treatment, *Am J Orthod* 26:521, 1940.
29. Breitner C: Further investigations of bone changes resulting from experimental orthodontic treatment, *Am J Orthod* 27:605, 1941.
30. Brown P: A cephalometric evaluation of high-pull molar headgear and facebow neck strap therapy, *Am J Orthod* 74:621, 1978.
31. Burstone CJ: *The biomechanics of tooth movement.* In Kraus BS, Riedel RA, editors: *Vistas in orthodontics,* Philadelphia, 1962, Lea & Febiger.
32. Charlier JP, Petrovic A, Hermann J: Effects of mandibular hyperpropulsion on the prechondroblastic zone of young rat condyle, *Am J Orthod* 55:71, 1969.
33. Christiansen RL, Burstone CJ: Centers of rotation within the periodontal space, *Am J Orthod* 55:353, 1969.
34. Creekmore TD: Inhibition or stimulation of the vertical growth of facial complex, its significance to treatment, *Angle Orthod* 37:285, 1967.
35. Creekmore TD, Radney LJ: Fränkel appliance therapy: orthopedic or orthodontic? *Am J Orthod* 83:89, 1983.
36. Cross JJ: Facial growth: before, during, and following orthodontic treatment, *Am J Orthod* 71:68, 1977.
37. Demisch A: Effects of activator therapy on the craniofacial skeleton in Class II, Division I, malocclusion, *Eur Orthod Soc Rep Congr* p. 295, 1972.
38. Demisch A: Long-term observation of the occlusal stability after distal bite therapy with the Bern activator, *Schweiz Monatsschr Zahnheilkd* 90:867, 1980.
39. Dietrich UC: Aktivator—mandibuläre Reaktion, *Schweiz Monatsschr Zahnheilkd* 83:1093, 1973.
40. Droschl H: The effect of heavy orthopaedic forces on the maxilla of the growing *Siamire sciureus* (squirrel monkey), *Am J Orthod* 63:449, 1973.

41. Elder JR, Tuenge RH: Cephalometric and histologic changes produced by extraoral high-pull traction to the maxilla of *Macaca mulatta*, *Am J Orthod* 66:599, 1974.

42. Elgoyhen JC, Moyers RE et al: Craniofacial adaptation to protrusive function in young rhesus monkeys, *Am J Orthod* 62:469, 1972.

43. Eschler J: Die Kieferdehnung mit funktionskieferorthopädischen Apparaten: der Funktionator, *Zahnaerztl Welt* 63:203, 1962.

44. Faulkner JA, Maxwell LC, White TP: *Adaptations in skeletal muscle*. In Carlson DS, McNamara JA Jr, editors: *Muscle adaptation in the craniofacial region. Monograph 8, Craniofacial growth series*, Ann Arbor, 1978, Center for Human Growth and Development, University of Michigan.

45. Forsberg CM, Odenrick L: Skeletal and soft tissue response to activator treatment, *Eur J Orthod* 3:247, 1981.

46. Fränkel R: Die Möglichkeiten einer basalen Nachentwicklung des Unterkiefers durch Bissverschiebung mit dem Funktionsregler, *Dtsch Stomatol* 21:198, 1971.

47. Fredrick DL: "Dentofacial changes produced by extraoral high-pull traction to the maxilla of the *Macaca mulatta;* a histologic and serial cephalometric study." Thesis, University of Washington, 1969.

48. Graber TM: *Dentofacial orthopedics*. In Graber TM, Swain BF, editors: *Current orthodontic concepts and techniques*, ed 2, Philadelphia, 1975, WB Saunders.

49. Graber TM, Chung DDB, Aoba JT: Dentofacial orthopaedics versus orthodontics, *J Am Dent Assoc* 75:1145, 1967.

50. Graber TM, Neumann B: *Removable orthodontic appliances*, Philadelphia, 1977, WB Saunders.

51. Haack DC, Weinstein S: Geometry and mechanics as related to tooth movement studied by means of two-dimensional model, *J Am Dent Assoc* 66:157, 1963.

52. Harvold EP: *The activator in interceptive orthodontics*, St Louis, 1974, Mosby.

53. Harvold EP, Vargervik K: Morphogenetic response to activator treatment, *Am J Orthod* 60:478, 1971.

54. Hasund A: The use of activators in a system employing fixed appliances, *Eur Orthod Soc Rep Congr* p. 329, 1969.

55. Häupl K, Psansky R: Experimentelle Untersuchungen über Gelenkstransformation bei Verwendung der Methoden der Funktionskieferorthopädie, *Dtsch Zahn Mund Kieferheilkd* 6:439, 1939.

56. Herren P: The activator's mode of action, *Am J Orthod* 45:512, 1959.

57. Herren P: Das Wirkungsprinzip des Distalbiss-Aktivators, *Fortschr Kieferorthop* 41:308, 1980.

58. Hotz RP: Application and appliance manipulation of functional forces, *Am J Orthod* 58:459, 1970.

59. Hotz RP: *Orthodontics in daily practice*, Bern, Switzerland, 1974, Hans Huber.

60. Howard RD: Skeletal changes with extraoral traction, *Eur J Orthod* 4:197, 1982.

61. Isaacson RJ, Zapfel RJ, Worms FW et al: Some effects of mandibular growth on the dental occlusion and profile, *Angle Orthod* 47:97, 1977.

62. Isaacson RJ, Zapfel RJ et al: Effects of rotational jaw growth on the occlusion and profile, *Am J Orthod* 72:276, 1977.

63. Jakobsson SO: Cephalometric evaluation of treatment effect on Class II, division 1, malocclusions, *Am J Orthod* 53:446, 1967.

64. Janson M: A cephalometric study of the efficiency of the Bionator, *Trans Eur Orthod Soc* 53:283, 1977.

65. Joho JP: The effects of extraoral low-pull traction to the mandibular dentition of *Macaca mulatta*, *Am J Orthod* 64:555, 1973.

66. Kloehn SJ: Guiding alveolar growth and eruption of teeth to reduce treatment time and produce a more balanced denture and face, *Angle Orthod* 17:33, 1947.

67. Korkhaus G: *German methodologies in maxillary orthopedics*. In Kraus BS, Riedel RA, editors: *Vistas in orthodontics*, Philadelphia, 1962, Lea & Febiger.

68. Kreiborg S, Leth Jensen B et al: Craniofacial growth in a case of congenital muscular dystrophy, *Am J Orthod* 74:207, 1978.

69. Kuhn RJ: Control of anterior vertical dimension and proper selection of extraoral anchorage, *Angle Orthod* 38:341, 1968.

70. Lagerström LO, Nielsen IL et al: Dental and skeletal contributions to occlusal correction in patients treated with the high-pull headgear-activator combination, *Am J Orthod* 97:495, 1990.

71. Luder HU: Effects of activator treatment—evidence for the occurrence of two different types of reaction, *Eur J Orthod* 3:205, 1981.

72. Luder HU: Skeletal profile changes related to two patterns of activator effects, *Am J Orthod* 81:390, 1982.

73. Marschner JF, Harris JE: Mandibular growth and Class II treatment, *Angle Orthod* 36:89, 1966.

74. McNamara JA Jr: *Neuromuscular and skeletal adaptations to altered orofacial function. Monograph 1, Craniofacial growth series*, Ann Arbor, 1972, Center for Human Growth and Development, University of Michigan.

75. McNamara JA Jr: Neuromuscular and skeletal adaptations to altered function in the orofacial region, *Am J Orthod* 64:578, 1973.

76. McNamara JA Jr: Functional determinants of craniofacial size and shape, *Eur J Orthod* 2:131, 1980.

77. McNamara JA Jr: Components of Class II malocclusion in children 8-10 years of age, *Angle Orthod* 51:177, 1981.

78. McNamara JA Jr, Carlson DS: Quantitative analysis of temporomandibular joint adaptations to protrusive function, *Am J Orthod* 76:593, 1979.

79. McNamara JA Jr, Connelly TG, McBride MC: *Histological studies of temporomandibular joint adaptations*. In McNamara JA Jr, editor: *Determinants of mandibular form and growth. Monograph 4, Craniofacial growth series*, Ann Arbor, 1975, Center for Human Growth and Development, University of Michigan.

80. McNamara JA Jr, Huge SA: The Fränkel appliance (FR-2); model preparation and appliance construction, *Am J Orthod* 80:478, 1981.

81. Meach CL: A cephalometric comparison of bony profile changes in Class II, division 1, patients treated with extraoral force and functional jaw orthopedics, *Am J Orthod* 52:353, 1966.

82. Meikle MC: The dentomaxillary complex and overjet correction in Class II, division 1, malocclusion: objectives of skeletal and alveolar remodeling, *Am J Orthod* 77:184, 1980.

83. Meldrum RJ: Alterations in the upper facial growth of *Macaca mulatta* resulting from high-pull headgear, *Am J Orthod* 67:393, 1975.

84. Melsen B: Effects of cervical anchorage during and after treatment: an implant study, *Am J Orthod* 73:526, 1978.

85. Merrifield LL, Cross JJ: Directional forces, *Am J Orthod* 57:435, 1971.

86. Mills CM, Holman RG, Graber TM: Heavy intermittent cervical traction in Class II treatment: a longitudinal cephalometric assessment, *Am J Orthod* 74:361, 1978.

87. Moyers RE, Riolo ML, Guire KE et al: Differential diagnosis of Class II malocclusions. I. Facial types associated with Class II malocclusions, *Am J Orthod* 78:477, 1980.

88. Nanda R, Goldin B: Biomechanical approaches to the study of alterations of facial morphology, *Am J Orthod* 78:213, 1980.

89. Oudet C, Petrovic AG: *Variations in the number of sarcomeres in series in the lateral pterygoid muscle as a function of the longitudinal deviation of the mandibular position produced by the postural hyperpropulsor*. In Carlson DS, McNamara JA Jr, editors: *Muscle adaptation in the craniofacial region. Monograph 8, Craniofacial growth series*, Ann Arbor, 1978, Center for Human Growth and Development, University of Michigan.

90. Pancherz H: Treatment of Class II malocclusions by jumping the bite with the Herbst appliance, *Am J Orthod* 76:423, 1979.

91. Pancherz H: The effect of continuous bite jumping on the dentofacial complex: a follow-up study after Herbst appliance treatment of Class II malocclusions, *Eur J Orthod* 3:49, 1981.

92. Pancherz H: The mechanism of Class II correction in Herbst appliance treatment, *Am J Orthod* 82:104, 1982.

93. Petrovic AG, Oudet CL, Shaye R: Unterkieferpropulsion durch eine im Oberkiefer fixierte Vorbissführung mit seitlicher Biss-sperre von unterschiedlicher Höhe hinsichtlich der täglichen Dauer der Behandlung, *Fortschr Kieferorthop* 43:243, 1982.

94. Petrovic A, Stutzmann J, Oudet CL: *Control processes in the post-natal growth of the condylar cartilage of the mandible.* In McNamara JA Jr: *Determinants of mandibular form and growth. Monograph 4, Craniofacial growth series,* Ann Arbor, 1975, Center for Human Growth and Development, University of Michigan.

95. Petrovic A, Stutzmann J, Gasson N: *The final length of the mandible: is it genetically predetermined? Is the functional maxipropulsion involving periodic forward repositioning the best procedure to elicit overlengthening?* In Carlson DS, Ribbins KA, editors: *Craniofacial biology. Monograph 10, Craniofacial growth series,* Ann Arbor, 1981, Center for Human Growth and Development, University of Michigan.

96. Pfeiffer JP, Grobéty D: Simultaneous use of cervical appliance and activator: an orthopedic approach to fixed appliance therapy, *Am J Orthod* 61:353, 1972.

97. Pfeiffer JP, Grobéty D: The Class II malocclusion: differential diagnosis and clinical application of activators, extraoral forces, and fixed appliances, *Am J Orthod* 68:499, 1975.

98. Pfeiffer JP, Grobéty D: A philosophy of combined orthopedic-orthodontic treatment, *Am J Orthod* 81:185, 1982.

99. Poulton DR: The influence of extraoral traction, *Am J Orthod* 53:8, 1967.

100. Pryputniewicz RJ, Burstone CJ: The effect of time and force magnitude on orthodontic tooth movement, *J Dent Res* 58:1754, 1979.

101. Pryputniewicz RJ, Burstone CJ, Bowley WW: Determination of arbitrary tooth displacements, *J Dent Res* 57:663, 1978.

102. Ricketts RM: The influence of orthodontic treatment on facial growth and development, *Angle Orthod* 30:103, 1960.

103. Ricketts RM: *Mechanisms of mandibular growth: a series of inquiries on the growth of the mandible.* In McNamara JA Jr, editor: *Determinants of mandibular form and growth. Monograph 4, Craniofacial growth series,* Ann Arbor, 1975, Center for Human Growth and Development, University of Michigan.

104. Ricketts RM, Bench RW, Gugino CF et al: *Bioprogressive therapy,* Denver, 1979, Rocky Mountain/Orthodontics.

105. Riolo ML, Moyers RE et al: *An atlas of craniofacial growth,* Ann Arbor, 1974, Center for Human Growth and Development, University of Michigan.

106. Root TL: JCO interviews: Dr. Terrell L. Root on headgear, *J Clin Orthod* 9:20, 1975.

107. Schudy FF: Vertical growth versus anteroposterior growth as related to function and treatment, *Angle Orthod* 34:75, 1964.

108. Schudy FF: The rotation of the mandible resulting from growth: its implications in orthodontic treatment, *Angle Orthod* 35:36, 1965.

109. Schudy FF: The association of anatomical entities as applied to clinical orthodontics, *Angle Orthod* 36:190, 1966.

110. Schulhof RJ, Engel GA: Results of Class II functional appliance treatment, *J Clin Orthod* 16:587, 1982.

111. Shaye R: JCO interviews: Dr. Robert Shaye on functional appliances, *J Clin Orthod* 17:330, 1983.

112. Slagsvold O: *Activator development and philosophy.* In Graber TM, Neumann B: *Removable orthodontic appliances,* Philadelphia, 1977, WB Saunders.

113. Sproule WR: "Dentofacial changes produced by extraoral cervical traction to the maxilla of the *Macaca mulatta;* a histologic and serial cephalometric study." Thesis, University of Washington, 1968.

114. Stöckli PW: Die Reaktionsfähigkeit des mandibulären Gelenkknorpels auf orthopädische Stimulation während der Wachstumsphase, *Schweiz Monatsschr Zahnheilkd* 82:335, 558, 1972.

115. Stöckli PW, Dietrich UC: Experimental and clinical findings following functional forward displacement of the mandible, *Trans Eur Orthod Soc,* p 435, 1973.

116. Stöckli PW, Willert HG: Tissue reaction in the temporomandibular joint resulting from anterior displacement of the mandible in the monkey, *Am J Orthod* 60:142, 1971.

117. Teuscher UM: Prinzipien extraoraler Kräfte, *Inf Orthod Kieferorthop* 8:9, 1976.

118. Teuscher UM: A growth-related concept for skeletal Class II treatment, *Am J Orthod* 74:258, 1978.

119. Teuscher UM: Sagittale und vertikale Gesichtspunkte bei der Distalbissbehandlung, *Fortschr Kieferorthop* 39:225, 1978.

120. Teuscher UM: Direction of force application for Class II, division 1, treatment with the activator-headgear combination, *Studieweek,* p 193, 1980.

121. Teuscher UM: Edgewise therapy with cervical and intermaxillary traction: influence on the bony chin, *Angle Orthod* 53:212, 1983.

122. Teuscher UM: An appraisal of growth and reaction to extraoral anchorage, *Am J Orthod* 82:113, 1986.

123. Teuscher UM: Quantitative Resultate einer wachstumsbezogenen Behandlungsmethode des Distalbisses bei jugendlichen Patienten, *Med Habilitationsschrift,* Universität Zürich, 1988, Heidelberg, Hüthig Verlag.

124. Thilander B, Filipsson R: Muscle activity related to activator and intermaxillary traction in Angle Class II, division 1, malocclusions: an electromyographic study of the temporal, masseter, and suprahyoid muscles, *Acta Odontol Scand* 24:241, 1966.

125. Thurow RC: Craniomaxillary orthopedic correction with en masse dental control, *Am J Orthod* 68:601, 1975.

126. Trayfoot J, Richardson A: Angle Class II, division 1, malocclusions treated by the Andresen method, *Br Dent J* 124:516, 1968.

127. Tuenge RH, Elder JR: Posttreatment changes following extraoral high-pull traction to the maxilla of *Macaca mulatta, Am J Orthod* 66:618, 1974.

128. Watson WG: A computerized appraisal of the high-pull facebow, *Am J Orthod* 62:561, 1972.

129. Watson WG: Functional appliances—a perspective. [Editorial.] *Am J Orthod* 79:559, 1981.

130. Watson WG: Functional appliances questioned. [Editorial.] *Am J Orthod* 82:519, 1982.

131. Weinstein S, Haack DC: Theoretical mechanics and practical orthodontics, *Angle Orthod* 29:177, 1959.

132. Wieslander L: The effect of orthodontic treatment on the concurrent development of the craniofacial complex, *Am J Orthod* 49:15, 1963.

133. Wieslander L: The effect of force on craniofacial development, *Am J Orthod* 65:531, 1974.

134. Wieslander L, Buck DL: Physiologic recovery after cervical traction therapy, *Am J Orthod* 66:294, 1974.

135. Wieslander L, Lagerström L: The effect of activator treatment on Class II malocclusions, *Am J Orthod* 75:20, 1979.

136. Williams S, Melsen B: Condylar development and mandibular rotation and displacement during activator treatment, *Am J Orthod* 81:322, 1982.

137. Williams S, Melsen B: The interplay between sagittal and vertical growth factors, *Am J Orthod* 81:327, 1982.

138. Witt E: Muscular physiological investigations into the effect of bimaxillary appliances, *Trans Eur Orthod Soc* p. 448, 1973.

139. Witt E, Komposch G: Intermaxilläre Kraftwirkung bi-maxillärer Geräte, *Fortschr Kieferorthop* 32:345, 1971.

140. Woodside DG, Reed RT et al: *Some effects of activator treatment on the growth rate of the mandible and position of the midface.* In Cook JT, editor: *Transactions of the Third International Orthodontic Congress,* St Louis, 1975, Mosby.

141. Worms FW, Isaacson RJ, Speidel RM: A concept and classification of rotation and extraoral force systems, *Angle Orthod* 43:384, 1973.

142. Yemm R: *The role of tissue elasticity in the control of mandibular resting posture.* In Anderson DJ, Matthews B, editors: *Mastication,* Bristol, 1976, John Wright & Sons.

143. Yemm R, Nordstrom SH: Forces developed by tissue elasticity as a determinant of mandibular resting posture in the rat, *Arch Oral Biol* 19:347, 1974.

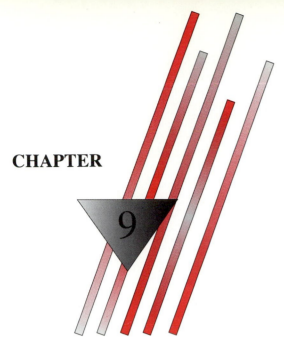

Mixed Dentition Treatment

JAMES A. McNAMARA, Jr.

CHAPTER

9

This chapter considers various aspects of mixed dentition treatment, defined as early orthodontic and orthopedic intervention provided during the mixed dentition and occasionally during the late deciduous dentition. The goal of early treatment is to correct existing or developing skeletal, dentoalveolar, and muscular imbalances to improve the orofacial environment before the eruption of the permanent dentition is complete. By initiating orthodontic and orthopedic treatment at a younger age, the overall need for complex orthodontic treatment involving permanent tooth extraction and orthognathic surgery presumably is reduced. This chapter provides an overview of early treatment and is adapted from a more extensive work on this subject by McNamara and Brudon.[88]

AN APPROACH TO EARLY TREATMENT

One of the dilemmas facing the orthodontist is whether to intervene before the eruption of the permanent dentition is complete. The argument is made that in many patients it is best to allow for the eruption of all permanent teeth (except for third molars) before initiating orthodontic treatment. With all teeth fully erupted, treatment often is provided in a relatively straightforward manner within a predictable period of time: 2 or 3 years. When dealing with the postpubescent patient in whom most growth has terminated, the clinician usually does not have to contend with unwanted changes associated with aberrant growth patterns. In some types of malocclusions, as for example in a Class III malocclusion characterized by mandibular prognathism, definitive orthodontic and surgical treatment is best deferred until the end of the active growth period.

Although deferring treatment of orthodontic problems to the adolescent age period is viewed as an advantage by some clinicians, it is viewed as a significant disadvantage by

others. Many clinicians seek to intervene in the mixed dentition and occasionally in the late deciduous dentition to eliminate or modify skeletal, muscular, and dentoalveolar abnormalities before the eruption of the permanent dentition occurs. On the surface, this concept seems reasonable because it appears more logical to prevent an abnormality from occurring rather than to wait until it has developed fully. Not all clinicians, however, employ early treatment protocol. The decision concerning whether to intervene before the eruption of the permanent dentition can be viewed on the basis of a number of interactive factors.

Factors in Decision-Making

Modification of Craniofacial Growth

During the last 25 years orthodontists and craniofacial biologists have had many discussions regarding the extent and location of therapeutically induced neuromuscular and skeletal adaptations throughout the craniofacial complex initiated during the mixed dentition. Most agree that the downward and forward growth of the maxillary complex can be affected by such therapeutic techniques as extraoral traction and activator therapy. Widening the transverse dimension of the maxilla through rapid maxillary expansion (RME) is not particularly controversial; however, the long-term stability of this form of treatment has not been evaluated thoroughly.

The question of whether the mandible can be increased in length in comparison to untreated controls also has been addressed in numerous experimental* and clinical studies.† At present the bulk of scientific evidence indicates that mandibular growth can be enhanced in growing individuals. The

---

*References 9, 21, 81, 82, 89, 90, 120-122, 140.
†References 36, 38, 42, 45, 87, 92, 108-110.

507

major question is whether this extra growth has clinical relevance. In contrast little evidence exists that the growth of the mandible can be diminished[141] either through the use of a chin cup or through orthopedic facial mask therapy; however, a redirection of mandibular growth to a more vertical vector has been observed after using a number of orthopedic techniques.[47]

Patient Cooperation

According to T.M. Graber[52] the *Achilles heel* of many early treatment protocols is patient cooperation. The ability to motivate a patient to comply is an essential ingredient of successful orthodontic therapy, whether therapy is initiated in the mixed or permanent dentition. Many orthodontists worry about beginning treatment in the mixed dentition because patient and parental cooperation may wane before fixed appliance therapy has been completed to the clinician's satisfaction. The goals and objectives of treatment must be established clearly to prevent unnecessary, prolonged treatment that may cause the patient to *burn out*.

In our opinion the most significant problem regarding patient cooperation, particularly in the mixed dentition patient, is in the mind of the orthodontist or the parent rather than in the mind of the young patient. Every effort must be made to incorporate the patient and parent in the treatment decision and to stress the importance of appliance wear according to the specific needs of the patient. Regimens requiring maximal patient cooperation should be used only after it has been determined that this type of appliance is the optimal appliance for a given skeletal and neuromuscular imbalance. The treatment time should be reasonably estimated and should be known to the patient and the parent at the beginning of the treatment period.

Management of Treatment

It is obvious that when patients begin treatment in the mixed dentition, the time from the onset of treatment to the completion of the final fixed appliance phase will extend well beyond the duration of a typical orthodontic treatment protocol initiated in the early permanent dentition. When many of the early treatment protocols were being developed in the late 1970s and early 1980s, there were many instances of prolonged treatments that not only had a negative effect on patient and parental enthusiasm but also became a nightmare from a practice management perspective. Thus more efficient early treatment protocols have evolved. These protocols have a defined duration and a reasonably predictable outcome.

In general terms an initial phase of treatment is provided that is approximately one year in duration, followed by intermittent observation during the transition from the mixed to the permanent dentition. The naturally occurring increases in arch space are incorporated into the overall treatment plan by anchoring the permanent first molars in position as the second deciduous molars are lost, usually by placing a transpalatal arch in the maxilla and a lingual arch

TABLE 9-1

Utility of Early Treatment Protocols

Angle classification	I	II	III
Deciduous	+	—	+ +
Early mixed	+ + +	(RME)	+ + +
Late mixed	+ +	+ + +	+
Early permanent	+	+ + +	—

Utility of early treatment protocols according to the type of malocclusion: + + +, most effective; + +, more effective; +, somewhat effective; —, usually not effective. Rapid maxillary expansion (RME) can be used in the early mixed dentition period in patients with Class II malocclusion to correct intra-arch problems before the later correction of the Class II sagittal relationship.

in the mandible. After all of the permanent teeth have erupted fully into occlusion (except for, perhaps, the second and third molars), fixed appliances then are used to align and fine-detail the occlusion. From a practice management point of view, separate charges are levied for the initial phase of early treatment and for the final comprehensive phase of treatment.

TIMING OF EARLY INTERVENTION

The timing of orthodontic intervention is of critical importance, and the initiation of our early treatment protocols varies according to the type of malocclusion being treated. For example, Class I tooth-size/arch-size discrepancy problems typically are treated when the patient is 8 or 9 years of age (Table 9-1). This treatment normally is initiated after the lower four incisors and the upper central incisors have erupted. In many instances, there is insufficient space to allow for the unimpeded eruption of the upper lateral incisors. Depending on the size of the permanent teeth, space maintenance, serial extraction, or orthopedic expansion protocols are used. (See Chapter 6.)

In the instance of a Class III malocclusion that is diagnosed either in the late deciduous or early mixed dentition, the onset of treatment may be earlier than it is for the Class I example (Table 9-1). The optimal time for the beginning of an early Class III treatment regimen (e.g., orthopedic facial mask, FR-3 appliance of Fränkel, chin cup) is coincident with the loss of the upper deciduous incisors and the eruption of the upper permanent central incisors. This earlier intervention in patients with a Class III malocclusion obviously will result in a longer period of time between the start of the initial phase of treatment and the end of the comprehensive treatment phase after the permanent dentition has erupted. Also, as will be discussed, the early treatment of Class III malocclusion may be characterized by more than one period of intervention during the mixed dentition.

The timing of treatment of mandibular deficiency in patients with Class II malocclusion differs slightly from that described previously for Class I and Class III malocclusions. Because there is a tendency toward earlier intervention in Class III problems than in Class I problems, we recommended delaying until the late mixed dentition period before using functional jaw orthopedics in patients with Class II malocclusion (characterized in part by mandibular skeletal retrusion [Table 9-1]). Both clinical and experimental studies have shown that there is a greater mandibular growth response with functional appliances when treatment is initiated during the circumpubertal growth period.[87,122] Ideally, functional appliance therapy (e.g., FR-2 of Fränkel, bionator) will be followed directly by a phase of fixed appliance therapy to align the permanent dentition. However, in patients who present with severe neuromuscular and skeletal problems, the initiation of treatment earlier in the mixed dentition is suggested.

In Class II patients who present with maxillary prognathism, the timing of treatment is less crucial. Extraoral traction can be employed in either the mixed or permanent dentition to satisfactorily treat this type of skeletal imbalance.[50,73,153,156]

It also should be noted that in many patients with Class II malocclusion identified in the 6- to 8-year-old age range, treatment may be initiated immediately to handle any intraarch problems (e.g, crowding, spacing, flaring); inter-arch discrepancies are addressed later. In other words, the same protocols (e.g., orthopedic expansion, serial extraction) that can be used for Class I patients also may be initiated in Class II patients with arch length discrepancies (Table 9-1); however, an attempt to correct mandibular deficiency is best delayed until the late mixed dentition period in patients with mild to moderate sagittal problems.

TREATMENT OF TOOTH-SIZE/ARCH-SIZE DISCREPANCY PROBLEMS

The most common type of malocclusion noted in the mixed dentition usually is described as *crowding*. These patients are referred by the general dentist or by the patient's parents because of obvious dentoalveolar protrusion or lack of sufficient space for permanent tooth eruption. Most commonly, this type of patient presents with a Class I molar relationship or a tendency toward either Class II or Class III malocclusion.

In the permanent dentition, discrepancies between tooth size and arch size usually are handled by one of three treatment modalities: extraction[10,11,150,151]; interproximal reduction[116,135,136]; or arch expansion.[56,57,155] Comparable treatment protocols in the mixed dentition are serial extraction and orthopedic expansion, with interproximal reduction usually being reserved for permanent dentition patients only. Additional methods of treating discrepancy problems in the mixed dentition that are not available for use in permanent dentition patients include techniques of space management (e.g., maintenance of leeway space). (See Chapter 6.)

SPACE MAINTENANCE DURING THE TRANSITION TO THE PERMANENT DENTITION

An integral part of any mixed dentition protocol is monitoring the transition from the mixed to the permanent dentition. As documented by Moyers and co-workers,[104] among others, there are significant differences in the sizes of the second deciduous molars and the succeeding second premolars. On the average, 2.5 mm of arch space per side can be gained in the mandibular arch and about 2 mm per side can be gained in the maxillary arch. However, there is wide variation in tooth size among patients,[74] and thus each patient must be evaluated radiographically to determine the relative size of the second deciduous molars and their successors. Simply maintaining available arch space during the transition of the dentition may be sufficient to resolve minor to moderate tooth-size/arch-size discrepancies, particularly if every reduction or other treatment procedure should be judicious interproximal reduction after the permanent dentition has erupted.

Two types of arches are used as holding appliances in the late transition of the dentition: the transpalatal arch and the lingual arch. These arches routinely are cemented in place before the loss of the second deciduous molars.

Transpalatal Arch

The transpalatal arch (TPA), as the name implies, extends from one maxillary first molar along the contour of the palate to the molar on the opposite side (Fig. 9-1). Although both fixed and removable types of transpalatal arches are avail-

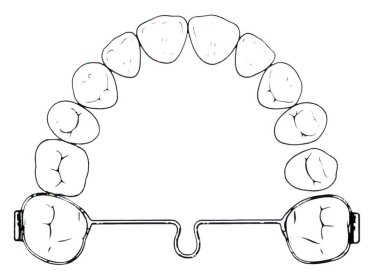

Fig. 9-1 Transpalatal arch. This arch can be used as both an active appliance and a stabilization appliance during the transition of the dentition. Note the net increase in available space following the transition from the second deciduous molar to the second premolar. (From McNamara JA Jr, Brudon WL: *Orthodontic and orthopedic treatment in the mixed dentition*, Ann Arbor, Mich, 1993, Needham Press.)

able, we routinely use the soldered transpalatal arch that is made from 0.036″ stainless steel wire and that is soldered to the molar bands at their mesiolingual line angles.

The major function of the transpalatal arch in the mixed dentition is to prevent the mesial migration of the upper first molars during the transition from the second deciduous molars to the second premolars. This appliance also is capable of producing molar rotations and changes in root torque[19,20] by sequential unilateral activation of the appliance.[88] The TPA also can be used for molar stabilization and anchorage. The transpalatal arch routinely is left in place until the final comprehensive phase of orthodontic therapy is completed.

Lingual Arch

The lingual arch, usually used in the mandible as part of our early treatment protocol, has a similar function to the transpalatal arch in the maxilla as a molar anchorage appliance. The lingual arch, also made out of 0.036″ stainless steel, extends along the lingual contour of the mandibular dentition from first molar to first molar (Fig. 9-2). Optional adjustment loops can be placed in the lingual arch in the region of the second deciduous molars.

The lower lingual arch is used less frequently than the transpalatal arch because there are many patients undergoing early orthodontic treatment who do not require the maintenance of arch space in the second premolar region. Thus the lower lingual arch is indicated only in patients in whom maximum molar anchorage is to be maintained. Not only is the lingual arch used in individuals with Class I malocclusion in whom arch space is to be stabilized, but it also is used in the treatment of patients with Class III malocclusion. In this instance, molar position is maintained to

prevent the forward movement of the molars (thus aggravating the Class III molar relationship) and to facilitate the more posterior eruption of the premolars. In contrast to the transpalatal arch, the lingual arch usually is removed after completion of the eruption of the second premolars and after the proper positioning of these teeth has been achieved.

SERIAL EXTRACTION

Another protocol that frequently is used in the treatment of tooth-size/arch-size discrepancies is serial extraction. This early treatment technique involves the sequential removal of deciduous teeth to facilitate the unimpeded eruption of the permanent teeth. Such a procedure often, but not always, results in the extraction of four premolar teeth. This protocol began in Europe in the 1930s and has been advocated by a number of individuals, including Hotz,[63,64] Kjellgren,[72] Terwilliger,[144] Lloyd,[75] and Palsson.[107] The sequence of serial extraction has been clarified further in a series of articles by Dewel[29-31] and in chapters on this topic by Graber,[51] Proffit,[125] and Moyers.[102] In addition, Chapter 6 explains the rationale and the protocol involved in serial extraction in detail, and thus this early treatment technique will be mentioned only briefly in this chapter.

Graber[51] states that serial extraction may be indicated when it is determined "with a fair degree of certainty that there will not be enough space in the jaws to accommodate all the permanent teeth in their proper alignment." Proffit[125] cites a predicted tooth-size/arch-size discrepancy of 10 mm or greater as an indication for serial extraction, whereas Ringenberg[128] cites a discrepancy of 7 mm or more.

In our opinion, the primary factor to be evaluated when making a treatment decision concerning serial extraction is the size of the individual permanent teeth. In instances in which tooth sizes are abnormally large (for example, as is indicated by the width of the upper and lower four permanent incisors), the initiation of serial extraction protocols may be appropriate. Another factor that must be considered is the anteroposterior positioning of the lower incisors relative to the adjacent skeletal elements and to the soft tissue, especially the lip musculature. Serial extraction in patients with crowded dentition, extreme bialveolar retrusion, and/or flat facial profiles obviously is not recommended because of potential unfavorable facial contour changes. Mild residual crowding of the lower incisors is preferable to creating a *dished-in* facial appearance. Similarly, a serial extraction protocol in patients with bialveolar protrusion is not indicated because maximum retraction of the incisors is desirable; maximum anchorage mechanics using fixed appliance therapy usually is the treatment of choice.[97]

Serial extraction may be combined with rapid maxillary expansion (RME) in certain patients with significant arch length discrepancy problems, who also present with a narrow tapered maxilla and with *negative space*[152] showing in the corners of the mouth while smiling. The use of RME is particularly appropriate in patients with broad facial con-

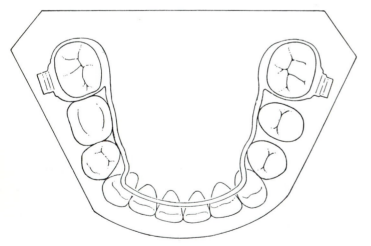

Fig. 9-2 Lower lingual arch. Note the maintenance of arch space following the loss of the second deciduous molar and the eruption of the second premolar on the left side. Adjustment loops can be placed in the arch and in the second premolar region if desired. (From McNamara JA Jr, Brudon WL: *Orthodontic and orthopedic treatment in the mixed dentition*, Ann Arbor, Mich, 1993, Needham Press.)

tours. The arches can be expanded first to *broaden* the smile, and then serial extraction procedures can be initiated subsequently to reduce or eliminate emerging tooth-arch imbalances.

It is well known that serial extraction is not a panacea in all patients who present with dental crowding in the mixed dentition.[128] Great care must be taken to avoid lingual tipping of the lower incisors and unfavorable changes in the sagittal position of the upper and lower dentitions. In addition, the initiation of serial extraction procedures may result in unwanted spacing in the dental arches. However, when appropriate, a protocol of sequentially extracting the deciduous dentition has proven to be an efficient, cost-effective, and satisfactory treatment for tooth-size/arch-size discrepancy problems.

ORTHOPEDIC EXPANSION

It is well documented that expansion of the dental arches can be produced by a variety of orthodontic treatments including those that employ fixed appliances. The types of expansion produced can be divided arbitrarily into three categories.

Orthodontic expansion. Orthodontic expansion that is produced by conventional fixed appliances or by various removable expansion plate and finger spring appliances usually results in lateral movements of the buccal segments that are primarily dentoalveolar in nature. The tendency is toward a lateral tipping of the crowns of the involved teeth and a resultant lingual tipping of the roots. The resistance of the cheek musculature and other soft tissue remains and provides forces that may lead to a relapse or rebound of the achieved orthodontic expansion.

Passive expansion. When the forces of the buccal and labial musculature are shielded from the occlusion, as with the FR-2 appliance of Fränkel,[45] a widening of the dental arches often occurs. This *passive* expansion is not a result of the application of extrinsic biomechanical forces but rather of intrinsic forces, such as those produced by the tongue. Brieden and co-workers,[17] in an implant study conducted in Fränkel patients, have demonstrated that bone deposition occurs primarily along the lateral aspect of the alveolus rather than at the mid-palatal suture. A related type of spontaneous arch expansion also has been observed following lip-bumper therapy.[13,106]

Orthopedic expansion. Rapid maxillary expansion (RME) appliances (Fig. 9-3) are the best examples of true orthopedic expansion because changes are produced primarily in the underlying skeletal structures rather than by the movement of teeth through alveolar bone.[56-59,147,148,155] RME not only separates the midpalatal suture but also affects the circumzygomatic and circummaxillary sutural systems.[139] After the palate has been widened, new bone is deposited in the area of expansion so that the integrity of the midpalatal suture usually is reestablished within 3 to 6 months.[57]

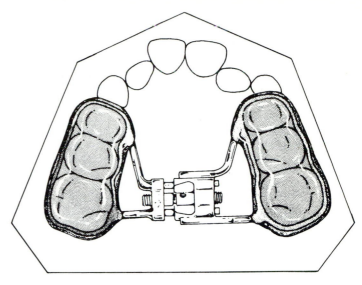

Fig. 9-3 An acrylic splint RME appliance that is bonded to the maxillary primary molars and the permanent first molars. The occlusal coverage of acrylic produces a posterior bite block effect on the vertical dimension. (From McNamara JA Jr, Brudon WL: *Orthodontic and orthopedic treatment in the mixed dentition*, Ann Arbor, Mich, 1993, Needham Press.)

Rationale for Early Orthodontic Expansion

The cornerstone of the early orthopedic expansion protocol used in the treatment of patients with arch length discrepancy problems is rapid maxillary expansion. Even though there will be a discussion of adjunctive treatments that produce tooth movement (e.g., Schwarz appliance, lip bumper, utility arch) as part of various mixed dentition protocols, rapid maxillary expansion is the essential component of this treatment approach. The use of this expansion protocol is based in part on our previous studies of the development of the dental arches in untreated individuals, both in the permanent dentition and in the mixed dentition.

Studies in the permanent dentition. Howe, McNamara, and O'Connor[65] carried out an investigation in which the dental casts of patients with severe crowding were compared to the dental casts of untreated individuals who were classified as having ideal (or near ideal) occlusions. The latter sample was gathered using serial dental casts from *The University of Michigan Elementary and Secondary School Growth Study.*[104] No statistically significant differences in tooth size were noted between the uncrowded and crowded populations, regardless of whether aggregate tooth size or the size of individual teeth were considered. In contrast, there were statistically significant differences in arch width and arch perimeter. Maxillary intermolar width was of particular importance as an easily measured clinical indicator. In the noncrowded dentition cases of males, the average distance between the upper first permanent molars (Fig. 9-4), measured at the point of the intersection of the lingual groove at the gingival margin was 37.4 mm (SD 1.7 mm)—

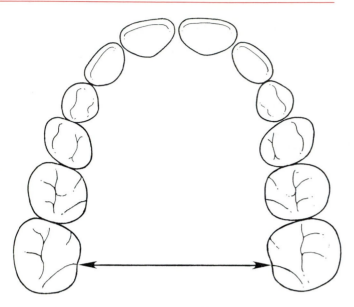

Fig. 9-4   Maxillary transpalatal width, as measured at the intersection of the lingual groove with the gingival margin. This distance is used as an indicator of maxillary bony base development. (From McNamara JA Jr, Brudon WL: *Orthodontic and orthopedic treatment in the mixed dentition,* Ann Arbor, Mich, 1993, Needham Press.)

a value that can be compared to a similar measure in the crowded cases of 31.1 mm (SD 4.1 mm). Note that the intermolar width in the patients with crowded dentitions was approximately 6 mm less than in the patients with noncrowded dentitions. Also the standard deviation was greater in individuals with crowded dentitions. Similar, but slightly smaller measures and differences were noted in the female sample. The average transpalatal width in the female group with noncrowded dentition was 36.2 mm (SD 1.92 mm) and in the group with crowded dentition was 30.8 mm (SD 2.40 mm).

The results of this study are similar to those of several other investigators. For example, Moorrees and Reed,[101] Mills,[98] McKeown,[80] and Radnzic[126] considered the relationship between tooth size, arch size, and crowding. These investigators found that arch size, particularly arch width, was associated strongly with the degree of crowding, whereas tooth size, in general, was not. Mills[98] found that the dental arches of those individuals with noncrowded dental arches were approximately 4 mm wider than they were in the patients with crowded arches. In contrast, Lundström[77] and Doris and co-workers[33] have reported associations between tooth size and dental crowding. Radnzic[126] suggests that although parameters appear to be interrelated, arch size, particularly arch length and arch perimeter, seem to be more important than tooth size as a cause of dental crowding.

Studies in Transitional Dentition

In the investigation previously described, Howe and co-workers[66] used the transpalatal width between the upper first

molars as an indicator of arch dimension. They concluded that a transpalatal width of 35 to 39 mm suggests a bony base of adequate size to accommodate a permanent dentition of average size (of course, a larger aggregate tooth size requires a larger bony base and *vice versa*). Because this study was conducted using data from individuals in the permanent dentition, it did not address the issue of the normal development of the dental arches. This question was considered in a second study[88,138] that examined the nature of normal changes in maxillary and mandibular transpalatal width from the early mixed dentition to the permanent dentition. Longitudinal changes in an untreated population from 7 to 15 years of age were evaluated, using the longitudinal records of 209 individuals from The University of Michigan Elementary and Secondary School Growth Study.[104] The average increase in transpalatal width between the upper first molars (Fig. 9-4) was 2.6 mm (Table 9-2). This sample was evaluated further by dividing it into three subgroups on the basis of initial transpalatal width. The *narrow group* had an initial transpalatal width of less than 31 mm; the *neutral group* had a transpalatal width of between 31 and 35 mm; and the *wide group* had an initial transpalatal width of greater than 35 mm (Table 9-3). The narrow subgroup had an increase in transpalatal of 3.3 mm between 7 and 15 years of age. That increase was greater than the neutral (2.5 mm) or the wide (1.7 mm) subgroups. A favorable finding was that the narrow group expanded to a greater extent without treatment than did the wider group. The unfavorable finding was the observation that, even with this greater amount of naturally occurring expansion, the narrow group reached an average transpalatal width of 32.7 mm, a dimension that was close to the transpalatal widths (31.1 mm in males and 30.8 mm in females) of the individuals with crowded dentitions in the study of Howe and co-workers.[66]

One of the conclusions that can be drawn from the studies cited above concerning dental arch development is that by providing some mechanism of widening the bony bases and increasing arch width and perimeter, more space can be obtained for the alignment of the permanent dentition. Of course, the dental arches cannot be widened *ad libitum,* as has been shown by many of the previously published studies of arch expansion. However, it seems logical to consider increasing arch size at a young age so that skeletal, dentoalveolar, and muscular adaptations can occur before the eruption of the permanent dentition.

Method of Orthopedic Expansion

The appliance of choice for use on mixed dentition patients is a bonded acrylic splint expander (Fig. 9-3). This appliance, which incorporates a Hyrax-type screw into a framework made of wire and acrylic, is used to separate the halves of the maxilla. It is widely recognized that maxillary expansion is achieved easily in a growing individual, particularly in individuals in the mixed dentition.[94-96] The acrylic-splint type of appliance that is made from 3 mm thick, heat-formed acrylic has the additional advantage of

TABLE 9-2
Transpalatal Arch Width Sexes Combined (mm)

Age	N	Mean	S.D.
7	119	32.7	1.4
8	171	33.2	1.5
9	181	33.2	1.4
10	179	33.7	1.5
11	159	34.5	1.4
12	128	35.2	1.4
13	116	35.4	1.5
14	93	35.2	1.4
15	74	35.3	1.4

Mean change in arch width, age 7 to 15
+2.6 mm

TABLE 9-3
Longitudinal Change in Transpalatal Arch Width (mm)

Age	Initial AW <31 mm Mean	S.D.	Initial AW 31-35 mm Mean	S.D.	Initial AW >35 mm Mean	S.D.
7	28.9	1.3	32.8	0.9	36.5	1.2
8	29.3	1.1	33.1	1.1	37.1	1.2
9	30.0	1.1	33.6	1.3	37.4	1.1
10	30.3	1.4	34.0	1.4	37.5	1.1
11	30.4	1.6	34.3	1.7	37.5	0.9
12	30.9	1.3	34.5	2.1	37.5	1.2
13	31.4	1.4	34.7	1.6	37.5	1.6
14	31.7	1.6	35.0	1.6	37.8	1.6
15	32.2	1.4	35.3	1.9	38.2	1.9

Mean change from age 7 to 15
+3.3 mm   +2.5 mm   +1.7 mm

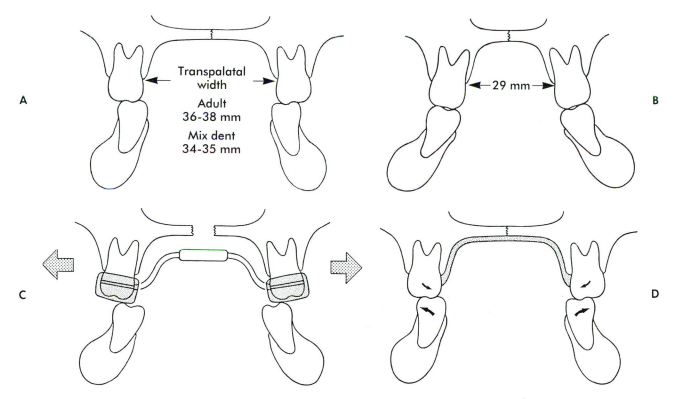

Fig. 9-5 Frontal cross-sectional view of transpalatal dimensions through the molar region. **A,** Ideal transpalatal width of the adult patient and the patient with mixed dentition. **B,** Patient with a constricted maxilla, as indicated by the intermolar width of 29 mm. **C,** The effect of the bonded acrylic splint RME appliance. Note that the lingual cusps of the upper posterior teeth approximate the buccal cusps of the lower posterior teeth. **D,** This same patient during the post-RME period. A removable palatal plate has been added to stabilize the intra-arch relationship. Note the slight spontaneous uprighting of the dentition. (Adapted from McNamara JA Jr, Brudon WL: *Orthodontic and orthopedic treatment in the mixed dentition,* Ann Arbor, Mich, 1993, Needham Press.)

acting as a bite block because of the thickness of the acrylic that covers the occlusal surfaces of the posterior dentition. The posterior bite block effect of the bonded acrylic splint expander prevents the extrusion of the posterior teeth, a finding often associated with banded rapid maxillary expansion appliances,[155] thus permitting the use of this type of expander in some patients with steep mandibular plane angles.

The treatment protocol that involves the use of a bonded expander is illustrated by the following example. The morphology of a patient in the mixed dentition with an idealized (e.g., 34 to 35 mm) transpalatal width (Fig. 9-5, *A*) can be compared to a patient with a narrow (e.g., 29 mm) transpalatal width (Fig. 9-5, *B*). A goal of the orthopedic treatment initiated in the mixed dentition is to reduce the need for extractions in the permanent dentition through the elimination of arch length discrepancies and the elimination of bony base imbalances. In instances of restricted transverse dimensions (Fig. 9-5, *B*), a bonded rapid maxillary expansion appliance is used (Fig. 9-5, *C*). The screw of the expander is activated ¼ turn (90°) per day (.22 mm) until the lingual cusps of the upper posterior teeth approximate the buccal cusps of the lower posterior teeth. In contrast to Haas,[60] who recommends full opening of the expansion screw to 10.5 to 11.0 mm, an action that usually produces a buccal crossbite, we advocate only as much expansion as is possible while contact is maintained between the upper and lower posterior teeth.

After the active phase of expansion is completed, the appliance is left in place for an additional 5 months to allow for a reorganization of the mid-palatal suture, as well as other sutural systems affected by the expansion, and to maximize the effect of the posterior bite block. At the end of the treatment time the RME appliance is removed and the patient is given a removable palatal plate to sustain the achieved result (Fig. 9-5, *D*). A recent study by Brust[18] examined patients treated with this type of expander. The findings indicate that there may be some slight uprighting of the lower posterior teeth during the postexpansion period. Little change in maxillary molar angulation is observed if a removable palatal plate is used for at least a year following RME treatment.

The active expansion of the two halves of the maxilla produces a midline diastema between the two upper central incisors. During the period following the active expansion of the appliance, a mesial tipping of the maxillary central and lateral incisors usually is observed. Such spontaneous tooth movement is typical following rapid maxillary expansion, and this movement often is interpreted as being evidence of *relapse* by the patient or the parents. The clinician should advise the family about the probability of such spontaneous tooth migration. Brackets often are placed on the upper incisors to close the midline diastema and align the anterior teeth 3 or 4 months following the initiation of RME treatment (Fig. 9-6). In certain instances a utility arch (Fig. 9-6) is used to retract, intrude, or protract the

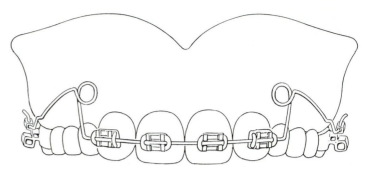

Fig. 9-6 The placement of brackets on the upper anterior teeth to achieve incisal alignment. In this illustration a retraction utility arch extends from the auxiliary tubes on the upper first molars to the incisors. A transpalatal arch (not shown) can be added to maintain transpalatal width. (From McNamara JA Jr, Brudon WL: *Orthodontic and orthopedic treatment in the mixed dentition*, Ann Arbor, Mich, 1993, Needham Press.)

upper incisors, depending on the needs of the individual patient.

Mandibular "Dental Decompensation"

In patients whose lower arches exhibit moderate crowding of the anterior teeth or in whom the posterior teeth are tipped lingually, two types of appliances can be used before rapid maxillary expansion: the removable Schwarz appliance and the lip bumper. The use of these *decompensating* (i.e., expanding, uprighting) appliances began as a result of our[88] initial experiences using the bonded RME appliances alone. We were able to produce the expected changes in maxillary transverse dimensions with the bonded expander quite readily, but we made no attempt to actively widen the lower dental arch. After evaluating RME in mixed dentition patients over a 5-year period, we discovered that in some patients, a spontaneous uprighting and *decrowding* of the lower teeth occurred, yet in others apparently there was no change in the position and alignment of the lower teeth.

Because one of the *cardinal rules* of orthodontics was that the clinician never should expand the lower arch, we were reluctant to do so. Yet, because expansion was observed in the lower arch on a sporadic basis using RME and because arch expansion was produced routinely by the FR-2 appliance of Fränkel,[40,41,45,79] we decided to attempt *orthodontic expansion* of the lower dental arch, using either the removable Schwarz appliance or the lip-bumper before *orthopedic expansion* of the maxilla. We assumed that expansion of the lower arch would not be stable unless the expansion was followed by maxillary orthopedic expansion.

Schwarz appliance. The Schwarz appliance is a horseshoe-shaped removable appliance that fits along the lingual border of the mandibular dentition (Fig. 9-7). The inferior border of the appliance extends below the gingival margin and contacts the lingual gingival tissue. A midline expansion screw is incorporated into the acrylic, and also

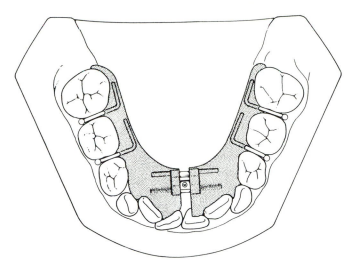

Fig. 9-7   The removable lower Schwarz appliance that is used for mandibular dental decompensation. This appliance produces an orthodontic tipping (uprighting) of the lower posterior teeth and may create additional arch space anteriorly. (From McNamara JA Jr, Brudon WL: *Orthodontic and orthopedic treatment in the mixed dentition*, Ann Arbor, Mich, 1993, Needham Press.)

ball clasps lie in the interproximal spaces between the deciduous and permanent molars.

The lower Schwarz appliance is indicated in patients with mild to moderate crowding in the lower anterior region or in instances in which there is significant lingual tipping of the posterior dentition. The appliance is activated once each week, producing about .25 mm of expansion in the midline of the appliance. Usually the appliance is expanded for 3 to 5 months, depending on the degree of incisal crowding, producing about 3 to 5 mm of arch length anteriorly.

Clinicians frequently have experienced difficulty understanding the reasoning underlying the use of the Schwarz appliance before rapid maxillary expansion. The following example illustrates the logic for this treatment decision. Fig. 9-8, *A*, is a schematic drawing of a bilateral posterior crossbite: a condition that easily is recognized clinically and for which rapid maxillary expansion is a generally accepted treatment regimen. In this example the mandibular bony base and dental arch are of normal width and there is normal posterior dental angulation, whereas the maxilla is constricted.

The example shown in Fig. 9-8, *B*, is from a patient who has maxillary constriction but in whom also there has been mandibular dentoalveolar *compensation* (i.e., the positions of the lower teeth have been influenced by the size and shape of the narrow maxilla). No obvious crossbite is present. Even though maxillary width is the same as in the previous example (Fig. 9-8, *A*), the lower posterior teeth have erupted with a more lingual inclination. The palate appears narrow (in this example a transpalatal width of 29 mm) and the arches are tapered in form. Mild-to-moderate lower incisor crowding also may be present. In such a pa-

tient, mandibular dental *decompensation* using a removable lower Schwarz appliance often is undertaken. The width and form of the mandibular dental arch is made more ideal before the time that rapid maxillary expansion is attempted. By decompensating the mandibular dental arch, greater arch expansion of the maxilla can be achieved than when RME is used alone.[18]

Simply stated, the purpose of the Schwarz appliance is to produce *orthodontic tipping* of the lower posterior teeth; thereby uprighting these teeth into a more normal inclination (Fig. 9-8, *C*). This movement is unstable if no further treatment is provided to the patient. A tendency toward a posterior crossbite is produced that is similar in many respects to the posterior crossbite shown in Fig. 9-8, *A*.

Usually the Schwarz appliance is left in place until the maxillary orthopedic expansion phase is completed (Fig. 9-8, *D*). As described earlier the maxilla is expanded using a bonded acrylic splint appliance until the upper lingual cusps barely touch the lower buccal cusps. Following a 5-month period of RME stabilization, allowing adequate time for the midpalatal suture and the adjacent sutural systems to reorganize and reossify, both appliances are removed and the patient is given a simple maxillary retainer (Fig. 9-9), with no retention provided in the mandible. If it is indicated, a simple mandibular retainer (e.g., Hawley design) also can be provided to the patient. In instances of severe anterior malalignment in either arch, a fixed appliance may be placed on the incisors to align these teeth.

Lip bumper.   The lip bumper (Fig. 9-10) is a removable appliance that also can be used for mandibular dental decompensation.[13,19,20,106] The lip bumper is particularly useful in patients who have tight or tense buccal and labial musculature. The lip bumper lies away from the dentition and shields the dentition from the forces of the adjacent soft tissue. The appliance usually is worn on a full-time basis and may be ligated in place. The lip bumper also should lie at the gingival margin of the lower central incisors. The lip bumper not only increases arch length through passive lateral and anterior expansion, but also serves to upright the lower molars distally, adding to the available arch length increase.

From a neuromuscular perspective the lip bumper appears to have a more desirable treatment effect than does the Schwarz appliance. The Schwarz appliance simply produces orthodontic tipping of the teeth through direct force application to the dentition and alveolus. On the other hand, the lip bumper shields the soft tissue from the dentition, allowing for spontaneous arch expansion.[13,106] However, we tend to favor the use of the Schwarz appliance over the lip bumper in most instances because of the predictability of the treatment outcome. Only in patients with constricted (tense) soft tissue is the lip bumper the appliance of choice.

Clinical Studies of Orthopedic Expansion

A substantial body of knowledge exists concerning the treatment effects produced by rapid maxillary expansion

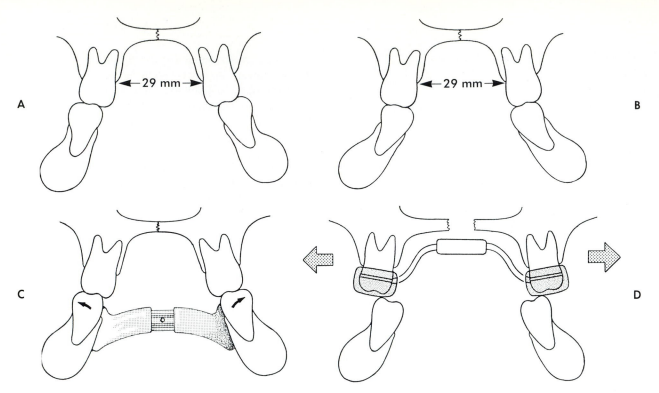

Fig. 9-8 Frontal cross-sectional view. **A,** Patient with a constricted maxilla, an uprighted lower posterior dentition, and a bilateral crossbite. **B,** A patient with a similar transpalatal width and with the mandibular corpus in the same position. Note the lower teeth are more lingually inclined, camouflaging the maxillary constriction. The uprighting of the lower posterior teeth: mandibular dental *decompensation,* is indicated before RME. **C,** The removable lower Schwarz expansion appliance orthodontically uprights the lower molars, producing a tendency toward a posterior crossbite. **D,** Rapid maxillary expansion following mandibular dental decompensation. The upper lingual cusps approximate the lower buccal cusps at the end of expansion. (Adapted from McNamara JA Jr, Brudon WL: *Orthodontic and orthopedic treatment in the mixed dentition,* Ann Arbor, Mich, 1993, Needham Press.)

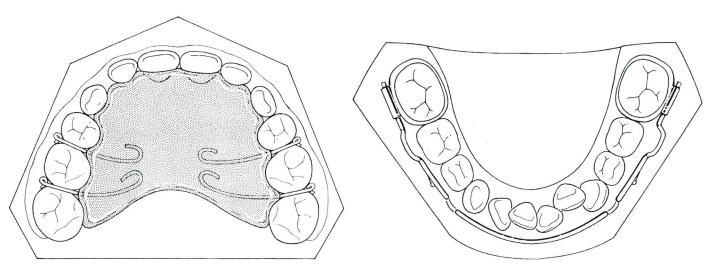

Fig. 9-9 Simple maxillary stabilization plate. This appliance usually is worn on a near full-time basis for at least 1 year following RME removal. (From McNamara JA Jr, Brudon WL: *Orthodontic and orthopedic treatment in the mixed dentition,* Ann Arbor, Mich, 1993, Needham Press.)

Fig. 9-10 Occlusal view of a mandibular lip bumper that inserts into buccal tubes on the lower first permanent molar bands. (From McNamara JA Jr, Brudon WL: *Orthodontic and orthopedic treatment in the mixed dentition,* Ann Arbor, Mich, 1993, Needham Press.)

(see McNamara and Brudon[88] for an extensive review of the literature), with much of the research devoted to a description of effects occurring during treatment and with less attention being paid to the long-term stability of RME. Most published studies have dealt with patients treated in the permanent dentition with little data available on the effect of RME in a mixed dentition population.

Studies in the mixed dentition. Since 1981, we have gathered serial dental casts on all our patients undergoing rapid maxillary expansion in the mixed dentition. Longitudinal cephalometric records also have been taken at appropriate time intervals. Two studies on the dental cast data have been conducted by Spillane[137] and Brust[18] and are described in McNamara and Brudon.[88]

The first study[137] reported the findings of 162 subjects who underwent rapid maxillary expansion during the mixed dentition before the eruption of the maxillary premolars and canines, using the protocol previously described. The expansion procedure was followed by a retention protocol that included the wearing of a removable palatal plate (Fig. 9-9) for at least 1 year, followed by full-time or part-time wear of the maintenance plate for an additional period of time. Spillane noted that the average increase in intermolar width was 5.94 mm (SD 1.59 mm). During the postretention period, the expanded maxillary dental arches were reasonably stable. For example, 90.5% of the original expansion was maintained after the first year (Fig. 9-11) with slightly less overall expansion being maintained (80.4%) at the end of the observation period (2.4 years postexpansion) at the time of *Phase II* records (before the final phase of compre-

hensive orthodontic treatment was initiated). Similar findings were observed during the transition from the primary molars to the premolars and from the primary canines to the permanent canines (Fig. 9-11).

The second study was conducted by Brust.[18] The initial sample group included 376 consecutive treated, mixed-dentition patients who received rapid maxillary expansion only with or in combination with lower expansion using a Schwarz appliance. Through the application of specific exclusionary criteria (see Brust[18] for details), a subsample of 146 patients, who received RME only and 36 patients who received RME following Schwarz appliance therapy, were studied. Serial dental casts of 50 untreated individuals from *The University of Michigan Elementary and Secondary School Growth Study*[103] were used as a matched control group. Longitudinal changes were analyzed using a recently developed digital imaging system (ELE Imaging Systems, Ann Arbor, Michigan) that had been adapted for the analysis of serial dental casts. Changes in arch width, arch perimeter, and molar angulation were evaluated preexpansion, immediately postexpansion, and at the time of Phase II records.

Changes in maxillary arch width. In the RME-only group, the transpalatal width (Fig. 9-4) was 31.9 mm (SD 2.8 mm) preexpansion and 37.7 mm (SD 2.8 mm) postexpansion, resulting in an average net change of 5.8 mm. At the time of Phase II records, the average transpalatal width was 36.8 mm (SD 3.1 mm), indicating that 85% of the original expansion was maintained at the time Phase II records were taken, with a residual expansion of 4.9 mm.

The initial transpalatal width in the RME-Schwarz group

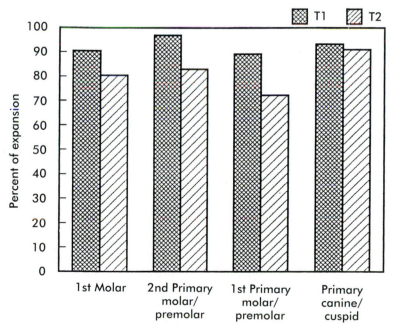

Fig. 9-11   Stability of arch dimensions following expansion with a bonded RME appliance. The amount of original expansion is indicated as 100%. The percentage of original expansion remaining at each posttreatment timepoint is shown: *T1:* One year after removal of the RME appliance. *T2,* At the time of eruption of the upper first premolars (2.4 years postexpansion). (Adapted from Spillane LM: Thesis, University of Michigan, 1990.)

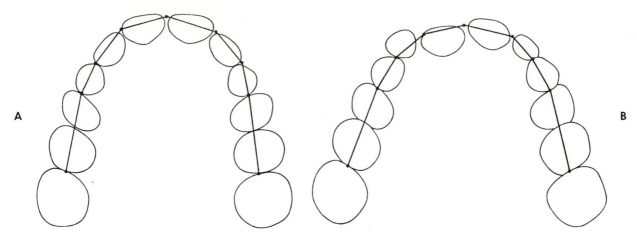

Fig. 9-12 Determination of maxillary arch perimeter. **A,** Idealized arch. **B,** Arch with malaligned teeth. (From McNamara JA Jr, Brudon WL: *Orthodontic and orthopedic treatment in the mixed dentition,* Ann Arbor, Mich, 1993, Needham Press.)

was slightly narrower than in the RME-only group (30.3 mm, SD 2.6 mm). At the time of expander removal, the transpalatal width was 36.9 mm (3.0 mm), indicating a 6.6 mm *increase* in transpalatal width. At the time that Phase II records were taken, there was an increase in transpalatal width to 37.5 mm (SD 3.6 mm), resulting in a residual expansion of 7.2 mm.

The control group had an initial transpalatal width of 32.2 mm (SD 2.5 mm) at the beginning of the observation period and a width of 33.1 mm (SD 2.6 mm) at the time interval corresponding to Phase II records. Thus, at the end of the observation period, residual expansion was greatest in the RME-Schwarz group (7.2 mm), whereas in the RME-only group it was 4.9 mm and in the control group 0.9 mm.

Changes in arch perimeter. In order to determine changes in arch perimeter, segments of a line were drawn between the contact points of adjacent teeth from the mesial midpoint of the first permanent molar to the corresponding point on the contralateral side of the maxillary or mandibular arch (Fig. 9-12). Arch perimeter was measured as a sum of the segments.

The initial maxillary arch perimeter was similar in the RME-only and control groups but was slightly reduced in the RME-Schwarz group (Table 9-4). In the RME-only group, maxillary arch perimeter increased 3.6 mm during the treatment period, with slightly over 70% of the increase remaining at the time of Phase II records. In the RME-Schwarz group, an initial increase of 4.1 mm was noted in maxillary arch perimeter, with an additional increase of 0.9 mm observed at Phase II records. Maxillary arch perimeter increased by 0.4 mm in the control group.

The major increase in mandibular arch perimeter was noted in the RME-Schwarz group (Table 9-5). A net increase of 2.3 mm was seen postexpansion, with 77% of that value (1.7 mm) still evident at the time of Phase II records. In contrast a slight increase (0.6 mm) was noted in the RME-

only group postexpansion, but this value decreased to −1.1 mm at the time of Phase II records. During the same time intervals, there was a net decrease (−1.6 mm) in the control group.

The results of the study by Brust[18] indicate that maxillary arch perimeter is increased following rapid maxillary expansion, with greater increases noted if mandibular dental decompensation using a Schwarz appliance has been performed before RME. Clinically relevant increases in mandibular arch perimeter were noted only in the RME-Schwarz group. When the net arch length *decrease* in the control group is compared to the net arch length *increase* in the RME-Schwarz group, the net gain is about 3.3 mm. On the basis of these findings, Brust[18] concluded that expansion therapy may alleviate the need for extraction in *borderline* cases displaying 3 to 4 mm of mandibular crowding. This type of orthopedic expansion treatment may be combined with other types of therapy to gain additional arch length (e.g., interproximal reduction, facebow, lip bumper). Patients with 6 mm or more of initial mandibular crowding or with vertical problems may be treated better using extraction therapy. Brust also concluded that RME-Schwarz therapy offered the clinician a greater amount of expansion in both the upper and lower arches when compared to RME-only treatment.

Studies in the permanent dentition. Because these types of treatment protocols using the bonded RME appliance have been used by us for slightly more than a decade, long-term studies of arch stability following early orthopedic expansion obviously do not exist. However, we have recently conducted a study[61] that has evaluated the long-term stability of the dental arches of adolescent patients who have undergone rapid maxillary expansion as part of their orthodontic treatment. The 83 patients on whom the Haas-type expander was used in conjunction with fixed appliances were compared to serial dental casts of 27 untreated individuals.

TABLE 9-4

Changes in Maxillary Arch Perimeter (mm)

Stage	N	Age	X	SD	Net change	% Ret
1. RME-Only Group						
Initial	146	8.5	75.6	4.3	0.0	—
Post-RME	142	9.3	79.2	4.1	3.6	100.0
Pre-Phase II	68	11.8	78.2	4.5	2.6	72.7
2. RME/Schwarz Group						
Initial	36	8.3	72.9	3.9	0.0	—
Post-RME	36	9.4	77.1	4.1	4.1	100.0
Pre-Phase II	12	12.7	77.9	4.7	5.0	121.5
3. Control Group						
Initial	50	8.6	75.8	3.2	0.0	—
Post-RME	49	9.6	76.3	3.1	0.5	—
Pre-Phase II	50	12.4	76.2	3.0	0.4	—

(From Brust.[18])

TABLE 9-5

Changes in Mandibular Arch Perimeter (mm)

Stage	N	Age	X	SD	Net change	% Ret
1. RME-Only Group						
Initial	146	8.5	68.6	3.4	0.0	—
Post-RME	115	10.2	69.2	3.2	0.6	100.0
Pre-Phase II	66	11.8	67.5	4.1	− 1.1	− 184.4
2. RME-Schwarz Group						
Initial	36	8.3	66.4	4.1	0.0	—
Post-RME	36	10.6	68.6	3.7	2.3	100.0
Pre-Phase II	12	12.5	68.1	4.3	1.7	77.1
3. Control Group						
Initial	50	8.6	67.6	2.6	0.0	—
Post-RME	49	9.6	67.5	2.7	− 0.0	—
Pre-Phase II	49	12.4	65.9	3.1	− 1.6	—

(From Brust.[18])

These two groups of individuals were approximately 11 years of age at the first interval studied (beginning of treatment), 14 years of age at the time of second records (end of treatment), and 21 years of age at the time the third set of records were taken (postretention). The most interesting findings were with regard to changes in arch perimeter.

The untreated individuals demonstrated a *net decrease* in maxillary arch perimeter of an average 3.8 mm and a *decrease* in mandibular arch perimeter of 4.4 mm from ages 11 to 21 years. In contrast the group that had undergone rapid maxillary expansion had a net *increase* in maxillary arch perimeter of 3.1 mm and a net *increase* in mandibular arch perimeter of 1.1 mm when the first and third sets of records were compared. When the decreases in arch perimeter seen in the control group are taken into consideration, the net treatment effect observed was an increase in maxillary arch perimeter of almost 6 mm and a 5 mm increase in mandibular arch perimeter. This long-term study indicates that when RME is undertaken in the early adolescent age period, significant long-term effects can be seen even at 6 years following fixed appliance removal.

SPONTANEOUS CORRECTION OF SAGITTAL MALOCCLUSIONS

The major focus of this section of the chapter thus far has been the resolution of intra-arch tooth-size/arch-size discrepancy problems. Interestingly, there is another phenomenon that has been a serendipitous finding, that is the *spontaneous* correction of mild Class II and Class III malocclusions.

Class II Tendency Patients

There are many patients in the mixed dentition who not only have intra-arch problems but also have a strong ten-

dency toward a Class II malocclusion. These patients have either an end-to-end molar relationship or a relationship more toward a full Class II molar position. Generally, these patients do not have severe skeletal imbalances but rather may be characterized clinically as having either slight mandibular skeletal retrusion or an orthognathic facial profile with minimal neuromuscular imbalances.

According to the routine protocol described previously, these patients undergo rapid maxillary expansion with or without prior mandibular dental decompensation. At the time of expander removal these patients have a buccal crossbite, with only the lingual cusps of the upper posterior teeth contacting the buccal cusps of the lower posterior teeth (Fig. 9-13, *A*). A maxillary maintenance plate is used to stabilize this relationship. When the patient returns (several appointments later), some interesting observations are noted: the tendency toward a buccal crossbite has disappeared (Fig. 9-13, *B*) and the patient now has a solid Class I sagittal occlusal relationship.

Clinicians traditionally have viewed a Class II malocclusion as primarily a sagittal and vertical problem.[1,73,134] Our experience with the post-RME correction of the Class II problem indicates that many Class II malocclusions have a strong transverse component. The overexpansion of the maxilla, which subsequently is stabilized through the use of a removable palatal plate, disrupts the occlusion. It appears that the patient becomes more comfortable by posturing his or her jaw slightly forward, thus eliminating the tendency toward a buccal crossbite and at the same time improving the sagittal occlusal relationship. In many respects, the teeth themselves act as an endogenous functional appliance, encouraging a change in mandibular posture and, ultimately, a change in the maxillomandibular occlusal relationship.

The correction for a patient with a Class II tendency is

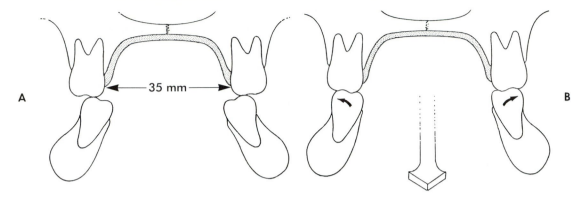

Fig. 9-13   Frontal cross-sectional view of patient during the post-RME period. **A,** The maxilla has been expanded so that the intermaxillary width is 35 mm, as measured between the upper first permanent molars. Note the tendency toward a buccal crossbite bilaterally. **B,** During the postexpansion period, note that the lower dentition has uprighted slightly and that there has been a forward sagittal movement of the mandible as the patient seeks to find a more stable position in which to occlude. (Adapted from McNamara JA Jr, Brudon WL: *Orthodontic and orthopedic treatment in the mixed dentition,* Ann Arbor, Mich, 1993, Needham Press.)

illustrated in Fig. 9-14. Fig. 9-14, *A,* shows the sagittal view of the skeletal and dentoalveolar structures of a patient with a Class II tendency who has excessive overjet and a narrow maxilla. The placement of a bonded maxillary expansion appliance immediately causes an increase in the vertical dimension of the face because of the posterior occlusal coverage. This change is beneficial in most patients because the increase in the vertical dimension prevents extrusion of the posterior teeth during the expansion process and also may result in an upward and slightly forward displacement (Fig. 9-14, *B*) of the maxilla (this phenomenon will be discussed subsequently in the discussion of the spontaneous correction of Class III). During the post-RME period (a removable palatal plate and anterior brackets may be worn [Fig. 9-14, *C*]) the mandible is postured forward by the patient because of the overexpansion of the maxilla. Thus the spontaneous correction of patients with a tendency toward a Class II malocclusion does not occur during the active expansion period but rather during the time that the maintenance plate is being worn.

This phenomenon of spontaneous occlusal correction following RME treatment occurs with sufficient frequency to become incorporated into our mixed dentition treatment plan. In patients with a Class II malocclusion and a reduced transpalatal width (e.g., <31 mm measured between the upper first molars), the maxilla will be widened using RME and then the maxillary arch of the patient will be stabilized with a maintenance plate. The patient will be monitored on a routine basis (e.g., every 4 months), with the decision concerning functional jaw orthopedics or extraoral traction being deferred until toward the end of the mixed dentition period.

Class III Tendency Patients

The use of a bonded rapid maxillary expansion appliance also can lead to a spontaneous occlusal correction in a patient with a tendency toward a Class III malocclusion. At first glance this phenomenon seems a paradox, given the previous discussion concerning the spontaneous correction of Class II tendency problems. However, the mechanism of Class III correction is distinctly different than that described above.

An examination of Fig. 9-14, *B,* provides some explanation for this phenomenon. The placement of an acrylic splint expander that opens the bite vertically 2 to 3 mm may provide an intrusive force against the maxilla caused by the stretch of the masticatory musculature; also a slight forward repositioning of the maxilla may occur. A slight forward movement of the maxilla following rapid maxillary expansion has been documented in clinical studies.[56,57,59] In addition, the placement of a bonded expander with acrylic coverage of the occlusion helps eliminate a tendency toward a pseudo-Class III malocclusion.

As with the patients with a Class II tendency who were described previously, patients in whom a borderline Class III malocclusion exists usually have a reasonably balanced facial pattern, often with only a slight tendency toward maxillary skeletal retrusion. Obviously, in patients in whom Class III malocclusion persists after expansion, more aggressive types of therapy are indicated, as will be discussed later.

When contrasting the spontaneous correction of patients with both Class II and Class III tendency, it must be emphasized that any spontaneous correction of a Class III malocclusion usually occurs during the *active* phase of treatment (within the first 30 or 40 days). The spontaneous correction

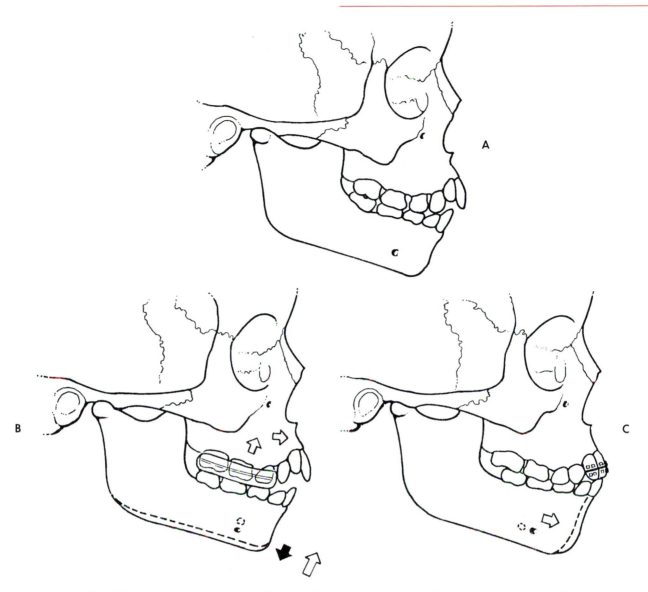

Fig. 9-14   Sequence of events leading to a spontaneous correction of a sagittal malocclusion. **A,** Pretreatment. The patient has excessive overjet and an end-to-end molar relationship. **B,** The placement of the appliance immediately creates a downward rotation of the position of the mandible because of the posterior occlusal acrylic. During treatment an intrusive (and slightly protrusive) force is produced on the skeletal and dental structures of the maxilla. **C,** During the postexpansion period, the upper dental arch has been widened. The lower jaw often is postured forward to achieve a more stable occlusal relationship. In this illustration, brackets have been placed on the upper anterior teeth to facilitate incisal alignment.

of Class II malocclusion usually is noted during the *retention* phase, after the bonded expander has been removed and the maintenance plate has been worn for 6 to 12 months. When planning the treatment for a patient with Class III tendency, facial mask hooks may be attached to the expansion appliance to facilitate the use of a facial mask if that treatment is deemed necessary at a later time.

THE TREATMENT OF CLASS II MALOCCLUSION

A number of treatments are available for correcting Class II malocclusion, including a variety of extraoral traction appliances, arch expansion appliances, extraction procedures, and functional jaw orthopedic appliances. Each treatment approach, however, differs in its effect on the skeletal structures of the craniofacial region, sometimes accelerating or limiting the growth of the various craniofacial structures involved.

COMPONENTS OF CLASS II MALOCCLUSION

Numerous studies have considered the components of Class II malocclusion, with most focusing on patients in the adolescent or adult age range.* These studies have shown that the term *Class II malocclusion* is not a single diagnostic entity but rather can result from numerous combinations of skeletal and dentoalveolar components.

One investigation of Class II malocclusion focused on individuals in the mixed dentition. In a study of 277 children with Class II malocclusion on whom lateral cephalograms were taken during the mixed dentition,[84] variations in the skeletal and dentoalveolar components of Class II malocclusion were noted. Mandibular skeletal retrusion was the most common single characteristic of the Class II sample. Wide variation also was noted in the vertical development of the face, with one third to one half of the sample having increased vertical facial dimensions. The anteroposterior position of the maxilla was on average neutral, with far

---

*References 16, 24, 34, 103, 158.

more instances of maxillary skeletal retrusion than maxillary skeletal protrusion being observed.

When measures independent of mandibular position were used for evaluation, the upper incisors of the Class II sample were, on average, in a normal anteroposterior position, with more instances of maxillary dentoalveolar retrusion than maxillary dentoalveolar protrusion being observed.[84] The lower incisors usually were well positioned anteroposteriorly, but instances of mandibular dental retrusion and protrusion also were noted.

CLASS II TREATMENT STRATEGIES

Once the skeletal and dentoalveolar components of an individual Class II malocclusion are identified through data gathered from the clinical examination, a cephalometric analysis, and the evaluation of study models, and appropriate treatment regimen is selected. This discussion will focus on the treatment of problems of Class II malocclusion that primarily are skeletally related, with specific emphasis on extraoral traction and functional jaw orthopedics—two of the most commonly used treatment approaches. It should be noted that in patients who have a forward positioning of the maxillary dentition relative to the bony base of the maxilla, either extraction protocols (i.e., utimately removing the upper first premolars) or dentoalveolar distalizing me-

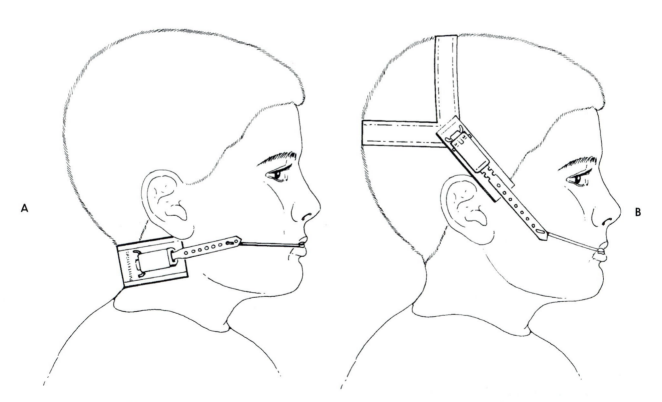

Fig. 9-15 Extra-oral traction. **A,** Low-pull (cervical) face bow with safety connector. **B,** High-pull face bow with safety connector. (From McNamara JA Jr, Brudon WL: *Orthodontic and orthopedic treatment in the mixed dentition,* Ann Arbor, Mich, 1993, Needham Press.)

chanics (e.g., distalizing magnets, NiTi coils, removable plates with finger springs) also can be used.

Extra-oral Traction

The most common treatment for true maxillary skeletal protrusion is extra-oral traction. Extra-oral traction appliances can be divided arbitrarily into two types: facebows and headgears. Facebows attach to tubes on the upper first molar bands, whereas headgears attach directly to the archwire or to auxiliaries connected to the archwire.[12]

Facebows. The cervical (low-pull) facebow (Fig. 9-15, *A*) is used most frequently in patients with decreased vertical facial dimensions. The inner bow of the facebow is anchored to tubes that are placed on the buccal surface of bands that are attached to the upper first molars. The outer bow is connected to a strap that extends to the cervical region and is anchored against the dorsal aspect of the neck. Usually the outer bow of the facebow lies above the plane of occlusion (e.g., 15° to 20°) so that the force is directed through the center of resistance in order to prevent distal tipping of the molars during treatment. Numerous clinical studies* have shown that the forward movement of the maxilla can be inhibited through the use of this type of appliance. Cer-

---

*References 50, 73, 124, 153, 156.

vical traction also can increase the vertical dimension through the extrusion of posterior teeth.

The direction of extra-oral force can be altered, depending upon the placement of the attached anchoring units. For example, a high-pull facebow (Fig. 9-15, *B*) is used in individuals in whom increases in vertical dimension are to be minimized or avoided. The facebow is attached to an occipital anchoring unit (headcap) to produce a more vertically directed force. As a growth guidance appliance, a high-pull facebow can decrease the vertical development of the maxilla, thereby allowing for autorotation of the mandible and maximizing the horizontal expression of mandibular growth.[151] A facebow also can be anchored simultaneously to a cervical neckstrap and a headcap—a combination that is often termed a *straight-pull* facebow.

Headgears. The forces produced by extraoral traction also can be attached anteriorly directly to the archwire through the use of J-hooks. Flared upper incisors can be retracted using either a straight-pull (Fig. 9-16, *A*) or a high-pull headgear (Fig. 9-16, *B*) combined with J hooks that are attached to the archwire anteriorly or by using a closing arch supported by headgear. Headgears with J hooks also are used to potentiate archwire mechanics by helping control forces incorporated into the archwire (e.g., torque, intrusion).[12]

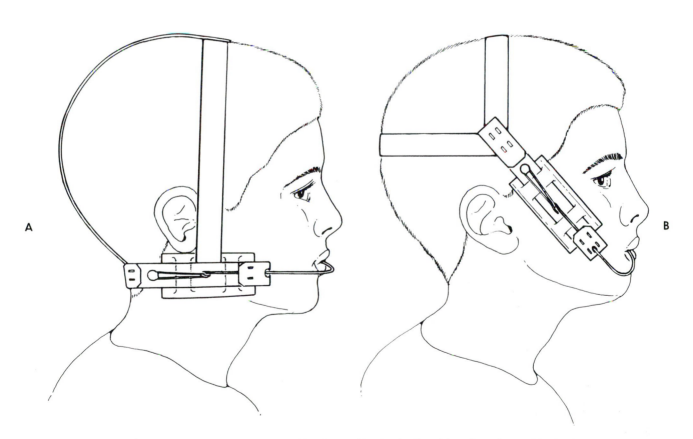

Fig. 9-16 Headgear. **A,** Straight-pull headgear with J hooks. **B,** High-pull headgear with J hooks. (From McNamara JA Jr, Brudon WL: *Orthondontic and orthopedic treatment in the mixed dentition,* Ann Arbor, Mich, 1993, Needham Press.)

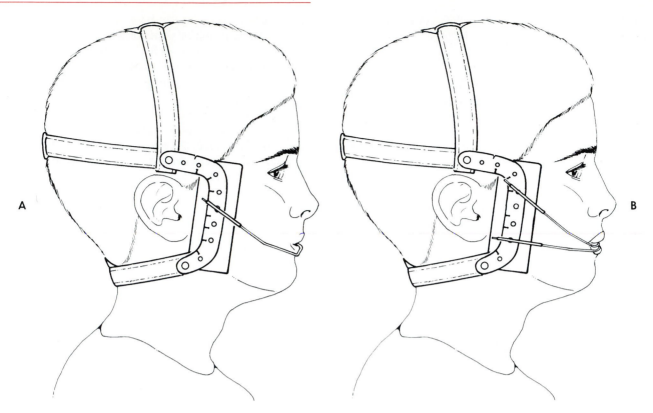

Fig. 9-17 Hickham-type headgear. **A,** Single pull to the maxillary dentition. **B,** Attachment of the J hooks to both the maxillary and mandibular dental arches. (From McNamara JA Jr, Brudon WL: *Orthodontic and orthopedic treatment in the mixed dentition,* Ann Arbor, Mich, 1993, Needham Press.)

The use of the Hickham-type headgear (Fig. 9-17) provides an additional treatment option with a variable direction of force. J hooks can be applied to the maxillary teeth in a variety of force vectors to retract and intrude the upper incisor teeth (Fig. 9-17, *A*). A similar type of retraction stabilization of the mandibular dental arch also can be achieved. It also is possible to attach to a high-pull headgear to the upper arch and a straight-pull headgear to the lower arch simultaneously (Fig. 9-17, *B*).

All of the extra-oral traction appliances described above restrict the normal downward and forward movement of the maxilla and also may help retract the maxillary and mandibular dentitions. These types of appliances are indicated in instances of maxillary skeletal protrusion, maxillary dentoalveolar protrusion, and mandibular dento-alveolar protrusion. The direction of force: low-pull, straight-pull, or high-pull, is in part determined by the pretreatment vertical dimensions of the patient.

Functional Jaw Orthopedic Appliances

Occlusal problems associated, at least in part, with mandibular skeleton retrusion often require some type of functional jaw orthopedic (FJO) appliance. Used infrequently in the United States until the mid 1970s, various appliance designs have been described, including the activator,[1] the bionator,[7,8] the Fränkel appliance,[36,42] the Bimler appliance,[14,15] and the Herbst appliance.[62,108]

It is not the purpose of this chapter to debate whether functional jaw orthopedic appliances do or do not enhance mandibular growth—a topic of great controversy during the last two decades. The question concerning whether the mandible can be increased in length in comparison to untreated controls has been addressed in numerous experimental studies.* In addition, a number of clinical studies of various appliances also have been conducted.† As mentioned earlier, the bulk of scientific evidence indicates that, in growing individuals, mandibular growth can be enhanced. The major question remaining is whether the extra growth has clinical relevance. It is our belief that the skeletal adaptations that are available combined with dentoalveolar changes can lead to a significant correction of Class II malocclusion using a variety of FJO treatment modalities.

Over the last 20 years a gradual evolution has occurred regarding the way in which functional jaw orthopedics is used in a contemporary orthodontic practice, especially con-

---

*References 9, 21, 81-83, 89, 90, 120-123, 140.
†References 25, 45, 47, 87, 92, 108, 110, 111, 127.

cerning appliance selection, the timing of intervention, and the need for preorthopedic orthodontic treatment.

Appliance selection. All functional jaw orthopedic appliances have one aspect in common: they induce a forward mandibular posturing as part of the overall treatment effect. Presumably, this alteration in the postural activity of the muscles of the craniofacial complex ultimately leads to changes in both skeletal and dental relationships.[45]

The FR-2 appliance of Fränkel. In the routine Class II malocclusion, characterized in part by mandibular skeletal retrusion, our appliance of choice is the function regulator (FR-2) appliance (Figs. 9-18 and 9-19) of Fränkel.[38,42,44,45] Of all the so-called *functional appliances* the FR-2 appliance is unique because it is primarily tissue-borne rather than tooth-borne. The base of operation is the maxillary and mandibular vestibules, and the appliance has a direct and primary effect on the neuromuscular system.

The orthopedic principles of Roux[130] have been incorporated into the design of the Fränkel appliance. The appliance first is used as an exercise device in retraining the associated musculature and indirectly producing changes in skeletal and dentoalveolar relationships by reprogramming the central nervous system. In contrast to virtually every other type of functional appliance, the FR-2 appliance interrupts abnormal patterns of muscle activity and ultimately produces an environment in which skeletal and dental arch changes occur spontaneously. Not only have increases in mandibular length been noted following FR-2 treatment,[44,45,87,92] but also changes in the transverse dimensions of the dental arches have been reported,* partly because of the shielding effect of the vestibular shields (Fig. 9-19) on the associated soft tissue.

*References 38, 42, 45, 79, 88.

In patients with mandibular skeletal retrusion who also show significant neuromuscular imbalances, such as hyperactive mentalis or hypertonic buccal musculature, the FR-2 appliance is particularly useful. For example, the lower labial pads (Fig. 9-18) help interrupt hyperactive mentalis activity—a clinical sign of lip incompetence. Fränkel and Fränkel[45] stress the importance of maintaining an adequate lip seal as a key element of successful orthopedic treatment. By balancing the neuromuscular environment, severe malocclusions can be treated successfully and the tendency toward relapse is minimized because the neural and soft tissue factors associated with a skeletal malocclusion have been addressed. Because the appliance is mostly tissue-borne rather than tooth-borne, maximum skeletal change can be achieved with minimal unwanted tooth movement. The bite registration usually is taken with the mandible 2 to 3 mm ahead of habitual occlusion. Fränkel and Fränkel[45] advocate a step-by-step advancement of the appliance to minimize unwanted dentoalveolar adaptations (e.g., lingual tipping of upper incisors, flaring of lower incisors).

The FR-2 appliance is especially effective in patients with either a neutral or short lower anterior facial height. The use of this appliance can lead to an increase in lower facial height during treatment, if indicated. This appliance also is used on patients with excessive vertical development, although care must be taken not to open the bite during treatment. In these patients in particular, a strict regimen of lip seal exercises[43,45,88] must be undertaken. Lip seal training is used as an adjunct to orofacial orthopedics in the same way as physical therapy is used in general orthopedics.

Treatment with the Fränkel appliance usually is initiated during the middle-to-late mixed dentition period, although earlier intervention is indicated in patients with severe neuromuscular problems. The duration of active treatment typ-

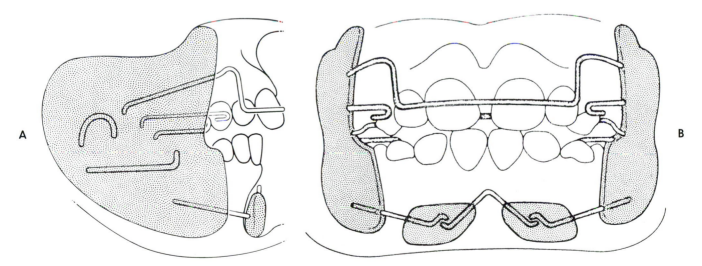

Fig. 9-18 The function regulator (FR-2) of Fränkel. **A,** Lateral view. **B,** Frontal view. The base of operation is the maxillary and mandibular vestibules. The appliance has a direct effect on the postural activity of the masticatory and perioral musculature, producing a change in mandibular postural position. (From McNamara JA Jr, Brudon WL: *Orthodontic and orthopedic treatment in the mixed dentition,* Ann Arbor, Mich, 1993, Needham Press.)

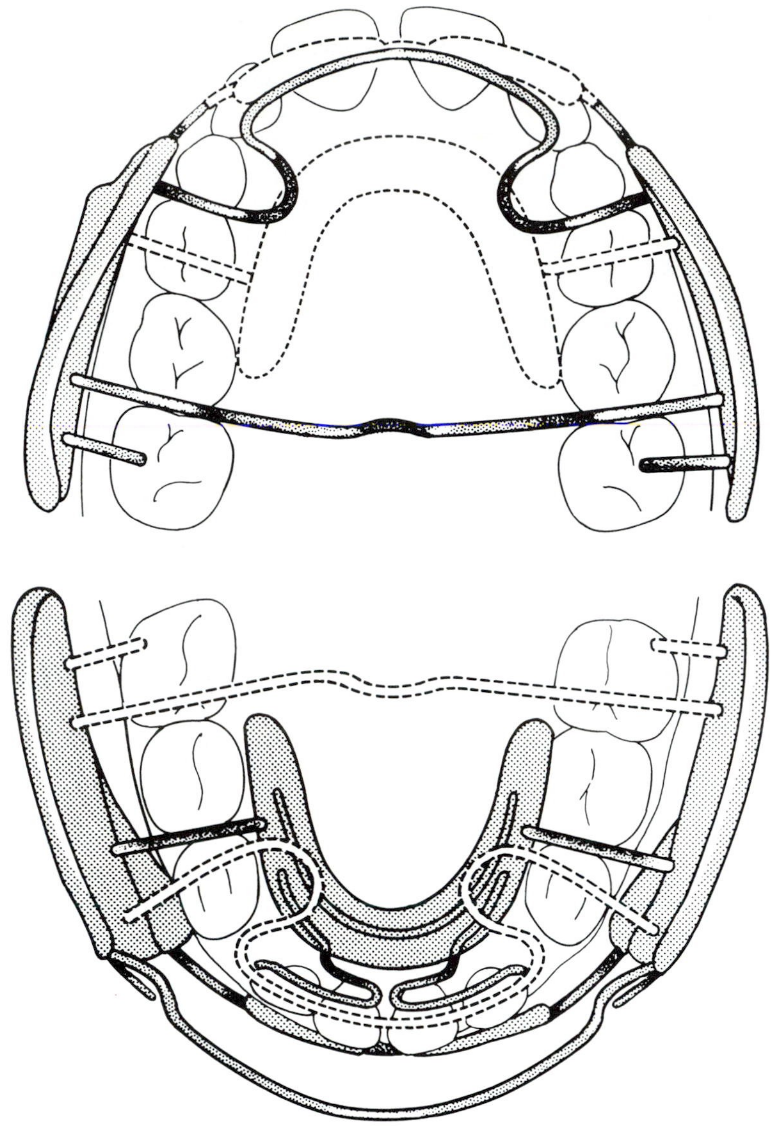

Fig. 9-19 The function regulator (FR-2) of Fränkel. **A,** Maxillary view. **B,** Mandibular view. Spontaneous expansion of the dental arches usually occurs because of the effect of the vestibular shields and the lower labial pads on the soft tissue.

ically is 18 to 24 months, and FR treatment usually is followed by a comprehensive phase of fixed appliance therapy to align and detail the permanent dentition. The description of the precise clinical management of the FR-2 appliance is found in Fränkel and Fränkel[45] and summarized in McNamara and Brudon.[88]

Bionator. Perhaps the most widely used functional appliance in the world today is the bionator.[3-8,70] The bionator is a generic term that refers to a family of appliances derived from the bulkier activator.[1] The acrylic parts of the bionator (Figs. 9-20 and 9-21) contact the teeth and supporting structures; thus changes are created in the skeletal, dentoalveolar, and muscular environments of the craniofacial region. However, this appliance does not affect the orofacial musculature in the same way as does the FR-2 appliance of Fränkel; therefore we use this appliance only occasionally in patients with Class II malocclusion.

The bite advancement produced by the appliance is a reflection of the bite registration. The bite should be ad-

vanced no more than 4 to 5 mm anteroposteriorly and 3 mm vertically. Some vertical opening is necessary anteriorly to accommodate the incisal cap that covers the lower incisors (Fig. 9-20). Posteriorly the acrylic can be configured as eruption facets or channels (Fig. 9-22, *A*) to guide the lateral and vertical eruption of the posterior teeth. Other designs of the bionator feature an occlusal table (Fig. 9-22, *B*) that prevents the downward and forward eruption of the upper posterior teeth and allows for increased eruption of the lower posterior teeth. Expansion screws can be placed sagittally in the appliance to allow for a step-by-step advancement of the appliance.

The belief among many clinicians is that the bionator is easier to use than is the FR-2. However, it has been our experience that once the technique of appliance management has been mastered, the FR-2 is no more difficult nor easier to use than the bionator. The bionator is indicated in patients with extremely short lower anterior facial height. In these patients there is not adequate vertical space for the posi-

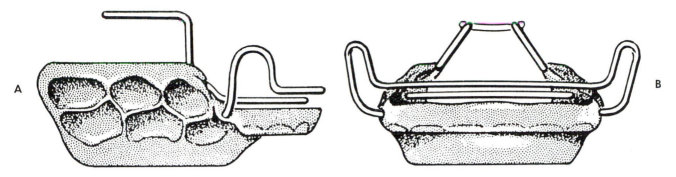

Fig. 9-20 The bionator. The so-called *California bionator* is an example of a bionator that can be used to correct Class II malocclusion. Eruption facets (channels) are present posteriorly to guide eruption and to produce expansion. **A,** Lateral view. **B,** Frontal view. (From McNamara JA Jr, Brudon WL: *Orthodontic and orthopedic treatment in the mixed dentition,* Ann Arbor, Mich, 1993, Needham Press.)

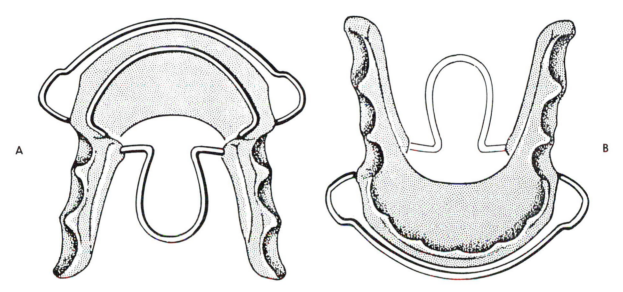

Fig. 9-21 The bionator. **A,** Maxillary view. **B,** Mandibular view. Wax relief is placed on the lingual surfaces of the lower incisors to prevent contact of this appliance against the lingual surfaces of the lower anterior teeth. (From McNamara JA Jr, Brudon WL: *Orthodontic and orthopedic treatment in the mixed dentition,* Ann Arbor, Mich, 1993, Needham Press.)

tioning of the lower labial pads of the FR-2, and thus a bionator is used not only to bring the mandible into a more forward position but also to increase the vertical dimension through the differential eruption of posterior teeth. In instances of excessive vertical face height the bionator can be used if the posterior teeth are prevented from further eruption by having acrylic placed interocclusally (Fig. 9-22, *C*).

Herbst appliance. An appliance that has proven satisfactory in the treatment of Class II malocclusion in the permanent dentition is the Herbst appliance: a fixed or removable functional appliance depending on the anchoring system used. The bite-jumping mechanism was developed by Herbst,[62] and the banded design of the appliance was reintroduced in the late 1970s by Pancherz.[108,109,111,112]

The acrylic splint design of the Herbst appliance[65,86,91] is constructed in a similar manner to the bonded acrylic splint expander described earlier (Figs. 9-23 and 9-24). Acrylic that is 3 mm thick is heated and forced over a metal framework using a thermal pressure machine. If the maxillary splint is removable, the canine is incorporated into the appliance (Fig. 9-23, *A*). If the maxillary part of the appliance is to be bonded in position, only the lingual surface of the maxillary canine is incorporated into the arch (Fig. 9-23, *B*). The maxillary splint covers the posterior dentition but does not contact the upper incisors.

The mandibular part of the appliance always is removable. A splint covers the entire posterior dentition and the lower anterior teeth (Fig. 9-24). The mandibular part of the

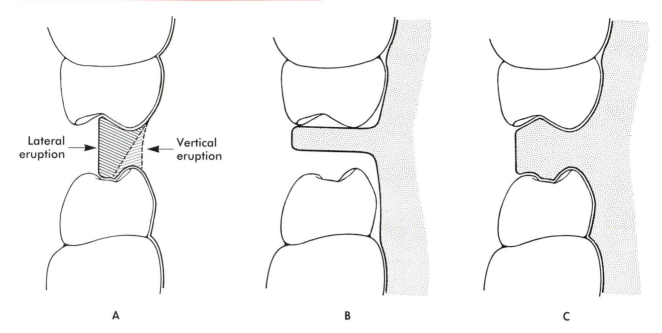

A   B   C

Fig. 9-22   Control of posterior vertical eruption. **A,** Eruption facets. If lateral eruption is desired, the acrylic is removed at an angle. If vertical eruption is desired, additional acrylic is removed. **B,** Occlusal table. The interocclusal acrylic is trimmed so that the maxillary posterior teeth touch the acrylic. The lower teeth remain free of the acrylic so that further eruption of these teeth can occur. **C,** Interocclusal acrylic. If no change in vertical eruption is desired, the interocclusal acrylic is left between the upper and lower posterior teeth. (Adapted from McNamara JA Jr, Brudon WL: *Orthodontic and orthopedic treatment in the mixed dentition,* Ann Arbor, Mich, 1993, Needham Press.)

appliance also covers the lingual surfaces of the anterior teeth and one third to one half of the labial surfaces of these teeth.

Clinical studies of the banded and acrylic splint designs of the appliance indicate that both skeletal and dentoalveolar adaptations are produced.[92,111] About 50% of the treatment effect is due to tooth movement, primarily the backward and upward movement of the posterior dentition. The primarily skeletal treatment effect produced is an increase in mandibular growth: 2.0 to 2.5 mm greater than normal values.[92,111]

There is no question that a Class I molar relationship can be achieved in most growing Class II patients following Herbst appliance treatment. However, it is our opinion that a Herbst appliance is not the appliance of choice in mixed dentition patients. After over a decade of using the Herbst appliance and after having followed patients originally treated in the mixed dentition for several years after Herbst therapy was completed but before the placement of fixed appliances was initiated, we have noted a significant tendency toward a relapse to the original malocclusion. This finding also has been noted by others.[112,157] This observation concerning Herbst patients treated in the mixed dentition may be partly due to the lack of direct effect on the orofacial musculature produced by the Herbst appliance (in contrast to the FR-2 appliance) and also may be related to the shape

of the deciduous teeth. The posterior deciduous teeth tend to be relatively flat and thus do not provide the same type of occlusal interdigitation as occurs in the permanent dentition.

Our lack of success using the Herbst appliance in the mixed dentition does not eliminate this appliance from consideration. Often we will initiate regimens in the early mixed dentition to address intra-arch space discrepancy problems (to be discussed below) and will postpone functional appliance treatment until after all deciduous teeth are lost and the succeeding teeth are erupted. This delayed intervention is particularly useful in patients who have excessive vertical facial development and steep mandibular plane angles. We have found that by intervening in the early permanent dentition using the Herbst appliance, satisfactory skeletal and dental adaptations have been noted overall. This appliance is used most effectively in patients who do not have profound neuromuscular imbalances.

Treatment Timing

As mentioned earlier, one of the major changes that has occurred during the last two decades has been an alteration in the timing of treatment using functional appliances. A study by McNamara and co-workers[87] that compared two groups of patients who were treated with the FR-2 appliance of Fränkel indicated that those patients who began treatment

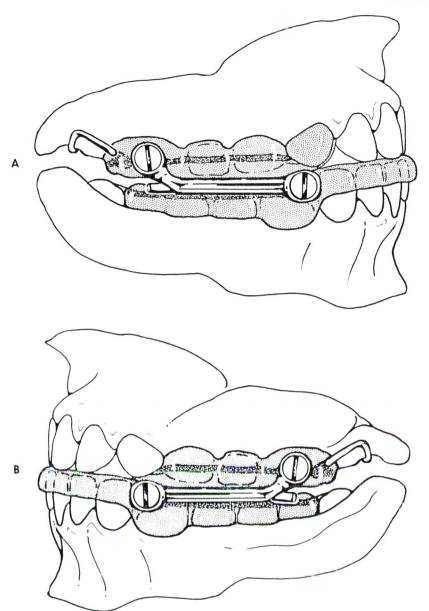

Fig. 9-23 The acrylic splint Herbst appliance. **A,** Right sagittal view. This drawing demonstrates full coverage of the maxillary canine: the design that is recommended when the maxillary splint is removable. **B,** Left sagittal view. This drawing demonstrates the design of the maxillary splint without coverage on the labial surface of the maxillary canine: the design that is recommended when the maxillary splint is bonded. (Adapted from McNamara JA Jr, Brudon WL: *Orthodontic and orthopedic treatment in the mixed dentition,* Ann Arbor, Mich, 1993, Needham Press.)

at an average of 11.5 years showed a greater mandibular growth response than did patients beginning treatment at approximately 8.5 years of age. The reason for this increased growth response may be related to the synergistic interaction between a change in function, produced by the functional appliance, and growth hormone and related substances that are in greater quantity during the circumpubertal growth period. The interaction between altered function and growth hormone has been demonstrated in the experimental studies of Petrovic and co-workers,[122] among others.

In general the onset of functional jaw orthopedic therapy in the mild to moderate Class II patient is delayed until the middle or the end of the mixed dentition. It is our intention to schedule FJO treatment so that this treatment will be followed immediately by a comprehensive phase of fixed appliance therapy. In instances of significant neuromuscular and skeletal imbalances, treatment is started earlier in the

mixed dentition, with the FR-2 appliance as the appliance of choice. Delaying treatment until the late mixed dentition does not mean that orthodontic treatment is not provided at an earlier time. In many patients a *preorthopedic phase* of treatment can be provided in the early mixed dentition as is described in detail below.

Phase I treatment. In the routine preparation of an adolescent or adult patient for orthognathic surgery, the orthodontist decompensates the dental arches in order to enable the surgeon to maximize the repositioning of the skeletal elements of the craniofacial complex. Often this type of treatment will involve the intrusion and/or flaring of the upper incisors and the intrusion and retraction of the lower incisors. Rapid maxillary expansion also can be used in younger patients who need surgery to eliminate transverse discrepancies in the maxilla before surgery.

In many respects the use of a functional jaw orthopedic

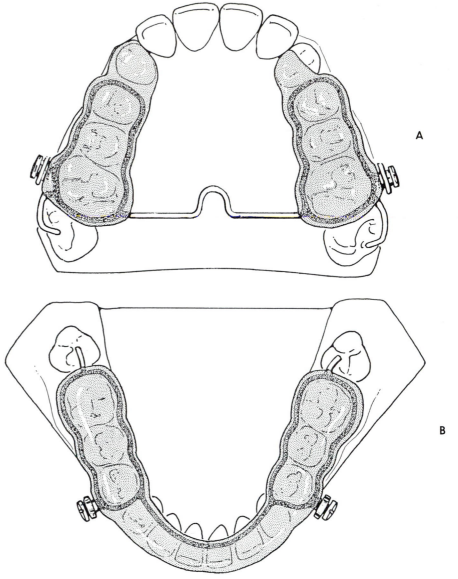

A

B

Fig. 9-24 The acrylic splint Herbst appliance. **A,** Maxillary view. The right side of the appliance demonstrates full canine coverage that is used when the splint is removable. On the left side, the acrylic extends only to the lingual aspect of the upper canines. This design is used when the upper splint is bonded. **B,** Mandibular view. The mandibular splint with full occlusal and incisal coverage is shown. The mandibular splint is always removable. (Adapted from McNamara JA Jr, Brudon WL: *Orthodontic and orthopedic treatment in the mixed dentition*, Ann Arbor, Mich, 1993, Needham Press.)

appliance mimics orthognathic surgery in that the clinician also is attempting to maximize the change in mandibular position during FJO treatment. As experience was gained using various functional and jaw orthopedic appliances, it became clear that some preparation of the dental arches was needed in a significant number of patients with mixed-dentition who had Class II malocclusion. In the study mentioned earlier[84] it was noted that over 30% of the Class II patients in the sample had upper incisors that were in a retroclined position. Thus one of the initial treatments of many Class II patients involves a flaring (and perhaps intrusion) of the upper incisors, using, for example, a protrusion utility arch (Fig. 9-25). Flared upper incisors can be retracted or intruded using a retraction utility arch (Fig. 9-26; see also Fig. 9-6) or a high-pull headgear with J-hooks (Fig. 9-17). The need for uprighting of the buccal segment, particularly in the lower arch, occasionally is noted, and a Schwarz appliance (Fig. 9-7) can be used in patients with this posterior dental configuration.

We increasingly appreciate the importance of the transverse dimension in the treatment of Class II malocclusion, and thus we use rapid maxillary expansion with a bonded acrylic splint appliance in the early mixed dentition. The widening of the maxilla into a slightly overcorrected position during the *early mixed dentition* often results in a spontaneous correction of a Class II relationship, occasionally even in a patient who has a full cusp Class II molar relationship. Thus the first major step in addressing a Class II problem may be the intervention in the transverse dimension. Only in the late mixed dentition is a direct attempt made to correct a Class II problem in mild to moderate cases.

Additional Comments Regarding Class II Treatment

There is no one ideal method for treating a Class II malocclusion in the mixed dentition. Following a thorough clinical examination, a precise analysis of both the cephalometric radiographs and the dental casts should be undertaken

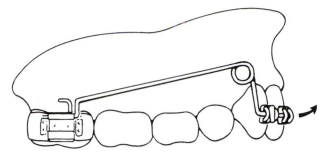

Fig. 9-25 The protrusion utility arch often is used to procline and intrude upper incisors before FJO treatment. When passive, the anterior part of the archwire lies 2 to 3 mm ahead of the incisor brackets. (From McNamara JA Jr, Brudon WL: *Orthodontic and orthopedic treatment in the mixed dentition,* Ann Arbor, Mich, 1993, Needham Press.)

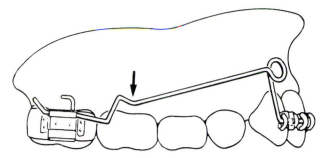

Fig. 9-26 A retraction utility arch is used to retract and intrude flared upper incisors. The arch is activated by pulling the wire posteriorly through the auxiliary tube on the first molar band and by turning the end of the wire superiorly and medially. Intrusion is produced by placing a gable bend in the vestibular segment of the wire *(arrow).* (From McNamara JA Jr, Brudon WL: *Orthodontic and orthopedic treatment in the mixed dentition,* Ann Arbor, Mich, 1993, Needham Press.)

to identify the components of malocclusion that make an individual patient unique. After a thorough diagnosis has been established, the clinician can select the appropriate treatment regimen from the wide variety of treatment modalities available.

Not all of the treatment modalities discussed are used by us with the same frequency. As true maxillary skeletal protrusion patients are observed relatively infrequently,[84] our use of extraoral traction is a less frequently used treatment option. Mandibular skeletal retrusion is a relatively common problem in Class II malocclusion; therefore our use of functional jaw orthopedics is the more frequently used treatment option. In recent years, following our experiences using rapid maxillary expansion and observing spontaneous correction of some Class II problems, even the use of FJO appliances has decreased over the frequency of use 5 to 10 years ago.

TREATMENT OF CLASS III MALOCCLUSION

One of the most difficult types of malocclusions to treat in the mixed dentition is the Class III malocclusion. The occurrence of an end-to-end incisor relationship or a frank anterior crossbite is identified easily by both the family practitioner and the parent as an abnormal occlusal relationship. Thus it is common for Class III patients to be referred for early treatment. However, the outcome of various early treatment protocols may or may not be successful, depending upon the severity of the problem, the family history of the patient, and the age at which treatment is initiated.

COMPONENTS OF CLASS III MALOCCLUSION

According to Mills,[99] Class III malocclusion occurs in about 5% of the North American population. This type of malocclusion is far more prevalent in other regions of the world, particularly in Asiatic countries. Thus, the treatment of Class III problems comprises a significant portion of orthodontic and orthopedic treatment in such countries as Japan and Korea.

Class III malocclusion does not encompass a single diagnostic entity. Guyer and co-workers[55] investigated the components of Class III malocclusion in 144 Michigan children between the ages of 5 and 15 years. A Class III malocclusion characterized simply by mandibular skeletal protrusion (mandibular prognathism), commonly called a major skeletal aberration in individuals with a Class III malocclusion, was found in less than 20% of the Michigan sample. A Class III relationship caused primarily by maxillary skeletal retrusion was found in 25% of the individuals studied, and a combination of maxillary skeletal retrusion and mandibular skeletal protrusion was found in approximately 22% of the Michigan sample. The remainder had no anteroposterior skeletal imbalances. In the younger ages studied, on average lower anterior facial heights were normal, with excessive vertical facial development observed only in adolescent Class III patients.

These findings are similar to those previously described by Sanborn,[133] Dietrich,[32] Jacobson and co-workers,[69] and Ellis and McNamara.[35] Thus as with all malocclusions that are considered by Angle classification, the Class III malocclusion includes a variety of skeletal and dental components that may vary from our concept of normal or ideal.

CLASS III TREATMENT STRATEGIES

Before discussing early treatment strategies, it is important to review briefly the usual approach to the correction of Class III malocclusion in an adolescent or adult patient. When a patient first is diagnosed as having a Class III malocclusion in the permanent dentition, treatment options are limited, particularly if there is a strong skeletal component to the Class III occlusal relationship. Such treatment usually includes comprehensive orthodontic therapy, either combined with extraction and/or orthognathic surgery. The orthognathic surgical procedure is designed to address the imbalance of the skeletal component (e.g., sagittal split osteotomy to posteriorly reposition the mandible in instances of mandibular prognathism, LeFort I advancement in instances of maxillary skeletal retrusion—both procedures may be used in instances of severe maxillomandibular skeletal imbalances). In other words the surgical procedure is designed to correct whatever skeletal imbalances are present. In patients in whom excessive skeletal growth is anticipated, the surgical procedure usually is deferred until the end of the active growth period. However, such patients still face the psychosocial problems during childhood that have been shown to be associated with this type of malocclusion.[49]

The treatment of Class III malocclusion in the mixed dentition (or late deciduous dentition) can be approached from a slightly different conceptual viewpoint. It is possible to select a treatment protocol that is intended to address the skeletal imbalance in a Class III mixed dentition patient. For example, Fränkel[42,45] recommends the function regulator (FR-3) appliance in patients whose malocclusion is characterized primarily by maxillary skeletal retrusion. On the other hand the orthopedic chin cup* has been used in patients whose malocclusions are characterized primarily by mandibular prognathism. More recently the orthopedic facial mask that has been popularized by Delaire[26-28] and refined by Petit[117,118] has been used. Each of these treatments has been shown to produce favorable (but unpredictable) effects in Class III patients; however, the stability of the treatment outcomes often have been unpredictable, particularly when these patients are evaluated from a long-term perspective. Also there are substantial differences with regard to the speed of correction and in the regions of the craniofacial complex that are affected.

Appliance Selection

A basic axiom of orthodontic treatment is that the treatment approach should be designed to address the specific nature of the skeletal and/or dentoalveolar imbalance. This axiom is illustrated by the selection of the specific surgical procedure or procedures used in the correction of a Class III malocclusion in an adolescent or adult patient. In patients with a Class II malocclusion it also is demonstrated by the selective use of extraoral traction in the correction of maxillary prognathism and of functional jaw orthopedics in the correction of mandibular retrusion. An exception to this rule may be the treatment of the developing Class III malocclusion.

The orthopedic facial mask.

Of the three mixed dentition treatment strategies discussed above, it is our opinion that the orthopedic facial mask has the widest application and produces the most dramatic results in the shortest period of time. Thus the orthopedic facial mask is our customary appliance of choice for most Class III patients seen in the early mixed dentition or late deciduous dentition. The use of this single regimen in most early Class III patients seems arbitrary and paradoxical at first glance, given the variety of combinations of skeletal and dental components of Class III malocclusion in patients with mixed dentition.[55] Because intervention using an orthopedic facial mask is undertaken at such an early age, the treatment effects produced by the facial mask ultimately are incorporated into the future craniofacial growth of the patient. The appliance system affects virtually all areas contributing to a Class III malocclusion (e.g., maxillary skeletal retrusion; maxillary dentoalveolar retrusion; mandibular prognathism; decreased lower anterior facial height); therefore this treatment protocol can be applied effectively to most developing Class III patients, regardless of the specific cause of the malocclusion. An exception to this use is in the patient who has an increased lower anterior facial height at the beginning of treatment.

The orthopedic facial mask system has three basic components: the facial mask, a bonded maxillary splint, and elastics. The facial mask (Fig. 9-27) is an extraoral device that has been modified by Petit[118] and now is available commercially (Great Lakes Orthodontic Products, Tonawanda, New York). In essence the facial mask is composed of a forehead pad and a chin pad that are connected by a heavy steel support rod. A crossbow (to which rubber bands are attached to produce a forward and downward elastic traction on the maxilla) is connected to this support rod. The position of the pads and crossbow can be adjusted simply by loosening and tightening set screws within each part of the appliance.

Although Petit[118] has recommended a number of different intra-oral devices, both fixed and removable, to which the elastics can be anchored, it is our strong preference to use a bonded maxillary expansion appliance that is similar in design to that discussed previously in the treatment of arch length discrepancy problems (see Fig. 9-3). The major modification in the splint design is the addition of facial mask hooks in the region of the upper first deciduous molar (Fig. 9-28). In patients in whom treatment is started before the eruption of the upper first molars, the appliance is designed to incorporate the first and second deciduous molars, as well as the deciduous canines.

Even though the orthopedic facial mask has been available for over 100 years,[68,123,142] surprisingly few studies have dealt with the treatment effects produced with the facial mask. Most published studies dealing with facial mask therapy have been anecdotal in nature.* It appears that the facial

---

*References 48, 54, 132, 141, 145.

*References 23, 85, 105, 129, 149.

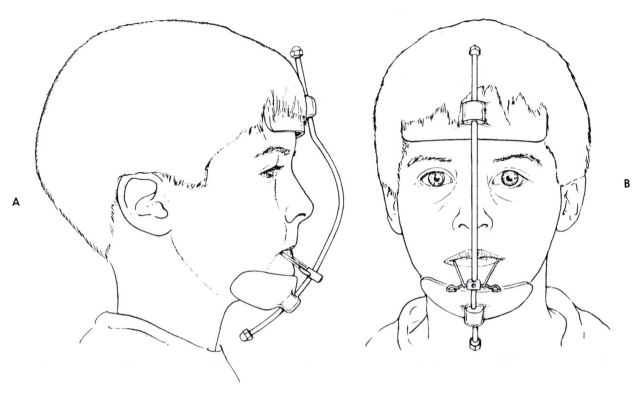

Fig. 9-27   The orthopedic facial mask of Petit. **A,** Lateral view. **B,** Frontal view. This appliance, best used in patients in the early mixed dentition, is worn on a full-time basis for about 6 months, after which it can be worn on a nighttime basis as a retention appliance. The elastics are connected to a bonded maxillary splint (see Fig. 9-28) to which hooks have been attached in the upper first deciduous molar region. (From McNamara JA Jr, Brudon WL: *Orthodontic and orthopedic treatment in the mixed dentition,* Ann Arbor, Mich, 1993, Needham Press.)

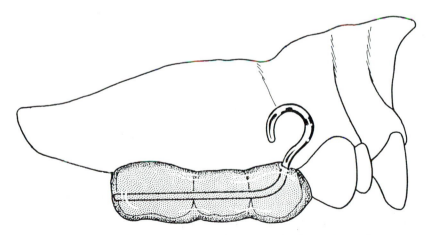

Fig. 9-28   The bonded maxillary acrylic splint (lateral view). The hooks for the elastics usually are placed adjacent to the upper first deciduous molars. (From McNamara JA Jr, Brudon WL: *Orthodontic and orthopedic treatment in the mixed dentition,* Ann Arbor, Mich, 1993, Needham Press.)

mask, especially when combined with a rigid maxillary anchorage unit (e.g., bonded acrylic splint expander), can produce one or more of the following treatment effects:

1. Correction of a CO-CR discrepancy; a shift in occlusal relationship that is immediate and usually is associated with pseudo-Class III patients
2. Maxillary skeletal protraction, with 1 to 2 mm of forward movement of the maxilla often (but not always) observed
3. Forward movement of the maxillary dentition
4. Lingual tipping of the lower incisors, particularly in patients with a preexisting anterior crossbite
5. Redirection of mandibular growth in a downward and backward direction, resulting in an increase in lower anterior facial height

In instances in which the patient begins treatment with a short lower anterior facial height, this change often is advantageous; in patients who have a long lower anterior facial height at the beginning of treatment, this treatment effect may be undesirable. There are no clinical studies that show that facial mask treatment leads to an inhibition of mandibular growth over the long term.

Once the decision has been made to use an orthopedic facial mask, the first step of the appliance therapy is the fabrication and bonding of the maxillary splint. (See McNamara and Brudon[88] for the technical details.) The splint is activated once per day until the desired increase in transverse width has been achieved. For patients in whom no increase in transverse dimension is desired, the appliance still is activated for 8 to 10 days to disjoin the maxillary sutural system and to promote maxillary protraction.[57]

After the patient has become accustomed to wearing the maxillary splint, facial mask treatment is initiated. A sequence of elastics of increasing force is used during the breaking-in period, until a heavy orthopedic force (14 oz. per side) is delivered to the maxillary complex. Normally, the facial mask is worn on a full-time basis (about 20 hours per day) for 4 to 6 months, and then it can be worn on a nighttime basis only for an additional period of time. It usually is unwise to have the splint remain bonded in place for more than 9 to 12 months because of the potential risk of leakage and subsequent decalcification of the underlying dentition.

The ideal stage of dental development during which to begin facial mask therapy is at the time of eruption of the upper permanent central incisors. Usually, the lower incisors already have erupted into occlusion. Achieving a positive horizontal and vertical overlap of the incisors during treatment is essential in providing an environment that will help maintain the achieved anteroposterior correction of the original Class III malocclusion. In patients with mild to moderate Class III problems, a positive overjet of 4 to 5 mm is achieved before the time that the facial mask is discontinued. It is anticipated that there will be some regression of the overjet relationship during the early posttreatment period. However, every effort should be made to maintain a positive

overbite and overjet relationship throughout the retention period.

After the facial mask and the rapid maxillary expansion appliance have been removed, the patient can be retained using a number of appliances, including a simple maintenance plate (Fig. 9-9), an FR-3 appliance of Fränkel, or a chin cup. Because the facial mask usually is used in the early mixed dentition, a substantial period of time may elapse before the final phase of fixed appliance treatment can be initiated.

The FR-3 appliance of Fränkel. An intra-oral appliance that has been used quite effectively in the treatment of Class III malocclusion in the mixed dentition is the functional regulator (FR-3) appliance of Fränkel,[39,42,44] McNamara and Huge,[93] Fränkel and Fränkel.[45] Of all the Fränkel appliances the FR-3 appliance (Fig. 9-29) perhaps is the easiest to manage clinically because no substantial postural change is produced in the maxillomandibular relationship. As with all Fränkel appliances the base of operation of the FR-3 appliance is the maxillary and mandibular vestibules. The appliance is designed to restrict the forces of the associated soft tissue on the maxillary complex (Fig. 9-29), transmitting these forces through the appliance to the mandible.

A major advantage in using the Fränkel appliance is that it is relatively inconspicuous, especially in comparison to the orthopedic facial mask. The FR-3 is worn intra-orally; wearing the appliance often improves the appearance of the patient by *filling out* the upper lip region in individuals with substantial maxillary skeletal retrusion. This appliance is worn easily by the patient. Interestingly, the treatment effects produced by the FR-3 appliance have been shown to be quite similar to those produced by the orthopedic facial

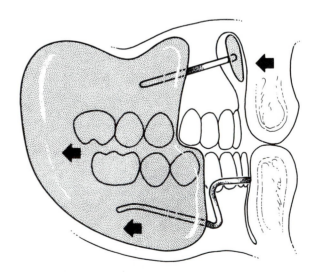

Fig. 9-29 The FR-3 appliance of Fränkel. The vestibular shields and the upper labial pads shield the maxillary alveolus from the forces of the surrounding soft tissue. These forces are transmitted through the appliance to the mandible. (From McNamara JA Jr, Brudon WL: *Orthodontic and orthopedic treatment in the mixed dentition,* Ann Arbor, Mich, 1993, Needham Press.)

mask. These effects include the relative forward movement of the maxilla and the maxillary dentition, a downward and backward redirection of mandibular growth, and some lingual tipping of the lower incisors.*

A major difference between the FR-3 appliance and the orthopedic facial mask is in the duration of treatment. In a routine Class III patient the orthopedic facial mask may produce a correction of the malocclusion within the first 6 months after initiating treatment. Normally, 12 to 24 months are necessary to produce a similar response with the FR-3 appliance. However, it is obvious that the FR-3 appliance has much more of an effect on the associated soft tissue, particularly on any existing hyperactivity in the muscles associated with the maxilla, than does the facial mask. This appliance was designed by Fränkel, again using the principles of Roux,[130] in that the primary action of the appliance is on the associated soft tissue, hopefully leading to a reprogramming of the central nervous system and a retraining of the craniofacial musculature.

When it is used as the primary appliance, the FR-3 is worn for about 20 hours per day, with the patients removing the appliance only during such activities as eating and playing contact sports. If the appliance is worn as a retainer

*References 39, 45, 71, 76, 93.

following either full-time FR-3 therapy or facial mask therapy, it usually is worn only during the nighttime hours.

The orthopedic chin cup. Perhaps the oldest of the orthopedic approaches to the treatment of Class III malocclusion is the chin cup. The effects of this appliance have been investigated thoroughly.* Much of the research has been conducted using Asian populations because of the higher incidence of Class III malocclusion in these groups.†

Although there are a wide variety of chin cup designs available commercially, in general these appliances can be divided into two types: the occipital-pull chin cup that is used in instances of mandibular prognathism, and the vertical-pull chin cup that is used in patients with steep mandibular plane angles and excessive lower anterior facial height.

The occipital-pull chin cup (Fig. 9-30, *A*) frequently is used in the treatment of Class III malocclusion. This type of chin cup is indicated for use in patients with mild to moderate mandibular prognathism. Success is greatest in those patients who can bring their incisors close to an edge-to-edge position when in centric relation. This treatment is particularly useful in patients who begin treatment with a

*References 2, 48, 54, 78, 145, 146.
†References 67, 78, 132, 141, 143.

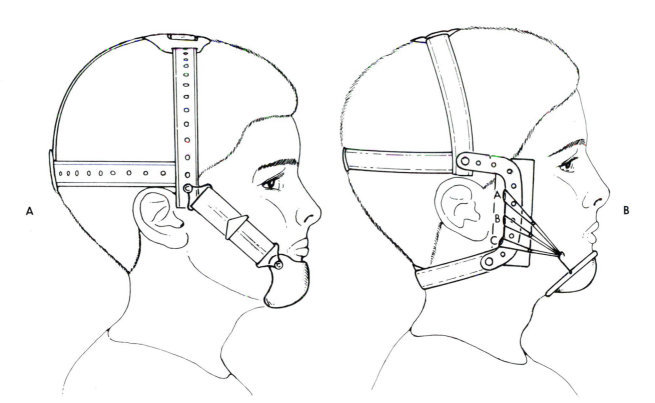

Fig. 9-30   The occipital-pull chin cup. **A,** Soft elastic appliance. The direction of force is determined by the position of the head cap. **B,** Hickham-type headgear is used as anchorage for a hard chin cup. The direction of pull can be adjusted according to the placement of the elastics *(A, B, C).* (Adapted from McNamara JA Jr, Brudon WL: *Orthodontic and orthopedic treatment in mixed dentition,* Ann Arbor, Mich, 1993, Needham Press.)

short lower anterior facial height, as this type of treatment can lead to an increase in this dimension. If the pull of the chin cup is directed below the condyle, the force of the appliance may lead to a downward and backward rotation of the mandible. If no opening of the mandibular plane angle is desired, the force should be directed through the condyle to help restrict mandibular growth. The use of a Hickham-type headcap combined with a hard chin cup (Fig. 9-30, *B*), allows for variable vectors of force to be produced on the lower jaw.

If no increase on lower anterior facial height is desired, the vertical-pull chin cup can be used (Fig. 9-31). Pearson[113-115] has reported that the use of a vertical-pull chin cup can result in a decrease in the mandibular plane angle and the gonial angle and an increase in posterior facial height in comparison to the growth of untreated individuals. This type of extraoral traction can be used in individuals who have Class III malocclusions and for those patients in whom an increase in the anterior vertical dimension is not desired.

It is difficult to create a true vertical pull in the mandible because of the problems encountered in anchoring the appliance cranially. One of the easiest of the vertically directed chin cups to manipulate clinically is shown in Fig. 9-31,

A. A padded band extends coronally and is secured to the posterior part of the head by a cloth strap. A spring mechanism is activated by pulling the tab inferiorly and attaching the tab to a hook on the hard chin cup.

Another type of chin cup that produces a vertical direction of force is shown in Fig. 9-31, *B*. This appliance incorporates a cloth headcap that curves around the crown of the head and is secured posteriorly with two horizontal straps. A throat strap also secures the appliance to the head of the patient. This particular design is useful in those patients in whom anchorage in the cranial region is difficult to achieve.

Both the occipital-pull and the vertical-pull chin cups create pressure on the temporomandibular (TM) joint region. Although this type of therapy has been used quite successfully for many decades, the increased sensitivity of the orthodontic specialist toward the diagnosis and treatment of temporomandibular joint problems should lead the clinician to monitor chin cup patients (also facial mask patients) on an ongoing basis for signs and symptoms of TM disorders. If any are noted, orthopedic treatment should be discontinued immediately.

One of the substantive concerns regarding chin cup therapy is whether the growth of the mandible can be retarded

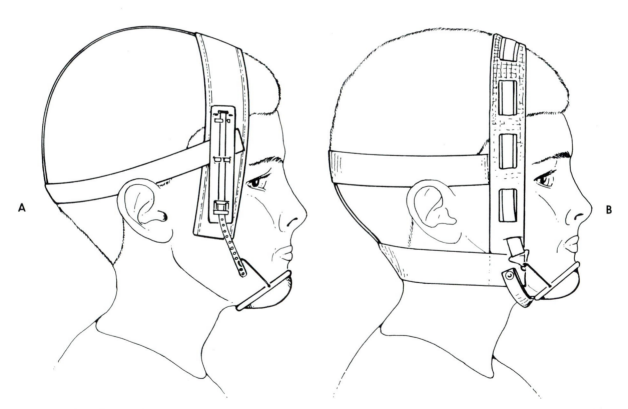

Fig. 9-31 The vertical-pull chin cup. **A,** Unitek design. A spring force design is used to create a vertical direction of pull. **B,** Summit design. A cloth head cap curves not only around the crown of the head but also is secured posteriorly with two horizontal straps. The force is produced by the stretch of the elastic material. In both of these examples a hard chin cup is shown. (From McNamara JA Jr, Brudon WL: *Orthodontic and orthopedic treatment in mixed dentition,* Ann Arbor, Mich, 1993, Needham Press.)

through wearing a chin cup. Sakamoto and co-workers[132] and Wendell and co-workers[154] have noted decreases in mandibular growth during treatment. When a group of Class III patients treated in the mixed dentition were examined, Wendell and associates noted that the mandibular length increases in the treated group were only about two thirds as great as those increases observed in the control group of mixed dentition individuals who received no treatment. However, Mitani and Fukazawa[100] noted no differences in mandibular length in Class III individuals who began treatment during the adolescent growth period in comparison to control values.

Changes in the vertical direction of mandibular growth have been noted. L.W. Graber[48] reported that in a sample of young Class III patients the predominantly horizontal mandibular growth pattern was redirected more vertically, indicating that the orthopedic chin cup can produce an increase in lower anterior facial height.

Additional Comments Regarding Class III Treatment

The Class III malocclusion is relatively easy to identify in a young patient; yet the treatment of this occlusal problem is fraught with many difficulties. Fortunately, the level of patient cooperation in the young patient with mixed dentition generally is excellent, and thus satisfactory compliance usually is achieved.

Of the three treatment modalities considered in this section, the orthopedic facial mask combined with a bonded maxillary splint seems most applicable in the routine Class III patient. This type of appliance produces treatment effects in both skeletal and dentoalveolar aspects of the craniofacial complex. Given a young patient, the resolution of the underlying Class III relationship occurs relatively quickly (4 to 9 months), and then the mask can be worn for a few additional months as a retainer at night before the bonded maxillary splint is removed. The FR-3 appliance of Fränkel can be used either as a primary interceptive appliance or as a retainer. This treatment regimen makes the most biologic sense because the primary focus of this therapy is on the soft tissue, particularly the musculature, that may in part have been the cause of the Class III relationships. The FR-3 appliance is less intrusive to the everyday life of the patient but may take two or three times as much treatment time to achieve correction of the malocclusion. The FR-3 appliance also can be used as a retention appliance following orthopedic facial mask or chin cup therapy.

The chin cup appliance is better suited to those patients for whom increases in lower face height are not desirable and in patients who exhibit true mandibular prognathism. The correction of the malocclusion may be relatively rapid using this treatment approach, depending upon the force level used, but long-term chin cup wear usually is indicated.

Our experience in treating Class III malocclusion in the mixed dentition during the last 20 years has led to some interesting observations. The most important observation is that perhaps 50% of the patients who undergo any type of early Class III intervention will need another phase of early treatment before the final phase of fixed appliance therapy. This may mean that chin cup therapy is resumed or that another phase of rapid palatal expansion, with or without facial mask therapy, may be indicated.

Because mandibular growth exceeds maxillary growth during adolescence, early Class III correction may be lost during the teenage years. The patients and parents should be advised of the possibility of surgical correction at the onset of interceptive treatment. The prudent clinician never makes predictions regarding the treatment of Class III malocclusion because the outcome of any individual Class III patient is difficult to estimate. We agree with T.M. Graber,[53] Sakamoto,[131] and Sugawara and co-workers[141] who advocate the treatment of Class III malocclusion as early as is practical.

CONCLUDING REMARKS REGARDING EARLY TREATMENT

An attempt has been made in this chapter to synthesize a coherent approach to orthodontic and orthopedic treatment in the mixed dentition. Although this topic has been addressed in many of the texts in orthodontics since the beginning of the century, early corrective orthodontic treatment generally has been considered as secondary or peripheral to full banded or bonded appliance therapy in the adolescent or adult patient. We have attempted to provide the reader with a conceptual framework on which the selection of various treatment modalities for the mixed dentition patient can be based.

A few concluding comments should be made on the basis of our own clinical experiences. Some of these comments are obvious, some are not.

1. That the overall treatment time of the patients will be extended from the normal 2 or 3 years treatment time generally needed for the adolescent patient is implicit in initiating mixed dentition treatment. However, initiating treatment in the mixed dentition does not imply that treatment will be provided continuously from the time of eruption of the permanent upper lateral incisors until the time that the permanent second molars are aligned with fixed appliances. We have tried to structure the treatment protocols so that typically a concentrated period of early treatment is initiated, generally in the early mixed dentition. There is a defined beginning of the treatment and a defined ending of the treatment that is known to the patient and the parents before the protocol is started.

2. Intermittent observation of the patient during the transition of the dentition is a prime component of early treatment. We generally prefer to see our patients every 4 to 6 months after the first phase of treatment is completed. The appliances used during this time are simple, usually only a removable palatal plate with

or without a labial wire that is worn full time for at least one year. Monitoring the patient on an intermittent basis allows the clinician to take advantage of the transition of the dentition, particularly in the second deciduous molar regions.

3. Passive holding arches (e.g., transpalatal arch, lingual arch) should be placed before the loss of the second deciduous molars in most early treatment patients. Not only will the leeway space be maintained: on the average of 2.5 mm unilaterally in the mandible and 2.0 mm unilaterally in the maxilla, but also maxillary molar rotation and uprighting can be achieved at the same time. The placement of these arches usually signals the beginning of Phase II treatment: the final stage of fixed appliance therapy.

4. Most patients undergoing early treatment will require a final phase of fixed appliances. Usually the treatment time is reduced to 12 to 18 months, as the majority of patients undergoing comprehensive therapy will be treated as nonextraction patients with Class I or near Class I molar relationships.

5. Initiating early treatment does not imply that all patients treated in the mixed dentition will avoid the extraction of permanent teeth. It has been our experience that even in those patients for whom orthopedic expansion protocols are initiated, the extraction of permanent teeth (usually premolars) is necessary in 5% to 10% of the patients. In some instances, orthopedic expansion of the maxilla is initiated to *broaden the smile* in patients with severe maxillary constriction,[152] and subsequently permanent teeth are extracted as part of the overall treatment protocol.

6. Initiating early treatment, particularly using either extra-oral traction or functional jaw orthopedics, will not eliminate the need for orthognathic surgery in all patients with severe skeletal and neuromuscular imbalances. Functional jaw orthopedics can be used alone or in combination with extraoral traction to minimize substantially the sagittal maxillomandibular imbalance, but it may be impossible to eliminate this imbalance entirely without compromising the facial esthetics of the individual. In these instances, orthognathic surgery in combination with fixed appliances is the treatment of choice. The need for orthognathic surgery also is obvious in patients with a Class III malocclusion characterized by significant skeletal imbalances, especially in those with a family history of significant Class III malocclusion.

7. Patient cooperation generally is excellent in patients treated in the mixed dentition, particularly if the appliance that is selected requires no or minimal patient cooperation other than that usually associated with a routine orthodontic treatment (e.g., good oral hygiene; wearing of retainers). By initiating treatment in the mixed dentition, many of the skeletal and dentoalveolar problems associated with malocclusion often are eliminated or reduced substantially, thereby lessening the need for prolonged fixed appliance therapy in the adolescent years.

In summary we have attempted to provide an overview of various early treatment protocols that may be appropriate for certain orthodontic patients within a given practice. As with all new technologies, each of these protocols should be evaluated with healthy skepticism and should be initiated slowly until the parameters of success and failure are clearly established. It is anticipated that some aspects of the protocols will be modified or additional protocols added as further experience is gained and as more long-term stability studies materialize. The protocols outlined in this chapter have been used routinely by us and have proven to be quite satisfactory if they are approached within a framework of common sense and with a thorough understanding of comprehensive orthodontic biomechanics. Routine fixed appliance therapy is characterized by a series of *midcourse corrections,* and early treatment is no different. Mixed dentition therapy should be undertaken with caution and should be only part of the total armamentarium of the practicing orthodontist.

Finally, it must be stressed that early treatment is not always necessary nor appropriate. In some instances early intervention does not change appreciably the environment of dentofacial development and permanent tooth eruption. In such instances early treatment may serve only to increase treatment time and cost and may result in a lack of patient cooperation in later years. However, if every effort is made to time the treatment appropriately so as to maximize the treatment benefit in the shortest period of time, and if the treatment protocol implemented has a reasonably predictable duration and outcome, early orthodontic intervention can be produced successfully for a wide variety of patients with mixed dentition.

ACKNOWLEDGMENTS

The author would like to thank Mr. William L. Brudon, Associate Professor Emeritus in the School of Art and the Department of Medical and Biological Illustration in the School of Medicine at The University of Michigan for providing the illustrations used in this chapter. Thanks also to Ms. Kelly Branish Spivy for her efforts in the preparation of this manuscript.

REFERENCES

1. Andresen V: The Norwegian system of gnatho-orthopedics, *Acta Gnathol* 1:4-36, 1936.
2. Armstrong CJ: A clinical evaluation of the chin cup, *Aust Dent J* 6:338-346, 1961.
3. Ascher F: Hemmung bei Anwendung moderner Aktivatoren, *Fortschr Kieferorthop* 25:490-501, 1964.
4. Ascher F: *Praktische Kieferorthopadie,* Munich, 1968, Urban & Schwazenberg.
5. Ascher F: Kontrollierte Ergebnisse der Rückbissbehandlung mit funktionskieferorthopädischen Geräten, *Kieferorthop* 32:149-159, 1971.
6. Ascher F: *Der Diagnolawinkel als Richtwert für Diagnose, Prognose*

und Therapie in der Kieferorthopadie. In: *Handlexikon der Zahnäzlichen Praxis*, Stuttgart, Germany, 1973, Medica Verlag.

7. Balters W: Die Technik und Übung der allgemeinen and speziellen Bionator-therapie, *Quintessenz* 1:77, 1964.

8. Balters W: *Die Einfügrund in die Bionator heilmethode*. In: *Äzusgewahite, Schriften und Vortraage*, Heidelberg, 1973, Druckerei Holzer.

9. Baume LJ, Derichsweiller H: Is the condylar growth center responsive to orthodontic therapy? An experimental study in *Macaca mulatta*, Oral Surg 14:347-362, 1961.

10. Begg PR: Light-wire technique: employing the principles of differential force, *Am J Orthod* 47:30-48, 1961.

11. Begg PR: *Begg orthodontic theory and technique*, Philadelphia, 1965, WB Saunders.

12. Berger EV: Personal communication, 1993.

13. Bjerregaard J, Bundgard AM, Melsen B: The effect of the mandibular lip bumper and maxillary bite plate on both movement, occlusion, and space conditions in the lower dental arch, *Eur J Orthod* 84:147-155, 1983.

14. Bimler HP: Indikation der Gebissformer, *Fortschritte der Kieferorthopäd* 25:212, 1964.

15. Bimler HP: *The Bimler appliance*. In Graber TM, Neumann B, editors: *Removable orthodontic appliances*, Philadelphia, 1984, WB Saunders.

16. Blair ES: A cephalometric roentgenographic appraisal of the skeletal morphology of Class I, Class II, division 1 and Class II, division 2 (Angle) malocclusion, *Angle Orthod* 24:106-119, 1954.

17. Brieden CM, Pangrazio-Kulbersh V, Kulbersh R: Maxillary, skeletal, and dental changes with Fränkel appliance therapy—an implant study, *Angle Orthod* 54:232-266, 1984.

18. Brust EW: "Arch dimensional changes concurrent with expansion in the mixed dentition." Unpublished Thesis, Department of Orthodontics and Pediatric Dentistry, The University of Michigan, 1992.

19. Cetlin NM: Personal communication, 1993.

20. Cetlin NM, TenHoeve A: Non-extraction treatment, *J Clin Orthod* 17:396-413, 1983.

21. Charlier JP, Petrovic A, Stutzmann JJ: Effects of mandibular hyperpropulsion on the prechondroblastic zone of young rat condyle, *Am J Orthod* 55:71-74, 1969.

22. Christie TE: Cephalometric patterns of adults with normal occlusions, *Angle Orthod* 47:129-135, 1977.

23. Cooke MS, Wreakes G: The face mask: a new form of reverse headgear, *Br J Orthod* 4:162-168, 1977.

24. Craig CE: The skeletal patterns characteristic of Class I and Class II, division 1 malocclusions, in *normalateralis, Angle Orthod* 21:44-56, 1951.

25. Creekmore TD, Radney LJ: Fränkel appliance therapy: orthopedic or orthodontic? *Am J Orthod* 83:89-108, 1983.

26. Delaire J: Confection du masque orthopedique, *Rev Stomat Paris* 72:579-584, 1971.

27. Delaire J: L'articulation fronto-maxillaire. Bases theroiques et principles generauz d'application de forces extra-orales posteroanterieures sur masque orthopedique, *Rev Stomat Paris* 77:921-930, 1976.

28. Delaire JP, Verson P, et al: Quelques resultats des tractions extraorales a appui fronto-mentonnier dans le traitement orthopedique des malformations maxillomandibulaires de Class III et des sequelles osseuses des fente labio-maxillaires, *Rev Stomat* Paris 73:633-642, 1972.

29. Dewel BF: Serial extractions in orthodontics; indications, objections, and treatment procedures, *Int J Orthod* 40:906-926, 1954.

30. Dewel BF: A critical analysis of serial extraction in orthodontic treatment, *Am J Orthod* 45:424-455, 1959.

31. Dewel BF: Serial extraction, its limitations and contraindications in orthodontic treatment, *Am J Orthod* 53:904-921, 1967.

32. Dietrich UC: Morphological variability of skeletal Class III relationships as revealed by cephalometric analysis, *Trans Eur Orthod Soc* pp. 131-143, 1970.

33. Doris JM, Bernard DW, Kuftinec M: A biometric study of tooth size and dental crowding, *Am J Orthod* 79:326-336, 1981.

34. Drelich RC: A cephalometric study of untreated Class II, division 1 malocclusion, *Angle Orthod* 21:44-56, 1948.

35. Ellis E, McNamara JA Jr: Components of adult Class II malocclusions, *Am J Oral Maxillofac Surg* 42:295-305, 1984.

36. Fränkel R: The theoretical concept underlying the treatment with functional correctors, *Trans Eur Orthod Soc* pp 244-254, 1966.

37. Fränkel R: The practical meaning of the functional matrix in orthodontics, *Trans Eur Orthod Soc* 45:207-219, 1969.

38. Fränkel R: The treatment of Class II, division 1 malocclusion with functional correctors, *Am J Orthod* 55:265-275, 1969.

39. Fränkel R: Maxillary retrusion in Class III and treatment with the functional corrector III, *Trans Eur Orthod Soc* pp 249-259, 1970.

40. Fränkel R: Guidance of eruption without extraction, *Trans Eur Orthod Soc* pp 303-315, 1971.

41. Fränkel R: Decrowding during eruption under the screening influence of vestibular shields, *Am J Orthod* 65:372-406, 1974.

42. Fränkel R: *Technik und Handhabung der Funktionsregler*, Berlin, 1976, VEB Verlag Volk und Gesundheit.

43. Fränkel R: Lip seal training in the treatment of skeletal open bite, *Eur J Orthod* 2:219-228, 1980.

44. Fränkel R: *Biomechanical aspects of the form/function relationship in craniofacial morphogenesis: a clinician's approach*. In McNamara Jr JA, Ribbens KA, Howe RP, editors: *Clinical alterations of the growing face, Monograph 14, Craniofacial Growth Series*, Ann Arbor, 1983, Center for Human Growth and Development, The University of Michigan.

45. Fränkel R, Fränkel C: *Orofacial orthopedics with the functional regulator*, Munich, 1989, S. Karger.

46. Gianelly AA: Personal communication, 1992.

47. Gianelly AA, Arena SH, Bernstein L: A comparison of Class II treatment changes noted with the light wire, edgewise, and Fränkel appliances, *Am J Orthod* 89:269-276, 1984.

48. Graber LW: Chin cup therapy for mandibular prognathism, *Am J Orthod* 72:23-41, 1977.

49. Graber LW: "Psycho-social implications of dentofacial appearance." Doctoral Dissertation, The University of Michigan, Ann Arbor, 1980.

50. Graber TM: Extra-oral force—facts and fallacies, *Am J Orthod* 41:490-505, 1955.

51. Graber TM: *Orthodontics: principles and practices*, Philadelphia, 1966, WB Saunders.

52. Graber TM: Personal communication, 1975.

53. Graber TM: *Extrinsic control factors influencing craniofacial growth*. In McNamara JA Jr, editor: *Determinants of mandibular form and growth, Monograph 4, Craniofacial Growth Series*, Ann Arbor, 1976, Center for Human Growth and Development, The University of Michigan.

54. Graber TM, Chung DD, Aoba JT: Dentofacial orthopedics versus orthodontics, *J Am Dent Assoc* 75:1145-1166, 1967.

55. Guyer EC, Ellis E et al: Components of Class III malocclusion in juveniles and adolescents, *Angle Orthod* 56:7-31, 1986.

56. Haas AJ: Rapid expansion of the maxillary dental arch and nasal cavity by opening the midpalatal suture, *Angle Orthod* 31:73-90, 1961.

57. Haas AJ: Treatment of maxillary deficiency by opening the midpalatal suture, *Angle Orthod* 65:200-217, 1965.

58. Haas AJ: Palatal expansion: just the beginning of dento-facial orthopedics, *Am J Orthod* 57:219-255, 1970.

59. Haas AJ: Long-term post-treatment evaluation of rapid palatal expansion, *Angle Orthod* 50:189-217, 1980.

60. Haas AJ: Personal communication, 1993.

61. Herberger TA, Reed PW, McNamara JA Jr: Long-term stability of rapid maxillary expansion in adolescent patients, In preparation, 1993.

62. Herbst E: *Atlas und Grundirss der Zahnärztlichen Orthopädie*, Munich, 1910, JF Lehmann Verlag.

63. Hotz R: Active supervision of the eruption of teeth by extraction, *Trans Europ Orthod Soc* pp. 134-160, 1948.

64. Hotz R: *Orthodontics in daily practice: possibilities and limitations in the area of children's dentistry,* Bern, Switzerland, 1974, Hans Huber.

65. Howe RP, McNamara JA Jr: Clinical management of the Herbst appliance, *J Clin Orthod* 17:456-463, 1983.

66. Howe RP, McNamara JA Jr, O'Connor KA: An examination of dental crowding and its relationship to tooth size and arch dimension, *Am J Orthod* 83:363-373, 1983.

67. Irie M, Nakamura S: Orthopedic approach to severe skeletal Class III malocclusion, *Am J Orthod* 67:377-392, 1975.

68. Jackson VH: *Orthodontia and orthopaedia,* 1904, JB Lippincott.

69. Jacobson A, Evans WG et al: Mandibular prognathism, *Am J Orthod* 66:140-171, 1974.

70. Janson I: *Bionator-Modifikationen in der Kieferorthopädischen Therapie,* Munich, 1987, Carl Henser Verlag.

71. Kerr WJS, TenHave TR, McNamara JA Jr: A comparison of skeletal and dental changes produced by functional regulators (FR-2 and FR-3), *Eur J Orthod* 11:235-242, 1989.

72. Kjellgren B: Serial extraction as a corrective procedure in dental orthopedic therapy, *Acta Odont Scand* 8:17-43, 1948.

73. Kloehn SJ: A new approach to the analysis and treatment of mixed dentition, *Am J Orthod* 31:161-186, 1953.

74. Leighton BC: The early signs of malocclusion, *Trans Eur Orthod Soc* pp. 353-368, 1969.

75. Lloyd ZB: Serial extraction, *Am J Orthod* 39:262-267, 1953.

76. Loh MK, Kerr WJ: The function regulator III: effects and indications for use, *Br J Orthod* 12:154-157, 1985.

77. Lundström A: The aetiology of crowding of the teeth (based on studies of twins and on morphological investigations) and orthodontic treatment (expansion or extraction), *Trans Eur Orthod Soc* pp. 176-189, 1951.

78. Matsui Y: Effect of chin cup on the growing mandible, *J Jap Ortho Soc* 24:165-181, 1965.

79. McDougall PD, McNamara JA Jr, Dierkes JM: Arch width development in Class II patients treated with the Fränkel appliance, *Am J Orthod* 82:10-22, 1982.

80. McKeown J: The diagnosis of incipient arch crowding in children, *N Z Dent J* 77:94-96, 1981.

81. McNamara JA Jr: *Neuromuscular and skeletal adaptations to altered orofacial function, Monograph 1, Craniofacial Growth Series,* Ann Arbor, 1972, Center for Human Growth and Development, The University of Michigan.

82. McNamara JA Jr: Neuromuscular and skeletal adaptations to altered function in the orofacial region, *Am J Orthod* 64:578-606, 1973.

83. McNamara JA Jr: Functional determinants of craniofacial size and shape, *Eur J Orthod* 2:131-159, 1980.

84. McNamara JA Jr: Components of Class II malocclusion in children 8-10 years of age, *Angle Orthod* 51:177-202, 1981.

85. McNamara JA Jr: An orthopedic approach to the treatment of Class III malocclusion in growing children, *J Clin Orthod* 21:598-608, 1987.

86. McNamara JA: The fabrication of the acrylic splint Herbst appliance, *Am J Orthod Dentofac Orthoped* 94:10-18, 1988.

87. McNamara JA Jr, Bookstein FL, Shaughnessy TG: Skeletal and dental adaptations following functional regulator therapy, *Am J Orthod* 88:91-110, 1985.

88. McNamara JA, Brudon WL: *Orthodontic and orthopedic treatment in the mixed dentition,* Ann Arbor, Mich, 1993, Needham Press.

89. McNamara JA Jr, Bryan FA: Long-term mandibular adaptations to protrusive function in the rhesus monkey *(Macaca mulatta), Am J Orthod Dentofac Orthop* 92:98-108, 1987.

90. McNamara JA Jr, Carlson DS: Quantitative analysis of temporomandibular joint adaptations to protrusive function, *Am J Orthod* 76:593-611, 1979.

91. McNamara JA Jr, Howe RP: The clinical management of the acrylic splint Herbst appliance, *Am J Orthod Dentofac Orthop* 94:142-149, 1988.

92. McNamara JA Jr, Howe RP, Dischinger TG: A comparison of Herbst and Fränkel treatment in Class II malocclusion, *Am J Orthod Dentofac Orthoped* 98:134-144, 1990.

93. McNamara JA Jr, Huge SA: The functional regulator (FR-3) of Fränkel, *Am J Orthod* 88:409-424, 1985.

94. Melsen B: A histological study of the influence of sutural morphology and skeletal maturation of rapid palatal expansion in children, *Trans Eur Orthod Soc* pp. 499-507, 1972.

95. Melsen B: Palatal growth studied on human autopsy material, *Am J Orthod* 68:42-45, 1975.

96. Melsen B, Melsen F: The post-natal development of the palatomaxillary region: studies on human autopsy material, *Am J Orthod* 82:329-342, 1982.

97. Merrifield LL, Cross JJ: Directional forces, *Am J Orthod* 57:435-464, 1970.

98. Mills LF: Arch width, arch length, and tooth size in young adult males, *Angle Orthod* 34:124-129, 1964.

99. Mills LF: Epidemiologic studies of occlusion IV: the prevalence of malocclusion in a population of 1,455 school children, *J Dent Res* 45:332-336, 1966.

100. Mitani H, Fukazawa H: Effects of chincap force on the timing and amount of mandibular growth associated with anterior reverse occlusion (Class III malocclusion) during puberty, *Am J Orthod Dentofac Orthop* 90:454-463, 1986.

101. Moorrees CFA, Reed RB: Biometrics of crowding and spacing of the teeth in the mandible, *Am J Phys Anthrop* 12:77-88, 1954.

102. Moyers RE: *Handbook of orthodontics,* ed 4, Chicago, 1988, Yearbook Medical.

103. Moyers RE, Riolo ML et al: Differential diagnosis of Class II malocclusions: Part I. Facial types associated with Class II malocclusions, *Am J Orthod* 78:477-494, 1980.

104. Moyers RE, van der Linden FPGM et al: *Standards of Human Occlusal Development: Monograph 5, Craniofacial Growth Series,* Ann Arbor, 1976, Center for Human Growth and Development, The University of Michigan.

105. Navarro CF, Arcovia CJ: Early management of maxillary dentofacial deficiency: three case reports, *Compend Contin Educ Dent* 12:708-716, 1991.

106. Nevant CT: "The effects of lip-bumper therapy on deficient mandibular arch length." Unpublished Thesis, Department of Orthodontics, Baylor University, Dallas, Texas, 1989.

107. Palsson F: Foregangare til den S.K. Serieextraktionen, *Orthod Rev* 7:118-135, 1956.

108. Pancherz H: Treatment of Class II malocclusion by jumping the bite with the Herbst appliance: a cephalometric investigation, *Am J Orthod* 76:432-442, 1979.

109. Pancherz H: The effect of continuous bite-jumping on the dentofacial complex: a follow-up study after Herbst appliance treatment of Class II malocclusion, *Eur J Orthod* 3:49-60, 1981.

110. Pancherz H: The mechanism of Class II correction and Herbst appliance treatment: a cephalometric investigation, *Am J Orthod* 83:104-113, 1982.

111. Pancherz H: The Herbst appliance—its biologic effects and clinical use, *Am J Orthod* 87:1-20, 1985.

112. Pancherz H: Dentofacial orthopedics in relation to somatic maturation, an analysis of 70 consecutive cases treated with the Herbst appliance, *Am J Orthod* 88:273-287, 1988.

113. Pearson LE: Vertical control in treatment of patients having rotational growth tendencies, *Angle Orthod* 48:132-140, 1978.

114. Pearson LE: Vertical control in fully-banded orthodontic treatment, *Angle Orthod* 56:205-224, 1986.

115. Pearson LE: Treatment of a severe openbite excessive vertical pattern with an eclectic nonsurgical approach, *Angle Orthod* 61:71-76, 1991.

116. Peck H, Peck S: An index for assessing tooth shape deviations as applied to the mandibular incisors, *Am J Orthod* 61:384-401, 1972.

117. Petit HP: Syndromes prognathiques: schemas de traitement "global" autour de masques faciaux, *Rev Orthop Dento Faciale* 16:381-411, 1982.

118. Petit HP: *Adaptation following accelerated facial mask therapy.* In McNamara Jr JA, Ribbens KA, Howe RP, editors: *Clinical alterations of the growing face, Monograph 14, Craniofacial Growth Series,* Ann Arbor, 1983, Center for Human Growth and Development, The University of Michigan.

119. Petit, HP: Normalisation morphogenetique, apport de l'orthopadie, *Orthod Fr* 62:549-557, 1991.

120. Petrovic A, Oudet C, Gasson N: Effets des appareils de propulsion et de retropulsion mandibulaire sur le nombre des sarcomeres en serie du muscle pterygoidien externe et sur la croissance du cartilage condylien du jeune rat, *Orthod Fr* 44:191-212, 1973.

121. Petrovic A, Stutzmann JJ, Gasson N: *The final length of the mandible: Is it genetically determined?* In Carlson DS, editor: *Craniofacial biology, Monograph 10,* Ann Arbor, 1981, Center for Human Growth and Development, The University of Michigan.

122. Petrovic A, Stutzmann JJ, Oudet C: *Control process in the postnatal growth of the condylar cartilage.* In McNamara JA Jr, editor: *Determinants of mandibular form and growth, Monograph 4,* Ann Arbor, 1975, Center for Human Growth and Development, The University of Michigan.

123. Potpeschenigg R: Deutsche Viertel Jahrschrift für Zahnheilkunde, 1885, Cited in *Monthly Rev Dent Surg III* pp. 464-465, 1974-1975.

124. Poulton D: The influence of extraoral traction, *Am J Orthod* 53:1-18, 1967.

125. Proffit WR: *Contemporary orthodontics,* St Louis, 1986, Mosby.

126. Radnzic D: Dental crowding and its relationship to mesiodistal crown diameters and arch dimensions, *Am J Orthod Dentofac Orthop* 94:50-56, 1988.

127. Righellis EG: Treatment effects of Fränkel activator and extraoral traction appliances, *Angle Orthod* 53:89-109, 1983.

128. Ringenberg QM: Serial extraction: stop, look, and be certain, *Am J Orthod* 50:327-336, 1964.

129. Roberts CA, Subtelny JD: Use of the face mask in the treatment of maxillary skeletal retrusion, *Am J Orthod Dentofac Orthop* 93:388-394, 1988.

130. Roux W: *Entwicklungsmechanik der Organismen, Bd. I und II,* Leipzig, Germany, 1895, W. Engelmann Verlag W.

131. Sakamoto T: Effective timing for the application of orthopedic force in the skeletal Class III malocclusion, *Am J Orthod* 80:411-416, 1981.

132. Sakamoto T, Iwase I et al: A roentgenocephalometric study of skeletal changes during and after chin cup treatment, *Am J Orthod* 85:341-350, 1984.

133. Sanborn RT: Differences between the facial skeletal patterns of Class III malocclusion and normal occlusion, *Angle Orthod* 25:208-222, 1955.

134. Schudy FF: Vertical growth vs. anteroposterior growth as related to function and treatment, *Angle Orthod* 34:75-93, 1964.

135. Sheridan JJ: Air-rotor stripping, *J Clin Orthod* 19:443-459, 1985.

136. Sheridan JJ: Air-rotor stripping, *J Clin Orthod* 21:781-788, 1987.

137. Spillane LM: "Arch dimensional changes in patients treated with maxillary expansion during the mixed dentition." Unpublished thesis, Department of Orthodontics and Pediatric Dentistry, University of Michigan, Ann Arbor, 1990.

138. Spillane LM, McNamara JA Jr: Arch width development relative to initial transpalatal width, *J Dent Res* IADR Abstracts, p. 374, 1989.

139. Starnbach H, Bayne D et al: Facioskeletal and dental changes resulting from rapid maxillary expansion, *Angle Orthod* 36:152-164, 1966.

140. Stöckli PW, Willert HG: Tissue reactions in the temporomandibular joint resulting from anterior displacement of the mandible in the monkey, *Am J Orthod* 60:142-155, 1971.

141. Sugawara J, Asanbo T et al: Long-term effects of chin cup therapy on skeletal profile in mandibular prognathism, *Am J Orthod Dentofac Orthop* 98:127-133, 1990.

142. Sutcliffe HW: Correction of a case of prognathism by the retraction of the mandible and the lower teeth, *Trans 6th Inter Cong,* London, 1914.

143. Suzuki N: Cephalometric observation on the effect of the chin cap, *J Jap Ortho Soc* 31:64-74, 1972.

144. Terwilliger GF: Treatment in the mixed dentition, *Angle Orthod* 20:109-113, 1950.

145. Thilander B: Treatment of Angle Class III malocclusion with chin cap, *Trans Eur Orthod Soc* pp. 384-398, 1963.

146. Thilander B: Chin-cap treatment for Angle Class III malocclusion: a longitudinal study, *Trans Eur Orthod Soc* pp. 311-327, 1965.

147. Timms DJ: An occlusal analysis of lateral maxillary expansion with midpalatal sutural opening, *Trans Eur Orthod Soc* pp. 73-79, 1968.

148. Timms DJ: Longterm follow-up of cases treated by rapid maxillary expansion, *Trans Eur Orthod Soc* pp. 211-215, 1976.

149. Turley PK: Orthopedic correction of Class III malocclusion with palatal expansion and custom protraction headgear, *J Clin Orthod* 22:314-325, 1988.

150. Tweed CH: A philosophy of orthodontic treatment, *Am J Orthod* 31:74-103, 1945.

151. Tweed CH: *Clinical orthodontics,* St Louis, 1966, Mosby.

152. Vanarsdall RL Jr: Personal communication, 1993.

153. Watson W: A computerized appraisal of high-pull headgear, *Am J Orthod* 62:561-579, 1972.

154. Wendell PD, Nanda R et al: The effects of chin cup therapy on the mandible: a longitudinal study, *Am J Orthod* 87:265-272, 1985.

155. Wertz RA: Skeletal and dental changes accompanying rapid midpalatal suture opening, *Am J Orthod* 59:411-466, 1970.

156. Wieslander L: Early or late cervical traction therapy in the mixed dentition, *Am J Orthod* 67:432-439, 1975.

157. Wieslander L: Personal communication, 1993.

158. Wylie WL: The assessment of anteroposterior dysplasia, *Angle Orthod* 17:97-109, 1947.

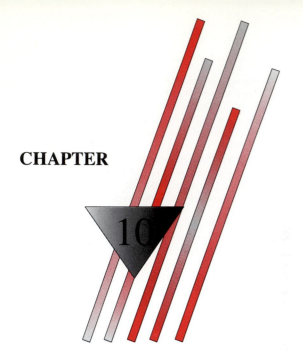

CHAPTER 10

Bonding in Orthodontics

BJÖRN U. ZACHRISSON

The introduction of the acid etch bonding technique has led to dramatic changes in the practice of orthodontics. The increased adhesion produced by acid pretreatment, using 85% phosphoric acid, was demonstrated in 1955 by Buonocore.[35] In 1965, with the advent of epoxy resin bonding, Newman[122] began to apply these findings to direct bonding of orthodontic attachments. Retief (cited in Reynolds[145]) also described an epoxy resin system designed to withstand orthodontic forces. In 1968 Smith introduced zinc polyacrylate (carboxylate) cement, and bracket bonding with this cement was reported.[118]

Around 1970 several articles appeared on bonding attachments with different adhesives.[145] Miura et al.[115] described an acrylic resin (Orthomite), using a modified trialkyl borane catalyst, that proved to be particularly successful for bonding plastic brackets and for enhanced adhesion in the presence of moisture. Also diacrylate resins, as both sealants and adhesives,[145] were introduced in orthodontics. The most widely used resin, commonly referred to as *Bowen's resin* or bisGMA (bisphenol A glycidyl dimethacrylate), was designed to improve bond strength and increase dimensional stability by cross-linking.

Thus in the early 1970s, a considerable number of preliminary reports were published on different commercially available direct or indirect bonding systems.[158] It was not until 1977, however, that the first detailed posttreatment evaluation of direct bonding, over a full period of orthodontic treatment, in a large sample of patients was published.[196] The clinical implication of this study, that acid etching and bonding had come to stay in orthodontics, has indeed been verified by clinicians worldwide. Today it is an exception to find an orthodontist who does not directly or indirectly bond some type of attachment to the teeth.[74]

The future of bonding is promising. Product development

in terms of adhesives, brackets, devices, and technical details is continually occurring at a rapid rate. It is, in fact, difficult for the practicing orthodontist to stay properly oriented. Also new avenues for bonding in orthodontics are opening up, and those approaches include lingual bonding, various types of bonded retainers and splints, semipermanent single-tooth replacements, resin buildups addressing tooth shape and size problems, and bonded space maintainers.

The purpose of this chapter is to attempt to update the current available information. Rapid developments in the field are likely to produce significant changes in several of the ideas, clinical suggestions, and even principles presented. Therefore the main emphasis in this chapter will be on *clinical* aspects. Attempts will be made to analyze important factors and offer advice (based on my own clinical and research experience and on the results published by others) that will help make the bonding of attachments and retainers efficient and trouble free.

To help organize the contents, the chapter is divided into four parts:

Bracket bonding
Debonding
Bonded retainers
Other applications of bonding

BRACKET BONDING

The simplicity of bonding can be misleading. The technique can undoubtedly be misused, not only by an inexperienced clinician but also by more experienced orthodontists who do not perform procedures with care. Success in bonding requires understanding of and adherence to accepted orthodontic and preventive dentistry principles.

542

Optimal performance in bonding of orthodontic attachments offers many advantages when compared to conventional banding:

1. It is esthetically superior (Fig. 10-1).
2. It is faster and simpler.
3. There is less discomfort for the patient (no band seating and separation) (Fig. 10-2).
4. Arch length is not increased by band material.
5. It allows more precise bracket placement (aberrant tooth shape does not result in difficult banding and poor attachment position).
6. Bonds are more hygienic than bands,[5,28] thus an improved gingival and periodontal condition is possible (Fig. 10-17) and there is better access for cleaning.
7. Partially erupted (or fractured) teeth can be controlled.
8. Mesiodistal enamel reduction is possible *during treatment*.
9. Interproximal areas are accessible for composite buildups.
10. Caries risk under loose bands is eliminated. Interproximal caries can be detected and treated. Dental invaginations on incisors can be controlled (Fig. 10-3).
11. There are no band spaces to close at the end of treatment.
12. No large inventory of bands is needed.
13. Brackets may be recycled, further reducing the cost.
14. Lingual brackets, *invisible braces,* can be used when the patient rejects visible orthodontic appliances (Fig. 10-1).
15. Attachments may be bonded to fixed bridgework, particularly when the facial surfaces of the abutment teeth are not in metal.

Probably the most important of these advantages are the *improved appearance*, the *hygiene*, the *decreased discomfort* of the patient, and the *ease of application* for the clinician.

However, several disadvantages of bonding are obvious or have emerged through its use:

1. A bonded bracket has a weaker attachment than a cemented band. Thus there is more chance that a bracket will come off rather than that a band will become loosened.
2. Some bonding adhesives are not sufficiently strong.
3. Better access for cleaning does not necessarily guarantee better oral hygiene and improved gingival condition, especially if excess adhesive extends beyond the bracket base (Figs. 10-15 and 10-18).
4. The protection against interproximal caries of well-contoured cemented bands[210] is absent.
5. Bonding is more complicated when lingual auxiliaries are required or where headgears are attached.
6. Rebonding a loose bracket requires more preparation than rebanding a loose band.
7. Debonding is more time-consuming than debanding, since removal of adhesive is more difficult than removal of cement.

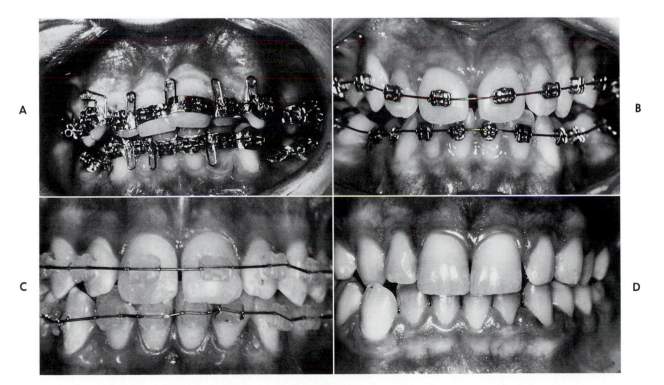

Fig. 10-1   Esthetic comparison between banded and bonded appliances. **A,** Full-banded dentition with multiloop archwires. **B,** Full-bonded appliance. **C,** Ceramic brackets. **D,** Lingual bonding.

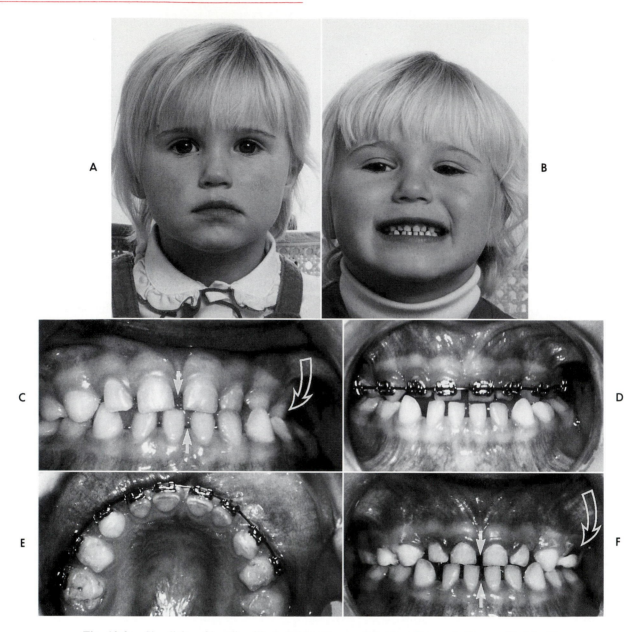

Fig. 10-2   Simplicity of bonding illustrated by the use of fixed appliances in 3-year-old girl with unilateral crossbite (*arrow* in **C**). **A** and **C,** Before treatment. **D** and **E,** During treatment. **B** and **F,** After treatment for 9 months. The left deciduous second molar is now erupting in good position. Note spontaneous midline correction.

The advantages and disadvantages of bonding versus banding must be weighed according to each practitioner's preferences, skill, and experience. It is obvious that neither bands nor bonded attachments completely fulfill all needs. *Bonding should be considered as only part of a modern preventive package* which also includes a strict oral hygiene, program,[4,193] fluoride supplementation,[37,150,194] and the use of simple yet effective appliances (Fig. 10-1, *B*). In other words, complicated mechanics with abundant use of coil springs, multilooped arches, etc. (Fig. 10-1, *A*), lends itself

less well to bonding and can easily compromise the integrity of tooth enamel and gingival tissues around brackets on small bonding bases.

Since bonding is still a fairly new procedure, it is not surprising that some clinicians have experienced problems.[188] The most commonly cited problems in this regard are the loosening of brackets, inaccurate bracket placement, decalcifications during treatment, and the time-consuming aspect of debonding. One of the main objectives of this chapter is *to demonstrate that such problems are unnec-*

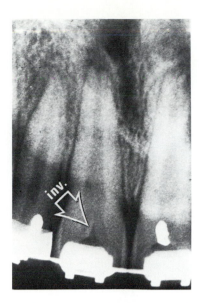

Fig. 10-3 An advantage of bonding is that invaginations *(arrow)* on incisors can be safely controlled. By contrast, with bands there is the risk that a loosened band may lead to caries and pulpal involvement.

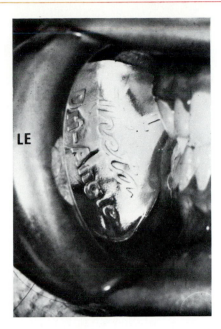

Fig. 10-4 Large Dri-Angle for restriction of saliva from the parotid duct. *LE,* Lip expander.

essary, and in most cases poor experiences in bonding are based on inadequate information.

Bonding procedure

The steps involved in direct and indirect bracket bonding on facial or lingual surfaces are as follows:

Cleaning
Enamel conditioning
Sealing
Bonding

Cleaning

Thorough cleaning of the teeth with a water slurry of pumice, or prophylaxis paste, is essential to remove plaque and the organic pellicle that normally covers all teeth.[1] *The teeth must be clean.* This requires rotary instruments, either a rubber cup or a polishing brush. A bristle brush cleans more effectively,[139,177] but care must be exercised to avoid traumatizing the gingival margin and initiating bleeding. Hence a *small* bristle brush is recommended. For increased patient comfort the cleaning should be done *before* placement of moisture-control devices like cheek and lip retractors, saliva ejectors, and cotton rolls.

The patient may rinse shortly afterward (this will be the last opportunity to rinse until completion of the bonding procedure), or the pumice and water residue can be eliminated with the vacuum evacuator.

Enamel Conditioning

Moisture control. After the rinse, salivary control and maintenance of a completely dry working field is absolutely essential. There are many devices on the market to accomplish this:

Lip expanders and/or cheek retractors
Saliva ejectors
Tongue guards with bite blocks
Salivary duct obstructors (Fig. 10-4)
Gadgets that combine several of these (Fig. 10-5)
Cotton or gauze rolls
Antisialogogues

These products are continually being improved, and the clinician must decide which ones work best. For simultaneous premolar-to-premolar bonding in both arches a technique using lip expanders, Dri-Angles to restrict the flow of saliva from the parotid duct, and a combined saliva ejector-tongue holder to remove moisture from the mouth (Fig. 10-5) works well. Dentists with limited experience may obtain better results by bonding one dental arch at a time. When bonding mandibular second and first molars, at any stage in treatment, the use of single or double hygroformic saliva ejectors is recommended (Fig. 10-6). For bonding on the lingual surfaces excellent saliva evacuator-bite blocks have been developed (Fig. 10-54).

With regard to antisialogogues, both tablets[40] and injectable solutions[30,191] of different preparations (Banthine, Pro-Banthine, atropine sulfate, etc.) are available. However, the excellent and rapid saliva flow restriction obtainable with Pro-Banthine injections[191] is no longer advised; the Council on Dental Therapeutics of the American Dental Association has recommended that this drug not be injected in patients who can take the oral form.

Present experience indicates that antisialogogues are gen-

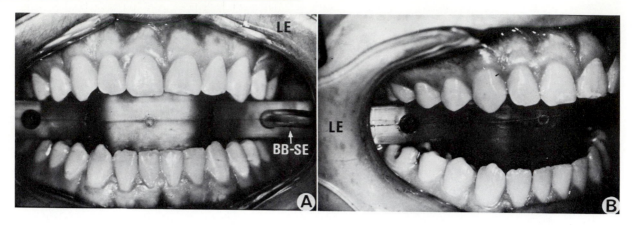

Fig. 10-5 Combined saliva ejector, tongue holder, and bite block *(BB-SE)* for moisture control during bracket bonding. *LE,* Lip expander.

erally not needed for most patients. When indicated, Banthine tablets (50 mg per 100 lb [45 kg] body weight) in a sugar-free drink, 15 minutes before bonding, may provide adequate results.[40]

Enamel pretreatment. After the operative field has been isolated, the teeth to be bonded are dried. The conditioning solution or gel (usually 37% phosphoric acid) is then lightly applied over the enamel surface with a foam pellet or brush for 15 to 60 seconds (see below). When etching solutions are used, the surface must be kept moist by repeated applications. To avoid damaging delicate enamel rods, care should be taken not to rub the liquid onto the teeth.

At the end of the etching period the etchant is rinsed off the teeth with abundant water spray. A high-speed evacuator (Fig. 10-7) is strongly recommended for increased efficiency in collecting the etchant-water rinse and to reduce moisture contamination on teeth and Dri-Angles. *Salivary contamination of the etched surface must not be allowed.* (If it occurs, rinse with the water spray or re-etch for a few seconds; the patient must not rinse.)

Next, the teeth are thoroughly dried with a moisture-and-oil-free air source to obtain the well-known dull, frosty appearance (Fig. 10-8). Teeth that do not appear dull and frosty white should be re-etched. Cervical enamel, because of its different morphology, usually looks somewhat different from the center and incisal portions of a sufficiently etched tooth[9] (Figs. 10-8 and 10-33). It should not be re-etched in attempts to produce a uniform appearance over the entire enamel surface.

This procedure probably reflects the general use of acid etching in orthodontics. There remain, however, both considerable discussion of and continuous debate over several aspects of enamel pretreatment:

1. Should the etch cover the entire facial enamel or only a small portion outside the bracket pad?
2. What is the optimal etching time? Is it different for young and old teeth?
3. Are gels preferable to solutions?

4. Is prolonged etching necessary when teeth are pretreated with fluoride?
5. Will incorporation of fluorides in the etching solution increase the resistance of enamel to caries attack?
6. Is etching permissible on teeth with internal white spots? Or is it more likely that the etchant will *open up* underlying demineralized areas?
7. How much enamel is removed by etching and how deep are the histologic alterations? Are they reversible? Is etching harmful?
8. Should other means than acid etching (e.g., crystal growth) be preferred?

Although these questions are of considerable theoretical interest, most debate concerning acid etching appears to be of somewhat limited clinical significance, at least as it has a bearing on bond strength. In other words, good bond strength apparently is much more dependent on (1) avoiding moisture contamination, (2) achieving undisturbed setting of the bonding adhesive, and (3) the use of a strong adhesive than upon variations in the etching procedures.

Some short answers to the foregoing questions are as follows:

1. Although it may seem logical to etch an area only slightly larger than the pad, clinical experience over more than 20 years indicates that etching the entire facial enamel with solution is harmless—at least when a fluoride mouthrinse is used regularly.
2. Recent studies[31,32,123,185] and my clinical experience indicate that 15 seconds is probably adequate for etching young permanent teeth. However, up to 60 seconds may be recommended for adult teeth. Longer periods provide no more, but actually less, retention because of the loss of surface structure.[52,160]
3. There is no apparent difference in the degree of surface irregularity after etching with an acid solution when compared with etching with an acid gel.[31] The gel provides better control for restricting the etched area but requires more thorough rinsing afterward.

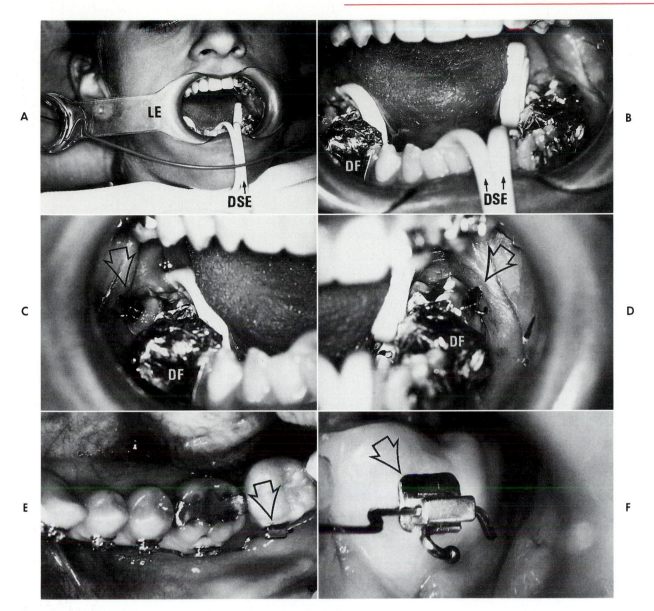

Fig. 10-6   In bonding second molars, the hygroformic saliva evacuator *(DSE)* is helpful to prevent moisture contamination. **A** and **B,** Overview of appliances. **C** and **D,** Working field at simultaneous bonding of both second molars. **E** and **F,** Optimal shape and base contour for my preferred (GAC no. 19-371-90 and 19-471-90) molar attachment *(open arrow)*. The rectangular buccal tube is off-set gingivally on a 3 × 4 mm base, and it has 0° torque and 15° distal off set. It has proven most useful for the bending of maxillary and mandibular first or second molars (or deciduous molars) in a number of different clinical situations.

4. Clinical and laboratory experience[31,32] indicates that extra etching time is not necessary when teeth have been pretreated with fluoride. When in doubt, check that the enamel looks uniformly dull and frosty white after the etch. If it does, surface retention is adequate for bonding.

5. Fluoridated phosphoric acid solutions and gels provide an overall morphologic etching effect similar to non-fluoridated ones, and give adequate bond strength in direct bonding procedures.[70] Further studies are needed to determine their clinical effectiveness and caries protection around bracket bases.

6. Caution should be exercised when etching over acquired and developmental demineralizations. It is best to avoid it. If this is impossible, a short etching time, the application of sealant, and the use of direct bonding with extra attention to not having areas of adhesive deficiency are important. The presence of voids,

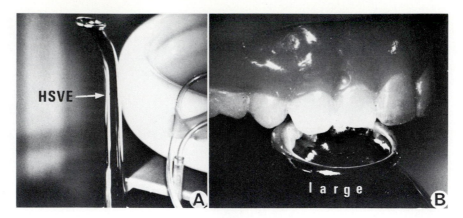

Fig. 10-7 A high-speed saliva evacuator *(HSVE)* with large opening is important for optimal collection of the etchant-water rinse.

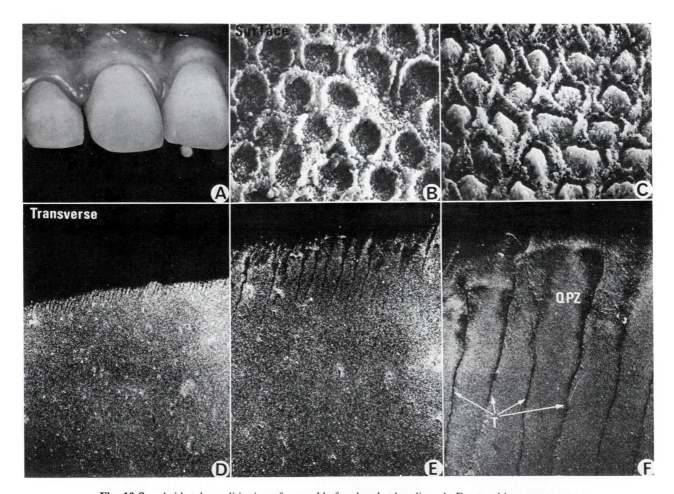

Fig. 10-8 Acid etch conditioning of enamel before bracket bonding. **A,** Frosty white appearance. **B** and **C,** Scanning electron micrograph of an enamel surface that has been etched with 37% phosphoric acid. (In **B** the prism centers have been removed preferentially whereas in **C** the loss of prism peripheries demonstrates the head-and-tail arrangement of the prisms.) **D** to **F,** Transverse section of an etched porous enamel surface showing two distinct zones, the qualitative porous zone *(QPZ)* and the quantitative porous zone. In the latter an even row of resin tags *(T)* may penetrate.

together with poor hygiene, can lead to metal corrosion[108] and indelible staining of underlying developmental white spots.[25]

7. A routine etching removes from 3 to 10 μm of surface enamel.[42,139,160,177] Another 25 μm reveals subtle histologic alterations,[36,78,159] creating the necessary mechanical interlocks (Figs. 10-8 and 10-9). Deeper localized dissolutions (Fig. 10-8) will generally cause penetration to a depth of about 100 μm or more.[36,52,160]

Although laboratory studies indicate that the enamel alterations are largely (though not completely) reversible,[162,173] it can be stated that the overall effect of applying etchant to healthy enamel is not detrimental. This is augmented by the fact that normal enamel is from 1000 to 2000 μm thick[52,207] (except as it tapers toward the cervical margin), abrasive wear of facial enamel is normal and proceeds at a rate of up to 2 μm per year,[110] and facial surfaces are self-cleaning and not prone to caries.[110] On the other hand, caution should be exercised when etching damaged teeth with exposed dentin, deep enamel cracks, external or internal demineralization.[42]

8. Crystal growth after use of polyacrylic acid with residual sulfate is reported[106] to provide retention areas in enamel similar to those after phosphoric acid etching (Fig. 10-46) with less risk of enamel damage at debonding.

This could potentially be advantegous when using ceramic brackets, but further clinical testing with this new technique is necessary.[12]

Sealing

After the teeth are completely dry and appear frosty white, a thin layer of sealant may be painted over the entire etched enamel surface. Sealant is best applied with a small foam pellet or brush with a single gingivoincisal stroke on each tooth. The sealant coating should be thin and even, for excess sealant may induce bracket drift and unnatural enamel topography when polymerized. Bracket placement should be started immediately after all etched surfaces are coated with sealant. The sealant surface layer will not polymerize. (In fact, the entire sealant layer may not cure when conventional autopolymerizing sealants are used.) It should not be removed, however, since it will cure with the adhesive in the next step.

Much confusion and uncertainty surround the use of sealants in orthodontic bonding. Research has been devoted to determining the exact function of the intermediate resin in the acid etch procedure. The findings are divergent. Some investigators conclude that an intermediate resin is necessary to achieve proper bond strength; some indicate that it is necessary to improve resistance to microleakage; others feel it is necessary for both reasons; still others do not think that the intermediate resin is necessary at all.[137,187]

A particular problem in orthodontics is that the sealant film on a facial tooth surface is so thin that oxygen inhibition of polymerization is likely to occur right through the film with autopolymerizing sealants[92,206] (Fig. 10-10). With acetone-containing[206] and light-polymerized[44,79] sealants, non-polymerization seems less a problem.

Why then should a sealant be of any value in bracket bonding? Although the sealant may not be necessary for strength and microleakage purposes, clinical evidence and laboratory studies[137] have not shown it to be a detrimental factor in achieving a good bond. The operator time in using it is minimal. If nothing else, sealing will permit a relaxation of moisture control, since this is no longer extremely important after resin coating. Sealants also provide enamel cover in areas of adhesive voids, which is probably especially valuable with indirect bonding. The caries protection of sealant around the bracket base is more uncertain,[44,79,187] and further studies are needed on the merits of fluoride-containing, light-cured sealants. Ceen and Gwinnett[44] found that light-polymerized sealants protect enamel adjacent to brackets from dissolution and subsurface lesions, whereas chemical-curing sealants polymerize poorly, exhibit drift, and have low resistance to abrasion.[43,206] Finally, sealants may at least theoretically permit easier bracket removal and protect against enamel tearouts at debonding, particularly when adhesives with small filler particles are used. Improved abrasion-resistant sealants with altered polymerization processes could become of value for orthodontic purposes when they are available.[91] Also unfilled resin mixed with compatible filled resin can lead to useful modifications of viscosity.[17]

Bonding

Immediately after all teeth to be bonded have been painted with sealant, the operator should proceed with the actual bonding of the attachments. At present, the majority of clinicians routinely bond brackets with the direct rather than the indirect technique.[74,77]

There are many different adhesives for direct bonding and

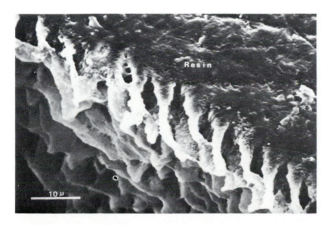

Fig. 10-9 Fitting surface of adhesive resin after the removal of enamel by demineralization. This surface shows an evenly distributed row of tags. (Courtesy ML Swartz.)

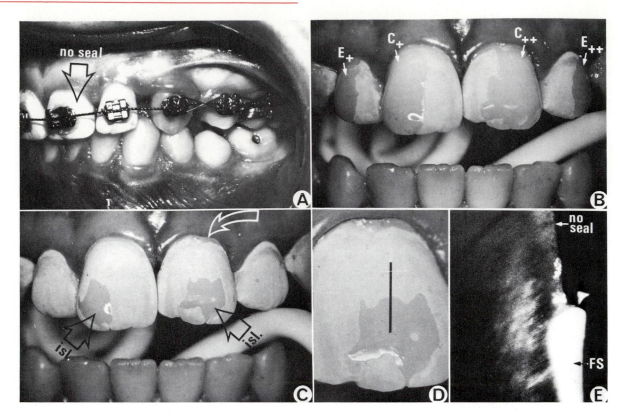

Fig. 10-10   Problems with conventional sealants on labial tooth surfaces. **A,** Shortly after bracket bonding. Subsequent to rinse and air spray, for a few seconds the enamel surface looks as if no sealant remains. **B,** Two brands of sealant applied on the distal halves of the maxillary incisors in thin *(+)* and thick *(+ +)* layers. **C,** After about 10 minutes' setting, followed by rinsing with abundant water and air spray and then air drying. Note that sealant *E* has not polymerized at all and sealant *C* has polymerized in bulky islands in the incisal region *(isl)* and in a rim *(arrow)* along the gingival margin. **D,** Enlargement of the left central incisor. The presence or absence of sealant tags in areas that gave an *etch-like* appearance at clinical inspection were studied in transverse ground sections, after a fluorescent dye had been added to the sealant. **E,** Area corresponding to the black line in **D.** There is no evidence of sealant tags in areas outside the fluorescent sealant island *(FS).*

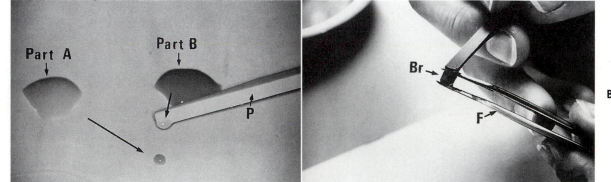

Fig. 10-11   Single tooth adhesive mixing. **A** and **B,** Small portions of prediluted adhesive pastes *A* and *B* are removed from master batches with opposite ends of a plastic instrument *(P)* and placed on the contact surface of the bracket *(Br).* Stainless steel instruments should not be used to mix adhesives with macrofillers since metal particles rub off and discolor the adhesive.

new ones appear continuously. However, the basic bonding technique is only slightly modified for varying materials according to each manufacturer's instructions. The easiest method of bonding is to apply a slight excess of adhesive to the backing of the attachment (Fig. 10-11) and then place the attachment on the tooth surface in its correct position.

When bonding attachments one at a time with a fresh homogeneous mix of relatively fast-setting adhesive the operator can work in a relaxed manner and obtain optimum bond strength for each bracket. There is no need to hurry, since plenty of time is available for placing the bracket in its correct position, checking it, and if necessary repositioning it within the working time of the adhesive. As soon as one attachment has been placed and adjusted to its correct position, the next bracket can be bonded while the previous one is setting. With fast-setting adhesives there is less time for moisture contamination, less risk for disruption of neighboring brackets, and less waiting for ligations to be made than when adhesives with long working times are used. An adhesive should have sufficient viscosity so that the bonded attachments do not drift out of position before the adhesive has set.

The recommended bracket bonding procedure[196,205] (with any adhesive) consists of the following steps:

1. Transfer
2. Positioning
3. Fitting
4. Removal of excess

Transfer. The bracket is gripped with a pair of cotton pliers or a reverse action tweezer and the mixed adhesive is applied to the back of the bonding base. The bracket is immediately placed on the tooth close to its correct position (Fig. 10-12).

Positioning. A placement scaler, such as the RM 349 (Fig. 10-12) or, preferably, one with parallel* edges (Fig. 10-13), is used to position the brackets mesiodistally and incisogingivally and to angulate them accurately. The placement scaler with parallel edges allows visualization of the bracket slot relative to the incisal edge and long axis of the teeth, with the scaler seated in the slot. Proper vertical positioning may be enhanced by different measuring devices or height guides on the brackets themselves. A mouth mirror

*LM-Dental, Turku, Finland.

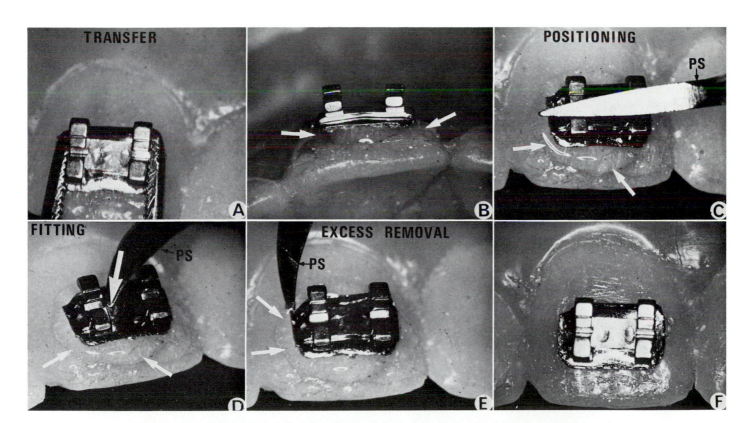

Fig. 10-12 Recommended direct bonding procedure. After the bracket is transferred to the tooth surface, orientation (angulation, height, mesiodistal position) is made with the placement scaler *(PS)*. Next, the scaler is used to seat the bracket firmly toward the tooth surface. This is important in securing maximal contact and optimal thickness of adhesive (*arrows* in **D**). Excess adhesive is then removed with the scaler along the pad periphery to produce the desired clean appearance in **F**.

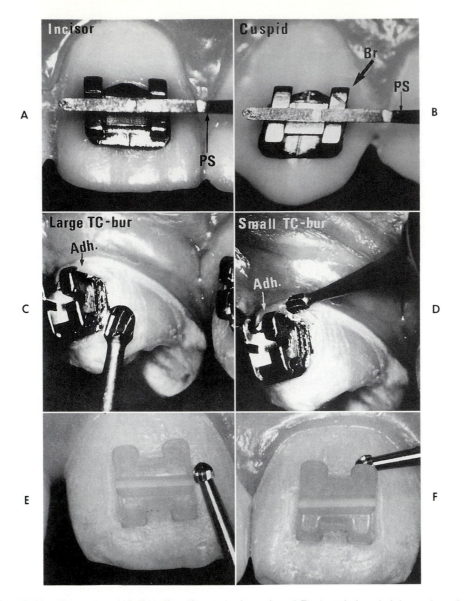

Fig. 10-13 Recommended direct-bonding procedure. **A** and **B,** Angulation, height, and mesio-distal position are determined with placement scaler *(PS)*. The parallel edges representing the bracket slot, the scaler can be held in the slot, while precise orientation relative to the incisal edge and long axis of the tooth is made. **C** and **D,** Use of *large* (no. 7006) and a *small* oval TC bur for removal of set adhesive *(Adh.)* around the bracket base and along the gingival margin, respectively. **E** and **F,** Small burs are also useful under ceramic bracket tie-wings.

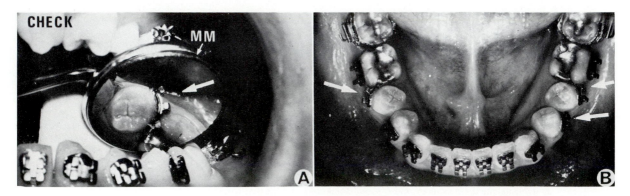

Fig. 10-14 Bracket position on difficult teeth *(arrows)* may be checked with a mouth mirror *(MM)*.

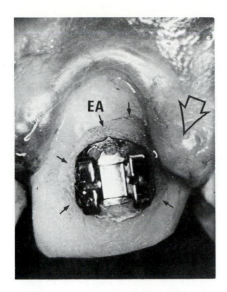

Fig. 10-15   Relationship between excess adhesive *(EA)* and gingival inflammation. Note the hyperplastic gingival changes on the distal aspect *(open arrow)*, where excess adhesive was close to the gingival margin. There is less reaction on the mesial aspect, where adhesive is further from the gingiva.

will aid in horizontal positioning, particularly on rotated premolars (Fig. 10-14).

Fitting. Next, the scaler is turned, and with one-point-contact with the bracket, it is pushed firmly toward the tooth surface[93] (Fig. 10-12). The tight fit will result in good bond strength, little material to remove on debonding, and reduced slide while excess material extrudes peripherally. It is important that the scaler be removed once the bracket is in correct position and no attempts be made to hold the bracket in place with the instrument. Even slight movement

may disturb the setting of the adhesive. *Totally undisturbed setting is essential for achieving adequate bond strength.*[205]

Removal of excess. A slight bit of excess adhesive is essential to minimize the possibility of voids and to be certain that it will be *buttered* into the entire mesh backing when the bracket is being fitted. The excess is particularly helpful on teeth with abnormal morphology. Excess will not be worn away by toothbrushing and other mechanical forces (Fig. 10-16); it must be removed (especially along the gingival margin) with the scaler before the adhesive has set (Fig. 10-12), or it must be removed with burs after setting.

To not disturb the bracket position during setting, it is now my preference to remove the excess after the adhesive has set. For this purpose, careful use of an oval (no. 7006, no. 2) or tapered (no. 1172) tungsten carbide (TC) bur* (Fig. 10-13) works well.

It is most important to remove the excess adhesive to prevent or minimize gingival irritation and plaque buildup around the periphery of the bonding base (Figs. 10-15 and 10-17). This will reduce periodontal damage and the possibility of decalcifications. In addition, removal of excess adhesive can improve esthetics by not only providing a neater and cleaner appearance but also by eliminating exposed adhesive that might become discolored in the oral environment (Fig. 10-18).

The benefits of careful excess removal are clearly demonstrated in Fig. 10-17, which shows excellent gingival health, even in the lower incisor region, with stippling evident near the termination of a full period of orthodontic treatment. On the other hand, clinically significant gingival hyperplasia and inflammation rapidly occur when excess

---

*Beavers Dental Products, Morrisburg, Ontario (also available from Unitek Corporation, Monrovia, Calif).

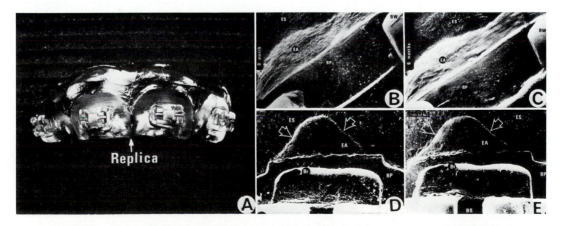

Fig. 10-16   Typical wear pattern of excess adhesive *(EA)*. Scanning electron micrographs of a replica model, **A,** at the time of bonding, **B** and **D,** and 6 months later, **C** and **E.** An example of abrasive wear of adhesive with large filler particles is shown in **B** and **C** and of adhesive with submicrometer-sized fillers in **D** and **E.** *Br,* Bracket; *BP,* bracket pad; *BS,* bracket slot; *BW,* bracket wing; *ES,* enamel surface.

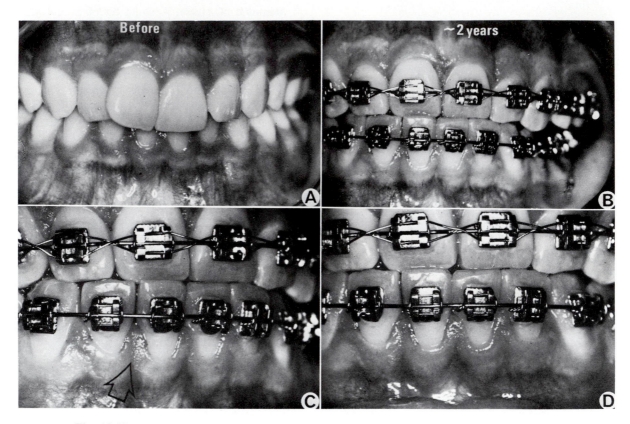

Fig. 10-17   When excess adhesive is carefully removed and good oral hygiene is maintained, the gingival condition is not adversely influenced by bonded appliances. **A,** Before treatment. **B,** Approximately 2 years later. **C** and **D,** Higher magnifications of **B.** Note the normal gingival condition with intact stippling *(open arrow)*.

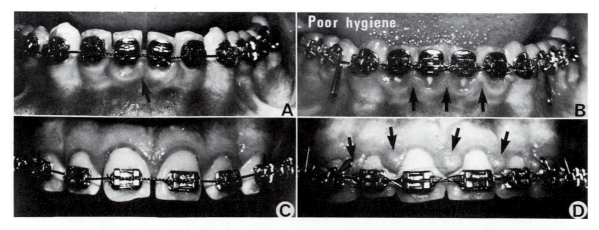

Fig. 10-18   Irrespective of the bonding technique, poor oral hygiene invariably results in marked hyperplastic gingival changes *(arrows* in **B** and **D**). This has occurred even though excess adhesive was carefully removed and polymerized sealant was scraped away from gingival margins. **A** and **C,** At start and, **A** and **D,** 6 months later.

adhesive comes close to the gingiva and is not properly removed[196,205] (Fig. 10-15).

When the procedure just described has been repeated for every bracket to be bonded, a careful check of position for each bracket is made (Fig. 10-14). Any attachment that is not in good position should be removed with pliers and rebonded immediately. After a leveling archwire is inserted, the patient is instructed how to brush properly around the brackets and archwires and is given a program to follow of daily fluoride mouthrinses (0.05% NaF).[194]

Types of adhesives

There are two basic types of dental resins currently in use for orthodontic bracket bonding. Both are polymers and are classified as *acrylic* or *diacrylate* resins.[145] The acrylic resins (Orthomite, Genie, etc.) are based on self-curing acrylics and consist of methylmethacrylate monomer and ultrafine powder. Most diacrylate resins are based on the acrylic modified epoxy resin mentioned in the introduction: bisGMA or Bowen's resin. A fundamental difference is that resins of the first type form linear polymers only whereas those of the second type may be polymerized also by cross-linking into a three-dimensional network. This cross-linking contributes to greater strength, lower water absorption, and less polymerization shrinkage.[145]

Both types of adhesive exist in either filled or unfilled forms. A number of independent investigations indicate that the filled diacrylate resins of the bisGMA type have the best physical properties and are the strongest adhesives for metal brackets.[39,93,206] Acrylic or combination resins have been most successful with plastic brackets. Some composite resins (including Concise) contain large coarse quartz or silica glass particles of highly variable size averaging 3 to 20 μm[33] (Fig. 10-19) that impart abrasion resistance properties. Others (Endur, Dynabond, etc.) contain minute filler particles of uniform size (0.2 and 0.3 μm) which, consequently, yield a smoother surface that retains less plaque[205] (Fig. 10-20) and is more prone to abrasion.[33] Reported failure rates for steel mesh-backed brackets direct-bonded with highly filled diacrylate resin may be as low as 1% to 4%.[205] Similarly, Buzzitta et al.[39] found that a highly filled diacrylate resin with large filler particles gave the highest values of in vitro body strength for metal brackets.

The clinical implication is that *adhesives with large-particle fillers are recommended for extra bond strength* (Fig. 10-21) *but careful removal of the excess is mandatory* since such adhesives accumulate plaque more easily than do others.[205]

There are several alternatives to chemically autopolymerizing paste-paste systems:

1. *No-mix adhesives.* These materials set when one paste under light pressure is brought together with a primer fluid on the etched enamel and bracket backing or when there is another paste on the tooth to be bonded. Thus one adhesive component is applied to the bracket base while another is applied to the dried etched tooth. As soon as it is precisely positioned, the bracket is pressed firmly into place and curing occurs usually within 30 to 60 seconds.

   Although the clinical bonding procedure may be

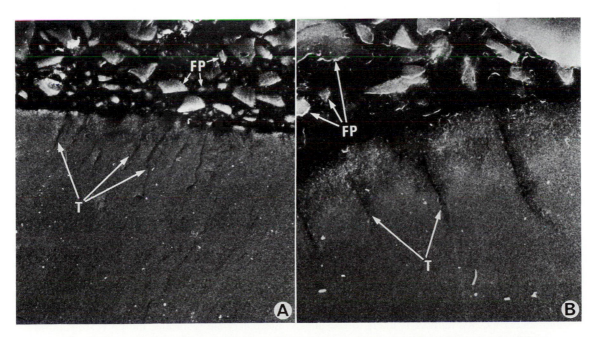

Fig. 10-19 Bonding adhesive with macrofillers. Because of size, these large filler particles *(FP)* cannot penetrate into the qualitative porous zone of etched enamel. (Fig. 10-8, **D** to **F**). Unfilled resin tags, *T*. (Magnification in **A** is 1000 × and in **B** 3000 × .) (Courtesy BO Brobakken.)

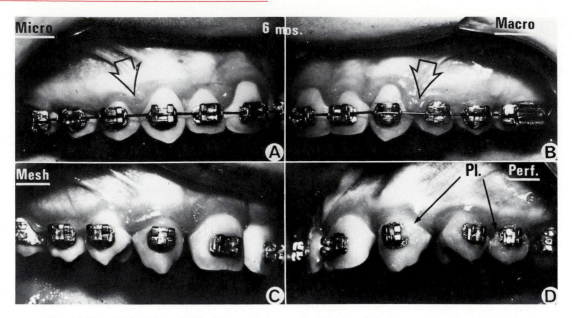

Fig. 10-20 Right-side and left-side comparisons of adhesives, **A** and **B,** and brackets, **C** and **D.**
Gingival irritation after 6 months is greater with the macrofilled than with the microfilled adhesive
(*open arrows* in **A** and **B**) and there is more plaque accumulation *(Pl)* on the perforated than on
the mesh-backed pads (**C** and **D**).

simplified with the no-mix adhesives, little long-term
information is available on their bond strengths when
compared with those of the conventionally mixed
paste-paste systems. Furthermore, little is known
about how much unpolymerized rest monomer remains in the cured adhesive,[176] and its eventual tox-
icity. In vitro tests have shown that liquid activators
of the no-mix systems are definitely toxic[66,176]; and
allergic reactions have been reported in patients, dental assistants, and doctors when such adhesives were
used[109] (Fig. 10-22).

2. *Visible-light polymerized adhesives.* These materials
may be cured by transmitting light through tooth structure and ceramic brackets. Ultraviolet light-polymerized resins were popular with plastic and perforated
metal brackets, but the inaccessibility of the light to
the resin under mesh-backed brackets turned most clinicians toward the autopolymerizing resins. Maximum
curing depth of light-activated resins is dependent on
the composition of the composite, the light source,
and the exposure time.[153] Visible light-activated adhesives have greater curing depths than UV-light-
activated adhesives.[153,181] By 1990, about 20% of
orthodontists in the United States were using light
curing routinely.[77] With the introduction of new techniques and adhesives, this number is likely to rise in
years to come.[186] Interesting in this development are
improved types of fluoride-releasing, visible light-curing adhesives, which are now becoming avail-

able.[113,127,146] However, further long-term clinical testing is necessary with this technique.

3. *Glass ionomer cements.* The glass ionomer cements
were introduced in 1972, primarily as luting agents
and direct restorative material, with unique properties
for bonding chemically to enamel and dentin, as well
as to stainless steel, being able to release fluoride
ions for caries protection. Several recent studies have
evaluated the use of glass ionomer cements in orthodontics.*

Such cements are now used routinely in my office for
cementing bands, because they are stronger than zinc phosphate and polycarboxylate cements, with less demineralization at the end of treatment.[101,117,147] But the present chem-
ically- or light-cured glass ionomers seem to have significantly lower in vitro bond strength than composite resins
for bonding brackets.† However, improved glass ionomer
cements may become an interesting alternative for bonding
of metal and ceramic brackets in the future, mainly because
of the caries prevention properties.

Selection of adhesives for direct bonding among the myriad alternatives available depends largely on factors like
handling characteristics, bond strength, and cost. However,
diacrylate resins do not bond with plastic brackets. Either
an acrylic monomer as a primer to enhance bonding between
the diacrylate resin and the polycarbonate bracket is necessary, or an acrylic resin adhesive must then be used.[145]

---

*References 101, 113, 117, 146, 147.
†References 47, 60, 67, 99, 113, 146.

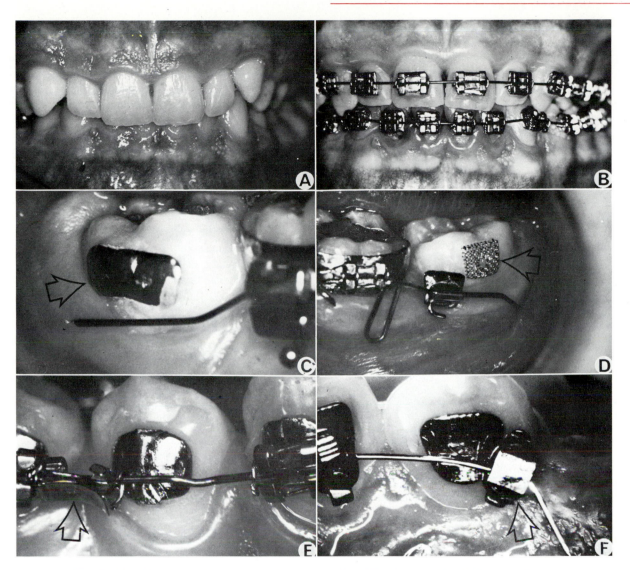

Fig. 10-21   Bond strength is of utmost importance. **A** and **B,** Deep overbite, before and after 2 years of treatment. No bite plate was used, and no bond failures occurred. **C** through **F,** Good bond strength between the bonding base and enamel. Failures have occurred between the brackets and the base *(open arrows).* **F,** Lingual bonding.

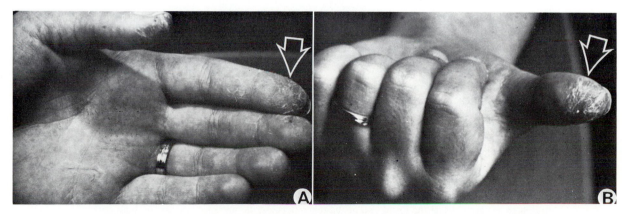

Fig. 10-22   Allergic reaction to bonding adhesive *(arrows).* Fingertips of a dental assistant.

As discussed in detail by Årtun and Zachrisson,[17] a modified restorative Concise is recommended for bonding brackets and retainers, etc. (p. 612). Since the original *restorative* Concise is somewhat too viscous, both pastes are diluted with the sealant resins (Fig. 10-23) as follows: 10 to 15 drops of liquid resin A are added to a *new* jar of the universal A paste and thoroughly incorporated; similarly, 10 to 15 drops of the liquid resin B are incorporated into a new jar

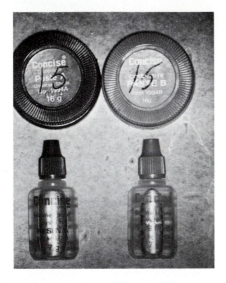

Fig. 10-23 Prediluted *15-drop* Concise. Each jar of restorative composite paste is diluted with about 15 drops of the corresponding liquid resin. Thus premixed, the paste-paste system is ready for use. The number of drops added is written on top of the jars.

of the catalyst B paste.* This gives an optimum consistency for routine direct bonding. (Each clinician can, of course, select any other viscosity by merely modifying the number of drops added.) Another advantage with this system is the possibility of hastening or slowing the setting time of the adhesive by varying the proportions of A and B pastes.[16,84] However, if the clinician wishes to hasten the set, more of the universal paste A is used. To slow the set, more of catalyst paste B is used. Thus the proportions may vary from 2:1 and 1:2 up to 5:1 and 1:5 without significantly influencing clinical bond strength.[84] It should be pointed out that the working time with any diacrylate resin is extremely dependent on office temperature. The use of a cold slab and refrigeration of the components will also slow the set and give the operator additional working time. Concise has the further advantage of a short *snap* time, which allows for almost immediate ligation.[196] It is the strongest adhesive for metal brackets[39,205] (Fig. 10-24), and no allergic reactions have been reported with it.[64] With this background and until more information becomes available on the alternatives, it seems safe to recommend an adhesive that has been working efficiently in direct bonding for the past 15 years.

In this connection it should be mentioned that *bond failures,* which are failures in the enamel-adhesive interface, are likely to be due to inadequate technique (e.g., moisture contamination or disturbed setting).

Failures in the adhesive-bracket interface are more likely caused by a weak adhesive.

---

*The *orthodontic* Concise is prediluted in a similar way; however, 75 to 80 drops (rather than the 10 to 15 drops suggested above) of the respective liquid resins are added, thus making it too fluid for direct bracket bonding.

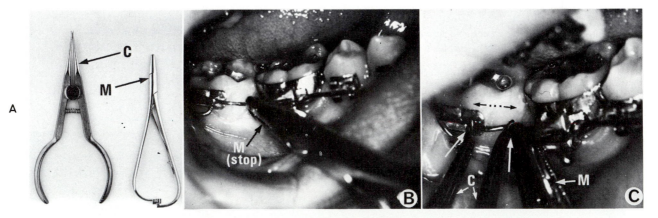

Fig. 10-24 The bond strength of macrofilled diacrylate adhesives is satisfactory for bonding lower second molars on a routine basis. A problem may be encountered, however, in archwire removal. This is solved with the following technique: **A,** A distally bent-over archwire from a bonded second molar tube is loosened by a Coon or Steiner tying pliers *(C)* and a Mathieu needle holder *(M).* The needle holder acts as a stop on the archwire a few millimeters from the mesial end of the buccal tube, **B.** The Coon pliers rests at the mesial part of the tube and at the stop. By closing the tying pliers the operator gently releases the archwire, often without even needing to straighten the archwire at the distal end of the tube. Because the pressure is equal on both ends of the buccal tube, the bond is not stressed unduly, **C.**

Summarizing the foregoing paragraphs, I would suggest that good success in bonding are in the following keys:

1. Develop a technique that ensures good moisture control.
2. Fit the brackets closely to the teeth.
3. Be sure that the setting of the adhesive is undisturbed.
4. Use a strong adhesive.

Brackets

Three types of attachments are presently available for orthodontic bracket bonding: plastic based, ceramic based, and metal (stainless steel) based. Of these, most clinicians prefer the metal attachments for routine applications, at least in children.[74,77,156]

Plastic brackets. Plastic attachments are made of polycarbonate and are used mainly for esthetic reasons[115] (Fig. 10-1). Pure plastic brackets lack strength to resist distortion and breakage (Fig. 10-25), wire slot wear (which leads to loss of tooth control), uptake of water, discoloration, and the need for compatible bonding resins.[145] Such plastic brackets may be useful in minimal force situations and for treatments of short duration, particularly in adults. New types of reinforced plastic brackets with and without steel slot inserts are presently being introduced. My clinical experience indicates that steel-slotted plastic brackets apparently are quite useful as an esthetic alternative to lingual orthodontics.

Ceramic brackets. Theoretically, porcelain brackets made of aluminum oxide (Figs. 10-26 and 10-27) could combine the esthetics of plastic and the reliability of metal brackets. Two forms are currently available: polycrystalline, made of sintered or fused aluminum oxide particles (e.g., GAC Allure, Unitek/3M Transcend 2000), and single-crystal form (e.g., "A"-company Starfire).[171] In contrast to current elastic ligatures both polycrystalline and single crystal brackets resist staining and discoloration. Steel ligatures can be used with caution.[64,65,171]

Ceramic brackets bond to enamel by two different mechanisms: (1) mechanical retention via indentations and/or undercuts in the base; and (2) chemical bonding by means of a silane coupling agent. With mechanical retention, the stress of debonding is generally at the adhesive-bracket interface, whereas the chemical bonding may produce excessive bond strengths, with the stress at debonding shifted towards the enamel-adhesive interface (see below under debonding). No-mix adhesives are not recommended for ceramic brackets[171]; however, chemically and, particularly, light-cured adhesives are useful.[126,171] With the latter, as much time as needed is available to position the brackets before polymerization. Brackets preloaded with light-cured paste can be applied to the teeth and pressed firmly in place in its approximate location. After adjusting the brackets and after excess adhesive has been removed, the brackets are tacked in place with a five-second exposure to the curing light; once all of the brackets are tacked, they are cured with a longer time exposure.

However, the ceramic brackets that are available at present are not optimal and show some significant drawbacks:

1. The frictional resistance between orthodontic wire and ceramic brackets is greater and less predictable than it is with steel brackets.* This makes it difficult to determine optimal force levels and anchorage control.
2. Ceramic brackets are not as durable as steel brackets and are brittle by nature. These brackets break easily during orthodontic treatment (Fig. 10-26, *A*), particularly when full-size (or close to full-size) stainless steel archwires are used for torquing purposes.[64,85]
3. Ceramic brackets are harder than steel and will rapidly induce enamel wear of any opposing teeth (Figs. 10-26, *C* and *D;* and 10-27, *B* through *E*.)
4. They are more difficult to debond than steel brackets, and wing fractures may easily occur during debracketing (see p. 570).
5. The surface is rougher and/or more porous than that of steel brackets and hence more easily attracts plaque and stain to the surrounding enamel.

---

*References 22, 72, 86, 100, 131, 172.

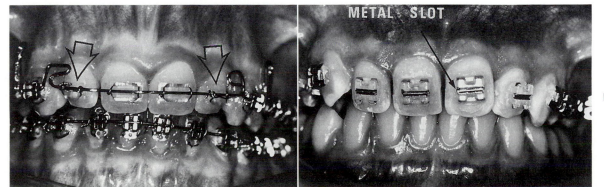

Fig. 10-25 Plastic brackets of different design. **A,** Pure polycarbonate. Note the wing breaks incurred during treatment *(open arrow).* **B,** Steel-slotted plastic bracket.

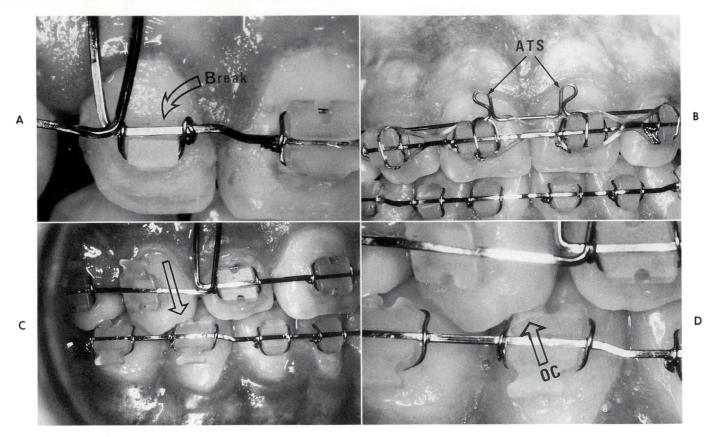

Fig. 10-26 Ceramic brackets. Care must be taken to counteract wing breakage, **A,** and to avoid wear of opposing teeth, **C** and **D. B,** Shows auxiliary torquing springs *(ATS)* which may be helpful to secure extra torque application.

Further improvements of currently available ceramic brackets are therefore required to help eliminate or reduce the disadvantages just mentioned. It may also be necessary to reduce the bond strength by altering the adhesive properties of the base, by changing the adhesive, or by adjusting the method of preparing the enamel surface.

Metal brackets. Although not as esthetically pleasing as ceramic and plastic brackets, small metal attachments are an improvement over bands (Fig. 10-1). Metal brackets rely on mechanical retention for bonding, and mesh gauze is the conventional method of providing this retention. Photo etched recessions or machined undercuts are also available.

When it comes to bond strength with mesh-backed brackets, the area of the base itself is probably not a critical factor. The use of small, less noticeable, metal bases (Fig. 10-28) helps avoid gingival irritation. For the same reason the base should be designed to follow the tissue contour along the gingival margin (Fig. 10-28). The base must not be smaller than the bracket wings, however, because of the danger of demineralization around the periphery. The mandibular molar and premolar bracket wings must be kept out-of-occlusion, or the brackets may easily come loose. There-

fore, *before bonding* it is recommended that (1) the patient be asked to bite together; the tooth area available for bonding should then be evaluated; (2) mandibular posterior brackets should be bonded out-of-occlusion whenever possible, which may necessitate adjustment bends in the archwires; and (3) any occlusal interferences on mandibular posterior attachments should be evaluated immediately *after bonding,* and those occlusal tie-wings that are in contact with maxillary molar/premolar cusps should be spot ground (with green stone, or similar). Using these procedures I have been successful in routinely bonding mandibular molar and premolar attachments in children and in adults for the past several years.

Corrosion of metal brackets is a problem, and black and green stains have appeared with bonded stainless steel attachments.[42,108] Crevice corrosion of the metal arising in areas of poor bonding may be due primarily to the type of stainless steel alloy (Type 304) used.[108] However, other factors such as galvanic action, bracket base design and construction, particular oral environment, and thermal recycling of brackets[83,111] may be contributing factors. Thus careful attention should be paid to any signs of corrosion in bonded brackets to avoid the possibility of enamel staining. The use

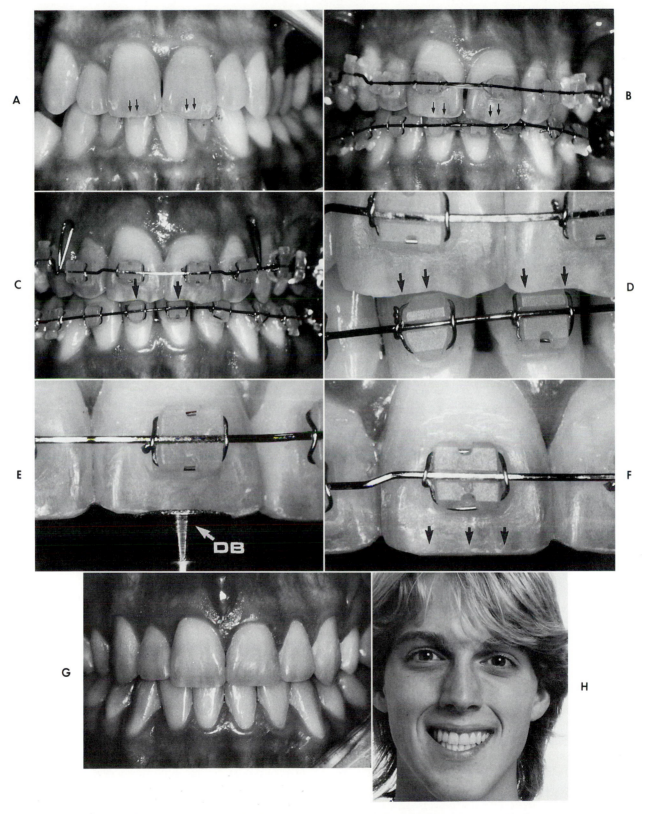

Fig. 10-27   Extreme wear of both maxillary central incisors occurred in this case because of contact with ceramic brackets in the mandible (compare **A** through **D**). Recontouring of the incisal edges by grinding with diamond bur: *DB* in **E,** provided satisfactory end result, **F** through **H.**

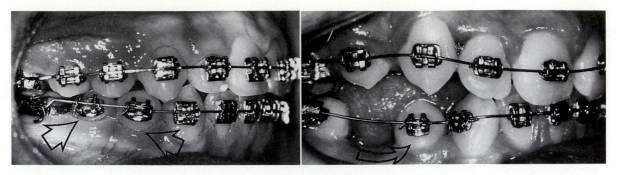

Fig. 10-28   The premolar base design should be such that it follows the contour of the marginal gingiva *(arrows)* thus minimizing irritation.

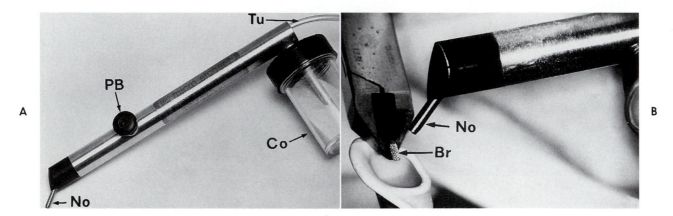

Fig. 10-29   The Micro-etcher is an FDA approved intra-oral sandblaster, which is most useful for preparing microretentive surfaces in gold and other metals, whenever needed. **A,** The appliance consists of a container *(Co)* for the aluminium oxide powder, a pushbutton *(PB)* for fingertip control, and a movable nozzle *(No),* where the abrasive particles are delivered. It is connected to compressed air via a plastic tubing *(Tu).* **B,** It is used also to improve the retentive surface of loose brackets (after grinding away the composite) before rebonding, and the inside of steel bands, which have come loose. See text for bonding brackets to gold and other metals.

of more corrosion-resistant stainless steel alloys would seem to be preferable in minimizing this problem.[108]

Bonding to crowns and restorations

Many adult patients have crown and bridge restorations fabricated from porcelain and nonprecious metals or gold. Banding becomes difficult, if not impossible, on the abutment teeth of fixed bridges. Recent advances in materials and techniques indicate, however, that effective bonding of orthodontic attachments to surfaces other than enamel may now be possible.

Bonding to gold. Until recently, bonding to gold and other metals was considered difficult. In the 1980s some adhesives (Enamelite 500,* Goldlink,† etc) and primers (Fusion)‡ were designed to allow such bonding; however,

---

*Lee Pharmaceuticals, South El Monte, California.
†Den-Mat Corp., Santa Maria, California.
‡Georg Taub Products, Jersey City, New Jersey.

published reports and clinical experience do not support their effectiveness.[192]

Roughening the gold surface with a green stone was found by Wood et al.[192] to significantly increase bond strengths to a highly filled resin system. However, the breakthrough came with intra-oral sandblasting. A handpiece abraded surface may look rough to the eye, but SEM studies indicate that the micromechanical retention of metals can be increased by at least 300% using intra-oral sandblasting.[56,167] In my hands the Micro-Etcher (Fig. 10-29), which uses 50 μm white aluminum oxide particles at approximately 7 kg/cm² pressure has been most advantageous for bonding to gold and other metals. During a quick 3-second blast with finger-tip control (and high-speed evacuator) the abrasive creates a retentive surface to which bonding with composite resin is greatly enhanced. Of course, the gold surface is easily repolished after debonding.

It appears that use of the Micro-Etcher followed by direct bonding with a highly filled composite, such as Concise, creates bond strengths that are clinically reliable over a full period of orthodontic treatment. It is highly likely that the bonds can be further strengthened by the use of intermediate primers (All-Bond* A and B)[53] and new 4-META adhesive resins,† which are claimed to bind chemically to precious and nonprecious metals.[51] Comparative studies are under way in our laboratory and clinic to test the usefulness of these materials.

Bonding to amalgam. Of course, microetching is also essential for bonding to amalgam and other nonprecious metals. Small amalgam restorations (e.g., buccal pit alloys) may not need to be sandblasted before bonding molar attachments, since the bond to the surrounding enamel is usually sufficiently strong. However, large amalgams should be sandblasted for about 3 seconds to provide an improved surface for bonding. Further clinical studies are needed on the merits of adhesives claimed to bond chemically to amalgam.

Bonding to acrylic and composite restoratives. With selected adhesives and/or pretreatments, brackets may be bonded to acrylic and composite crowns or build-ups. Before bonding, the surface should be roughened with sandpaper disks (or similar) to increase the retention for the bonding adhesive. An acrylic adhesive resin is preferred for bonding metal, plastic, or ceramic brackets to acrylic crowns.

The bond strength obtained, with the addition of new composite to mature composite, is substantially less than the cohesive strength of the material.[29] However, brackets bonded to a fresh, roughened surface of old composite restorations appear to be clinically successful in most instances.

Bonding to porcelain. In 1986 Wood et al.[192] showed that roughening the porcelain surface, adding a porcelain primer, and using a highly filled adhesive resin when bonding to glazed porcelain added progressively to bond strength. Their in vitro findings indicated that the bond strength to porcelain equalled or surpassed those obtained after bonding to acid-etched enamel of natural teeth, and therefore they expressed warnings that the bond strengths were high enough to damage the porcelain tooth surface during debondings. Similar concerns have been expressed by others.[58,95,96,166]

Several studies have reported that roughening of porcelain and silane treatment may produce in vitro bond strengths that should also be clinically successful[58,64,65,166]; however, these claims have not been verified by clinical investigations or by my own experience. Furthermore, other authors have claimed that the composite-porcelain bond is mostly micromechanical and that the contribution of the silane application for a chemical bond is negligible.[56,164] Therefore, the concept of etching porcelain with hydrofluoric or other acids to provide an even more retentive surface is interesting but needs verification.

Cracks or fractures occurring in porcelain crowns or laminate veneers during in vitro debonding may not reflect the clinical situation adequately. It is possible to clinically debond both metal and ceramic brackets much more gently than is done with laboratory machines and to secure an adhesive-bracket separation with all adhesive remaining on the tooth surface. Detaching metal brackets can be achieved by using a 45-degree peripheral force or by squeezing the bracket wings (see p. 571); ceramic brackets that do not come off easily can be ground away with diamond instruments.[184]

Conventional acid-etching is ineffective in the preparation of porcelain surfaces for mechanical retention of brackets. However, several porcelain etchants have been developed.[56,164] The most commonly used etchant is 9.6% hydrofluoric acid in gel form* for 2 to 4 minutes. This is a strong acid, which requires an isolated work space and great caution. Other studies indicate that 1.23 or 4% APF (acidulated phosphate fluoride) solution or gel,† containing sodium fluoride, phosphoric acid, and hydrofluoric acid, may provide equivalent bond strengths, in spite of a more superficial action and with less prominent morphologic changes.[56]

Although the clinical use of hydrofluoric acid for 2 minutes is quite promising for bonding brackets and retainer wires to porcelain crowns, further laboratory and clinical studies are presently being done by us using different porcelain etchants and silane primers, with and without intraoral sandblasting to roughen the porcelain. The refinishing of the porcelain to its original smoothness[58,166] also needs further study.

Lingual attachments

A drawback when bonding brackets on the labial, as compared to banding, is that conventional attachments for control during tooth movement (e.g., cleats, buttons, sheaths, and eyelets) are not included. In selected instances such aids may be bonded to the lingual surfaces to supplement the appliance (Figs. 10-30 and 10-31). However, there is a risk that bonded lingual attachments may be swallowed or aspirated if they come loose, since generally nothing else is holding them. Special snap-in or *safety* lingual cleats that stay attached to the appliances when they become loose are available (Fig. 10-31) and may be useful on canines and premolars for rotation control, intermaxillary elastics, pulling down impacted canines, etc. Alternatively, the cleats may be *closed* with an instrument over the elastic module or steel ligature.

The bonding of brackets to the lingual surfaces of teeth will be discussed separately (p. 568).

Ligation of bonded brackets

In contrast to brackets on bands, bonded brackets will not withstand heavy pull into archwires. Thus it is important

---

*Bisco Inc., Itasca, Illinios.
†Super-Bond C&B, Sun Medical Company, Ltd., Kyoto, Japan.

*Pulpdent Corp., Watertown, Maine.
†Chameleon Dental Products, Inc., Kansas City, Kansas.

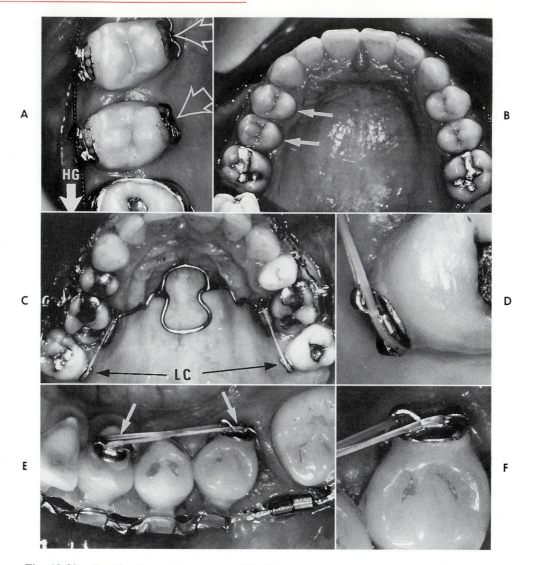

Fig. 10-30 Bonding lingual cleats. **A** and **B,** Cleats *(open arrows)* may be needed in addition to brackets when the maxillary first molars have been distalized with headgear and the premolars *follow* the molar. **C** and **F** shows other clinical situations when bonding cleats are useful.

to learn a few clinical tips on correct ligation. Although elastic modules are time saving and have been used successfully by many clinicians, steel ties are safer and more hygienic.[65,205] The rule of thumb in ligation is that the ligature wire should be twisted with the strand that crosses the archwire closest to the bracket wing. This will tighten the ligature when the end is tucked under the archwire.

To perform *active* ligations without pulling off any brackets, the operator should push the archwire into the bottom of the bracket slot using the fingers (for flexible wires) or (for stiffer wires) a Weingart plier, ligature director, etc. and then make a *passive* ligation (Fig. 10-32). If full engagement is not possible, the ligature can be retied at the next visit and/or elastomers can be added.

Ligature-less brackets are also available, and presently at least two different principles are involved: Orec* and Forestadent.† Such brackets may offer the advantages of saving time and probably increasing patient comfort.

Indirect bonding

Several techniques for indirect bonding are available.‡ Most are based on the procedures described by Silverman and Cohen.[157,158] In these techniques the brackets are attached to the teeth on the patient's models, transferred to the mouth with some sort of tray into which the brackets become incorporated, and then bonded simultaneously (Fig. 10-33).

---

*Hanson speed bracket, Orec Corporation, San Clemente, California.
†Bernhard Förster GmbH, Pforzheim, Germany.
‡References 2, 120, 156, 164, 174.

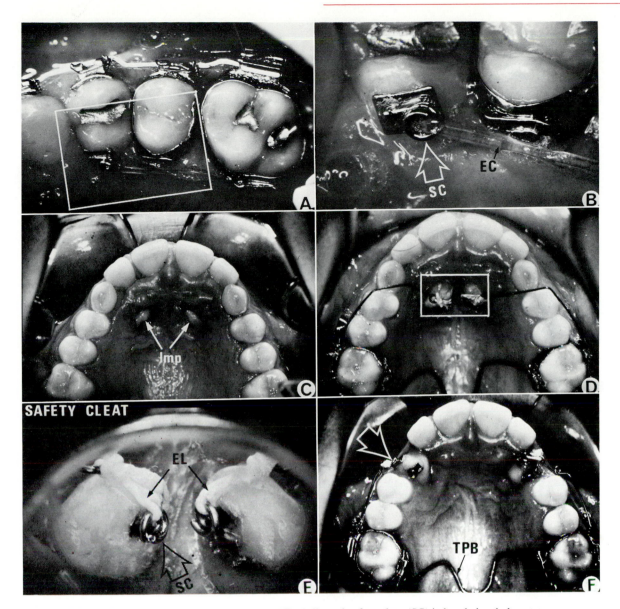

Fig. 10-31 Bonding safety cleats. **A** and **B,** A lingual safety cleat *(SC)* is bonded to help rotate a first premolar by means of elastic chain *(EC)*. **C** through **F,** Two impacted canines *(Imp)*. Snap-in cleats *(SC)* were used during orthodontic correction. **E,** Boxed area in **D.** *EL,* Elastic ligature; *TPB,* transpalatal bar.

The main advantage of indirect as compared to direct bonding is that the brackets can be more accurately positioned in the laboratory and the clinical chair time is decreased. However, the chairside procedure is more critical, at least for inexperienced clinicians; removal of excess adhesive is more difficult and more time consuming; the risk for adhesive deficiencies under the brackets is greater; and the failure rates seem to be slightly higher.[205]

Reasons for differences in bond strength between the two techniques,[205] if any,[2] may be as follows: (1) the bracket bases may be fitted closer to the tooth surfaces with one-point fitting by a placement scaler (Fig. 10-12) than when a transfer is placed over the teeth; and (2) a totally undis-turbed setting is more easily obtained with direct bonding when the scaler is released from the bracket (p. 553).

However, *when correct technique is used, failure rates with both direct and indirect bonding fall within a clinically acceptable range.*

Neither technique has reached its ultimate stage. In direct bonding there is a need for improved instruments to give exact bracket positioning. In indirect bonding, new techniques for the transfer that provide less disturbance during adhesive polymerization and easier removal of excess would be desirable. At present the individual practitioner may use either method based on practice routine, auxiliary personnel, and clinical ability. For instance, indirect bonding is more

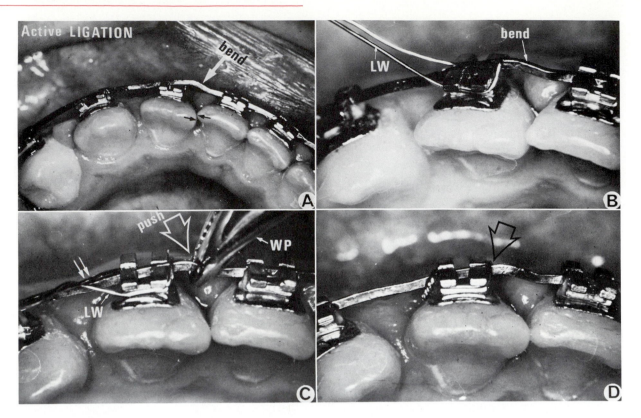

Fig. 10-32   Technique for active ligation to bonded brackets. **A,** A bend in the 0.016 × 0.022 archwire made to overcorrect a contact point in the mandibular incisor region *(small arrows).* **B through D,** A Weingart pliers *(WP)* is used to push the archwire toward the base of the bracket slot before a passive ligation is made. The ligature wire should be twisted so the strand that goes over the archwire *(double arrows* in **C)** is closest to the bracket wing. When not complete, as in **D,** the ligature is tightened at the next appointment.

likely to be used when all brackets are placed at one time at the start of orthodontic treatment rather than with a progressive strap-up over several months. Also, in lingual orthodontics the indirect technique is a prerequisite for good bracket alignment[3] because there are evident difficulties in direct visualization.

Clinical procedure

As mentioned, several indirect bonding techniques have proved reliable in clinical practice. They differ in the way the brackets are attached temporarily to the model (caramel candy, laboratory adhesive, bonding resin), the type of transfer tray or other mechanism used (silicone, vacuum-formed, acrylic with transfer arms, etc.), the adhesive or sealant employed, whether segmented or full bonding is used, and the way the transfer is removed so as not to exert excessive force on a still maturing bond.

Probably the two most popular techniques are the silicone impression material (Fig. 10-33) and the double sealant.

Indirect bonding with silicone transfer trays
(Fig. 10-33)

1. Take an impression and pour up a stone (not plaster) model. The model must be dry. It may be marked for long axis and incisal or occlusal height on each tooth.
2. Select brackets for each tooth.
3. Apply a small portion of water-soluble adhesive on each base or tooth.
4. Position the brackets on the model. Check all measurements and alignments. Reposition if needed.
5. For silicone tray fabrication, mix material according to the manufacturer's instructions. Press the putty onto the cemented brackets. Form the tray allowing sufficient thickness for strength.
6. After the silicone putty has set, immerse the model and tray in hot water to release the brackets from the stone. Remove any remaining adhesive under running water.

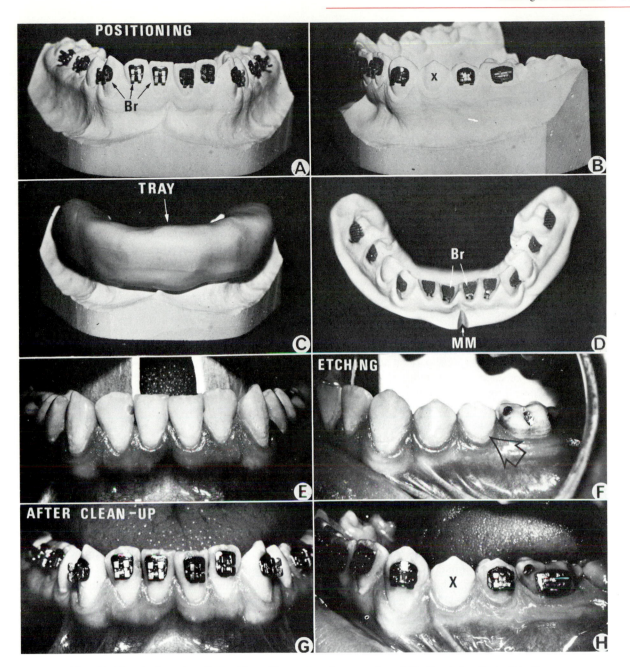

Fig. 10-33 Indirect bonding with a silicone transfer tray. **A** and **B,** Brackets attached to the plaster model. **C** and **D,** Tray (hard Optosil). Note the brackets *(Br)* and the orientation mark in midline *(MM)*. **E** and **F,** Etching of the right and left sides simultaneously. Note the difference in appearance between central and cervical portions of the enamel *(open arrow* in **F).** **G** and **H,** Final appearance subsequent to careful cleanup with instruments and a TC bur. The first premolars *(X)* were referred for extraction at this stage. (Courtesy BO Brobakken.)

7. Trim the silicone tray and mark the midline.
8. Prepare the patient's teeth as for a direct application (p. 545).
9. Mix adhesive, load it in a syringe, and apply a sufficient portion to the bonding bases.
10. Seat the tray on the prepared arch and hold with firm and steady pressure for about 3 minutes.

11. Remove the tray after 10 mintues. The tray may be cut longitudinally or transversely to reduce the risk of bracket debonding when it is peeled off.
12. Complete the bonding by careful removal of excess adhesive flash. Use oval (no. 7006 and no. 2) or tapered (no. 1172 or no. 1171) TC bur to clean the area properly around each bracket. *If this step is*

neglected, gingival irritation with redness, hyperplasia, and bleeding will develop within a short time and remain throughout treatment. This is not acceptable! Also inspect around the bracket pad for adhesive voids (from too little adhesive, tray slide on the teeth, delayed seating, etc.) and fill in with a small mix of adhesive if needed.

Indirect bonding with the double-sealant technique.[175] In this technique the bonding adhesive pastes, rather than a water-soluble temporary adhesive, are used to attach the brackets to the patient's stone model. Small portions of catalyst and universal adhesive pastes are dispensed side by side on a mixing pad. On a *per tooth* basis, enough adhesive for one attachment is mixed and applied to the back of the bonding base. The bracket is placed on the model, and the excess adhesive is removed from the periphery of the base. This step is repeated until all brackets are bonded to the stone model.

After at least 10 minutes (enough time for the bonding material to set) a placement tray is vacuum-formed for each arch. Models with trays attached are placed in water until thoroughly saturated. Then trays are separated and trimmed so the gingival edge of each tray is within 2 mm of the brackets. The midline is marked with indelible ink. The embedded bonding bases are lightly abraded with a stone point, after which the placement tray is ready for clinical use.

The clinical procedure is begun with the customary prophylaxis, isolation, and etching of the patient's teeth. The lingual sides of the bonding bases are painted with catalyst sealant resin (part B) 6 drops per arch. The dry etched teeth are painted with the universal sealant resin (part A). It is important that this use of the sealant liquids not be reversed. The tray is then inserted into the patient's mouth, seated, and held in place for at least 3 minutes. It is removed by peeling from the lingual toward the buccal. Excess flash of sealant is carefully removed from the gingival and contact areas of the teeth. A definite advantage of this technique is that the cleanup is simple, since little flash is present and consists of unfilled sealant only. Although laboratory tests are favorable,[114] there are no published data on bond strength with this technique as compared to other bonding techniques.

Lingual bracket bonding—*invisible braces*

When it became apparent in the late 1970s that bonding of brackets was a viable procedure and that esthetic plastic and ceramic brackets were a compromise, placing the brackets on the lingual surfaces of the teeth appeared to be the ultimate esthetic approach (Figs. 10-1 and 10-34). The technique rapidly gained popularity in the early 1980s, but most clinicians experienced considerable difficulties, particularly in the finishing stages,[11] and abandoned the technique for routine use.

The development was pioneered in Japan by Fujita,[68] who worked on the *mushroom* arch, and by several American

orthodontists: Kurz (Alexander et al.[3]), Kelly,[98] and Paige,[133] and more recently, Creekmore.[49] Although it appears possible to treat malocclusions successfully from the lingual side,[11,68,76] a combined lingual and buccal segmental approach may offer a number of options with no great esthetic compromises in most patients.

Somewhat surprisingly, the problem with lingual orthodontics is not that brackets become loose but rather that some pronunciation difficulties occur immediately after insertion (although the difficulties vary individually and may disappear within a few weeks[68]). Furthermore, the technique is difficult and time consuming and the working position is awkward.[68,181]

More precision is necessary for the adjustment of lingual archwires, with reduced interbracket distance. If the lingual treatment is to become more important in the future, additional improvements in bracket design and technical aids are needed.

Rebonding

Bonded brackets that become loose during treatment consume much chair time, are poor publicity for the office, and are a nuisance to the orthodontist. The best way to avoid loose brackets is to adhere strictly to the rules for good bonding mentioned on p. 559. It is also important to use a quick technique for rebonding loose brackets.

The same direct-bonding technique with fast-setting prediluted Concise just described[16] (p. 558) may be used. The loose bracket is removed from the archwire. At the same time the ligatures on two neighboring brackets are cut and the archwire is placed on top of these brackets. The adhesive remaining on the tooth surface is removed with a TC bur. If a new bracket is not to be used, the adhesive remaining on the loose bracket is removed, taking care not to burnish the mesh backing, and the bracket is then sandblasted (Fig. 10-29), although better bond strength is probably achieved with a new bracket.[87] The tooth is then etched for 15 seconds and sealed, and the bracket is rebonded. Sometimes positioning of the bracket can be accomplished by sliding the archwire back into the slots, but the risk then is that an undisturbed setting of adhesive is not obtained. The neighboring brackets are re-ligated first, and then the bracket is rebonded.

Recycling

Several methods of recycling debonded attachments for repeat use, either by commercial companies or by a duplicated procedure in office, have become available.[103] The main goal of the recycling process is to remove the adhesive from the bracket completely without damaging or weakening the delicate bracket backing or distorting the dimensions of the bracket slot. At present it appears that about 30% of orthodontists in the United States recycle at least some of their metal and/or ceramic brackets.[77]

Commercial processes employ either heat (about 450° C), to burn off the resin, followed by electropolishing to remove

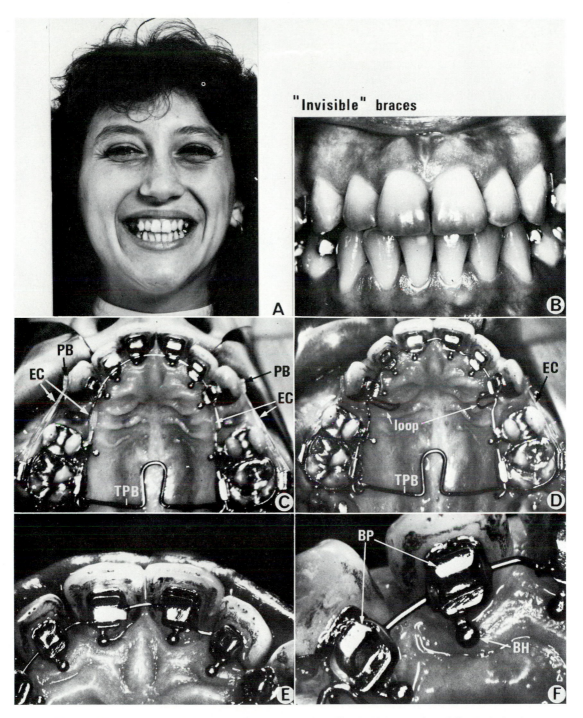

Fig. 10-34 Lingual orthodontics with one type of appliance (Ormco). **A** and **B,** Esthetics is excellent since the appliance is almost invisible. **C** and **D,** Subsequent to the first premolar extraction. Distalization of the canines is done with elastic chains to a plastic button *(PB)* and the lingual ball hook on a continuous archwire. **D,** The anterior segment is retracted on a loop archwire and labial elastics. **E** and **F,** Higher magnifications of the lingual bracket details. *BH,* Ball hook; *BP,* bite plane on the bracket; *TPB,* transpalatal bar.

the oxide buildup (e.g., Esmadent), or solvent stripping combined with high-frequency vibrations and only flash electropolishing (e.g., Ortho-Cycle). The electropolishing is needed for removal of any tarnish or oxide formed during elimination of the adhesive from the clogged pad.

Buchman[34] published photomicrographs showing microstructural changes after thermal treatment that were correlated with a decrease in corrosion resistance and hardness. Changes in torque angle and slot size after one or two recyclings were below clinical significance.[34,82]

Long-term clinical studies are needed to evaluate (1) the importance of any reduction in retentive strength after repeated recyclings of metal and ceramic brackets; and (2) the corrosion potential for recycled brackets, whether heated or not and whether electropolished for varying lengths of time or not electropolished at all.

Concluding Remarks

Bonding of brackets has changed the practice of orthodontics and has passed to a routine clinical procedure in a remarkably short time.[139] Modifications of technical devices, sealants and adhesives, attachments, and procedures are continuing. Careful study of the available information by the orthodontist will be mandatory in keeping up with progress. However, cautious interpretation of in vitro studies is recommended, since the in vivo results do not always reflect and verify the laboratory findings. Long-term follow-up studies are needed in several areas.

At present I am routinely using *bonded* brackets on all teeth except maxillary first molars. In most routine situations, *banding* maxillary first molars provides a stronger attachment and availability of lingual sheaths (for transpalatal bars, elastics, headgear, etc.) and may give some interproximal caries protection. Finally, the procedure described for bonding mandibular second molars has, somewhat surprisingly, proved to be quite successful in clinical use over many years. This is particularly true in adolescents, when teeth are erupting during the course of treatment. The mandibular second molar is better suited for bonding than for banding since gingival emergence of the buccal surface precedes emergence of the distal surface.

DEBONDING

The objectives of debonding are to remove the attachment and all the adhesive resin from the tooth and to restore the surface as closely as possible to its pretreatment condition without inducing iatrogenic damage. To obtain these objectives, a correct technique is of fundamental importance. Debonding may be unnecessarily time consuming and damaging to the enamel if performed with improper technique or in a careless manner.

Since several aspects of debonding are controversial and the procedure is considered difficult or complicated by some clinicians,[74] it will be discussed in detail as follows:

Clinical procedure

Characteristics of normal enamel
Influence on surface enamel of different debonding instruments on surface enamel
Amount of enamel lost in debonding
Enamel tearouts
Enamel cracks (fracture lines)
Adhesive remnant wear
Reversal of decalcifications

Clinical Procedures

Although several methods have been recommended in the literature for bracket removal and adhesive cleanup* and some discrepancy of opinion still exists, the techniques to be described have proved successful in my experience. Its rationale will be mentioned throughout the ensuing discussion.

The clinical debonding procedure may be divided in two stages:

1. Bracket removal
2. Removal of residual adhesive

Bracket removal—steel brackets. Several different procedures for debracketing with pliers are available. An original method was to place the tips of a twin-beaked pliers against the mesial and distal edges of the bonding base and to cut the brackets off between the tooth and the base (Fig. 10-35, *A* and *B*). Several pliers are available for this purpose. A gentler technique is to squeeze the bracket wings mesiodistally (Fig. 10-35, *C* and *D*) and lift the bracket off with a peel force. This technique is particularly useful on brittle, mobile, or endodontically treated teeth. The brackets are easily deformed and less suitable for recycling when the latter method is used. The recommended technique, in which brackets are not deformed, is illustrated in Fig. 10-36.

These techniques all use a peeling-type force, which is most effective in breaking the adhesive bond. The break is likely to occur in the adhesive-bracket interface, thus leaving adhesive remnants on the enamel. Attempts to remove the bracket by shearing it off (as is done in removing bands) can be traumatic to the patient and potentially damaging to the enamel.

Bracket removal—ceramic brackets. With the introduction of ceramic brackets, a new concern over enamel fracture and loss from debonding has arisen.[141] Because of differences in bracket chemistry and in bonding mechanisms, various ceramic brackets behave differently on debonding. For example, ceramic brackets using mechanical retention appear to cause fewer problems in debonding than do those using chemical retention.[141,183,190] It is important in this regard to have some knowledge about the *normal* frequency, distribution, and orientation of enamel cracks in young and in older teeth (see p. 578).

The ceramic brackets most easy to debond are the GAC Allure brackets, which contain two rows of *holds,* where a

---

*References 33, 38, 41, 80, 130, 141, 144, 184, 204.

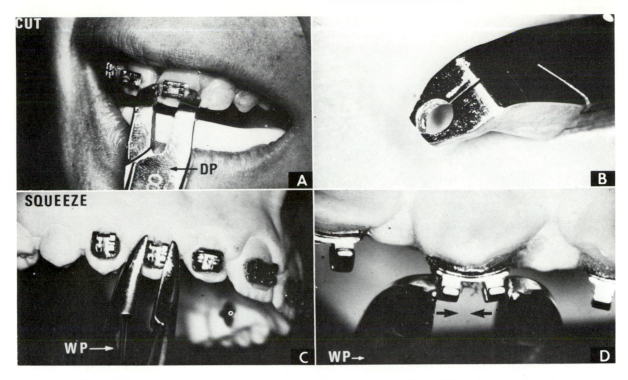

Fig. 10-35   Bracket removal with cut, **A** and **B**, and squeeze, **C** and **D**, techniques. **A** and **B** show how brackets are removed with a debonding pliers between the bracket pad and enamel. **C** and **D**, Debracketing is done by means of squeezing the bracket wings with Weingart pliers *(WP)*. This is a gentle technique, but the brackets are easily destroyed and cannot be recycled.

predominantly mechanical bond can be predictably and safely broken in the adhesive-bracket interface when a peripheral force was applied. The recommended debracketing instrument with these brackets, is the ETM 346 RT (Fig. 10-37, *D*). The jaws are placed occlusogingivally and the brackets are lifted off with peripheral force application, much the same as for steel brackets (Fig. 10-37, *C* and *D*).

Much of the concern with ceramic bracket debonding originates from early problems with those brackets that relied on a predominantly chemical bond, such as Transcend.[90] The recommended tool was a wrench-type instrument that required a torquing force. Rotating the instrument distributed force over the entire base area, which increased the risk for bracket fracture and enamel damage.[171] However, the next generation: Transcend 2000, relies more on mechanical bonding[190] and comes supplied with a reciprocal-action, pistol-type debracketing tool (Fig. 10-37, *A* and *B*). It is positioned horizontally over the brackets, with the jaws aligned occlusogingivally over the tie-wings, and then is squeezed harder until the brackets separate from the tooth (Fig. 10-37). Several tie-wings may still fracture, which in practice requires grinding away the rest of the bracket.[141] *Cutting* the brackets off with gradual pressure from the tips of twin-beaked pliers oriented mesiodistally close to the bracket/adhesive interface is *not* recommended because it might introduce horizontal enamel cracks. The grinding is generally done with low- or high-speed of diamond burs.

Low-speed grinding of ceramic brackets with no water coolant may cause permanent damage or necrosis of dental pulps.[184] Therefore, water cooling of the grinding sites is necessary. Also high-volume suction and eye protection is recommended to reduce the number of ceramic particles spread about the operatory area.[184]

Finally, thermal debonding is an option that appears to be increasingly available. Electrothermal debracketing instruments are presently not available for all types of ceramic brackets, and the technique is still at an introductory stage.[26,94,152]

Removal of residual adhesive. Because of the color similarity between present adhesives and enamel, complete removal of all remaining adhesive is not easily achieved. There is reason to believe that many patients are left with incomplete resin removal[63] (Fig. 10-48), which is not acceptable. Abrasive wear of present bonding resins is limited,[33] and remnants are likely to become unesthetically discolored with time (Fig. 10-47).

The removal of excess adhesive may be accomplished by (1) scraping with a supersharp band or bond-removing pliers or with a scaler[196] or by (2) using a suitable bur and contra-angle.

Although the first method (Fig. 10-38, *A* and *B*) is fast and frequently successful on curved teeth (premolars, canines), it is less useful on flat anterior teeth. There is also a risk of creating significant scratch marks.

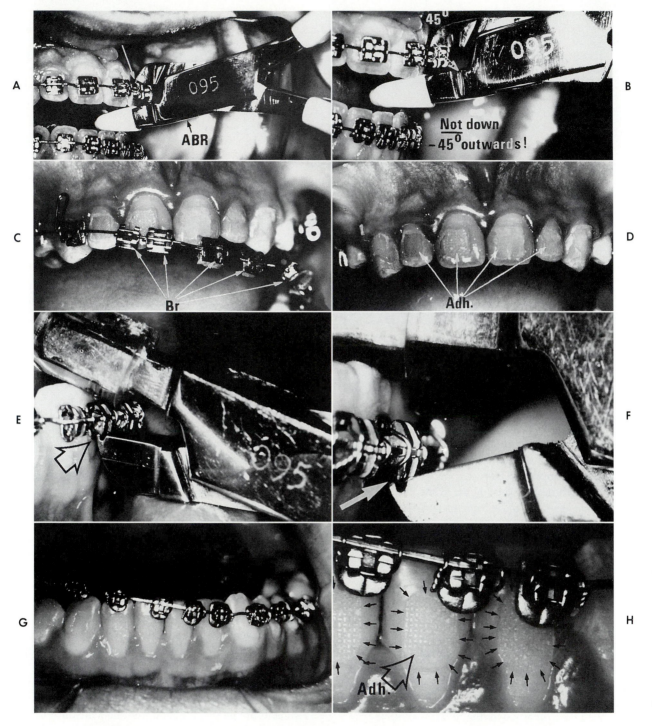

Fig. 10-36 Recommended technique for removal of steel brackets in the maxilla, **A** through **D,** and mandible, **E** through **H.** Still ligated in place, the brackets are gripped one by one with an 0.095 Orthopli, bracket removing plier *(ABR)* and lifted *outwardly* at a 45° angle. The indentation in the pliers fits into the gingival tie-wings *(arrows in **E** and **F**)* for a secure grip. This is a quick and gentle technique that leaves the brackets *(Br)* intact and fit for recycling, if so desired. The bond breaks in the adhesive-bracket interface, and the pattern of the mesh-backing is visible on the adhesive remaining on the teeth, **D** and **H.**

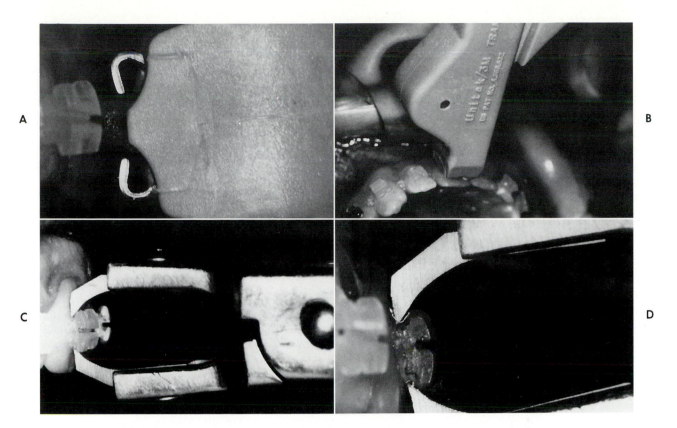

Fig. 10-37 Transcend 2000 ceramic brackets are recommended to be removed with the Transcend debonding plier, a reciprocal action pistol-type instrument, **A** and **B.** The debonding of GAC Allure ceramic brackets should be made with peripheral force application to the gingival tie-wings with an ETM 346 RT, or similar, plier, **C** and **D.**

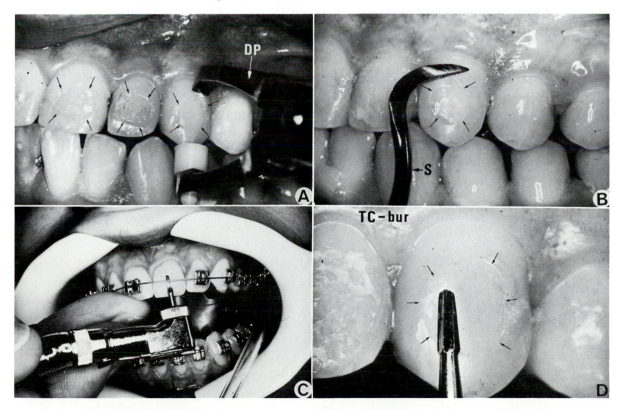

Fig. 10-38 Adhesive that remains after debracketing is removed by, **A** and **B,** scraping with debanding or debonding pliers *(DP)* or a scaler *(S)*. Whatever cannot be easily scraped off is removed with a tungsten carbide bur at about 30,000 rpm, **C** and **D.**

A preferred alternative for incisors is to use a suitable dome-tapered tungsten carbide (TC) bur (no. 1172, 1171, or 1171L) in a contra-angle handpiece (Fig. 10-38, *C* and *D*). It is important that adequate speed be used. Clinical experience and laboratory studies[204] indicate that approximately 30,000 rpm is optimal for rapid adhesive removal without enamel damage. Light *painting* movements of the bur should be used so as not to scratch the enamel. Water cooling should not be employed when the last remnants are removed, because it lessens the contrast with enamel. Higher speeds than 30,000 rpm may be useful for bulk adhesive removal but are contraindicated closer to the enamel because of the risk of marring the surface.[80,204] Slower speeds (10,000 rpm and less) are ineffective, and the increased jiggling vibration of the bur may be uncomfortable to the patient.

When all adhesive has been removed, polishing of the tooth surface may be performed with pumice (or a commercial prophylaxis paste) in a routine manner. However, in view of the normal wear of enamel, this step may be optional.

Characteristics of normal enamel

Apparently not every clinician is familiar with the dynamic changes that continuously take place throughout life in the outer, most superficial enamel layers.[110,162] Because a tooth surface is not in a static state, the *normal* structure differs considerably between young, adolescent, and adult teeth.[110] Normal wear must be considered in any discussion of tooth surface appearance after debonding. The characteristics are visible on both the clinical and the microscopic level.

The most evident clinical characteristics of *young* teeth that have just erupted into the oral cavity are the perikymata* that run around the tooth over its entire surface (Fig. 10-39). By scanning electron microscopy (SEM), the open enamel prism ends are recognized as small holes.[204] In *adult* teeth the clinical picture reflects wear and exposure to vary-

---

*The use of the enamel surface terms *perikymata* and *imbrications/imbrication lines* in the dental literature is inconsistent and confusing. The present terminology is based on recent recommendations (Risnes S: Rationale for consistency in the use of enamel surface terms: perikymata and imbrications, *Scand J Dent Res* 92:1, 1984).

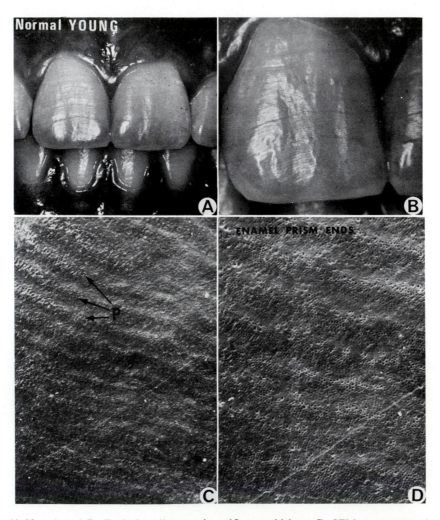

Fig. 10-39 A and **B,** Typical perikymata in a 10-year-old boy. **C,** SEM appearance. (×50.) **D,** Enlargement of the central portion in **C,** showing numerous small pits (the typical signs of enamel prism ends) and a crack. *P,* Perikymata.

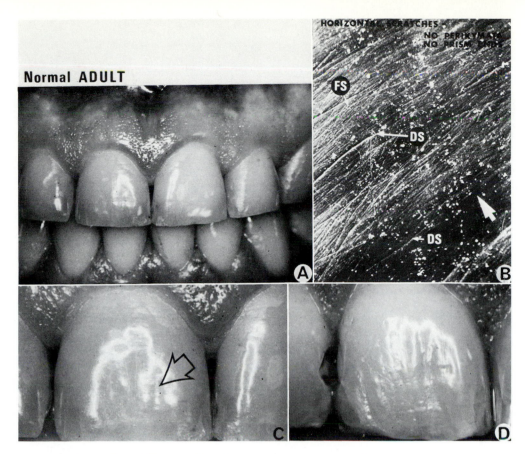

Fig. 10-40 **A, C,** and **D,** In adult teeth the perikymata remain in developmental grooves (*open arrow* in **C**). Note the other irregularities: vertical and horizontal scratches, pits, internal white spots, vertical cracks, **B,** SEM. (×50.) There are neither perikymata nor prism end openings. However, note the severe horizontal scratches. Most are fine *(FS)* but some are coarser and deeper *(DS)*.

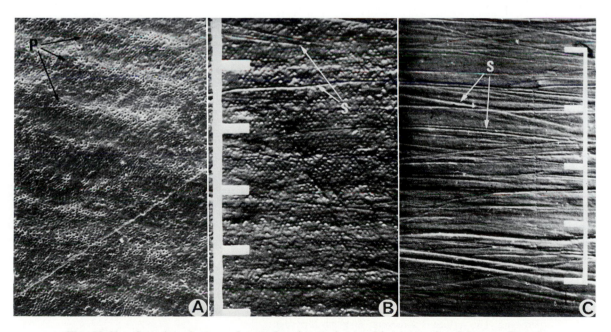

Fig. 10-41 Scanning electron micrographs of normal enamel in young, **A,** adolescent, **B,** and adult, **C,** teeth. Note the gradual transition from virgin tooth with perikymata *(P)* and open prism ends to a gradually increasing scratched *(S)* appearance. (Scale division is 0.1 mm.) (**B** and **C** courtesy F Mannerberg.)

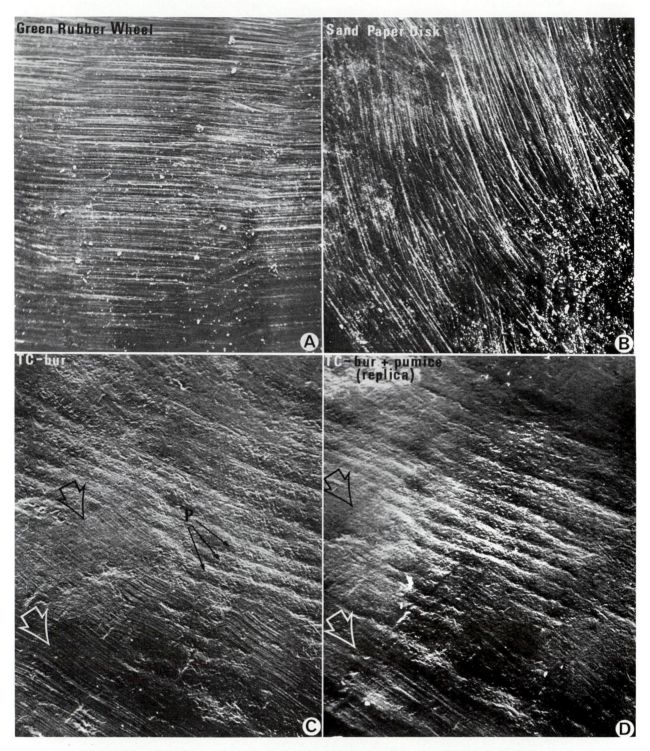

Fig. 10-42   Comparison of the effect of three debonding techniques on the enamel surface. **A** to **C,** SEM after adhesive removal without subsequent polishing. ($\times 50$.) Note that the scratches are of similar appearance in **A** and **B,** but that in **C** there is only slight faceting with fine scratches *(open arrows)* intermingled with the perikyma ridges *(P)*. **D,** Same area as in **C** in replica after pumicing. The surface is somewhat smoother *(arrows)*.

ing mechanical forces (toothbrushing habits, abrasive foodstuffs, etc.). In other words, the perikyma ridges are worn away and replaced by a scratched pattern (Fig. 10-40). Frequently, cracks are seen. By SEM there is no evidence of prism ends or perikymata; instead deep and finer scratches run across the surface[110,204] (Figs. 10-40 and 10-41). Teeth in *adolescents* reflect an intermediate stage (Fig. 10-41). According to Mannerberg, at 8 years of age practically all teeth show evident perikymata on from one third to two thirds of the tooth surface; at age 13 the number is reduced to 70% to 80%; and at age 18 only 25% to 50% of teeth demonstrate such ridges. Using a replica technique to study the gradual removal of artificial scratch marks on the teeth, Mannerberg found the normal wear to range from 0 to 2 μm per year. For comparison, a sandpaper disk that touches the enamel only a fraction of a second will leave scratch marks at least 5 μm deep.

Influence on enamel by different debonding instruments

By proposing an enamel surface index (ESI) with five scores (*0* to *4*) for tooth appearance and using replica scanning electron microscopy and step-by-step polishing, Zachrisson and Årtun[204] were able to compare different instruments commonly used in debonding procedures and to rank their degrees of surface marring on young permanent teeth.

The study demonstrated that (1) diamond instruments were unacceptable (score *4*); even fine diamond burs produced coarse scratches[139] and gave a deeply marred appearance; (2) medium sandpaper disks and a green rubber wheel produced similar scratches (score *3*) (Fig. 10-42) that could not be polished away; (3) fine sandpaper disks produced several marked and some even deeper scratches and a surface appearance largely resembling that of adult teeth (score *2*); (4) plain cut and spiral fluted TC burs operated at about 25,000 rpm were the only instruments that provided a satisfactory surface appppearance (score *1*) (Figs. 10-42 and 10-43); but (5) none of the instruments tested left the virgin tooth surface with its perikymata intact (score *0*).

The *clinical implication* of the study is that tungsten carbide (TC) burs produce the finest scratch pattern with the least enamel loss and are superior in their ability to reach difficult areas (Fig. 10-43)—pits, fissures, along the gingival margin, etc. A drawback remaining with present TC burs, however, is that they wear rapidly. For optimum efficiency the bur must be replaced when it becomes blunt (in clinical practice this generally means that the bur should be discarded after debonding an average patient with 15 to 20 bonded attachments). Increased-diameter burs or high-speed equipment may also be used for bulk removal.

The oval TC bur is useful for removing adhesive remnants after debonding retainers and brackets on the lingual surfaces of teeth.

An ultrasonic scaler may be an alternative. Although it has the advantage of patient comfort and its use can be delegated to auxiliary personnel, it also has several disadvantages: (1) water coolant results in poor contrast between adhesive and enamel; (2) the technique is slow; (3) ultrasonic tips need improvement in design; (4) gouges (10 to 20 μm deep) may remain on the tooth surface.[38]

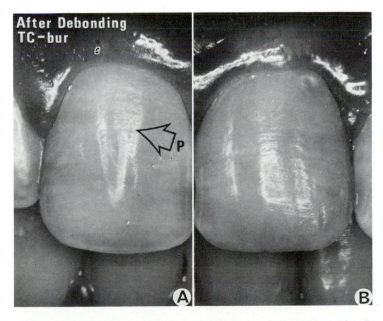

Fig. 10-43 After debonding with a tungsten carbide bur at low speed. (×2.) Gentleness of technique is reflected by the evident perikymata-like pattern *(P)* on debonded teeth *(arrow)*. Same case as in Fig. 10-66.

Amount of enamel lost in debonding

There is discussion in the orthodontic literature on how much enamel is actually removed in routine bonding and debonding. The amount is related to several factors, including the instruments used for prophylaxis and debonding and the type of adhesive resin employed.[52,139,177,204] It appears that the removal of unfilled resin is easier and may require less surface altering procedures than the removal of filled resins.

An initial prophylaxis with bristle brush for 10 to 15 seconds per tooth (which is, in fact, much longer than most clinical routines) may abrade away as much as 10 μm of enamel whereas only about 5 μm may be lost when a rubber cup is used.[139,177]

Cleanup of *unfilled resins* may be accomplished with hand instrumentation only, and this procedure generally results in a loss of 5 to 8 μm of enamel. Depending on the instruments used for prophylaxis, total enamel loss for unfilled resins may be 20 to 40 μm.[139,177]

Adequate removal of *filled resin* generally requires rotary instrumentation and the enamel loss is then 10 to 25 μm. Pus and Way[139] found a high-speed bur and green rubber wheel removes approximately 20 μm, and a low-speed TC bur removes around 10 μm, of enamel. Total enamel loss for filled resins may be 30 to 60 μm, depending on the instruments used for prophylaxis and debonding.[26,139,177]

The foregoing measurements are based on in vitro micrometer studies using an optical system of a profile projector and steel reference markers. Obviously this technique may be more accurate than judging enamel loss by SEM observations of damaged perikyma morphology, which gives an impression of a more limited enamel loss when TC burs are used carefully.[204] It has been claimed that many teeth can show perikymata-like structures after as much as 30 μm of enamel has been lost.[172] Additional deep-reaching enamel tearouts down to a depth of 100 μm and localized enamel loss of 150 to 160 μm have also been reported.[52]

In a *clinical perspective* the enamel loss encountered with routine bonding and debonding procedures, exclusive of deep enamel fractures or gouges resulting from injudicious use of hand instrument or burs, is not significant in terms of total thickness of enamel. The surfaces usually bonded have a thickness of 1500 to 2000 μm. Also the claim that removal of the outermost layer of enamel (which is particularly caries resistant and fluoride rich) may be harmful is not in full accordance with recent views on tooth surface dynamics and with clinical experience over many years. The facial tooth surfaces are left smooth and self-cleansing after debonding. It has been demonstrated that caries will not develop in such sites even if the entire enamel layer is removed.[119,120] Similarly, no histologic or clinical evidence of adverse effects was experienced after marked recontouring of canines that had been ground to resemble lateral incisors as long as the surfaces were left smooth and sufficient water cooling was used.[180,207] In that case about half the enamel thickness was removed.

Enamel Tearouts

Localized enamel tearouts have been reported to occur associated with bonding and debonding both metal[52] and ceramic brackets.[141] They may, at least in part, be related to the type of filler particles in the adhesive resin used for bonding and to the location of bond breakage. When comparisons were made between tooth surface appearance after debonding metal brackets attached with either macrofilled (10 to 30 μm) or microfilled (0.2 to 0.3 μm) adhesives, there was a difference when the resin was scraped off with pliers (Fig. 10-44).

It is likely that small filler particles may penetrate into the etched enamel to a greater degree than macrofillers may penetrate (Fig. 10-19). For instance, the *holes* corresponding to the dissolved enamel prism cores in the central etch type (Fig. 10-8, *B*) are 3 to 5 μm in diameter. Upon debonding, the small fillers would reinforce the adhesive tags. The macrofillers, on the other hand, would create a more natural breakpoint in the enamel-adhesive interface. Similarly, with unfilled resins there would be no *natural* breakpoint.

Ceramic brackets using chemical retention appear to cause enamel damage more often than those using mechanical retention.[141] This damage occurs probably because the location of the bond breakage is at the enamel-adhesive rather than at the adhesive-bracket interface.[141] Until more knowledge is gained to reduce the possibility of enamel damage, the *clinical implication* of these observations must be: (1) to use brackets that have mechanical retention, and debonding instruments and techniques, which primarily attack the adhesive-bracket interface, and to leave all or the majority of composite on the tooth (Figs. 10-35, *C* and *D*, and 10-36, *D* and *H*); and (2) to avoid scraping away adhesive remnants with hand instruments when unfilled or microfilled adhesive resins are used on anterior teeth. Although this technique may take a little extra time, it will eliminate the risk of developing detectable enamel tearoffs (Fig. 10-44).

Enamel cracks

Cracks, occurring as split lines in the enamel, are common but are often overlooked at clinical examination because most are difficult to distinguish clearly without special technique; generally they do not show up on routine, intra-oral photographs (Fig. 10-45). Thus finger shadowing in good light or, preferably, fiberoptic transillumination is needed for a proper impression of the crack[208] (Fig. 10-45). The origin of cracks is multicausal. Different forms of mechanical[140] and thermal insult may fracture the enamel cap after eruption; this is due to the marked difference in rigidity between enamel and dentin.

It is a distinct possibility that the sharp sound sometimes heard upon removal of bonded orthodontic brackets with pliers could be associated with the creation of enamel cracks. The occurrence of cracks in debonded, debanded, and orthodontically untreated teeth was discussed in our study.[208]

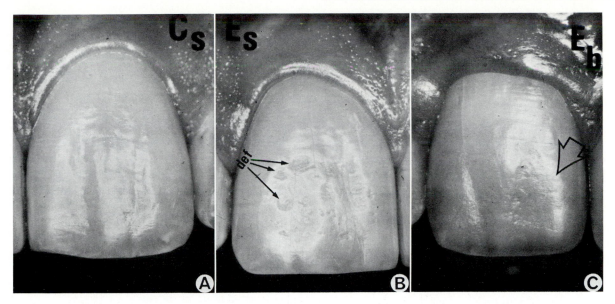

Fig. 10-44   Area after debonding. ($\times 2$.) **A,** Macrofilled adhesive scraped off *(C_s)*. **B,** Microfilled adhesive scraped off *(E_s)*. Note the localized enamel defects *(def)*. **C,** Microfilled adhesive removed with a TC bur *(E_b)*. Note the intact enamel surface with perikymata-like appearance *(arrow)*.

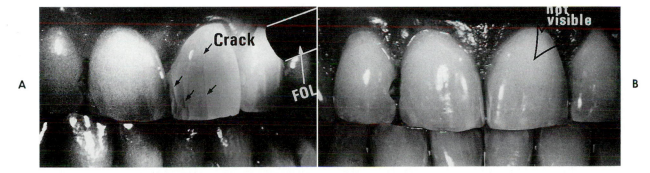

Fig. 10-45   Enamel cracks generally are not visible on intra-oral photographs. Several cracks clearly seen on the left central incisor with fiberoptic transillumination *(arrows* in **A**) are undetectable by routine photography, **B.** Note the vertical orientation of the cracks.

Using fiberoptic light technique, we examined more than 3000 teeth in 135 adolescents. The prevalence of cracks, their distribution per tooth, their location on the tooth surface, and the type (pronounced versus mild, horizontal versus vertical) were described. The most important findings were that (1) *vertical* cracks are common (in fact, more than 50% of all teeth studied had such cracks) however, there is great individual variation; (2) few *horizontal* and oblique cracks are observed normally; (3) there is no significant difference between the three groups with regard to prevalence and location of cracks; and (4) the most notable cracks (i.e., those visible under normal office illumination) are on the maxillary central incisors and canines.

The *clinical implication* of these findings is that if an orthodontist (1) observes several distinct enamel cracks on a patient's teeth after debonding, particularly on teeth other than maxillary canines and central incisors, or (2) detects cracks in a predominantly horizontal direction this is an indication that the bonding and/or debonding technique used may need improvement. For instance, wrong technique or too much force used in removal of the bracket and residual adhesive may be suspected.

Another clinical implication may be the need for pretreatment examination of cracks, notifying the patient and/or parents if pronounced cracks are present. The reason for this examination is that patients may be overly inspective after appliance removal and may detect cracks that were present before treatment, of which they were unaware. They may question the orthodontist about the cause of the cracks. Without pretreatment diagnosis and documentation (most cracks are not visible on routine intra-oral slides), it is almost impossible to prove that such cracks are indeed unrelated to the orthodontic treatment.

Adhesive remnant wear

Whether the base is cut off or the bracket is merely *lifted* away during bracket removal, large amounts of adhesive will generally remain on the enamel surface (Figs. 10-36 and 10-46). Frequently adhesive has been found on the tooth surface, even after attempts to remove it with mechanical instruments (pliers, scaler, abrasive wheels, burs, stones, ultrasonics, scalpel, etc.).[38,41,52,80] This is true for unfilled and for different types of filled resins. Because of color resemblance to the teeth, particularly when wet, residual adhesive may easily remain undetected.[62] In other instances adhesive may be left on purpose, since the operator expects that it will wear off with time.

Abrasive wear depends to a large extent on the size, type, and amount of reinforcing fillers in the adhesive.[33] Thus unfilled or lightly filled resins with small filler particles may abrade away more readily than adhesives with larger reinforcing filler particles. Brobakken and Zachrisson[33] studied the resistance of some commonly used bonding materials to abrasive wear over a specific time. Somewhat surprisingly, the degree of abrasion was minimal not only for diacrylate adhesives with macrofillers (Concise, Solo-Tach) but also for an adhesive resin with submicrometer-sized filler particles (Endur). When, at the time of debonding, varying amounts of adhesive were purposely left on the teeth assumed to be the most exposed to toothbrushing forces (i.e., the maxillary left canine and one neighboring tooth), the abrasion over a 12-month period was almost insignificant in clinical terms. Only thin films of residual adhesive showed any reduction in size (Fig. 10-47).

The *clinical implications* of leaving residual adhesive after debonding are not clear. Gwinnett and Ceen[79] reported that small remnants of unfilled sealant did not predispose to plaque accumulation and did begin to wear away with time. However, this finding cannot automatically be transferred to different types of filled adhesives, some of which have much greater wear resistance and accumulate plaque more readily.[205] The presence of extremely thin films of adhesive may not be of esthetic or other concern since any color change in the films probably cannot be perceived. In some instances it may even be advantageous to *seal* surface irregularities like pits and grooves to protect against demineralization. Nonetheless, in light of Brobakken and Zachrisson's findings,[33] it would seem to be too optimistic to believe that residual filled adhesive will quickly disappear by itself after debonding (Fig. 10-48); it appears irresponsible to leave large accumulations of adhesive.

Reversal of decalcification

White spots or areas of demineralization are carious lesions of varying extent. The incidence and severity of white spots after a full term of orthodontic treatment have been studied by several authors.* The general conclusion was that individual teeth, banded or bonded, may exhibit significantly more white spot formation than may untreated control teeth (Fig. 10-49). In a multibonded technique (with lack of any preventive fluoride program) Gorelick et al.[75] found that 50% of the patients experienced an increase in white spots. The highest incidence was in the maxillary incisors, particularly the laterals. This obvious degree of iatrogenic damage suggested the need for preventive programs using fluoride associated with fixed appliance orthodontic treatment.

Extensive overviews of the different methods of *ortho-*

---

*References 75, 116, 128, 210, 211.

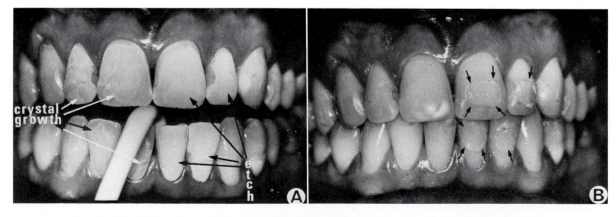

Fig. 10-46 Comparison of debonding after acid etch (left side) and crystal growth (right side). **A,** Clinical view subsequent to enamel conditioning. **B,** After debracketing with the squeeze technique (Fig. 10-35). The right side is virtually free of residual adhesive whereas the left shows obvious breaks in the adhesive-bracket mesh interface *(arrows)*.

dontic fluoride administration have been presented.[37,194] Daily rinsing with dilute (0.05%) sodium fluoride solution throughout the periods of treatment and retention, plus regular use of a fluoride dentifrice, is recommended as a routine procedure for all orthodontic patients.[194] In addition, painting a fluoride varnish over caries-susceptible sites at each visit may be useful in patients with hygiene problems.[33] The

weak fluoride mouthrinse is effective yet has few risks, and most patients can easily manage to use it for a 1- or 2- year period. Also, definite responsibility must be given to the patient to avoid decalcifications during treatment.

Much evidence now exists from both in vivo and in vitro studies to support the claim that small carious lesions can *heal,* a process usually referred to as *remineraliza-*

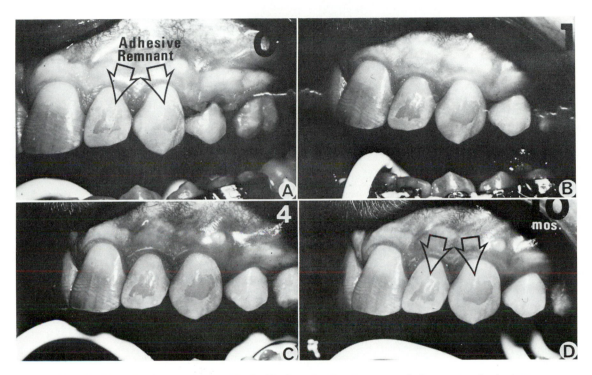

Fig. 10-47   Abrasive wear of residual adhesive after bracket removal. Remnants of submicrometer-sized filled resin purposely left on the maxillary left canine and lateral incisor. Standardized intra-oral photographs after quick etching (10 sec) show the condition at the time of debonding, **A,** and 1, 4, and 10 months later, **B, C,** and **D.** There is remarkably little change caused by mechanical abrasion throughout the year. Clearly, this kind of abrasive wear must be regarded as clinically insignificant.

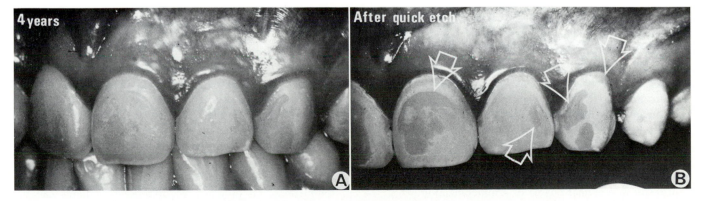

Fig. 10-48   Insignificant abrasive wear of residual macrofilled adhesive (Concise) left on enamel after bracket removal as long as 4 years earlier. **A,** Clinical view. **B,** After quick etch (10 sec) for better visualization of adhesive remnants *(open arrows).*

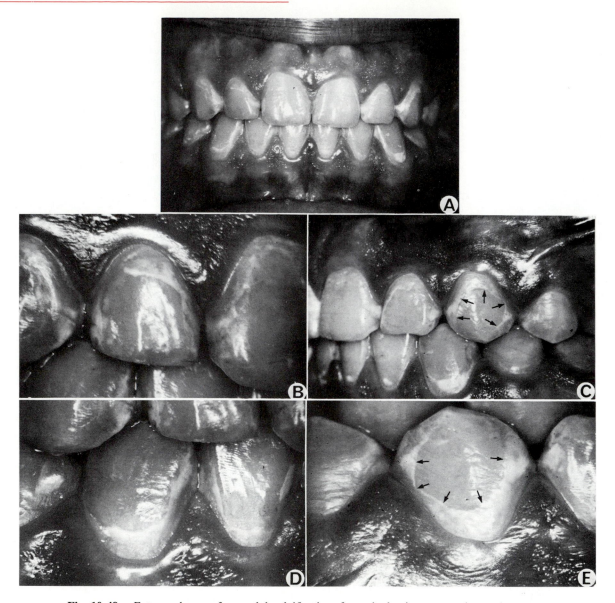

Fig. 10-49 Extreme degree of enamel decalcification after orthodontic treatment in a caries-prone patient. Note that white spot lesions occur on multiple teeth, **A.** In fact, the contour of the bonded brackets can be seen on several teeth (*arrows* in **C** and **E**).

tion.[18,129,162] Dental caries may not be a process of simple continuing demineralization. Rather, caries may be the result of a dynamic series of events, with remineralization occurring naturally during the formation of a carious lesion. Fluoride ions greatly enhance the degree of remineralization (incorporation of calcium and phosphate from the saliva) and reduce the time required for this mechanism to occur.[61,162,173] Only lower levels of fluoride are required to trigger the mechanism; raising the fluoride level further does not result in a greater degree of remineralization.[162]

Recent evidence also supports the contention that one of the chief mechanisms whereby fluoride reduces caries incidence is remineralization.[57,61,162] Other fluoride effects may

be on plaque adhesion (both quantitively and qualitatively),[150] although the more traditional theory: that fluoride increases enamel resistance, is probably not too significant. Thus fluoride ion may be concentrated into demineralized areas, which thereby act as reservoirs promoting remineralization from the saliva.

Although there is sufficient clinical evidence to prove that the process of white spot formation can be reversed, at least in part, more information is necessary before the optimal remineralization program for orthodontic patients can be established.

Årtun and Thylstrup[15] found that removal of the cariogenic challenge after debonding results in arrest of further demineralization, and a gradual regression of the lesion at the clinical level takes place primarily because of surface abrasion with some redeposition of minerals. However, Øgaard et al.[129] observed that remineralization of surface softened enamel (like under a loose band or bracket from one visit to another) and remineralization of subsurface lesions are completely different processes. The surface softened lesions remineralize faster and more completely than subsurface lesions, which remineralize extremely slowly, probably because of lesion arrest by widespread use of fluoride. Visible white spots that develop during orthodontic therapy should therefore *not* be treated with concentrated fluoride agents immediately after debonding, since this procedure will arrest the lesions and prevent complete repair. It is to be expected that in the future, more effective methods for caries reversal will become available.

At present it seems advisable to recommend a period of 2 to 3 months of good oral hygiene but without fluoride supplementation associated with the debonding session. This should reduce the clinical visibility of the white spots. More fluoride may tend to precipitate calcium phosphate onto the enamel surface and block the surface pores. This would limit remineralization to the superficial part of the lesion, and the optical appearance of the white spot would not be reduced.

BONDED RETAINERS

Permanent maintenance of the achieved orthodontic result after successful treatment of malocclusion is undoubtedly a great, if not the greatest, problem for clinicians treating young patients. This is especially true for adult patients. Therefore the relative scarcity of literature on the subject is surprising.

The use of fixed bonded retainers is increasing,[77] and the various forms allow more differentiated retention than before. Bonded retainers also have other advantages:

1. Completely invisible from in front (Figs. 10-50 and 10-62)
2. Reduced caries risk under loose bands
3. Reduced need for long-term patient cooperation
4. Prolonged semipermanent, and even permanent, retention when conventional retainers do not provide the same degree of stability

The term *differential retention,* as introduced by James L. Jensen,[89] implies that special attention is directed toward the strongest or most important predilection site for relapse in each and every case. Thus the most appropriate mode of retention for the postorthodontic situation in question should be employed; it should be based upon a careful evaluation of the pretreatment diagnostic records, habits, patient cooperation, growth pattern, and age. Implicit in the intro-

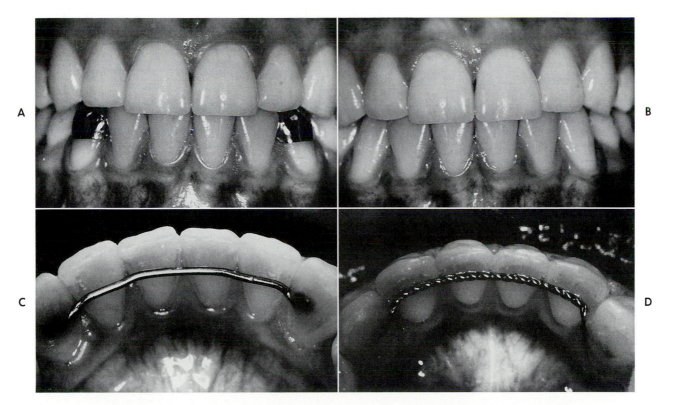

Fig. 10-50 Conventional, **A,** and bonded, **B** through **D,** retainers. **C,** The adhesive covers a terminal loop, whereas **D** shows the thick, twisted wire bonded on the canines only.

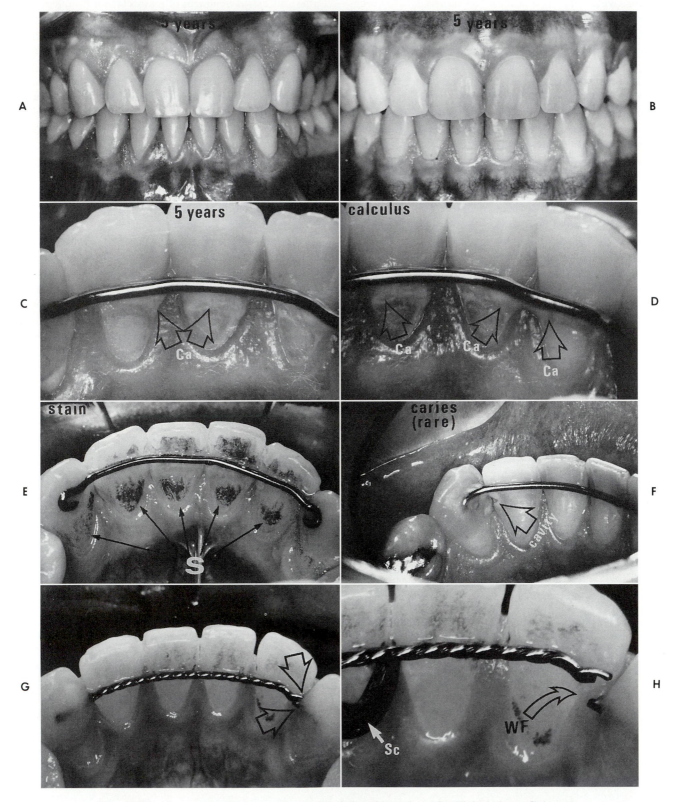

Fig. 10-51 Long-term appearance of some bonded retainers. **A** and **B,** Clinical views. **C** through **E.** At 5-year follow-up the accumulation of calculus *(Ca)* and stain *(s)* is common whereas in **F,** caries *(open arrow)* is extremely rare. **G** and **H,** Fatigue fracture of the wire mesial to right canine. **I** through **L,** Two types of failure of bonded lingual retainers.

duction of the acid etch technique for direct-bonded retainers is the provision of a variety of new methods for retention. This discussion will review the current level of technical expertise regarding bonded retainers.

Since the technique is comparatively new, any discussion of it is weakened by the evident lack of published clinical and long-term research findings with various types of retainers and splints. For this reason it will, to a large part, be based on my own experiences. The following subdivisions are used:

Mandibular canine-to-canine (3-3) retainers
Mandibular premolar-to-premolar retainers
Direct contact splinting
Flexible spiral wire (FSW) retainers
 Retainers that prevent space from reopening
 Hold retainers for individual teeth

In the following pages, two basically different types of multistrand wire will be discussed—a *thick* one (0.032 inch) and a *thin* one (0.0215 inch)—with entirely different indications and modes of bonding.

Bonded lingual canine-to-canine retainers

In 1977 promising short-term clinical results (1 to 2½ years) with 43 bonded lingual canine-to-canine (3-3) retainers were reported.[197] These retainers were made of 0.032 to 0.036 inch round stainless steel wire, with loops at the terminal ends, and they were direct bonded with a wear-resistant restorative composite material (Concise). Our later clinical experience has confirmed that long-term results are also encouraging. It is now clear that bonded 3-3 retainers can provide excellent results[14,25,75,199] (Fig. 10-51) if meticulous construction and bonding techniques are followed, along with some modifications of the original design.

In differential retention philosophy the purpose of a bonded 3-3 retainer is (1) to prevent incisor recrowding; (2) to hold the achieved lower incisor position in space; and (3) to keep the rotation center in the incisor area when there is a mandibular anterior growth rotation tendency. It may be particularly indicated in persons with a flat functional occlusal plane[89] (p. 589), open bite, Class II with rotation center in the premolar area (Björk's anterior rotation Type III[27]), or Class III growth tendency.

The standard appliance is bonded to the lingual surfaces of the canine teeth. Supplementary bonding of incisors is *not* recommended with thick wire diameters (0.032 inch and over) since such bonds tend to break and they complicate oral hygiene procedures. The bar, which was originally constructed from plain blue Elgiloy wire* with a loop at each

---

*Rocky Mountain/Orthodontics, Denver, Colorado.

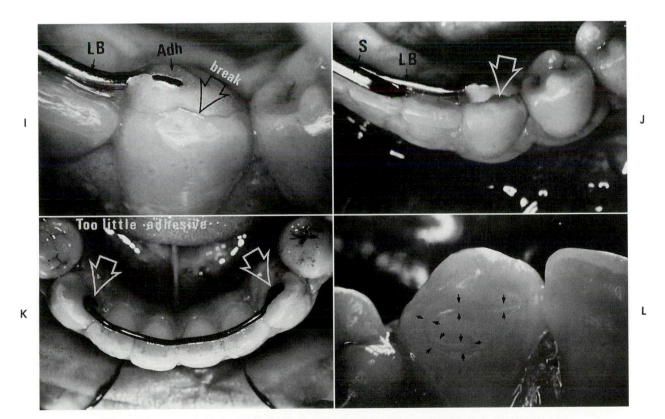

Fig 10-51, cont'd　I and J, Type I, in the enamel-adhesive interface. K and L, Type II, in the adhesive-retainer interface. Note the impression of the terminal loop in the adhesive in L *(arrows)*.

terminal end for added retention[197] (Fig. 10-50) has more recently been replaced by a similar-diameter multistrand wire* (Figs. 10-50 and 10-51). Retainers made of this wire are neater since there is adequate retention of the adhesive in the wire spirals. Bonding is still done with microfilled composite because such adhesives provide the strongest bonds[205] and show comparatively little abrasion over extended periods.[33] Thus the retainers can be made optimally strong and neat and can be expected to remain so for a long time.

Some companies supply preformed lingual 3-3 retainers with bonding pads (Fig. 10-52). These may be more difficult to fit and bond tightly. At the same time it may also be more difficult to obtain maximum contact on the lingual surfaces of all four incisors. The short- and long-term success of preformed retainers with pads has not been reported, whether bonded directly or indirectly (Fig. 10-52).

Failure Analysis

Initial failures with bonded lingual 3-3 retainers were classified into two types.[199] *Type I failure* was related to separation at the tooth-adhesive interface (Fig. 10-51, *I* and *J*) and occurred with the highest frequency. It was most

---

*Unitek Corporation, Monrovia, California.

commonly the result of moisture contamination or movement of the lingual bar during the initial polymerization of the composite. *Type II failure* occurred at the adhesive-retainer wire interface (Fig. 10-51, *K* and *L*) and was due to inadequate bulk of adhesive for sufficient strength (or abrasive wear of the adhesive). *It is important to notice that with adequate technique, both types of failure can be avoided.* In other words, a clinician who experiences discouraging failure rates should reevaluate and improve the technique of making bonded lingual retainers.

Technical procedure

The following clinical recommendations (Fig. 10-53) represent our present approach. This approach is suggested to counteract the aforementioned reasons for bond breakage. The basic principles have been tested clinically over several years. *Although it may seem possible to take shortcuts, this is strongly discouraged;* strict adherence to a meticulous technique has been found to be the key to long-term success.

1. While the orthodontic appliances remain in place, take a snap impression of the patient's teeth and pour a working model of hard stone (plaster is inadequate, since it may abrade during wire fabrication; then the retainer will not fit in the mouth).

2. Use 0.032 spiral wire perfectly fitted to the lingual

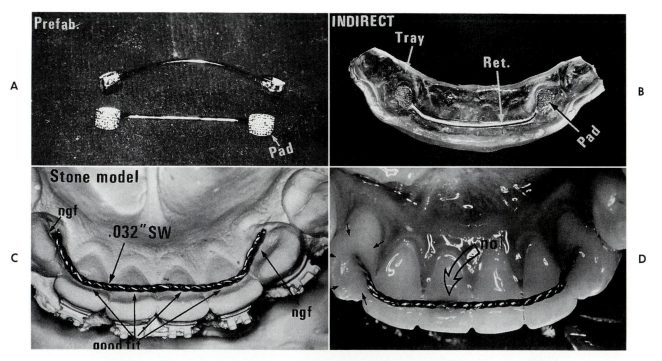

Fig. 10-52 Failure rates for a prefabricated 3-3 retainer with distal pads, **A,** and indirect bonding of such retainers, **B,** have not been reported. My preference, **C** through **F,** in a 3-3 retainer incorporates a good fit of wire to the lingual surface for all four incisors but not for the canines (*ngf*), where the wire will be covered with adhesive. **D,** With the thick (0.032 inch) spiral wire (*SW*) only the terminal ends should be included. Bonds, like the one to the incisor (*arrow*) with this wire, are prone to break since physiologic tooth movement is not possible.

surfaces of all incisors, with the working model as a guide. Make offsets in the wire as needed; use of the Tweed pliers is recommended for the thick spiral wire. In our experience it is almost impossible to get as intimate an adaptation to the critical areas of all teeth when a direct approach (no working model) is used. Cut the wire to required length.

3. Clean the lingual surfaces of both canines with a TC bur or pumice.

4. Check the position of the wire in the mouth. When optimal, fix with steel ligatures around the bracket wings of two or three incisors (Fig. 10-53, *B*).

5. The lingual saliva evacuator-bite block-tongue holder provides a dry working field with good overview (Fig. 10-53, *A* and *B*). One to three cotton rolls can be placed in the labial lower incisor region (but the lip expander is not used).

6. With retainer wire in place, etch the lingual surfaces of the canines with 37% phosphoric acid for 60 seconds. Rinse and dry completely. (Use a high-speed

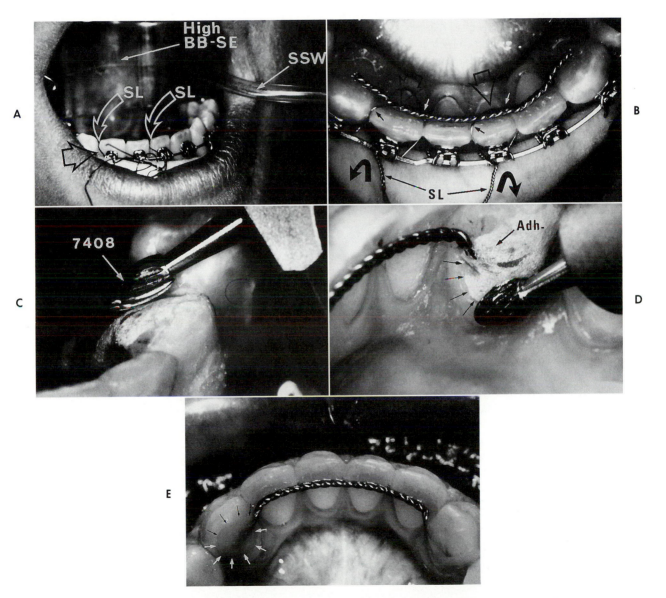

Fig. 10-53 Making the bonded 3-3 retainer. **A,** Lingual saliva ejector with high bite block *(BB-SE)* secures an optimally dry working field with no interfering appliances. **B,** The 0.032 inch spiral wire is positioned by means of two or three steel ligatures *(SL)*. A small amount of fast-setting adhesive is used for tacking. In **C** and **D,** trimming with 7408 TC bur provides optimal contour of the adhesive, while avoiding contact with the gingival tissue. **E,** Final result. Adhesive at the terminal ends *only*.

vacuum evacuator.) Sealant is not needed on lingual surfaces, partly because of the reduced risk of decalcification. This fast and efficient procedure reduces the risk of moisture contamination.

7. Bond the retainer using a two-step procedure:

   A. *Tacking:* Tack the wire to both canines with a *small* amount of fast-setting mix of prediluted (10- to 15-drop) Concise paste A and liquid resin B in a 2:1 volume ratio (Fig. 10-53, *B*). This initial tacking is vital for strength. Since the wire must not now be displaced, the bulk of adhesive can be added in a totally undisturbed setting.

   B. *Bulk of adhesive:* Bond the retainer wire to the right and left canines with a slow-setting mix of the 10- to 15-drop Concise.[16] It takes some experience to find the right consistency. If too much liquid is added, the adhesive will drift away from where it is placed and may flow interdentally or contact the gingiva.

8. Check with a mouth mirror to see that enough adhesive is used, and add more adhesive wherever required (often the distogingival corners). It is important to have *abundant* adhesive in both a mesiodistal and an incisogingival direction (Fig. 10-52, *C* through *E*).

9. Trim along the gingival margin and contour the bulk with oval TC burs (no. 7408 and 7006) (Fig. 10-53, *C* and *D*). *This step is mandatory.* It is not possible to obtain neat, yet strong appliances without the use of burs. Trim the adhesive so it has a *smooth gentle contour* in an incisogingival direction (Fig. 10-53). The same bur is ideal on the lingual surface at the time of retainer debonding. Interdentally, a smaller bur (no. 2) is used.

10. Instruct the patient in proper oral hygiene and use of dental floss (Fig. 10-54). It is possible to direct the floss under a 3-3 retainer wire without aids, but a floss threader facilitates the procedure. Patients are instructed to floss once daily to prevent accumulation of calculus and plaque.

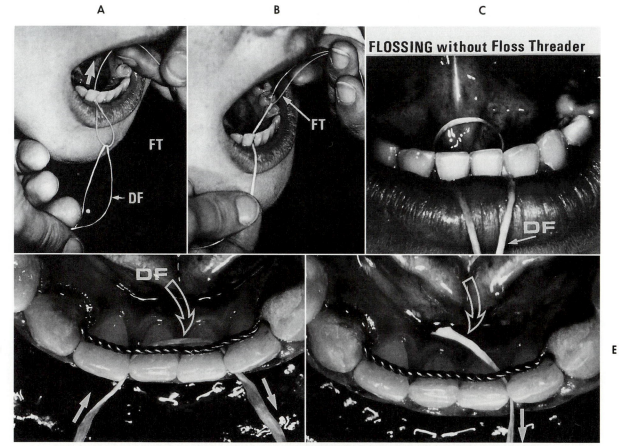

Fig. 10-54 Interdental cleaning under a bonded 3-3 retainer. **A** and **B**, A floss threader *(FT)* may be used to gain access under the wire. **C**, If a floss threader is not available, a loop is formed over two incisors. **D**, The loop is moved under the retainer bar *(arrow)*. **E**, When one end of the floss is pulled in, the other will snap free *(open arrow)* and can be grabbed with the fingers. Patients are instructed to move the floss over the interproximal surfaces once daily.

Long-Term Experience

Experience with bonded 3-3 retainers over 10 to 15 years is excellent, provided careful bonding technqiue is used.[200] The 3-3 retainers made of 0.32-inch spiral wire are neat, clean, and extremely safe for long-term use, since patients will immediately notice any loosening. For several years, it has been my preferred routine mandibular retainer for children and also for many adults. However, many patients apparently have difficulties keeping the area clean, despite patient instruction in hygiene, and accumulations of supragingival calculus (Fig. 10-51, *C* and *D*) and stain (Fig. 10-51, *E*) are often noted alongside and beneath the retaining wire.

Decalcification and caries are only exceptionally observed (Fig. 10-51, *F*). Thus in 60 children who had worn such a retainer for an average of 24 months, Gorelick et al.[75] reported no white spot formation at all on the lingual surfaces of bonded canines or on the lingual surfaces of the incisors against which the wire had rested. Also clinical data indicate no significant difference in plaque and calculus accumulation between the round and thick spiral retainer wires.[10,14]

The presence of even large amounts of calculus around mandibular retainers need not be alarming in young, healthy patients with no periodontal pockets. Gaare et al.[69] recently compared the effect of toothbrushing after professional prophylaxis in patients with large amounts of calculus (removal requiring an average removal time of 1 hour per patient) with the effect of toothbrushing as the sole hygiene method. They found no significant benefit of the calculus removal, which supports the hypothesis that it is not the calculus but the plaque that forms on it that has pathogenic potential. The effects of calculus accumulations on retainers in adults with existing periodontal problems are unknown at present.

The improved 0.32-inch wire now available is twisted more tightly than before, which is an advantage from a stability point of view. In the future, it could be interesting to test larger diameters of spiral wire, since in some cases accidental distortion over the long span from canine-to-canine may occur. However, at present such wires are not available.

Since the retainers are invisible, there may be a problem in deciding when to remove them. Extended retention periods (about 6 years) are recommended by some clinicians,[76,81] and we too have found them favorable in many patients, while waiting for the patient's third molars to erupt. However, as an alternative, the bonded retainer may be replaced after some years with a removable one for long-term or permanent nighttime wear.

Bonded lingual premolar-to-premolar retainers

In certain postorthodontic situations it may be desirable to extend the traditional mandibular canine-to-canine retainer posteriorly to include fixation and attachment to the first or second premolar teeth.[148]

The purpose of the premolar-to-premolar retainer in differential retention terms is to: (1) maintain lower incisor intrusion and anteroposterior changes, (2) prevent lower incisor crowding, and (3) hold expansion of the mandibular

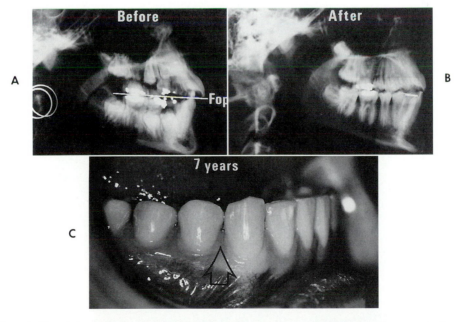

Fig. 10-55 A bonded premolar-to-premolar retainer may be useful in preventing reextrusion of the mandibular anteriors in a patient with a deep overbite when the incisors are high above the functional occlusal plane *(FOP)* before treatment. **A** and **B,** Cephalograms before and after orthodontic treatment. **C,** Stable contact between the first premolar and canine 2 years after the bonded 4-3/3-4 retainer was removed (years posttreatment).

first premolars.[148] This retainer may be indicated particularly for deep overbites in which the incisors are high above the functional occlusal plane.[89] (Fig. 10-55), since a 3-3 retainer will not prevent extrusion of the anterior segment, and whenever expansion has been made over the first premolar area.[148]

Technical Procedure

The clinical procedures involved in the bonding of the 4-3/3-4 and 5-3/3-5 (where first premolars have been extracted) retainers are similar to those mentioned previously. The retainer is bonded at four locations (Fig. 10-56); as a

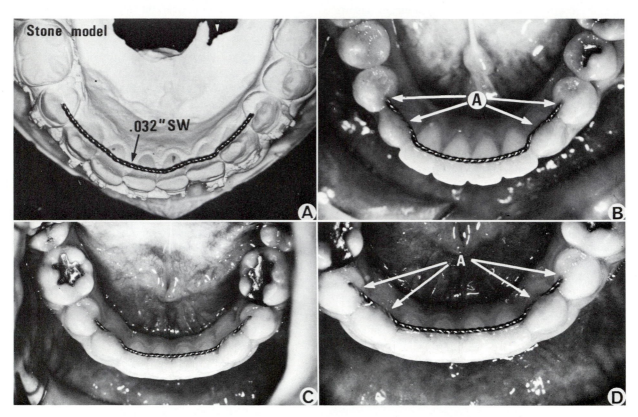

Fig. 10-56   Making the bonded 4-3-3-4 retainer **A,** Precision fitting of thick (0.032) spiral wire *(SW)* on the stone model. **B,** Wire bonded with adhesive at four sites *(arrows)*. **C** and **D,** Typical appearance. *A,* Adhesive.

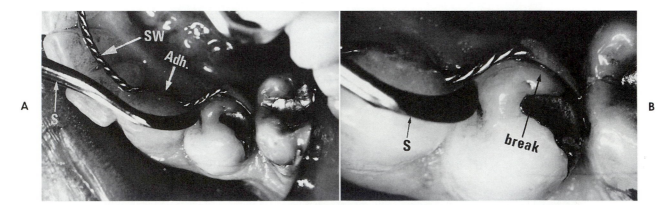

Fig. 10-57   **A** and **B,** Bonded trial 4-3-3-4 retainers to the lingual surfaces of the premolars *(arrows)* were not successful. **B,** Bond breakage *(arrows)*. A scaler *(S)* is inserted only to visualize the break area.

rule the occlusal fossa of the premolars is used rather than the lingual surface. The reason for this is the rather poor strength of retainer wire bonded on the lingual surfaces of premolars and molars (Fig. 10-57).

When bonding to the premolars, only the mesial portion of the occlusal fossa is used to avoid occlusal interferences.

Long-Term Experiences

Clinical experimentation over the past several years has been only partially encouraging. The bonds to the *occlusal fossae* are *durable* but prone to abrasive wear, and it is difficult to clean satisfactorily between the canine and premolar.

Direct contact splinting

In the late 1970s several preliminary and short-term clinical reports were published on direct contact splinting of segments of teeth. They appeared mostly in the orthodontic and periodontic literature and represented attempts to prevent postorthodontic space reopening between teeth and to provide stability against traumatic jiggling (so-called periodontal splints). Other reports[154] suggested adding an artificial tooth where one incisor was missing and securing it with splinting of the contact, either unilaterally or bilaterally. A variety of techniques and adhesive resins were used.[102,151] Although some degree of clinical success was

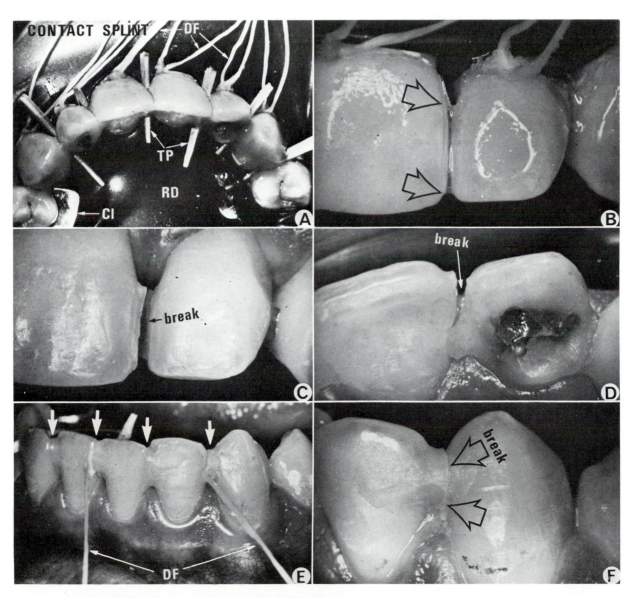

Fig. 10-58 Direct contact splinting. **A,** Working field with rubber dam *(RD)*, toothpicks *(TP)*, dental floss *(DF)*, and clamp *(Cl)*. **B,** Contact splint using UV-light polymerized sealant. Note the wide contact area in the incisoapical direction *(open arrows)*. **C,** Break after 2 months of splinting. **D** to **F,** Breaks *(arrows)* in different splints where restorative composite was used. Dental floss *(DF)* is inserted in **E** to show the location of the failures.

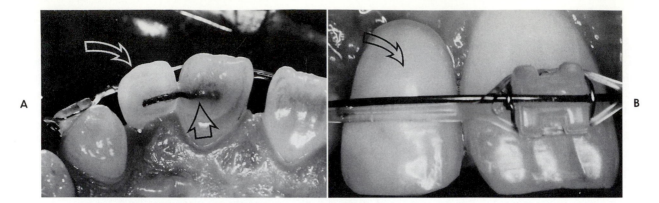

Fig. 10-59 Missing lateral incisor case where an acrylic pontic was direct-splinted to the central incisor during the orthodontic treatment. Note braided rectangular wire reinforcement.

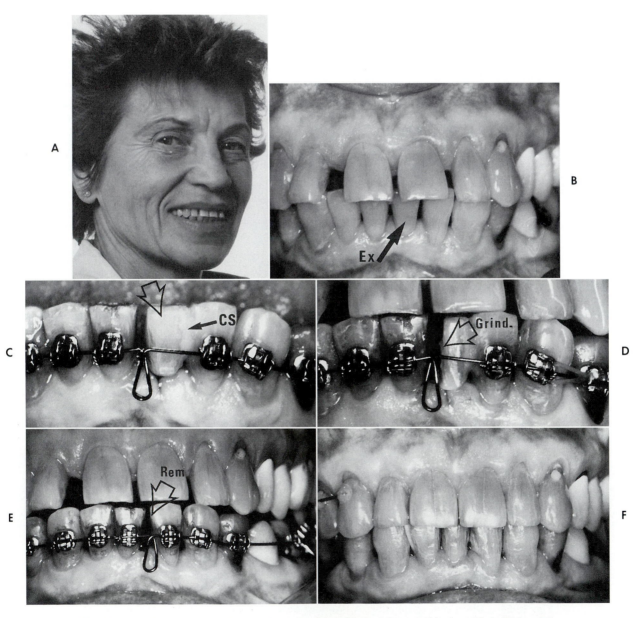

Fig. 10-60 Direct contact splinting of extracted mandibular left central incisor (*Ex* in **B**) in adult woman, where the protruding lower incisors had caused multiple spacing of maxillary incisors, **A** and **B.** The patient was anxious not to show the extraction space. During treatment, **C** through **E**, the natural pontic *(open arrow)* was gradually ground and finally removed, **E.** Final result is shown in **F.**

experienced, follow-up results indicated a high percentage of bond breakage.[88,151,170,195]

Bond breakage was clearly illustrated in some experiments on postorthodontic splinting[195] (Fig. 10-58). Careful technique involved the use of rubber dam for moisture control, toothpicks to avoid interdental flow of adhesive, and bonding adhesive applied in a wide incisogingival area (Fig. 10-58). A number of clinical situations calling for specific retention were addressed: closed median diastema, closed extraction spaces, ectopic incisors, impacted canines, holding of six mandibular anterior teeth after decrowding, and labial expansion or retraction. Two different restorative-type composite resins and one UV light-polymerized sealant were tested.[195] The results were consistently discouraging; breakage or fracture of the adhesive occurred within a few weeks or months whenever larger segments than two teeth were splinted (Fig. 10-58).

This is in clear contrast to our experience with the FSW retainers (p. 596). *The apparent reason for the bond breakage is the need for independent physiologic tooth movement during function.* Unfortunately, the rigidity of the contact splints does not facilitate individual tooth movements, and it is therefore *not* recommended as a mode of bonded retention.

Long-Term Experience

Based on the foregoing and other studies, the following can generally be stated: (1) contact splinting without some form of wire reinforcement should no longer be considered a method of choice, since wire supplementation greatly reduces bond failure rates; (2) whenever wire reinforcement is used, it should allow proper cleaning and some slight physiologic mobility of the bonded teeth.

When contact splinting on pontics is used to hide *empty spaces* after extractions of premolars in children or lower incisors in adults, it is recommended that the splint be reinforced with a small piece of braided wire (Figs. 10-59 through 10-61). If the splint breaks, this wire will keep the pontic in position.

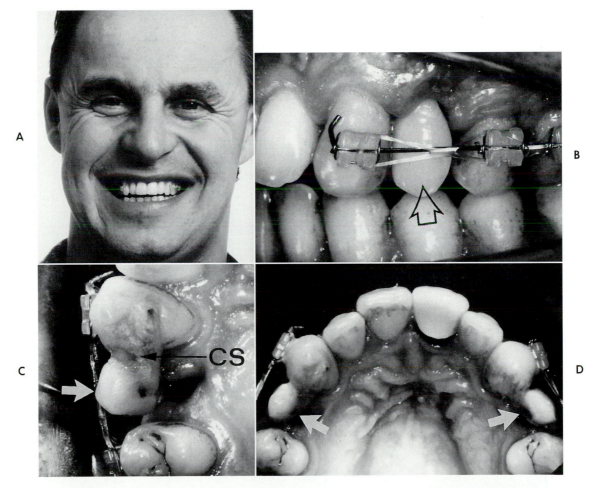

Fig. 10-61 Direct contact splinting of acrylic pontics to hide the premolar extraction spaces in adult male patient, **A,** concerned not to show *empty spaces.* Both contact splints *(CS)* were reinforced with a braided rectangular wire, which kept the pontics in place during the canine retraction period despite resin fracture in both contact points. The pontics were ground on the distal surfaces *(arrows in* **D***)* to accommodate to the space conditions.

Flexible spiral wire (FSW) retainers

Clinical experience and differential retention philosophy have demonstrated the need for two types of bonded wire retainer:

1. Thick wire (0.032-inch diameter)
2. Thin wire (0.0215-inch diameter)

The thick wire is used for 3-3 and 4-3/3-4 retainers and bonded on the terminal dental units only (p. 585), whereas the thin spiral wire is used for various retainers in which *all* teeth in a segment are bonded. As mentioned, bond breakage occurs too easily when other than terminal anchor teeth are bonded to the thick spiral wire diameter.

In discussing the FSW retainer the following subdivisions will be used:

1. Principle and general background
2. Advantages and disadvantages
3. Long-term experience
4. Technical procedures
5. Indications
6. Case presentations

In 1977 our preliminary results indicated that bonded retainers using thin multistrand flexible wire (0.015- to 0.020-inch diameter) appeared to be suitable for preventing space reopening in different clinical situations[197] (Fig. 10-62). Long-term (up to 6 years) results are now available for different wire types, verifying that the combination of thin spiral wire with wear-resistant bonded composite can provide a useful mode of retention for a variety of post-orthodontic situations[50,199,200,202] (Fig. 10-63).

Advantages and Disadvantages

FSW retainers have several *advantages:*

1. They may allow safe retention of treatment results when proper retention is difficult, or even impossible, with traditional removable appliances.
2. They allow slight movement of all bonded teeth and segments of teeth. Apparently this is the main reason for the excellent long-term results.
3. They are invisible.
4. They are neat and clean.
5. They can be placed out of occlusion in most instances. If not, there remains the possibility of hiding the wire under a slight groove in the enamel.
6. They can be used alone or in combination with removable retainers.

However, there are some *disadvantages* with such retainers. Good oral hygiene of the patients is mandatory. Flossing is recommended in each interdental space incisal to the wire once daily and using a dental floss threader gingival to the wire is recommended several times weekly. The gingival reaction is, of course, also dependent on careful removal of excess adhesive at the time of retainer bonding.[200] Also side effects in the form of undesirable movement of bonded teeth may occur if the wire is too thin and/or

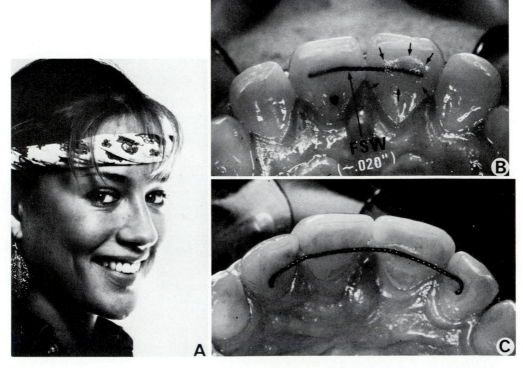

Fig. 10-62 Flexible spiral wire retainer in which thin wire (approximately 0.020 inch diameter) is used. **A,** Bonded retainer, invisible. **B,** Two-unit and, **C,** four-unit retainers.

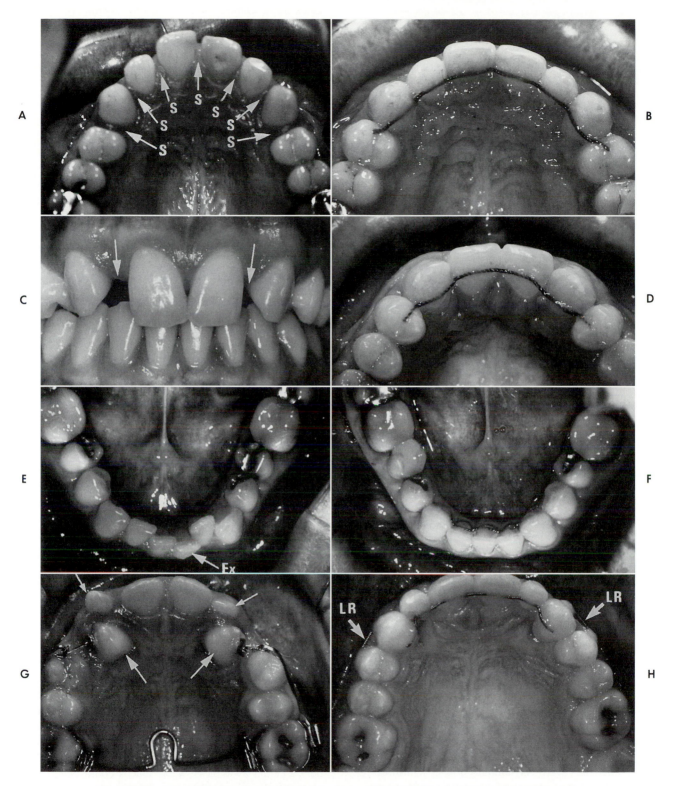

Fig. 10-63   Four different clinical situations, where a lingual FSW retainer is used for improved retention. The cases represent multiple spacing of maxillary incisors, **A** and **B,** bilaterally missing maxillary lateral incisors, and **D,** one lower incisor extraction *(Ex)* in Class III plus open bite tendency case **E** and **F,** and two palatally impacted maxillary canines, **G** and **H.** In **B,** the 8-unit retainer is bonded in the occlusal fossa of the first premolars, whereas in **H,** a short labial retainer *(LR)* is used bilaterally to stabilize the mesially rotated and palatally displaced canines.

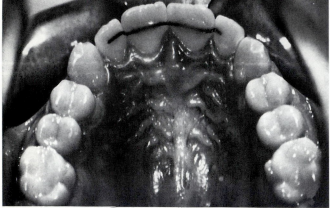

Fig. 10-64 Unexpected side effect of a 2-unit bonded retainer. **A,** The two central incisors have moved in opposite directions. (Courtesy JL Jensen.) Such side-effects are eliminated when a 0.0215 inch wire is bonded over four incisors, **B.**

not entirely passive while bonding (Fig. 10-64). Finally these retainers are more subject to mechanical stress and are thus less indicated in deep overbite cases when the wire cannot be placed out of occlusion.

Long-Term Experience

In the late 1970s and early 1980s, experiments were performed with different sizes (0.015- to 0.020-inch diameter) and types of multistranded wires.[197,200,201] Early findings were that the incidence of wire breakage appeared to decrease with increasing wire diameter,[200,201] that undesirable side effects and tooth movements occurred when short segments of 0.015-inch wire was used (Fig. 10-64), and that there was an unacceptable incidence of bond failures when the wires were bonded to the lingual surfaces of premolars.[196,200,201] More recently, bond failures and other clinical features of lingually bonded retainers were reported by Dahl and Zachrisson.[50] The observation periods were an average of 6 years for maxillary and mandibular 0.0215-inch three-stranded wire* and 3 years for the same diameter five-stranded wire.†

The failure rates were considerably lower than those reported in other recent studies of lingual retainers over periods of 2 to 3 years.[15,20] The results with the five-stranded

---
*Rocky Mountain Triflex wire, GAC Wildcat wire.
†Penta-One, Masel Orthodontics, Bristol, Pennsylvania.

Penta-One wire were particularly encouraging. The failure rates for loosening were 8% in the maxilla and 6% in the mandible; for wire fracture the failure rates were 3% in the maxilla and were nonexistent in the mandible.[50]

Long-Term Experience

The discrepancies between this and other studies can probably be explained by fewer occlusal interferences (with less contact with opposing teeth to allow for more wear) and by technical factors (such as adequate buccolingual width of composite over the wire, quite smooth contouring of the adhesive, completely undisturbed setting of the adhesive in every case, careful adaptation of the wire to the lingual contours of the teeth, etc.). The reduction of wire breakage compared with earlier results is probably related to the increased flexibility of five smaller wires occupying the same diameter as the three larger wires in previous retainers (Fig. 10-72). Since the most common mode of failure with bonded FSW retainers is due to abrasion of composite and subsequent loosening of bonds between wire and composite,[15] it is advisable to avoid occlusal contact and/or to add a relatively thick layer of adhesive over the wire. Even the absence of tooth contact, such as in the mandible, mechanical forces: tongue activity, chewing, and toothbrushing, may cause notable abrasion over years.

It is necessary, therefore, to have enough bulk of adhesive buccolingually also over the mandibular wires, and failure to do so results in loosening (Fig. 10-65). A recent study[82] showed that posterior composites may have higher hardness and better wear resistance than anterior composites like Concise, but there was no difference in surface hardness between several self-cured and light-cured composite resins. Studies are now under way to compare the abrasion rate, handling properties and failure incidence in retainers bonded with different anterior and posterior chemical- and light-cured composite resins.

Patient acceptance of the FSW retainer is excellent.[19,50] In addition, adults especially appreciate that the stability of the treatment result is not dependent on their cooperation, which is the case when removable retainers are worn continuously or worn at night (Fig. 10-66).

When patients with previous multiple spacing of anterior teeth were in the retention phase of treatment, it was often found that after approximately 6 months small spaces (1 to 2 mm) opened up distal to the terminal ends of the retainer wire. Since these spaces apparently did not open further, it was concluded that they illustrated a settled occlusion with the FSW retainer in place in a new state of physiologic equilibrium.[19,50,200] Depending on the occlusion and the patient's dental awareness, such spaces could be filled with mesiodistally extended fillings or crowns or allowed to remain (Fig. 10-71).

At present little is known about the length of time that the bonded FSW retainer should be left in place. The type of original malocclusion and the patient's age and ability to

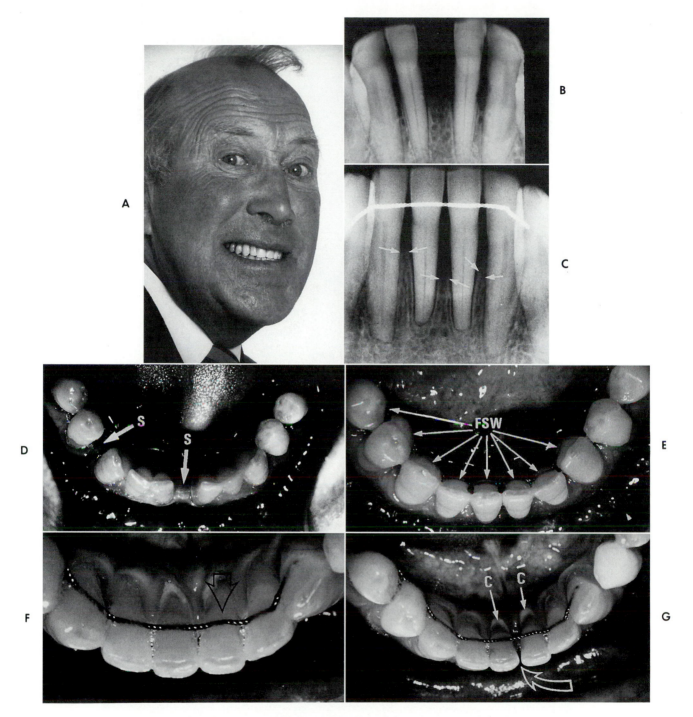

Fig. 10-65   Bonded lingual retainer for stabilization of the treatment result in 64-year-old male patient, **A** with lower incisor migration, **B** and **D** caused by periodontal break-down. The spaces (*S* in **D**) were retained with an 8-unit FSW retainer from the right second premolar to the left canine, **E** through **G**. Note abrasion of the adhesive, particularly on the left central incisor (*arrow* in **F**), which 2 years later had caused loosening between composite and wire with slight space reopening (*open arrow* in **G**). Also note calculus *(C)* in **F** and **G**.

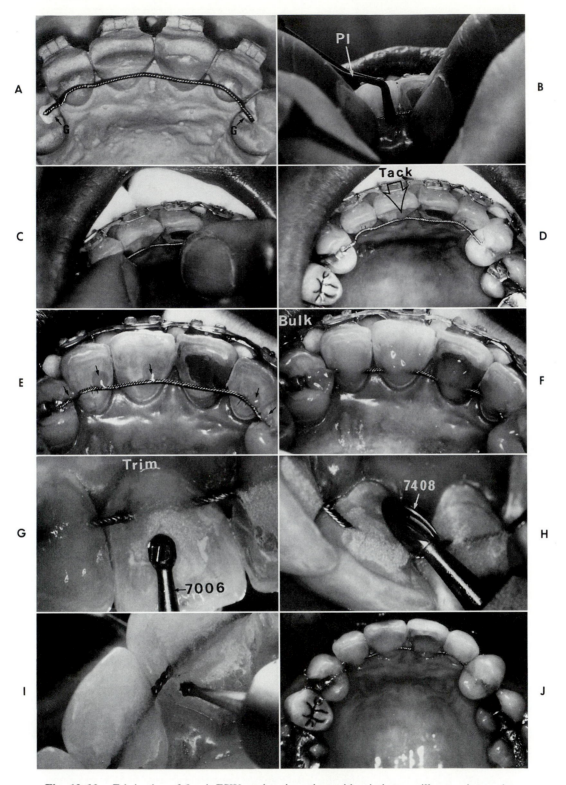

Fig. 10-66 Fabrication of 6-unit FSW retainer in patient with missing maxillary canines, where the first premolars have been moved mesially. **A,** The Penta-One wire is carefully adapted passively to the lingual contour of the incisors. A small groove *(G)* has been prepared with bur in the occlusal fissure of the premolars. The initial tacking to one central incisor, **B** through **D,** is made with the wire finger-held in the optimal position. This initial tacking (*Tack* in **D**) allows direct check of position and fit of the retainer wire and is the key to good bond success. When correct, the remaining teeth are next tacked with a small amount of fast-setting composite, **E,** before the bulk of adhesive is added in a gingival-occlusal movement, **F.** A thin mix of adhesive is then added with explorer to fill in the bond mesially and distally on each tooth. Trimming is made with TC burs, **G** through **I.** The 7006 bur is ideal incisal to the wire to avoid occlusal interference, whereas the contour gingival to the wire is made with the 7408 bur. **J** shows the final result.

keep the retainer clean may be decisive factors. As long as the retainer is intact, the treatment result is maintained; and as long as the patient performs adequate plaque control, there is no real reason to remove the retainer.

Accumulations of calculus in mandibular retainers may not be too alarming. In selected cases retainers may be used as an alternative (actually preferred) to crown-and-bridge or similar therapy for permanent stabilization. Advanced periodontal cases probably also need permanent retention (Fig. 10-65). Obviously, further follow-up research is needed for semipermanent and permanent use of bonded retainers. As discussed for the 3-3 retainers (p. 585), it is probably more practical in some cases to use the bonded lingual retainer for a *normal* or prolonged retention period and then replace it with a removable retainer for nighttime wear on a more permanent basis.

Technical Procedure

Based on clinical experience with the FSW retainer over the past 15 years, the following clinical direct-bonding procedure is now advocated for its fabrication and bonding[50] (Fig. 10-66).

1. Toward the end of orthodontic treatment, take a snap impression and pour a working model in stone.
2. Using fine, three-pronged wire bending pliers and marking pen, adapt the 0.0215-inch Penta-One wire* closely and passively to the critical areas of the lingual surface of the teeth to be bonded. Cut the wire to the required length.
3. Check the retainer wire in the mouth for good fit in an entirely passive state, and adjust if necessary.
4. Clean and etch the surfaces to be bonded in the routine manner.
5. Use a four-handed approach (or similar) for initial tacking (Fig. 10-66, *B* through *D*). The wire is hand-

---

*Masel Orthodontics, 2701 Bartram Road, Bristol, Pennsylvania 19007.

held in the optimal position while it is tacked to one incisor with a small amount of a fast-setting mix of Concise paste A and liquid resin B in a 2:1 volume ratio (see p. 588). Check the wire for passive tension after tacking (Fig. 10-66, *D*). If it is passive, then tack the remaining teeth; if not, then remove the wire and start over.

6. The initial tacking (Fig. 10-66, *E*) is vital to securing wire passiveness and optimal bond strength, for the *tacked* wire must not be displaced and cause disturbed setting when the bulk of adhesive is added. Use a double-ended metal instrument for adding a slow-setting mix of prediluted Concise (p. 589). Check with a mouth mirror to be sure that enough adhesive is used. Add more whenever it is required. It is important for strength that the adhesive cover a large buccolingual area over the wire. Fig. 10-67 shows the optimal amount.
7. Contour the bulk of adhesive and remove away any excess along the gingival margin. These are mandatory steps if optimal results (like those shown in Figs. 10-66 and 10-67) are to be attained. Use oval TC burs (no. 7006 and 7408) to obtain correct amount and contour of adhesive (Fig. 10-67), and remove interdentally with small, round burs (nos. 1 and 2).
8. Instruct the patient in proper oral hygiene and use of dental floss over the contact points (Fig. 10-68) and in each interdental area with a floss threader. Alternatively to this direct-bonding procedure, an indirect method using Xantopren-Optosil transfer trays,[20] or acrylic or vacuum-formed splints,[21] will also allow precise bonding of lingual retainers.

Repair

The most common problem subsequent to wire fracture or the loosening of bonding site(s) in FSW retainers is unwanted movement of one or more teeth. At this stage, the

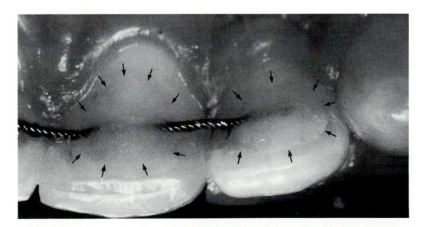

Fig. 10-67 The optimal contour of adhesive on a bonded retainer should include a relatively thick buccolingual thickness in the middle portion, tapering towards the peripheries *(small arrows)*.

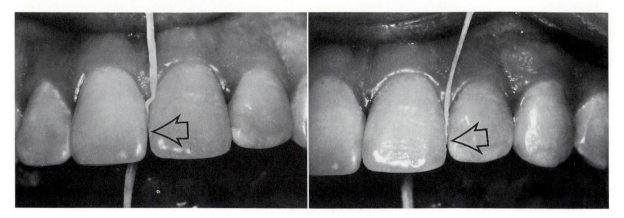

Fig. 10-68 Daily flossing of the contact points incisal to the bonded retainer *(arrows)* is quick and easy, whereas the use of floss threader (see Fig. 10-54, *A* and *B*) under each interdental region requires more cooperation.

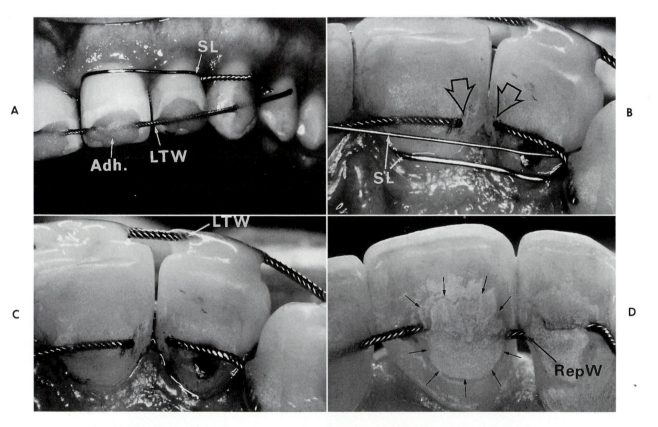

Fig. 10-69 Repair of broken retainer (fatigue fracture of wire between left central and lateral incisor), using labial temporary wire *(LTW)* for stabilization during rebonding. When the loose teeth have been pulled together with steel ligatures *(SL* in **A** and **B)** to close a small space, the temporary wire is bonded with adhesive *(Adh.)* following a quick 5-second etch labially. After setting, the steel ligatures can be removed to provide a nice working field, **C,** where the repair wire *(RepW)* can be bonded with no disturbed setting gingival to the main retainer wire, **D.**

teeth are not firmly seated in their sockets and can, therefore, generally be forced back into position using heavy pull with one or two steel ligatures, etc. (Fig. 10-69, *A* and *B*).

When the repair is then made, either a temporary contact splint, using composite resin, or a temporary bonded labial wire have proven to be of considerable value. The latter normally provides better stability, and it will allow a good working area with undisturbed setting of the repair adhesive (Fig. 10-69, *C* and *D*). After the repair the temporary labial wire (or contact splint) is removed with TC burs.

Indications

There are at least two indications or suggestions for using bonded FSW retainers:
1. Prevention of space reopening
   a. Median diastemas
   b. Spaced anterior teeth
   c. Adult periodontal conditions with the potential for postorthodontic tooth migration
   d. Accidental loss of maxillary incisors requiring the closure and retention of large anterior spaces
   e. Mandibular incisor extractions
2. *Holding* of individual teeth
   a. Severely rotated maxillary incisors
   b. Palatally impacted canines

In these and other situations the bonded *thin* spiral wire retainer can be used alone or in combination with a removable retainer. Some details of specific interest relative to the retention in this list of treated malocclusions will be briefly discussed.

Closed median diastemas. The bonded FSW retainer is ideal for short- or long-term retention of closed median diastemas. It should preferably be bonded over four units (Figs. 10-64, *B*). Its main advantages, as compared to several other types of bonded retainer suggested in recent years,* are its neatness (e.g., no pads or similar fixtures that should fit the lingual surfaces) and its excellent durability (partly because it allows physiologic movement).

With routine use it is fairly easy to make and bond the retainer wire passively. As mentioned, any activity in the wire at the time of bonding will, of course, result in subsequent tooth movement. Also trauma that causes permanent deformation of thin spiral wires may induce such movement[63] (Fig. 10-64). The use of 0.0215 five-stranded wire over four teeth apparently reduces the risk of untoward side effects.[50,200]

Multiple spacing of anterior teeth. Unimaxillary or bimaxillary spacing of teeth in adolescents and adults is gen-

---

*References 45, 46, 54, 59, 71, 97, 105, 132, 143.

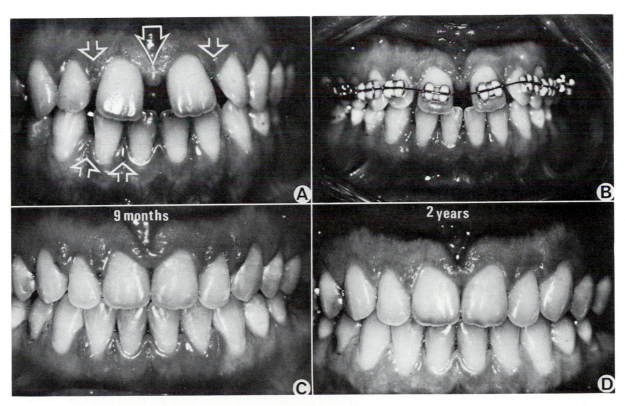

Fig. 10-70 **A,** Excessive spacing in both dental arches *(arrows)* before orthodontic treatment. Note the particularly wide median diastema. **B,** At the start of therapy. **C,** At 9 months and, **D,** at 2 years posttreatment. Note the improvement in gingival contour in **D.** (See also Fig. 10-71).

erally easy to treat but difficult to retain. There may be a great tendency for space reopening, even despite long periods of retention with conventional appliances. For this reason a number of experimental approaches have been reported recently, including the use of splints,[59,102] staples,[45,46] and mesh.[71,151]

None of these methods, however, seems to have gained wide acceptance. Although good conditions for adequate plaque removal are definitely necessary in any type of dental replacement therapy, this principle does not seem to have been adhered to in several of the suggested bonded splinting appliances. When compared to the neat FSW retainer, they

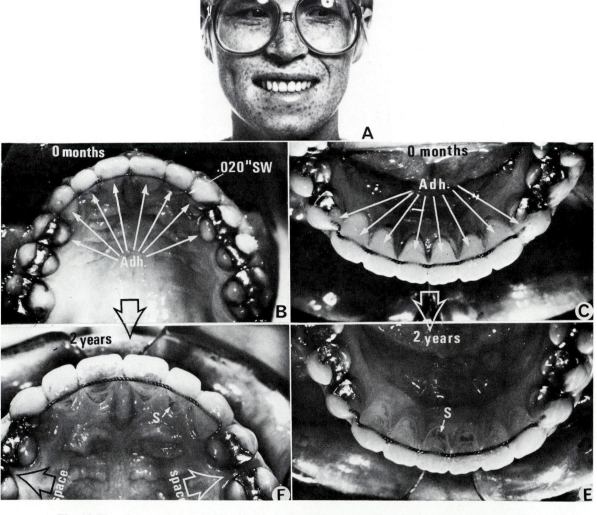

Fig. 10-71 Same patient as in Fig. 10-70. **A,** Invisible retainer. **B** and **C,** At the end of treatment a thin spiral wire was bonded to eight anterior teeth *(Adh)* in both arches, **F** and **E,** Two years later. Note that slight spaces have opened up behind the terminal ends of the maxillary retainer *(open arrows)*. In the mandible the result is stable and the retainer intact. The situation was almost identical at follow-up visits several years later.

may appear unnecessarily bulky and complicated. As discussed[50,200,201] and illustrated (Figs. 10-70 and 10-71) the bonded FSW retainer is to be preferred.

Periodontal conditions with tooth migration. The bonded FSW retainer is well suited for stabilizing and maintaining teeth in their new position after orthodontic treatment of adults with periodontal problems (Fig. 10-65). Its main advantage over removable retainers worn part time is that jiggling is completely avoided. It may also be used for periodontal splinting when teeth exhibit increased mobility or when the mobility is of a magnitude that disturbs masticatory function or patient comfort.[104,125]

Recently, extracoronal splinting, using acid etching and composite resins, has been suggested, either alone or incorporating ligature wire, a perforated cast form, fiberglass,[132] or grid material.[151] Direct contact splinting is not durable enough; composite over wire ligation creates unnecessary bulk and compromises esthetics; and the cast splints require expensive and time-consuming techniques. Rosenberg[151] reported that the use of orthodontic grid-material-splints is a completely reversible procedure. The splints are easy to construct and inexpensive, and they require minimal chairside time. However, all these advantages

are also present in the bonded FSW retainer, which in addition has a considerably neater and more hygienic appearance (Figs. 10-70 and 10-71). Clinical studies may be needed to compare the durability and effectiveness of different types of splints in the hands of other operators.

In order to reduce failures in terms of wire fracture (Fig. 10-72) or loosening, it is important that the patient try to avoid biting on a bonded maxillary retainer. In some instances, a deep overbite will only result in abrasive wear of the composite and wire, without loosening (Fig. 10-73). But several studies indicate the direct biting on the retainer wire is the most common reason for retainers coming loose. Subsequent to abrasion of the adhesive, loosening occurs between composite and the wire. Thus it is recommended in cases of deep overbite to bond the retainer wire gingivally to the contact line, or, if this is not possible, to hide the wire in a small groove in the enamel (Fig. 10-74).

Accidental loss of maxillary incisor(s). Most accidents in which maxillary central incisors are knocked out of the mouth occur in the age period from 8 to 10 years.[6]

When orthodontic space closure is selected as the treatment alternative (a discussion on indications is presented elsewhere[136,168,198,209]) the canines and premolars frequently

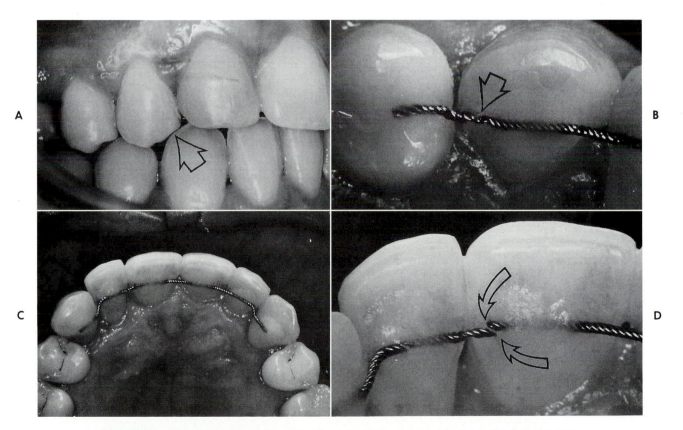

Fig. 10-72 Fatigue fracture of lingual retainer wire in two patients. **A,** A missing lateral incisor situation. The mandibular right canine hits the wire in the occlusal fossa of the first premolar (*arrow* in **A**), with resultant fracture (*arrow* in **B**). **C** and **D,** A wire fracture has occurred between the right lateral and central incisors (*arrows* in **D**).

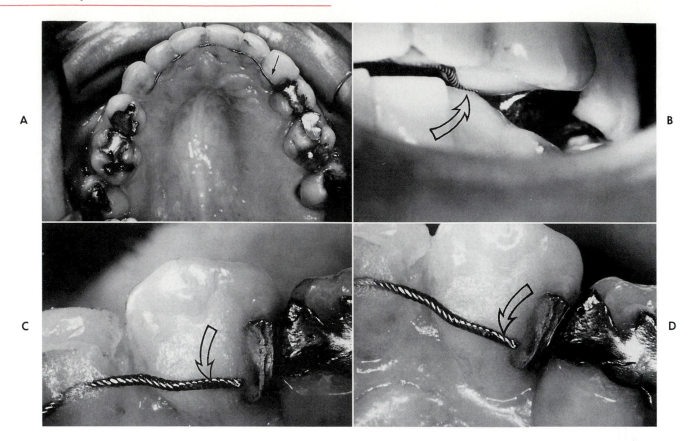

Fig. 10-73 Marked abrasive wear of bonded lingual retainer in the maxillary left canine area (**A, C,** and **D**) caused by occlusal contact with the mandibular canine, **B.** Note excessive wear of the composite resin; the round wire has been worn flat. When a state of equilibrium is reached, such retainers may still be kept in place for several years because of the retentive potential of the wire spirals.

have not yet erupted and a two-stage orthodontic treatment is indicated. In the first stage the lateral incisors are brought mesially, to prevent bone resorption and to allow mesially directed eruption of the canines (Fig. 10-75, *B*). Then there is usually a waiting period of 1 to 3 years until all permanent teeth have erupted, at which time the second stage of orthodontics can be performed. When removable retainers are used in the waiting period between the two stages, more often than not the patient perceives the experience as a prolonged and tiring orthodontic treatment over too many years. As shown in Fig. 10-75, the FSW retainer is excellent in these situations. When it is bonded to the lingual surfaces of the approximated lateral incisors, the patient soon forgets about its existence, and consequently the patient is fresh and cooperative when the final stage of orthodontics begins.

Of course, a similar approach can be chosen in other two-stage operations.

Mandibular incisor extractions. As discussed by Joondeph and Riedel (Chapter 16), Tuverson,[182] and others, sometimes one or two lower incisors will be extracted as part of orthodontic treatment. For instance, this may be true

in some adult patients, as well as in patients with an open bite Class III tendency or a periodontal problem involving excessive gingival recession on the most protruding incisor, etc. Whatever the reason for the extraction, clinical experience indicates that there is a high risk for space reopening with conventional retainers, whether removable plates or fixed 3-3 retainers. By contrast, an FSW retainer bonded to the three remaining incisors (or extended further distally) will safely maintain the treatment result for as long as it is kept in place.

Rotation of maxillary incisors. It is a well-known clinical problem that severely rotated maxillary incisors in different types of malocclusion have a great tendency to relapse. This is particularly undesirable because the upper anterior region is the most esthetically important one for the patient.

Several techniques can be used to improve the stability—including overrotation, fiberotomy, and extended retention periods. Still another aid may be the placement of a bonded FSW retainer.

Whenever a removable plate is used in the maxilla together with a bonded six-unit retainer, a modified design is

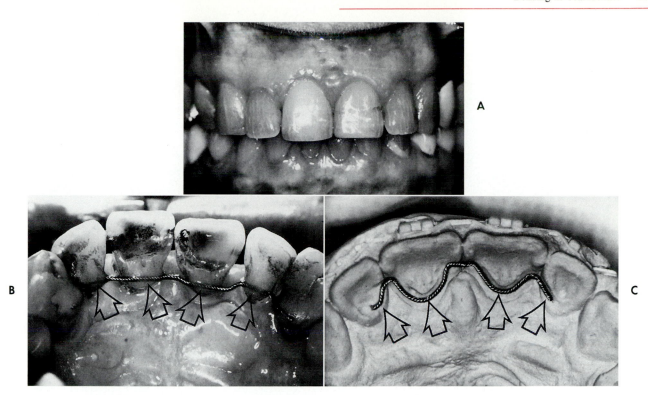

Fig. 10-74   If a deep overbite situation remains after treatment, the risk of loosening of a bonded lingual retainer is obvious. To avoid occlusal interference, the retainer wire may be bonded gingival to the contact line **B** or in exceptional cases even hidden in a small groove in the enamel, **C**.

necessary to avoid wire fracture caused by the plate's labial wire (Figs. 10-76 and 10-77).

21-12 retainer. The FSW retainer can also be bonded to the four mandibular incisors (Fig. 10-78) as an alternative to a bonded 3-3 retainer. The indications are primarily when the operator is uncertain of the optimal intercanine distance or wants the canines to settle undisturbed for other reasons. However, since the long-term results are excellent for six-unit mandibular retainers,[50] there is little reason to use the four-unit solution in my opinion.

Palatally impacted canines. Canines that have erupted into the palate may also display great relapse tendency in a lingual direction, particularly when there is no interlocking lateral overbite. In such instances an FSW retainer bonded to the lingual or buccal of the teeth has proved to be an excellent retainer (Fig. 10-79). Its main advantage is that it allows more undisturbed bone and soft tissue healing over long periods than can be obtained with removable retainers.

Concluding Remarks

When it comes to finding simple, reliable, and neat retainers and splints for a variety of clinical situations, the bonded FSW retainer opens up a range of new possibilities. The one limitation to its design and use in difficult or unusual circumstances is the imagination and alertness of the op-

erator. Clinical experience with it over the past 10 to 15 years has been excellent when meticulous technique was employed; otherwise results can be discouraging. Again, we caution against using shortcuts in fabrication.

Direct-Bonded Labial Retainers

Clinical experimentation with short labial retainers was started in the late 1980s in order to try to improve the long-term results in some specific retention situations. Typical problems were:

1. Inability to prevent some space reopening in closed extraction sites in adults
2. A tendency for some lingual relapse of previously palatally impacted canines
3. Space reopening when molars and premolars had been moved mesially in cases with excess space

Common to these situations was that some support in the premolar area for 1 to 2 years would appear advantageous to improve the stability. The background for bonding retainer wires labially was based on unsatisfactory results when the orthodontist bonded wires to the lingual surface of premolars.[200-203] The alternative: to bond the wire occlusally in the premolars, presents other problems. In most instances antagonistic contact cannot be avoided, unless a groove is prepared. This would probably not be acceptable

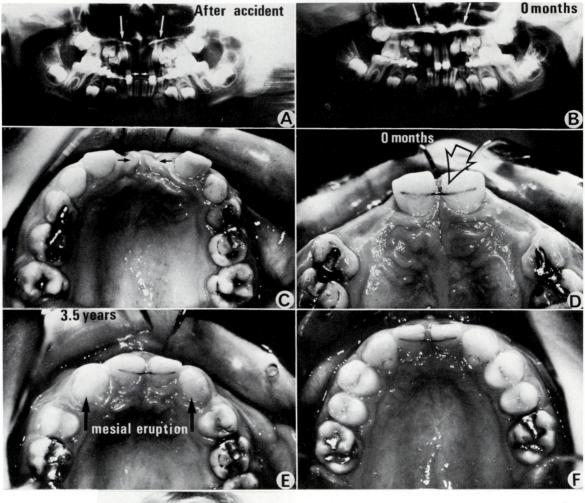

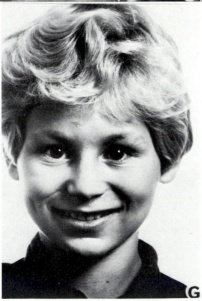

Fig. 10-75 A bonded lingual FSW retainer was useful for the long wait necessary between two periods of orthodontic treatment in this 9-year-old trauma victim. **A** and **C,** Panoramic and occlusal views of the dentition at the time of injury. **B** and **D,** Corresponding views at the end of the first orthodontic treatment period. Note in **B** the changed eruption path of the maxillary canines as compared to **A** *(arrows).* **E,** After 3 years, 6 months of waiting (with no appliances except a bonded retainer), the canines (and first premolars) had erupted in a desired mesial position *(arrows).* The second orthodontic period was begun. **F** and **G** show the status 1 year, 2 months after the end of treatment, with the bonded retainer still intact. The patient was now referred for composite buildups on the lateral incisors.

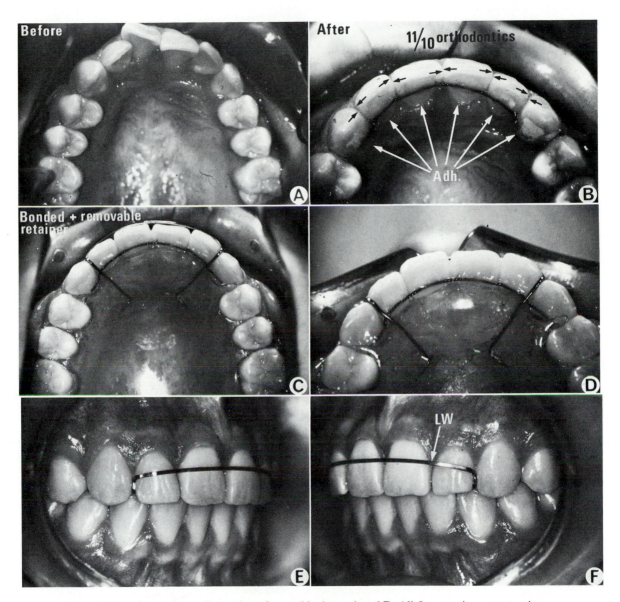

Fig. 10-76 Correction and retention of rotated incisors. **A** and **B,** All five anterior contact points were slightly overcorrected (so-called 11/10 orthodontics) during treatment (*arrows* in **B**), and a six-unit FSW retainer was bonded lingually with the four incisors still overcorrected. **C** through **F,** In addition, a removable retainer without molar clasps was used at night. *LW,* Labial rectangular wire.

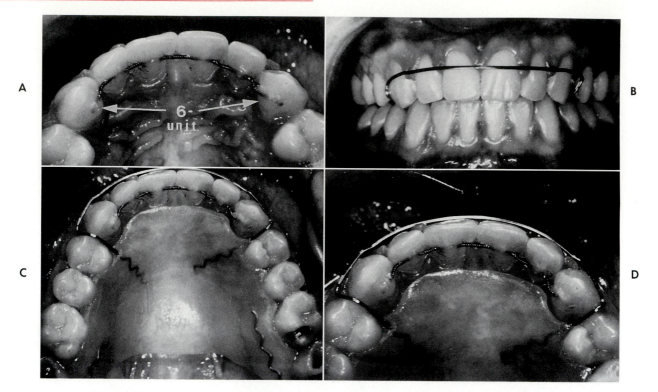

Fig. 10-77 Recommended version of removable plate to be used together with a 6-unit bonded lingual retainer. The rectangular (0.019 × 0.026 inch) labial wire of this plate extends distal to the bonded retainer, to not risk retainer wire fracture (compare Fig. 10-76 *C* and *D*). The acrylic of the plate can be ground away from the teeth involved in the bonded retainer, **C** and **D**.

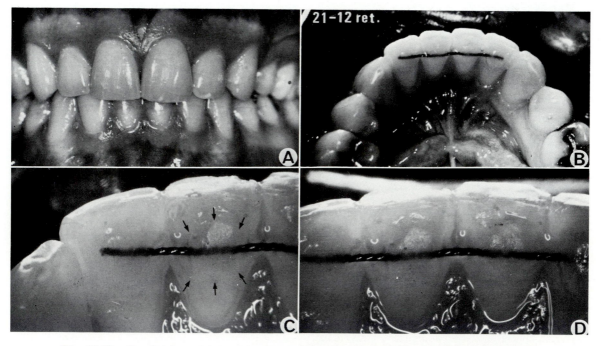

Fig. 10-78 Bonded lingual 2-1/1-2 retainer. A thin wire (approximately 0.020) should be used when several incisors are bonded. It allows slight physiologic tooth movement, which evidently prevents bond breakage (Fig. 10-52).

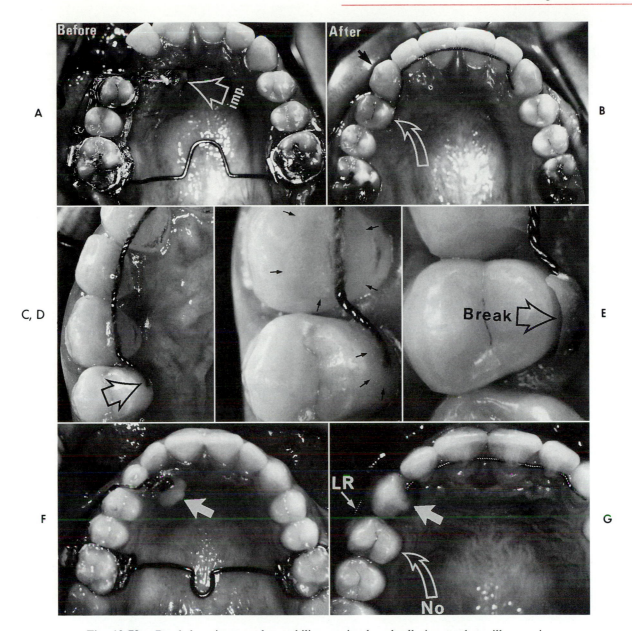

Fig. 10-79 Bonded retainers used to stabilize previously palatally impacted maxillary canines. **A** through **E** shows our old approach with bonding the retainer wire to the lingual surface of the first premolar, **C** and **D.** As illustrated in **E,** this approach frequently results in fracture in the enamel-composite interface *(arrow)*. Improved results have been obtained when the bonded lingual retainer is ended at the corrected canine *(arrow* in **G**), and a short (2 teeth) labial retainer *(LR* in **G**) is used in addition. See also Fig. 10-63, *G* and *H.*

in routine situations. It was therefore decided to bond short retainer wires labially to examine the success rates and the patient reactions.

Technical Procedure

In principle the fabrication of labial retainers is similar to the technique used for direct-bonding of lingual retainers (p. 589). Fig. 10-80 illustrates the procedure.

1. A straight piece of 0.0215-inch Penta-One wire is cut to desired length.

2. After etching, the retainer wire is tacked on the teeth after both ends are dipped in the fast-setting mix of composite on a plastic spatula (Fig. 10-80, *C*).
3. After the adhesive sets, a bulk of adhesive is added.
4. Contour trimming of excess is done with TC burs (nos. 7408 and 7006) and interdental trimming is done with small round burs (nos. 1 or 2). Care is taken to avoid contact between composite and gingival margin at the bonding sites, as well as contact between the interdental papillae and the retainer wire.

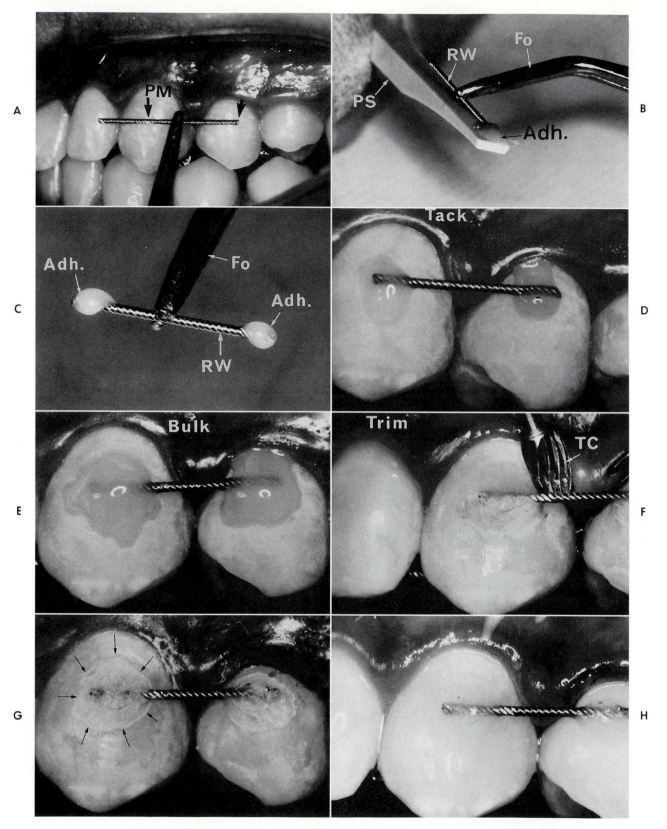

Fig. 10-80 Fabrication of the short labially bonded retainer. During trial, **A,** the distal end should not extend beyond the midbuccal portion of the premolar, and a pen mark *(PM)* is made mesially. Held in forceps *(Fo),* the small wire *(RW)* is dipped in the adhesive *(Adh.)* on a plastic spatula *(PS)* in both ends, so that there is an adhesive portion on either side, **C,** for tacking, **D.** Bulk of adhesive is added, **E,** and trimming is done with TC burs, **F,** so that the adhesive is kept well away from the gingival margin, **G.** Final result is shown in **H.**

Long-Term Results

The first follow-up study of direct-bonded labial retainers as reported recently by Axelsson and Zachrisson[19] demonstrated excellent results for short segments (2 teeth), with regard to bond success rate and, somewhat surprisingly, to patient acceptance. The failure rates for retainers of 2 teeth was about 4% over an average period of 2 years. The re-

tainers were placed over closed extraction sites in adults (Figs. 10-81, 10-82, and 10-83) for added retention of previously palatally impacted canines (Fig. 10-79).

When longer retainers (3 to 4 teeth) were placed labially in the mandible (Figs. 10-84 and 10-85), however, the bond failures increased markedly.[19]

Further clinical testing with these labial retainers and/or

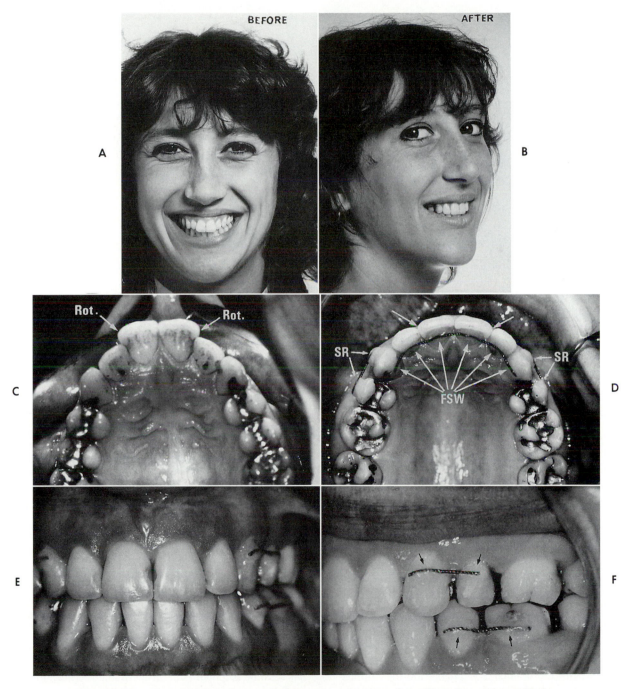

Fig. 10-81   Short labial retainers to help prevent reopening of maxillary first and mandibular second premolar extraction sites in adult bimaxillary protrusion female patient. **A** and **C,** Before treatment. **B** and **D** through **F,** After treatment. The short labial retainers *(SR)* were used in addition to upper and lower lingual retainers *(FSW)* and a maxillary removable plate. Same patient as in Fig. 10-34.

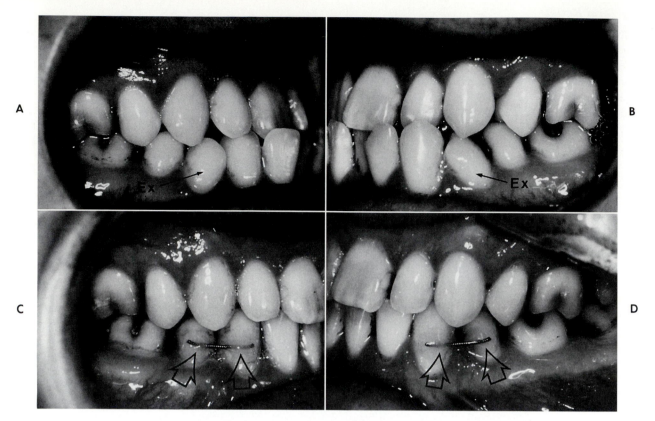

Fig. 10-82 Short labial retainers (*arrows* in **C** and **D**) after extraction *(Ex)* of first premolars and orthodontic treatment in the mandible only.

tooth-colored alternatives will be interesting in years to come.

OTHER APPLICATIONS OF BONDING IN ORTHODONTICS

Numerous other clinical possibilities of interest to orthodontists exist in which the acid etch technique and bonding has proved useful:

Space maintainers
Semipermanent single-tooth replacements
Trauma fixation
Resin buildups for tooth size and shape problems

Bonded space maintainers

Several approaches to bonded space maintainers have been described,[13,122,163] with varying degrees of short-term success reported. Long-term results on a group of patients are not available for any design. Analogous to the encouraging results with the bonded 3-3 retainer are the findings of Årtun and Marstrander,[13] who compared the durability of 64 space maintainers when either a round 0.032-inch wire with terminal loops (Fig. 10-86, *A*) or a twisted stainless steel wire of 0.032 inch diameter without loops (Fig. 10-86, *B)* was bonded with composite resin (Concise). A

utility wire design was used to reduce the influence of occlusal forces. Although the failure rate after 6 months was significantly higher for the first alternative, it was in the 10% range for the second (an acceptable level). The main reason for the difference was thought to be the fact that the thick spiral wire allowed less bulk (and thus less occlusal interference) and was easier to individualize. Simonsen[163] reported bonding space maintainers on the lingual sides of teeth, apparently with good success.

More studies are needed on designs of bonded space maintainer on the labial or lingual aspects before a variant for routine use can be universally accepted (Fig. 10-87).

Bonded single-tooth replacements

Because of the well-known problems with fixed bridgework and removable appliances of the *spoon denture* type in young patients, acid etching and bonding offers a range of esthetic techniques for the solution of the problem with anterior teeth.[51,149,154] The use of resin bonded bridgework has become accepted as a semipermanent procedure. Failure rates are over a 10-year period and may be in the 30% range,[189] particularly if cases are selected so that there would be no or only limited occlusal contact on the restoration. Higher failure rates have been experienced when there is occlusal contact, particularly in children.[155]

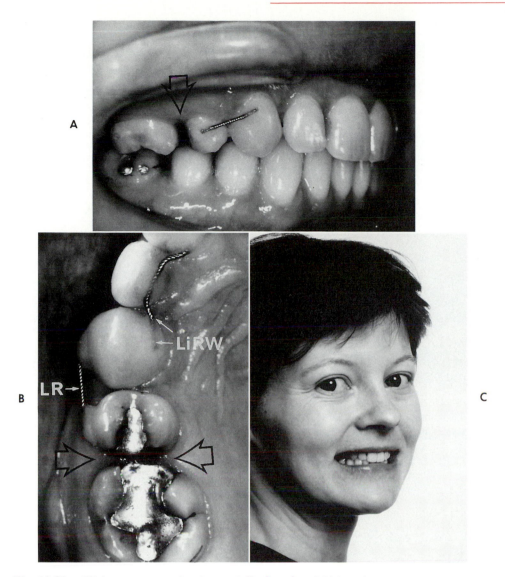

Fig. 10-83 Slight space reopening *(arrows)* distal to short labial retainer *(LR)* in adult female, upper first premolar extraction case. The reopening evidently reflects a tooth size discrepancy, which can be taken care of when remaking the amalgam fillings. Note in **C** that the labial wire is inconspicuous upon smiling.

A cheaper, simpler, and perhaps more durable alternative than the cast variants for anterior tooth replacement was proposed in 1984 by Årtun and Zachrisson.[17] We used an acrylic prosthetic tooth and inserted into it two flexible braided rectangular (0.016 × 0.022) and one round (0.0195) spiral wire for support (Fig. 10-88).

The following properties were aimed at:

1. Possibility for physiologic movement of the bridge units within the periodontal tissues
2. Avoidance of direct occlusal contact on metal
3. Avoidance of metal shine through
4. Uncomplicated repair
5. Access to the pulp cavity and root canal in cases where endodontic treatment might be indicated

Clinical results with the 3-wire design in a nonselected material without concern for the degree of overbite in 51 adolescents were promising but not entirely satisfactory.[17] Bond failure rates were 26% after 2 years and 39% after 3 years. Most breakage occurred on central incisors in direct occlusal contact during protrusive mandibular movements, and were seen as wire fracture. The failure rates were much lower when there was no antagonistic contact with the pontic during functional movements. None of the lateral incisors had come loose (Fig. 10-89).

Later modifications have included an improved 4-wire design, using two rectangular braided wires on either side (Fig. 10-90, *C* through *G*). In cases where direct occlusal contact could not be avoided, a small groove was prepared

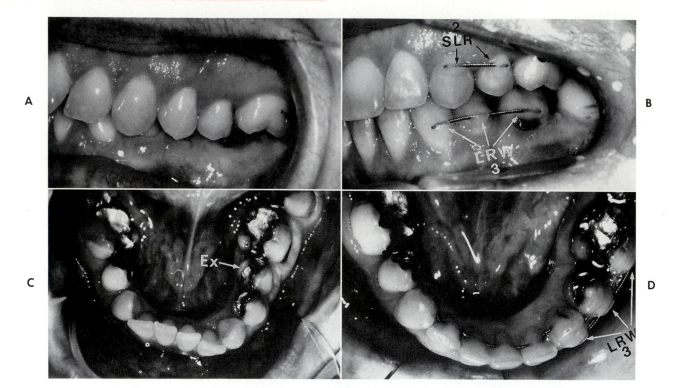

Fig. 10-84 Maxillary short *(SLR)* and mandibular long *(LRW)* labial retainers in adult female patient with marked scissors bite and some crowding, **A** and **C.** The orthodontic treatment involved extraction of the left maxillary first and mandibular second premolars.

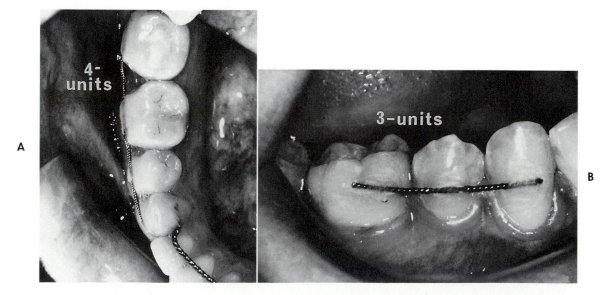

Fig. 10-85 Long labial mandibular retainers in two different patients. **A** shows a 4-unit and **B,** a 3-unit variant. As discussed in the text, the failure rates for these long labial retainers in the mandible is presently uncomfortably high.

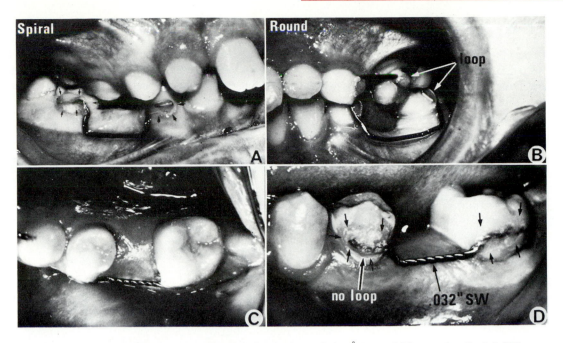

Fig. 10-86 Bonded space maintainer design in the study by Årtun and Marstrander. **B,** A 0.032 inch round wire with terminal loops is used, whereas in **A** the wire is 0.032 inch spiral. Note the utility design to minimize occlusal interference. **C** and **D** show the recommended bonded space maintainer design with a thick (0.032) spiral without loops. *Small arrows* in **D** denote the optimal amount of adhesive.

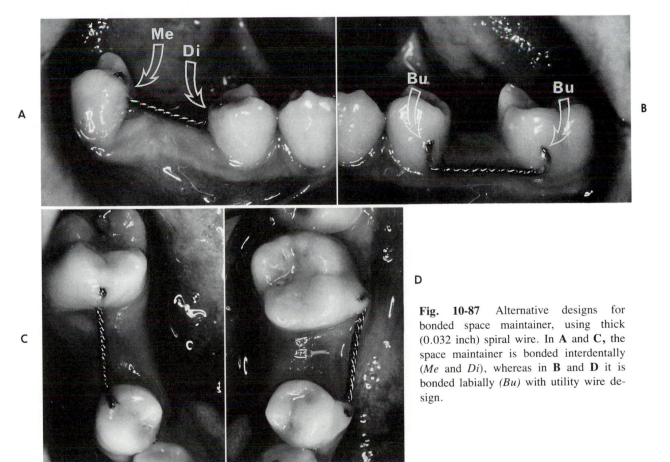

Fig. 10-87 Alternative designs for bonded space maintainer, using thick (0.032 inch) spiral wire. In **A** and **C,** the space maintainer is bonded interdentally (*Me* and *Di*), whereas in **B** and **D** it is bonded labially *(Bu)* with utility wire design.

to hide the incisal wire(s) (Fig. 10-90, *B*). In a nonselected sample of 36 bridges, the failure rate over a 4-year period with the 4-wire design was about 20%.[179]

Despite these failure rates, this type of replacement has several advantages for use in children and adolescents. Of particular interest is the fact that similar types of replacement can be used during orthodontic treatment. Acrylic teeth can be attached to neighbors to avoid empty-looking spaces in adults when incisor or premolar extractions are needed (Figs. 10-59, 10-60, and 10-61). Without doubt, further evaluation of the clinical efficacy of these promising and exciting alternatives is necessary.

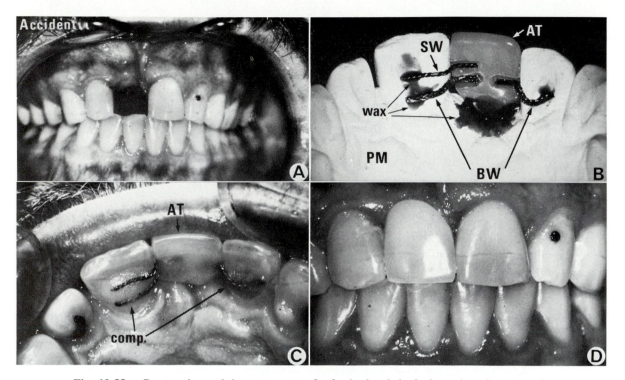

Fig. 10-88 Construction and the appearance of a 3-wire bonded, single-tooth replacement. **A,** Maxillary right central incisor knocked out in an automobile accident. **B,** Acrylic tooth *(AT)* fitted on a plaster working model *(PM)* and temporarily attached with sticky wax. Two braided 0.016 × 0.022 inch wires *(BW)* are contoured along the gingival margin of the supporting incisors, and one round (0.020) spiral wire provides additional support. The wires are bonded to the artificial crown with cold cure acrylic. **C,** Acrylic tooth *(AT)* bonded with restorative composite *(comp)*. **D** Final result. Right central incisor made slightly shorter than the intact left central to avoid excessive load in eccentric mandibular movements. (Courtesy J Årtun.)

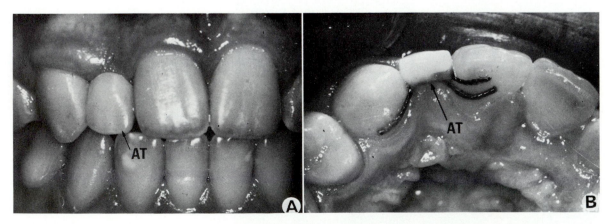

Fig. 10-89 A bonded, single-tooth replacement is particularly indicated for missing maxillary lateral incisors. Same technical procedure as in Fig. 10-88.

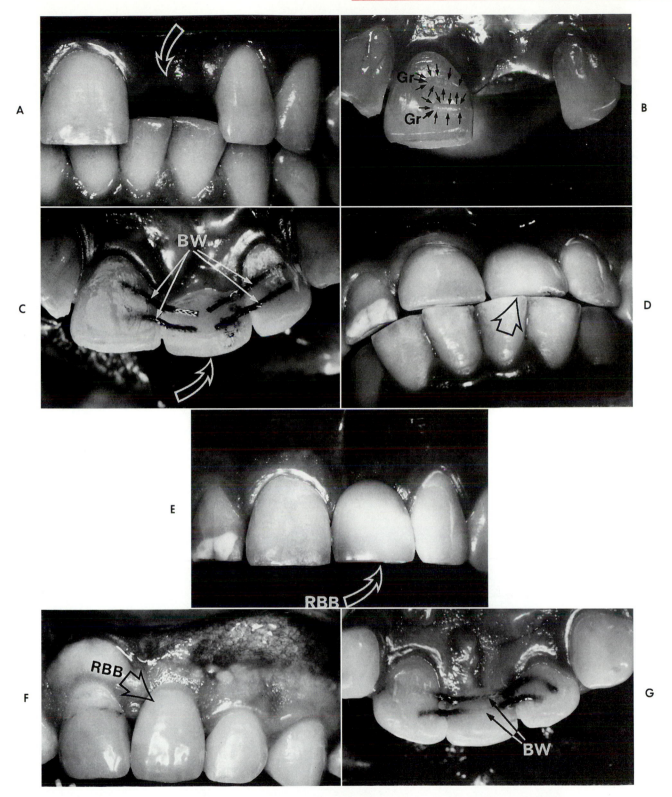

Fig. 10-90 Alternative designs for single-tooth replacement. In **A** through **E,** a 4-wire design *(BW)* is used including, small grooves prepared with bur in the enamel of the right central incisor *(Gr* in **B**), and the bite is carefully checked in occlusion and mandibular excursions *(arrow* in **D**). As in Fig. 10-88, the left central incisor in the resin-bonded bridge *(RBB)* is made slightly shorter than the intact right central incisor to avoid excessive functional loads. **F** and **G,** An improved version of the resin-bonded bridge *(RBB)* with 4-wire design, where the two braided wires *(BW)* run continuously through the pontic. Note the attempts to achieve *clean* interdental conditions in **F** and **G.**

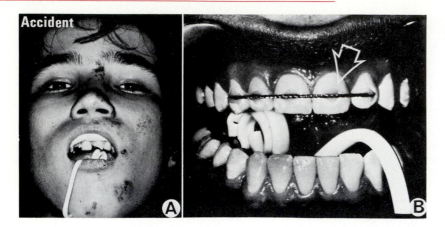

Fig. 10-91 Temporary fixation of several loose maxillary incisors after injury. Spiral wire bonded to five units. This procedure is simple, neat, and clean.

Fig. 10-92 **A,** Composite buildup on a peg-shaped maxillary lateral incisor *(arrow)*. Light polymerized composite *(comp)* was added on the mesial and distal aspects. **B,** Labial and, **C,** lingual appearances. **E** shows a porcelain laminate veneer *(PLV)* on a maxillary left lateral incisor, which was peg-shaped at the beginning of the orthodontic treatment, **D.**

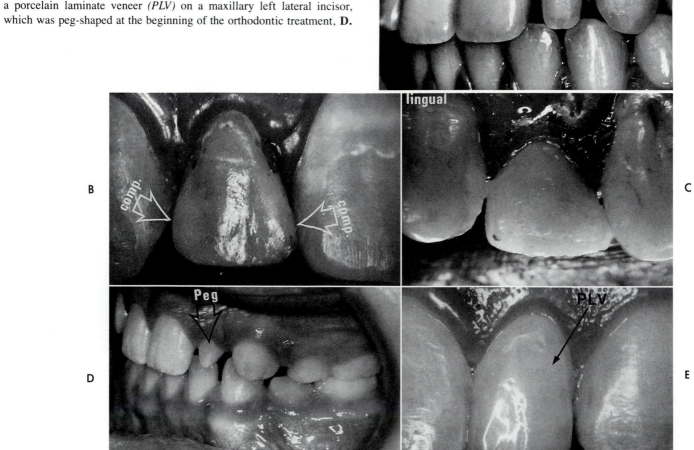

Splinting of traumatic injuries

The goal of splinting traumatized teeth is to stabilize and to allow healing and to prevent further damage to the pulp and periodontal structures. Several types of traumatic splinting devices are conventionally used,[6] but for various reasons none of these splints is optimal.[151] Thus clinical experiments using different bonded wires are interesting. Short-term studies have demonstrated clinical success with bonded plastic wire[7] and *thick* (0.032 inch) stainless steel spiral wire.[23] Such splints are demonstrated in Fig. 10-91.

Since there is an increasing tendency to avoid too rigid splinting (except possibly for root fractures), future studies should be directed toward the use of thin flexible wire retainers for this purpose.

Composite buildups and porcelain laminate veneers. The addition of composite resin or porcelain laminates to noncarious teeth during or after orthodontic treatment may be indicated on single or multiple teeth to solve tooth shape and/or size problems. There is a range of situations in which buildup techniques may provide esthetic improvement of the orthodontic result.

For example, small or peg-shaped maxillary lateral incisors (Fig. 10-92), as well as canines brought into contact with maxillary centrals when the laterals are congenitally missing (Fig. 10-93) may need such esthetic improvement. Fields[63] described the addition of bonded resin to the interproximal surfaces of maxillary anterior teeth to increase their mesiodistal widths, after careful case planning and distribution of the space available and after discussion of the pros and cons of this procedure.

Later reports[168,179,180,198] demonstrated that tooth shape can be enhanced when maxillary canines substitute for lateral incisors by careful tooth positioning, selective grinding, and the addition of composite resin to the crowns of the canines (Fig. 10-93). Occasionally, first premolars in lateral incisor position also need the addition of resin (Fig. 10-94). Other

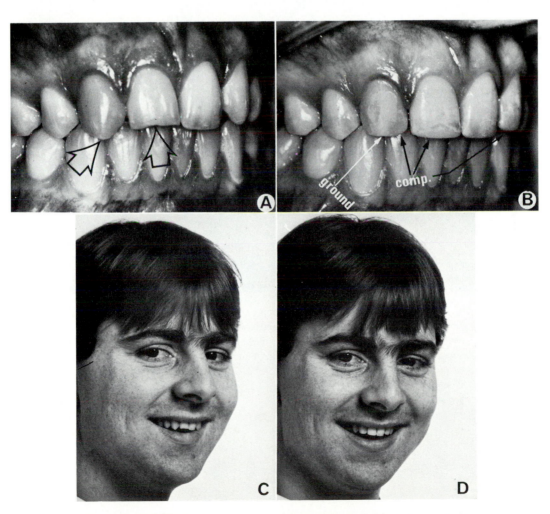

Fig. 10-93 Composite buildup leading to esthetic improvement postorthodontically for a patient in whom the maxillary lateral incisors were missing. **A,** After space closure. Note the unfavorable appearance of both canines and the traumatically injured right central incisor *(arrows)*. **B,** Combination grinding of the canines and composite buildup on the mesial aspects of the canines and the incisal edge of the central incisor. **C** and **D,** Results of this quick procedure.

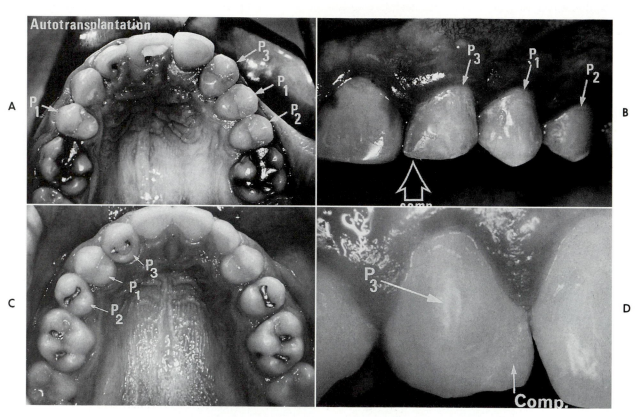

Fig. 10-94 **C** and **D,** Another premolar autotransplantation case, where a mandibular premolar *(P3)* was transplanted to the maxillary right lateral incisor region. The patient had congenital absence of both maxillary canines and the right lateral incisor. After orthodontic space closure, **C,** a composite build-up *(Comp.)* was made on the mandibular premolar *(P3)* to simulate *lateral incisor* appearance.

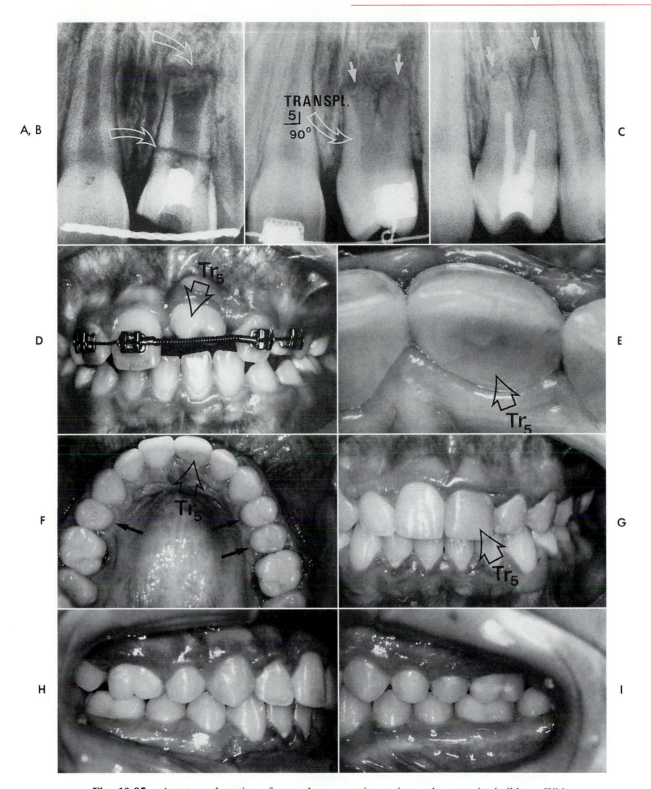

Fig. 10-95   Autotransplantation of premolar to anterior region and composite build-up. With hopeless prognosis *(arrows)* after traumatic injury, the left central incisior in **A** was replaced with the maxillary right second premolar *(Tr$_5$)* turned 90 degrees, **B** and **D**. Root development continued *(arrows in **B** and **D**)*, but because of rapid pulp obliteration, preventive endodontics was done, **C**. After grinding, **E**, a composite build-up was made, **G**, and orthodontic treatment was continued to result, **H** and **I**. Note that the 90° rotated maxillary second premolar is somewhat wide mesiodistally in the cervical region, **B**, **C**, and **G**, and its gingival contour differs from that of the intact right central incisor, **G**. Still, the result is satisfactory.

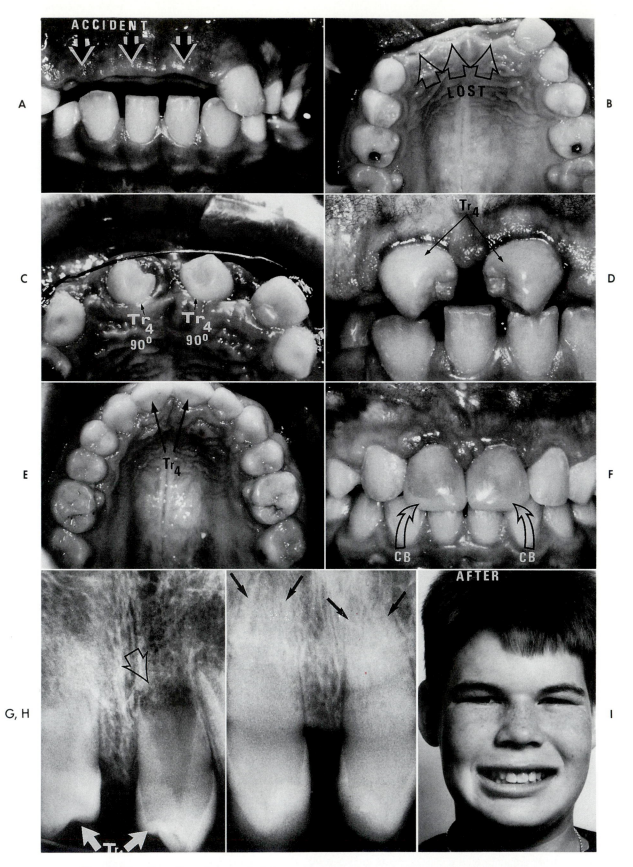

Fig. 10-96 Complicated traumatic injury case, where three maxillary incisors were accidentally lost (*arrows* in **A** and **B**). Two first premolars *(Tr₄)* were autotransplanted from the mandible to the maxillary central incisor region, and turned 90°. Root development continued, and the root canals were evident in the parts of the roots that were formed after the transplantation, **G** and **H**. After grinding, composite build-ups *(CB)* were made, and orthodontic space closure was continued to completion, **F** and **I**. Final result is shown in **F** and **I**.

situations that require buildups include those that involve premolars being autotransplanted to the anterior region[168] (Figs. 10-95 and 10-96).

The esthetic result with present light-cured composite resins is not as desirable as those obtained with porcelain laminate veneers, but the reversible and nondestructive nature of the buildup technique makes it an attractive alternative in young patients.

Summary

The present chapter represents an update on the use of the acid etch technique and resin bonding in orthodontics. Four parts deal with bracket bonding, debonding, differential retention with bonded retainers, and other applications of bonding in orthodontics (space maintainers, single-tooth replacements, trauma fixation, resin buildups). Emphasis is placed on the *clinical* application, and attempts are made to base the clinical recommendations on available scientific background data, when such information is available, and on my own clinical experience.

REFERENCES

1. Aboush YEY, Tareen A, Elderton RJ: Resin-to-enamel bonds: effect of cleaning the enamel surface with prophylaxis pastes containing fluoride or oil, *Br Dent J* 1991:171, 207.
2. Aguirre MJ, King GJ, Waldron JM: Assessment of bracket placement and bond strength when comparing direct bonding to indirect bonding techniques, *Am J Orthod* 82:269, 1982.
3. Alexander M, Alexander RG, Gorman JC et al: Lingual orthodontics: a status report, *J Clin Orthod* 16:225, 1982.
4. Alexander CM, Jacobs JD, Turpin DC: Disease control in an orthodontic office, *Am J Orthod* 71:79, 1977.
5. Alexander SA: Effects of orthodontic attachments on the gingival health of permanent second molars, *Am J Orthod* 100:337, 1991.
6. Andreasen GF, Stieg MA: Bonding and debonding brackets to porcelain and gold, *Am J Orthod* 93:341, 1988.
7. Andreasen JO: *Traumatic injuries of the teeth*, ed 2, Philadelphia, 1992, WB Saunders.
8. Antrim DD, Ostrowski JS: A functional splint for traumatized teeth, *J Endod* 8:328, 1982.
9. Arakawa V, Takahashi Y, Sebata M: The effect of acid etching on the cervical region of the buccal surface of the human premolar, with special reference to direct bonding techniques. *Am J Orthod* 76:201, 1979.
10. Årtun J: Caries and periodontal reactions associated with long-term use of different types of bonded lingual retainers, *Am J Orthod* 86:112, 1984.
11. Årtun J: A post-treatment evaluation of multibonded lingual appliances in orthodontics, *Eur J Orthod* 9:204, 1987.
12. Årtun J, Bergland S: Clinical trials with crystal growth conditioning as an alternative to acid-etch pretreatment, *Am J Orthod* 85:333, 1984.
13. Årtun J, Marstrander PB: Clinical efficiency of two different types of direct bonded space maintainers, *J Dent Child* 50:197, 1983.
14. Årtun J, Spadafora AT et al: Hygiene status associated with different types of bonded, orthodontic canine-to-canine retainers, *J Clin Periodontol* 14:89, 1987.
15. Årtun J, Thylstrup A: Clinical and scanning electron microscopic study of surface changes of incipient caries lesions after debonding, *Scand J Dent Res* 94:193, 1986.
16. Årtun J, Urbye KS: The effect of orthodontic treatment on periodontal bone support in patients with advanced loss of marginal periodontium, *Am J Orthod* 93:143, 1988.
17. Årtun J, Zachrisson BU: Improving the handling properties of a composite resin for direct bonding, *Am J Orthod* 81:269, 1982.
18. Årtun J, Zachrisson BU: New technique for semipermanent replacement of missing incisors, *Am J Orthod* 85:367, 1984.
19. Axelsson S, Zachrisson BU: Clinical experience with direct-bonded labial retainers, *J Clin Orthod* 26:480, 1992.
20. Banthleon HP, Droschl H: A precise and time-saving method of setting up an indirectly bonded retainer, *Am J Orthod* 93:78, 1988.
21. Becker A, Goultschin J: The multistranded retainer and splint, *Am J Orthod* 85:470, 1984.
22. Bednar JR, Gruendeman GW, Sandrik JL: A comparative study of frictional forces between orthodontic brackets and archwires, *Am J Orthod* 100:513, 1991.
23. Bell O, Størmer K, Zachrisson BU: Ny metode for fiksering av traumatiserte tenner, *Nor Tannlaegeforen Tid* 94:49, 1984.
24. Belostoky L: "Cure-on-touch" bonding with a preloaded bracket delivery system, *J Clin Orthod* 16:450, 1982.
25. Benvenga MN: Clinical evaluation of bonded orthodontic retainers, *Orthodontia* 13:46, 1980.
26. Bishara SE, Trulove TS: Comparisons of different debonding techniques for ceramic brackets: an in vitro study, *Am J Orthod* 98:263, 1990.
27. Björk A: Prediction of mandibular growth rotation, *Am J Orthod* 55:585, 1965.
28. Boyd RL: Periodontal considerations in the use of bonds or bands on molars in adolescents and adults, *Angle Orthod* 62:117, 1992.
29. Bradburn GB, Pender N: An in vitro study of the bond strength of two light-cured composites used in the direct bonding of orthodontic brackets to molars, *Am J Orthod* 102:418, 1992.
30. Brandt S, Servoss JM, Persily KB: Atropine sulphate—an effective antisialagogue, *J Clin Orthod* 15:629, 1981.
31. Brännström M, Malmgren O, Nordenvall KJ: Etching of young permanent teeth with an acid gel, *Am J Orthod* 82:379, 1982.
32. Brännström M, Nordenvall KJ, Malmgren O: The effect of various pretreatment methods of the enamel in bonding procedures. *Am J Orthod* 74:522, 1978.
33. Brobakken BO, Zachrisson BU: Abrasive wear of bonding adhesives: studies during treatment and after bracket removal, *Am J Orthod* 79:134, 1981.
34. Buchman DJ: Effects of recycling on metallic direct bond orthodontic brackets, *Am J Orthod* 77:654, 1980.
35. Buonocore MG: A simple method of increasing the adhesion of acrylic filling materials to enamel surface, *J Dent Res* 34:849, 1955.
36. Buonocore MG: Adhesives in the prevention of caries, *J Am Dent Assoc* 87:1000, 1973.
37. Buonocore MG, Vezin JC: Orthodontic fluoride protection, *J Clin Orthod* 14:321, 1980.
38. Burapavong V, Marshall GW, Apfel DA: Enamel surface characteristics on removal of bonded orthodontic brackets, *Am J Orthod* 74:176, 1978.
39. Buzitta VAJ, Hallgren SE, Powers JM: Bond strength of orthodontic direct-bonding cement-bracket systems as studied in vitro, *Am J Orthod* 81:87, 1982.
40. Carter RN: Salivary control, *J Clin Orthod* 15:562, 1981.
41. Caspersen I: Residual acrylic adhesive after removal of plastic orthodontic brackets: a scanning electron microscopic study, *Am J Orthod* 71:637, 1977.
42. Ceen RF, Gwinnett AJ: Indelible iatrogenic staining of enamel following debonding, *J Clin Orthod* 14:713, 1980.
43. Ceen RF, Gwinnett AJ: Microscopic evaluation of the thickness of sealants used in orthodontic bonding, *Am J Orthod* 78:523, 1980.
44. Ceen RF, Gwinnett AJ: White spot formation associated with sealants used in orthodontics, *Pediatr Dent* 3:174, 1981.
45. Chan KC, Andreasen GF: Conservative retention for spaced maxillary central incisors, *Am J Orthod* 67:324, 1975.

46. Clark KC, Williams JK: The management of spacing in the maxillary incisor region, *Am J Orthod* 69:72, 1976.

47. Compton AM, Meyers CE, Hondrum SD, Lorton L: Comparison of the shear bond strength of a light-cured glass ionomer and a chemically cured glass ionomer for use as an orthodontic bonding agent, *Am J Orthod* 101:138, 1992.

48. Coreil MN, McInnes-Ledoux P et al: Shear bond strength of four orthodontic bonding systems, *Am J Orthod* 97:126, 1990.

49. Creekmore T: Lingual orthodontics—its renaissance, *Am J Orthod* 96:120, 1989.

50. Dahl EH, Zachrisson BU: Long-term experience with direct-bonded lingual retainers, *J Clin Orthod* 25:619, 1991.

51. Deguchi T, Amari M: Adhesive fixed partial dentures (bridges) as posttreatment retention in missing tooth cases, *Am J Orthod* 92:511, 1987.

52. Dickinson GL, Stevens JT et al: Comparison of shear bond strengths of some third-generation dentin bonding agents, *Oper Dent* 16:223, 1991.

53. Diedrich P: Enamel alterations from bracket bonding and debonding: a study with the scanning electron microscopy, *Am J Orthod* 79:500, 1981.

54. Eade P: A modified direct bond lingual retainer technique, *Br J Orthod* 7:125, 1980.

55. Eames WB, Rogers LB et al: Bonding agents for repairing porcelain and gold, *Oper Dent* 2:118, 1977.

56. Edris AA, Jabr AA et al: SEM evaluation of etch patterns by three etchants on three porcelains, *J Prosthet Dent* 64:734, 1990.

57. Ekstrand J, Øgaard B, Rolla G: Moderna aspekter på fluorens kariostatiska verkningsmekanismer, *Tandl Tidn* 79:97, 1987.

58. Eustaquio R, Garner LD, Moore BK: Comparative tensile strengths of brackets bonded to porcelain with orthodontic adhesive and porcelain repair systems, *Am J Orthod* 94:421, 1988.

59. Evans CA, Shaff HA: Acid-etch technique adapted for splinting of anterior teeth: a report of marked root resorption, *Am J Orthod* 71:317, 1977.

60. Fajen VB, Duncanson MG et al: An in vitro evaluation of bond strength of three different glass ionomer cements, *Am J Orthod* 97:316, 1990.

61. Fejerskov O, Thylstrup A, Joost-Larsen M: Rational use of fluorides in caries prevention: a concept based on possible cariostatic mechanisms, *Acta Odontol Scand* 39:241, 1981.

62. Fields HW: Orthodontic-restorative treatment for relative mandibular anterior excess tooth size problems, *Am J Orthod* 78:176, 1981.

63. Fields HW: Bonded resins in orthodontics, *Pediatr Dent* 4:51, 1982.

64. Flores DA, Caruso JM et al: The fracture strength of ceramic brackets: a comparative study, *Angle Orthod* 60:269, 1990.

65. Forsberg CM, Brattström V et al: Ligature wires and elastomeric rings: two methods of ligation and their association with microbial colonization of *Streptococcus mutans* and lactobacilli, *Eur J Orthod* 13:416, 1991.

66. Fredericks HE: Mutagenic potential of orthodontic bonding materials, *Am J Orthod* 80:316, 1981.

67. Fricker JP: A 12-month clinical evaluation of a glass polyalkenoate cement for the direct bonding of orthodontic brackets, *Am J Orthod* 101:381, 1992.

68. Fujita K: Multilingual-bracket and mushroom arch wire technique, *Am J Orthod* 82:120, 1982.

69. Gaare D, Rölla G et al: Improvement of gingival health by toothbrushing in individuals with large amounts of calculus, *J Clin Periodont* 17:38, 1990.

70. Garcia-Godoy F, Hubbard GW, Storey AT: Effect of a fluoridated etching gel on enamel morphology and shear bond strength of orthodontic brackets, *Am J Orthod* 100:163, 1991.

71. Gazit E, Lieberman MA: An esthetic and effective retainer for lower anterior teeth, *Am J Orthod* 70:91, 1976.

72. Ghafari J: Problems associated with ceramic brackets suggest limiting use to selected teeth, *Angle Orthod* 62:145, 1992.

73. Ghasseim-Tary B: Direct bonding to porcelain: an in vitro study, *Am J Orthod* 76:80, 1979.

74. Gorelick L: Bonding—the state of the art: a national survey, *J Clin Orthod* 13:39, 1979.

75. Gorelick L, Geiger AM, Gwinnett AJ: Incidence of white spot formation after bonding and banding, *Am J Orthod* 81:93, 1982.

76. Gorman JC, Smith RJ: Comparison of treatment effects with labial and lingual fixed appliances, *Am J Orthod* 99:202, 1991.

77. Gottlieb EL, Nelson AH, Vogels DS: 1990 JCO study of orthodontic diagnosis and treatment procedures: part I: results and trends, *J Clin Orthod* 25:145, 1991.

78. Gwinnett AJ: The bonding of sealants to enamel, *J Am Soc Prev Dent* 3:21, 1973.

79. Gwinnett AJ, Ceen RF: An ultraviolet photographic technique for monitoring plaque during direct bonding procedures, *Am J Orthod* 73:178, 1978.

80. Gwinnett AJ, Gorelick L: Microscopic evaluation of enamel after debonding, *Am J Orthod* 71:651, 1977.

81. Haas AJ: Long-term posttreatment evaluation of rapid palatal expansion, *Angle Orthod* 50:189, 1980.

82. Helvatjoglou–Antoniadi M, Papadogianis Y et al: Surface hardness of light-cured and self-cured composite resins, *J Prosthet Dent* 65:215, 1991.

83. Hixson ME, Brantley WA et al: Changes in bracket slot tolerance following recycling of direct-bond metallic orthodontic appliances, *Am J Orthod* 81:447, 1982.

84. Hocevar RA: Direct bonding metal brackets with the Concise-Enamel bond system, *J Clin Orthod* 11:473, 1977.

85. Holt MH, Nanda RS, Duncanson MG: Fracture resistance of ceramic brackets during arch-wire torsion, *Am J Orthod* 99:287, 1991.

86. Ireland AJ, Sheriff M, McDonald F: Effect of bracket and wire composition on frictional forces, *Eur J Orthod* 13:328, 1991.

87. Jassem HA, Retief DH, Hamison HC: Tensile and shear strengths of bonded and rebonded orthodontic attachments, *Am J Orthod* 79:661, 1981.

88. Jenkins CBG: Etch-retained anterior pontics: a 4-year study, *Br Dent J* 144:206, 1978.

89. Jensen JL: Personal communication, 1993.

90. Joseph VP, Rossouw PE: The shear bond strength of stainless steel and ceramic brackets used with chemically and light-activated composite resins, *Am J Orthod* 97:121, 1990.

91. Joseph VP, Rossouw PE: The shear bond strengths of stainless steel orthodontic brackets bonded to teeth with orthodontic composite resin and various fissure sealants, *Am J Orthod* 98:66, 1990.

92. Joseph VP, Rossouw PE, Basson NJ: Do sealants seal: An SEM investigation, *J Clin Orthod* 26:141, 1992.

93. Jost–Brinkman PG, Schiffer A, Miethke RR: The effect of adhesive layer thickness on bond strength, *J Clin Orthod* 26:718, 1992.

94. Jost–Brinkman PG, Stein H et al: Histologic investigation of the human pulp after thermodebonding of metal and ceramic brackets, *Am J Orthod* 102:410, 1992.

95. Kao EC, Boltz KC, Johnston WM: Direct bonding of orthodontic brackets to porcelain laminate veneers, *Am J Orthod* 94:458, 1988.

96. Kao EC, Johnston WM: Fracture incidence on debonding of orthodontic brackets from porcelain veneer laminates, *J Prosthet Dent* 66:331, 1991.

97. Kaswiner B: A new method of retention, *J Clin Orthod* 7:744, 1973.

98. Kelly VM: JCO interviews: Dr. Vincent M. Kelly on lingual orthodontics, *J Clin Orthod* 16:461, 1982.

99. Klockowski R, Davis EL et al: Bond strength and durability of glass ionomer cements used as bonding agents in the placement of orthodontic brackets, *Am J Orthod* 96:60, 1989.

100. Kusy RP, Whitley JQ, Prewitt MJ: Comparison of the frictional coefficients for selected arch wire-bracket slot combinations in the dry and wet states, *Angle Orthod* 61:293, 1991.

101. Kvam E, Broch J, Nissen-Meyer IH: Comparison between a zinc

phosphate cement and a glass ionomer cement for cementation of orthodontic bands, *Eur J Orthod* 5:307, 1983.

102. Laag B: Retention-fixering med emaljbundet plastmaterial, *Tandläkartidn* 69:1083, 1977.
103. Lew KKK, Chew CL, Lee KW: A comparison of shear bond strengths between new and recycled ceramic brackets. *Eur J Orthod* 13:306, 1991.
104. Lindhe J, Nyman S: The role of occlusion in periodontal disease and the biological rationale for splinting in treatment of periodontics, *Oral Sci Rev* 10:11, 1977.
105. Lubit EC: The bonded lingual retainer, *J Clin Orthod* 13:311, 1979.
106. Maijer R, Smith DC: A new surface treatment for bonding, *J Biomed Mater Res* 13:975, 1979.
107. Maijer R, Smith DC: Variables influencing the bond strength of metal orthodontic bracket bases. *Am J Orthod* 79:20, 1981.
108. Maijer R, Smith DC: Corrosion of orthodontic bracket bases, *Am J Orthod* 81:43, 1982.
109. Malmgren O, Medin L: Överkänslighetsreaktioner vid användning av bondingmaterialer inom ortodontivård, *Tandläkartidn* 73:544, 1981.
110. Mannerberg F: Appearance of tooth surface, *Odontol Rev* 11(suppl 6): 1960.
111. Mascia VE, Chen SR: Shearing strengths of recycled direct-bonding brackets, *Am J Orthod* 82:211, 1982.
112. Maskeroni AJ, Meyers CE, Lorton L: Ceramic bracket bonding: a comparison of bond strength with polyacrylic acid and phosphoric acid enamel conditioning, *Am J Orthod* 97:168, 1990.
113. McCourt JW, Cooley RL, Barnwell S: Bond strength of light-cure fluoride-releasing base-liners as orthodontic bracket adhesives, *Am J Orthod* 100:47, 1991.
114. Milne JW, Andreasen GF, Jakobsen JR: Bond strength comparison: a simplified indirect technique versus direct placement of brackets, *Am J Orthod* 96:8, 1989.
115. Miura F, Nakagawa K, Masuhara E: New direct bonding system for plastic brackets, *Am J Orthod* 59:350, 1971.
116. Mizrahi E: Enamel demineralization following orthodontic treatment, *Am J Orthod* 82:62, 1982.
117. Mizrahi E: Glass ionomer cements in orthodontics—an update, *Am J Orthod* 93:505, 1988.
118. Mizrahi E, Smith DC: Direct cementation of orthodontic brackets to dental enamel, *Br Dent J* 127:371, 1969.
119. Mjör IA: Histologic studies of human coronal dentine following cavity preparation and exposure of ground facets in vivo, *Arch Oral Biol* 12:247, 1967.
120. Mjör IA, Kvam E: Dental pulp reactions following the exposure of coronal dentine in vivo, *Acta Odontol Scand* 27:145, 1969.
121. Moin K, Dogon IL: Indirect bonding of orthodontic attachment, *Am J Orthod* 72:261, 1977.
122. Newman GV: Epoxy adhesives for orthodontic attachments: progress report, *Am J Orthod* 51:901, 1965.
123. Newman G: A posttreatment survey of direct bonding of metal brackets, *Am J Orthod* 74:197, 1978.
124. Nordenvall KJ, Brännström M, Malmgren O: Etching of deciduous teeth and young and old permanent teeth: a comparison between 15 and 60 seconds of etching, *Am J Orthod* 78:99, 1980.
125. Nyman S, Lindhe J: Persistent tooth hypermobility following completion of periodontal treatments, *J Clin Periodontol* 3:81, 1976.
126. Ødegaard J, Segner D: The use of visible light-curing composites in bonding ceramic brackets, *Am J Orthod* 97:188, 1990.
127. Øgaard B, Rezk-Lega F et al: Cariostatic effect of fluoride release from a visible light-curing adhesive for bonding of orthodontic brackets, *Am J Orthod* 101:303, 1992.
128. Øgaard B: Prevalence of white spot lesions in 19-year-olds: a study on untreated and orthodontically treated persons 5 years after treatment, *Am J Orthod* 96:423, 1989.
129. Øgaard B, Rolla G et al: Orthodontic appliances and enamel de-

mineralization, part 2: prevention and treatment of lesions, *Am J Orthod* 94:123, 1988.
130. Oliver RG: A new instrument for debonding clean-up, *J Clin Orthod* 25:407, 1991.
131. Omana HM, Moore RN, Bagby MD: Frictional properties of metal and ceramic brackets, *J Clin Orthod* 26:425, 1992.
132. Orchin JD: Permanent lingual bonded retainers, *J Clin Orthod* 24:229, 1990.
133. Paige SF: A lingual light-wire technique, *J Clin Orthod* 16:534, 1982.
134. Palmer ME: Bonded space maintainers, *J Clin Orthod* 13:176, 1979.
135. Pameijer CH, Stallard RE: The fallacy of polishing composite restorations, *Dent Survey* 49:33, 1973.
136. Paulsen HU, Zachrisson BU: *Autotransplantation of teeth and orthodontic treatment planning.* In Andreasen JO, editor: *Atlas of replantation and transplantation of teeth,* Fribourg, Switzerland, 1992, Medoglobe SA, p. 257.
137. Prevost AP, Fuller JL, Peterson LC: The use of an intermediate resin in the acid etch procedure: retentive strength, microleakage, and failure mode analysis, *J Dent Res* 61:412, 1982.
138. Proffitt WR, Fields HW et al: *Contemporary orthodontics,* St Louis, 1986, Mosby.
139. Pus MD, Way DC: Enamel loss due to orthodontic bonding with filled and unfilled resins using various clean-up techniques, *Am J Orthod* 77:269, 1980.
140. Ravn JJ: Follow-up study of permanent incisors with enamel cracks as a result of acute trauma, *Scand J Dent Res* 89:117, 1981.
141. Redd TB, Shivapuja PK: Debonding ceramic brackets: effects on enamel, *J Clin Orthod* 25:475, 1991.
142. Reinhardt JW, Denehy GE, Chan KC: Acid-etch bonded cast orthodontic retainers, *Am J Orthod* 75:138, 1979.
143. Retief DH: Failure at the dental adhesive-etched enamel interface, *J Oral Rehabil* 1:265, 1974.
144. Retief DH, Denys FR: Finishing of enamel surfaces after debonding of orthodontic attachments, *Angle Orthod* 49:1, 1979.
145. Reynolds IR: A review of direct orthodontic bonding, *Br J Orthod* 2:171, 1975.
146. Rezk-Lega F, Øgaard B: Tensile bond force of glass ionomer cements in direct bonding of orthodontic brackets: an in vitro comparative study, *Am J Orthod* 100:357, 1991.
147. Rezk-Lega F, Øgaard B, Arends J: An in vitro study on the merits of two glass ionomers for the cementation of orthodontic bands, *Am J Orthod* 99:162, 1991.
148. Ricketts RM, Bench RW, Gugino CF et al: *Bioprogressive therapy,* Denver, 1979, Rocky Mountain/Orthodontics.
149. Rochette AL: Attachment of splint to enamel of lower anterior teeth, *J Prosthet Dent* 30:418, 1973.
150. Rölla G: Effects of fluoride on initiation of plaque formation, *Caries Res* 11:243, 1977.
151. Rosenberg S: A new method for stabilization of periodontally involved teeth, *J Periodontol* 51:469, 1980.
152. Rueggeberg FA, Lockwood P: Thermal debracketing of orthodontic resins, *Am J Orthod* 98:56, 1990.
153. Ruyter IA, Øysaed H: Conversion in different depths of ultraviolet and visible light activated composite materials, *Acta Odontol Scand* 40:179, 1982.
154. Scheer B, Silverstone LM: Replacement of missing anterior teeth by etched retained bridges, *J Int Assoc Dent Child* 6:17, 1975.
155. Shaw MJ, Tay WM: Clinical performance of resin-bonded cast metal bridges (Rochette bridges), *Br Dent J* 152:378, 1982.
156. Sheykholeslam Z, Brandt S: Some factors affecting the bonding of orthodontic attachments to tooth surface, *J Clin Orthod* 11:734, 1977.
157. Silverman E, Cohen ML: The twenty minute full strap up, *J Clin Orthod* 10:764, 1976.
158. Silverman E, Cohen M et al: A universal direct bonding system for both metal and plastic brackets, *Am J Orthod* 62:236, 1972.
159. Silverstone LM: Fissure sealants: laboratory studies, *Caries Res* 8:2, 1974.

160. Silverstone LM: *The acid etch technique: in vitro studies with special reference to the enamel surface and the enamel-resin interface.* In Silverstone LM, Dogon L, editors: *Proceedings of an international symposium on the acid etch technique,* St Paul, Minn, 1975, North Central.

161. Silverstone LM: Remineralization phenomena, *Caries Res* 11:59, 1977.

162. Silverstone LM: The effect of fluoride in the remineralization of enamel caries and caries-like lesions in vitro, *J Public Health Dent* 42:42, 1982.

163. Simonsen RJ: Space maintenance utilizing acid etch bonding, *Dent Survey* 54:27, 1978.

164. Simonsen RJ, Calamia JP: Tensile bond strength of etched porcelain, *J Dent Res* 61:279, 1983.

165. Smaha CN, Voth ED: A positioning device for direct bracket attachment, *Am J Orthod* 62:394, 1972.

166. Smith GA, McInnes-Ledoux P et al: Orthodontic bonding to porcelain—bond strength and refinishing, *Am J Orthod* 94:245, 1988.

167. Sorensen JA, Kang SK, Avera SP: Porcelain-composite interface microleakage with various porcelain surface treatments, *Dent Material* 7:118, 1991.

168. Stenvik A, Zachrisson BU: Orthodontic closure and transplantation in the treatment of missing teeth: an overview, *Endod Dent Traumatol* 9, 1993, (in press).

169. Stephens CD, Jenkins CBG: Crown modification using composite resin to achieve incisor overbite, *Br J Orthod* 4:121, 1977.

170. Stoller NH, Green PA: A comparison of a composite restorative material and wire ligation as methods of stabilizing excessively mobile mandibular anterior teeth, *J Periodontol* 52:451, 1981.

171. Swartz M: Ceramic brackets, *J Clin Orthod* 22:82, 1988.

172. Tanne K, Matsubara S et al: Wire friction from ceramic brackets during simulated canine retraction, *Angle Orthod* 61:285, 1991.

173. Ten Cate JM, Arends J: Remineralization of artificial lesions in vitro, *Caries Res* 11:277, 1977.

174. Thayer KE, Doukoudakis A: Acid-etch canine riser occlusal treatment, *J Prosthet Dent* 46:149, 1981.

175. Thomas RG: Indirect bonding: simplicity in action, *J Clin Orthod* 13:93, 1979.

176. Thompson IR, Miller EG, Bowles WH: Leaching of unpolymerized materials from orthodontic bonding resin, *J Dent Res* 61:989, 1982.

177. Thompson RE, Way DC: Enamel loss due to prophylaxis and multiple bonding/debonding of orthodontic attachments, *Am J Orthod* 79:282, 1981.

178. Thompson VP, Livaditis GJ: Etched casting acid etch composite bonded posterior bridges, *Pediatr Dent* 4:38, 1982.

179. Thordarson A, Zachrisson BU: Improved design of the "Oslobridge"—long-term (5 yrs) results, *Nordic Orthod Soc* p. 28, 1991, (abstract).

180. Thordarson A, Zachrisson BU, Mjör IA: Remodeling of canines to the shape of lateral incisors by grinding: a long-term clinical and radiographic evaluation, *Am J Orthod* 100:123, 1991.

181. Tirtha R, Fan PL et al: In vitro depth of cure of photo-activated composites, *J Dent Res* 61:1184, 1982.

182. Tuverson DL: Anterior interocclusal relations, *Am J Orthod* 78:361, 1980.

183. Viazis AD, Cavanaugh G, Bevis RR: Bond strength of ceramic brackets under shear stress: an in vitro report, *Am J Orthod* 98:214, 1990.

184. Vukovich ME, Wood DP, Daley TD: Heat generated by grinding during removal of ceramic brackets, *Am J Orthod* 99:505, 1991.

185. Wang WN, Lu TC: Bond strength with various etching times on young permanent teeth, *Am J Orthod* 100:72, 1991.

186. Wang WN, Meng CL: A study of bond strength between light- and self-cured orthodontic resin, *Am J Orthod* 101:350, 1992.

187. Wang WN, Tarng TH: Evaluation of the sealant in orthodontic bonding, *Am J Orthod* 100:209, 1991.

188. Wertz RA: Beginning bonding—state of the art, *Angle Orthod* 50:245, 1980.

189. Williams VD, Thayer KE et al: Cast metal, resin-bonded prostheses: a 10-year retrospective study, *J Prosthet Dent* 61:436, 1989.

190. Winchester LJ: Bond strengths of five different ceramic brackets: an in vitro study, *Eur J Orthod* 92:293, 1991.

191. White LW: Effective saliva control for orthodontic patients, *J Clin Orthod* 9:648, 1975.

192. Wood DP, Jordan RE et al: Bonding to porcelain and gold, *Am J Orthod* 89:194, 1986.

193. Zachrisson BU: Oral hygiene for orthodontic patients: current concepts and practical advice, *Am J Orthod* 66:487, 1974.

194. Zachrisson BU: Fluoride application procedures in orthodontic practice: current concepts, *Angle Orthod* 44:72, 1975.

195. Zachrisson BU: *The acid etch technique in orthodontics: clinical studies.* In Silverstone LM, Dogon L, editors: *Proceedings of an international symposium on the acid etch technique,* St Paul, Minn, 1975, North Central.

196. Zachrisson BU: A posttreatment evaluation of direct bonding in orthodontics, *Am J Orthod* 71:173, 1977.

197. Zachrisson BU: Clinical experience with direct-bonded orthodontic retainers, *Am J Orthod* 71:440, 1977.

198. Zachrisson BU: Improving orthodontic results in cases with maxillary incisors missing, *Am J Orthod* 73:274, 1978.

199. Zachrisson BU: Differential retention with bonded retainers, *Pac Coast Soc Orthod Bull* 51:62, 1979.

200. Zachrisson BU: The bonded lingual retainer and multiple spacing of anterior teeth, *J Clin Orthod* 17:838, 1983.

201. Zachrisson BU: JCO interviews on excellence in finishing, *J Clin Orthod* 20:460 and 536, 1986.

202. Zachrisson BU: *Adult retention: a new approach.* In Graber LW, editor: *Orthodontics: state of the art; essence of the science,* St Louis, 1986, Mosby, p. 310.

203. Zachrisson BU: *Finishing and retention procedures for improved esthetics and stability.* In Nanda R, editor: *Fourth international orthodontic symposium,* Hartford, 1993, University of Connecticut (in press).

204. Zachrisson BU, Årtun J: Enamel surface appearance after various debonding techniques, *Am J Orthod* 75:121, 1979.

205. Zachrisson BU, Brobakken BO: Clinical comparison of direct versus indirect bonding with different bracket types and adhesives, *Am J Orthod* 74:62, 1978.

206. Zachrisson BU, Heimgard E et al: Problems with sealants for bracket bonding, *Am J Orthod* 75:641, 1979.

207. Zachrisson BU, Mjör IA: Remodelling of teeth by grinding, *Am J Orthod* 68:545, 1975.

208. Zachrisson BU, Skogan Ø, Høymyhr S: Enamel cracks in debonded, debanded, and orthodontically untreated teeth, *Am J Orthod* 77:307, 1980.

209. Zachrisson BU, Thilander B: *Treatment of dento-alveolar anomalies.* In Thilander B, Rönning O, editors: *Introduction to orthodontics,* Tandläkarforlaget, Stockholm, 1985, p. 135.

210. Zachrisson BU, Zachrisson S: Caries incidence and oral hygiene during orthodontic treatment, *Scand J Dent Res* 79:394, 1971.

211. Zachrisson BU, Zachrisson S: Caries incidence and orthodontic treatment with fixed appliances, *Scand J Dent Res* 79:183, 1971.

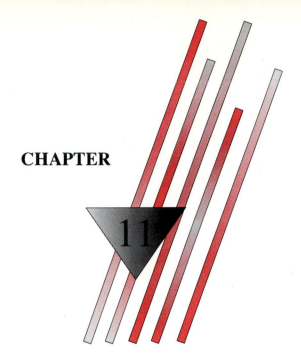

CHAPTER

11

The Tweed-Merrifield Edgewise Appliance: Philosophy, Diagnosis, and Treatment

JAMES L. VADEN

JACK G. DALE

HERBERT A. KLONTZ

"Nothing worthwhile ever departs."

HISTORICAL PERSPECTIVE

It was an obsession for order that motivated Edward Hartley Angle (Fig. 11-1) to create the Angle System in 1887. This system ultimately resulted in the introduction of the edgewise multibanded appliance 41 years later in 1928—2 years before his death. A man of great vision, he created The Angle School of Orthodontia in 1900. It was the first school of its kind in orthodontics. Being a postgraduate institution, the objective was to train highly selected and gifted dentists to ensure that Angle's "worthwhile" system would never "depart."

Before the Angle System, orthodontics was being practiced in a highly individualistic manner. There were hundreds of different ways to treat patients. Many practitioners made the appliances by hand from raw materials. Treatment was awkward, fragmentary, time-consuming, empirical and, in a word, chaotic. Individuals began nowhere and ended nowhere. They often created what Angle referred to as appliance monstrosities (Fig. 11-2).

What was orthodontics like before the Angle System, and why was it referred to as being in a chaotic condition?

The first scientific attempt at tooth movement occurred in 1728 when the French physician, Pierre Fauchard, made use of a flat strip of metal, pierced with holes suitably placed. The strip was formed into an arch. Various *crooked* teeth were secured to it by means of threads passing around them and through the holes. The threads were then tied to apply a force to the teeth (Fig. 11-3). The anchorage that it employed was simple anchorage, for it accomplished only simple tooth-tipping movement. Thus the first expansion arch was introduced into orthodontics. Unfortunately, it lacked stability; there was no effective way to firmly fix it in position on the teeth.

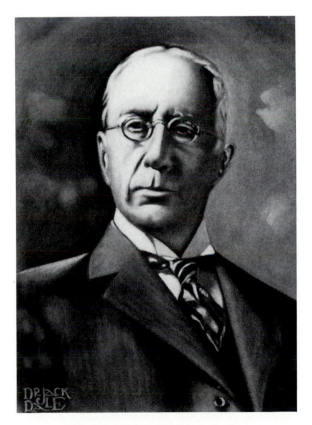

Fig. 11-1   Dr. Edward H. Angle.

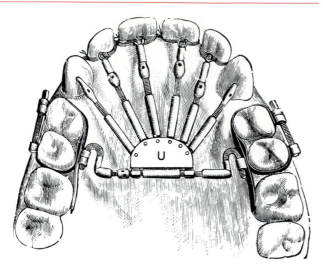

Fig. 11-2   An appliance used before the Angle system, often referred to by Dr. Angle as a monstrosity. (From Angle EH: *Treatment of malocclusion of the teeth,* Philadelphia, 1907, SS White Dental Manufacturing, p. 176.)

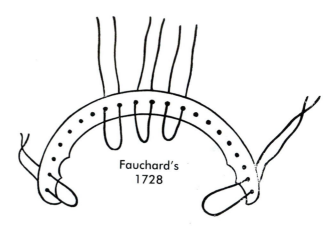

Fig. 11-3   Pierre Fauchard's orthodontic appliance, 1728. (From Angle EH: *Treatment of malocclusion of the teeth,* Philadelphia, 1907, SS White Dental Manufacturing, p. 196.)

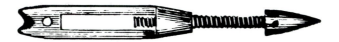

Fig. 11-4   Dwinelle's jack-screw, 1849. (From Steiner CC: *The Angle orthodontist,* Brooklyn, NY, 1933, E.H. Angle Society of Orthodontia, p. 281.)

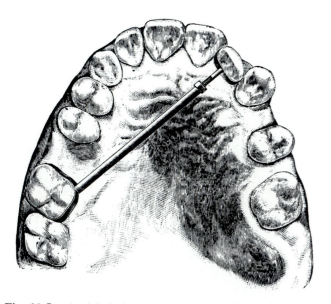

Fig. 11-5   Angle's jack-screw. (From Goddard CL: *The American text-book of operative dentistry,* Philadelphia, 1897, Lea Brothers, p. 580.)

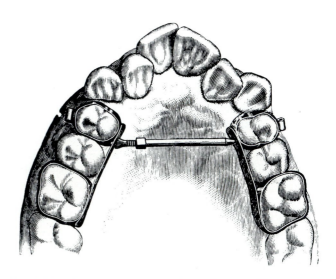

Fig. 11-6   Angle's jack-screw. (From Goddard CL: *The American text-book of operative dentistry,* Philadelphia, 1897, Lea Brothers, p. 567.)

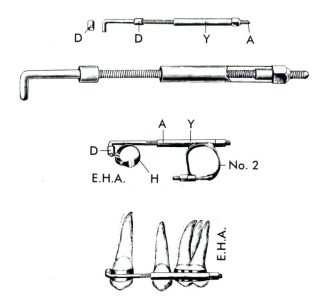

Fig. 11-7 Angle's retraction screw, 1887. (From Angle EH: *Treatment of malocclusion of the teeth,* Philadelphia, 1907, SS White Dental Manufacturing, p. 186.)

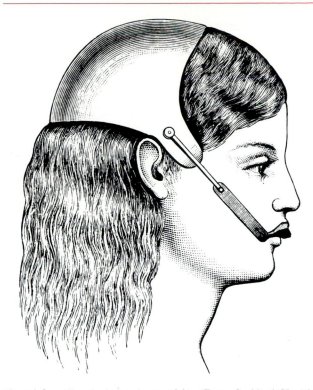

Fig. 11-8 Kingsley's headgear, 1861. (From Goddard CL: *The American text-book of operative dentistry,* Philadelphia, 1897, Lea Brothers, p. 642.)

Schange, another Frenchman, invented the adjustable clamp band with the introduction of a lingual screw, in 1841. In the intervening 113 years many removable appliances were made. Through the use of vulcanite the dentist attempted to gain greater stability but without much success. Angle was never impressed with removable contemporary appliances.

The practice of orthodontics was altered forever in 1870 with an invention that most orthodontists have not seriously associated with treatment. It was the invention of dental cement by Magill of Erie, Pennsylvania. Indeed, without adhesives, orthodontic practice as we know it today would not be possible.

In 1849 in New York, Dwinelle invented the regulating jack screw (Fig. 11-4). It delivered a pushing force on the teeth. Angle improved the jack screw by making it more delicate, and by increasing its range of action (Figs. 11-5 and 11-6). After tedious experimentation he replaced gold with a fine quality nickel silver. In this instance reciprocal anchorage was employed. He also developed the regulating retraction screw (Fig. 11-7). This screw delivered a pulling force on the teeth. Stationary anchorage was now possible in treatment. Instead of taking anchorage from the crest of the alveolar process alone, it could now be secured throughout the entire length of the tooth root (Fig. 11-7). Soldering was introduced at this time to provide for the attachment of the jack screws and the retraction screws to bands.

The orthodontic appliance now had the archwire, bands, cement, and soldered attachments. It had the jack screw and the retraction screw to provide a push and a pull force to the teeth, and it was now possible to employ simple, reciprocal and stationary anchorage. It is important to point

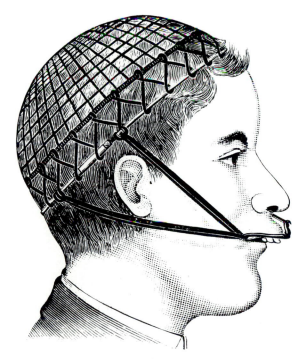

Fig. 11-9 Dr. Angle's headgear *(cap).* (From Goddard CL: *The American text-book of operative dentistry,* Philadelphia, 1897, Lea Brothers, p. 627.)

out that these components were made on fine machinery by skilled machinists.

In 1861 Kingsley (1829-1913) introduced the headgear to apply extra oral force and provide occipital anchorage (Fig. 11-8). Angle respected Kingsley so much that he immediately incorporated Kingsley's headgear into his evolving system (Fig. 11-9).

In 1861 Coffin introduced flexible piano wire. In 1887 Angle developed the prototype of the first bracket attachment: a delicate metal tube soldered to the band. These two inventions that took place 26 years apart enabled the orthodontist to apply a rotation force to teeth (Fig. 11-10).

Although Tucker described the use of rubber elastics in Boston in 1846, the new invention did not become significant until Case and Baker used it to provide intermaxillary force and intermaxillary anchorage. Intermaxillary anchorage became known as Baker Anchorage (Fig. 11-11).

Edward Angle, following graduation from dental school in 1878 and before his introduction of the Angle System in 1887, experienced many technical problems and frustrations in treatment, which irritated, motivated, and inspired him to develop a standard appliance. He believed that an orthodontic appliance must have five properties:

1. Simple: must push, pull, and rotate teeth
2. Stable: must be fixed to the teeth
3. Efficient: must be based on Newton's third law and anchorage
4. Delicate: must be accepted by the tissues and must not cause inflammation and soreness
5. Inconspicuous: must be esthetically acceptable

He designed a standard appliance composed of a specific number of basic components (Fig. 11-12). He had these components mass produced so they could be assembled into a simple, stable, efficient, delicate, and inconspicuous treatment device—without difficulty, in less time, and with minimal pain and discomfort to the patient. This universal application enabled practitioners to treat more patients and to reach a higher level of excellence, with less expense than

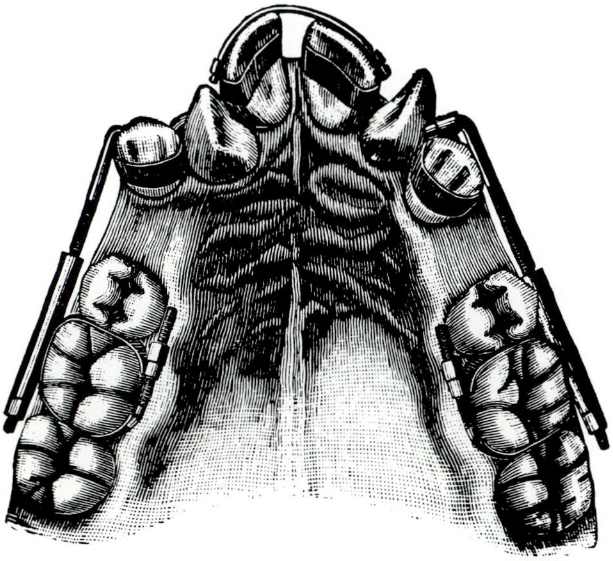

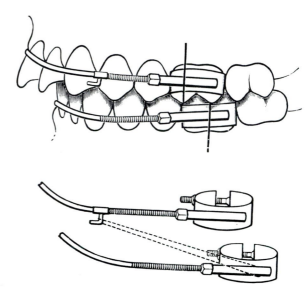

Fig. 11-11 Baker's intermaxillary anchorage. (From Steiner CC: *The Angle orthodontist,* Brooklyn, NY, 1933, EH Angle Society of Orthodontia, p. 283.)

Fig. 11-10 Dr. Angle's appliance, 1887, illustrating adjustable clamp bands, retraction screws, cemented bands, soldered attachment (retraction screw to clamp band), soldered tubes (prototype of first bracket on incisors and cuspids), and rotation spring on incisors. (From Angle EH: *Treatment of malocclusion of the teeth,* Philadelphia, 1907, SS White Dental Manufacturing, p. 590.)

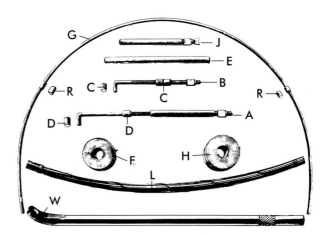

Fig. 11-12 The basic components of Dr. Angle's standard appliance, illustrating traction screws, *A* and *B,* attachment tubes, *C* and *D,* jack-screws, *E* and *J,* lever wires, *L,* band material, *F* and *H,* archwire, *G,* and wrench, *W.* (From Angle EH: *Treatment of malocclusion of the teeth,* Philadelphia, 1907, SS White Dental Manufacturing, p. 188.)

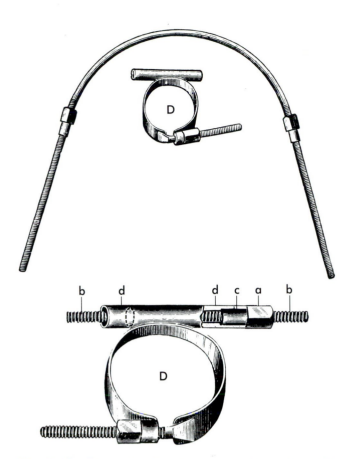

Fig. 11-13   Dr. Angle's E arch appliance. (From Angle EH: *Treatment of malocclusion of the teeth*, Philadelphia, 1907, SS White Dental Manufacturing, p. 199.)

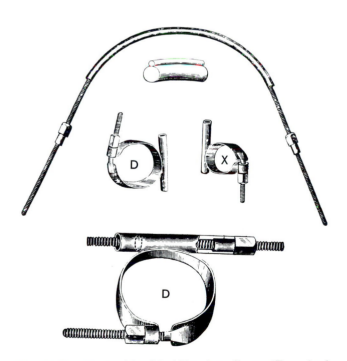

Fig. 11-14   Dr. Angle's ribbed E arch appliance. (From Angle EH: *Treatment of malocclusion of the teeth*, Philadelphia, 1907, SS White Dental Manufacturing, p. 200.)

they had done previously. In effect it was the beginning of a relationship between the manufacturers, the suppliers, and the orthodontists—it was the **Angle System.**

THE DEVELOPMENT OF THE EDGEWISE APPLIANCE
The E Arch Appliance

By the time that the seventh and final edition of Angle's book was published in 1907, he had virtually discontinued the use of jack screws. He now used a heavy, ideal expansion arch attached by solder to two first molar clamp bands (Fig. 11-13). It employed crown movements of teeth and simple anchorage. Brass ligature wire and stationary anchorage in the molar area were used to expand all the teeth into normal alignment and occlusion. The heavy archwire was supplied in four different designs, depending on the treatment planned:

1. The basic E arch as seen in Fig. 11-13. It was used in the mandible in Baker (Case) Anchorage (Fig. 11-11).
2. The ribbed E arch as seen in Fig. 11-14. It was used in expansion by tying brass ligatures to the arch (Fig. 11-15).
3. The E arch without threaded ends that fit into the molar sheaths, with an attached ball for the high-pull headgear in the incisor area (Figs. 11-16, *A,* and 11-17).
4. The E arch with hooks, as seen in the maxilla (Fig. 11-11). The entire maxillary dentition was moved distally, and the mandibular dentition was moved mesially by the action of intermaxillary elastics. This approach also had a maxillo-mandibular growth guidance effect which was to be recognized later.

With the basic and ribbed E arch, the dentition was enlarged in all dimensions by the ligatures; retention appliances were worn as long as the patient would tolerate them, and when they were discarded, various degrees of malocclusion recurred.

With the use of the E arch in conjunction with the high-pull headgear, the protruding maxillary anterior teeth were

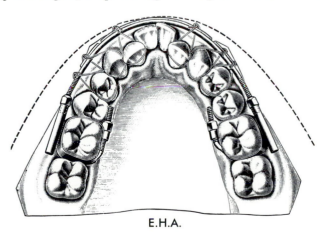

E.H.A.

Fig. 11-15   Dr. Angle's ribbed E arch appliance in use. (From Angle EH: *Treatment of malocclusion of the teeth*, Philadelphia, 1907, SS White Dental Manufacturing, p. 249.)

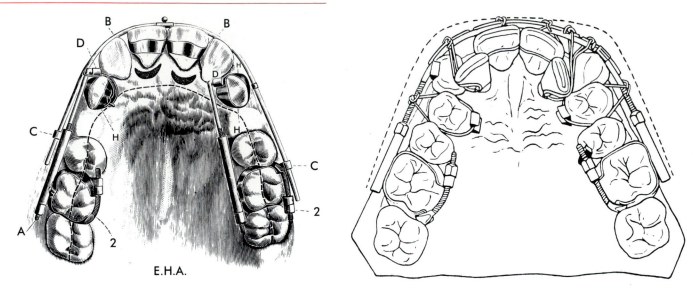

Fig. 11-16 Dr. Angle's E arch appliance, illustrating the ball joint attachment for the headgear and retraction screws. (From Angle EH: *Treatment of malocclusion of the teeth,* Philadelphia, 1907, SS White Dental Manufacturing, p. 602.)

retracted into spaces provided by the extraction of permanent first premolar teeth—that's correct: *the extraction of teeth* (Figs. 11-16 through 11-18).

> *By studying this device in its entirety it will be seen how nearly ideal the plan is for the distribution of force for the reduction of the permanent teeth; how as the arch receives pressure from the ball and socket joint. It is moved distally, not only carrying the protruding teeth with it, but compelling their regular arrangement, all being retracted until the spaces made vacant by the ex-traction of the first premolars are closed, without any displacement of the posterior teeth.*
>
> **Edward H. Angle,**
> *The Malocclusion of the Teeth,*
> *Seventh Edition, 1907, p. 193.*

Angle discontinued extracting teeth, for the most part, when he began using intermaxillary elastic forces and Baker Anchorage (Fig. 11-11). He used a maxillary E arch with threaded ends and with intermaxillary hooks. This permitted the correct orientation of the teeth of both arches into proper occlusion without extraction. The maxillary dentition was retracted, and the mandibular dentition was moved forward. Unfortunately, there was a serious problem: the correction of the axial relationships of the teeth could not be accomplished. He concluded from his failures that it was necessary to move teeth bodily to produce stable results.

The Pin and Tube Appliance

In response to this necessity, Angle developed the pin and tube appliance (Fig. 11-19). The new appliance served its purpose admirably. However, the ideal arch of the E arch appliance had to be sacrificed in order to fit each tooth with the pin and tube attachment. The arches had to be altered as tooth movement was carried out—always progressing toward ideal arch form. To accomplish tooth movement, pins had to be expertly soldered, fitted perfectly into the tubes on the bands, removed, moved along the archwire, soldered again; and fitted once more into the tubes on the bands. This precise and delicate maneuver had to be carried out with each appointment. At the same time the axial inclination of the pins had to be altered and the square ends of the archwire had to be fitted properly into the square tubes on the molar bands. Patients were required to come into the office for activation every few days. The pin and tube appliance was an exceedingly difficult appliance to manipulate; only a few operators could use it. Nevertheless, it was the first appliance with a mechanism for root movement.

The Ribbon Arch Appliance

Because the pin and tube appliance was difficult to use, Angle, in 1915, developed the ribbon arch appliance (Fig. 11-20). Brackets were introduced with this new appliance. It was a much simpler appliance to construct and to activate. It was characterized by brackets with a vertical slot. The archwire, which initially conformed to the malocclusion, was held in place in the brackets by brass pins. The teeth were free to move along the archwire like a string of beads. The appliance had force control and a degree of stationary anchorage. The Begg technique is based on this appliance with the bracket placed upside down.

En masse movement of teeth was necessary, particularly

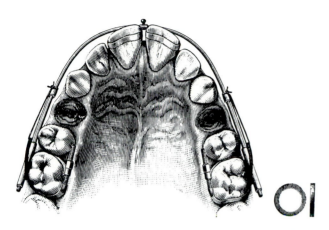

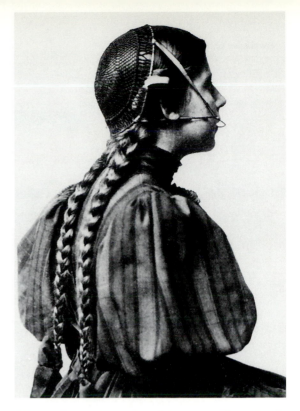

Fig. 11-17 Dr. Angle's E arch appliance, illustrating the ball joint attachment for the headgear and elastic traction. (From Angle EH: *Treatment of malocclusion of the teeth*, Philadelphia, 1907, SS White Dental Manufacturing, p. 190.)

Fig. 11-18 Dr. Angle's high-pull headgear, illustrating the cap and the elastic traction. (From Angle EH: *Treatment of malocclusion of the teeth*, Philadelphia, 1907, SS White Dental Manufacturing, p. 192.)

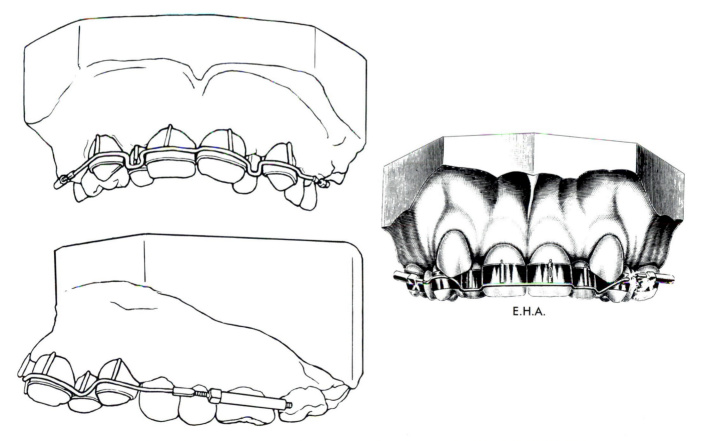

E.H.A.

Fig. 11-19 Dr. Angle's pin and tube appliance. (From Steiner CC: *The Angle orthodontist*, Brooklyn, NY, Philadelphia, 1933, EH Angle Society of Orthodontia, p. 284.)

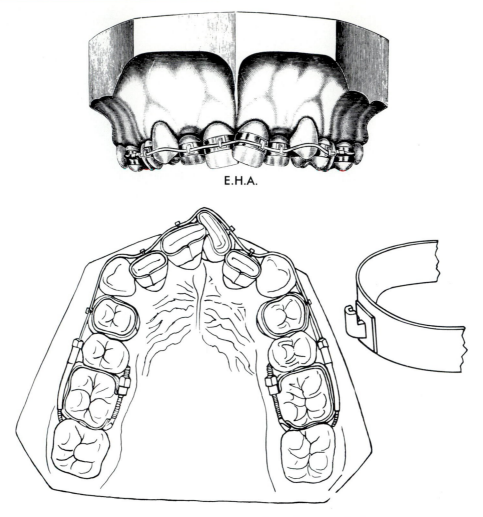

E.H.A.

Fig. 11-20 Dr. Angle's ribbon arch appliance. (From Steiner CC: *The Angle orthodontist*, Brooklyn, NY, 1933, EH Angle Society of Orthodontia, p. 284.)

in an anteroposterior direction in a significant number of patients. The ribbon arch appliance was not generally suitable for this type of movement. Anterior teeth could only be retracted at the expense of the anchorage provided by the posterior teeth. Mesial and distal tipping bends could not be incorporated into the archwire, and the premolar teeth could not be moved bodily.

The Edgewise Appliance

With the knowledge born from his experience, Angle set out once again to devise an appliance that would not only overcome these difficulties but would better relate possibilities to ideals of treatment than did its predecessor (Fig. 11-21). He changed the form of the brackets by locating the slot in the center and by placing it in a horizontal plane, instead of in a vertical plane. The archwire was held in position, first by a brass ligature and later by a delicate stainless steel wire ligature. The ribbon arch appliance

bracket had only two walls within the bracket itself; the third wall was the band surrounding the wall, and the slot opened vertically. The new edgewise bracket consisted of a rectangular box with three walls within the bracket, 0.022 inch × 0.028 inch in dimension; its slot opened horizontally (Fig. 11-22). This new design provided more accuracy and thus a more efficient torquing mechanism.

Angle introduced the edgewise bracket 2 years before he died. He had little time to teach its manipulation, to develop it further, or to improve its use—and he knew it.

CHARLES H. TWEED (Fig. 11-23)

When Tweed graduated from an improvised Angle course given by George Hahn in 1928, he was 33 years of age, and Angle was 73. Angle was bitterly disappointed in the reception that had been accorded the edgewise appliance. He was infuriated and bitter about the modifications that were being made by several of his graduates, particularly

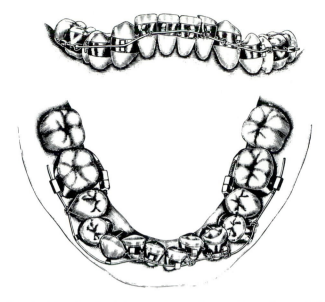

Fig. 11-21 Dr. Angle's edgewise appliance. (From Steiner CC: *The Angle orthodontist,* Brooklyn, New York 1933, EH Angle Society of Orthodontia.

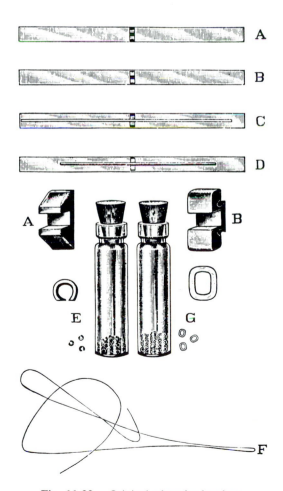

Fig. 11-22 Original edgewise brackets.

Spencer Adkinson. It was obvious that something had to be done if this appliance was to survive intact. Angle decided that an article describing the appliance must be published in *Dental Cosmos.* Since Tweed had just finished the *course,* and since Angle admired and respected Tweed's ability, he asked Tweed to help with the article. For 7 weeks they worked together and in the process became close friends. It was during this time that Angle advised Tweed that he could never master the edgewise appliance unless he limited his practice solely to its use. And so, with the completion of the article for *Dental Cosmos,* Charles Tweed returned to Arizona and established (in Phoenix) the *first pure edgewise specialty practice in the United States.*

For the next 2 years, the two men worked closely together. Tweed diagnosed and treated his patients, while Angle acted as his advisor. Dr. Angle was pleased with the results, and he was instrumental in making it possible for Tweed to participate in several programs. During these 2 years and in a series of over 100 letters (now housed in the Tweed Foundation library), Angle urged his young disciple to carry out two vital requests: (1) to dedicate his life to the development of the edgewise appliance; and (2) to make every effort to establish orthodontics as a specialty within the dental profession.

Dr. Tweed acted upon these requests. He secured the passing of the *first orthodontic specialty law in the United States.* He accomplished this task by canvassing patients, by persuading dentists, by influencing politicians, by arousing patients, by speaking at meetings, by having petitions

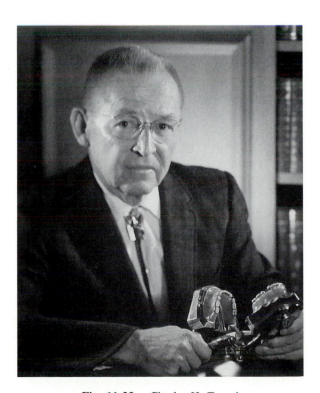

Fig. 11-23 Charles H. Tweed.

signed, and even by taking patients before the legislature. In short it was a one-man blitz. His untiring and relentless efforts were successful, and in 1929 the Arizona legislature passed the *first law limiting the practice of orthodontics to specialists.* Dr. Tweed received Arizona's Certificate No. 1 and became the *first certified specialist in orthodontics in the United States.*

On August 11, 1930, Dr. Edward Hartley Angle died at the age of 75. There is a strange antithesis to be found between the first printed lines of Dr. Angle, wherein he states: "We are reminded that there is still much to be accomplished before this great subject of orthodontics is unfolded to us in a manner in which we may comprehend it in all its requirements," and his words, spoken so shortly before death, "I have finished my work, it is as perfect as I can make it." The intervening years were spent in unceasing effort, constant work, illness, and considerable bitterness. Happily, toward the end, with the help of his beloved wife, Anna Hopkins Angle, he achieved success and witnessed the fulfillment of his cherished goals. Nevertheless, everyone knew he, who was always experimenting; always selecting and discarding; never satisfied with the results at hand; always pondering over possible improvement, would be the last to accept perfection (even if he had attained it), until he and the world had proved it beyond all reasonable doubt. Angle must have known, even when he made his last statement on his death bed, that his work must go on. He must have been at peace with the knowledge that he had found the right man to carry on his beautiful work.

In 1932 Dr. Tweed published his first article in the Angle Orthodontist. It was titled: *Reports of Cases Treated with Edgewise Arch Mechanism.*[25] Tweed held to Angle's firm conviction that the practitioner must never extract teeth. This conviction lasted for 3 years.

What Tweed began to observe in his patients during retention was discouraging to him. It was so discouraging, in fact, that he almost gave up orthodontic practice. He knew he had the appliance and he knew he had the ability, but his results were unsatisfactory. He devoted the next 3 years of his life to a study of his successes and his failures. During this 3-year period he made a most important observation: upright mandibular incisors were frequently related to successful treatment. In order to upright incisors, he concluded that the clinician must prepare anchorage and extract teeth. He then selected his failures, extracted four first premolar teeth from them, and retreated them. He did this without charging a fee.

In 1936 Dr. Tweed delivered and subsequently published his first paper[26,27] on the extraction of teeth for orthodontic treatment to the membership of the Angle Society. "Mother" Angle who was also an orthodontist, the editor of the Angle Orthodontist, and a member of the Angle Society, refused to attend the lecture. George Hahn, the man who went out of his way to create the opportunity for Tweed to take the Angle course, criticized him severely. Angle disciples considered Charles Tweed to be a traitor to the greatest man

orthodontics had ever known. Tweed was crushed by the response; however, he returned home determined to continue his research.

He worked even harder than before. By 1940 he had produced case reports (four sets of records) of 100 consecutively treated patients, who were first treated nonextraction and later with extraction therapy. He presented a paper and displayed his case reports at the next meeting of the Angle Society in Chicago.

Dr. Strang, one of Angle's students in the early years, described the event this way:

I noted that Dr. Charles Tweed was scheduled to be on the program of the meeting in Chicago. I planned to be there with the objective of lacing into him for violating Dr. Angle's sacred principle of nonextraction in treatment.

Previous to reading his paper, Dr. Tweed had placed on tables before and after models and photographs of one hundred consecutively treated cases. The results in all of these one hundred cases were magnificent and beyond criticism. I also met Dr. Tweed and noted that he was a most modest, unassuming and friendly chap.

Dr. Tweed read his well-written and illustrated paper. He explained his objective of keeping the teeth over basal bone, which made it necessary to extract teeth in many patients; however, it did produce stable results. Then he sat down. There was no applause. The room filled with shouted demands from the floor. For at least an hour, Charlie got the worst tongue-lashing that you can possibly imagine and not one word of praise for the beautiful results of treatment. Here was a student of Dr. Angle's violating the most fixed and rigid rule in his instruction— never extract teeth.

During all this vicious attack, my mind took a complete turnover. I could visualize nothing but that marvelous exhibit of treated cases. Not one individual in the room had complimented the essayist. They were all ripping him to pieces for extracting teeth. Finally, I obtained the floor and complimented and defended him to the best of my ability. When I sat down, I, too, took a tongue-lashing that compared very favorably with the one Charlie had just received. Subsequently, I took his course, and practiced, taught and published his techniques in my textbook. Dr. Tweed's work was so outstanding as to elevate him, in my mind, to the position of the best clinical orthodontist in the world.[24]

Tweed's many contributions to the specialty established a benchmark in orthodontic thought and treatment. Most notable among his many contributions were the following:

1. Emphasized the four objectives of orthodontic treatment with emphasis and concern for facial esthetics
2. Developed the concept of uprighting teeth over basal bone with emphasis on the mandibular incisors
3. Made the extraction of teeth for orthodontic correction acceptable, and popularized the extraction of the first premolars[28]

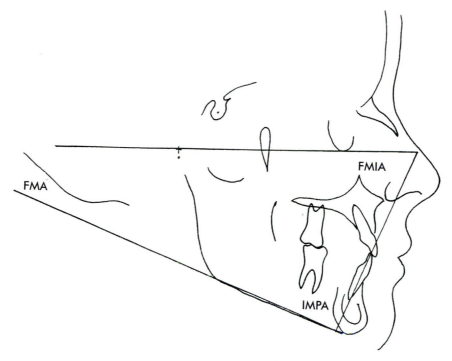

Fig. 11-24 Tweed's diagnostic facial triangle.

4. Enhanced the clinical application of cephalometrics
5. Developed the diagnostic facial triangle[30] to make cephalometrics a diagnostic tool, as well as a guide in treatment and an evaluation of treatment results (Fig. 11-24)
6. Developed a concept of orderly treatment procedures and introduced anchorage preparation as a major step in treatment[29,31]
7. Developed a fundamentally sound and consistent preorthodontic guidance program using and popularizing serial extraction of primary and permanent teeth

In addition to his many clinical contributions to the specialty, Tweed gave guidance, inspiration, and leadership to more orthodontists than anyone else in the world. Because of Charles Tweed and his disciples, the edgewise appliance became universally popular and the practice of clinical orthodontics was regarded more as a necessary service requested by the public.

Angle gave orthodontics the edgewise *bracket,* but Tweed gave the specialty the *appliance.* Tweed was considered the premier edgewise orthodontist of his day. Many who admired his results wished to learn his techniques. The orthodontic world journeyed to Tucson to take Tweed's course to learn his method of treatment with the edgewise appliance. *The Tweed Philosophy was born.*

Dr. Tweed, one of orthodontics' most brilliant innovators, kept his promise to his mentor. He devoted 42 years of his life (from 1928 until his death on January 11, 1970) to the advancement of the edgewise appliance.

LEVERN MERRIFIELD

In 1960 Tweed selected one of his most outstanding students, Levern Merrifield (Fig. 11-25), Ponca City, Oklahoma, to continue his work on the edgewise appliance and to be the co-director of his course. Merrifield took Tweed's course in 1953 and became a member of Tweed's staff in 1955. He became the course director at the time of Tweed's death in 1970. Merrifield has devoted the past 40 years of his life to the study of orthodontic diagnosis and to the use of the edgewise appliance. Merrifield's contributions have been popularized and are now being taught at the *Tweed Course* in Tucson. These include:

1. The fundamental concept of *Dimensions of the Denture*[9]

The differential diagnostic concepts of:

2. Dimensions of the lower face
3. Total space analysis[12,13]
4. Guidelines for space management decisions to:
   A. Facilitate maximum orthodontic correction
   B. Define areas of skeletal, facial, and dental disharmony

The treatment concepts of:

5. Directional control during treatment[14]
6. Sequential tooth movement
7. Sequential mandibular anchorage preparation[15]
8. The organization of treatment into four orderly steps, which have specific objectives

Merrifield's innovations in diagnosis and his experience in the use of the edgewise appliance have improved on

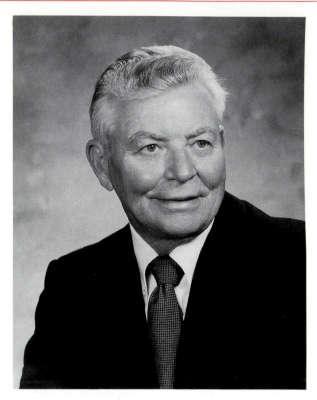

Fig. 11-25   Levern Merrifield.

Tweed's contributions and concepts to give the modern orthodontist a more accurate, reliable, precise, efficient, and practical protocol of diagnosis and treatment. Adherence to this protocol allows the clinician to: (1) define objectives for the face, the skeletal pattern, and the dentition; (2) properly diagnose the malocclusion; and (3) treat with the edgewise appliance to efficiently reach the predetermined objectives.

These universally accepted objectives enable the clinician to position and arrange the teeth for:

1. Maximum stability and esthetics
2. Functional efficiency
3. Health of the teeth, the jaws, the joints, and the surrounding tissues
4. Facial balance and harmony

They also allow him or her to:

5. Position and arrange the teeth in the immature patient, to harmonize the correction with normal growth processes, and to maximize the compensation for the less-than-normal pattern
6. Position the dentition so that it is in a continual state of maximum harmony with its environment (This final objective can be realized only if the first five objectives are successfully attained.)

DIMENSIONS OF THE DENTURE

The clinical practice of orthodontics has always been based on the various dimensions of the dentition. There are three dimensions: height, width, and length (vertical; transverse; sagittal). These dimensions allow the teeth to be moved in six directions: mesially, distally, facially, lingually, intrusively, and extrusively. All of these movements, which are routinely accomplished with orthodontic appliances, are limited and restricted by the physical environment of bone, muscle, and soft tissue, which exert an influence on the teeth and the jaws. Since the beginning of the orthodontic specialty, an effort has been made to determine the extreme limits of this environment. It appears that each engineering change in appliance fabrication brings about a new challenge to the physical limitations of the dentition's environment. *Dimensions of the denture* include four basic premises—*provided that the musculature is normal:*

Premise 1: There is an anterior limit. The teeth must not be placed forward of basal bone. If the teeth are too far forward, all of the aforementioned objectives of treatment are compromised.

Premise 2: There is a posterior limit. Teeth can be positioned distally off the maxillary tuberosity and/or impacted into the area behind the mandibular first molar in the mandibular arch just as they can be moved too far forward of basal bone.

Premise 3: There is a lateral limit. If the teeth are moved buccally into the masseter and buccinator muscles, relapse is likely to result over the long term.

Premise 4: There is a vertical limit. Vertical expansion is disastrous to facial balance and harmony in the sagittal plane, except in deep bite cases.

In summary, orthodontists must recognize their limitations and design their treatment to conform to these dimensions *when normal muscle balance exists.*

DIFFERENTIAL DIAGNOSIS

Merrifield, in his effort to establish a sound diagnostic basis for his *Directional Force* treatment, using multibanded mechanotherapy, introduced analyses that allow clinicians to determine which teeth should be removed when extractions are necessary. His work enables the clinician to arrive at a differential diagnosis instead of treating all extraction problems by removing four first premolars, as did Dr. Tweed.

Attainment of the previously stated objectives requires a thorough and accurate diagnosis that specifically identifies the major areas of disharmony. Webster defines diagnosis as "a determination of a disease from symptoms, data, or tests, and the decisions and judgments made prior to treatment." Merrifield's diagnostic philosophy can be outlined as follows:

1. Recognize and treat within the dimensions of the denture. This means *nonexpansion* in malocclusions with normal muscular balance.
2. Recognize the dimensions of the lower face, and treat for maximum facial harmony and balance.
3. Recognize and understand the skeletal pattern. Diagnose

and treat in harmony with normal growth and developmental patterns, and optimize the less than normal pattern. Once the major areas of disharmony are identified, all necessary and practical means should be expended to correct the problem.

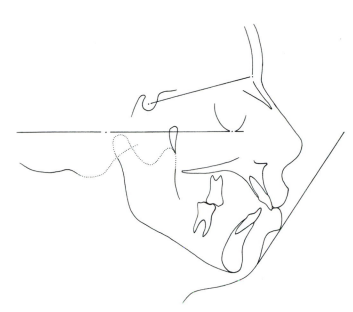

Fig. 11-26   Profile line drawn on a protrusive face.

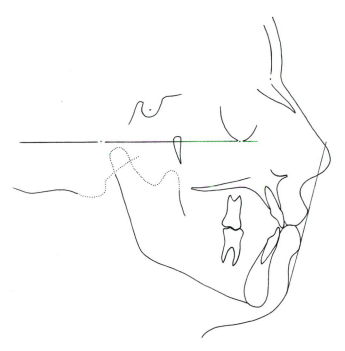

Fig. 11-27   Profile line drawn on a facial profile that exhibits balance and harmony.

The Face

The dimension of the lower face is vitally important to the achievement of esthetic and harmonious facial balance. The profile line is universally used to give the orthodontic practitioner an idea of lip procumbency and balance (Fig. 11-26). The ideal relationship of the profile line to soft tissue is to be tangent to the chin, to the vermilion border of both lips, and to bisect the nose (Fig. 11-27). For centuries it has been a premise that this type of relationship of the profile line to the lips, the chin, and the nose results in a pleasing and balanced appearance. Integral to the diagnosis of facial balance is an observation of the relative thickness of the upper lip and the total chin (Fig. 11-28). Upper lip thickness should equal total chin thickness. If these two values are different (particularly if total chin thickness is less than upper lip thickness), a compensation must be made in anterior retraction that will result in a more ideal facial balance and harmony.

Similarly, on frontal view the face should be balanced. The vermilion border of the lower lip should bisect the distance between the bottom of the chin and the ala of the nose. The vermilion border of the upper lip should also bisect the distance from the vermilion border of the lower lip to the ala of the nose. These relationships are universally accepted orthodontic standards for facial balance and harmony.

The Skeletal Pattern

An analytical observation of the skeletal pattern is an integral part of any diagnosis. A careful cephalometric analysis must include (but is not limited to) a study and an understanding of the following information (Figs. 11-29 and 11-30):

FMIA—Tweed established a standard of 68° for individuals with an FMA of 22° to 28°. The standard should be 65° if the FMA is 30° or above, and the FMIA will increase if the FMA is lower. Tweed believed that this value was

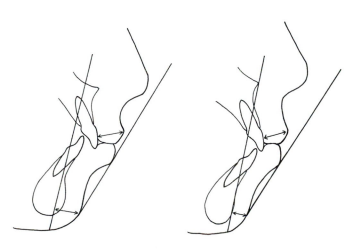

Fig. 11-28   Drawing of relative lip thickness.

significant in establishing balance and harmony of the lower face.

FMA—The FMA is probably the most significant value for skeletal analysis because it defines the direction of lower facial growth in both the horizontal and vertical dimension. The standard or normal range of 22° to 28° for this value projects a skeletal pattern with normal growth direction. An FMA greater than the normal range indicates excessive vertical growth, and an FMA less than the normal range indicates deficient vertical growth.

IMPA—The IMPA defines the axial inclination of the mandibular incisor in relation to the mandibular plane. It is

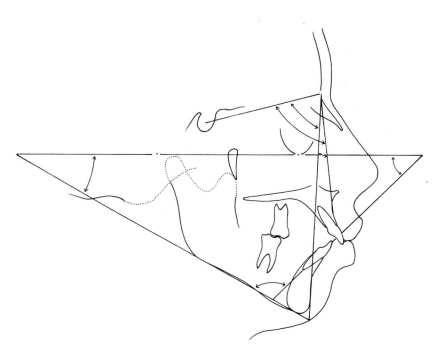

Fig. 11-29   Cephalometric tracing with all values and planes.

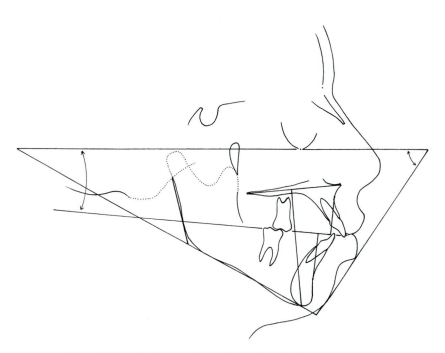

Fig. 11-30   Cephalometric tracing with all values and planes.

a good guide to use in maintaining or positioning these teeth in their relationship to basal bone. The standard of 88° indicates an upright position, and with a normal FMA, this position reflects optimum balance and harmony of the lower facial profile. If the FMA is above normal, the orthodontist must compensate by further uprighting the mandibular incisors. If the FMA is below the normal range, compensation can be made by leaving the mandibular incisors at their pretreatment position or by positioning them more to the labial. Labial inclination of the mandibular incisors is generally limited to 94° in patients with normal muscular balance because of tissue health and stability.

SNA—This angle indicates the relative horizontal position of the maxilla to the cranial base. The range at the termination of growth is 80° to 84° for a Caucasian sample.

SNB—This angle expresses the horizontal relationship of the mandible to the cranial base. A range of 78° to 82° indicates a normal horizontal mandibular position. If the value is below 74°, and a large maxillo-mandibular discrepancy exists, orthognathic surgery should be considered as an adjunct to orthodontic treatment. The same concern should be accorded a value of over 84°.

ANB—The normal range for this angle is 1° to 5°. This value expresses a favorable horizontal relationship of the maxilla to the mandible. Class II malocclusions become proportionally more difficult with higher ANB angles. A case with an ANB above 10° usually will require surgery as an adjunct to proper treatment. The negative ANB angle is even more indicative of facial disproportion in the horizontal dimension. A negative ANB angle of −3° or more, when the mandible is in its habitual occlusion, indicates a possibility of the need for surgical assistance in Class III orthodontic correction.

AO-BO—This relationship indicates the horizontal relationship of the maxilla to the mandible and is perhaps more sensitive to mal-relationships than the ANB angle because it is measured at the occlusal plane. Orthodontic treatment becomes more difficult when the AO-BO is greater than the normal range of 0 to 4 mm. The AO-BO changes in direct proportion to the occlusal plane angle.

Occlusal plane—This angular value expresses a dental-skeletal relationship of the occlusal plane to the Frankfort horizontal plane. A range of 8° to 12° is normal with variations of about 2° between males and females. The angle for the female averages approximately 9° and for the male approximately 11°. Values above and below the normal range indicate more difficulty in treatment. In most orthodontic corrections the original value should be maintained or decreased. An increase of the occlusal plane angle during treatment indicates a loss of control. An increase is usually unstable because the occlusal plane is determined by muscular balance, primarily the muscles of mastication. The occlusal plane angle frequently returns to its pretreatment value when it is increased, resulting in a detrimental relapse of the *corrected* interdental relationship.

Z angle—The chin/lip soft tissue profile line related to the Frankfort horizontal plane has a normal range of 70° to 80°. The ideal value is 75° to 78°, depending on age and sex. This angle was developed to further define facial esthetics and is an adjunct to the FMIA. It is more indicative of the soft tissue profile than FMIA and is responsive to maxillary incisor position. Maxillary incisor retraction of 4 mm allows 4 mm of lower lip retraction and approximately 3 mm of upper lip response. Horizontal mandibular repositioning will also affect this value. Vertical facial height increase, both anterior and posterior, can influence the Z angle. This angle enables the clinician to make a critical facial analysis.

Posterior facial height—This is a linear measurement in millimeters of ramus height from articulare to the mandibular plane, tangent to the posterior border of the ramus. The value is related to facial form, both vertically and horizontally. An increase in ramus height is essential for downward and forward mandibular response. The relationship of posterior facial height to anterior facial height determines the FMA and lower facial proportion. In the growing child with a Class II malocclusion, ramal growth change and its relationship to anterior facial height in both proportion and in volume is critical.

Anterior facial height—This is a linear measurement in millimeters of the vertical distance between the palatal plane and menton. The line is perpendicular to the palatal plane. A value of about 65 mm for a 12-year-old patient indicates a normal anterior facial height. This vertical value must be monitored carefully if it is more than 5 mm above or below normal. In Class II malocclusion correction it is essential to limit an increase in AFH. This is accomplished by controlling maxillary and mandibular molar extrusion and by using an anterior high-pull force on the maxilla.

Facial height index—André Horn[5] has recently studied the relationship of anterior to posterior facial height. After developing the Facial Height Index, he found that normal posterior facial height is 0.69 or 69% of anterior facial height. The normal range of PFH to AFH is 0.65 to 0.75. If the value is below or above this range, the malocclusion is more complex and it will be difficult to correct. An index of 0.80 is severe and indicates a low FMA malocclusion that is caused by either too much posterior growth or too little growth in the anterior. As the index approaches 0.60, the skeletal pattern demonstrates too little posterior height and/or too much anterior height.

Facial height change ratio—This ratio is valuable in the evaluation of the treatment interval changes. A ratio of 2 times as much posterior facial height increase as anterior facial height increase during treatment is ideal for the correction of Class II, division 1, and dentoalveolar protrusion malocclusions. However, even more important is the volume of change. For example, a 6 mm posterior facial height increase with a 3 mm anterior facial height increase is much more beneficial than a 2 mm posterior facial height increase coupled with a 1 mm anterior facial height increase, even though both values reflect a 2:1 ratio.

Radziminski,[20] Gebeck and Merrifield,[4,17] Isaacson,[6] Pearson,[18,19] and Schudy[23] have described the important relationship between vertical dimension control and successful treatment of Class II malocclusions. Following an evaluation of successfully and unsuccessfully treated Class II malocclusions, Merrifield and Gebeck concluded that successfully treated patients exhibited favorable mandibular changes. This occurred primarily because AFH was controlled and PFH increased. Unsuccessful treatment results were more likely to occur in patients where an increase was observed in AFH but not in PFH. Merrifield and Gebeck reported a 2-to-1 ratio of increase in PFH to AFH in their sample of successfully treated Class II malocclusions; that is, on the average PFH increased twice as much as AFH.

The Dentition

Total space analysis—Along with a consideration of the face and the skeletal pattern, the orthodontist must consider the dentition. Available space can neither be created nor destroyed by tooth movement. Therefore, orthodontic treatment is a space management procedure. Space management is a process of determining whether, when, and which teeth need to be extracted. This is differential diagnosis. The extraction of teeth is a treatment procedure, just as appliance construction and wire manipulation are treatment procedures. Often, diagnosis and treatment are confused. Diagnosis is an attempt to balance tooth material most advantageously with present and future available space. All 32 teeth, as well as the anterior, posterior, vertical, and lateral limits of the denture must be considered. *Total Space Analysis* as described by Merrifield[13] is divided into three parts:

1. Anterior
2. Midarch
3. Posterior

This division is made for the following two reasons:

1. Simplicity in identifying the area of space deficit or space surplus
2. Accuracy in differential diagnosis

1. Anterior denture area
   a. Teeth width

   $$3\ 2\ 1 \mid 1\ 2\ 3$$

   b. Available space
   c. Tooth arch disc
   d. Headfilm correction
   e. Soft tissue modification

2. Mid-arch denture area
   a. Teeth width

   $$6\ 5\ 4 \mid 4\ 5\ 6$$

   b. Available space
   c. Tooth arch disc
   d. Curve of Spee

3. Posterior denture area
   a. Teeth width

   $$8\ 7 \mid 7\ 8$$

   b. Available space
   c. Tooth arch disc
   d. Estimated increase

Denture total

_____

_____
_____
_____
_____

Deficit _____ Surplus _____

_____

_____
_____
_____

Deficit _____ Surplus _____

_____

_____
_____
_____

Deficit _____ Surplus _____
Deficit _____ Surplus _____

Headfilm correction

FMA 21° to 29°, the FMIA should be 68°
FMA 30° or greater, the FMIA should be 65°
FMA 20° or less, the IMPA should not exceed 94°
0.8 × the FMIA difference = correction

Increase in posterior denture area

3 mm per year for girls, until age 14
3 mm per year for boys, until age 16

Fig. 11-31 Total dentition space analysis.

Anterior Space Analysis (Fig. 11-31, *A*)

Anterior space analysis includes the measurement in millimeters of the space available in the mandibular arch from canine to canine and a measurement of the mesiodistal dimension of each of the six anterior teeth. The difference is referred to as a surplus or deficit. The Tweed diagnostic facial triangle is also used to further analyze this area. Lateral headfilm discrepancy is the amount of mandibular incisor uprighting that is needed to reach facial balance. This value is added to the anterior space measurement. The total (if a deficit) is referred to as anterior discrepancy. Anterior discrepancies are the overriding consideration of the malocclusion. They are correctly resolved by the removal of the first premolar teeth. The resulting space is used to move the canines distally in order to obtain the space to upright and align the incisors.

Midarch Analysis (Fig. 11-31, *B*)

The midarch area includes the mandibular first molars and the first and second premolars. Careful analysis of this area may show mesially inclined first molars, rotations, spaces, a deep curve of Spee, crossbites, missing teeth, habit abnormality, blocked out teeth, and occlusal disharmonies. This is an extremely important area of the denture. Because it is in the center of the arch, this area allows the easiest and most direct method of space management for malocclusion correction when it can be so used. Crowding, a deep curve of Spee, and end-on or full step Class II occlusions, not accompanied by anterior discrepancy, indicate a need for second premolar extraction in the mandibular arch. Careful measurement of the space from the distal of the canine to the distal of the first molar should be recorded as available midarch space. An equally accurate measurement of the mesiodistal width of the first premolar, the second premolar, and the first molar must also be recorded. To this is added the space required to level the curve of Spee. From these measurements the practitioner can determine the space deficit or surplus in this area.

Many diagnosticians have suggested that they extract second premolar teeth to eliminate facial retrusion. This is faulty reasoning. As a rule these cases have little anterior discrepancy, and the mandibular second premolars are removed because the resulting space is most advantageously located for the correction of midarch problems. The midarch space analysis is vital to proper differential diagnosis.

Posterior Space Analysis (Fig. 11-31, *C*)

The posterior denture area is of great importance. There is a posterior limit to the denture. Regardless of age, this posterior limit appears to be the anterior border of the ramus. The required space in the posterior space analysis is the mesiodistal width of the second molars and the third molars in the mandibular arch. The available space is more difficult to ascertain on the immature patient. It is a linear measurement in millimeters of the space distal to the mandibular first molars. The measurement is made from the distal of the mandibular first molar to the anterior border of the ramus along the occlusal plane. It is recognized that the posterior limit may be 2 to 3 mm distal to the anterior border of the ramus because of the lingual shelf that exists to accommodate the mandibular molars. However, these teeth on the lingual shelf are not generally in good functional occlusion. An estimate of posterior arch length increase based on both age and sex is added to this value.

Certain variables must be considered in estimating the increase in posterior available space. These variables are:
1. Rate of mesio-occlusal migration of the mandibular first molar
2. Rate of resorption of the anterior border of the ramus
3. Time of cessation of molar migration
4. Time of cessation of ramus resorption
5. Sex
6. Age

A review of the literature[2,9,21] reveals that a consensus of researchers suggest that 3 mm of increase in the posterior denture area occurs each year until age 14 for girls and age 16 for boys. This is an increase of 1.5 mm on each side per year, after the full eruption of the first molars. In the mature patient (girls beyond 15 years and boys beyond 16 years) a measurement from the distal of the first molar to the anterior border of the ramus at the occlusal plane is a valuable determination of the space available in the posterior area. It is of extreme importance to diagnosis and treatment planning to know whether there is a surplus or deficit of space in this area. It is not prudent to create a posterior discrepancy while making adjustments in other areas: the midarch or the anterior area. It is equally imprudent not to use a posterior space surplus to help alleviate midarch and anterior deficits. The most easily recognizable symptom of a posterior space deficit on the young patient is the late eruption of the second molar. If space is not available for this tooth by the age of its normal eruption, it should be obvious that there is a posterior space problem. A good lateral jaw x-ray examination can immediately confirm the clinical observation by using the above-mentioned guidelines.

In summary a *Total Space Analysis* (Fig. 11-31) is a valuable diagnostic tool that enables the orthodontic specialist to treat within the dimensions of the denture. The *Total Space Analysis,* when it is used with a skeletal analysis and a facial analysis, can lead the orthodontic clinician to make correct differential diagnostic decisions. Diagnosis, by definition, is both subjective and objective. When diagnostic guidelines or decisions are suggested, they can appropriately be called *one person's opinion.* The following diagnostic space management guidelines are suggested for use and should not be considered as rules. Some suggested diagnostic choices are outlined for (1) tooth/arch discrepancies, and (2) skeletal disharmonies.

DIAGNOSTIC SPACE MANAGEMENT GUIDELINES

Total Space Analysis—Tooth Arch Discrepancies

A. Anterior surplus or deficit:

+ to −2 mm	**Space management** Nonextraction	
3 mm to 5 mm without crowding	Extract:	$\dfrac{8 \mid 8}{8 \mid 8}$
3 mm to 5 mm with crowding	Extract:	$\dfrac{5 \mid 5}{5 \mid 5}$
5 mm to 7 mm with less than 3 mm anterior crowding	Extract:	$\dfrac{4 \mid 4}{5 \mid 5}$
5 mm to 7 mm with more than 3 mm anterior crowding	Extract:	$\dfrac{4 \mid 4}{4 \mid 4}$
7 mm to 15 mm anterior deficit	Extract:	$\dfrac{4 \mid 4}{4 \mid 4}$
16 mm and above	Extract:	$\dfrac{\times 4 \mid 4\times}{\times 4 \mid 4\times}$

B. Midarch surplus or deficit: Anterior deficits override midarch deficits

+ to 3 mm	Nonextraction	
3 mm to 5 mm without crowding	Extract:	$\dfrac{8 \mid 8}{8 \mid 8}$
3 mm to 5 mm with Class II molar	Extract:	$\dfrac{4 \mid 4}{5 \mid 5}$
5 mm to 7 mm with maxillary anterior protrusion	Extract:	$\dfrac{4 \mid 4}{5 \mid 5}$
5 mm to 7 mm	Extract:	$\dfrac{5 \mid 5}{5 \mid 5}$
8 mm to 15 mm deficit	Extract:*	$\dfrac{\times 4 \mid 4\times}{\times 5 \mid 5\times}$
Over 15 mm deficit	Extract:	$\dfrac{\times 4 \mid 4\times}{\times 5 \mid 5\times}$

C. Posterior surplus or deficit: The space analysis in this area is of great importance, although in corrective procedures anterior and mid-arch deficits are overriding. The posterior space must be carefully measured and projected. No orthodontic treatment is complete until all decisions and treatment procedures are completed in this area.

+ to −5 mm with good position
of the third molars
Await full development
of the third molars

+ to −5 mm with poor position of the third molars	Extract:	$\dfrac{8 \mid 8}{8 \mid 8}$

Note: Wait for maxillary third molars until age 16. Have the mandibular third molars out immediately if other treatment is necessary.

5 mm to 15 mm deficit	Extract:	$\dfrac{8 \mid 8}{8 \mid 8}$

Note: Determine the timing of these extractions in relationship to other treatment that is necessary.

D. Skeletal disharmonies

1. Horizontal—Class II malocclusions
   Confirm with AO-BO measurement
   Sella must be in a normal position
   ANB: 3° to 5°

3° −5°	Extract:	$\dfrac{8 \mid 8}{8 \mid 8}$

*Use × for all molars (first; second; third).

3° −5°	Extract:	$\dfrac{4 \mid 4}{}$
3° −5°	Extract:	$\dfrac{4 \mid 4}{5 \mid 5}$
3° −5° subdivision	Extract:	$\dfrac{4 \mid 4}{5 \mid 4}$
ANB: 5° to 8°	Extract:	$\dfrac{7 \mid 7}{8 \mid 8}$
ANB: 9° to 12°	Extract:	$\dfrac{6 \mid 6}{8 \mid 8}$

ANB: 12° and above — Surgery and Orthodontics:
SNB 10° below normal; consider surgery on mandible
SNA 10° above normal; consider maxillary surgery
Both SNA and SNB abnormal; consider maxillary and mandibular surgery

2. Horizontal—Class III malocclusions; confirm with AO-BO measurement
   ANB: 0° to −5°
   Nonextraction if space is available for shifting through tipping and torquing
   Lower incisor extraction if growth is complete

Space deficit	Extract:	$\dfrac{5 \mid 5}{4 \mid 4}$

   ANB: Greater than −5°
   Evaluate carefully for orthognathic surgery along with orthodontics

3. Vertical disharmonies—open bites
   Mild — Intrusive directional force treatment
   First premolar extractions are advantageous
   Medium — Molar extractions and intrusive directional force treatment
   Severe — Surgery and orthodontics

4. Vertical disharmonies—closed bites
   Mild — Extrusive directional force treatment: second order distal tipping forces
   Second premolar extractions are advantageous
   Severe — Bite plates—vertical elastics and other extrusive directional forces
   Surgery

5. Facial disharmonies
   Chin-lip relationships
   Mild — These can be compensated by tooth positioning, and the deficit is added to the anterior discrepancy as a soft tissue modification
   Severe — Plastic surgery along with directional force orthodontics

A consideration of the three areas: the face, the skeletal pattern, and the dentition, enables the practitioner to identify the major areas of disharmony and to diagnose the case in a manner that will result in the correction of the greatest number of problems with which the patient presents.

THE TWEED–MERRIFIELD EDGEWISE APPLIANCE
The Brackets and Tubes

An appliance is the basic instrument that is used to reach orthodontic goals. As E. H. Angle stressed, the appliance must have certain characteristics—simplicity, efficiency, and comfort. It must also be hygienic, esthetic, and above all, it must have a wide range of versatility. The neutral 0.022 slot edgewise appliance consists of bands, or mesh pads, with single, double width 0.022 brackets on the six anterior teeth, intermediate single width brackets on the premolar bands, twin brackets on the first molars, and heavy edgewise 0.022 tubes with mesial hooks on the second molars (Fig. 11-42, A). The bands also have lingual hooks attached on the molars and lingual cleats on the premolars and canines. The lingual hooks increase versatility and are especially necessary to correct and control rotations. Each of the brackets and tubes is placed at right angles to the long axis of the tooth. They are precisely positioned in relation to the incisal edges of the incisor teeth and to the cusps of the remaining teeth. There are no tips, no torque, nor any variations in thickness in the bracket or the neutral slot. The slot size of 0.022 allows the clinician to use a multiplicity of archwire dimensions.

Archwires

Resilient edgewise archwire is used with the Tweed–Merrifield 0.022 edgewise appliance. The dimensions of the wire commonly used are 0.017 × 0.022, 0.018 × 0.025, 0.019 × 0.025, 0.020 × 0.025, and 0.0215 × 0.028. These wire dimensions give a great range of versatility with the 0.022 × 0.028 bracket slot and allow the sequential application of forces as needed for various treatment objectives. There is no need for archwire reduction, except in one stage of treatment, and this improves accuracy and consistency. Many patients can be treated with three mandibular archwires and three to four maxillary archwires. The objective is to enhance both tooth movement and control with the proper edgewise archwire. If bonded brackets are used, the initial dimension of the archwires may need to be one size smaller.

First, Second, and Third Order Bends and Their Interaction

Knowledge of the action, the interaction, and the reaction of teeth to bends in the archwire is critical to the use of any orthodontic appliance. It is fundamental and drastically affects clinical results.

First order bends

The action and reaction of first order bends affects expansion or contraction. These actions are most easily monitored and are routinely used to move individual teeth. The interaction of the bends can affect the third order position of the teeth if expansionary forces are used.

Third order bends

Third order bend reaction in the mandibular archwire is complementary to all the teeth if properly placed. The objective is to have some degree of lingual crown torque on all mandibular teeth. Therefore the posterior and anterior

segments work together in action, reaction, and interaction. The ideal third order bends in the mandibular archwire are: incisors (−7°), canines and first premolars (−12°), second premolars and molars (−20°).

Conversely, third order bends in the maxillary archwire are antagonistic. The anterior segment needs no torque (0°) or slight lingual root torque, and the posterior segment needs lingual crown torque: canines and first premolars (−7°), second premolars and molars (−12°). It is not wise to apply active torque force simultaneously in segments with opposite actions. In the maxillary arch it is prudent to apply active third order bends sequentially and in only one direction at any given time.

Second order bends

Second order bends in the posterior segment of the mandibular arch are antagonistic to the teeth in the anterior segment. Without excellent directional control and a careful application of these second order forces in a sequential manner, all control of the anterior teeth will be lost. The anterior teeth cannot support the simultaneous tipping of all the posterior teeth, so the placement of compensating bends in the initial archwire before compensation is needed is incorrect. Only after tipping of the teeth should the compensation bends be placed.

Second order bends in the posterior segment of the mandibular archwire also affect the third order force on the mandibular anterior teeth in a negative manner. These teeth generally require lingual crown torque. Posterior tipping bends apply labial crown torque force to the incisors. This fact must be given careful consideration in archwire fabrication and force application.

In the maxillary arch, second order bends in the posterior segments are generally desirable or complementary to the teeth in the anterior segment. The reaction to the tipping forces intrudes the maxillary incisors and gives a lingual root torque effect to these teeth. This is generally positive or complementary to treatment objectives.

The Auxiliaries

The auxiliaries routinely used with the Tweed–Merrifield edgewise force system are elastics and directionally oriented headgears. Primarily, the high pull J hook headgear and the straight pull J hook headgear furnish the extra-oral force in a directional manner. Patient compliance is absolutely imperative.

Variations of the Appliance

Many variations of the edgewise appliance have been introduced in the last 20 years. Most notable of the variations is the *Straight Wire Appliance* introduced in 1972 by Andrews.[1] The *Straight Wire Appliance* incorporates first, second, and third order bends into the bracket, with the theory being that these bends will not have to be placed in the archwire. Another variation is a change in slot size from 0.022 to 0.018 and even to 0.016. Various orthodontic suppliers market numerous variations of the *Straight Wire Appliance* with different tip and torque to suit the individual operator's desires. Other modifications have been extensively described by Burstone,[3] Lindquist,[10] and Roth.[22] (See Chapter 11.)

TREATMENT WITH THE TWEED–MERRIFIELD EDGEWISE APPLIANCE

The treatment protocol must complement the diagnostic philosophy. Using Tweed's treatment concepts as a foundation, Merrifield has developed force systems that simplify the use of the edgewise appliance. For example, Tweed used 12 sets of archwires during the treatment of each patient. Today, with the modern edgewise appliance and under the guidance of Merrifield and other colleagues, only four to five sets of archwires are used. Merrifield's *Sequential Directional Force Technology*[16] is simple, straightforward, and fundamentally sound. From the Tweed era and into the era of Merrifield, the key to quality with the edgewise appliance continues to be directionally controlled precision archwire manipulation. There are essentially five concepts composing the treatment philosophy:

1. Sequential banding or bonding
2. Sequential and/or individual tooth movement
3. Sequential mandibular anchorage preparation
4. Directional forces including control of the vertical dimension, which will enhance mandibular response
5. Proper timing of treatment

Sequential Banding or Bonding

The application of the appliance to the patient is important. The second molars, the second premolars, and the canines are banded. The central incisors can be either banded or bonded (Fig. 11-37). This procedure of sequential appliance placement is less traumatic to the patient. It is easier and less time consuming for the orthodontist. It allows greater efficiency in the action of the archwire during the first months of treatment because it gives the archwire much longer interbracket length. This creates a power storage that accomplishes treatment objectives more rapidly. Sequential appliance placement also gives the orthodontist the opportunity to insert a wire of larger dimension that is less subject to occlusal or bracket engagement distortion.

After the banded or bracketed teeth respond to the forces of the archwire and auxiliaries, additional teeth are banded or bonded in sequence so that the forces can be most efficient. The maxillary first molars are banded after one appointment (Fig. 11-39). The mandibular first molars are banded after the second appointment (Fig. 11-40), and the lateral incisor bands or bonds are placed at either the third or fourth appointment, depending upon the progress of the treatment (Fig. 11-41).

Sequential Tooth Movement

Tooth movement is sequential. It is not en masse movement that was introduced by Tweed. Teeth are moved rapidly and with precision because they are moved individually or in small units.

Sequential Mandibular Anchorage Preparation

Tweed attempted, with varying degrees of success, to prepare mandibular anchorage with Class III elastics. All the compensation bends were placed in the archwire at one time. The normal sequelae of this force system were labially flared and intruded mandibular incisors (Fig. 11-32). Se-

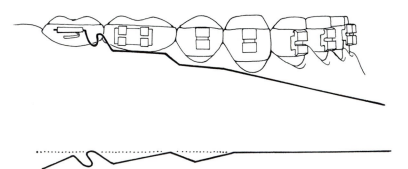

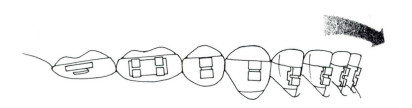

Fig. 11-32   Tweed en masse anchorage.

quential mandibular anchorage preparation, developed by Merrifield, is the system that allows mandibular anchorage to be prepared quickly and easily by tipping only two teeth at a time to their anchorage prepared position. This system uses the high pull headgear for support rather than Class III elastics. In the initial step of treatment, denture preparation, the second molar is tipped to its desired anchorage position (Fig. 11-43). After space is closed, a compensating bend is placed mesial to the second molar to maintain its tip, and the mandibular first molar is tipped to an anchorage position (Fig. 11-48). After the first molar is tipped, a compensation bend is placed mesial to the molar to maintain its tip, and the second premolar is tipped distally to its anchorage prepared position (Fig. 11-49). The anchorage preparation is accomplished by using 10 teeth as *anchorage units* to tip two teeth. If is often referred to as the *Merrifield 10-2 system*. This method of mandibular anchorage preparation is sequential and precise. Unlike the en masse anchorage of the Tweed era, it is controlled.

Directional Force

The hallmark of modern Tweed–Merrifield edgewise treatment is the use of directional force systems to move the teeth. Directional forces can be defined as controlled forces which place the teeth in the most harmonious relationship with their environment. It is critical to employ a force system that controls the mandibular posterior teeth and the maxillary anterior teeth. The resultant vector of all forces should be upward and forward so that the opportunity for a favorable skeletal change is enhanced, particularly in dentoalveolar protrusion Class II malocclusion correction (Fig. 11-33). An upward and forward force system requires that the mandibular incisor be upright over basal bone so that the maxillary incisor can be moved distally and superiorly

(Fig. 11-34). In order for the upward and forward force system to be a reality, vertical control is critical. To control the vertical dimension, the clinician must control the mandibular plane and the occlusal plane (Fig. 11-33). If point *B* drops down and back, the face becomes lengthened, the mandibular incisor is tipped forward off basal bone, and the maxillary incisor drops down and back instead of being moved up and back (Fig. 11-35). The unfortunate result of this procedure is a patient with a lengthened face, a gummy smile, incompetent lips, and a more recessive chin.

Timing of Treatment

The timing of the treatment is an integral part of the philosophy. Treatment should be initiated at the time when treatment objectives can be most readily accomplished. This may mean interceptive treatment in the mixed dentition, selected extractions in the mixed dentition, or waiting for second molar eruption before initiating active treatment. Diagnostic discretion is the determinant.

STEPS OF TREATMENT

Tweed–Merrifield Edgewise Directional Force Treatment can be organized into four force systems: *Denture Preparation*, *Denture Correction*, *Denture Completion*, and *Denture Recovery*. During each step of treatment, there are certain objectives that must be attained.

Denture Preparation

Denture preparation prepares the malocclusion for correction. Objectives include: (1) leveling; (2) individual tooth movement and rotation correction; (3) retraction of both maxillary and mandibular canines; and (4) preparation of

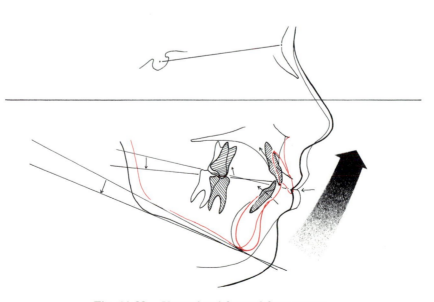

Fig. 11-33   Upward and forward force system.

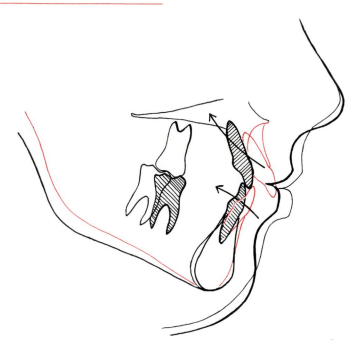

Fig. 11-34   Upright mandibular incisor; maxillary incisor moved up and back.

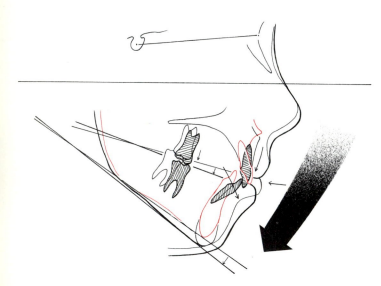

Fig. 11-35   Downward and backward force system.

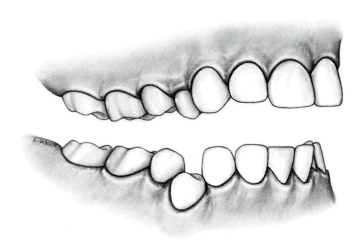

Fig. 11-36

the terminal molars for stress resistance. The denture preparation stage of treatment takes approximately 6 months. One mandibular archwire and one maxillary archwire are used to complete this step.

The teeth of the original malocclusion (Fig. 11-36) are sequentially banded or bonded. After the placement of the appliance (Fig. 11-37, *A* and *B*), an 0.018 × 0.025 resilient mandibular archwire and 0.017 × 0.022 resilient maxillary archwire are placed in each arch (Fig. 11-38, *A* and *B*).

The loop stops are flush with the second molar tubes in each arch. The mandibular second molar receives an effective distal tip of 15° from this initial archwire. In the maxillary arch, there is enough tip in the wire distal to the loop to have an effective 5° distal tip on the second molar. The objective in each arch is to maintain the maxillary molar in its already distally tipped position and to begin tipping the mandibular second molar to an anchorage prepared position. There is a second premolar offset bend mesial to the second

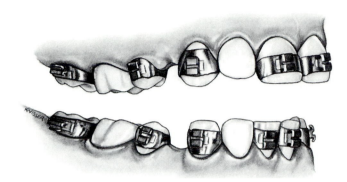

Fig. 11-37, A

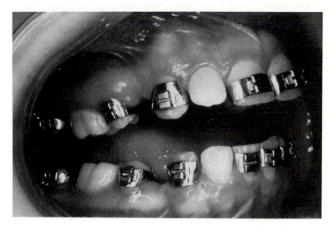

Fig. 11-37, B

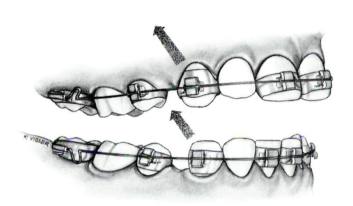

Fig. 11-38, A

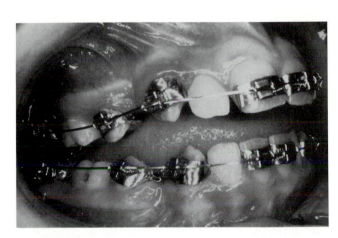

Fig. 11-38, B

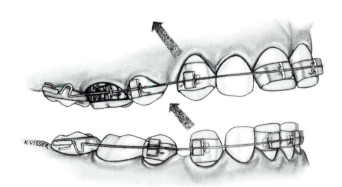

Fig. 11-39, A

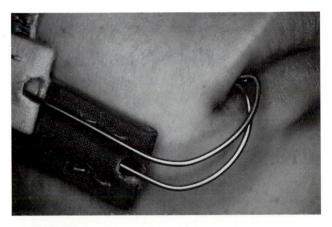

Fig. 11-39, B

premolar bracket in each archwire. The purpose of this bend is to keep the canines from expanding out of the alveolar trough as they are retracted with the headgear. The third order bends in each archwire are passive. High-pull J hook headgear are used to retract both maxillary and mandibular canines. After each month of treatment both archwires are removed and the terminal molar tip in the mandibular archwire is increased to maintain an effective 15° tip as the tooth tips distally. After the first month of treatment the

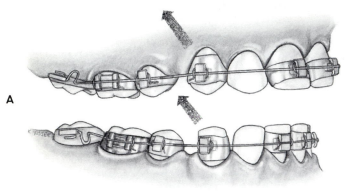

A

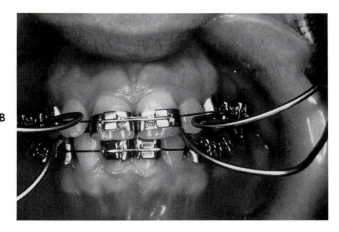

B

Fig. 11-40, A and B

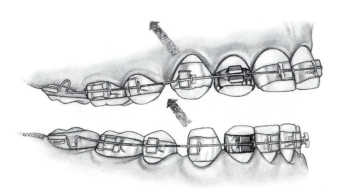

Fig. 11-41

maxillary first molars are banded. The J-hook headgear continues canine retraction. (Fig. 11-39, *A* and *B*), and after the second month of treatment the *mandibular first molars are banded* (Fig. 11-40, *A* and *B*). As the canines retract and as the arches are leveled, the *lateral incisors are banded or* bonded (Fig. 11-41), and power chain force to aid canine retraction can be used (Figs. 11-42, *A* and *B*). It is important to remember that at each visit during denture preparation, the archwires are removed, carefully coordinated, checked for proper first, second, and third order bends, and re-ligated. Canine retraction is continued with power chain and headgear force (Fig. 11-42, *A* and *B*). At the end of the denture preparation stage of treatment the dentition should be fully bracketed and level, the canines should be retracted, all rotations should be corrected, and the mandibular terminal molars should be tipped distally into an anchorage prepared position (Fig. 11-43, *A* and *B*).

Denture Correction

The second step of treatment is called denture correction. During denture correction the spaces are closed with maxillary and mandibular closing loops which are supported by J hook headgear attached to hooks soldered between the maxillary and mandibular central and lateral incisors. The mandibular archwire is a 0.019 × 0.025 working archwire with 6 mm vertical loops distal to the lateral incisor brackets. The 0.020 × 0.025 maxillary archwire has 6.5 mm vertical

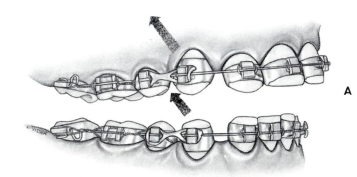

A

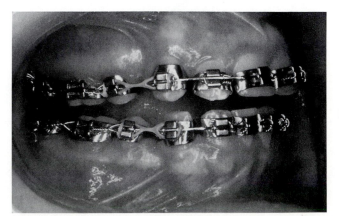

B

Fig. 11-42, A and B

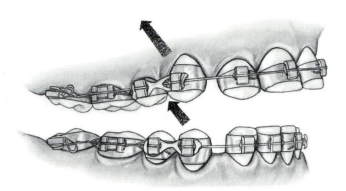

Fig. 11-43, A

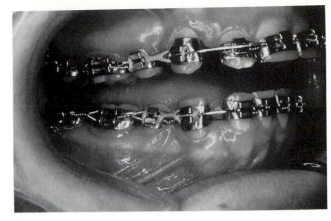

Fig. 11-43, B

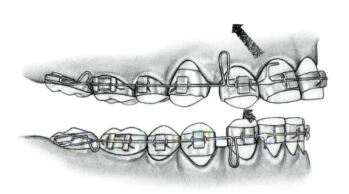

Fig. 11-44, A

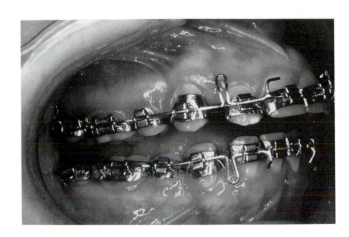

Fig. 11-44, B

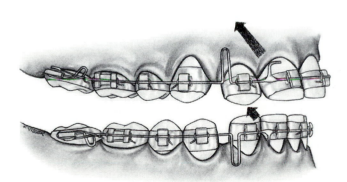

Fig. 11-45, A

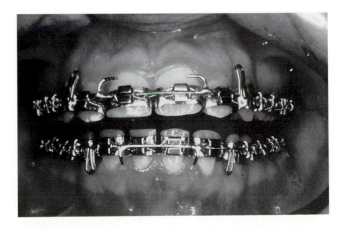

Fig. 11-45, B

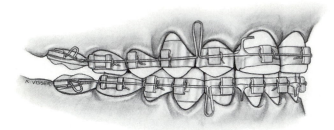

Fig. 11-46, A

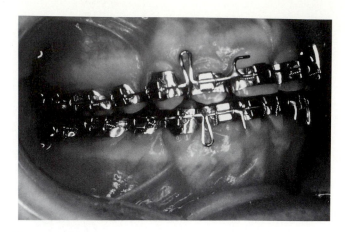

Fig. 11-46, B

loops distal to the lateral incisor brackets. In both arches the loop stops are immediately distal to the brackets of the first molars (Fig. 11-44, *A* and *B*). The loop stop in the mandibular archwire incorporates a *compensation* to maintain the 15° terminal molar tip (Figs. 11-44, *A* and *B*). After each activation the archwire is removed and the compensating height of the distal leg of the loop stop in the mandibular archwire is reduced so that the archwire remains passive to the previously tipped second molar (Fig. 11-45, *A* and *B*). The maxillary archwire is coordinated with the mandibular archwire and activated each month until all maxillary space is closed. At the end of space closure (Fig. 11-46, *A* and *B*) the curve of occlusion in the maxillary arch should have been maintained, and the mandibular arch should have been completely leveled, with the 15° distal tip of the second molar maintained. The case is now ready for mandibular anchorage preparation. This step positions the teeth in the mandibular midarch area and in the posterior area into axial inclinations that will allow final coordination with the maxillary teeth for normal functional occlusion.

Sequential Mandibular Anchorage Preparation

Sequential mandibular anchorage preparation is based on sequential tooth movement. The concept is that the archwire exerts an active force on only two teeth while remaining passive to the other teeth in the arch. Thus the remaining teeth act as stabilizing or anchorage units as two teeth are tipped. It is referred to as the *10-2 anchorage system,* and this system allows a quickly controlled response without serious reaction. It is further supported and activated by the high-pull headgear worn on vertical spurs soldered distal to the mandibular lateral incisors.

Sequential mandibular anchorage preparation is initiated during the denture preparation step of treatment by tipping the second molar to a 15° distal inclination. After the mandibular space is closed during the denture correction step of treatment, the arch is checked to make sure (1) that it is

level; (2) that the second molars are tipped to a 15° distal angulation (Fig. 11-47, *A* and *B*). This procedure is referred to as *Readout.*[7] At this time the second step of sequential mandibular anchorage preparation, first molar anchorage, is initiated. Another 0.019 × 0.025 archwire with the loop stops bent flush against the second molar tubes is fabricated. First and third order bends are ideal. Gingival headgear hooks are soldered distal to the lateral incisors. To tip the first molars to an anchorage prepared position, a 10° distal tip is placed 1 mm mesial to the first molar brackets. A compensating bend that maintains the 15° of terminal molar tip is placed just mesial to the loop stop. The archwire is now passive to the second molar and *crosses the twin brackets of the first molar* at a 10° angle (Fig. 11-48). The second molars are now part of the 10 stabilizing units, and the first molars are the two teeth that receive the action of the directional forces and the archwire. For an ideal response a high-pull headgear is applied to the anterior vertical spurs. After 1 month the archwire is removed, and a readout should show a +5° to +8° distal inclination of the first molars. The second molars should continue to readout +15°.

The third and final step of sequential mandibular anchorage preparation is to place a *5° distal tip 1 mm mesial to the second premolar brackets.* A compensating bend is placed in the embrasure between the second premolars and the first molars to maintain the first molars in their anchorage prepared position (Fig. 11-49). This bend allows the archwire in the second premolar area to be on a bias to the second premolar bracket when the archwire is seated in the second molar tubes and in the first molar brackets. The archwire must be passive in the brackets of the first molars and in the second molar tubes. The archwire is ligated and again the high-pull headgear is worn to the vertical spurs. Usually, headgear that is worn during sleeping hours only is effective. During this step of anchorage preparation, the first and second molars and the six anterior teeth are part of the 10 stabilizing units, and the two premolars are the recipients of the *10-2 directional force system.* At the end

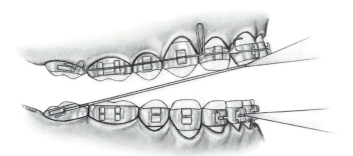

Fig. 11-47, A

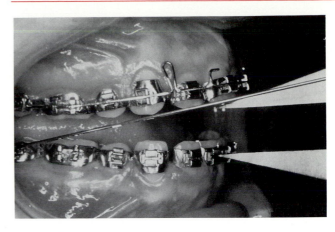

Fig. 11-47, B

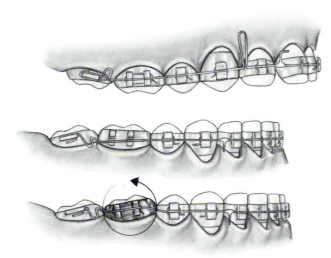

Fig. 11-48

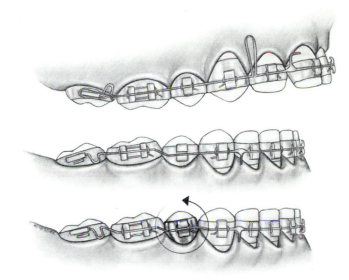

Fig. 11-49

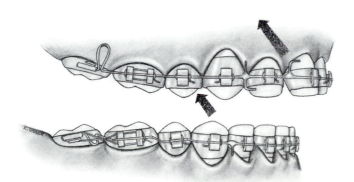

Fig. 11-50, A

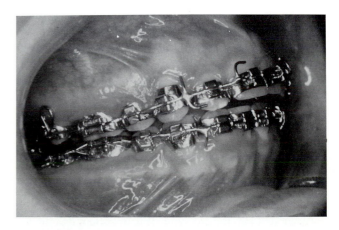

Fig. 11-50, B

of mandibular anchorage preparation, a readout will show that the second molars have a distal axial inclination of 15°, the first molars have a distal axial inclination of 5° to 8°, and the second premolars have a distal axial inclination of 0 to 3° (Fig. 11-50, *A* and *B*).

The denture correction step of treatment should now be complete for the Class I malocclusion. The objectives of the denture correction step of treatment for the correction of the Class I malocclusion are (1) complete space closure in both arches; (2) sequential anchorage preparation in the mandibular arch; (3) an enhanced curve of occlusion in the maxillary arch; and (4) a Class I intercuspation of the canines and premolars. The mesiobuccal cusp of the maxillary first molar should fit into the mesiobuccal groove of the mandibular first molar. The distal cusps of these teeth should be discluded as should those of the second molars.

The Class II Force System

For cases with an *end-on* or a full step Class II relationship of the buccal segments, a new system of forces must be used to complete denture correction. A careful study of the cusp relationships will determine the force system that is required. It is absolutely necessary to make a final diagnostic decision for Class II correction based on (1) the ANB relationship; (2) a maxillary posterior space analysis; and (3) patient cooperation. The following guidelines are used:

1. If the maxillary third molars are missing or if the ANB is 5° or less and the patient is cooperative, the system to be described will accomplish the best result. If the third molars are present and are approaching eruption, they should be removed to facilitate distal movement of the maxillary arch.

2. If the ANB relationship is 5° to 8° and a Class II cusp relationship exists with a cooperative patient, the extraction of the maxillary second molars will be the most advantageous. The force system to be described is used to distalize the maxillary arch into the second molar extraction space.

3. If the ANB is above 10° and/or if the patient's compliance is questionable, either the first molars should be removed, or surgical correction should be considered. Facial balance and harmony after correction should also be carefully considered before making either recommendation.

The Class II force system cannot be used unless compliance requirements are strictly followed by the patient. If an attempt is made to use the Class II force system without cooperation, the maxillary anterior teeth will be pushed forward off basal bone. Patient cooperation must therefore be assured before the use of the Class II force system.

At the end of sequential mandibular anchorage preparation, a mandibular 0.0215 × 0.028 stabilizing archwire is fabricated. Ideal first, second, and third order bends are incorporated into the archwire. It is important that the loop stop be 0.5 mm short of the molar tubes and that the wire

be passive to all the brackets. Gingival spurs are soldered distal to the mandibular lateral incisors. The wire is seated and ligated, and the terminal molar is cinched tightly to the loop stop.

A 0.020 × 0.025 maxillary archwire with closed bulbous loops bent flush against the second molar tubes is fabricated. This archwire has ideal first and second order bends. There is 7° of progressive lingual crown torque in the molar segment. Gingival high-pull headgear hooks are soldered distal to the central incisors. Class II hooks are soldered occlusal and distal to the lateral incisors (Fig. 11-50, *A* and *B*). The closed bulbous loops are opened 1 mm on each side, and the archwire is ligated in place. Eight ounce Class II elastics are worn from the hooks on the mandibular second molar tubes to the Class II hooks on the maxillary archwire. Anterior vertical elastics are worn from the spurs on the mandibular archwire to the high-pull headgear hooks on the maxillary archwire. The high-pull headgear is also worn on these same maxillary hooks (Fig. 11-51).

This force system is employed for approximately 1 month to sequentially move the maxillary second molars distally. At the next appointment, the mandibular archwire is removed and checked. The maxillary archwire is also removed so that the bulbous loops can again be activated 1 mm. *Sliding 0.030 jigs are fabricated and placed on the maxillary archwire* so that the distal eyelets contact the mesial bracket of the maxillary first molars and the mesial eyelets are midway between the canine and premolar brackets. The mesial eyelet has an extension for a Class II elastic. The archwires are re-ligated. At this time, 6 oz Class II elastics are worn 24 hours each day from the hook on the mandibular second molar tube to the sliding jig, and a second 6 to 8 oz Class II elastic is worn from the mandibular second molar hook to the Class II hook on the maxillary archwire. In addition, an anterior vertical elastic is worn 12 hours each day. The high-pull headgear is worn to the maxillary archwire 14 hours per day (Fig. 11-52, *A* and *B*). This is an efficient force system with excellent directional control. It is sequential because the maxillary second molars, the maxillary first molars, and the rest of the maxillary teeth are receiving individual distal force. Four months of treatment with

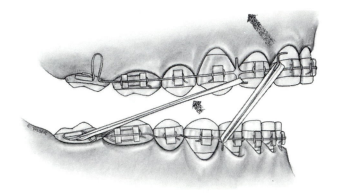

Fig. 11-51

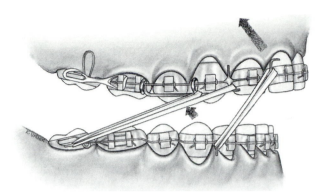

Fig. 11-52, A

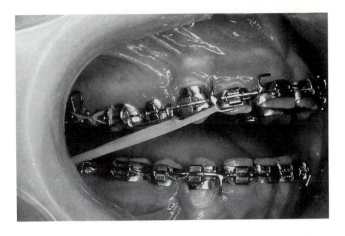

Fig. 11-52, B

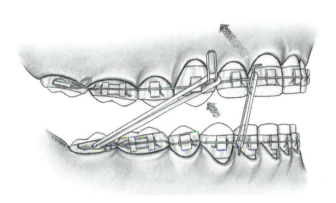

Fig. 11-53, A

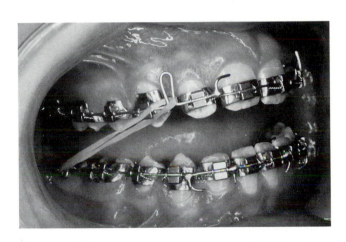

Fig. 11-53, B

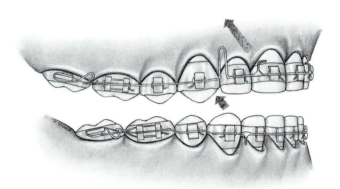

Fig. 11-54, A

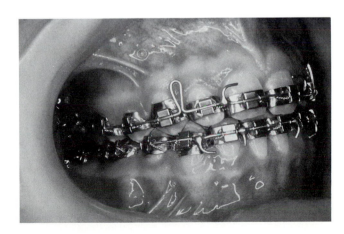

Fig. 11-54, B

monthly reactivation should position the posterior teeth in an overtreated Class I relationship. This system will not strain the mandibular denture if the anterior vertical elastics are worn and if sufficient space is available in the maxillary posterior denture area.

After overcorrection of the Class II relationship of the posterior teeth, a 0.020 × 0.025 maxillary archwire with 6½ mm closing loops distal to the lateral incisors is fabricated. This archwire has ideal first, second, and third order bends. Gingival headgear hooks are soldered distal to the central incisors (Fig. 11-53, *A* and *B*). The closing loops are opened 1 mm per visit by cinching the loop stops to the molar tube. The Class II force should be milder: 4 to 6 oz instead of 6 to 8 oz. The anterior vertical elastic and the maxillary high-pull headgear are used in conjunction with these light Class II elastics. After all the maxillary space is closed (Fig. 11-54, *A* and *B*), the step of denture correction has been completed, and the case is ready for the next step of treatment: denture completion.

Denture Completion

The third step of treatment is identified as denture completion. Ideal first, second, and third order bends are placed in the mandibular and maxillary 0.0215 × 0.028 resilient archwires. The mandibular archwire duplicates the anchorage preparation archwire in a Class I case or the previously used mandibular stabilizing archwire if a Class II force system was used. Hooks for the high-pull headgear, for anterior vertical elastics, and for Class II elastics are soldered to the archwires as previously described. Supplemental hooks for vertical elastics are soldered as needed for denture completion (Fig. 11-55, *A* and *B*). The forces used during denture completion are based on a critical study of the arrangement of each tooth in each arch. The relationship of one arch to the other and the relationship of the arches to their entire environment are also studied. Necessary second and third order adjustments are made in each archwire as needed. A progress cephalogram and tracing can be eval-

uated to determine the final mandibular incisor position and any minor control of the palatal, occlusal, and mandibular planes that may be needed. Study of the tracing may also reveal to the clinician the requirement for lingual root torque in the maxillary incisors. Visual clinical observations permit evaluation of the lip line, the maxillary incisor relationship, and the amount of cusp seating and artistic positioning of the incisors that is necessary. Denture completion can be considered as *mini* treatment of the malocclusion. During this treatment step, the orthodontist repeats the systems of forces that are necessary, until the original malocclusion is overcorrected. After overcorrection, the final artistic bends and cusp seating forces that give detail and quality to the overcorrected malocclusion are added. At the end of the denture completion stage of treatment, the following characteristics should be readily observed: (1) the incisors must be aligned; (2) the occlusion must be overtreated to a Class I relationship; (3) the anterior teeth must be edge-to-edge; (4) the maxillary canines and second premolars must be locked tightly into a Class I relationship; (5) the mesiobuccal cusp of the maxillary first molar must occlude in the mesiobuccal groove of the mandibular first molar; (6) the distal cusps of the first molars and the second molars must be out of occlusion; and (7) all spaces must be closed tightly from the second premolars forward (Fig. 11-56, *A* and *B*).

Denture Recovery

The orthodontist must not strive for the ideal final result at the end of treatment. The ideal result will occur after all treatment mechanics are discontinued and after uninhibited function and other environmental influences, active in the post-treatment period, stabilize and finalize the position of the total dentition. All bands, except for those on the four canines and the four first molars, are removed. The first molars are ligated to the canines in both arches.

In the mandibular arch, the canines are ligated to each other. In the maxillary arch a power chain is placed from one canine bracket to the canine bracket on the opposite

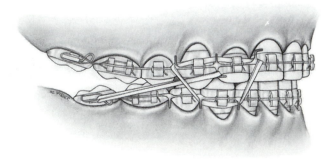

Fig. 11-55, A

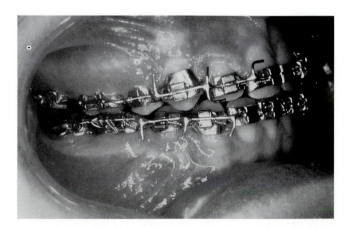

Fig. 11-55, B

side (Fig. 11-57). In 7 days the remaining bands are removed, and the retainers are placed (Fig. 11-58, *A* and *B*).

When all bands are removed and the retainers are placed, the most critical phase occurs. This is the recovery period, and the forces involved are those of the surrounding environment, primarily the muscles and the periodontium. If mechanical corrective procedures minimally achieve normal relationships of the teeth, there will be inevitable relapse. Any change is likely to be away from ideal occlusion toward malocclusion. Denture recovery, based on the concept of overcorrection, is predicated on clinical experience and clinical research. Certain tooth and denture changes effected during treatment will tend to revert toward their original position. For instance, in overbite and rotation correction, approximately one half of the correction is lost in subsequent *settling*. During recovery, function settles these teeth into their most efficient, healthy, and stable positions (Fig. 11-59).

The Tweed-Merrifield edgewise appliance correction of four different types of malocclusions will now be discussed:

(1) a Class II—four first premolar extraction case; (2) a Class II—maxillary first premolar, mandibular second premolar extraction case; (3) a Class II—nonpremolar extraction case; and (4) a Class II—premolar and molar extraction case (maxillary and mandibular first premolars; maxillary second molars; mandibular third molars).

The objective of showing the records of these patients is to illustrate differential diagnosis and edgewise treatment. The four patients have been treated by Herbert Klontz. Dr. Klontz took the Tweed course in 1963 and again in 1965. He became the course coordinator of the Tweed course in 1976. In 1983 he was elevated to his current position of director of the teaching program of the Tweed Foundation. His superb clinical skills, developed over 25 years, are evident, and verify that all six treatment objectives can be routinely attained in the treatment of difficult and wide-ranging malocclusions if the force systems presented in this chapter are used.

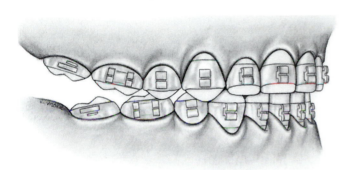

Fig. 11-56, A

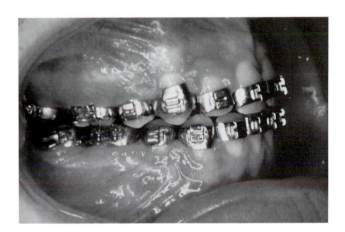

Fig. 11-56, B

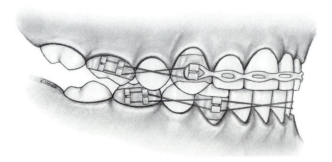

Fig. 11-57

CASE STUDIES

CASE I

Diagnosis

The first patient will be discussed in detail to demonstrate the diagnosis, treatment planning, and treatment results. Orthodontic records include profile and full-face photographs (Fig. 11-60, *A*) that show a lack of facial balance because of the receding chin and the unsightly forward roll of the lower lip. The anterior view of the casts (Fig. 11-61, *A* through *D*) shows a deep overbite, a midline deviation, and irregular teeth. The occlusal views show anterior crowding. (Note the lingual inclination of the mandibular second molars.) The right side of the casts illustrates the Class II canine and molar relationship, while the left side illustrates the Class I relationship.

The pretreatment cephalometric tracing (Fig. 11-62) demonstrates the skeletal Class II pattern. An FMIA of 52°, FMA of 36°, and IMPA of 92° indicate the need to upright the mandibular incisors. The ANB of 7° and the AO-BO of 4 mm confirm the Class II skeletal pattern. The higher-than-normal occlusal plane—

Frankfort plane angle of 17°—made correction difficult. The face was analyzed by measuring the Z-angle. The patient's Z-angle of 58° was approximately 20° less than the normal of 78°—an indication of poor balance of facial proportions. Upper lip thickness equaled total chin thickness, so no soft tissue modification was indicated.

The total space analysis (Fig. 11-63) was calculated for the patient. In the anterior denture area the tooth arch discrepancy plus the headfilm discrepancy yielded an anterior denture deficit of 15.4 mm. In the midarch area, the tooth-arch discrepancy was 4 mm. The tooth-arch discrepancy in the posterior denture area, after considering the estimated increase, was 7 mm. The sum of the anterior, midarch, and posterior deficits was 26.4 mm. The decision was made to extract the maxillary and mandibular first premolars to correct this difficult malocclusion.

Treatment

The treatment steps of this patient have been previously outlined in this chapter. Treatment was completed by using the force system exactly as it has been illustrated.

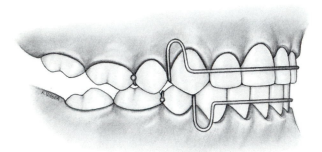

Fig. 11-58, A

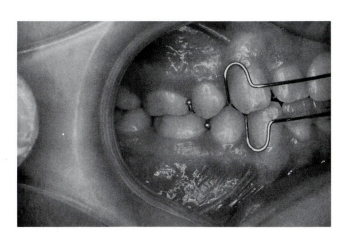

Fig. 11-58, B

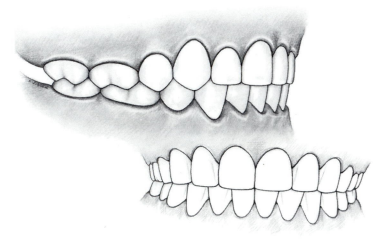

Fig. 11-59

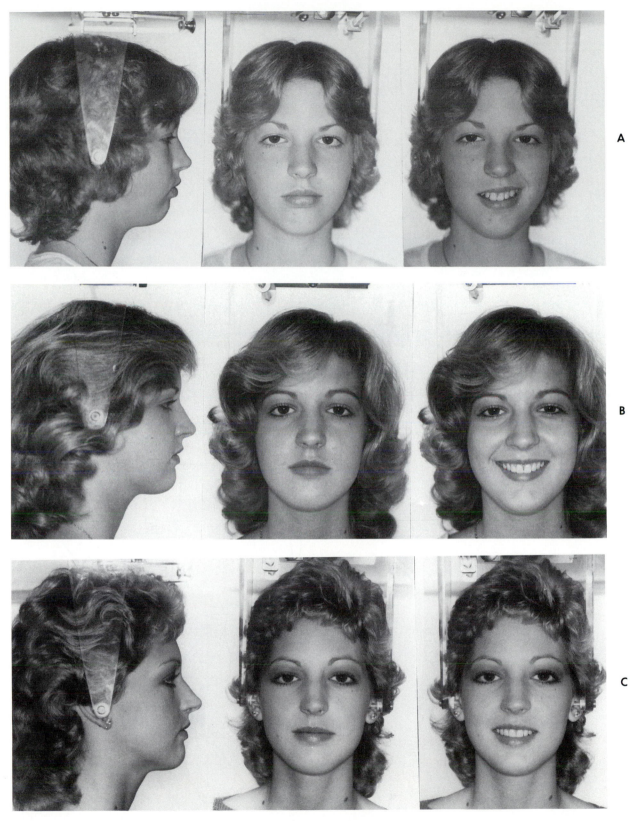

Fig. 11-60   *Case I:* **A,** Pretreatment facial photographs. **B,** Posttreatment facial photographs.
C, Recall facial photographs.

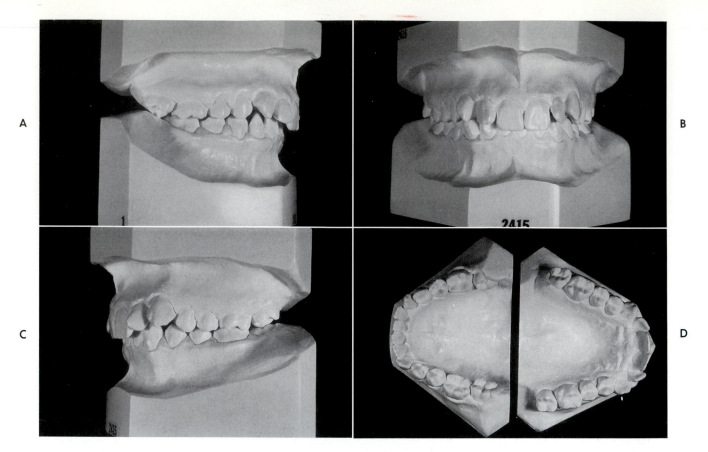

Fig. 11-61 *Case I:* Pretreatment casts.

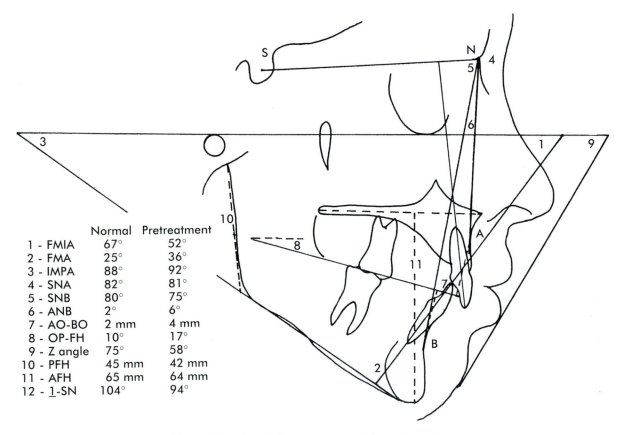

	Normal	Pretreatment
1 - FMIA	67°	52°
2 - FMA	25°	36°
3 - IMPA	88°	92°
4 - SNA	82°	81°
5 - SNB	80°	75°
6 - ANB	2°	6°
7 - AO-BO	2 mm	4 mm
8 - OP-FH	10°	17°
9 - Z angle	75°	58°
10 - PFH	45 mm	42 mm
11 - AFH	65 mm	64 mm
12 - 1-SN	104°	94°

Fig. 11-62 *Case I:* Pretreatment cephalometric tracing.

A. Anterior denture area

    a. Teeth width   3 2 1   1 2 3   37
    b. Available space   34
    c. Tooth arch disc   3
    d. Headfilm correction   10.4
    e. Soft tissue modification   2
                                           Deficit <u>15.4</u> Surplus _____

B. Mid-arch denture area

    a. Teeth width   6 5 4   4 5 6   55
    b. Available space   53
    c. Tooth arch disc   2
    d. Curve of Spee   2
                                           Deficit <u> 4 </u> Surplus _____

C. Posterior denture area

    a. Teeth width   8 7   7 8   41
    b. Available space   30
    c. Tooth arch disc   11
    d. Estimated increase   4
                                           Deficit <u> 7 </u> Surplus _____

                        Denture total Deficit <u>26.4</u> Surplus _____

Fig. 11-63 *Case I:* Total dentition space analysis.

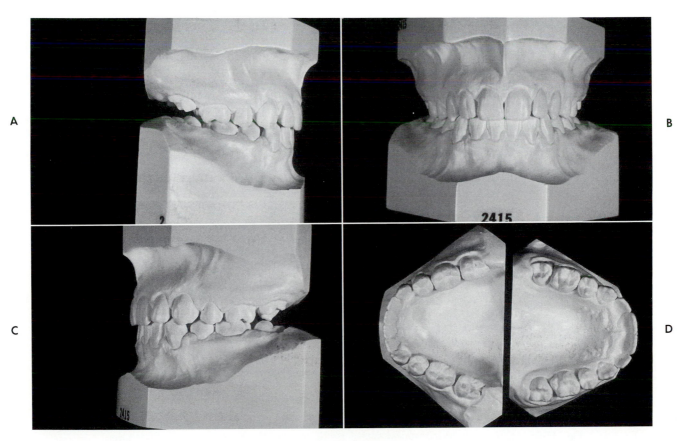

Fig. 11-64 *Case I:* Posttreatment casts.

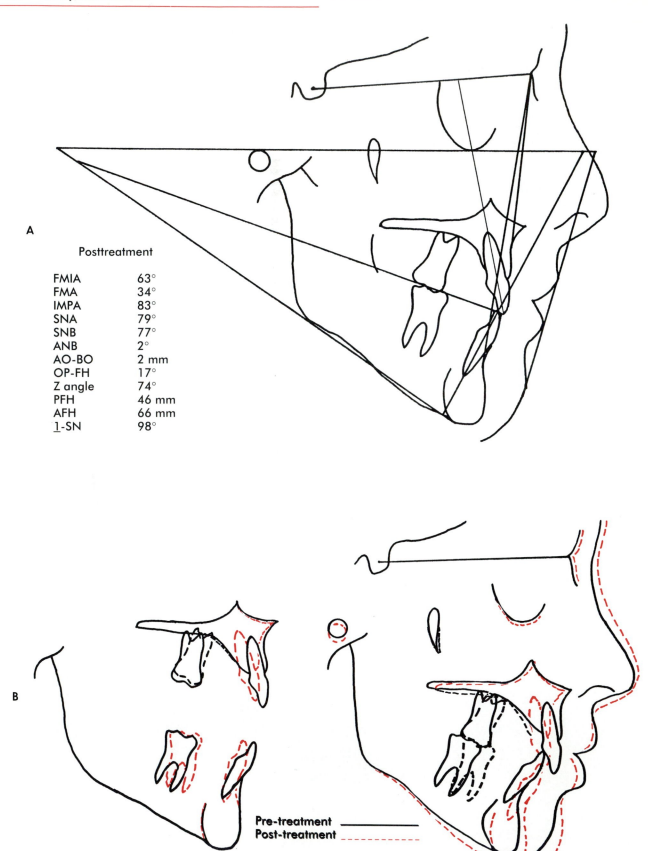

A

Posttreatment

FMIA	63°
FMA	34°
IMPA	83°
SNA	79°
SNB	77°
ANB	2°
AO-BO	2 mm
OP-FH	17°
Z angle	74°
PFH	46 mm
AFH	66 mm
1-SN	98°

B

Pre-treatment ————————
Post-treatment – – – – – –

Fig. 11-65 *Case I:* **A,** Posttreatment cephalometric tracing. **B,** Pretreatment—posttreatment composite.

Results

The posttreatment facial photographs show a pleasing facial change, a balanced facial profile, and a favorable smile line (Fig. 11-60, *B*).

The posttreatment dental casts (Fig. 11-64, *A* through *D*) show the Class I interdigitation of the buccal segments, the overbite and midline correction, and the *treatment* occlusion. The posttreatment cephalometric tracing (Fig. 11-65, *A*) confirms that the mandibular incisors were uprighted from 92° to 83°. The FMA was reduced from 36° to 34°. The FMIA increased to a more normal 63°. Reflecting vertical control, the occlusal plane remained at 17°, while ANB was reduced to 2°. The Z-angle improved from 58° to 74°.

The pretreatment and posttreatment composite cephalometric tracings (Fig. 11-65, *B*) illustrate the downward and forward movement of the mandible relative to cranial base. This type of mandibular response, when in harmony with growth and development, is vital to correct the difficult, high FMA angle, Class II malocclusion. Note the upright mandibular incisors and the upward and backward movement of the maxillary anterior teeth.

Stability

Four-year postretention records were made. The facial photographs (Fig. 11-60, *C*) show a balanced profile with an attractive smile. The casts (Fig. 11-66, *A* through *D*) illustrate that the occlusion has settled. There is a stable buccal segment correction, and the mandibular incisor area is stable. The composite cephalometric tracings (Fig. 11-67), superimposed on SN at Sella, show continued downward and forward movement of the facial complex, as well as the stability of the upright mandibular incisors and the intruded maxillary incisors.

CASE II

Diagnosis

Profile and full-face photographs (Fig. 11-68, *A*) indicate a protrusion. The casts (Fig. 11-69, *A* through *D*) exhibit labially flared mandibular incisors and a Class II posterior relationship of the buccal segments. The pretreatment cephalometric tracing (Fig. 11-70) shows an ANB of 7° and an AO-BO of 7 mm—a reflection of the Class II problem. The FMA is a low 20°, but an IMPA of 108° and an FMIA of 52° indicate dental protrusion. A 62° Z-angle is indicative of a face that can be favorably changed only if the mandibular incisors are uprighted.

The total space analysis values are as follows: Anterior deficit: 7 mm; midarch deficit: 0 mm; posterior deficit: 6 mm. The total denture deficit is 13 mm.

The extraction choice for this patient is the maxillary first premolars and mandibular second premolars. The maxillary first premolars were extracted to reduce the protrusion, and the mandibular second premolars were extracted to gain space for Class II molar correction.

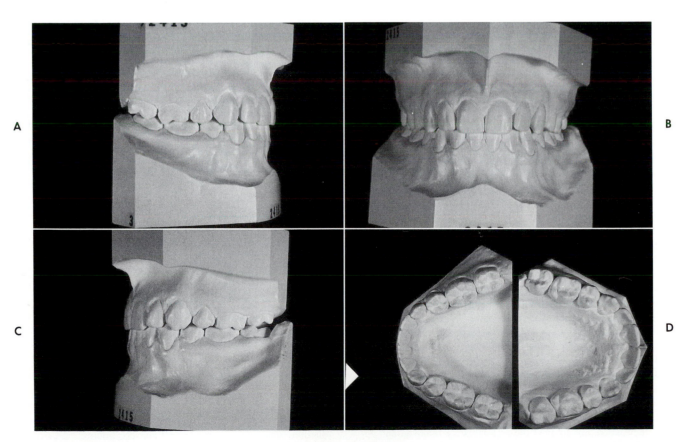

A   B   C   D

Fig. 11-66 Recall casts.

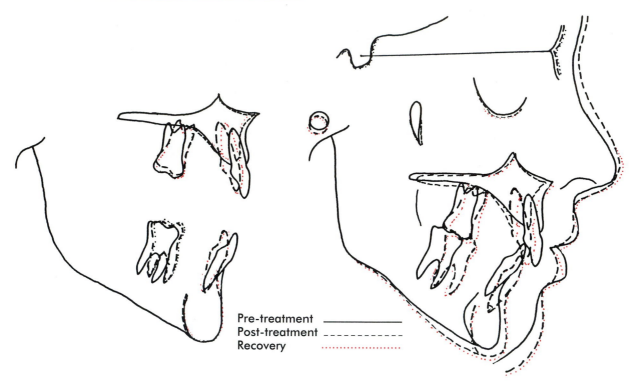

Pre-treatment ——————————
Post-treatment – – – – – – – – –
Recovery ·····················

Fig. 11-67 Pretreatment; posttreatment; recall cephalometric tracings.

Treatment

Klontz designed the force system[8] used to correct the Class II molar relationship in this type of malocclusion. He altered the denture preparation and denture correction steps of the protocol.

Denture Preparation

Denture preparation for the maxillary arch includes leveling, rotation control, bracket engagement, maxillary canine retraction, and molar positioning. In the mandibular arch, denture preparation includes all the above along with the upright mesial movement of the mandibular first molars.

The appliance is applied sequentially. Initially, the maxillary central incisors, canines, second premolars, and second molars are banded. Mandibular central incisors, canines, and first premolars are banded. The mandibular first molars are banded with a buccal tube attachment on the band (Fig. 11-71, *A* and *B*).

The initial archwires are fabricated from resilient edgewise wire—0.017 × 0.022 for the maxillary arch, and 0.018 × 0.025 for the mandibular arch. Ideal first, second, and third order bends are placed, and the archwires are ligated. If necessary, adjustments are made for canine bracket engagement. The high-pull headgears are adjusted to hook directly over the archwires against each canine. A good procedure is to fit the mandibular high-pull headgear first, then place the maxillary high-pull headgear on top of the mandibular headgear. The headgears should be checked and adjusted at each appointment for proper fit, comfort, and compliance.

At the second appointment the archwires are removed and adjusted. Maxillary first molar offsets are placed in the maxillary archwire, and the maxillary first molars are banded with regular Siamese twin brackets. At the third visit the archwires are untied, and the maxillary and mandibular laterals are banded. The archwires are adjusted and retied. Headgear wear is continued for 12 to 14 hours per day on the maxillary arch and as necessary on the mandibular arch.

After total bracket engagement has been accomplished (usually three to four adjustments), the mandibular archwire is replaced with an 0.018 × 0.025 closing loop archwire. The loop is placed just distal to the first premolar bracket, and a shoe horn loop tie back is bent into the archwire just distal to the closing loop (Fig. 11-72). After two or three activations of the loop, the mandibular first molars will have been moved mesially to close most of the extraction space. Nighttime wear of the high-pull headgear is continued to the maxillary canines. After five or six visits, using one archwire in the maxillary arch and two archwires in the mandibular arch, the denture preparation treatment objectives have been met. In the maxillary arch, there has been complete canine retraction, maintenance of, or a slight increase in the terminal molar inclination, and maintenance of the gentle curve of Spee. Objectives accomplished in the mandibular arch include second premolar extraction space closure by mesial first molar movement, a flattened occlusal plane, and maintenance of the first molar inclination (Fig. 11-73).

Denture Correction

Denture correction includes maxillary anterior protrusion reduction, space closure, posterior tooth positioning, and overbite-overjet correction. Denture correction treatment in the mandibular

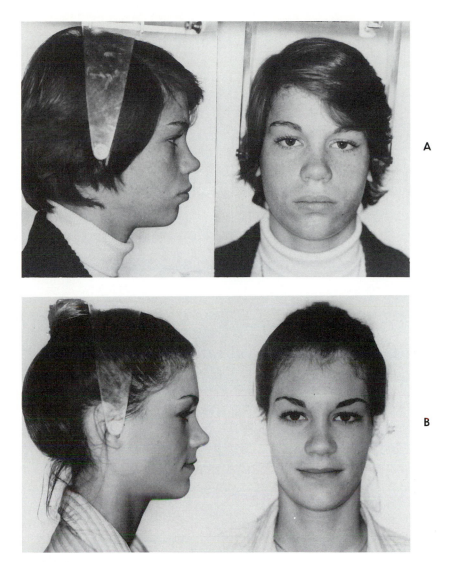

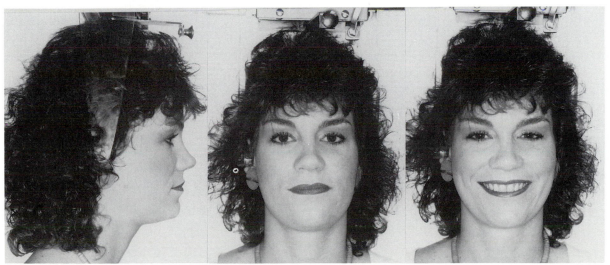

Fig. 11-68 *Case II:* **A,** Pretreatment facial photographs. **B,** Posttreatment facial photographs. **C,** Recall facial photographs.

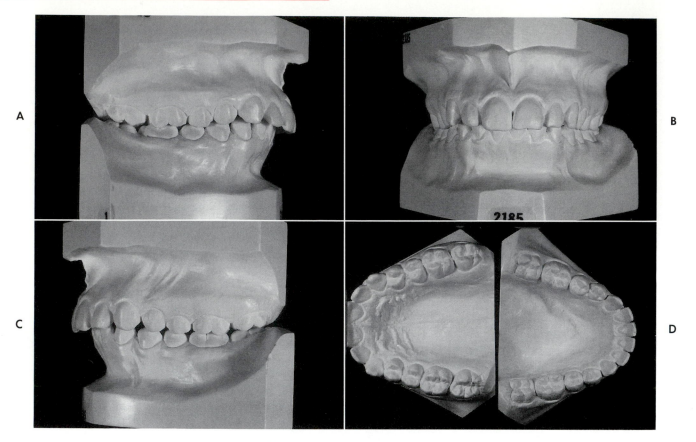

Fig. 11-69 *Case II:* Pretreatment casts.

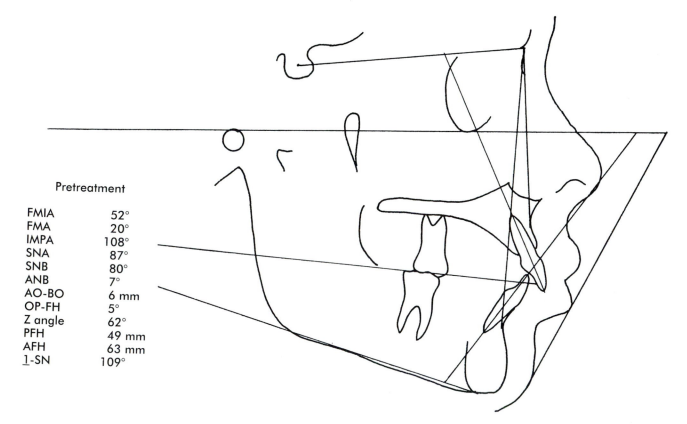

Pretreatment

FMIA	52°
FMA	20°
IMPA	108°
SNA	87°
SNB	80°
ANB	7°
AO-BO	6 mm
OP-FH	5°
Z angle	62°
PFH	49 mm
AFH	63 mm
1-SN	109°

Fig. 11-70 *Case II:* Pretreatment cephalometric tracing.

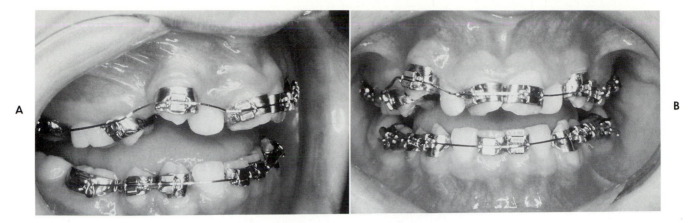

Fig. 11-71   *Case II:* **A,** Photo of denture preparation archwires. **B,** Photo of denture preparation archwires.

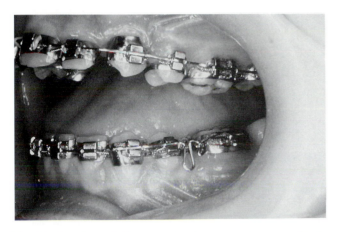

Fig. 11-72   *Case II:* Photo of *shoe horn* loop in the mandibular archwire.

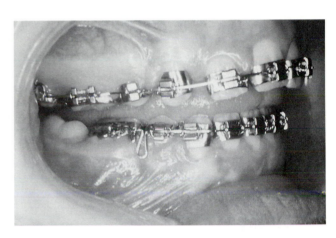

Fig. 11-73   *Case II:* Photo of mandibular arch after mesial molar movement.

arch includes incisor positioning, mandibular anchorage preparation, and root paralleling for stabilization.

Terminal molar anchorage is now prepared in the mandibular arch. The first molar bands with the buccal tube attachments are removed, and the second molars are banded. A 0.019 × 0.025 archwire with loop stops flush against the second molar tubes is fabricated. Proper first and third order bends are placed. Fifteen degrees of active distal tip is placed on the mandibular second molars. A 0.020 × 0.025 maxillary archwire with 6.5 mm closing loops distal to the lateral incisors is fabricated. The loop stop is immediately distal to the first molar bracket. Gingival headgear hooks are soldered distal to the central incisors (Fig. 11-74).

The archwires are ligated, the maxillary closing loop activated, and headgears applied. The maxillary high-pull headgear is attached to the hook between the central and lateral incisors. The mandibular headgear is attached over the wire directly against the canines. As the mandibular second molar begins to upright, the first molar can be banded. The mandibular archwire should be adjusted by placing a first molar offset and a vertical height ad-

justment to prevent first molar extrusion. The second molar distal tip is increased so the effective tip remains at 15°.

In the maxillary arch space closure is continued, while in the mandibular arch the second molar is gradually depressed and tipped to a 15° distal inclination. When (1) the mandibular arch has been completely leveled, and (2) the mandibular second molar has a 15° distal inclination, a new 0.019 × 0.025 mandibular archwire is fabricated. If any mandibular extraction space is left, a 6 mm closing loop is placed distal to the first premolar, and the loop stop is placed so that it will be flush with the buccal tube after all the space is closed (Fig. 11-75). A high-pull headgear hook is soldered to the archwire between the mandibular central and lateral incisors. The first step is to close any second premolar extraction space that remains by activating the closing loop. The high-pull headgear is worn only during sleeping hours. The second step with this archwire is anchorage preparation of the first molar. A 10° distal tip is placed just mesial to the first molar bracket, and a compensating bend is placed mesial to the loop stop to maintain the distally tipped second molar.

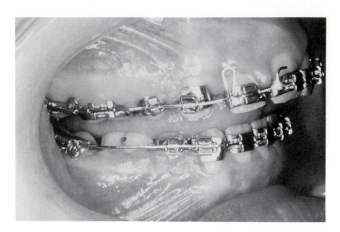

Fig. 11-74 *Case II:* Continuous mandibular archwire, maxillary closing loop archwire.

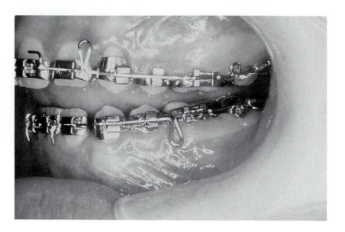

Fig. 11-75 *Case II:* Mandibular closing loop archwire.

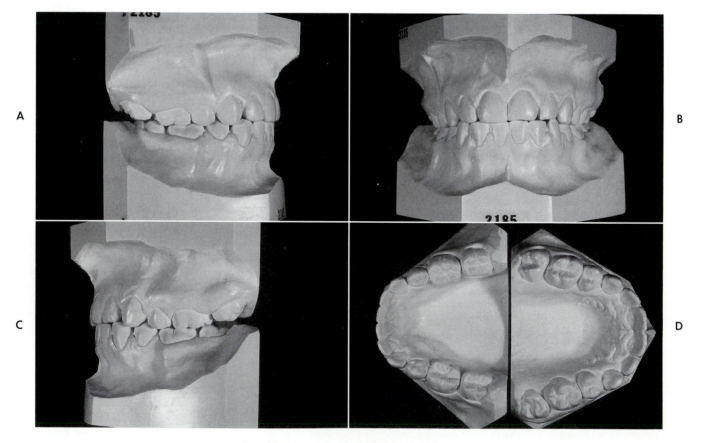

Fig. 11-76 *Case II:* Posttreatment casts.

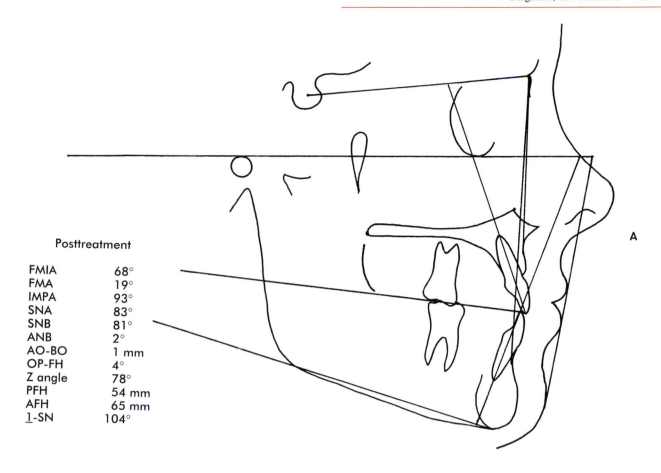

Posttreatment	
FMIA	68°
FMA	19°
IMPA	93°
SNA	83°
SNB	81°
ANB	2°
AO-BO	1 mm
OP-FH	4°
Z angle	78°
PFH	54 mm
AFH	65 mm
1-SN	104°

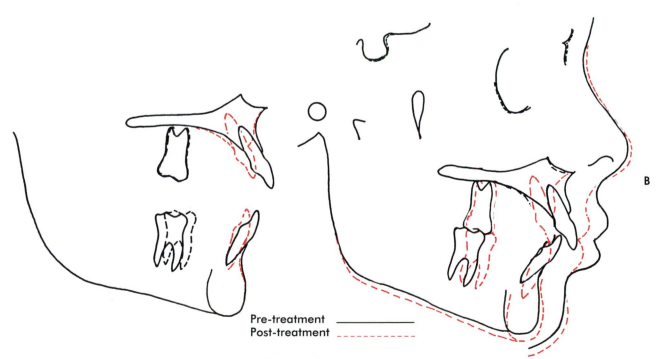

Pre-treatment _____
Post-treatment _ _ _ _ _ _ _ _ _

Fig. 11-77   *Case II:* **A,** Posttreatment cephalometric tracing. **B,** Pretreatment—posttreatment composite.

If all the space has been closed in the extraction site, this archwire may be fabricated as a continuous archwire without the closing loop. The same archwire adjustment procedures are used to prepare mandibular anchorage. The terminal molar distal tip of 15° must be maintained. The first molar is distally tipped 8° to 10°, and the first premolar is distally tipped 3°. The canines and anteriors are upright. Treatment is now completed in the manner that has been previously described.

Results

The posttreatment facial photographs (Fig. 11-68, *B*) show a dramatic facial change. The posttreatment dental casts (Fig. 11-76, *A* through *D*) show the Class I intercuspation of the buccal segments and the overbite correction. The posttreatment cephalometric tracing (Fig. 11-77, *A*) confirms that the mandibular incisors were uprighted from 108° to 93°. FMIA improved from 52° to 68°. ANB was reduced to 2°, and the Z-angle increased from 62° to 78°. The pretreatment and posttreatment composite cephalometric tracings (Fig. 11-77, *B*) confirm that the mandibular incisors were uprighted and that the maxillary incisors were retracted and intruded. The mandible moved forward and downward, enhancing the Class II correction.

Stability

Ten year postretention records were made. The facial photographs (Fig. 11-68, *C*) show a well balanced profile with a pleasing smile. The casts (Fig. 11-78, *A* through *D*) confirm the stability of the correction and the settling of the occlusion. The composite tracings (Fig. 11-79) show the pretreatment, posttreatment, and 10-year postretention skeletal and dental changes.

CASE III

Diagnosis

The third patient will demonstrate a diagnostic differentiation for a less severe malocclusion. The pretreatment profile, full face, and smile photographs (Fig. 11-80, *A*) exhibit a pleasing facial appearance that must be maintained. The cast analysis (Fig. 11-81, *A* through *D)* reveals a Class II relationship on the left side, an end to end relationship on the right side, a diastema between the maxillary central incisors, a midline shift, and a deep overbite.

A pretreatment ANB of 5 degrees confirms the Class II skeletal pattern. On the cephalometric tracing (Fig. 11-82), most cephalometric values are within normal range. There is no deficit in the anterior, midarch, or posterior denture areas. No premolars were extracted.

Treatment

Treatment of the nonpremolar extraction case, either Class II or Class I, with Merrifield edgewise sequential directional forces is similar to the treatment systems previously discussed. It is important, however, to understand that Class II malocclusion correction generally requires more anchorage preparation than Class

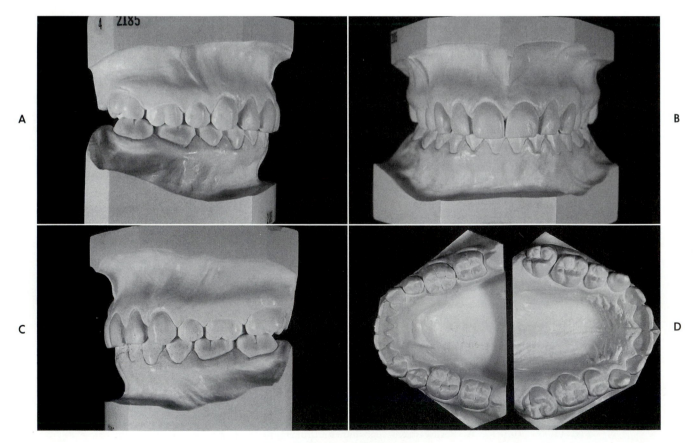

Fig. 11-78 *Case II:* Recall casts.

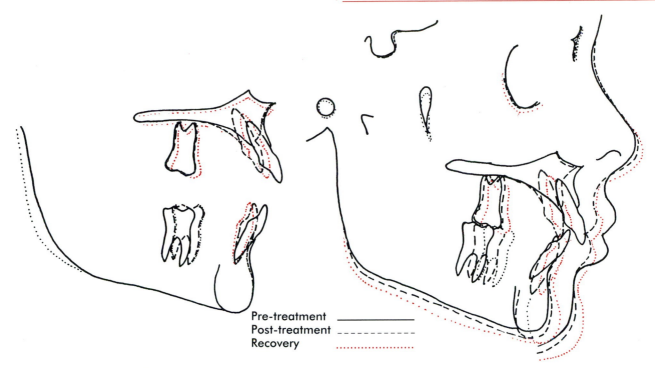

Fig. 11-79   *Case II:* Pretreatment; posttreatment; recall cephalometric composite tracings.

I malocclusion correction because Class II elastics are generally used. The overall objectives of proper denture position and excellent facial esthetics are the same, whether the case is treated by extraction or without extraction of premolars. In most nonpremolar extraction cases, treatment requires more attention to anchorage conservation than is necessary with premolar extraction treatment. The posterior part of the denture must be analyzed carefully because there must be space in the mandibular arch for anchorage preparation. In most cases, to have space for mandibular anchorage preparation and for proper dental positioning requires that the mandibular third molars be extracted before treatment if feasible.

Likewise, space must be available in the posterior part of the maxillary arch for Class II correction. Diagnosis and treatment planning is critical in this area because, frequently, the maxillary third molars should be extracted before the Class II correction step of treatment. During the treatment of certain types of nonpremolar extraction cases, consideration is given to the extraction of the maxillary second molars if the third molars are properly forming. The extraction of the maxillary second molars creates space for effective distalization of the remaining maxillary teeth into a Class I relationship. The maxillary third molars, after eruption, function with the mandibular second molars. The treatment of the nonpremolar extraction case is divided into the same four steps of treatment that have been previously outlined: denture preparation, denture correction, denture completion, and denture recovery.

Denture Preparation

The dentition is sequentially banded and/or bonded. An 0.018 × 0.025 mandibular archwire with arch curvature and with 5 mm bulbous loops bent flush against the second molar tubes is used.

There should be approximately 5° of effective distal tip against the second molars when the wire is ligated. The maxillary archwire is 0.017 × 0.022, with 7 mm bulbous loops bent flush against the second molar tubes. The effective distal tip on the molars is approximately 5°. Hooks are soldered to each wire distal to the lateral incisors for the attachment of J hook headgear (Fig. 11-83, *A* and *B*). A useful addition to the nonpremolar extraction Class II malocclusion correction is the simultaneous use of high-pull headgear on both maxillary and mandibular archwires during denture preparation. The purpose of both headgears is not to correct the molar relationship but to prevent downward and forward migration of the anterior teeth during sequential banding in the maxillary arch and forward tipping of the anterior teeth during sequential banding and posterior anchorage preparation in the mandibular arch. After each month of treatment, the archwires are removed, the bulbous loops are activated 1 mm, and additional teeth are banded or bonded (Figs. 11-84, *A* and *B*). As the archwires are adjusted the effective distal tip of the mandibular archwire on the second molar is increased to a full 15° as the second molar tips distally.

While in the stage of denture preparation, a new 0.019 × 0.025 mandibular working archwire is constructed. Anchorage preparation is initiated after all teeth are banded and after the second molars have been tipped to a 15° distal inclination. This archwire has ideal first and third order bends, and the loop stops are bent flush with the second molar tubes. Using this 0.019 × 0.025 mandibular archwire, anchorage is prepared by placing a compensation bend mesial to the loop stop to insure that the wire is passive in the buccal tube and then by tipping the first molar 10°. After the first molar is tipped, a compensation bend is placed mesial to the first molar, and the second premolar is tipped 5°. These steps have been previously outlined.

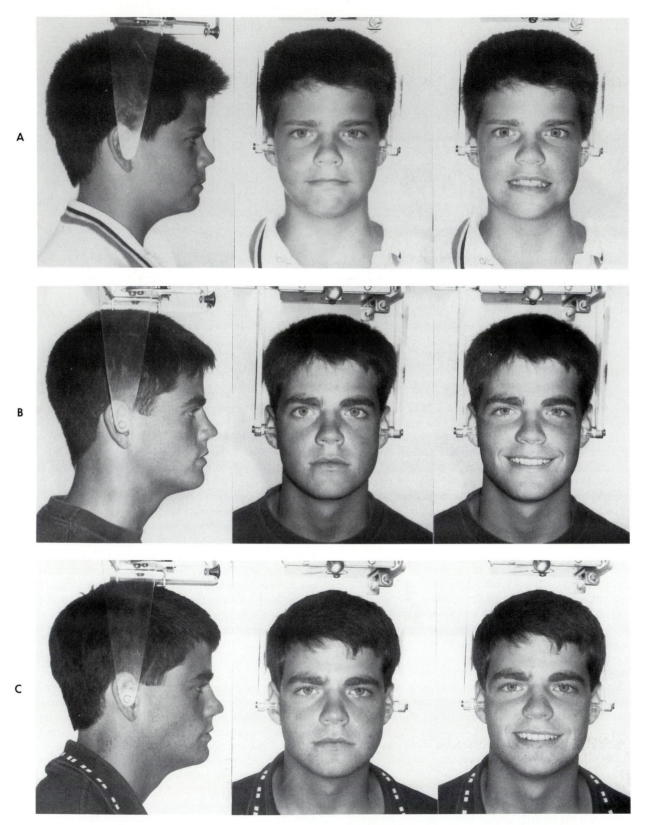

Fig. 11-80 *Case III:* **A,** Pretreatment facial photographs. **B,** Posttreatment facial photographs. **C,** Recall facial photographs.

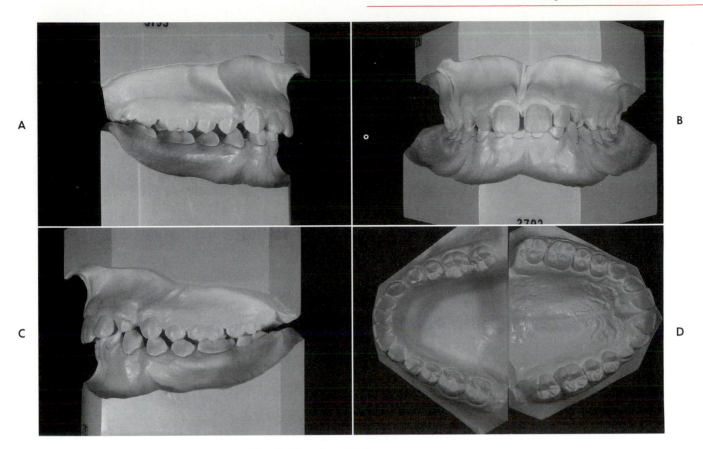

Fig. 11-81   *Case III:* Pretreatment casts.

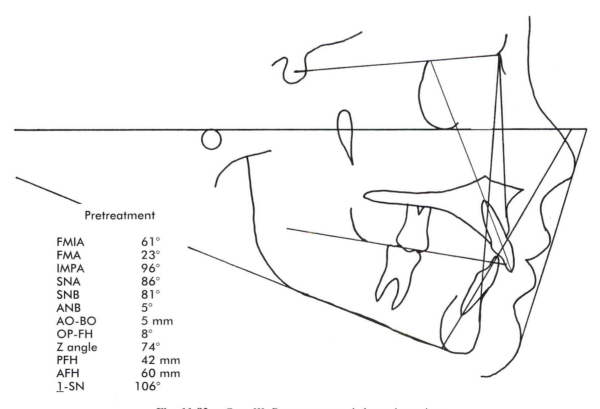

Pretreatment	
FMIA	61°
FMA	23°
IMPA	96°
SNA	86°
SNB	81°
ANB	5°
AO-BO	5 mm
OP-FH	8°
Z angle	74°
PFH	42 mm
AFH	60 mm
1̲-SN	106°

Fig. 11-82   *Case III:* Pretreatment cephalometric tracing.

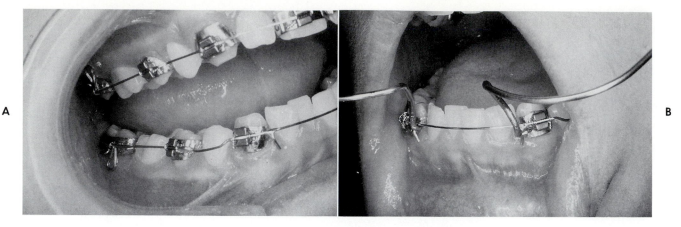

Fig. 11-83 *Case III:* **A,** Initial archwires. **B,** Headgear attachment photo.

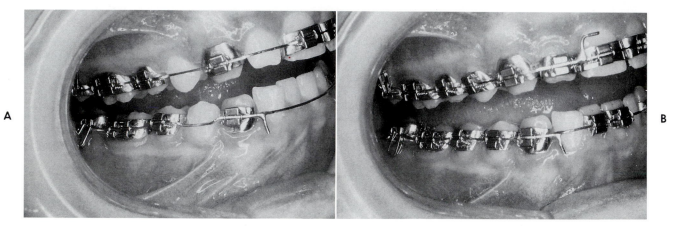

Fig. 11-84 *Case III:* Sequential banding of the nonpremolar extract case.

Denture Correction

A 0.0215 × 0.028 stabilizing archwire is used in the mandibular arch. The archwire has ideal first order and third order bends. The loop stops are bent 0.5 mm anterior to the molar tubes. Gingival 0.025 spurs for up and down elastics are soldered distal to the lateral incisors.

A 0.020 × 0.025 working archwire is used in the maxillary arch. The first order and third order bends are ideal. There is 7° of progressive lingual crown torque in the posterior area. Seven millimeter bulbous loops are placed in contact with the second molar tubes. Gingival high-pull headgear hooks are soldered between the central and lateral incisors, and Class II hooks are soldered between the lateral incisors and the canines.

The Class II forces that are used are the mechanics that have been previously described in the technique section of this chapter. The bulbous loops are opened 1 mm each month to move the second molars distally. Jigs are added to move the first molars distally along the wire. If the second premolars, first premolars, and canines do not follow the molars, 1 month of power chains will close any space that is opened. As the maxillary buccal seg-ments move distally, it may be necessary to slightly widen the archwire to prevent buccal crossbite. The mandibular archwire is checked and the terminal molar ties are cut and recinched at each monthly interval. After maxillary posterior tooth distalization, a 0.020 × 0.025 closing loop archwire is fabricated. The closing loops are 1 mm distal to the lateral incisor brackets. The closing loops are activated 1 mm per month by ligating the omega loop to the buccal tube. The auxilaries that are worn to complement this force system are a high-pull headgear to the hooks that are soldered gingival to the wire between the central and lateral incisors. Eight oz Class II elastics are worn 24 hours per day. Anterior vertical elastics are also worn when the headgear is in use.

Denture Completion

The previous 0.0215 × 0.028 mandibular stabilizing wire is removed and checked for ideal first, second, and third order bends. A 0.0215 × 0.028 maxillary archwire with ideal first, second, and third order bends is fabricated and coordinated carefully with the mandibular archwire. The omega loops in both archwires are placed in contact with the molar tubes. Cusp seating spurs and hooks for the headgear and elastics are soldered. The force system can be any combination of elastics and headgear. The case is treated to completion (Fig. 11-85). After appliance removal, the maxillary and mandibular Hawley retainers are constructed and placed.

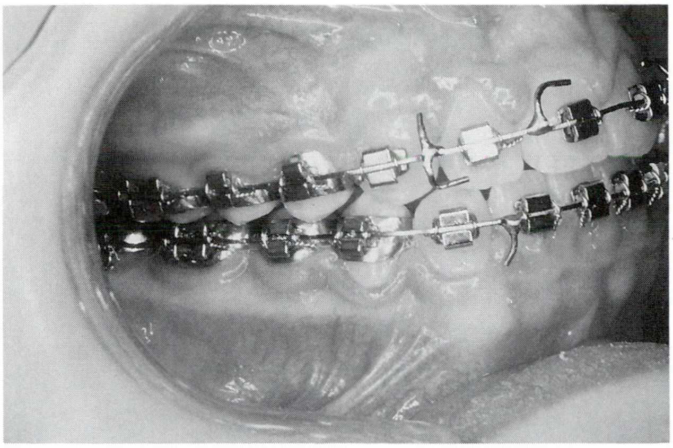

Results

The posttreatment facial photographs (Fig. 11-80, *C*) show the maintenance of the pretreatment facial balance. The dental casts (Fig. 11-86, *A* through *D*) exhibit the Class I treatment occlusion. The overbite, overjet, and midline have been corrected. The posttreatment cephalometric tracing (Fig. 11-87, *A*) shows uprighting of the mandibular incisors, a reduction of the ANB to 2° and an 81° Z-angle. The pretreatment and posttreatment composite cephalometric tracings (Fig. 11-87, *B*) exhibit the maintenance of tooth position and the good mandibular response which helped correct the Class II dental relationship.

Stability

The retention records demonstrate facial balance (Fig. 11-80,*C*), the maintenance of the dental correction through recovery (Fig. 11-88, *A* through *D*), and continued mandibular response (Fig. 11-89).

Fig. 11-85 *Case III:* Denture completion—nonpremolar extraction case.

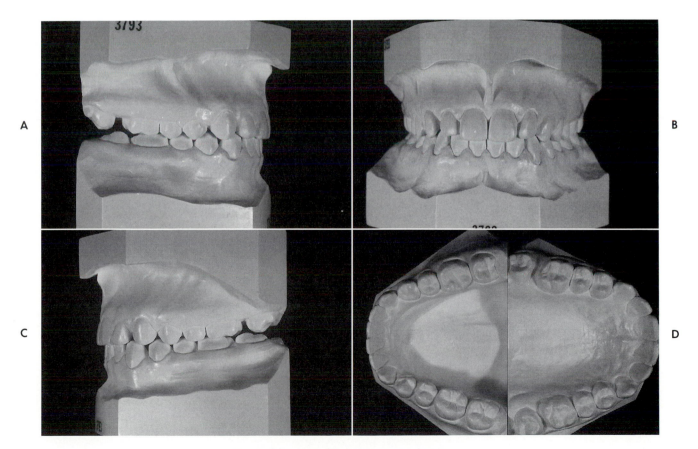

Fig. 11-86 *Case III:* Posttreatment dental casts.

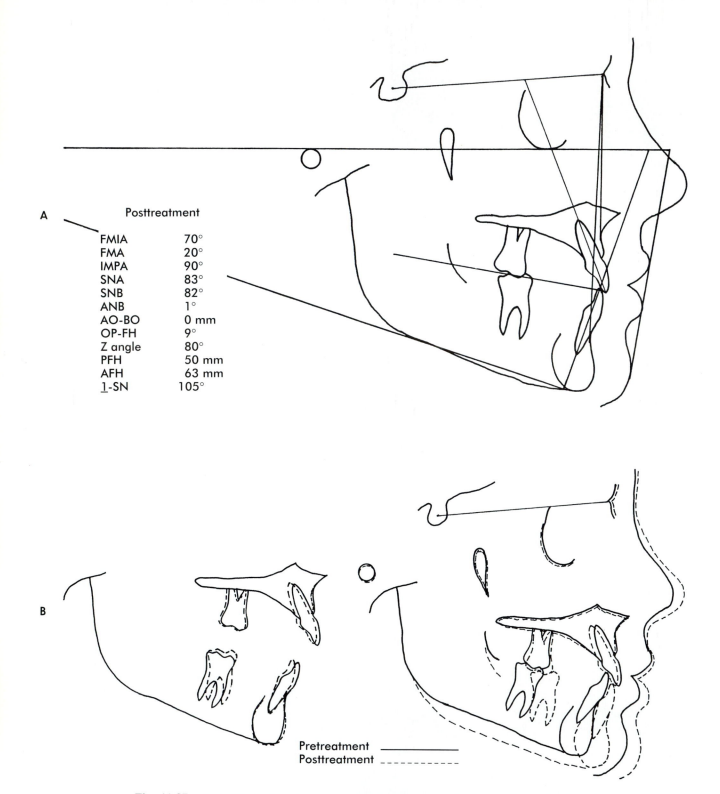

A Posttreatment

FMIA	70°
FMA	20°
IMPA	90°
SNA	83°
SNB	82°
ANB	1°
AO-BO	0 mm
OP-FH	9°
Z angle	80°
PFH	50 mm
AFH	63 mm
1-SN	105°

B

Pretreatment ——————
Posttreatment - - - - - - -

Fig. 11-87 *Case III:* **A,** Posttreatment cephalometric tracing. **B,** Pretreatment—posttreatment cephalometric composite tracings.

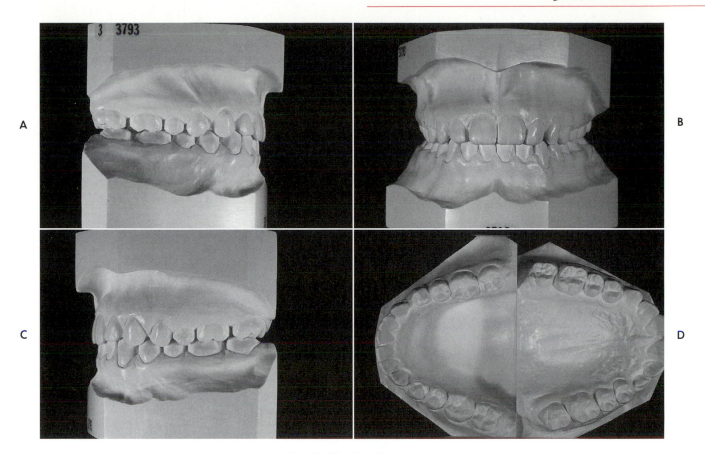

Fig. 11-88   Recall casts.

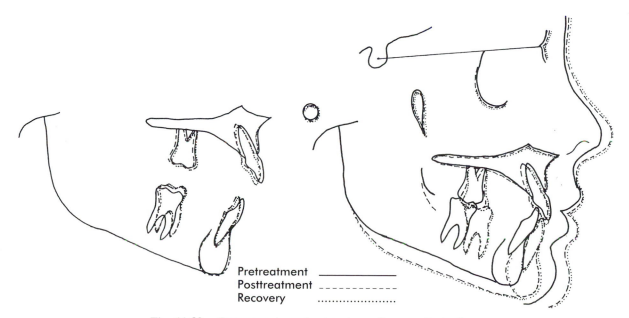

Pretreatment _____
Posttreatment ------------
Recovery ....

Fig. 11-89   Pretreatment; posttreatment; recall composite tracing.

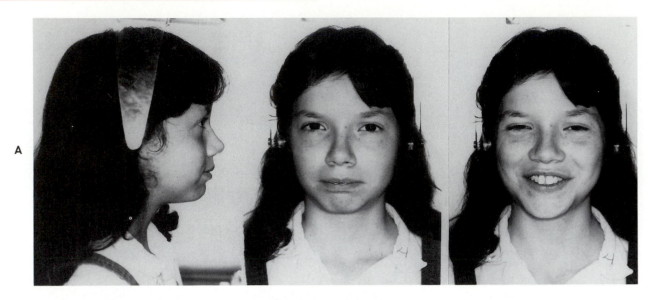

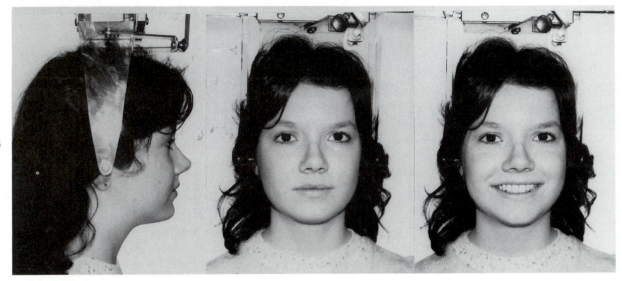

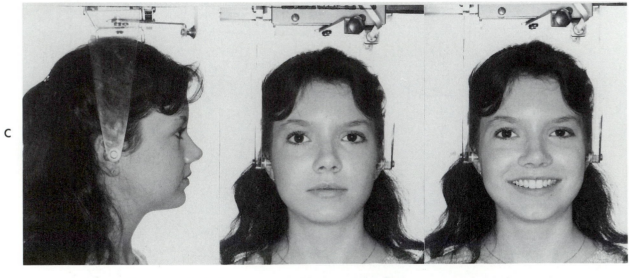

Fig. 11-90 *Case IV:* **A,** Pretreatment facial photographs. **B,** Posttreatment facial photographs. **C,** Recall facial photographs.

CASE IV

Diagnosis

The facial photographs (Fig. 11-90, *A*) show a protrusion and a lack of facial balance. The casts (Fig. 11-91, *A* through *D*) through *D*) exhibit full a Class II step malocclusion on both right and left sides, protrusion, and crowding of the anterior teeth. The pretreatment cephalometric tracing (Fig. 11-92) demonstrates the Class II skeletal and dental relationship. Mandibular incisor flaring is confirmed by an IMPA of 98°. The FMIA of 55° and the Z-angle of 60° reflect the protrusion.

Total space analysis confirms an anterior deficit of 14.4 mm, a midarch deficit of 4 mm, and a posterior deficit of 8 mm, yielding a 26.4 mm total denture deficit for this difficult case.

To correct the crowding and protrusion, four first premolars were extracted. Even after first premolar removal, a space deficit of 3.4 mm existed, along with the 10 mm Class II correction requirement. Therefore, it was necessary to study the posterior denture area. The mandibular third molars were extracted so that maximum anchorage could be prepared during treatment. After maxillary space closure and mandibular anchorage preparation, the malocclusion was evaluated, and the maxillary second molars were extracted to provide space for maxillary posterior distal tooth movement.

Treatment

The archwire sequence for this patient was the same sequence employed for the first patient described. The only difference was that after the maxillary second molars were extracted, the bracketed first molar bands were changed to bands with buccal tubes, and a 0.0215 × 0.028 archwire with 7 mm bulbous loops bent flush against the molar tubes was fabricated (Fig. 11-93). The first molars were distalized into the space created by the extraction of the second molars. The second premolars were retracted with power chains and jigs. The canines were retracted with headgear and power chains. A 0.020 × 0.025 maxillary closing loop archwire with vertical loops distal to the lateral incisors was fabricated and anterior spaces were closed using the force systems previously described (Fig. 11-94).

Results

The post-treatment facial photographs (Fig. 11-90, *B*) show the pleasing facial change. The post-treatment dental casts (Fig. 11-95, *A* through *D*) exhibit the Class I intercuspation of the buccal segments, overbite and overjet correction, and no crowding. The post-treatment cephalometric tracing (Fig. 11-96, *A*) confirms mandibular incisor uprighting and an ideal FMIA of 65°. The ANB is reduced to 2°, and the Z-angle is increased to 77°. Pretreatment and posttreatment composite tracings (Fig. 11-96, *B*) illustrate the downward and forward movement of the mandible. Note the uprighting of the mandibular incisors and the intrusion and distal movement of the maxillary incisors.

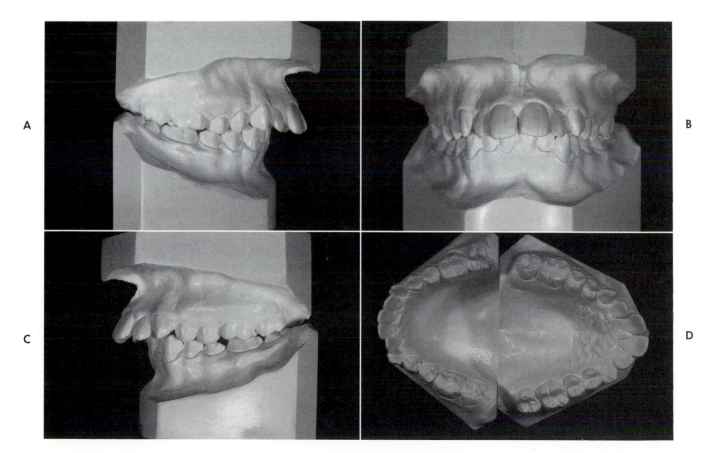

Fig. 11-91   *Case IV:* Pretreatment casts.

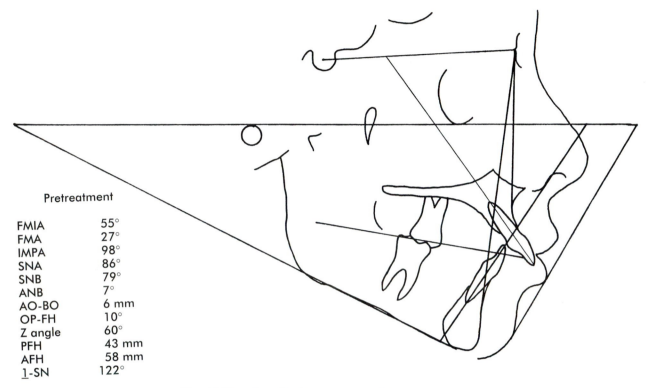

Pretreatment	
FMIA	55°
FMA	27°
IMPA	98°
SNA	86°
SNB	79°
ANB	7°
AO-BO	6 mm
OP-FH	10°
Z angle	60°
PFH	43 mm
AFH	58 mm
1̲-SN	122°

Fig. 11-92   *Case IV:* Pretreatment cephalometric tracing.

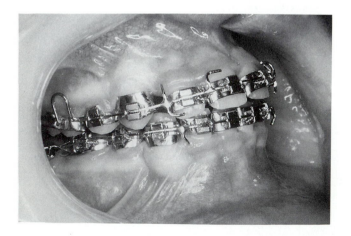

Fig. 11-93   *Case IV:* Maxillary bulbous loop archwire.

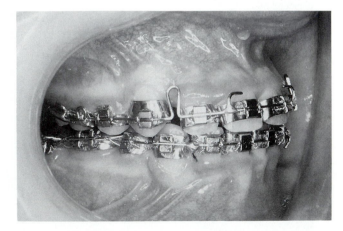

Fig. 11-94   *Case IV:* Denture completion.

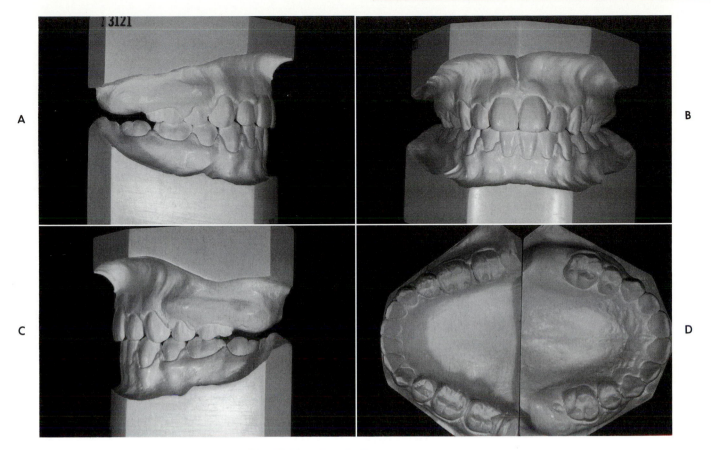

Fig. 11-95   *Case IV:* Posttreatment casts.

Stability

Five-year retention records confirm a stable treatment result that continued to improve. The 5-year recovery records show a balanced face (Fig. 11-90, *C*). The casts (Fig. 11-97, *A* through *D*) illustrate the eruption of the maxillary third molars and the settling of the occlusion. The cephalometric tracing superimpositions (Fig. 11-98) confirm the maintenance of the correction.

The treatment of these four patients shows the versatility of the modern Tweed-Merrifield edgewise appliance. All four patients illustrate Merrifield's differential diagnosis and sequential directionally controlled force systems. Proper treatment in each instance required correct diagnostic decisions and precision archwire manipulation, and each required a slightly different alteration to the basic mechanical force system. In all patients the resultant force vector was directionally controlled to achieve an improved skeletal and dental position.

Summary

The edgewise appliance has endured the test of time. This "worthwhile" invention has evolved from its inventor, Edward H. Angle, who was determined to use it to correct malocclusions while preserving "the full complement of teeth," through 42 years of development and improvement with Charles H. Tweed who, after countless failures, introduced the extraction of four first premolars and anchorage preparation to produce facial balance. It continues through 40 years of achievements to date with Levern Merrifield who introduced (1) differential diagnosis, which led to the removal of the teeth that would best produce balance, harmony, and facial proportion within the craniofacial complex; (2) directional force technology; and (3) sequential wire manipulation treatment, which has become the most precise and most efficient instrument for the routine correction of major malocclusions that exists in the world today.

Although the Tweed-Merrifield edgewise appliance is the direct descendent of the appliance that was invented 66 years ago (1928) by Edward Angle, it is used with a totally different philosophy of treatment.

With the magnitude of effort that is being directed toward the further sophistication of the appliance; with the comprehensive nature of the clinical research that is being carried on by the Tweed Foundation and others, and with the intense world-wide interest in the Foundation, its objectives, and its courses, it is difficult to imagine that this "worthwhile" invention will ever "depart."

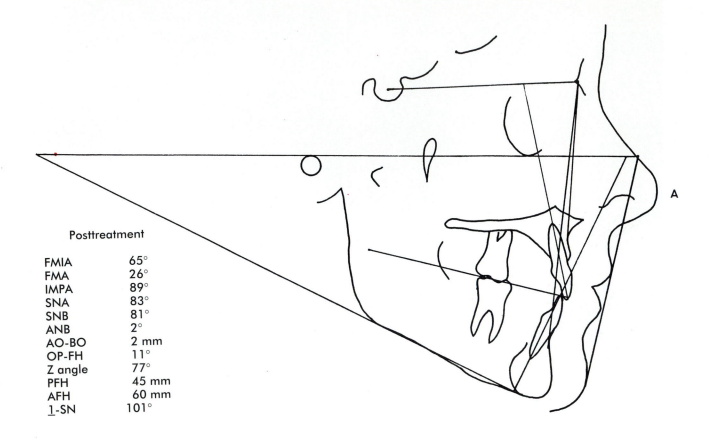

Posttreatment

FMIA	65°
FMA	26°
IMPA	89°
SNA	83°
SNB	81°
ANB	2°
AO-BO	2 mm
OP-FH	11°
Z angle	77°
PFH	45 mm
AFH	60 mm
1-SN	101°

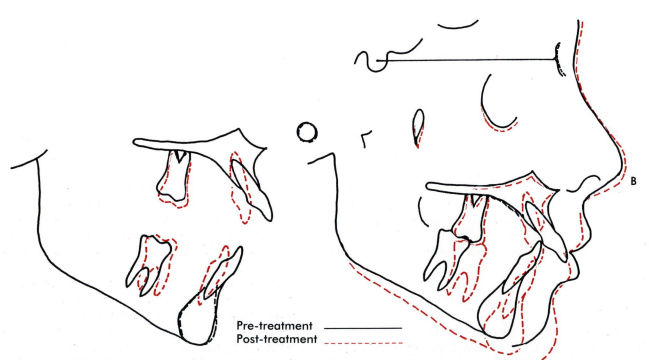

Pre-treatment ──────────
Post-treatment ─ ─ ─ ─ ─

Fig. 11-96 *Case IV:* **A,** Posttreatment cephalometric tracing. **B,** Pretreatment—posttreatment composite tracing.

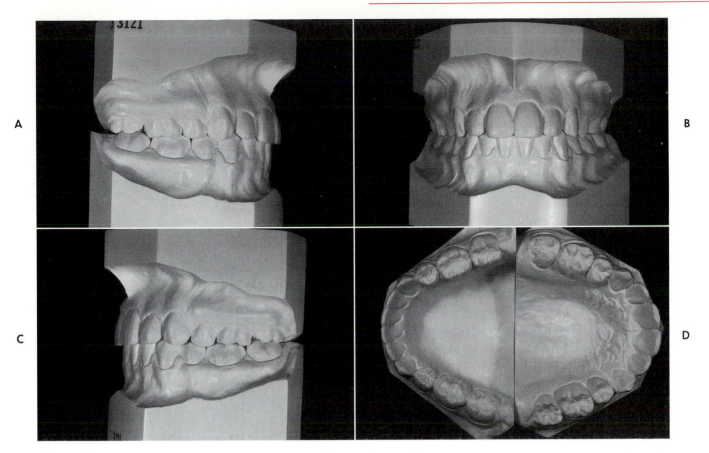

Fig. 11-97   *Case IV:* Recall casts.

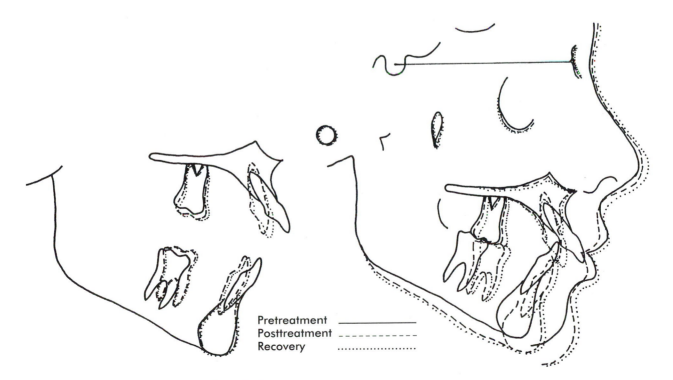

Pretreatment ——————
Posttreatment – – – – – –
Recovery ....

Fig. 11-98   *Case IV:* Pretreatment; posttreatment; recall cephalometric tracings.

REFERENCES

1. Andrews LF: The six keys to normal occlusion, *Am J Orthod* 62:296-309, 1972.
2. Bjørk A, Jensen E, Palling M: Mandibular growth and third molar impaction. *Eur Orthod Soc Trans* 32:164, 1956.
3. Burstone CJ: *Application of bioengineering to clinical orthodontics.* In Graber TM, Swain B, editors: *Orthodontics: current principles and techniques,* St Louis, 1985, Mosby, pp. 193-227.
4. Gebeck TR, Merrifield LL: Analysis: concepts and values. Part I, *J Chas Tweed Found* 17:19-48, 1989.
5. Horn AJ: Facial height index, *Am J Orthod Dentofac Orthop* 102(2)180-186, 1992.
6. Isaacson RJ: The geometry of facial growth and its effect on the dental occlusion and facial form, *J Chas Tweed Found* 9:21-38, 1981.
7. Klontz HA: Readout, *J Chas Tweed Found* 13:53-64, 1985.
8. Klontz HA: Diagnosis and force systems utilized in treating the maxillary first premolar and mandibular second premolar extraction case, *J Chas Tweed Found* 15:19-57, 1987.
9. Ledyard BC: A study of the mandibular third molar area, *Am J Orthod* 39:366-374, 1953.
10. Lindquist JT: *The edgewise appliance.* In Graber TM, Swain B: *Orthodontics: current principles and techniques,* St Louis, 1985, Mosby, pp. 565-639.
11. Merrifield LL: The dimensions of the denture. Unpublished paper presented at each Tweed Course-Charles Tweed Memorial Center, Tucson, Ariz, 1993.
12. Merrifield LL: The profile line as an aid in critically evaluating facial esthetics, *Am J Orthod* 52(11):804-822, 1966.
13. Merrifield LL: Differential diagnosis with total space analysis, *J Chas Tweed Found* 6:10-15, 1978.
14. Merrifield LL, Cross JJ: Directional force, *Am J Orthod* 57:435-464, 1970.
15. Merrifield LL, The systems of directional force, *J Chas Tweed Found* 10:15-29, 1982.
16. Merrifield LL: Edgewise sequential directional force technology, *J Chas Tweed Found* 14:22-37, 1986.
17. Merrifield LL, Gebeck TR: Analysis: concepts and values, part II, *J Chas Tweed Found* 17:49-64, 1989.
18. Pearson LE: Vertical control in treatment of patients having backward rotational growth tendencies, *Angle Orthod* 43:132-40, 1978.
19. Pearson LE: Vertical control in fully-banded orthodontic treatment, *Angle Orthod* 56:205-224, 1986.
20. Radziminski G: The control of horizontal planes in Class II treatment, *J Chas Tweed Found* 15:125-140, 1987.
21. Richardson ME: Development of the lower third molar from ten to fifteen years, *Angle Orthod* 43:191-193, 1973.
22. Roth Ron H: *Treatment mechanics for the straight wire appliance.* In Graber TM, Swain BF, editors: *Orthodontics: current principles and techniques,* St Louis, 1985, Mosby, pp. 665-716.
23. Schudy FF: Sound biological concepts in orthodontics, *Am J Orthod* 63:376-397, 1973.
24. Strang RH: Highlights of sixty-four years in orthodontics, *Angle Orthod* 44:101-112, 1974.
25. Tweed CH: Reports of cases treated with the edgewise arch mechanism, *Angle Orthod* 2(4):236-243, 1932.
26. Tweed CH: The application of the principles of the edgewise arch in the treatment of Class II, division 1: part I. *Angle Orthod* p. 208, 1936.
27. Tweed CH: The application of the principles of the edgewise arch in the treatment of Class II, division 1: part II. *Angle Orthod* p. 256, 1936.
28. Tweed CH: Indications for the extraction of teeth in orthodontic procedures, *Am J Orthod Oral Surg* 30:405-428, 1944.
29. Tweed CH: A philosophy of orthodontic treatment, *Am J Orthod Oral Surg* 31:74-103, 1945.
30. Tweed CH: The Frankfort-mandibular incisor angle (FMIA) in orthodontic diagnosis: treatment planning and prognosis, *Am J Orthod Oral Surg* 24:121-169, 1954.
31. Tweed CH: *Clinical orthodontics,* vols 1, 2, St Louis, 1966, Mosby.

ADDITIONAL READINGS

Andrews LE: *Straighwire: the concept and appliance,* San Diego, 1989, LA Wells.

Angle EH: *The malocclusion of the teeth,* Philadelphia, 1907, SS White Dental Manufacturing.

Burstone CJ: Variable-modulus orthodontics, *Am J Orthod* 80:1-16, 1981.

Burstone CJ, Goldberg AJ: Maximum forces and deflections from orthodontic appliances, *Am J Orthod* 84:95-103, 1983.

Dale J, Rushton J: *A half century of care: a future of caring,* Tucson, Ariz, 1982, Charles H. Tweed International Foundation for Orthodontic Research.

Goddard CL: *The American text-book of operative dentistry,* Philadelphia, 1897, Lea Brothers.

Graber TM: *Orthodontics: principles and practice,* ed 3, Philadelphia, 1961, WB Saunders.

Graber TM: *Orthodontic principles and practice,* Philadelphia, 1972, WB Saunders.

Graber TM: *Current orthodontic concepts and techniques,* vol 1, Philadelphia, 1969, WB Saunders.

Johnston L, editor, Merrifield LL: *New vistas in orthodontics: the sequential directional force edgewise technique,* Philadelphia, 1985, Lea & Febiger, pp. 184-208.

McKay FS: *A memorial meeting of the late Edward Hartley Angle,* The Eastern Association of Graduates of the Angle School of Orthodontia, New York, Jan. 26, 1931, Vanderbilt Hotel.

Merrifield LL, Klontz HK: *Tweed course syllabus,* Tucson, Arizona, 1993, The Charles Tweed Foundation.

Steiner CC: Is there one best orthodontic appliance? *Angle Orthod* 3:277-298, 1933.

Thompson WM: Dr. Robert H. W. Strang, 1881-1982. *Angle Orthod* 53:5, 1983.

Weinberger BW: *Orthodontics: an historical review of its orgin and evolution,* St Louis, 1926, Mosby.

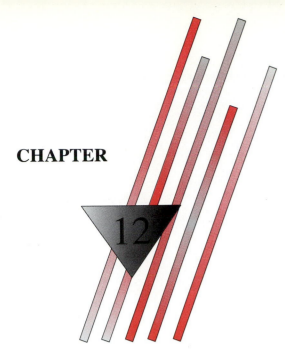

Treatment Mechanics for the Straight Wire Appliance

CHAPTER 12

RONALD H. ROTH

It has been over 20 years since the Andrews *straight wire appliance* first became commercially available. Since that time it has remained somewhat controversial, and certainly it has been misunderstood.

Andrews routinely upgraded the results achieved by orthodontists throughout the world: he provided the *six keys* to occlusion research and built tooth positioning into his appliance (thus starting a trend among orthodontic appliance manufacturers); however, his appliance has captured only a small percentage of the marketplace because of the misunderstanding that preadjusted edgewise, with adjustments milled into the face of the brackets, is the same appliance as the Andrews *straight wire appliance*.

A *true straight wire appliance* captures three dimensions (tip; torque; in-out) of tooth positioning for each tooth. The appliance creates a base that is contoured occlusogingivally and mesiodistally so that the stem of the bracket is parallel to the occlusal plane when the base is placed correctly on the tooth crown and when the tooth is positioned correctly in the three dimensions of space. The bracket slot then can be cut parallel to the stem. When all the teeth are in their proper positions, the bracket slots are parallel to each other around the arch. Thus the archwire has no offset bends and is parallel to the occlusal plane around the arch.

The appliance of choice as far as I am concerned is the A Company straight wire appliance as developed by Lawrence Andrews (Fig. 12-1, *A* through *D*). The reason for selecting this one as the appliance of choice is that it is *the only straight wire appliance at the present time that is truly a straight wire appliance from the standpoint of a level slot lineup*. All the slots of the brackets are at the same height and level in all three dimensions when the teeth are in the correct positions. This is accomplished by the contours for torque, rotation, and in-out being built into the base of the

brackets—a patented feature that only *A* Company had permission to use in the manufacture of appliances. This factor separates the appliance from all other so-called straight wire appliances on the market.

It has been said (and it may be true) that the tooth doesn't *know* if the torque is built into the face of the bracket or into the base of the bracket. However, the tooth next to it *knows,* since all the teeth are being tied together with one wire. To have a true straight wire appliance, there must be *level slot lineup* when the teeth are all in the correct positions. It is physically impossible to achieve this level slot lineup with any appliance that does not have the compound contoured base with torque in the base.

Over a time and through clinical testing, the values built into the original Andrew's straight wire appliance have been modified into what is currently known as *the Roth Rx* (Figs. 12-2 and 12-3, *A* through *C*). The purpose of the Roth Rx was to provide idealized tooth positions before appliance removal that would in most instances allow the teeth to settle to what was found in the nonorthodontic normals that were studied by Andrews. The basic underlying assumptions were that (1) with appliances in place, it would be virtually impossible to position the teeth precisely into the occlusion shown by the nonorthodontic normal sample because of bracket interference; and (2) after appliance removal (no matter how well treated the patient may be) the teeth will shift slightly from the positions they occupied at the time the appliances were removed. This being the case, I altered the prescription of the Andrews straight wire appliance to what I believed would allow the teeth to be placed in a slightly overcorrected position in all three planes of space but not so far overcorrected that the teeth would not *settle* into an idealized position. It was also taken into account that, since the nonorthodontic normals had a

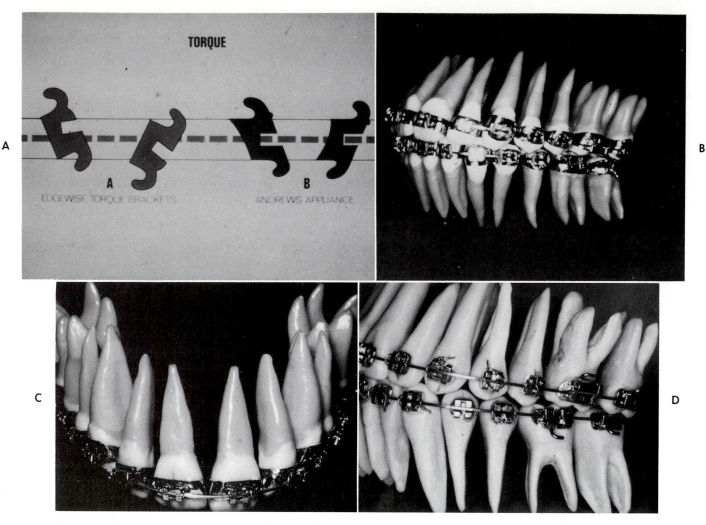

Fig. 12-1   **A,** Difference between preadjusted edgewise brackets and Andrews straight wire brackets with torque in the varying thickness compound contour base. **B,** Andrews straight wire appliance on extracted teeth. Full archwire with only archform. **C,** Maxillary root positions. **D,** Typodont teeth, full-sized archwire.

slight curve of Spee, bracket placement should be altered to allow the placement of a flat, full-sized, unbent (other than arch form) rectangular wire to completely level the curve of Spee and attain my *end of appliance therapy goals* (Fig. 12-4).

The Roth Rx is available in both 0.018 and 0.022 slot brackets. My preference has been the 0.022 slot Siamese brackets. The clinician can argue the advantages and disadvantages of the 0.018 versus the 0.022 slot. In my opinion the 0.018 slot brackets are too restrictive in wire size selection; and after having worked with both 0.018 and 0.022 slot brackets, I prefer the 0.022 slot based on the type of treatment mechanics I use plus I am also using a true *straight wire appliance*. There are certain techniques in which 0.018 slot is definitely advantageous. If I were to use the pure Tweed technique or the pure Bioprogressive technique, my preference would be the 0.018 slot. However, with the treat-

ment mechanics I prefer, the 0.022 slot bracket offers more advantages in wire size selection, in stabilizing arches as anchor units for orthognathic surgery, and in controlling torque in the buccal segments (which is important from the standpoint of functional occlusion). The other argument that seems to crop up in discussions of appliance configuration is about the single wing bracket with rotation arms (e.g., the Steiner wings or the Lang antirotation arms) versus the twin bracket. It has been argued that the single wing brackets offer greater interbracket span and are therefore more advantageous in terms of force delivery to the teeth. This again may be true with certain types of treatment mechanics. However, keep in mind that I am using a true straight wire appliance that has many resilient and *space age* wires in the treatment sequence; it is not necessary therefore to have the interbracket span that may be essential in some other treatment mechanics techniques. The Roth Rx also incorporates

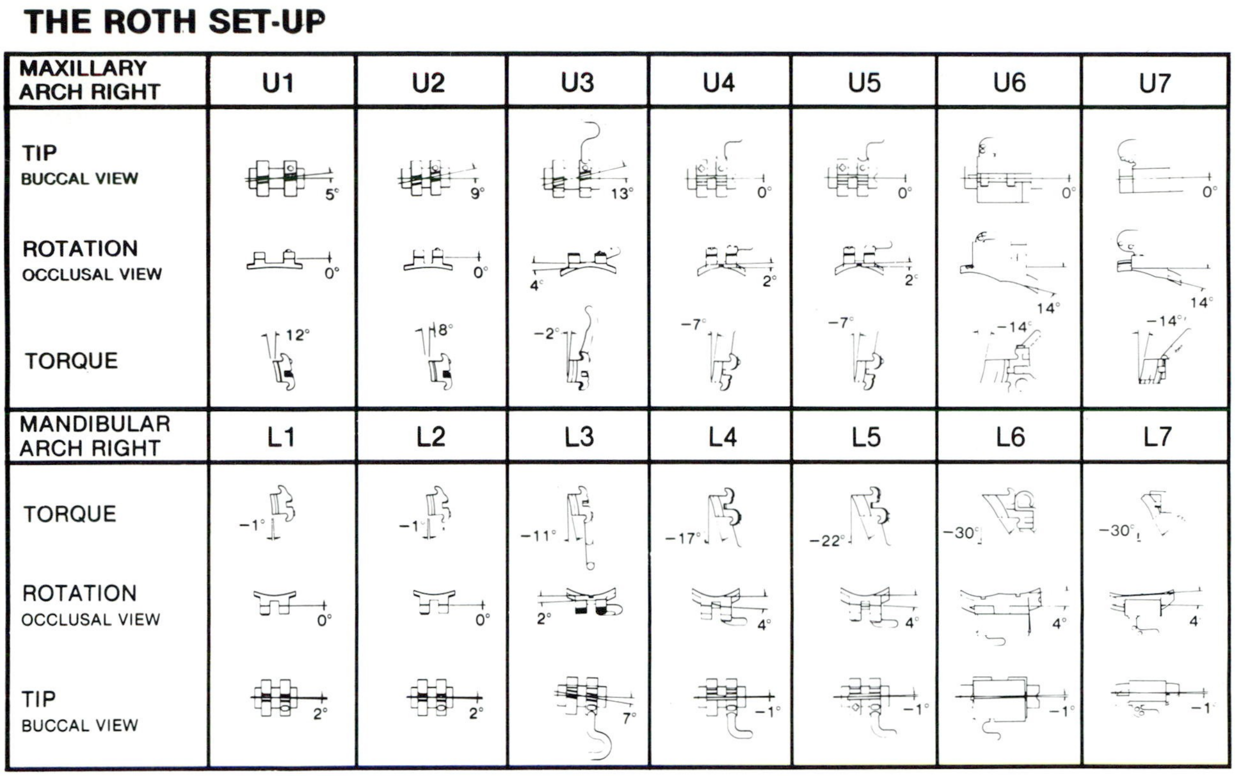

THE ROTH SET-UP

MAXILLARY ARCH RIGHT	U1	U2	U3	U4	U5	U6	U7
TIP BUCCAL VIEW	5°	9°	13°	0°	0°	0°	0°
ROTATION OCCLUSAL VIEW	0°	0°	4°	2°	2°	14°	14°
TORQUE	12°	8°	−2°	−7°	−7°	−14°	−14°

MANDIBULAR ARCH RIGHT	L1	L2	L3	L4	L5	L6	L7
TORQUE	−1°	−1°	−11°	−17°	−22°	−30°	−30°
ROTATION OCCLUSAL VIEW	0°	0°	2°	4°	4°	4°	4
TIP BUCCAL VIEW	2°	2°	7°	−1°	−1°	−1°	−1

Fig. 12-2 Angulations for the Roth bracket setup based on the contoured straight wire appliance. When used with other edgewise brackets, different values will result.

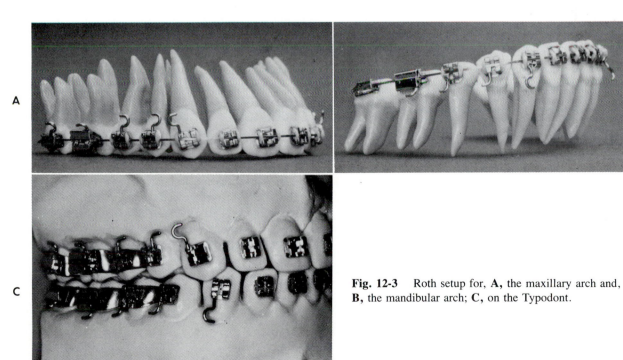

Fig. 12-3 Roth setup for, **A,** the maxillary arch and, **B,** the mandibular arch; **C,** on the Typodont.

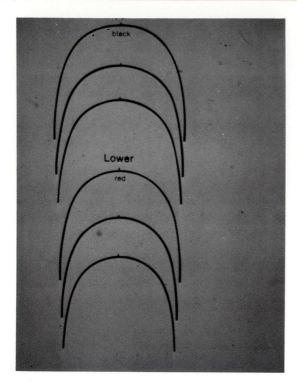

Fig. 12-4 Roth arch form.

a number of hooks for various types of elastic configurations, with double and triple tubes for the use of auxiliary wires. It has its own specific requirements for bracket placement that vary slightly from the positions advocated by Andrews.

A plethora of *preadjusted edgewise* and *essentially-the-same-as straight wire appliances* have flooded the market. At least 85% of all orthodontists think they are using a true straight wire appliance when, in fact, they are not.

I refer the reader to Andrews'[2] recent book for a thorough thesis regarding the true *straight wire appliance* and for information that explains the *fully programmed* appliance, comparing it with the *partially programmed appliances* or with the *preadjusted edgewise* appliance.

My aim in using the appliance has been to attain specific treatment goals and tooth positions in the most efficient and least time-consuming manner possible.

Within the Andrews straight wire system, I introduced a prescription that changed some of the values, anterior bracket positions, and attachments to produce a universal prescription that could be used in a high percentage of cases. The prescription eliminated the necessity of putting offset bends into the finishing wires to attain a subtle *overcorrection* of tooth positions at the end of appliance therapy. From these mildly *overcorrected* tooth positions, the teeth will *settle* into the nonorthodontic normal positions unaided and with a high percentage of regularity. In other words, the prescription is for tooth positions at the conclusion of fixed appliance therapy. The goal is for *specific* overcorrected tooth positions before appliance removal, and it has proved

to function effectively. It was introduced in 1975 and has not been changed since. Thousands of cases have been treated successfully with this prescription to meet the aforementioned goals. The reader is referred to several *Journal of Clinical Orthodontics* articles[6,7] for a more thorough discourse.

Erwin C. Pletcher recently developed a form of the *straight wire appliance* called *Activa*. Activa is a *self-locking* edgewise bracket, made with compound-contoured, torque-in-base straight wire technology by the *A* Company of San Diego, California.

Dr. Pletcher has designed many types of self-locking edgewise brackets over the years. His latest design is a self-locking bracket that could be made in the true straight wire design.

When Pletcher designed the bracket, he fabricated quadrants of typodont-style arches of teeth that were 10 times normal size and he fashioned brackets out of plastic for prototypes. He constructed enlarged versions of archwires and springs, as well as various instruments (along with typodonts) to test the various bracket designs. The current self-locking appliance is the result.

I became interested in the appliance about 4 years ago. I had always been interested in self-locking brackets from the standpoint of mechanical advantage and speed. I have used most if not all of the various self-locking brackets that were made for the edgewise slot. However, after using these brackets I was not impressed with the results because control was minimal and they were not easy to use. Many times I would be in mid-treatment with these various appliances and would need tie-wings to get a better purchase on a tooth or would want a way to detail the tooth positions without having to employ first, second, or third order archwire bends.

Because of many disappointing experiences with self-locking brackets, I was hesitant to try the new Activa brackets.

It was because of the dissatisfaction with both steel ligatures and Alastics and the concern over fingers becoming *stuck* receiving puncture wounds with steel ligature wires, that I decided to try the new brackets.

For the better part of 4 years, 98% of my patients were started with Activa brackets. Although the appliance works well through the gross movement stages of treatment and presents the advantages of speed of movement, with less force and less chairtime, some problems exist.

Overall, I believe the appliance has the great mechanical potential to significantly reduce force levels used in treatment, to reduce treatment time, and to reduce the necessity of extra-oral force and both inter- and intra-arch elastics. I have spent the last 3 years working out some treatment mechanics sequences with the appliance. Some details of the appliance need to be worked out in regard to ease in obtaining a finely tuned finish when compared with the standard size twin straight wire brackets.

The features (see Figs. 12-5, *A* through *C*, through 12-11) of these brackets and their benefits are as follows:

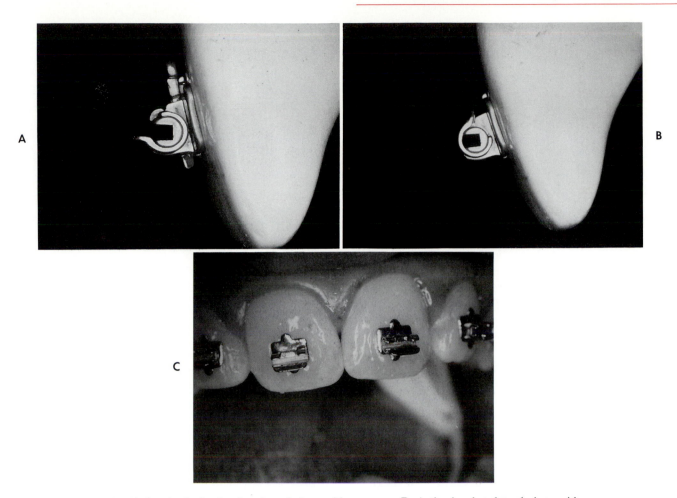

Fig. 12-5 **A,** Activa bracket, lateral view, with cap open. **B,** Activa bracket, lateral view, with cap closed. **C,** Activa bracket on upper centrals, with caps opened. (Courtesy of *A* Company, Johnson & Johnson.)

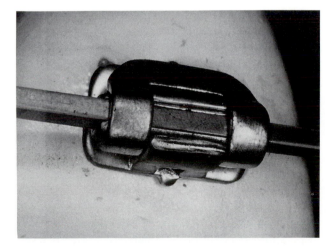

Fig. 12-6 Activa bracket closed, with rectangular archwire in place, showing vertical slot from the occlusal.

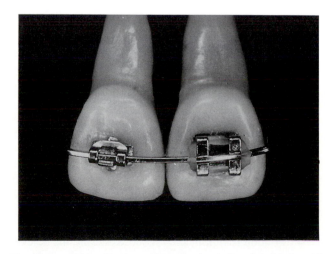

Fig. 12-7 Activa bracket and standard twin bracket side-by-side for size comparison.

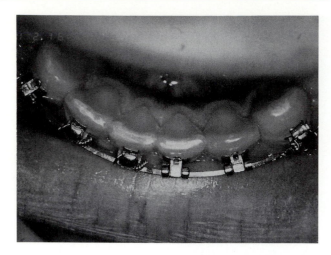

Fig. 12-8   Occlusal view of lower arch, showing a 0.022 × 0.028 archwire in place with Activa and a variety of straight wire brackets in place, and showing contact points of teeth aligned properly.

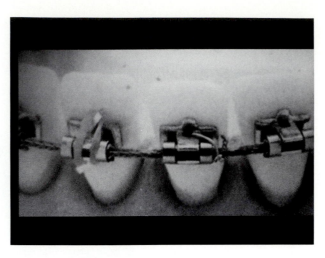

Fig. 12-9   Different ways that Activa brackets can be ligated.

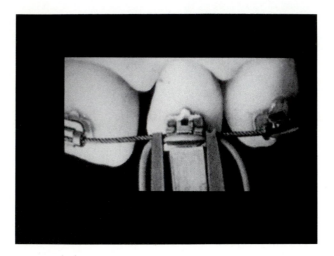

Fig. 12-10   Power thread being placed over the archwire and cap being closed with Activa archwire seating key.

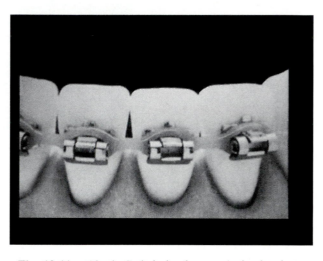

Fig. 12-11   Alastic C-chain in place on Activa brackets.

Advantages

1. Self locking—a locking cap rotates open or closed and snaps closed or open over a built-in detent; many times no special instruments are required to open or close the caps.
2. All brackets have vertical slots that are 0.020 square for use with hooks, uprighting and rotation springs or Pletcher coils for retraction.
3. The brackets are smaller (vertically) than twin or mini-twin brackets; therefore, they are more esthetic to the patient. The brackets are as wide as twin brackets but appear small because they are *in-line* with the archwire and are not as noticeable.
4. Friction is significantly reduced because the brackets are like a series of tubes once the caps are closed; there is no binding of the wire because of ligature ties or Alastics. Studies at the University of Detroit by Kumar[4] show a dramatically reduced static and dynamic resistance caused by friction when compared with steel brackets that have steel ties; an even more dramatic reduction when compared with Alastic ties and ceramic brackets.
5. The brackets are *true* straight wire and will integrate with any of the straight wire brackets made by *A* Company within the same arch. For example, within one arch, standard twins or mini-twins could be used and the clinician will still achieve a *"straight wire"* finish. There is 100% compatibility.
6. Since it is easy to get a purchase on the bracket to tie a tooth to the archwire through the vertical slot

or the main archwire slot, the clinician never has the feeling that he or she *needs* a tie-wing.

7. Since all that is required to change archwires is simple opening and closing of the caps, archwire changes are faster and easier. New bases, with proper clinical crown long-axes referents, need to be produced by the manufacturer.

8. The reduced friction causes teeth to move dramatically faster with less force. The clip breakage problem must be solved by the manufacturer.

9. It is possible to immobilize a tooth or a group of teeth so that they will not move, by placing an elastic over the archwire in the slot of any bracket and then closing the cap over the elastic. This feature makes anchorage control easy and places it in the hands of the operator. When changing bracket positions in the later stages of treatment for detailing, it is necessary to drop back into much smaller size wires and to then level back up to the finishing wires. This slows treatment considerably. The clinician also must use some means to keep spacing from occurring in the arches because of the low friction of the appliance during the releveling process.

10. The appliance will accept C-chain Alastics.

11. Although the appliance can be used with any kind of mechanics, sliding mechanics work well with Activa brackets.

12. The appliance provides excellent patient comfort and acceptance.

Disadvantages

1. Rotations and tip may not be completely reduced unless the bracket slots are filled or tied through the vertical slots and over the archwire on the mesial or distal of the brackets.

2. Proper bracket placement must first be learned.

3. Some of the brackets will need more overcorrection built into them because of the difference between these brackets and conventional edgewise brackets, regarding archwire engagement in the slots during treatment.

4. The practitioner will probably desire to change mechanics to take advantage of the sliding ability of the appliance. Most notably, this means eliminating C-chains as much as possible.

5. The orthodontist may need to retrain auxiliary personnel to use the new appliance.

6. It will take time to learn how to use the appliance most effectively.

PREPARATION

There is no doubt that getting started with a new appliance is at best a learning and growing experience and at worst a time consuming and costly clinical adventure.

It has been my observation after teaching for many years that for most orthodontists change is a painful experience and only the most adventurous will stick with something new until they learn how to work with it.

Most will attempt use of the new appliance without changing anything but the appliance and will give it up after a few inconveniences.

It is helpful at first to admit to yourself that you will not be completely efficient with a new appliance and realize that it requires time to gain proficiency; however, it will be worth the time, effort, and cost in the long run.

The Activa appliance is a *true straight wire* appliance in that it is truly a fully programmed appliance with the proper tooth positions built into a special bracket for each tooth. Each bracket has the features built into it to position a particular tooth properly in all three planes of space without having to place offset bends in the archwires. It is important to place the brackets correctly to get the maximum results from the appliance.

In the use of any appliance, if the orthodontist wants to obtain a well-detailed result on a consistent basis, it is important to position the brackets properly. I have never seen an orthodontist consistently position teeth beautifully with poorly placed brackets, whichever appliance is used. In the *straight wire appliance*, if the time and effort is taken to position brackets well, the clinician's efforts will be rewarded by rarely having to put offsets in the archwires to detail the positions of the teeth.

The Activa brackets are easier to place if they are handled with the latches open. An identification color on the underside of the latch identifies each bracket. The example follows:

Upper central—blue
Upper lateral—pink
Upper cuspid—green
Upper bicuspids—light purple
Lower incisors—yellow
Lower cuspid—light blue
Lower first bicuspid—white
Lower second bicuspid—red

The latches close to the gingival: the uppers close up and the lowers close down.

A 0.020 square vertical slot, which can be used for a variety of purposes, is in each bracket. Custom hooks are made for these slots, which are easily placed or removed as necessary. (See Figs. 12-12, *A* and *B,* and 12-13.)

Incisal and gingival points on the bracket pad should be aligned with the *long axis of the clinical crown* of each anterior tooth for proper angulation and mesiodistal placement of the bracket. However, these points were not properly located for canines and upper incisors. This problem is being remedied by the manufacturer in the form of a new base design. The premolars have a rectangular pad and the edge of the pad can be placed like a *band margin* to locate the bracket so that it is aligned with the long axis of the clinical crown.

As with all other true straight wire appliances, the brackets should be placed at the *middle of the clinical crown* of

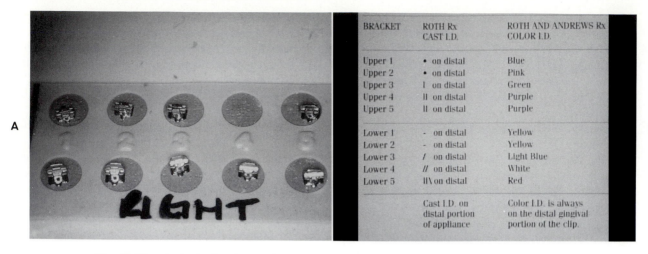

BRACKET	ROTH Rx CAST I.D.	ROTH AND ANDREWS Rx COLOR I.D.
Upper 1	• on distal	Blue
Upper 2	• on distal	Pink
Upper 3	I on distal	Green
Upper 4	II on distal	Purple
Upper 5	II on distal	Purple
Lower 1	- on distal	Yellow
Lower 2	- on distal	Yellow
Lower 3	/ on distal	Light Blue
Lower 4	// on distal	White
Lower 5	II\ on distal	Red
	Cast I.D. on distal portion of appliance	Color I.D. is always on the distal gingival portion of the clip.

Fig. 12-12 **A,** Activa brackets on bonding tray with caps open. **B,** ID chart for Activa brackets.

the posterior teeth from a height standpoint. A specific incisal edge or cusp tip measurement to the middle of the bracket is inappropriate for these appliances, since the taller, the crowns, the more gingival would be the center of the bracket from the incisal edge or cusp tip.

The primary important relationship in the *true straight wire appliance* is the relationship of each tooth's bracket to the adjacent tooth; it is not the relationship of the absolute height of each bracket from the incisal edge or cusp tip.

For instance, if we were to take average-height teeth and measure from the center of the bracket slots to the buccal cusp tips and incisal edges, the measurements would be something like this:

U_1	4.0 mm	L_1	4.0 mm
U_2	4.0 mm	L_2	4.0 mm
U_3	5.0 mm	L_3	4.5 mm
U_4	4.0 mm	L_4	3.5 mm
U_5	3.5 mm	L_5	3.5 mm
U_6	3.0 mm	L_6	3.0 mm
U_7	2.5 mm	L_7	3.0 mm

If the crowns were 1 mm longer than normal, all the bracket heights would be 1 mm more gingival. If the crowns were 1 mm shorter than normal, all the bracket heights would be more occlusal by 1 mm. The bicuspid placements will also be somewhat varied, depending on whether the premolars look more like canines than premolars, whether the case is an extraction case, and whether there is a significant size discrepancy between first and second premolars. These factors will generally alter the bracket heights within 1 mm, one way or the other.

Initially, the Activa bracket bases were occasionally distorted because of the fixture used to place the *clips* or locking cap. This problem has been rectified, as was a minor problem with the adjustment of the tension of the clip. However, the clip brittleness is still a problem.

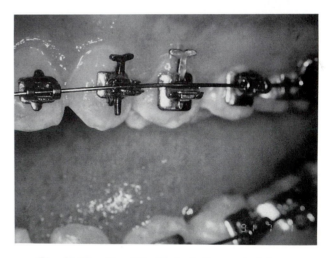

Fig. 12-13 New T-hooks in Activa vertical slots.

If a clip breaks it can be replaced. Beading wax should be placed over the *barrel* of the bracket on the mesial and distal after the old clip has been completely removed. If the new clip is then lined up as shown in the diagram, a plugger can be used to snap it into position. The critical part is getting the new clip properly aligned so that the open portion can slide over the barrel of the bracket. This procedure takes some practice; however, once it is learned, it can be done quickly. (See Fig. 12-14, *A* through *D*.)

In my hands the most effective materials for bonding and cementation are the fluoride-releasing glass ionomer cement, and the resin-filled fluoride releasing light bond sealant with the Phase II self-cure, two paste adhesive.

Light bonding with any metal bracket seems to result in too many instances of the adhesive not being completely cured under the bracket, regardless of the material. If the clinician studies the number of loose brackets occurring with

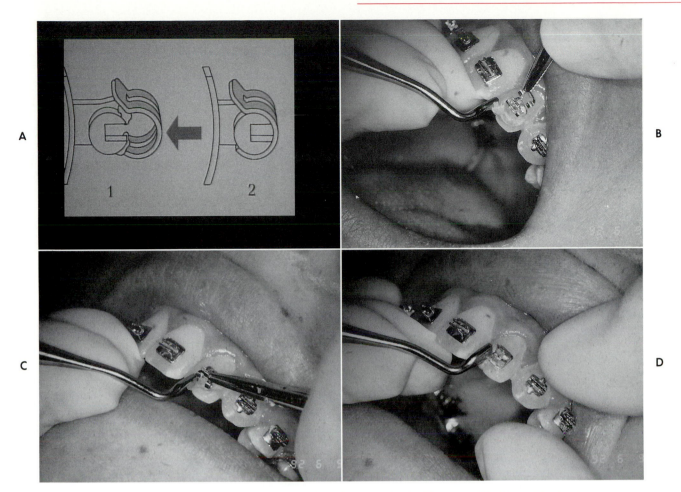

Fig. 12-14 **A,** Diagram for replacement of Activa cap or latch. (Courtesy of Dr. Erwin Pletcher.) **B,** Clinical procedure to replace Activa cap. *Step one* is to place beading wax on barrel of bracket, and bring cap to bracket, using a small instrument. **C,** *Step two* is to angle cap correctly relative to the bracket, and let beading wax hold the cap. **D,** *Step three* is to rock cap into place with plugger, until it snaps on the barrel of the bracket.

light bond sealant as opposed to self-cure sealant, it will become evident that there are significantly more loose brackets with light bond. The bond failure occurs between the adhesive and the bracket base, regardless of the material. This was a conclusion drawn after avidly working with a light bond technique for 3 years, using a variety of materials, techniques, and light guns.

This subject arises because when Activa was first introduced, light bonding was also becoming popular. Several colleagues tried light bonding and Activa at the same time and blamed the appliance for the bond failures. However, when the same failures occurred with tie-wing type brackets, the appliance was exonerated and light bonding was blamed.

The Activa brackets appear to stand out further from the tooth surface than twin brackets; however, that is only an illusion. In a twin bracket the stem of the bracket is covered from view by the tie-wings. The stem on an Activa bracket is not covered. Therefore, it looks as if it is longer. In Fig.

12-8 the arch has a variety of straight wire brackets in one arch, with a 0.022 × 0.028 archwire in place. Note that the teeth line up contact point-to-contact point.

When learning to place the brackets, it is strongly recommended that the orthodontist pour an extra set of stone models and then draw the *crown long-axis* on each tooth with a pencil, using this set of models at the chair as an aid in getting the brackets properly aligned with the *crown long axes* intra-orally.

INSTRUMENTATION

The following special instruments (see Figs. 12-15 through 12-18) are to be used with the Activa appliance.

Activa archwire seating key. This instrument is used to push the archwire into the bracket slot and hold it there until the latch has been closed with the second prong of the instrument. The instrument is double ended, and the other

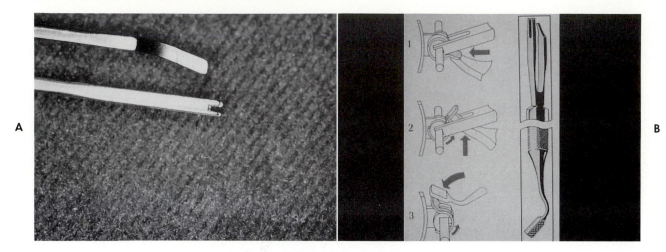

Fig. 12-15   **A,** Close up of Activa archwire seating key. **B,** Sequential steps in using the archwire seating key.

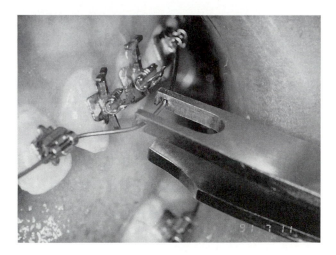

Fig. 12-16   Activa archwire placement instrument will pull wire away from tooth, the wire then can be seated into the bracket slot, and the cap can be closed.

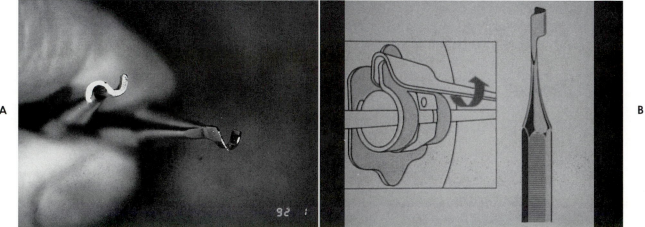

Fig. 12-17   **A,** Broussard Tyer and Activa cap opening tool. **B,** Diagram of showing use of the Activa cap opening instrument.

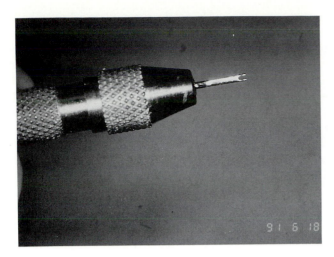

Fig. 12-18   Pletcher spring activator.

end has a serrated plugger tip for nonslip snapping of the Activa cap to its final closure.

Activa archwire placement tool. This instrument is used with light flexible wire and pulls the archwire from the tooth, tips the archwire so that it will line up with the slot, seats the wire, and closes the cap. It is a modification of the Archwire seating key and is also doubled ended, with a plugger tip on the opposite end.

Activa cap opening tool. This instrument resembles half of the ligature twisting end of a Broussard ligature tyer and is used to open the Activa caps. It is double ended and has the *mirror image* tip at the other end so that one end is for upper left and lower right quadrants and the other end is for upper right and lower left quadrants.

Pletcher spring activator. This instrument is made from a springwinder handle and has a tiny two pronged tip that

is used to wind the straight end of a Pletcher coil spring to reactivate it.

In addition, a ligature director can be used to seat the archwire in the bracket slots on initial or early archwires. A sickle scaler can also be used to open the caps.

FEATURES OF THE APPLIANCE

The appliance has a special bracket for each tooth: right and left; upper and lower. Each bracket has mesial and distal contours that are built into the base and that will take into account rotation, torque, and tip. Each is constructed to fit the bracket site on the face of the tooth. In addition, the brackets have various thicknesses to establish the proper in-out relationships between the facial surfaces of the teeth.

The archwire can be *forced* into the slot just as the orthodontist *ties* a wire into the slot of a tie-wing bracket. (See Fig. 12-19, *A* and *B*.) However, the cap should never be forced. For instance, in the early stages of treatment, the wire (e.g., 0.016 nickel titanium) can be pushed into the bracket slot of a tipped and rotated tooth with a ligature director, then the cap can be gently rolled closed with finger pressure. Once the cap closes partially, the wire is trapped in the slot and need not be held while the cap is completely locked with a plugger.

In seating large rectangular wires or steel rectangular wires, the Activa seating key should be used to push the wire into the slot and hold it there, while the opposite prong of the instrument rolls the cap partially closed. The plugger end of the instrument is then used to snap the cap closed.

It is, in fact, easier to seat archwires on crowded cases with Activa than it is to seat them with tie-wing brackets. In the majority of instances even severe rotations will allow the seating of the initial wires and allow the cap to be closed.

If it is impossible (for some reason) to close the cap on any given bracket, that particular tooth can be tied to the

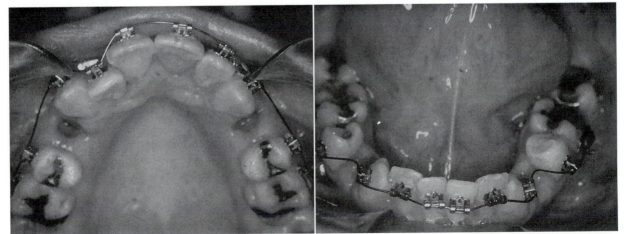

Fig. 12-19   A, Initial NiTi archwire in crowded upper arch. **B,** Initial NiTi archwire in crowded lower arch.

archwire by placing a ligature wire in the main archwire slot, closing the cap, and then tying to the archwire with a steel ligature wire; or the tooth can be tied to the main archwire with a steel ligature wire placed through the vertical slot. In other words, the orthodontist is never never at a loss to get a positive purchase on a tooth.

If a tooth is severely rotated (45° or more), a hook can be placed on a nearby tooth, a Pletcher coil positioned over the hook, and the coil can be stretched to the rotated tooth, placing the end of it in the vertical slot or hooking the end of it over the closed cap in the main archwire slot to rotate the tooth. (See Fig. 12-20, *A* through *C.*)

Each bracket has a rectangular vertical slot (0.020 inches square). Each bracket has a cap that rolls closed and snaps shut over a closing detent. An opening detent also holds the cap open; however, it is not as strong as the closing detent.

Mesial and distal undercuts are located behind each bracket's edgewise slot, allowing the use of Alastics or C-chains. However, the Alastic chains must be placed before the archwire is seated—an obvious disadvantage when using C-chains if the operator intends to change C-chains without changing the archwires. However, the appliance offers a better way to close spaces and extraction sites, as we shall see later. Therefore, Alastic chain is used on a limited basis by this operator in using this appliance (a blessing, in my opinion).

The bracket slot is the standard edgewise configuration and size and is the same length as that of a standard twin bracket. However, when the cap is closed, the bracket literally becomes a tube. This feature explains the significant reduction in friction with the appliance. Sliding mechanics will work effectively and efficiently with light forces, thus reducing the necessity of headgear wear and use of interarch elastics.

When a *series of tubes* is used around the arch (the Activa appliance is a *series of tubes* when the caps are closed), the archwire will not be seated to the base of the bracket slot until a full-sized rectangular wire is placed. For full seating, but with greater friction, an approach would be to tie through the vertical slot to the mesial and distal of each tooth around the archwire, thus making the wire *bottom out* in the bracket slot. Therefore to gain the advantage of less friction and no ligature ties, the practitioner gives up full seating until engaging the finishing wires.

Everything is a *trade-off* so to speak; that which is gained in reduction of friction must be paid for with some loss of control. When the Activa appliance is compared with a

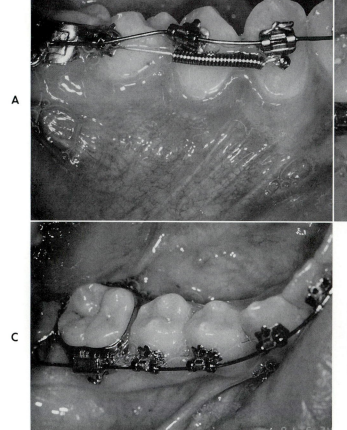

Fig. 12-20 **A,** Hook in vertical slot of canine bracket with Pletcher coil attached and placed in vertical slot of severely rotated lower second bicuspid. **B,** Occlusal view of the same situation. **C,** Rotation is corrected, and next archwire is placed 1 month later.

standard size straight wire twin bracket, loss of control is minimal, meaning a little more tipping and rotation of teeth into the extraction site may occur, unless the orthodontist *prepares* the tooth positions properly before space closure. Also some loss of torque control of upper anterior teeth may be apparent when compared with the standard twin bracket. However, certain archwires can easily compensate for loss of torque control, and that will be discussed later.

The loss of a small amount of torque, rotation, and tip control versus that of the standard twin straight wire appliance is a beneficial trade off for the great reduction in friction that the Activa appliance offers, and the reduction of friction is so dramatic that the movement of teeth can be seen in days versus weeks when compared with tie-wing brackets! However, this low friction may become a disadvantage in the finishing stages of treatment.

The ability to use the vertical slots quickly and conveniently for hooks, springs, etc. on all teeth is another plus. If hooks are not needed, they can be removed easily and the appliance is streamlined for easy hygiene care.

Patients enjoy the comfort and the esthetics of the appliance, and the archwire changes are made quickly and easily. Treatment time is reduced as well—significantly so in extraction cases.

Teeth can be grouped into *anchor units* by using an auxiliary wire through the vertical slots; or an elastic or power thread can be placed in any bracket over the archwire and the cap can be closed over the power thread or elastic to get a *brake* effect (see Fig. 12-21) so that a particular tooth or teeth will not move. *Stationary anchorage* can be created and reciprocal forces can be used with no extra-oral traction or interarch elastics.

The operator has total control over which teeth move where. In these days of reduced patient cooperation, this is a bonanza.

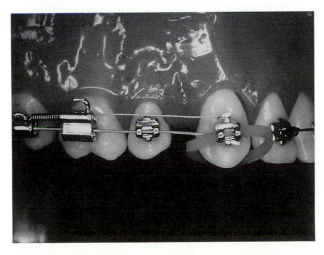

Fig. 12-21 Typodont with elastic placed in canine slot over the archwire with cap closed to immobilize the canine with the wire, while Pletcher coil moves upper posterior teeth mesially.

MECHANICS

Any mechanics that will work with edgewise brackets will work with the Activa appliance. However, the orthodontist would be well advised to take advantage of the reduced friction by using sliding mechanics.

I have spent the last 3½ years learning the most efficient ways to use Activa; I have devised a system that seems to work well. My prescription has extra-uprighting and distal rotation in the buccal segments, extra-torque of upper molars and incisors, and counter rotation built into it. The same prescription, therefore, is used on most cases.

Until a first molar Activa bracket becomes available, a lower second molar tube on the lower first molar will be used (both attachments normally have the same prescription anyway). The sliding of the archwire is enhanced by making placement easier because both attachments are the same size occlusogingivally.

The mechanics can be divided into four categories as follows:
1. Nonextraction cases
2. Maximum anchorage extraction cases
   Extreme crowding
   Extreme protrusion
3. Medium anchorage extraction cases
4. Minimum anchorage extraction cases

(See Figs. 12-22 through 12-38 for treatment sequences.)

The mechanics can be divided into the following stages:
1. Initial tooth alignment
2. Leveling and overbite correction
3. Overcorrection of torque and overbite on extraction cases
4. Extraction space closure
   Maximum retraction cases
      Start upper canines
      Start lower canines
      After complete canine retraction retract lower incisors
      Retract and intrude upper incisors
   Medium retraction cases
      Start upper canines
      Start lower canines
      After partial canine retraction
      Consolidate lower spaces
      Consolidate upper spaces and intrude upper anteriors
   Minimum retraction cases
      Align
      Use lower six anteriors to slip premolars
      Then use lower six anteriors and premolars to slip molars
      Repeat in the upper arch
5 Relevel as necessary after extraction site closure
6. Finish lower arch
7. Retract, intrude, and torque upper anteriors PRN
8. Detail

Text continued on p. 709.

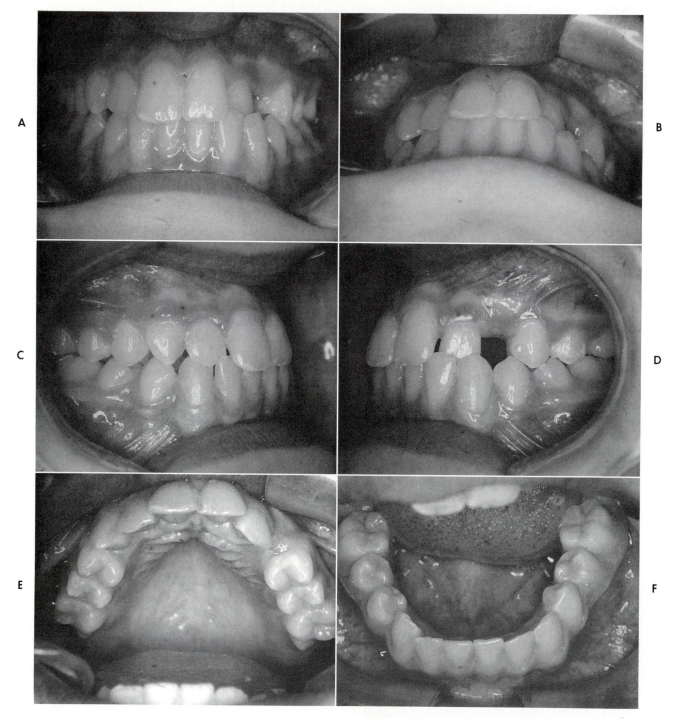

Fig. 12-22 **A,** Pretreatment nonextraction case frontal view. **B,** Overjet view. **C,** Right lateral view. **D,** Left lateral view. **E,** Upper arch. **F,** Lower arch.

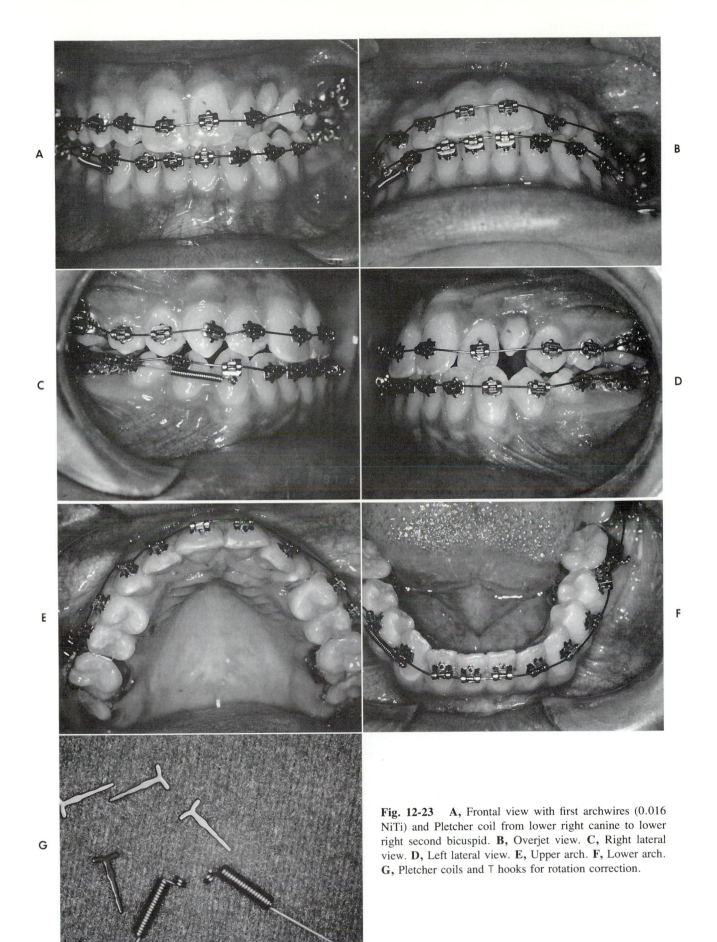

Fig. 12-23 **A,** Frontal view with first archwires (0.016 NiTi) and Pletcher coil from lower right canine to lower right second bicuspid. **B,** Overjet view. **C,** Right lateral view. **D,** Left lateral view. **E,** Upper arch. **F,** Lower arch. **G,** Pletcher coils and T hooks for rotation correction.

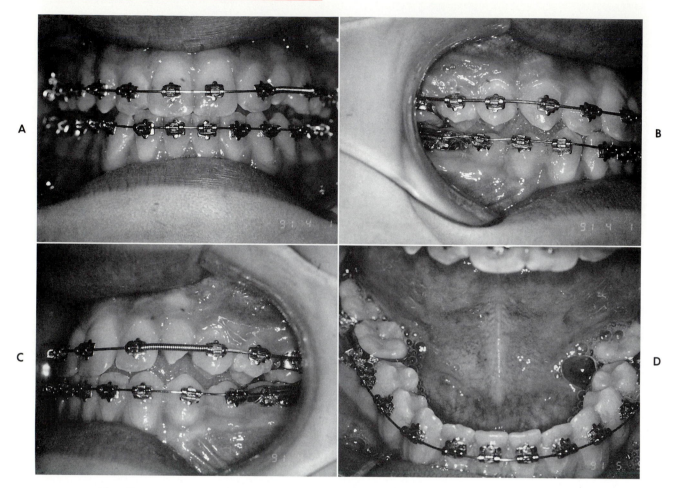

Fig. 12-24 **A,** Frontal view with 0.019 × 0.025 NiTi upper arch with compressed coil between upper left lateral and upper left first premolar. **B,** Right lateral view. **C,** Left lateral view. **D,** Lower arch with lower right second premolar bracket engaged on the archwire.

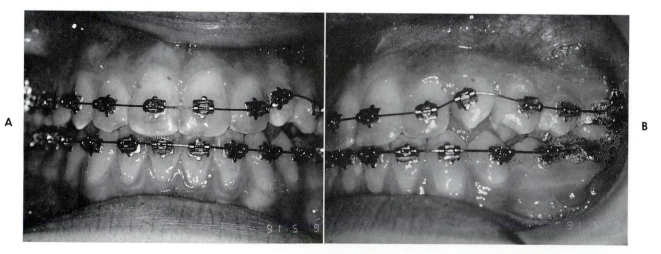

Fig. 12-25 **A,** Frontal view with upper left canine bracketed and 0.016 NiTi arch engaged. **B,** Left lateral view.

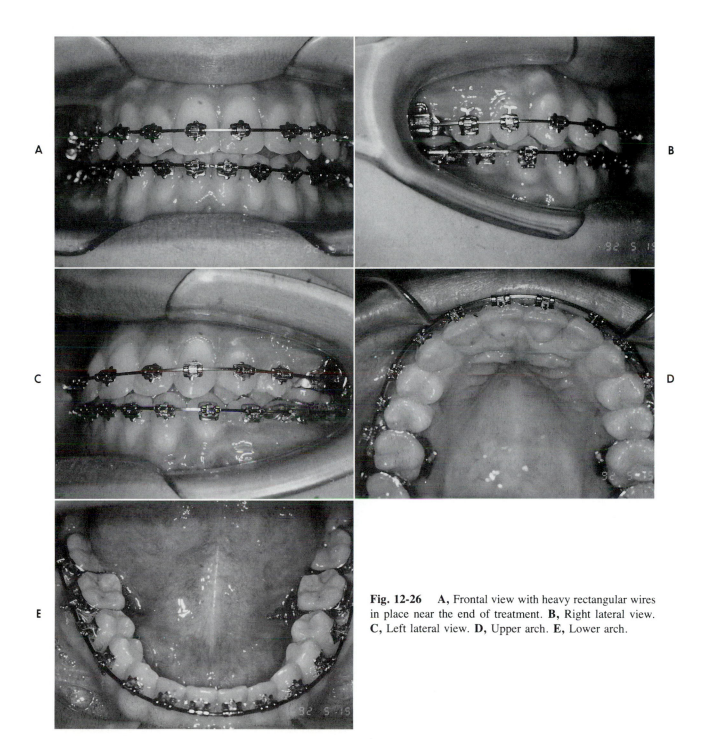

Fig. 12-26   **A,** Frontal view with heavy rectangular wires in place near the end of treatment. **B,** Right lateral view. **C,** Left lateral view. **D,** Upper arch. **E,** Lower arch.

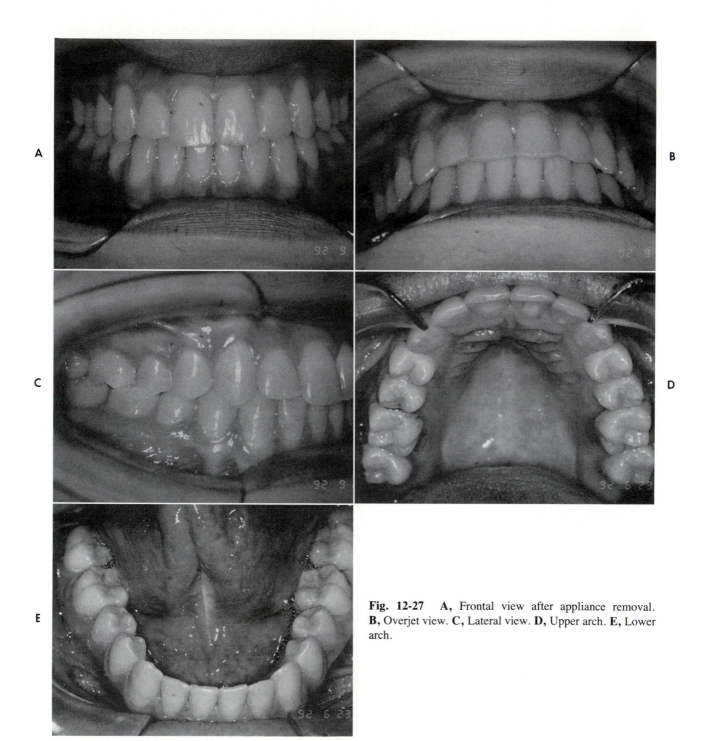

Fig. 12-27   **A,** Frontal view after appliance removal. **B,** Overjet view. **C,** Lateral view. **D,** Upper arch. **E,** Lower arch.

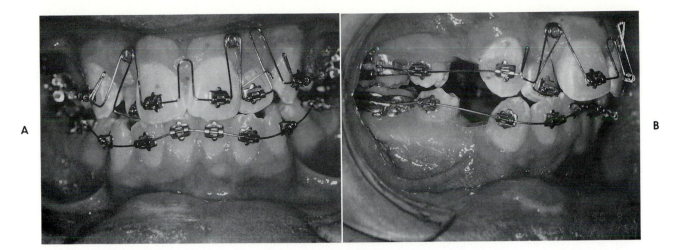

Fig. 12-28 **A,** Frontal view of maximum anchorage case, with Jarabak helical loops in upper and 0.016 NiTi in lower. Initial archwires. **B,** Lateral view, same archwires.

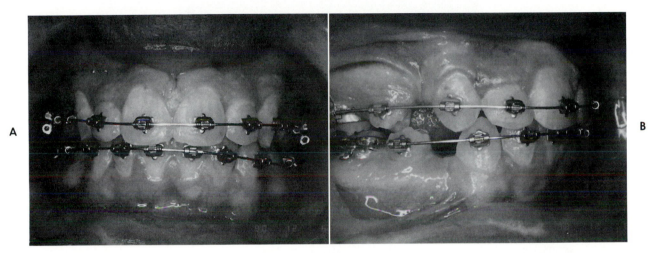

Fig. 12-29 **A,** Frontal view, 3 months later, with 0.019 × 0.025 upper and lower NiTi rectangular wire. Canines have moved back into the extraction sites. **B,** Lateral view, same archwires.

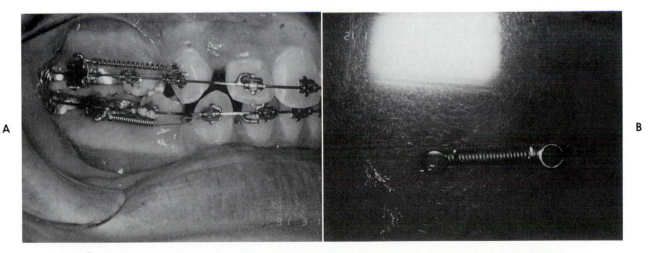

Fig. 12-30 **A,** Lateral view of same case, with upper Wonder Wire of 0.021 × 0.025 in the anterior and 0.018 posteriorly; lower 0.019 × 0.025 posted hook arch, elastic in the lower premolar bracket to guard lower anchorage; *double ringed* 9 mm nickel titanium coil to the upper canine; a Pletcher coil to the lower canine for retraction. There are twin transpalatal bars to the upper first and second molars to hold upper anchorage. **B,** Close up of the "double ringed" nickel titanium 9 mm coil.

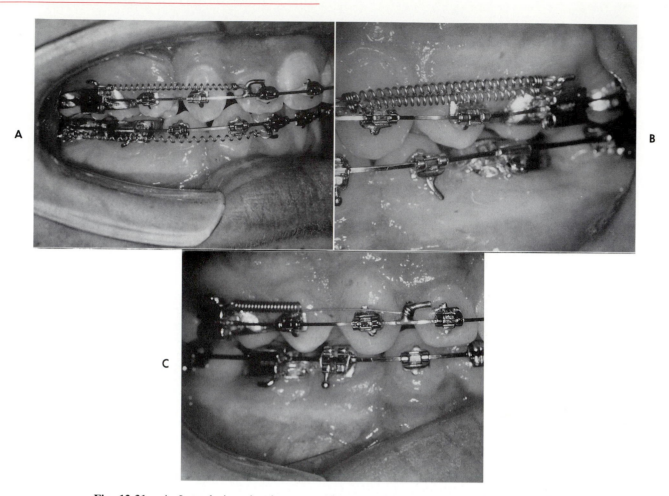

Fig. 12-31 **A,** Lateral view showing upper 15 mm and lower 12 mm nickel titanium coils to posted hook arches to retract the incisors. **B,** Doubled nickel titanium coils (9 mm) for upper incisor retraction. **C,** Pletcher coil to posted hook for incisor retraction.

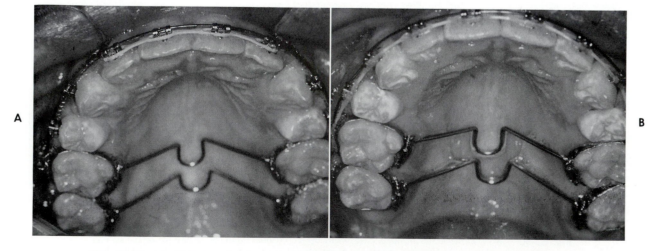

Fig. 12-32 **A,** Upper occlusal view, showing twin transpalatal bars to hold upper anchorage while upper anteriors are retracted with 15 mm nickel titanium coils. (Note incisor spacing is held with Alastic C-chain.) **B,** Spaces are now closed, and C-chain is being used around the arch with a nickel titanium archwire, until a large rectangular steel wire can be placed and cinched back.

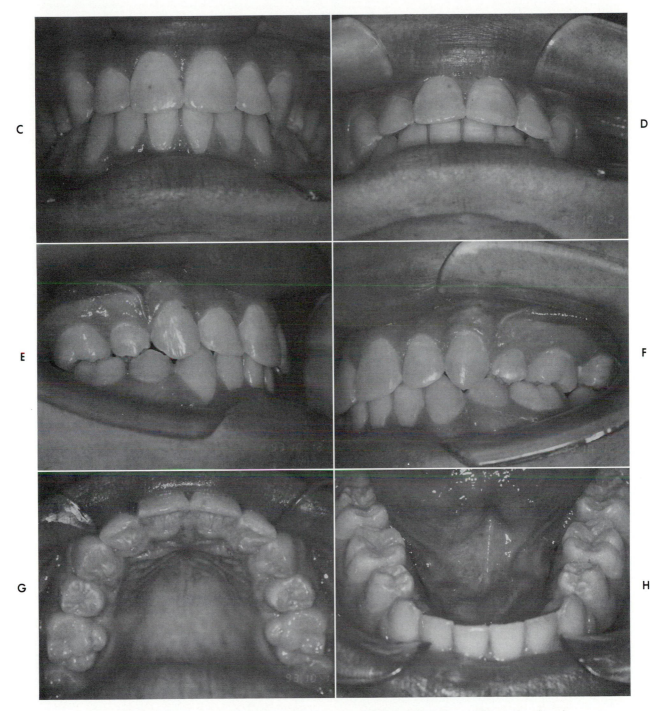

Fig. 12-32, cont'd   C through **H,** Finished case as finished with Activa appliance showing six intra-oral views.

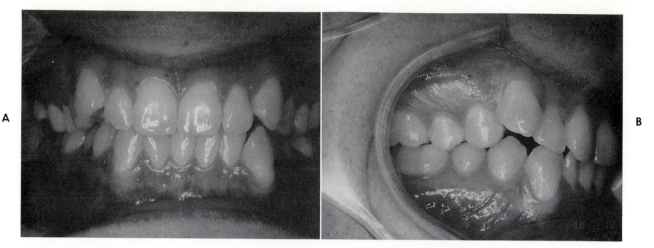

Fig. 12-33 **A,** Frontal view of minimum anchorage extraction case. **B,** Lateral view of same case.

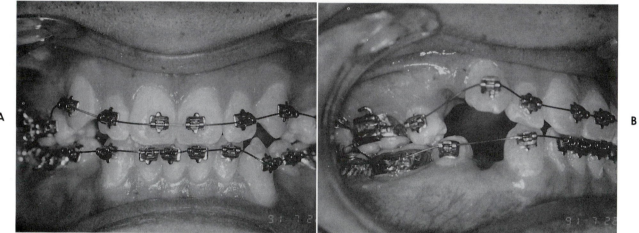

Fig. 12-34 **A,** Frontal view, after extractions and placement of appliances and first 0.016 NiTi archwires. **B,** Lateral view, same time.

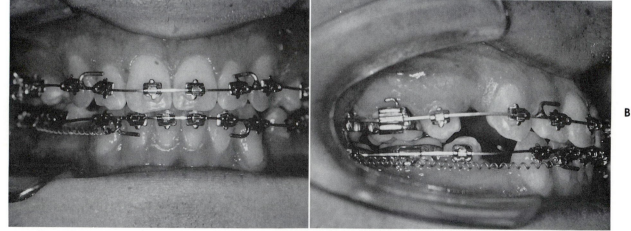

Fig. 12-35 **A,** Frontal view, several months later, after case has been leveled to 0.019 × 0.025 steel-posted hook archwires. **B,** Lateral view, showing 12 mm nickel titanium, double ringed coil in place to slip anchorage.

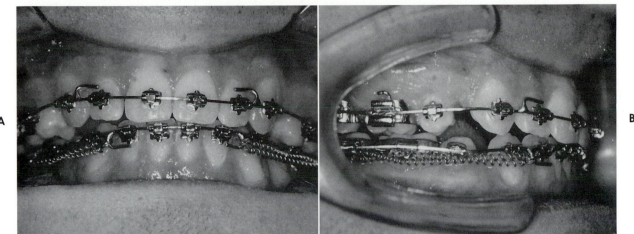

Fig. 12-36   A, Frontal view, showing double nickel titanium coils used to close remaining lower space. **B,** Lateral view, same appointment. Note how much upper space has closed without closing mechanics to the upper arch. There is so little friction that the upper anteriors retract to the lowers with lip pressure, and the upper posteriors move forward as the lower posteriors move forward.

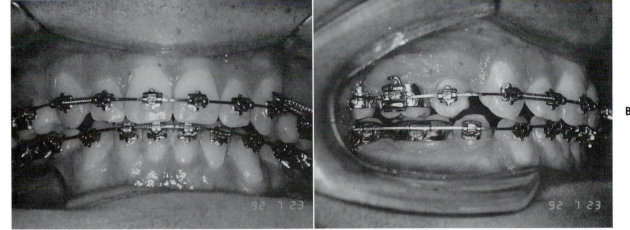

Fig. 12-37   A, Frontal view, showing coils being used to center the upper midline. **B,** Lateral view, showing lower arch closed; the remaining space can be closed with some loss of upper anchorage.

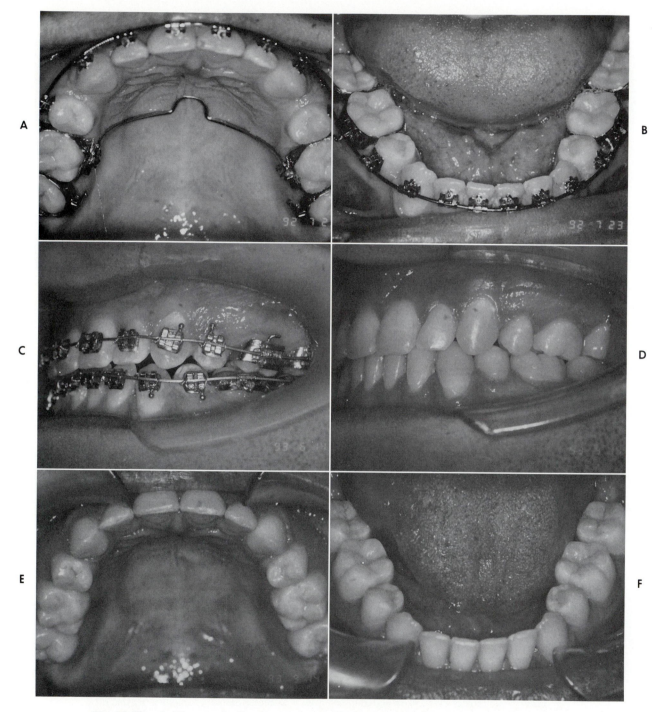

Fig. 12-38 **A,** Upper arch, showing transpalatal bar used to guard upper anchorage during space closure. **B,** Lower arch, with space closed ready to go into larger rectangular steel wire for detailing and final archform. **C-F,** Same case switched to standard size twin straight wire brackets with 0.019 × 0.025 nickel titanium wires in place and the finished result.

NONEXTRACTION

The nonextraction case requires relatively simple mechanics. Correction usually requires leveling of the curve of Spee and retraction of the upper incisors and/or torque of the upper incisors. True Class II correction must be accomplished orthopedically or surgically if there is a true skeletal discrepancy. In many cases, however, the Class II molar relation (if dentoalveolar in nature) will be corrected by distal rotation of upper first molars and/or loss of anchorage in the lower arch.

1. Bracket engagement and alignment are initially done with light nickel titanium wires such as 0.016 or 0.014. Usually I will use the largest gauge nickel titanium that can be placed comfortably for the patient.

2. As the teeth align, bracket positioning is checked and brackets are reset as needed when the patient presents for wire changes.

3. Severe rotations, where the wire cannot be engaged in the bracket slot, are handled with Pletcher coils, until the wire can be engaged in the slot. This is necessary only on rare occasions and usually where there is a severe distal rotation of a second bicuspid. Most other rotations will allow placement of the wire into the bracket slot and closing of the cap.

4. Once the brackets are aligned, then heavier wires are used, such as 0.019 × 0.025 nickel titanium and then 0.019 × 0.025 stainless steel.

5. Spaces in the lower arch can be consolidated using a posted hook, 0.019 × 0.025 heat-treated blue elgiloy wire with reverse curve of Spee with 12 or 15 mm nickel titanium coils that are attached from the hooks on the lower second molars to the posted hooks on the archwires.

6. Depending on the situation the upper arch could be a 0.021 × 0.025 × 0.018 wonder wire with 0°, 5°, 10°, 15°, or 20° torque; or it could be 0.019 × 0.025 posted hook arch of heat-treated blue elgiloy, with compensating curve.

7. The lower arch can then be leveled to 0.021 × 0.025 stainless steel archwire by first going to nickel titanium of that size and/or TMA of that size.

8. Once into a 0.021 × 0.025 stainless steel archwire in the lower arch, the curve of Spee should be level. At this time bracket placement should be carefully checked for details of positioning and any brackets that need to be reset should be done; a 0.021 × 0.025 nickel titanium wire should be placed, until the following appointment, when steel wire can be placed once again.

9. Short Class II elastics can be used to an upper arch, as previously described, or transpalatal bars can be used to the upper first and/or second molars (for anchorage), and nickel titanium springs from the upper molars to the posted hooks can be used to retract the upper anteriors.

10. After retraction and space closure in the upper arch, a 0.021 × 0.025 nickel titanium wire can be placed. Before the same size steel wire is placed, check bracket positions for details, and reset as necessary.

11. Next, 0.022 × 0.028 super elastic NiTi wires are placed for full bracket expression and correction of any minor rotations. These can be followed by stainless steel of the same size as needed.

12. Final archwires can be 0.022 × 0.028 super elastic NiTi, or wires of smaller dimension can be used to allow optimum settling to occlusal intercuspation.

MAXIMUM ANCHORAGE EXTRACTION CASES WITH SEVERE CROWDING

1. The same steps are followed as in the initial steps of nonextraction treatment. Usually, by the time alignment of brackets is attained, little space remains.

2. Space closure can then be done on 0.019 × 0.025 posted-hook arches of blue elgiloy, with reverse and compensating curves and 12 or 15 mm nickel titanium coils from the molars to the posted hooks, or with J-hook headgear as necessary.

3. The sequence would be to close the lower spaces first and then the upper ones, using elastic, nickel titanium coils, or J-hook headgear as necessary.

4. Finishing, after all space closure, would follow the steps as previously outlined to obtain full bracket engagement thus allowing the *straight wire* features engineered into the brackets to detail the tooth positions.

MAXIMUM ANCHORAGE EXTRACTION CASES WITH EXTREME PROTRUSION

In a maximum anchorage situation, retraction of the anterior teeth distally through the extraction sites is the goal. Of course, the retraction of the anterior teeth could be accomplished with J-hook headgear. However, it is more desirable to retract the anterior teeth without headgear if possible. The elimination of extra-oral traction can be accomplished as follows, while maintaining the posterior anchorage.

1. Align as described above.

2. After 0.019 × 0.025 nickel titanium wires, go to heat treated blue elgiloy 0.019 × 0.025 posted hook archwires, with reverse and compensating curves. These are placed and cinched back distal of the second molars. Power thread is placed in the second premolar brackets over the archwire and the bracket cap is closed; creating a frictional stop that does not allow the posterior teeth to move forward, much like a brake pad on an automobile. T hooks are placed in the canine vertical slots, and transpalatal arches are placed on the upper first and/or second molars for anchorage control. Nickel titanium springs (9 mm) are then used to start retracting the upper canines.

3. Once the canines are in Class I, springs can be hooked to the lower canines, and they can start to be moved distally.

4. Once all the canines have been retracted, the hooks can be removed from the canines and the elastics can be removed from the premolar slots; 12 or 15 mm coils can be used from the second molars to the posted hooks on the lower arch.

5. Once the space is closed in the lower arch, the lower wire can be increased in size to 0.021 × 0.025 nickel titanium, TMA or steel in that progression until the curve of Spee has been adequately leveled.

6. At this point the upper anteriors can be retracted, using coils from the upper molars to the posted hooks with transpalatal bars as anchorage.

7. After all space is closed, finishing can proceed as described under nonextraction treatment.

MEDIUM ANCHORAGE EXTRACTION CASES

The mechanics, again, are the same initially until the 0.019 × 0.025 heat treated blue elgiloy posted hook archwires are in place. At that point, instead of individually retracting canines, go to 12 or 15 mm coils from the molars to the posted hooks, and do not retract canines separately. Close all spaces, and then level to 0.021 × 0.025 stainless steel. Close the upper space using the same method. Remove palatal bars when you wish to slip anchorage.

MINIMUM ANCHORAGE EXTRACTION CASES

Initially the minimum anchorage extraction case is handled as are the others. However, instead of progressing to 0.019 × 0.025 heat treated blue elgiloy wires, the practi-

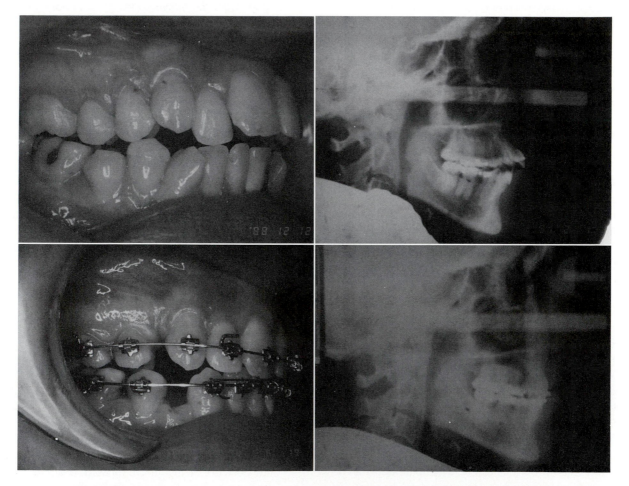

Fig. 12-39 Lateral intra-oral views and accompanying cephalometric headfilms showing only lip retraction of anterior teeth with no closing mechanics applied.

tioner would go to upper and lower heat treated wonder wire with posted hooks and some reverse and compensating curve. These wires would have labial crown torque in the anterior section as necessary (up to 20°). The anteriors would be held together with a *piggyback* sectional 0.020 steel segment going through the vertical slots from canine to canine; there would be power thread in the bracket slots of all four canines. Coils of 9 mm would be used to first bring the premolars forward and then the molars. Finishing would then proceed as described in the nonextraction sequence.

Summary

If the orthodontist uses these descriptions as guidelines, it will be easy to improvise along these lines to fit any given situation. The idea here is to use fairly simple mechanics that have a broad range of applicability and to use the engineering of the appliance to control anchorage as needed, without resorting to extra-oral traction. The appliance succeeds rapidly if the mechanics outlined are followed in principle.

In some instances, because of the reduced friction of the appliance, the patient's lips will literally retract the anterior teeth, while they align and level as shown in the accompanying example.

The Activa appliance is easy to use, incorporating the benefits of reduced treatment time, reduce chairtime, and in most instances eliminating or minimizing extra-oral traction and inter-arch elastics.

Although the clinician routinely can achieve a good result with the appliance (Fig. 12-32, *C* through *H*), the most precise result may be more difficult and take longer to attain in the finishing stages of treatment than it does with the standard size twin straight wire brackets. This is particularly true in extraction cases.

As a result, after struggling for a couple of years with extraction case finishing with Activa, I started rebracketing the extraction cases from second premolar to second premolar, upper and lower, with the Roth Rx in the standard size twin straight wire appliance. I found I could finish the cases as desired in much less time (2 to 3 months) just by ligature tying large NiTi wires in on the day of re-bracketing and then going to large steel wires, followed by 0.025 multistrand braided rectangular finishing wires. (See Fig. 12-38, *C* through *F*.)

Using the Activa brackets for most of the tooth movement and then switching the brackets to do the fine finishing is worth the effort because of the following:

1. Reset the brackets to attain the finish on all cases, rather than bending offsets in the wire to overcome incorrect bracket positions.
2. The mechanics and time-saving features of Activa (both chairtime and treatment time) for gross tooth movement is still reduced significantly over tie brackets. This is probably kinder to the tissues.
3. The change-over of the appliance is simple to work into the routine and does not require more than 30 minutes.

Perhaps the changes that will be coming from the manufacturer will make the change-over of the appliance unnecessary in the future, but even if it doesn't, the reduced treatment time, reduced chairtime, and less demand for cooperation may be worth it. At the present time, this aspect of the appliance system is still under consideration.

REFERENCES

1. Activa Premier Club Bulletin, 2:2 A Company, San Diego, Calif, 1992.
2. Andrews LF: *Straight wire: the concept and appliance*, San Diego, CA, 1989, LA Wells.
3. Andrews LF: The six keys to normal occlusion, *Am J Orthod* 63:296, 1972.
4. Kumar P: Thesis. University of Detroit, 1991.
5. Pletcher E: Mechanics with the Activa appliance. Personal communication, 1993.
6. Roth RH: The straight wire appliance 17 years later, *J Clin Orthod* 21:9, 1987.
7. Roth RH: Five year clinical evaluation of the Andrews straight wire appliance, *J Clin Orthod* 10:836, 1976.

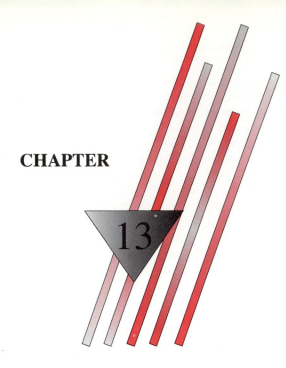

CHAPTER 13

Periodontal/Orthodontic Interrelationships

ROBERT L. VANARSDALL

No matter how talented the orthodontist, a magnificent orthodontic correction can be destroyed by failure to recognize periodontal susceptibility (Fig. 13-1, A through I). The short- and long-term successful outcome of orthodontic treatment is influenced by the patient's periodontal status before, during, and after active orthodontic therapy. The long-term prognosis of the natural dentition depends to a significant extent upon optimal responses and systemic resistance or predisposition of the patient to different clinical forms of periodontal diseases. Periodontal pathogenesis is a multifactorial etiologic process, and the orthodontist must recognize the clinical forms of inflammatory periodontal diseases. At the 1989 World Workshop in Clinical Periodontics a classification of the various types of periodontal infections was established (microbial combinations) even though there are still difficulties in distinguishing them by their clinical features.[34]

Types of Inflammatory Diseases

Gingivitis—the reversible lesion. Allowing microorganisms to accumulate around teeth can cause gingival redness, bleeding and edema, changes in gingival morphology, reduced tissue adaptation to the teeth, increased flow of gingival crevicular fluid, and other clinical signs of inflammation.[11,17] Obviously, mechanical plaque removal can reduce chronic gingivitis, but many orthodontic patients, young and older, may not be motivated to remove the plaque; therefore plaque removal must be done by the referring office or with other professional removal, with scaling and thorough tooth cleaning during orthodontic treatment. Removal of supragingival bacteria has been shown to have an effect on the formation of subgingival plaque; therefore antibiotic rinses for specific problem patients

(mouthbreathing, medication-influenced gingival overgrowth,[37] hormone-influenced gingivitis, etc.) are recommended. One of the most effective antiplaque, antigingivitis agents has been chlorhexidine digluconate; however, the side effects of reversible staining, tissue response, and taste alterations must be monitored. Exaggerated gingival overgrowth and responses to plaque have been reported with hormonal changes in pregnancy, with puberty, during the menstural cycle, and in response to steroid therapy and birth control medications.[49]

Gingivitis (without attachment loss) has been classified according to initial, early, and established stages. The initial lesion occurs in 1 to 2 days after plaque is allowed to remain on teeth, while the established lesion occurs weeks later, when inflammation has advanced to proliferation of epithelium into the connective tissue. Only the established lesion can be observed as clinical gingivitis. The important point is that alveolar bone loss has not as yet occurred and hopefully the lesion can be prevented from spreading into the supporting tissues for an extended period. Therefore, it is critical to establish the appropriate plaque control interval for the orthodontic patient that will prevent destructive alveolar bone loss. Pseudo-pockets or gingival overgrowth/enlargement (e.g., with phenytoin, cyclosporin) of the gingival margin and papilla, be it drug induced or primarily plaque related, is exacerbated by poor oral hygiene. Constant professional reinforcement is necessary.

Periodontitis—the irreversible or destructive lesion. Though gingival inflammation may be a prerequisite, the actual mechanisms responsible for conversion of gingivitis to periodontitis are still being debated.[47] All forms of periodontitis exhibit loss of connective tissue attachment and usually gingival inflammation. The episodic burst type of

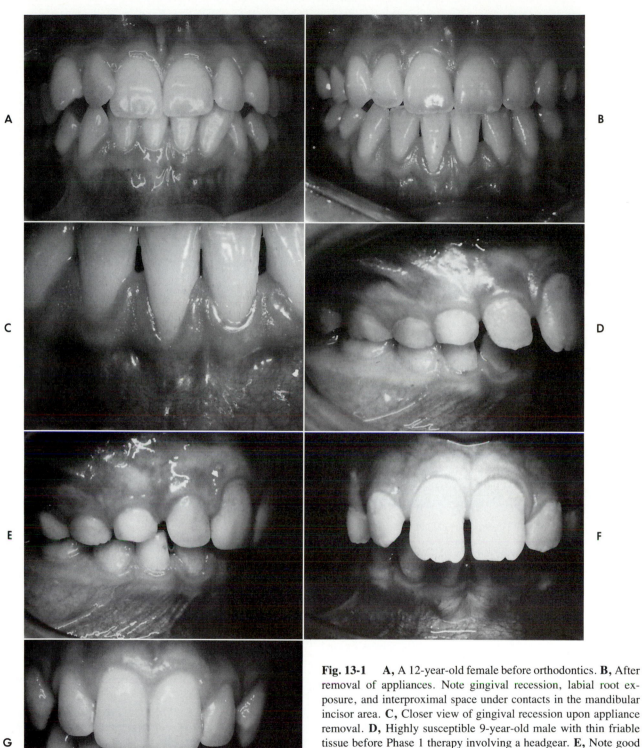

Fig. 13-1 **A,** A 12-year-old female before orthodontics. **B,** After removal of appliances. Note gingival recession, labial root exposure, and interproximal space under contacts in the mandibular incisor area. **C,** Closer view of gingival recession upon appliance removal. **D,** Highly susceptible 9-year-old male with thin friable tissue before Phase 1 therapy involving a headgear. **E,** Note good cooperation resulting in distalization of the maxillary dentition. **F,** Anterior view before placement of orthodontic appliances. **G,** Anterior view at the end of Phase 1. Excessive exposure of the anatomical crowns and beginning root exposure on all lower anterior teeth.

Continued.

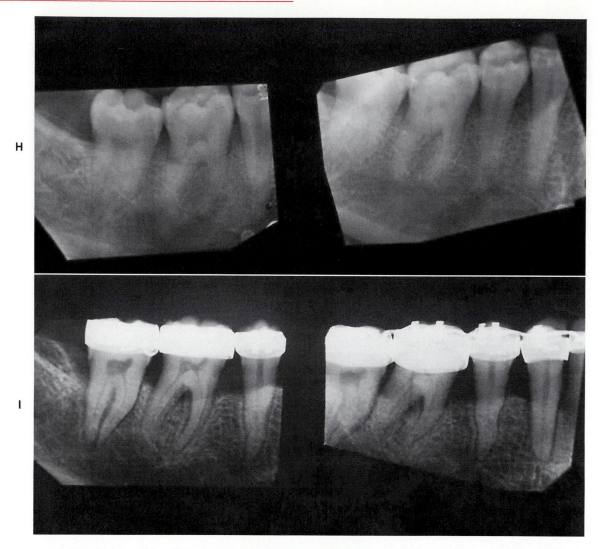

Fig. 13-1, cont'd **H,** Preorthodontic periapical radiographs of an adult female before placement of orthodontic appliances. **I,** Several months later progress films are taken because of excessive tooth mobility. Observe radiographic evidence of accelerated bone loss.

disease usually progresses in short intervals with significant attachment loss being followed by periodic remission and an indefinite period of inactivity.[48]

Adult periodontitis is the most common form of periodontitis, and studies in the United States show that about 50% of 18- to 19-year-old individuals exhibit at least one site with 2 mm or more of attachment loss.[32] Prevalence increases to about 80% for those who are 35 to 39 years of age, 87% for persons who are 45 to 49 years, and exceeds 90% for subjects who are 60 years and older. Organisms most frequently reported that have been associated with adult periodontitis are *Porphyromonas gingivalis, Prevotella intermedia,* and *Bacteroides forsythus;* these organisms can be tested for rather easily.

Prepubertal periodontitis is a rare form that appears soon after eruption of the primary teeth and is characterized by severe gingival inflammation, rapid bone resorption, and possibly tooth loss.[50] This disease can present as a localized condition that affects only several primary teeth or as a more generalized form that affects both the primary and permanent dentition.

Localized and generalized juvenile (early-onset) periodontitis arises in the circumpubertal period.[4] Localized juvenile periodontitis has a familial tendency and exhibits severe, rapidly progressing alveolar bone loss affecting primarily the permanent first molars and incisors.[8] These patients (even though they have significant disease) form little dental plaque and calculus and may respond well to local debridement supplemented with tetracycline or appropriate antibiotic therapy. The generalized juvenile periodontitis (sometimes called rapidly progressive periodontitis) is considered a problem of young adults; but it may begin at or around puberty. Here marked gingival inflammation may be present, with heavy accumulations of plaque and calculus seen around many teeth. Most periodontists use mechanical debridement in conjunction with antibiotic therapy to resolve the infection.

Rapidly progressive periodontitis is seen in young adults and the cause and pathogenesis appears to share many of the features of generalized juvenile periodontitis, such as rapid loss of bone and, in some subjects, depressed neutrophil functions.[36]

Refractory periodontitis is a disease classification used to define sites in patients who continue to be infected with periodontal pathogens and who experience a high rate of attachment and tooth loss, despite intensive periodontal treatment to prevent bone loss. Any periodontal patient can undergo changes that affect host defenses, or systemic disease may cause a lesion or sites to become recalcitrant. It may be more important to emphasize the category *refractory,* since any of the periodontal diseases can become refractory. This is the category in which orthodontic patients who have individual sites with recurrent inflammatory episodes are usually classified.

Periodontitis can also be *associated with systemic diseases* such as diabetes mellitus, cyclic neutropenia, Down's syndrome, Papillon–Lefevre syndrome, inflammatory bowel disease, Addison's disease, and combined and acquired immunodeficiency diseases.[22]

In general it should be recognized that children can develop severe forms of periodontitis but at much less prevalence of destruction than in adults. Severe bone loss in a child or adolescent might also be an early sign of systemic disease and thereby may indicate the need for a medical evaluation.

As is described in Chapter 14 on "Adult Orthodontics: Diagnosis and Treatment," the orthodontic patient may be at greater risk of attachment loss once teeth have become mobile because of tooth movement (Fig. 13-1, *H* and *I*). The clinical signs of inflammation and tooth mobility must be recognized and controlled during treatment to prevent extensive bone loss. Periodic monitoring of the periodontal status with probing, microbiologic assessment by immunologic assays, DNA probes, and culturing, as well as clinical findings are useful in determining scaling intervals and in detecting potential sites of increased risk of attachment loss. These methods may be used to assess the endpoint of the effectiveness of scaling and root planing before orthodontic treatment to insure that no putative pathogens remain. Genetic studies offer potential to identify high-risk individuals, such as family members of localized juvenile periodontitis patients with neutrophil chemotactic abnormalities, who are 10 times more likely to develop periodontal disease than most family members.

High-risk factors. An assessment must be made on an individual patient basis to determine if periodontal factors exist that may place the patient at greater risk than normal for developing periodontal disease during orthodontic ther-

apy. The clinician must identify the susceptible patient and develop strategies to prevent loss of attachment and gingival recession.

Significant past dental history could be unsuccessful orthodontic treatment at an earlier age. In addition, the patient who has had a history of previous periodontitis will obviously be more susceptible to the disease process. Although it is difficult to predict which sites may progress from gingival inflammation to periodontitis, the group with previous disease is more vulnerable to further bone loss. In fact it has been reported that for individuals who have shown a history of previous bone loss, gingivitis may be a greater threat to further bone loss.[27] No one should begin orthodontics with active destructive sites, and a person who has had periodontal disease previously should be more closely monitored to prevent development of new bursts of active sites that may result in rapid bone loss. A small percentage of adolescents (10%) and a much larger group of susceptible adults (50%) must be treated differently. Other risk factors include gingival bleeding upon probing, tooth mobility and thin, friable gingival tissue. Each of these factors are discussed in Chapter 14. In addition, tobacco use and diabetes have been shown to be risk factors for a higher prevalence of periodontal disease.[14a,17a]

A risk marker would be a characteristic that would identify patients who are likely to have periodontal disease. In this regard the transverse skeletal pattern may be the most critical evaluation when assessing the potential for facial gingival recession. In a study on patients from two private orthodontic practices conducted at the University of Pennsylvania, 55 patients (ages 8 to 13 at the time of treatment with a Haas expander) were recalled 8 to 10 years after rapid palatal expansion (consisting of 10 to 10.5 mm of expansion over a 3 week period) and compared with 30 control patients (matched for age) from the same practices, who were evaluated for stability and clinical crown height after edgewise nonexpansion.[58] The patients were assessed from models, kodachrome slides, P/A cephalograms before treatment and at the end of orthodontic treatment; they were recalled 10 years later for examination and new records. Results indicated that of the expanded cases, although extremely stable, (Fig. 13-2, *A* and *B*), 20% exhibited unusual facial gingival recession on one or more teeth as opposed to only 6% gingival recession in the nonexpanded control patients (Fig. 13-3). Skeletally, 9 of the 11 patients, who had undergone expansion and experienced facial gingival recession, had maxilla transverse deficiency along with mandibular transverse excess and the other 2 patients had excessively large mandibles (Fig. 13-4, *A* through *I*). Therefore, in the adolescent patient who has a small maxilla and a large mandible, there is potential to move teeth beyond the *envelope of the alveolar process* and predispose a patient to gingival recession. The *envelope of discrepancy* for the transverse dimension is much more critical from a stability and periodontal standpoint (see Chapter 14). Untreated susceptible adults with significant transverse skeletal discrep-

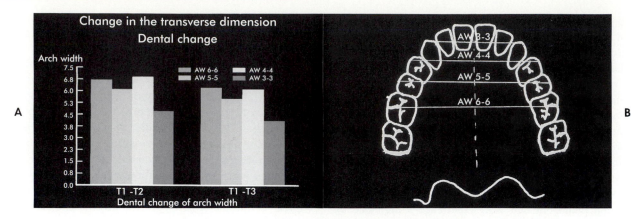

Fig. 13-2 **A,** The histogram of maxillary dental change, with rapid palatal expansion from T_1 (before expansion) until T_2 (at the completion of expansion). The second group of bars represents the expansion that was maintained until T_3 (the final time period 10 years after expansion). **B,** Diagram to illustrate how maxillary arch dental width was measured with electronic digital calipers for each tooth in the 55 expanded cases.

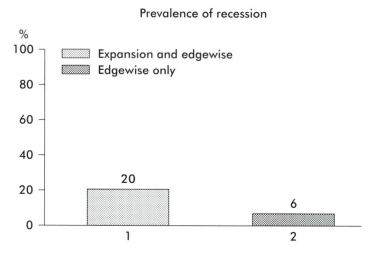

Fig. 13-3 Twenty percent (11 out of 55) of the expanded cases experienced gingival recession, as compared with only 6% in the edgewise-only treatment group. The hypothesis that recession is evenly distributed across expanded and edgewise groups was rejected (p value 0.0025).

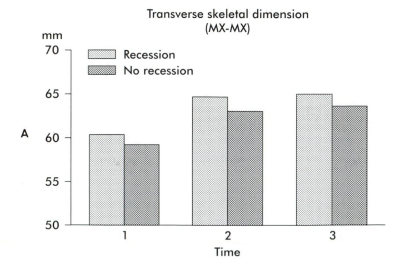

Fig. 13-4 **A,** From the histogram, observe that all of the 55 expanded patients at T_1 had a maxillare (MX to MX) transpalatal dimension of approximately 60 mm (deficient) and were expanded at the bony base 4 to 5 mm at T_2 and at T_3 (final time period). The basal skeletal increase remained stable and only increased with time 0.33 mm. There was little difference in the maxillary skeletal dimension for the (11 [dark screen]) patients who experienced recession and the patients (44 [lighter screen]) that did *not* experience recession. The relationship between maxillary and mandibular widths was critical to evaluate, and this proportional evaluation identified the 11 individuals with problems.

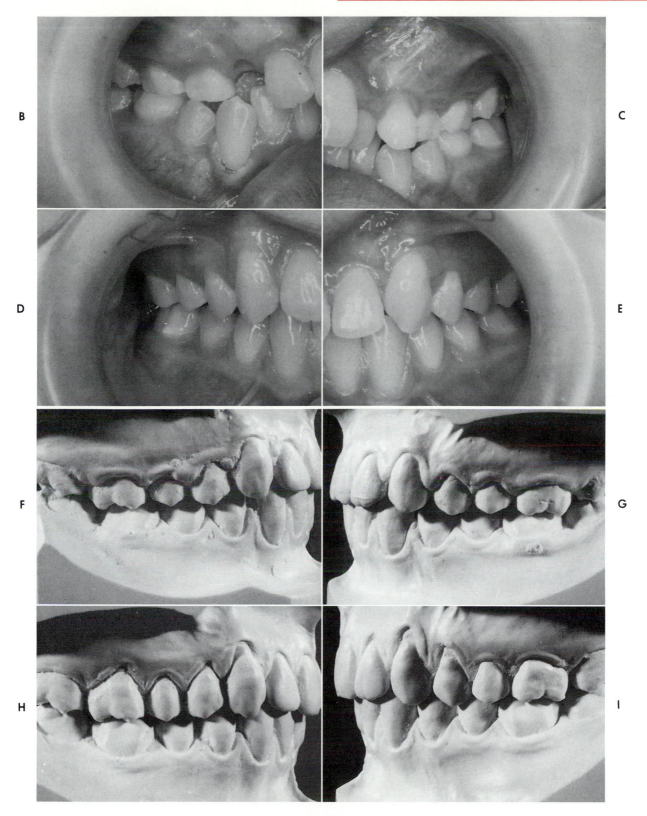

Fig. 13-4, cont'd   **B** and **C,** Buccal views of a 9.4-year-old, Class I, division 1, female with a 9 mm narrow maxilla and an excessive mandible in the transverse dimension. **D** and **E,** Observe buccal segments after completion of treatment. **F** and **G,** Models taken at the time of appliance removal. **H** and **I,** Models; 10.8 years after completion of treatment. Note gingival recession in maxillary buccal segments observed years after the patient is out of appliances.

ancy exhibit advanced stages of destructive periodontal disease. Hundreds of adult orthodontic retreatment patients have been given excellent stability following surgically assisted rapid palatal expansion to correct transverse skeletal discrepancy. Growth in the transverse dimension is severely slowed by 15 years and has been reported to be essentially completed.[5,7] Therefore, early orthodontic treatment in the deciduous or early mixed dentition is ideal to correct transverse skeletal abnormalities orthopedically, while growth is significantly active and palatal separation is most effective. It has been well established that expansion of buccal segments with fixed appliances has limitations and will tend to be unstable, regressing toward pretreatment widths.[40] Orthopedic expansion of the palate has been studied with the use of implants. This study confirmed 50% dental movement and 50% skeletal movement in young children. In adolescents, however, only 35% movement was skeletal and 65% of the movement was dental.[20] Therefore as the young patient becomes older, there is greater dental tipping, which,

as we have previously reported, places teeth at higher risk for gingival recession (Fig. 13-5, A and B). Lindhe has stated that when, "during orthodontic treatment a tooth is moved through the envelope of the alveolar process . . . at sites with thin and inflamed gingiva," there is "a risk that gingival recession may occur."[24] The labial plate of bone in the maxilla is extremely thin on the facial surfaces of the teeth (Fig. 13-6, A). The buccal plate in the mandible is thin in the coronal thirds from the first molar area, moving anteriorly, and is considerably thinner in the premolar/incisor areas (Fig. 13-6, B and C). Facial movement of the teeth into thin tissues has been tested in monkeys. Extensive bodily movement of incisors in a labial direction through the alveolar bone (Fig. 13-7, A and B) resulted in small apical displacement of the gingival margin, which appeared to be thinned by the tooth movement, and the alveolar bone height was reduced.[64] Therefore less tooth movement and greater orthopedic changes in the transverse could be obtained by a surgical adjunct, which has not been shown to

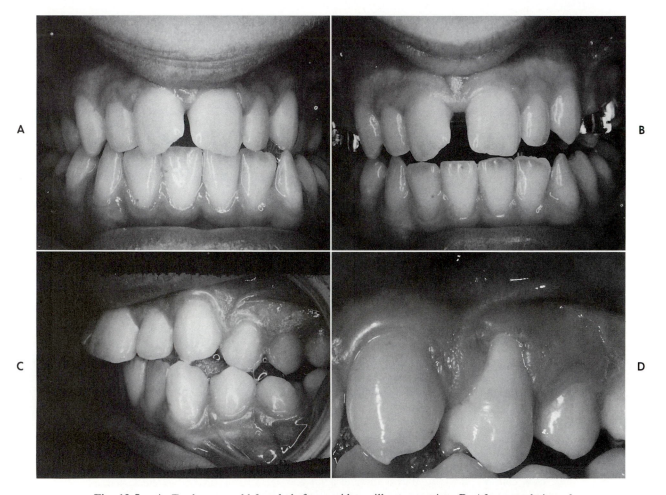

Fig. 13-5   **A,** Twelve-year-old female before rapid maxillary expansion. **B,** After completion of active expansion. Observe mid-line diastema and tissue level on the left first premolar. **C,** Note tissue level on the maxillary left first premolar before expansion. **D,** Several weeks post-expansion. Observe 3 to 4 mm of recession on the first premolar that has been reported as an initial complication with RPE treatment.

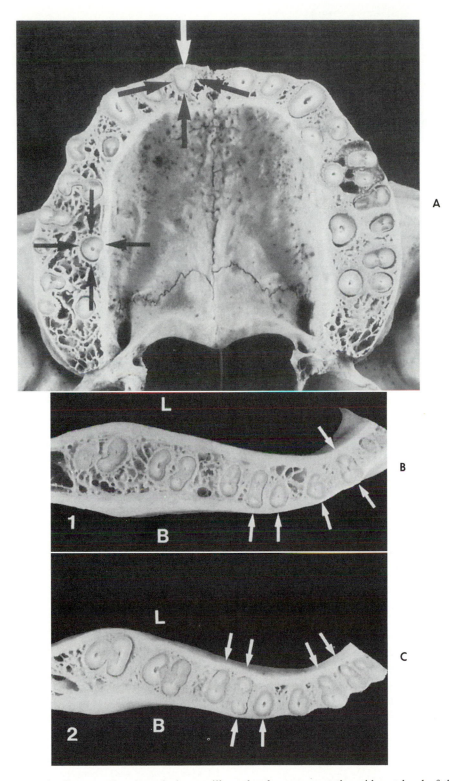

Fig. 13-6   **A,** Cross section through the maxillary alveolar process at the mid-root level of the teeth. This illustration exemplifies how extremely thin the buccal bone is in the maxillary arch. **B,** Cross sections through the mandibular alveolar process at the coronal and the apical thirds of the roots. The art illustrates the thin labial bone on the mandibular teeth in the crestal two-thirds. (From Lindhe J: *Textbook of clinical periodontology,* Copenhagen, 1989, Munksgaard.) **C,** Note thin facial bone over the sockets from which the maxillary teeth were removed.

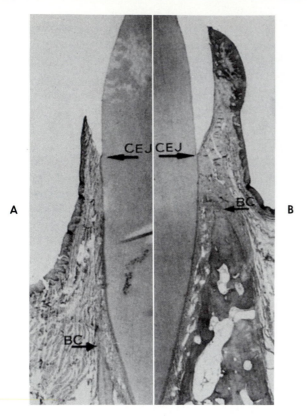

Fig. 13-7 **A** and **B**, Histologic specimens demonstrating *(A)* reduced alveolar bone height *(BC*—bone crest) at an incisor that has been bodily moved in a labial direction, and *(B)* normal alveolar bone height at an unmoved control tooth. Observe that the connective tissue attachment has been maintained; however, there has been a reduced height of the free gingival tissue on the labially displaced incisor *(A)*. (From Lindhe J: *Textbook of clinical periodontology,* Copenhagen, 1989, Munksgaard.)

create the adverse gingival changes seen with orthopedic expansion in severe skeletal transverse maxillary deficiency problems. The decision to use a surgical adjunct is based upon comparing the maxillomandibular proportions to individual normal variations. Correction of the transverse skeletal discrepancy is accomplished (1) to prevent periodontal problems; (2) for greater dental/skeletal stability (Fig. 13-8, *A* through *C*) found in adult retreatment cases; and (3) for improved dentofacial esthetics by eliminating or improving lateral *negative space,* which accompanies maxillary transverse deficiency (Fig. 13-8, *D* through *H*).

Tissue Response to Certain Types of Tooth Movement

Age-related changes occur in the skeleton and alveolar bone with increasing age, and there is an increased lag period or delayed response to mechanical force in adults that is greater than that seen in younger patients.[39] However, teeth move equally well in adults as they do in children, and there is no evidence that teeth move at a slower rate

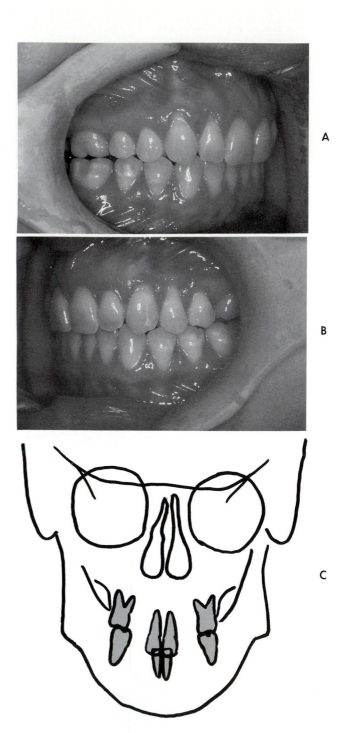

Fig. 13-8 A case in which orthodontic treatment was done and the transverse skeletal discrepancy was camouflaged. **A,** Post-treatment right lateral view. The case is unstable and has significant gingival recession in buccal segments and poor dental esthetics with *negative space* between cheeks and the buccal segments. **B,** Gingival recession on maxillary and mandibular premolars. **C,** The skeletal pattern is normal in the sagittal and vertical dimension. On the posteroanterior cephalometric tracing, note maxillary and mandibular widths. The MX to MX maxillary distance (57.8) and the AG to AG mandibular distance (92.0) can only be evaluated from the PA cephalometric radiograph.

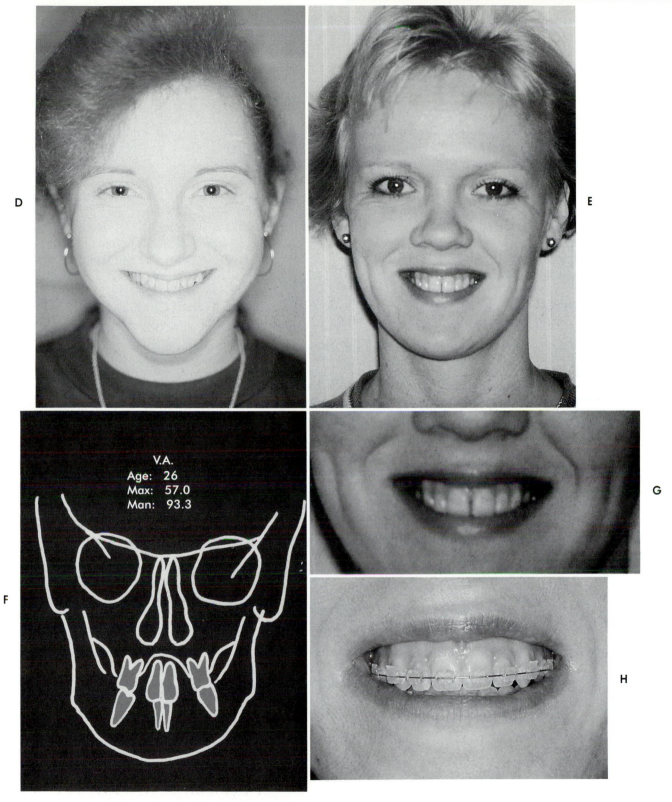

Fig. 13-8, cont'd   **D,** A 15-year-old patient with a severe Class III, and *normal transverse* skeletal dimension—with a full smile there is no *negative space*. **E,** Note large *negative spaces* in the corners of the buccal segments of a 26-year-old female with transverse maxillary deficiency and mandibular excess. **F,** PA cephalometric tracing of patient. Notice maxillary and mandibular widths. **G,** Pretreatment *negative space*. **H,** Negative space is eliminated by surgically assisted RPE to correct the transverse skeletal dysplasia. Excessive gingiva was removed, with the gingival retention procedure at appliance removal.

for adults. Regardless of the direction a tooth is moved in a healthy periodontium, the bone around the tooth remodels without the supporting tissues experiencing damage. The bone should follow the tooth in changes of position, and this principle is used to create favorable alveolar changes in patients with periodontal defects. Significant evidence exists that uprighting of mesially inclined molars will reduce pocket depth and improve altered bony morphology[9,66] (Fig. 13-9, A through D). The bone on the mesial is erupted as the molar is tipped distally. Every dentist has seen teeth erupt, and as a tooth moves occlusally, the healthy alveolar process moves with it (Fig. 13-10, A). In chronic inflammation as a tooth erupts the alveolar bone is lost and the tooth appears to extrude out of the periodontal tissues (Fig. 13-10, B). In molar uprighting the connective tissue attachment on the mesial of the molar and to the crestal bone creates tension and allows for remodeling of the bone (Fig. 13-9, C and D).

Clinically, there are ranges of force that are biologically acceptable to the periodontium. It is helpful to remember that (because tooth movement is primarily a periodontal ligament-induced phenomenon) identical forces do not place the same stress on the supporting tissues of different teeth. Root length and configuration, quantity of bone support, point of force application, and center of rotation come into play to determine stress areas in the periodontal ligament. To prevent potential tissue damage, it is important to consider areas of maximal stress that might occur in the periodontal ligament. Bone loss risk is increased as a result of inflamed connnective tissue located apical to crestal alveolar bone[61] and certain types of forces may aggravate the progression of inflammatory periodontal disease.[25] Periodontal disease in the periodontal ligament under stress has been shown in rats (between M1 and M2) where infectious inflammatory infiltration spreads from the epithelical aspect into the transseptal ligament (Fig. 13-11, A). These animals

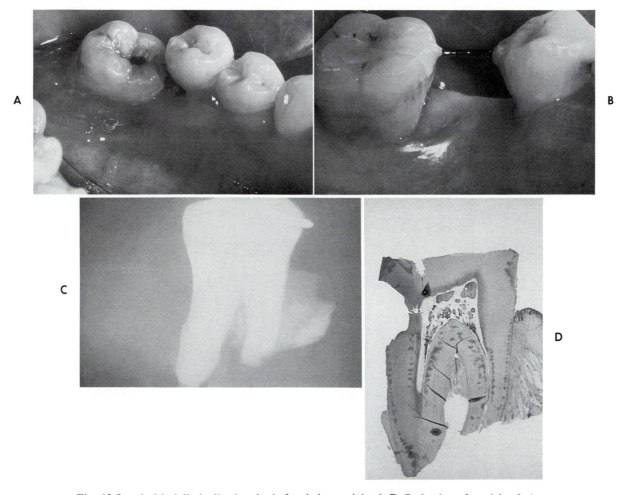

Fig. 13-9 **A,** Mesially inclined molar before being uprighted. **B,** Reduction of mesial soft tissue pocket depth. The extrusive component of uprighting allows for eversion of the pocket epithelium. **C,** Radiograph of human clinical case after uprighting. **D,** Histologic slide of the same tooth. Observe new bony spicules on the mesial where the alveolar crest has remodeled from the tension of the connective tissue attachment. There is no evidence of reattachment or increase in new attachment. (Courtesy Dr. I.S. Brown, Philadelphia, Pennsylvania.)

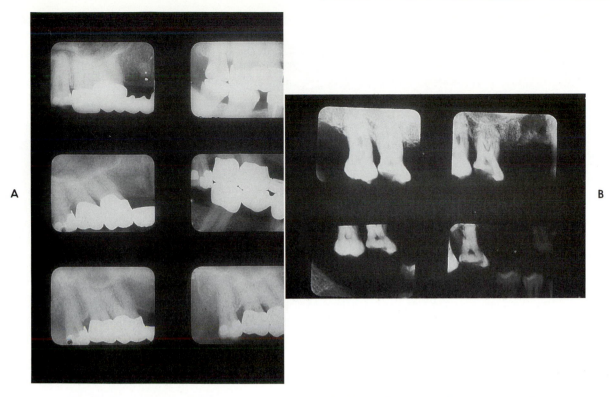

Fig. 13-10 **A,** Periapical films (over an 18-year period); the maxillary third molar erupts naturally. The area was kept clean and the bone follows the tooth. **B,** Radiograph of unopposed tooth erupting in the presence of periodontal disease. The bone does not follow the tooth. (Courtesy of Dr. Morton Amsterdam, Philadelphia, Pennsylvania.)

demonstrated complete destruction of the transseptal ligament within 28 days.[41]

Therefore, in an effort to prevent aggravated loss of attachment or tissue damage, it is critical to determine maximal stress areas, which can occur crestally or in the periodontal ligament. While most tooth movement involves combinations of movements, clinicians tend to view movement more simply in terms of intrusion, extrusion, tipping, translation, and torque.

Eruption of teeth. Eruption or extrusion of a tooth or several teeth along with clinical crown height reduction has been reported to reduce intrabony defects and decrease pocket depth.[18,60] Single tooth eruption should be distinguished from overbite correction and control of vertical dimension during routine orthodontic correction. Extrusion of an individual tooth is used specifically for correction of isolated periodontal osseous lesions. Studies have shown eruption in the presence of gingival inflammation will reduce bleeding upon probing, decrease pocket depth and even produce new bone formation at the alveolar crest as teeth were erupted, with no occlusal factor present and while controls remained unchanged.[59] Eruption or uprighting of molars without scaling and root planing in human patients has been shown to reduce pathogenic bacteria.[57] During clinical treatment however, inflammation should always be controlled to ensure that the supracrestal connective tissue

remains healthy and that crestal alveolar bone height remains at its original level.

In the double-blind molar uprighting study at Pennsylvania,[57] bacterial samples were taken from the mesial pockets of molars to be uprighted (experimental tooth) and from the contralateral mesially inclined molar that served as the control in each subject. Indirect immunofluorescence was used to identify *Bacteroides forysthus*, *Bacteroides gingivalis*, *Bacteroides intermedius*, and *Actinobacillus actinomycetemcomitans*. During the study no scaling, root planing, or subgingival inflammatory control was employed. The study revealed that in all experimental sites (mesial to molar) that exhibited the above microorganisms at the time of bonding, there was a significant decrease in their numbers at the end of treatment. However, Hawley bite plates were worn by all patients to disarticulate the molars during molar uprighting. In a similar study of 10 patients over a 12-week period, assessing the effects of molar uprighting on the microflora of human adults using DNA probes, it was found that Bacteroides pathogens exhibited a decrease at the experimental site with uprighting.[33]

Eruption of a tooth is the least hazardous type of movement to solve osseous morphology defects on individual teeth created by periodontal disease or tooth fractures. It is understood that extrusion of anterior segments in skeletal open bite patterns with muscular problems have been shown

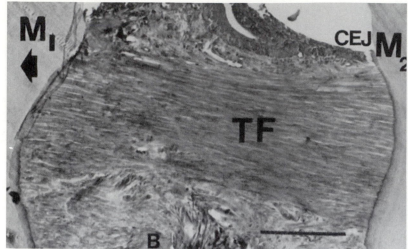

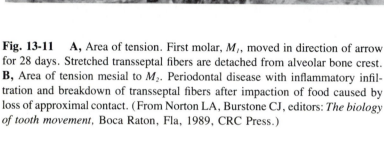

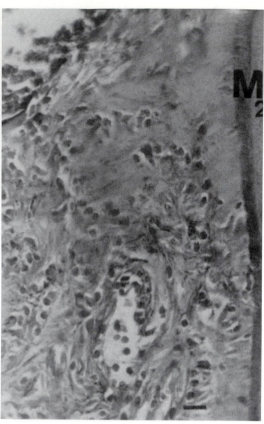

Fig. 13-11   A, Area of tension. First molar, M_1, moved in direction of arrow for 28 days. Stretched transseptal fibers are detached from alveolar bone crest. **B,** Area of tension mesial to M_2. Periodontal disease with inflammatory infiltration and breakdown of transseptal fibers after impaction of food caused by loss of approximal contact. (From Norton LA, Burstone CJ, editors: *The biology of tooth movement,* Boca Raton, Fla, 1989, CRC Press.)

to exhibit shortening of the roots. If teeth have normal bone support or if bone loss has been horizontal (alveolar crests and cementoenamel junctions are level), then movement should involve intrusion or extrusion as necessary to correct the orthodontic deformity.

Intrusion of teeth. Conflicting evidence has been reported regarding the benefits of intrusion of individual teeth. One study has reported intrusion of individual teeth that did not result in development of pockets.[31] This same investigator reported earlier that intrusion in monkeys induced increased new attachment levels following flap operations to excise pocket epithelium and to place an experimental notch on the root.[30] It is well known in periodontal research that dogs and monkeys exhibit new attachment during normal healing after surgical flap procedures without tooth movement (Fig. 13-12, *A* and *B*), and this has been described.[55] Others have observed that intrusion may result in root resorption, pulpal disturbances, and incomplete root formation in younger individuals.[45] Clinicians have cautioned that intrusion of anterior teeth during leveling of the occlusal plane to correct deep overbite can deepen infrabony defects (Fig. 13-13, *A* through *C*) on individual teeth.[28] These conflicting reports indicate that intrusion can be a *more* hazardous type of movement; since the force is concentrated at the apex, root resorption has been a well known sequela and light forces have been recommended (Chapter 2).

Intrusion has been reported to create altered cemento-

enamel junction and angular crest relationships along with only epithelial attachment to roots; therefore the periodontally susceptible patient is at greater risk for future periodontal breakdown (Fig. 13-13, *B* and *C*). Tooth movement, when properly executed, will improve periodontal conditions and be beneficial to periodontal health; extrusion is much more *predictable* than intrusion to accomplish this purpose. Whenever new connective tissue attachment or periodontal regeneration to restore lost supporting periodontal tissues is the treatment objective, the use of guided tissue regeneration (e.g., barrier membranes) is the predictable way to manipulate cells that lead to new attachment. Guided tissue regeneration procedures should always precede orthodontic tooth movement and should be part of initial therapy before active orthodontic treatment is begun.

Tipping Movement

When a single force is applied to the crown of the tooth, the tooth can rotate around its center of resistance (for an incisor, approximately the midpoint of the root) and there is increased compression (pressure) at the crest and at the root apex. In this instance, one half of the periodontal ligament has the potential to receive high pressure from essentially light force.

Experiments in the beagle dog demonstrated that with tipping and intruding movements, forces were capable of causing a gingival lesion to be converted to a lesion asso-

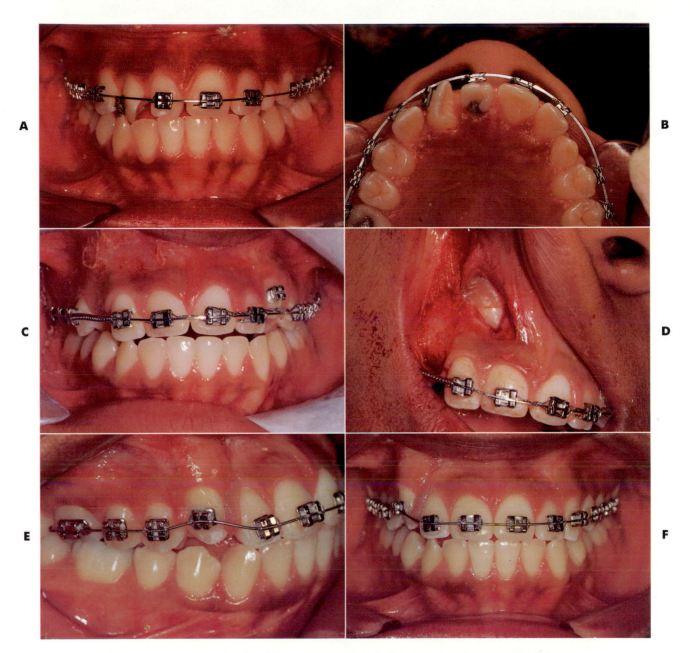

Plate 1 **A,** Young female with a supernumerary incisor between the two central incisors. **B,** Palatal view of supernumerary to the right of the midline. **C,** The supernumerary was removed. The right central and lateral incisors were properly positioned. **D,** The maxillary right canine was surgically uncovered. Pedical graft is placed on the labial. **E,** Observe the tissue health as the tooth is being moved into position. **F,** Anterior view of maxillary right canine.

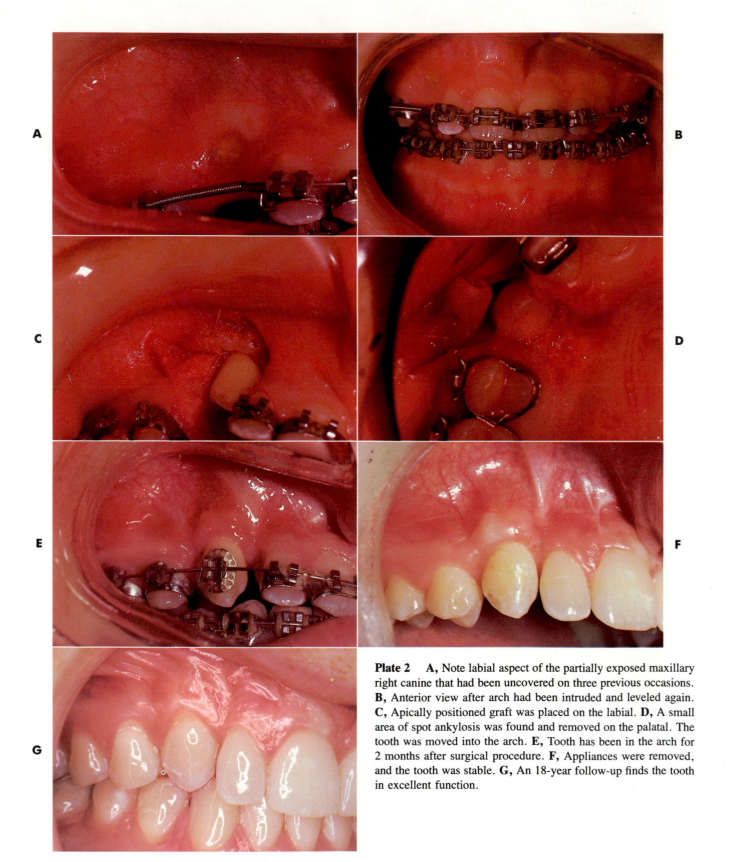

Plate 2 **A,** Note labial aspect of the partially exposed maxillary right canine that had been uncovered on three previous occasions. **B,** Anterior view after arch had been intruded and leveled again. **C,** Apically positioned graft was placed on the labial. **D,** A small area of spot ankylosis was found and removed on the palatal. The tooth was moved into the arch. **E,** Tooth has been in the arch for 2 months after surgical procedure. **F,** Appliances were removed, and the tooth was stable. **G,** An 18-year follow-up finds the tooth in excellent function.

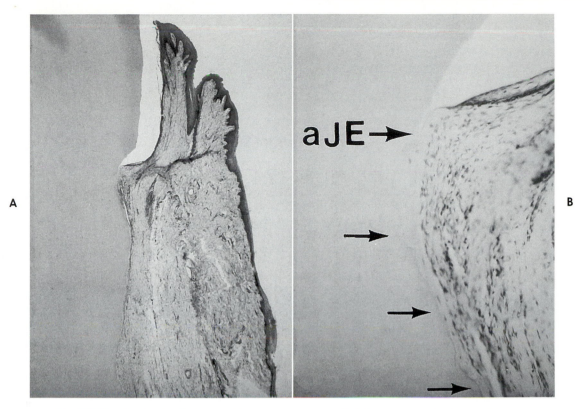

Fig. 13-12 **A,** Healing following flap surgery in a dog. **B,** Microphotograph of normal healing following flap surgery in a dog (without tooth movement). A new connective tissue attachment is formed and extends coronally from the apical border of the notch prepared at the surgically created bone crest to the apical termination of the *aJE*. (Courtesy of Dr. J. Lindhe, Gothenburg.)

ciated with attachment loss.[13] In tipping movements the force should be light and the area kept clean to prevent the formation of angular bony defects.

Bodily Movement into a Defect

It has been suggested that movement into infrabony defects can result in healing and regeneration of the attachment apparatus.[15] In addition, periodontists have believed that in the presence of a wide osseous defect adjacent to a tooth, if the tooth were moved in order to narrow the defect, better healing potential may be possible. Unfortunately, a more recent study has shown that if infrabony defects are created in the lower incisor area of rhesus monkeys (undergoing good plaque control) and if the tooth then is moved into and through the original defect, a long epithelial-attachment to the roots is created, with no *new* attachment apparent.[38] The results, however, indicated that even though movement into infrabony periodontal defects did not result in regeneration of attachment, no further loss of connective tissue attachment occurred.

The most recent study performed in four beagle dogs found angular bony defects were created and plaque was allowed to accumulate. Teeth were translated into inflamed, infrabony pockets, and additional attachment loss occurred on the teeth moved into the infrabony pockets.[65] Therefore it was concluded that bodily tooth movement may increase the rate of destruction of the connective tissue attachment at teeth with inflamed, infrabony pockets.

At Pennsylvania, teeth have been moved into defects with the patients' contralateral side serving as their own control (Fig. 13-14, *A* through *L*). Radiographs revealed that loss of attachment has occurred where a tooth has been moved into a defect in an edentulous area (Fig. 13-14, *E* through *F*). It is possible to move the tooth away from a defect and, with sufficient eruption, to eliminate or reduce a bony defect, and this is usually the treatment of choice to improve the osseous architecture.

A study involving closing edentulous spaces in the mandible was performed on a group of 11- to 17-year-old patients and compared with a group of 23- to 46-year-old adults.[46] The results indicated that the older adults had more loss of crestal bone and greater root resorption than the younger patient group.

MUCOGINGIVAL CONSIDERATIONS

During tooth movement the periodontal tissues should maintain a stable relationship around the cervical area of

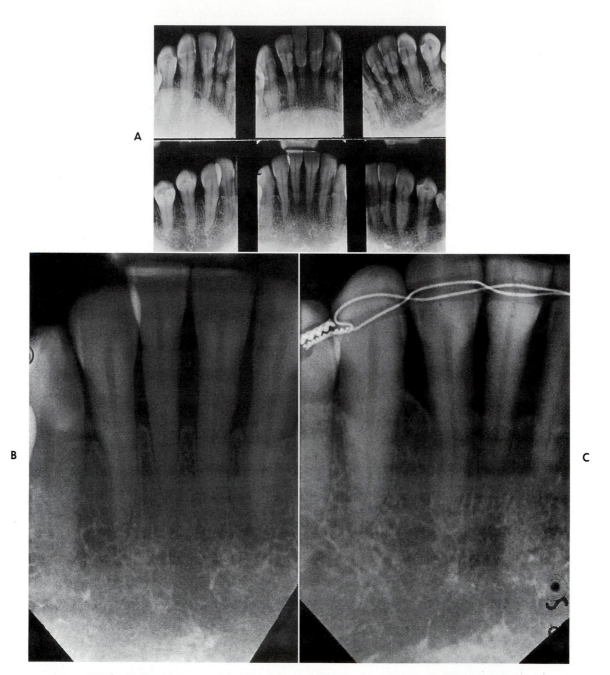

Fig. 13-13 **A,** Radiographs of lower anteriors, with loss of bone before scaling. Lower radiographs were taken after scaling. Note that the bone loss is horizontal (level alveolar crests) between the cuspid and incisor group. The ideal way to decrease overbite would be to reduce the crowns with a high-speed bur and improve the crown to the root ratio, keeping the bone level between adjacent teeth. Instead teeth were banded according to the incisal edge and intruded. **B,** Preorthodontic periapical radiograph of lower anteriors before intrusion. Note the level alveolar crest between the canine and the lateral incisor. **C,** Periapical radiograph of lower anterior area after intrusion. Note CEJ is no longer level between the canine and lateral incisor; however, a large angular crest has been created between the canine and the lateral incisor. An angular crest has been described as a predilected site to periodontal breakdown. (From Marks MH, Corn H, editors: *Atlas of adult orthodontics*, Philadelphia, 1989, Lea & Febiger.)

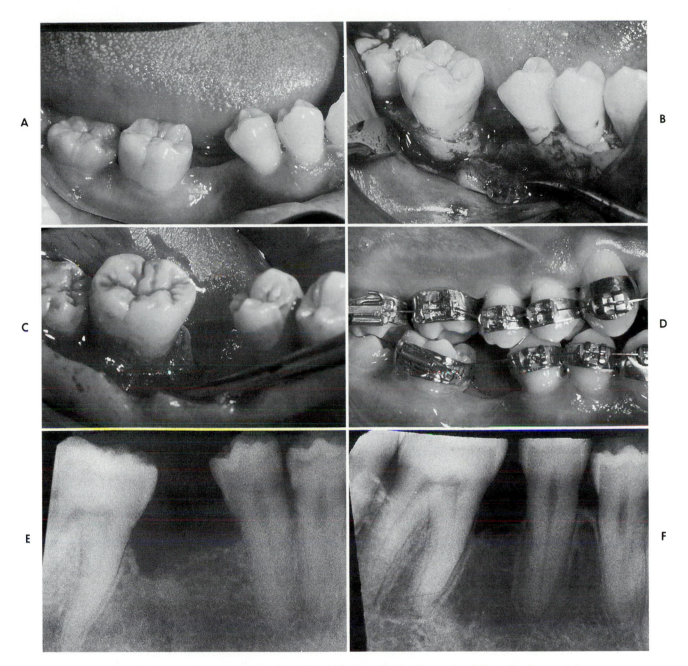

Fig. 13-14   **A,** A 37-year-old male, with missing mandibular first molars bilaterally. Lower right preoperative (test side) view of side with defect in edendulous area. **B,** Lower right edentulous ridge area, with tissue reflected. Note defect mesial to the second molar. **C,** Another view of osseous defect before tooth movement. **D,** Appliance placement on right side to begin space closure. **E,** Preorthodontic periapical radiograph. Note mesial attachment level radiographically. **F,** Post-orthodontic periapical radiograph. Observe evidence of bone loss on the mesial of the second molar during space closure.   *Continued.*

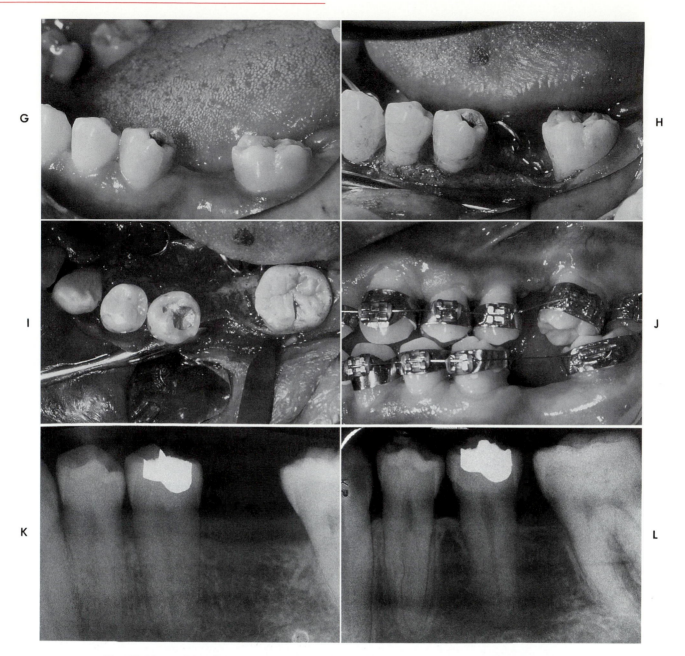

Fig. 13-14, cont'd   G, Lower left preorthodontic view of side *without* a vertical defect in the ridge. **H,** Tissue reflected in lower left (control side). Note there is no defect in the osseous ridge mesial to the second molar. **I,** Occlusal view of osseous ridge area, with no osseous defect. **J,** Appliance placement on left side to begin space closure. **K,** Periapical radiograph of lower left before space closed. Note mesial attachment on second molar. **L,** Periapical radiograph after space closure. There is no radiographic evidence of bone loss on the mesial of the second molar on control side.

the tooth. An adequate amount of attached gingiva is necessary to be compatible with gingival health and to allow appliances (functional, orthopedic) to deliver orthodontic treatment without creating bone loss and gingival recession. Clinical experience and animal studies have clearly established that more pronounced, clinically recognizable inflammation occurs in regions where there is a lack of attached gingiva (Fig. 13-15, *A*) than in areas with a wider zone of attached gingiva (Fig. 13-15, *B*). Histologically, however, the teeth lacking gingiva were thinner in the buccolingual dimension than those with a wide zone of attached gingiva; but investigators reported that inflammatory cell infiltrate and its apical extrusion (degree of inflammation) were similar.[62,63] Two studies have indicated that as teeth are moved

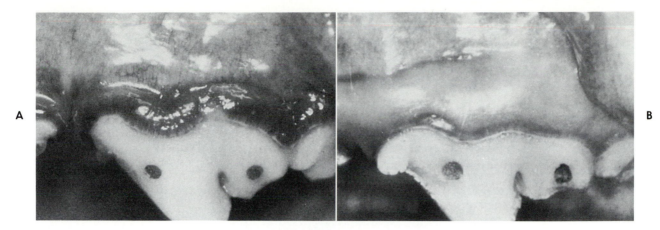

Fig. 13-15   Teeth in a dog after 40 days of plaque accumulation. The clinical signs of inflammation are more pronounced at the site with the narrow band of gingiva, **A,** than at the site with the wide zone of attached gingiva, **B.** It was believed that the vascular system was more readily visible in its thinner units that lack gingiva. (From Lindhe J: *Textbook of clinical periodontology,* Copenhagen, 1989, Munksgaard.)

labially and as tension is created on the marginal tissue, the thickness of the gingival tissue on the pressure side becomes important. With labial bodily movement, incisors exhibited apical displacement of the gingival margin, but no loss of connective tissue attachment was apparent where there were no signs of inflammation. Where inflammation was present, loss of connective tissue attachment occurred.[64] Therefore if the tooth movement is expected to result in a reduced volume of soft tissue thickness and where an alveolar bone dehiscence may have occurred in the presence of inflammation, gingival recession is a risk. Obviously, all orthodontic cases will have gingival inflammation, and bodily facial movement can predispose to gingival recession; to prevent this a gingival graft can be used.

The free gingival graft is the most versatile, most widely used, and most predictable procedure for gingival augmentation.[42] When it is performed before recession occurs, it is considered to be less traumatic and highly predictable and will prevent recession during orthodontics. However, many periodontists still feel with younger patients that a *wait and see* attitude is acceptable because so many predictable ways of correcting recession have become available. Root exposure is most likely to be progressive in a younger patient, since labial bone loss may be impossible to correct. It is *essential* to prevent it. Therefore, clinical judgment and animal studies support the need for creating a *thicker* gingiva that can better withstand the inflammatory insult during tooth movement.

The thin, delicate tissue is far more prone to exhibit recession during orthodontics than is normal-to-thick tissue. If there is a minimal zone of attached gingiva or thin tissue (Fig. 13-16, *A* through *C*), particularly on abutment teeth, a free gingival graft that enhances the type of tissue around the tooth will help control inflammation; this should be done before beginning orthodontic movement. Differences in al-

veolar housing also should be evaluated. It is not necessarily true that a thin, soft tissue is associated with a thin labiolingual osseous support. All combinations are seen, such as thick, soft tissue with a thin labial plate of bone. It is difficult to change the labial osseous thickness (especially the thin type) that is characteristic for the individual patient; however, it is not difficult or traumatic to improve the soft tissue with a free graft. Obviously the decision concerning *prophylactic* periodontal procedures must be made with consideration for, among other things, growth and development, tooth position, type and direction of anticipated tooth movement, oral physiotherapy, integrity of the mucogingival junction, tissue type, inflammation, muscle pull, frenum attachment, mucogingival and osseous defects, anticipated tissue changes, and profile considerations (see box below).

 DIAGNOSTIC CONSIDERATIONS IN CASE SELECTION FOR GRAFTING BEFORE ORTHODONTIC TREATMENT

- Growth and development
- Tooth position
- Oral physiotherapy
- Type of hard and soft tissue
- Inflammation
- Integrity of the mucogingival junction
- Mucogingival and osseous defects
- Type and direction of anticipated tooth movement
- Tissue changes associated with tooth movement
- Profile considerations
- Mechanotherapy to be used
- Patient cooperation

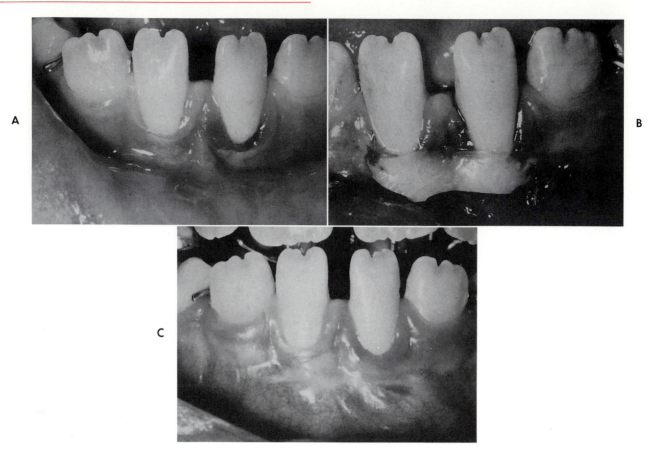

Fig. 13-16 **A,** Inadequate attached gingiva on lower central incisors of an 8-year-old female. Pronounced signs of inflammation, especially on the left central; a free graft should be placed before early treatment protocols. **B,** Donor tissue from the palate is in place. **C,** Postoperative result before beginning treatment.

Critical evaluation of the periodontium before orthodontic treatment begins can prevent, minimize, or at least not aggravate an exisiting periodontal condition. Other areas that frequently involve conflicting periodontal management are frenum considerations, gingival hyperplasia, mouth breathing, and ectopically positioned teeth.

FRENUM CONSIDERATIONS, GINGIVAL HYPERPLASIA, GINGIVAL RETENTION AND MOUTH BREATHING
Mandibular Midline Frenum

When a frenum is associated with a mucogingival problem, it most frequently relates to an inadequate zone of attached gingiva. Therefore the use of frenectomy to correct mucogingival problems is considered obsolete. The high frenum insertion contributes to movement of the marginal gingiva where the keratinized tissue has been lost or detached or where mechanical trauma exists. This problem is most prevalent in the lower anterior area.

Maxillary Midline Frenum

It has been recommended that a frenectomy procedure be done in the maxillary midline for young children because of the belief that the midline diastema is caused by the maxillary labial frenum. Many believe that this frenum prevents mesial migration of the maxillary central incisors and that removal should precede orthodontic therapy. Others have suggested that if the frenum is removed, the space can be orthodontically closed more easily. However, the practitioner must remember that a physiologic space will normally be present between the maxillary central incisors until eruption of the canines in the adolescent dentition. In addition, a frenectomy procedure may cause scar tissue that could prevent orthodontic space closure. With extremely large diastemas (6 to 8 mm) in the early transitional dentition a frenectomy is usually recommended to facilitate space closure, regain space at the midline, and prevent ectopic eruption of the lateral incisors or canines. These interceptive early treatment problems require complete orthodontic supervision, usually additional mechanotherapy, and several stages of treatment.

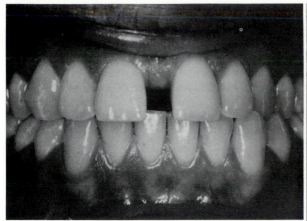

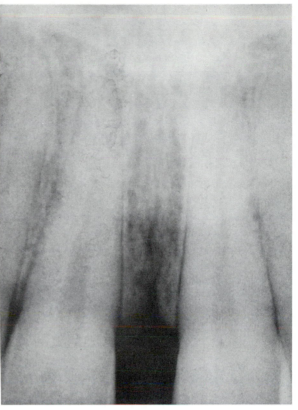

Fig. 13-17   A, Clinical appearance of a persistent midline diastema in a 20-year-old female. **B,** Radiographic appearance of mid-line interdental bone before orthodontics, exhibiting a V-shaped suture, which is the diagnostic key to potential relapse.

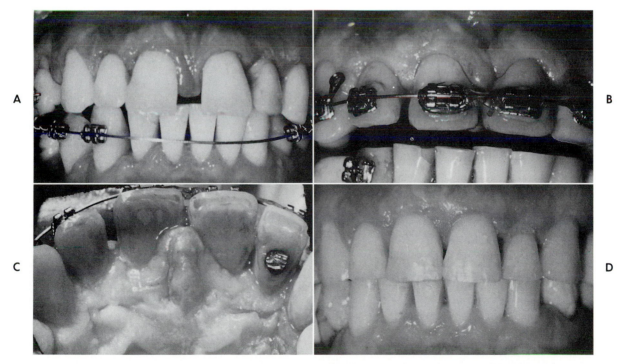

Fig. 13-18   A, Preorthodontic diastema of a 40-year-old adult male with significant periodontal disease and loss of posterior support. **B** and **C,** During midline diastema closure the soft tissue became enlarged and sore and prevented complete space closure. Therefore, a frenectomy was done to remove the frenum before completion of tooth movement. **D,** Mid-line area after completion of tooth movement and reestablishing posterior support.

A U- or V-shaped roentgenographic appearance of the interproximal bone between the maxillary central incisors is a diagnostic key to the persistent midline diastema (Fig. 13-17, *A* and *B*). This roentgenogram of the mature midline suture with firm teeth preorthodontically indicates that relapse will follow even excellent orthodontic treatment (no occlusal discrepancies, muscular habits or problems, tooth-size discrepancies, and ideal axial inclinations, overbite, and overjet). The patient should be informed before orthodontic treatment of the need of indefinite retention with bonding of the central incisors after treatment to prevent return of the maxillary midline diastema.

Generally, surgical removal of a maxillary labial frenum should be delayed until after orthodontic treatment, unless the tissue prevents space closure or becomes painful and traumatized (Fig. 13-18, *A* through *D*). Removal may be indicated after treatment to change irreversible hyperplastic tissue to normal gingival form and to enhance posttreatment stability. This is particularly helpful on incisors during Phase I of early treatment problems.

Gingival Hyperplasia

Mild gingival changes associated with orthodontic appliances seem to be transitory, and the periodontal tissues sustain little permanent damage.[14] Usually this condition will resolve itself or will respond to plaque removal, curettage, or both. Should the gingival tissue or enlargement interfere with tooth movement, however, it must be surgically removed. Otherwise, it is preferable to wait until appliances are removed to correct surgically abnormal gingival form[51] and use the procedure to enhance post-treatment stability.

Gingival Retention and Esthetic Considerations

Frequently, tissue will show an exaggerated response to local factors, and gingival reflection with internal bevel incision (gingivectomy) can be done to promote stability, as well as optimal esthetics and gingival topography (see Chapter 14). In adults with altered passive eruption, the gingival tissue fails to recede, and the patient thinks that his or her teeth are *short* (Fig. 13-19, *A, B,* and *C*). Many such patients have thick buccal alveolar bone that must be thinned by minor osteoplasty, and if necessary, a normal 1.5 mm relationship between the osseous crest and the CEJ should be established. This will prevent the return of the tissue incisally onto the anatomic crown during healing. The internal bevel gingivectomy and gingival reflection procedures should not be done on the labial aspect of anterior teeth that have thin gingival tissue. Also, tissue on bell-shaped anterior teeth should only be reflected on the lingual or palatal aspects. The interdental tissue in these two instances may not heal back to the level of contact points, creating an unesthetic result. Spaces below the contact points are disturbing to the patient.

Fiberotomy[1,12]

This procedure should be done after correction of any preorthodontically rotated teeth, especially maxillary and mandibular anterior teeth, such as maxillary lateral incisors in Class II, division 2, problems. The procedure should be done before debonding after mild (3° to 5°) overcorrection. The overcorrection is removed 1 week after the surgical procedure and before impressions for retainers (Fig. 13-20,

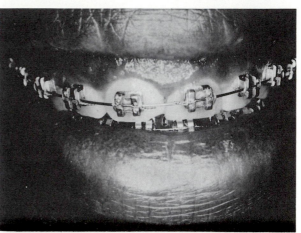

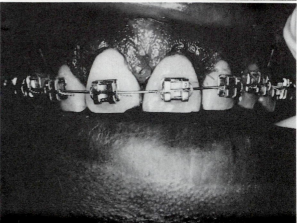

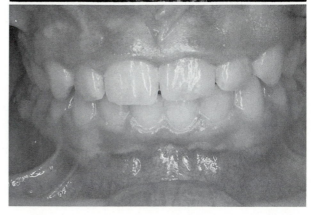

Fig. 13-19 **A,** A 37-year-old female complains of short teeth. She has a normal vertical dimension and upper lip length. **B,** Note normal-sized anatomical crowns at the time of internal bevel gingivectomy for esthetics and stability. **C,** A 14-year-old male with short clinical crowns.

A through *D*). Internal bevel gingivectomy or labiolingual flap reflections with interproximal sutures (see Chapter 12) enhance alignment and reduce labiolingual and vertical dental relapse. These procedures should be done before fixed appliances are removed.

Mouth Breathing

A significant problem in the orthodontic patient is the added periodontal insult of mouth breathing. The drying effect on the exposed tissue in the susceptible patient is associated with enlarged, erythematous labial gingiva particularly in the maxillary and mandibular anterior regions. With a short upper lip, a demarcation line can usually be seen where the lip contacts the labial tissue (Fig. 13-21, *A* and *B*). The mouth breather will usually exhibit dry, cracked lips as well. Although orthodontic retraction of anterior segments may help to provide a better lip seal, extra-oral

appliances and lip bumpers will exacerbate the problem or may even cause mouth breathing in the normal patient. The patient who exhibits symptoms of an inability to breathe properly (tongue posture, enlarged adenoid tissue, narrow high palatal vault, allergies) should be referred for evaluation of nasal obstruction and adenoid tissue. Although the plaque index is not significantly higher in mouth breathers, it has been reported that there is an increase in the gingival index.[19] This increased inflammation should be reduced to a minimum before fixed appliances are placed and is usually accomplished by scaling and curettage.

Considerations with Ectopically Positioned and Unerupted Teeth

Many orthodontic patients exhibit teeth that have not penetrated the oral mucosa or will not erupt. Certain teeth demonstrate eruption that has been delayed significantly

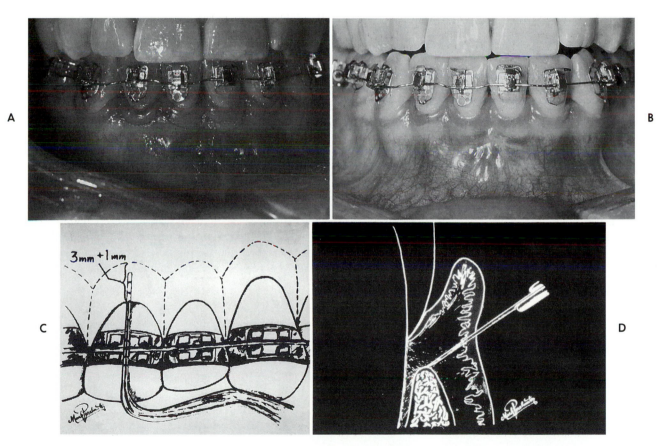

Fig. 13-20 A, Mild overcorrections have been done for the mandibular incisors. Sounding-type incisions are made through the incisal papilla to bone and angled toward the tooth. The interproximal incisions are joined labially in an attempt to sound out the osseous crest. Incisions are made on the lingual aspect as well. In this case the mandibular frenum (frenotomy) was released so that the tissue would not be retracted on the labial aspect of the central incisors. **B,** Two weeks postoperatively. Overcorrections will be removed. **C,** Diagramatic representation of probing to establish bleeding points. **D,** Diagram to illustrate sounding incision made at 45° angle to the long axis of the tooth. (From Ahrens DG, Shapiro Y et al: *Am J Orthod* 80:83-91, 1981.)

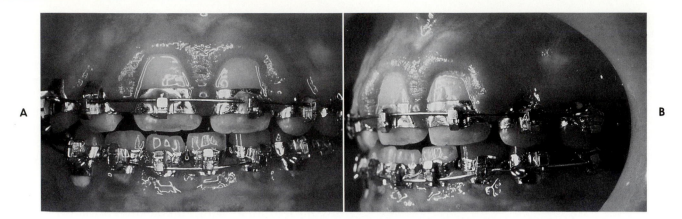

Fig. 13-21 **A,** Exaggerated response to mouth breathing. Note lip line over central incisors, where the lip covers the labial gingiva. **B,** Enlarged gingival tissue harbors dentobacterial plaque, and the increased pseudopocket depth acts as a reservoir for retention of subgingival plaque.

beyond the time when normal dental eruption for a particular patient should have occurred. Clinical orthodontists that have treated cases involving unerupted teeth have all faced the problems of devitalization, reexposure or reuncovering of the tooth, ankylosis, external root resorption, and injury to adjacent teeth when an unerupted tooth has been surgically uncovered from the wrong side of the ridge. The marginal bone loss, gingival recession, and sensitivity problems that are seen once the roots are exposed for an individual are complications that invariably result in prolonged treatment time, esthetic deformities, and, in many cases, loss of teeth (Fig. 13-22, *A* through *G*). Most of these problems: reexposure, gingival recession, and bone loss, can be prevented. Proper management of the periodontal tissues is critical in preventing loss of attachment. When the teeth are uncovered, it is not recommended to use electrosurgery or lasers—techniques that have attracted a lot of attention recently; these instruments are used strictly to remove the overlying tissue. Excision of the surrounding tissue on the

unerupted tooth leaves inadequate keratinized tissue (Fig. 13-22, *D* through *F*).

As far as labial impactions are concerned, they should *not* be uncovered and a free gingival graft placed on them. Free gingival grafts do not survive on enamel. The surgical procedure is primarily an apically or laterally positioned pedicle graft.[56] The maxillary incisors can be done nicely from an orthodontic standpoint. When a tooth is uncovered, space in the arch should be created before uncovering the tooth if it is on the labial. The edentulous space created in the arch provides a tissue area to act as a donor site so that an adequate zone of attached gingiva can be taken for the partial thickness of the apically or laterally positioned graft (Fig. 13-23, *A* through *J*). If space is unavailable between the teeth in the arch, a free graft may be placed at the mucogingival junction and then converted into a pedicle graft to be placed on the unerupted tooth. Whenever the tissue for a particular patient is so thin that it could not be dissected away as a partial thickness graft, a free graft can

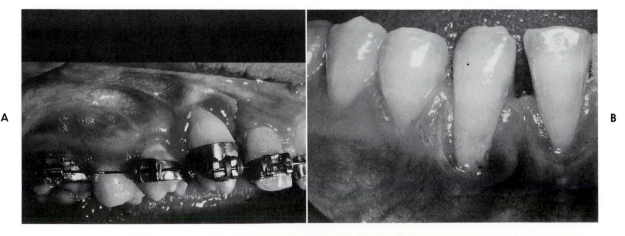

Fig. 13-22 For legend see opposite page.

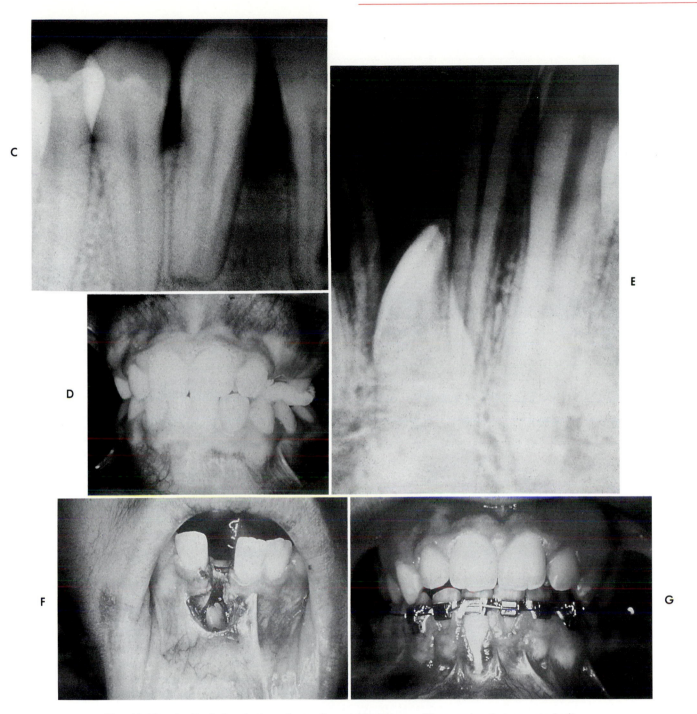

Fig. 13-22   **A,** Typical esthetic and recession problem on maxillary canine that was surgically uncovered without keratinized tissue being placed on the tooth. **B,** Clinical appearance of a previously unerupted and surgically uncovered mandibular canine. The tooth exhibits absence of attached gingiva and gingival recession, and is an esthetic concern of the patient. **C,** Periapical radiograph reveals marginal bone loss of a third of the alveolar support and root blunting. These complications could have been prevented. **D,** A young child with retained mandibular right primary central incisor. **E,** Note unerupted central incisor on periapical film. **F,** Surgical uncovering involved extraction of primary tooth and removal of all overlying soft and hard tissue. The surgery did not provide for attached gingiva over the labial of the tooth. **G,** An undesirable response, with recession and loss of attachment as the tooth is guided into the arch.

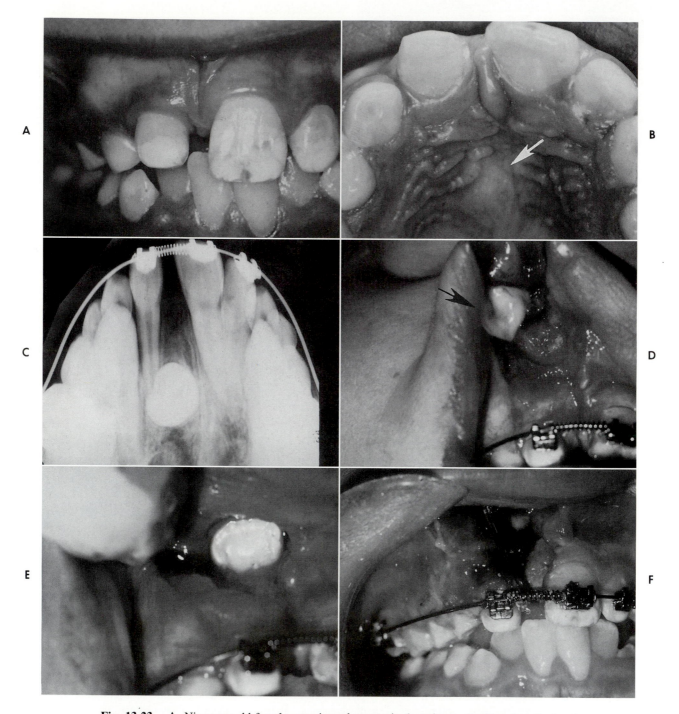

Fig. 13-23 A, Nine-year-old female experienced trauma in the primary dentition that displaced the right central incisor palatally and towards the eye. **B,** An occlusal view to the distal and to the right of the incisal papilla. Observe the bulge (*arrow*) caused by the dilacerated root of the displaced central. **C,** After the base arch is placed, the occlusal radiograph illustrates vertical position of the central incisor crown. **D,** Partial thickness graft is dissected away to get to the maxillary labial bone. **E,** After removal of the labial bone, observe that the incisor crown is upside down; therefore, the graft was placed on the labial enamel, on the palatal side of the tooth. **F,** One week later. The tooth was bonded on the palatal aspect and activated with elastomeric thread.

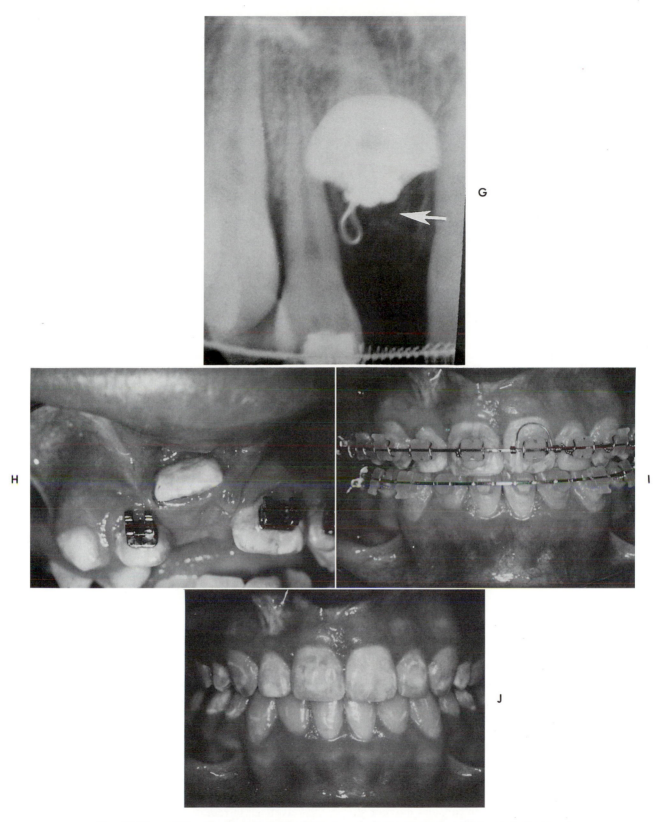

Fig. 13-23, cont'd   G, Several months later. A periapical radiograph, with bonded attachment on the palatal aspect of the crown, and the dilacerated root that is vertical to the crown. **H and I,** Once the crown is horizontal, the palatal attachment is removed and a labial attachment is placed to flip the tooth into the arch. **J,** Postorthodontically, it is difficult to detect which incisor was displaced.

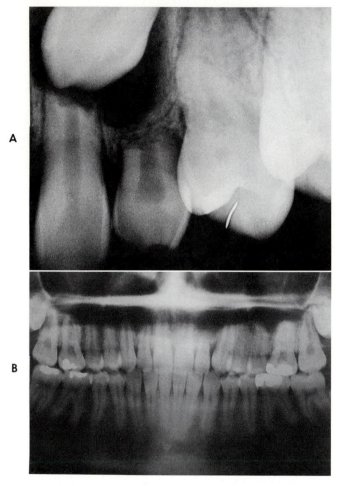

Fig. 13-24 **A,** Periapical radiograph demonstrates over 50% resorption of the lateral incisor root. The crown of the canine had to be surgically uncovered and kept in contact with the oral cavity. **B,** Panoramic radiograph shows that the finished case has no further resorption of the lateral root.

be placed at the mucogingival junction. Grafts should be partial thickness; this preference should be expressed to the oral surgeon because full thickness grafts would be thick and unesthetic. Large dental follicles frequently occur, especially on maxillary canines in 9- or 10-year-old individuals, before the teeth have erupted out of the palate. When these enlarged dental follicles are resorbing hard tooth structure in the arch (roots of teeth in the arch), they must be uncovered (Fig. 13-24, *A* and *B*). Even though they may not have more than 50% root formation at that point, the canine should be uncovered and a bonded attachment placed. The canine should be moved in contact with the palatal mucosa, the attachment taken off, and the root allowed to continue to develop on the canine. If the canine is not uncovered and brought in contact with the oral cavity, the enlarged follicle will usually continue to resorb the roots of the incisor teeth. If it is allowed to recover-up by the palatal tissue, it will begin to resorb tooth structure again.

The question often arises whether a tooth will erupt into the arch. The real key is the incisal edge. If it is headed away from the occlusal plane or if the tooth is upside down, it will not erupt into the oral cavity. If a tooth is erupting slowly or if it is holding up treatment time, then it should be surgically uncovered and orthodontically positioned into the arch. The *most difficult canine* is the canine that erupts between the roots of a premolar—particularly the maxillary first premolar that has a bifurcated root (Fig. 13-25, *A* through *F*). The periapical radiograph should be evaluated closely for this type of premolar root form. When the canine erupts and lodges between the roots of a bifurcated first premolar, it is difficult to uncover it without getting into the apicies of the premolar. This is true whether the canine is uncovered from the palatal or the labial side of the arch. This situation is one in which the premolar would have to be extracted in order to salvage the maxillary canine (Fig. 13-25, *E* and *F*). The labial impactions are much less difficult to manage if a soft tissue grafting procedure is used (see Plate 1 p. 724a).

With the maxillary palatally positioned canines, which occur 3 times more frequently, the problem is different. The palate is all masticatory mucosa, therefore a graft is not placed on the teeth. These teeth are uncovered by reflecting the palatal tissue, by placing a window, and then by replacing the tissue over the palate (Fig. 13-26, *A* and *B*). A periodontal dressing is placed for 7 to 10 days before being removed, at which time a bonded attachment is placed, and tooth movement is begun.

A major orthodontic principle that applies to palatal canines is the use of a sufficient-sized base arch (at least an 0.018 or a rectangular stainless steel base arch). The base arch must be large enough to prevent deflection of teeth in the maxillary arch into the opposing occlusion each time the patient closes his or her mouth. The devitalization of lateral incisors often occurs because a very flexible, multistranded base arch or light nitinol base arch has been used so that when the palatally impacted tooth is activated over a long period of time it deflects teeth (particularly maxillary lateral incisors) into the opposing occlusion, and laterals can be devitalized by occlusal trauma. For adults the primary teeth are left in place until the palatally displaced tooth is moved close to the arch; then the primary tooth is taken out. Once the primary tooth is removed, an acrylic pontic is placed on the archwire for esthetics. Palatally impacted teeth as well must be constantly evaluated for bleeding around the crown or for active bleeding around the tooth; ideally, this is done with a curette. If there is *excessive bleeding* the patient should be referred back to the general dental office or to the periodontal office for periodic scaling and curettage to remove the bacteria from the subgingival area. This occurs because of the palatal tissue depth around unerupted teeth. Otherwise, there is a small chance of loss of attachment on a palatally impacted tooth. Any tooth that has been surgically uncovered should always be checked at each visit for *excessive mobility*. In many instances the den-

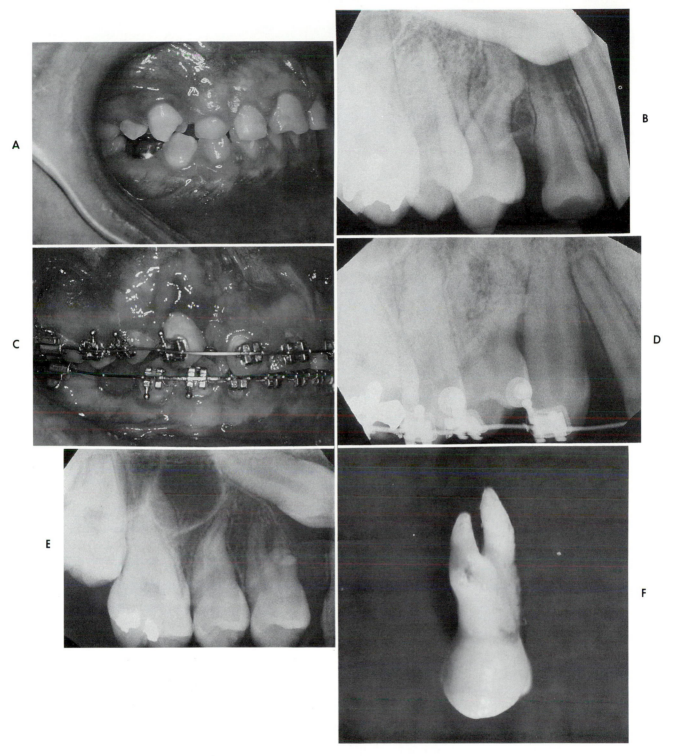

Fig. 13-25 A, Right clinical view of primary canine still in position before appliances were placed. **B,** On preoperative periapical radiograph, note the bifurcated first premolar root with the maxillary right canine lodged between the roots. **C,** Several years later the tooth has been guided anteriorly from the labial into the arch. This is an adolescent male whose oral hygiene, despite constant reinforcement, remained inadequate; note significant gingival hyperplasia. **D,** Progress periapical film indicates possible loss of attachment, though probing depth is minimal. **E,** Young female with unerupted maxillary right canine. Pretreatment periapical radiograph indicates bifurcated first premolar. **F,** The premolar was extracted. This root form can complicate and prolong treatment.

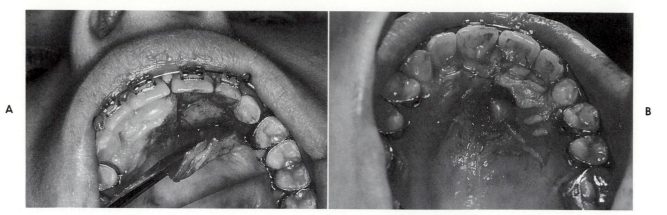

Fig. 13-26   **A,** The ectopically positioned palatal canine can rarely be palpated. The palatal soft tissue must be reflected and osseous surgery is required to enter the follicular space. Inadequate exposure will not only prolong treatment but may also cause injury to the tooth as well because of the inadequate field of vision. **B,** The palatal tissue is placed back in position and a soft tissue window is created in the orientation of the long axis of the anatomical crown.

tal follicle can grow aggressively around the erupting tooth that has been uncovered and can displace or detach the graft from the crown on labial impactions, and it can cause bone loss around the entire tooth as the tooth is moved into the arch. When excessive mobility is observed, the patient must be referred to the periodontist to find out if bone is following the erupting tooth. An x-ray examination should be made to evaluate the presence of osteoid tissue and to ensure that the periodontal attachment is following the tooth as it is being guided into the arch. To aid eruption of a deeply positioned palatal impaction, a 0.012 or a 0.014 S.S. wire should be spun until taut directly across the palate, from the canine or premolar area to the premolar area on the opposite side of the arch. An explorer is used to tighten the wire with a Spanish windlass technique; then the attachment is placed on the palatally positioned tooth, and a power thread is tied from the tooth to the wire that goes across the palate. The force is directed so as to erupt the tooth into the palate out of the palatal soft tissues (Fig. 13-27, *A* through *D*). Then the tooth is rotated and moved directly into the arch. If the tooth is moved, covered by soft tissue through the palatal tissue, and erupted into the arch, treatment time will be prolonged by many months. Therefore, it should be erupted within 7 to 10 days after the surgical procedure has been done. It should be erupted down through the thick tissue and brought to the level of palatal contour. At this point it can be determined if the tooth is backward and if it needs to be rotated; rotational movement should be initiated immediately (even in the center of the palate) as it is moved toward its proper position in the arch.

After canines the second premolar is the tooth that most frequently requires surgical uncovering. As it is with mandibular premolars, apically repositioned grafts are necessary. If the tooth is located on the lingual, the graft is placed on the lingual only. If the tooth is in the center of the arch

(an occlusal radiograph is needed to locate these teeth before uncovering), an apically positioned graft on the lingual, as well as on the facial, is required (Fig. 13-28, *A* through *J*). Ideally, the surgeon should be given as much assistance from the orthodontist as possible in determining the location of teeth and also given any special information about the surgical uncovering. With the mandibular molars as well, it is necessary to do a buccal and a lingual graft when these teeth are located in the middle of the ridge. Osseous surgery needs to be done that will allow the graft to be placed onto the enamel, both on the buccal and lingual aspects of the anatomical crown. Less frequently, a mandibular incisor (or several mandibular incisors) may need to be uncovered. With mandibular incisors, both a labial and a lingual graft must be done; these grafts have to be extended beyond the line angle of each individual crown (Fig. 13-29, *A* through *F*). If the grafts are not placed beyond the line angle of the unerupted tooth, a mucogingival defect may be created on the line angle, whether it be on the lingual or the facial, even when teeth are in the center of the ridge.

As patients get older the teeth tend to become ankylosed particularly as the patients age into their 30s and 40s; the radiograph can reveal this complication. A radiograph of a tooth that appears to fade into the bone indicates ankylosis (Fig. 13-30, *A* and *B*). Teeth with this radiographic appearance should be considered hopeless; no attempt should be made to bring them into the oral cavity; all unerupted teeth cannot be salvaged, and the prognosis here may be poor. There are certain impacted teeth, even the canines that should be extracted. However, the number of successfully treated unerupted teeth can be increased by proper management of the tissues attached to them. Few esthetic deformities and more favorable long-term prognoses for these teeth will result from protecting the marginal integrity of the attachment apparatus and from preventing an

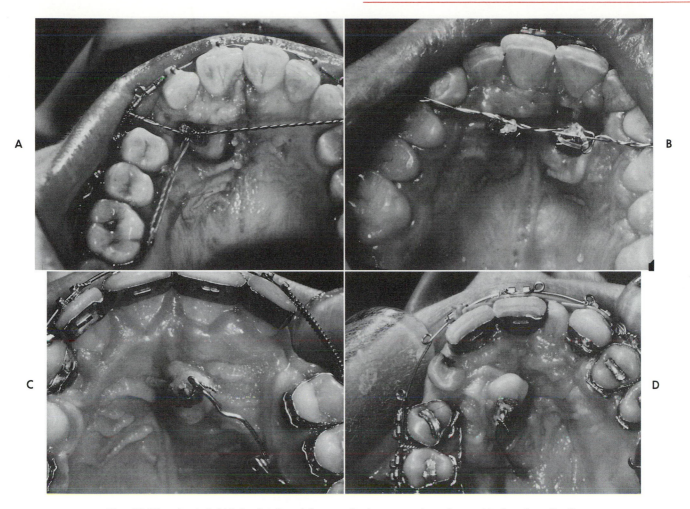

Fig. 13-27   A, A 0.014 dead soft stainless steel wire across the palate, with thread to distally erupt the canine towards the tongue. **B,** A 0.012 stainless steel wire is used to tie elastomeric thread to each canine to erupt both teeth to the level of the palatal vault. They then can be guided towards the arch. **C,** Note auxiliary spring soldered to the molar tube to erupt the canine. **D,** An Australian stainless steel auxiliary spring is being used because of its long range of action. A variety of different types of devices may be designed to move the canine to the level of palatal tissue so that it can be more effectively erupted.

apical shift of the dentogingival junction; this can be done most effectively by using a pedicle graft as has been described.

Ankylosis and External Root Resorption

In addition to the surgical procedure and orthodontic management of unerupted teeth, there are other, more perplexing problems with impacted teeth.[54] Most clinicians have been confronted with ankylosis of both deciduous and permanent molars that occur in the primary and transitional dentition. Some permanent teeth that have been exposed to the oral cavity are ankylosed. The most frequent cause of ankylosis is generally believed to be trauma to a tooth. External root resorption is commonly associated with tooth replantation.

Many reports have discussed the possible causative factors associated with ankylosis.[6,21,35,54]

All too often the clinical orthodontist has ordered extraction of teeth, with the expectation of bringing an unerupted tooth into the arch. The unerupted tooth is exposed by the oral surgeon, and later the orthodontist finds that the tooth will not move. After repeated attempts at luxation, with ankylosis returning, the tooth is removed by the surgeon. The statement, "one in the mouth is worth two in the gums" may seem to apply.

A high incidence of tooth ankylosis and external root resorption reportedly has been associated with impacted teeth that have been uncovered and ligated with dead soft stainless steel at the cementoenamel junction area[52,53] (Fig. 13-31, *A* through *I*). This procedure[23] was first reported in

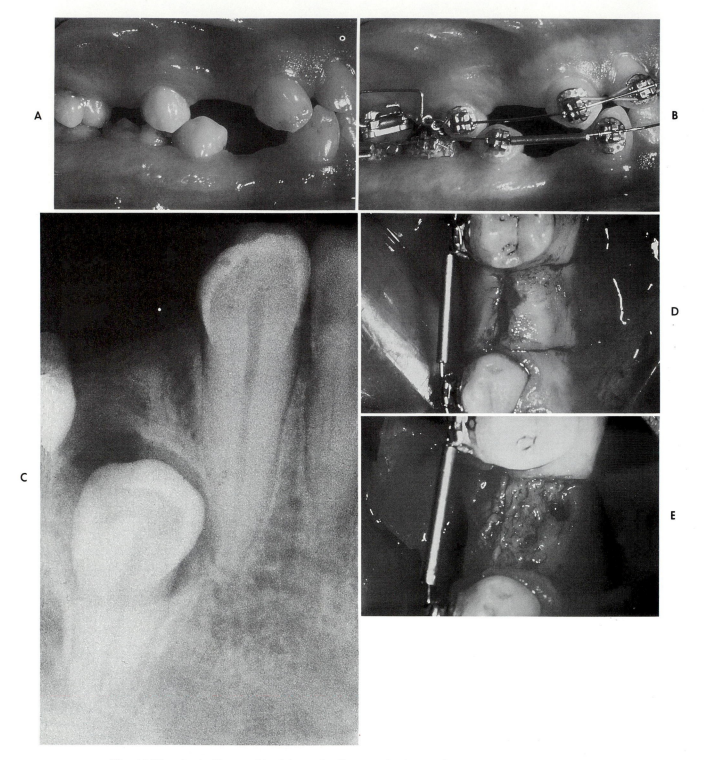

Fig. 13-28 **A,** A 37-year-old adult needs alignment in the maxillary right posterior segment before restorative dentistry. The lower right first premolar is impacted and ankylosed. The patient was advised to have the tooth extracted, but she elected to have orthodontic treatment. **B,** Appliances were placed to align maxillary arch and to allow for immediate orthodontic force to be activated upon the lower premolar, once it was luxated. **C,** Preoperative radiograph of the ankylosed first premolar before it was uncovered. **D,** Initial releasing incisions to mobilize a pedicle graft for the lingual and the facial of the unerupted premolar. **E,** With the tissue reflected it can be seen that the premolar is totally covered by bone.

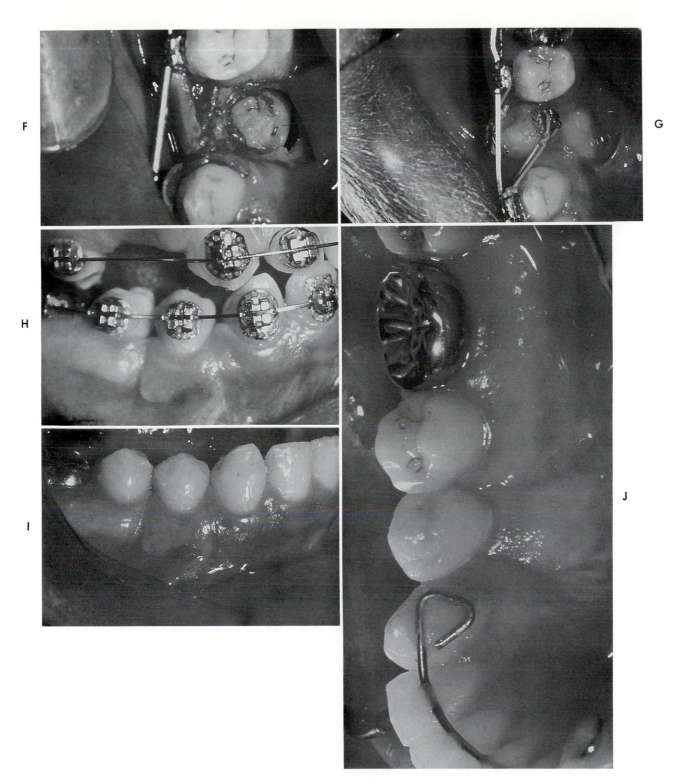

Fig. 13-28, cont'd **F,** Osseous surgery is performed to uncover the tooth, which is located towards the lingual. The tooth is carefully luxated (moved occlusogingivally) until area of fusion is broken. A bonded attachment is placed (bonding would be done only on an ankylosed tooth at the time of surgery) and power thread must be activated within 24 hours and reactivated every 10 days, or it will reankylose. **G,** Two points of attachment are needed to effectively rotate the premolar. **H,** Note that as the tooth moves towards the occlusal plane, the facial gingiva moves with it. **I,** One year after the tooth was positioned into the arch, it had not reankylosed. **J,** On the lingual aspect, observe how more gingiva has been created as the tooth was erupted. When the tissue attaches to the bone and the tooth (as eruption occurs), more gingiva is created. (From Hösl E, Zachrisson BU, Baldauf A, editors: *Orthodontics and periodontics,* Chicago, 1985, Quintessence.)

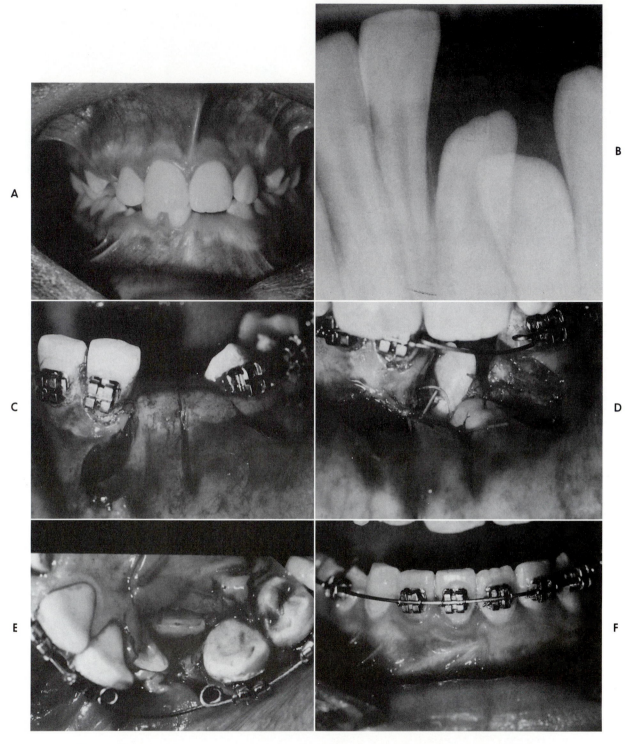

Fig. 13-29 **A,** An 11-year-old female in whom the mandibular left central and lateral incisors will not erupt. **B,** Preoperative radiograph of the unerupted mandibular incisors. **C,** Initial incisions to establish individual pedicle grafts for each incisor on the labial and on the lingual of the two teeth. **D,** The mandibular arch was bonded and the archwire was placed before the surgical procedure. Individual apically positioned pedicle grafts are placed on the labial surface of each incisor. **E,** Occlusal view showing apically positioned pedicle grafts that were placed on the lingual aspect of each mandibular incisor. Margins of grafts are placed on the enamel coronal to the CEJ area. **F,** Observe incisors with grafts attached to the enamel on the left central and lateral incisors exhibiting normal gingival contour. (From Schatz JP, Joho J, editors: *Minor surgery in orthodontics*, Chicago, 1992, Quintessence.)

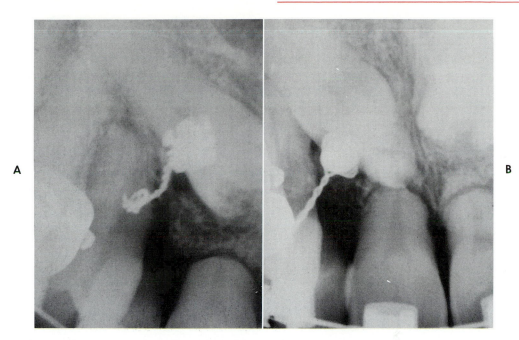

Fig. 13-30   A, Periapical radiograph of a 50-year-old female does not exhibit a well-defined root, and there is no evidence of a periodontal ligament space. Pulp appears to be obliterated. **B,** Both crowns seem to fade or blend into the bone. Note the resorption areas on the anatomical crowns of canine and bonded incisors. This canine is ankylosed and cannot be moved into the arch.

1942 and is still being used today.[2,16] The use of the wire loop has been called the "simplest and most often used means of attachment . . . of an unerupted tooth."[10]

However, it would require an extreme amount of surgical finesse to tighten a wire placed in the cervical third of an impacted tooth and not impinge on the normal cemento-enamel junction (CEJ)-alveolar bone relationship. This form of attachment can cause permanent crestal bone loss at the time the tooth is ligated. In addition, the wire may damage the tooth and act as an irritant on the tooth side of the periodontal ligament space; this could create injury or an environment (in a susceptible patient) that is prone to ankylosis (Fig. 13-31, C through I). Recent studies in periodontal wound healing have clarified the biologic response that allows for replacement resorption and ankylosis. The wire can damage the cells on the tooth side of the periodontal ligament and prevent apical downgrowth of epithelium, which can protect the root against resorption and ankylosis. It is now known that granulation tissue derived from bone induces resorption and ankylosis. Ankylosis, however, always occurs at the crestal area where the wire is positioned. It has been hypothesized that the circumferential destruction of the periodontal ligament extending from the cementum to the bone may be a necessary prerequisite for ankylosis.[3] Several researchers have suggested that ankylosis can occur because of the repopulation of the periodontal ligament from the adjacent bone marrow.[26,29]

The mechanism of injury and ankylosis is becoming better understood[43]; however, there is one common denominator that patients with this problem predictably exhibit—all demonstrate rapid healing clinically. In periodontics, supracrestal external root resorption has been reported to occur when fresh hip marrow with cancellous bone was used as osseous autograft material. The wire loop may also allow inflammation to be established in the area of resorption. The replacement resorption may be arrested by removal of the bone, or the tooth will become extensively resorbed at the crestal area.

Usually, when teeth that exhibit external root resorption are exposed (if one assumes that ankylosis has been allowed to exist for a short period of time), only a small area (1 to 2 mm) will be involved. The bone can be removed with a chisel, and the tooth can be orthodontically positioned into the arch, with continuous force being placed one day after the tooth is uncovered surgically and freed up (Fig. 13-32, A through C). (See Plate 2 p. 724b.) If the force is allowed to dissipate (for any period of time), the tooth may become reankylosed. Once the tooth has been freed from the bone by osseous surgery or luxation (so that the tooth has a vertical component to the mobility), the force must be reactivated every 10 days.

Many teeth that are ankylosed do not have crestal external root resorption or crestal ankylosis that can be seen upon tissue reflection, permitting the ankylosed spot to be removed. These teeth can merely be freed by luxation, and an immediate continuous force can be used to position the tooth orthodontically into the arch. Multirooted molars or canines with dilacerated roots have a poorer prognosis for

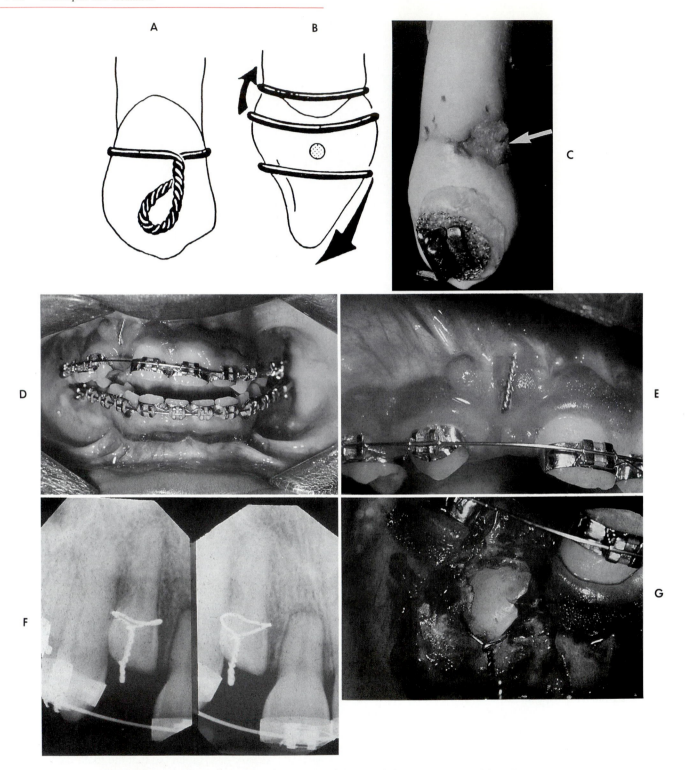

Fig. 13-31 **A,** Diagramatically, the ligature tied around the cementoenamel junction area (if it were to stay above the contact area) will move incisally and come off of the tooth. **B,** When the tooth is ligated below the contact area, it tends to move apically and impinge upon the cementoenamel area to damage the root surface. **C,** An extracted canine from an orthodontic case that was surgically uncovered and ligated with a wire loop. Bone invading the root has spread from the cementoenamel junction area into the root and the anatomic crown. **D,** This 16-year-old female had the lateral incisor uncovered and a wire looped attachment placed by the surgeon; ankylosis occurred. The lateral has caused an open bite by intruding the maxillary arch as wire changes have continued. **E,** Wire that penetrates the alveolar mucosa was tied to the base arch by elastomeric thread. **F,** Observe radiographic appearance of bone invading the root apical to the wire loop. **G,** Upon reflection of the soft tissue, observe the bone over the wire loop and invading the tooth.

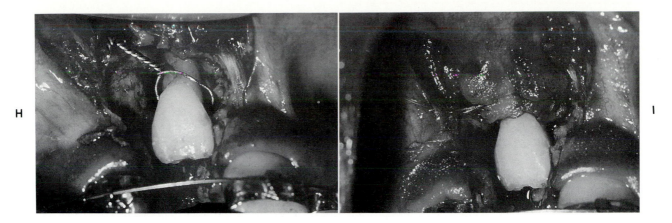

Fig. 13-31, cont'd   H, Osseous surgery is done to create sound tooth structure. All bone attached to the root is removed. **I,** A pedicle graft is placed on the tooth, and the tooth was salvaged.

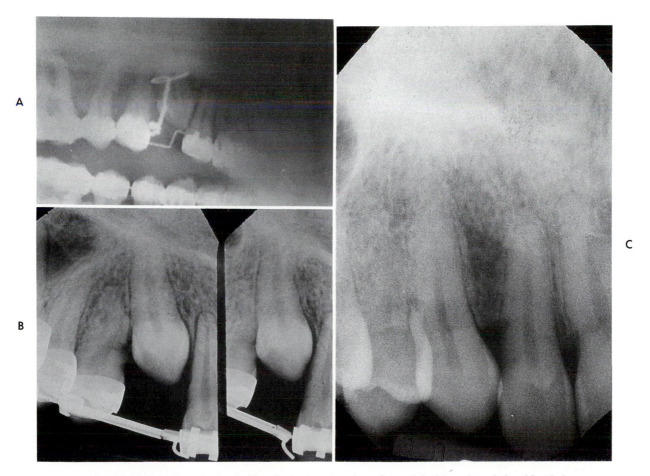

Fig. 13-32   Same patient as in Plate 2. **A,** Anterior view after arch had been intruded and leveled again. **B,** Periapical radiograph at the time the tooth was uncovered. **C,** Periapical radiograph—18 years later.

movement after luxation than normally shaped, single-rooted teeth. Because of crestal replacement resorption or ankylosis, tooth extraction may be prevented by osseous surgery to free it, orthodontic movement into the arch, and reestablishment of a normal anatomic crown for the tooth, using restorative dentistry.

It should be understood that all ectopically positioned or ankylosed teeth cannot be successfully treated. However, a higher percentage of success can be achieved with unerupted teeth by attending normal development, supporting tissue, atraumatic surgery, bonded attachments, control of gingival inflammation, and the use of minimal orthodontic forces.

CONCLUSIONS

No attempt has been made in this chapter to provide a complete discussion of orthodontic and periodontal inter-relationships. The intent has been to highlight frequent problem areas. Gingival retention procedures, management of adult patients, and correction of periodontal problems can be reviewed in Chapter 14. Research information and documented periodontal problems (gathered from clinical observation, clinical trials, animal research, and retrospective analysis) are sufficient to allow the formulation of clinical guidelines for achievement of orthodontic objectives in problem cases; the ultimate objective is that the patient will be better off, rather than not, for treatment. Periodontal problems have not been eliminated for all patients, but significant progress has been made toward prevention of many adverse responses.

Ten percent of adolescents, as well as patients with special problems, and adult patients, will remain a periodontal challenge for the future. The prerequisite for effective orthodontic treatment will be the orthodontist's possession of a periodontal knowledge base sufficient to prevent periodontal injury.

REFERENCES

1. Ahrens DG, Shapiro Y, Kuftinec M: An approach to rotational relapse, *Am J Orthod* 80:83, 1981.
2. Alling CC: Impacted canine teeth, *Dent Clin North Am* 23:446-447, 1979.
3. Atrizodeh F, Kennedy J, Zander H: Ankylosis of teeth following thermal injury, *J Periodont Res* 6:159, 1971.
4. Baer PN: The case for periodontosis as a clinical entity, *J Periodontol* 42:516, 1971.
5. Baumrind S, Korn EL: Transverse development of human jaws between the ages of 8.5 and 15.5 years, studied longitudinally with use of implants, *J Dent Res* 69:6, 1298-1306, 1990.
6. Biederman W: The ankylosed tooth, *Dent Clin North Am* 493-508, 1964.
7. Bjørk A: Growth of the maxilla in three dimensions as revealed radiographically by the implant method, *Br J Orthod* 4:53-64, 1975.
8. Boughman JA, Astemboski FA, Blitzer MG: Early-onset periodontal disease: a genetics perspective, *Crit Rev Oral Biol Med* 1:89, 1990.
9. Brown IS: Effect of orthodontic therapy on periodontal defects, *J Periodontol* 44:742, 1973.
10. Buchanan G: Surgical intervention as an aid to orthodontics, *Ann Austral Col Dent Surg* 1:73, 1967.
11. Cimasoni G: *Crevicular fluid updated*. In Myers HM, editor: *Monographs in oral science*, vol 12, Basel, Switzerland, 1983, S. Karger.
12. Edwards JG: A surgical procedure to eliminate rotational relapse, *Am J Orthod* 57:35, 1970.
13. Ericsson I, Thilander B et al: The effect of orthodontic tilting movements on the periodontal tissues of infected and non-infected dentitions in dogs, *J Clin Periodontol* 4:278-293, 1977.
14. Geiger AM: *Gingival response to orthodontic treatment*. In McNamara JA, Ribbens KA, editors: *Malocclusion and the periodontium*, Monograph 15, Craniofacial growth series, Ann Arbor, 1984, Center for Human Growth and Development, The University of Michigan.
14a. Genco RJ, Loe H: *The role of systemic conditions and disorders in periodontal disease: Periodontology 2000*, vol 2, Copenhagen, 1993, Munksgaard.
15. Geraci TF: Orthodontic movements of teeth into artificially produced infrabony defects in the rhesus monkey: a histological report, *J Periodontol* 44-116, 1973.
16. Goodsell JF: Surgical exposure and orthodontic guidance of the impacted tooth, *Dent Clin North Am* 23:386-387, 1979.
17. Greenstein G: The role of bleeding upon probing in the diagnosis of periodontal disease: a literature review, *J Periodontol* 55:684, 1984.
17a. Grossi SG et al: Evaluation of risk indicators for periodontal disease, *J Periodont* (in press).
18. Ingber JS: Forced eruption: a method of treated one- and two-wall infrabony osseous defects-rationale and case report, *J Periodontol* 45:199, 1974.
19. Jacobsen L: Mouth breathing and gingivitis, *J Periodont Res* 8:269, 1973.
20. Krebs A: Midpalatal suture expansion studied by the implant method over a seven year period, *Trans Eur Orthod Soc* 40:131-142, 1964.
21. Kronfeld R: *Bony union (ankylosis) of roots and alveolus*. In: *Histopathology of the teeth and their surrounding structures*, ed 2, Philadelphia, 1939, Lea & Febiger.
22. Leggott PJ, Robertson PB et al: Oral manifestations of primary and acquired immunodeficiency diseases in children, *Pediatr Dent* 9:98-104, 1987.
23. Leslie SW: A new method of treating unerupted teeth by means of surgery and orthodontia, *J Can Dent Assoc* 8:364-369, 1942.
24. Lindhe J: *Clinical periodontology*, ed 2, Munksgaard, Copenhagen, 1989,
25. Lindhe J, Svanberg G: Influences of trauma from occlusions on progression of experimental periodontitis in the beagle dog, *J Clin Periodontol* 1:3-14, 1974.
26. Line SE, Polson A, Zander HA: Relationship between periodontal injury selective cell repopulation and ankylosis, *J Periodontol* 45:725, 1974.
27. Loe H, Anerud A et al: Natural history of periodontal disease in man: rapid, moderate, and no loss of attachment in Sri Lankan laborers, 14 to 46 years of age, *J Clin Periodontol* 13:431, 1986.
28. Marks MH, Corn H: *Atlas of adult orthodontics*, Philadelphia, 1989, Lea & Febiger, pp. 134-135.
29. Melcher AH: Repair of wounds in the periodontium of the rat: influence of periodontal ligament on osteogenesis, *Arch Oral Biol* 15:1183, 1970.
30. Melsen B: Tissue reaction following application of extrusion and intrusive forces to teeth in adult monkeys, *Am J Orthod Dentofac Orthop* 89:469-475, 1986.
31. Melsen B, Agerbaek N, Markenstam G: Intrusion of incisors in adult patients with marginal bone loss, *Am J Orthod Dentofac Orthop* 96:232-241, 1989.
32. Miller AJ, Brunelle JA et al: *Oral health of United States adults*, NIH publication No. 97-2868, Bethesda, Maryland, 1987, National Institute of Dental Research.
33. Morenzi V: "Assessment of the effects of orthodontic molar uprighting on the microflora of human adult periodontal tissues using recombinant DNA technology." Unpublished thesis, Philadelphia, 1989, University of Pennsylvania.
34. Nevins M, Becker W, Kornman K, editors: *Proceedings of the world*

workshop in clinical periodontics, Chicago, 1989, American Academy of Periodontology.

35. Noyes FB: "Submerging" deciduous molars, *Angle Orthod* 2:77, 1932.

36. Page RC, Altman LC, Ebersole JL et al: Rapidly progressive periodontitis: a distinct clinical condition, *J Periodontol* 54:197, 1983.

37. Pihlstrom B: Prevention and treatment of dilantin-associated gingival enlargement, *Compend-Cont Educ Dent* 14:506, 1990.

38. Polsen A, Caton J et al: Periodontal response after tooth movement into infrabony defects, *J Periodontol* 55:197-202, 1984.

39. Reitan K: Tissue reaction as related to the age factor, *Dent Rec* 74:271-279, 1954.

40. Riedel RA: Retention and relapse, *J Clin Orthod* 10:454-472, 1976.

41. Rygh P: The periodontal ligament under stress. In Norton LA, Burstone CJ, editors: *The biology of tooth movement,* Boca Raton, Florida, 1989, CRC Press, pp. 9-27.

42. Seibert J: In Robinsin P, Guernsey L, editors: *Clinical transplantation in dental specialties,* St Louis, 1980, Mosby, p. 131.

43. Sirirat M: Potentials for root resorption during periodontal wound healing, *J Clin Periodontol* 11:41-52, 1984.

44. Steiner GG, Pearson JK, Aincomo J: Changes in the marginal periodontum as a result of labial tooth movement in monkeys, *J Periodontol* 52:314-320, 1981.

45. Stenvik A, Mjör I: Pulp and denture reactions to experimental tooth intrusion, *Am J Orthod* 57:370-385, 1976.

46. Stepovich ML: A clinical study on closing edentulous spaces in the mandible, *Angle Orthod* 49:227, 1979.

47. Socransky SS: Microbiology of periodontal disease: present status and future considerations, *J Periodontol* 48:497, 1977.

48. Socransky SS: Haffajee AD et al: New concepts of destructive periodontal disease, *J Clin Periodontol* 11:21, 1984.

49. Sooriyamoorthy M, Gower DB: Hormonal influences on gingival tissue: relationship to periodontal disease, *J Clin Periodontol* 16:201, 1989.

50. Sweeney EA, Alcoforado GAP et al: Prevalence and microbiology of localized prepubertal periodontitis, *Oral Microbiol Immunol* 2:71, 1987.

51. Vanarsdall RL: *Periodontal considerations in corrective orthodontics.* In Clark JW, editor: *Clinical dentistry,* vol 2, Hagerstown, Md, 1978, Harper & Row.

52. Vanarsdall RL: *Periodontal problems associated with orthodontic treatment,* Annual Conference on Orthodontics, Philadelphia, May 1978, University of Pennsylvania.

53. Vanarsdall RL: *Management of ankylosed teeth,* Special Interest Clinics, American Association of Orthodontists annual session, Washington, DC, May 5, 1979.

54. Vanarsdall RL: *Periodontal problems associated with orthodontic treatment.* In Barrer H, editor: *Orthodontics: the state of the art,* Philadelphia, 1981, University of Pennsylvania Press.

55. Vanarsdall RL: La Reaction Des Tissus Parodontaux Aux Movements Orthodontiquic, *L'Orthodont Francaise, Orthodontic De L'adulte, S.I.D., Vanves* 57:421-433, 1986.

56. Vanarsdall RL, Corn H: Soft-tissue management of labially positioned unerupted teeth, *Am J Orthod* 72:53-64, 1977.

57. Vanarsdall R, Hamlin J: "The effects of molar uprighting on the microbiological flora of the periodontium." Unpublished thesis. Philadelphia, 1987, University of Pennsylvania.

58. Vanarsdall RL, Herberger TA: "Rapid palatal expansion: long-term stability and periodontal implications." Unpublished thesis. Philadelphia, 1987, University of Pennsylvania.

59. VanVenroy J, Vanarsdall RL: Eruption: correlation of histologic and radiographic findings in the animal model with clinical and radiographic findings in humans, *Int J Adult Orthod Orthognath Surg* 235-247, 1987.

60. VanVenroy JR, Yukna RA: Orthodontic extrusion of single-rooted teeth affected with advanced periodontal disease, *Am J Orthod* 67:74, 1985.

61. Waerhaug J: The infrabony pocket and its relationship to trauma from occlusion and subgingival plaque, *J Periodontol* 50:355-365, 1979.

62. Wennström JL, Lindhe J: Plaque-induced gingival inflammation in the absence of attached gingiva in dogs, *J Clin Periodontol* 10:266-276, 1983.

63. Wennström JL, Lindhe J: The role of attached gingiva for maintenance of periodontal health. Healing following excisional and grafting procedures in dogs, *J Clin Periodontol* 10:206-226, 1983.

64. Wennström JL, Lindhe J et al: Some periodontal tissue reactions to orthodontic tooth movement in monkeys, *J Clin Periodontol* 14:121-129, 1987.

65. Wennström J, Stokland BL et al: Periodontal tissue response to orthodontic movement of teeth with infrabony pockets, *Am J Orthod Dentofac Orthop* 103:313-319, 1993.

66. Wise RJ, Kramer GM: Predetermination of osseous changes associated with uprighting tipped molars by probing, *Int J Periodontol Rest Dent* 3:69, 1983.

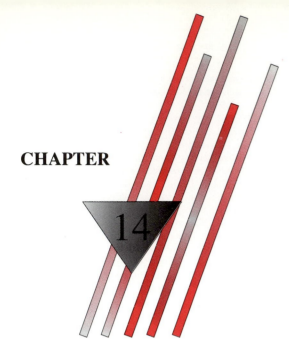

Adult Orthodontics: Diagnosis and Treatment

ROBERT L. VANARSDALL
DAVID R. MUSICH

CHAPTER

14

PURPOSES OF THIS CHAPTER

1. To discuss how the continued increase of adult patients into modern orthodontic practices has altered the scope of orthodontic treatment procedures
2. To define specific orthodontic treatment objectives that apply to adult patients and require careful consideration throughout their treatment
3. To identify diagnostic considerations that are particularly important in the clarification of adult patients' orthodontic problems
4. To describe factors in treatment planning that differentiate adolescents from adults
5. To describe methods of adult patient management that clinicians can incorporate into their practices to enhance their success rate in the treatment of adults
6. To introduce a classification system of adult case types that will enable the clinician to focus on the patient's major treatment needs rather than to be limited by the traditional morphological classification system
7. To demonstrate the usefulness of this classification system and present examples of successfully treated patients
8. To present the concept of treatment sequencing and to explain why proper sequencing in adult patients is fundamental to achieving desired goals
9. To discuss adult retention measures and to describe the indications for variations of the *basic* retention protocols.

HISTORY OF ADULT PATIENTS IN ORTHODONTIC PRACTICES

In 1880 Kingsley indicated an early awareness of the orthodontic potential for adult patients. After the treatment of a 40-year-old patient for an anterior crossbite prior to restorative dentistry, he stated:

It may be regarded as settled that there are hardly any limits to the age when movement of teeth might not succeed.

Kingsley also pointed out that some differences existed between tooth movement in adolescent patients and tooth movement in older patients:

But at 17, 18, and 19, the action is slower, growing more and more difficult, and in cases where a considerable number of teeth are to be moved, the results become more and more doubtful with advancing years.

Although benefits of orthodontic treatment for adult patients were demonstrated as early as the turn of the century, the published statements regarding adult orthodontic treatment were mostly negative. Significant caution and even avoidance of adult orthodontic therapy were often recommended. In 1901 MacDowell[61] wrote:

Impossible Age. After the age of 16 years, a complete and permanent change in transition of the occlusion the author believes to be almost impossible. There may be a case or two of rare exceptions, but as a rule the change cannot be accomplished successfully owing to the development of the adult glenoid fossa and the density of the bones and muscles of mastication.

In 1912 Lischer[58] summarized the contemporary (at the turn of the century) orthodontic view regarding the optimal age for treatment:

Recent experiences of many practitioners have led us to a keener appreciation of the "golden age of treatment," by which we mean that time in an individual's life when a change from the temporary to the permanent dentition takes place. This covers the period from the sixth to the fourteenth year.

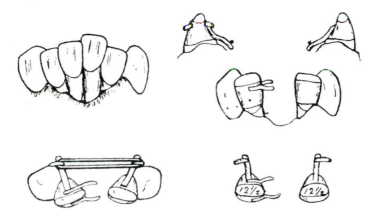

Fig. 14-1 Schematic illustration of an adult treated by Dr. Case because of mandibular crowding and periodontal disease. Case's illustration also shows a carefully designed appliance for bodily space closure after the removal of diseased teeth.

However, not all authorities in the early 1900s were negative when they discussed orthodontic therapy for adult patients. In 1921 Case demonstrated that value of orthodontic therapy for a patient with *pyorrhea* in the lower anterior area. Because of the significant advancement of periodontal disease, treatment required extraction of the two lower central incisors. In his text Case showed an appliance that he had designed to close the extraction space and he made the following statement (Fig. 14-1):

The space was closed with the apparatus, as shown, and the disease was completely eradicated and terminated in the most satisfactory restoration of the surrounding tissues. This case is a fair illustration of many similar cases older than forty years which were corrected with equal success in the author's practice.

Since there were so few orthodontists in the early 1900s and so many adolescents who could benefit from the orthodontic therapy available at the time, it is understandable that there was little tendency to encourage treatment of the more complicated and demanding adult group. For these reasons, as well as a variety of other influential factors, growth and development became the principal area of clinical activity and research for the orthodontic specialist. It is conceivable also that the emphasis on treatment involving craniofacial growth and development delayed the study of treatment problems specifically related to the slow-growing adult patient group. As a result the emergence of orthodontic treatment for the adult patient was delayed.

In the past two decades, however, a major reorientation of orthodontic thinking has occurred regarding adult patients. The following list cites several reasons for the increased interest by orthodontists in the adult as a patient, as well as several reasons for increased interest shown by adults in orthodontic treatment.

1. Improved appliance placement techniques[28,31,39,102]
2. More sophisticated and successful management of the symptoms associated with joint dysfunction[4,69,87,100]
3. More effective management of skeletal jaw dysplasias, using advanced orthognathic surgical techniques[12,81]
4. Increased desire of patients and restorative dentists for treatment of *dental mutilation* problems, using tooth movement and fixed restorations rather than removable prostheses[8,68]
5. Reduced vulnerability to periodontal breakdown as a result of improved tooth relationships and occlusal function[42,79]

In 1971 Lindegaard et al[57] stated that three main factors determine which problems should be treated from both a medical and an orthodontic point of view:

1. A disease or abnormality must be present.
2. The need for treatment must be understood; this need for treatment should be determined by the clinical gravity of the disorder, the available resources for orthodontic care, the prognosis for successful treatment, and the priority for orthodontic care based on personal and professional judgment.
3. In addition to the above factors, the patient must have a strong desire for treatment.

In this context, the past 20 years have seen a major change in orthodontic practices. The demand for orthodontic services by the 12-year-old population has decreased. Proportionately, however, changed lifestyles and patient awareness have increased the demand for adult orthodontic treatment, and multidisciplinary dental therapy has allowed better management of the more complicated and unique requirements of the adult patient population, thereby greatly improving quality of care and treatment prognosis. Department chairmen of several teaching institutions participating in a round table discussion concerning the future of orthodontics[16] made significant statements regarding adult orthodontic therapy. At this conference in 1976, Reidel and Dougherty most accurately predicted the current status of adult orthodontic treatment today. Reidel was supportive regarding the future of adult therapy, adding that the clinician should not forget adjunctive orthodontic services provided by peri-

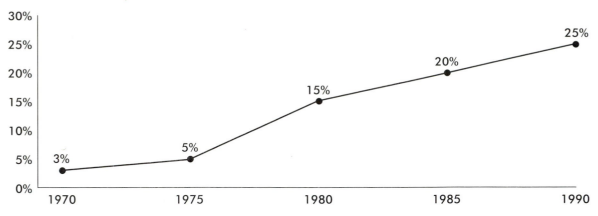

Fig. 14-2   The percentage of adult patients who have received orthodontic treatment has increased significantly in the last two decades. This graph illustrates an 800% increase of adult patients having orthodontic treatment from 1970 to 1990.

odontists and restorative dentists. Dougherty claimed that "orthodontics is total discipline and it makes no difference whether the patient is young or old."

Adult Practice Today

In addition to the recent improvements in treatment techniques and the recent changes in treatment philosophies, there have been important statistical reasons for orthodontists to become more involved in the management of the adult patient (Fig. 14-2).

There is a decline in the average share of the adolescent orthodontic market, owing to an increase in the number of orthodontists and nonorthodontists who are doing orthodontics, combined with a relatively static number of annual births.

Practices that grew, reported a higher percentage of adult patients than those that didn't grow. Treatment of adults was rated significantly higher as a practice-building method by growing practices than by declining practices.

SCOPE OF PROCEDURES

As the volume (percentage) of adult patients increased in orthodontic practices, the skills required of the orthodontist changed. Musich's 1986 paper demonstrated the scope of treatment planning considerations (Fig. 14-3). Of the almost 1400 consecutively examined adults in Musich's study, almost 30% of the sample required multidisciplinary management to attain optimal treatment outcomes.

When treating adults, the orthodontist needs to be prepared to do the following:
1. Diagnose different stages of periodontal disease and their associated risk factors
2. Diagnose TMJ dysfunction before, during, or after tooth movement

3. Determine which cases require surgical management and which ones require incisor re-angulation to camouflage the skeletal base discrepancy
4. Work co-operatively with a team of other specialists to give the patient the best outcome

Other sections of this chapter will describe more completely the appropriate methods required to fulfill the above responsibilities for our adult patient group.

Adult Orthodontic Treatment Objectives

The traditional adolescent orthodontic treatment objectives of (1) dentofacial esthetics; (2) stomatognathic function; (3) stability; and (4) static and dynamic Class I occlusion often may not be realistic or necessary for all adult patients. Treatment in which adolescent goals are not achieved is not necessarily compromised; rather the mechanotherapy should satisfy the objective of providing the minimal dental manipulation appropriate for the individual case. Many of the Class I occlusal goals can be considered overtreatment for patients who also require restorative dentistry, prosthetics, plastic surgery, or other multidisciplinary dentofacial corrections.

The following is a list of additional objectives particularly useful for adult problems requiring tooth replacement but not requiring surgical skeletal correction. While it is clear that the correction of severe dentofacial skeletal problems calls for a multidisciplinary solution; not every adult with mild or moderate skeletal Class I, Class II, or Class III disharmony will need to undergo orthognathic surgery.
1. Parallelism of abutment teeth
2. Most favorable distribution of teeth
   a. Intra-arch
   b. Inter-arch
3. Redistribution and redirection of occlusal and incisal forces

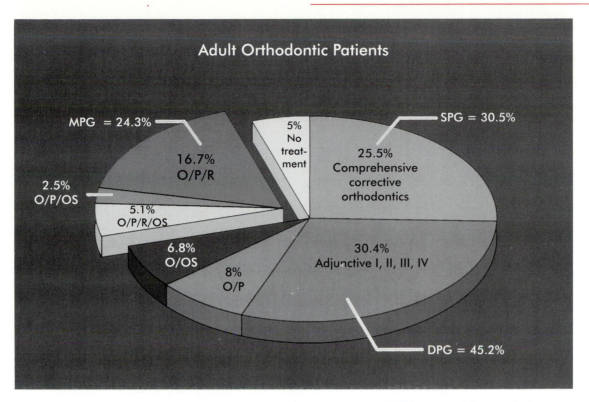

Fig. 14-3   A summary diagram of findings from Musich's study of 1370 consecutively examined adults:

    30.5%—Solo provider group (SPG)—25.5% required conventional corrective orthodontics.

    45.2%—Dual provider group (DPG)—within this group two primary providers were required to complete the treatment:

Orthodontist/restorative (O/R)	30.4%
Orthodontist/periodontist (O/P)	8.0%
Orthodontist/oral surgeon (O/OS)	6.8%

    24.3%—Multiple provider group (MPG)

    Note: 5% required no orthodontic treatment, and 65% required dual or multiple provider therapy.

4. Adequate embrasure space and proper tooth position
5. Acceptable occlusal plane and potential for incisal guidance at satisfactory vertical dimension
6. Adequate occlusal landmark relationships
7. Improved lip competency and support
8. Improved crown/root ratio
9. Improvement or correction of mucogingival and osseous defects
10. Better self-maintenance of periodontal health
11. Esthetic and functional improvement
12. Attainment of traditional orthodontic treatment objectives

Parallelism of abutment teeth. The abutment teeth must be placed parallel with the other teeth to permit insertion of multiple unit replacements and to allow for restorations that involve both anterior and posterior teeth. A restoration will have a better prognosis if the abutment teeth are parallel before tooth preparation,[26] since that will avoid excess cutting or devitalization during abutment preparation and also allow for a better periodontal response. For full arch splints,

the posterior teeth should be reasonably parallel to anterior abutments. Parallel abutments allow for better restorative retention and help prevent cement washout and caries (Fig. 14-4).

Most favorable distribution of teeth. The teeth should be distributed evenly for replacement of fixed and removable prostheses in the individual arches (Fig. 14-5). In addition, they should be positioned so that occlusion of natural teeth can be established bilaterally between arches.[9]

Redistribution of occlusal and incisal forces. Cases with significant bone loss (60% to 70%) require that occlusal forces be directed vertically along or on the long axis of the roots to maintain the occlusal vertical dimension (Fig. 14-6). When the posterior teeth are missing, the anterior teeth can be positioned to allow for more axially directed transfer of force, and can then be reshaped to function as posterior teeth (supporting the vertical dimension).[9]

Adequate embrasure space and proper root position. This allows for better periodontal health especially when the placement of restorations is necessary (Fig. 14-7). The anatomic relation of the roots is important in the pathogen-

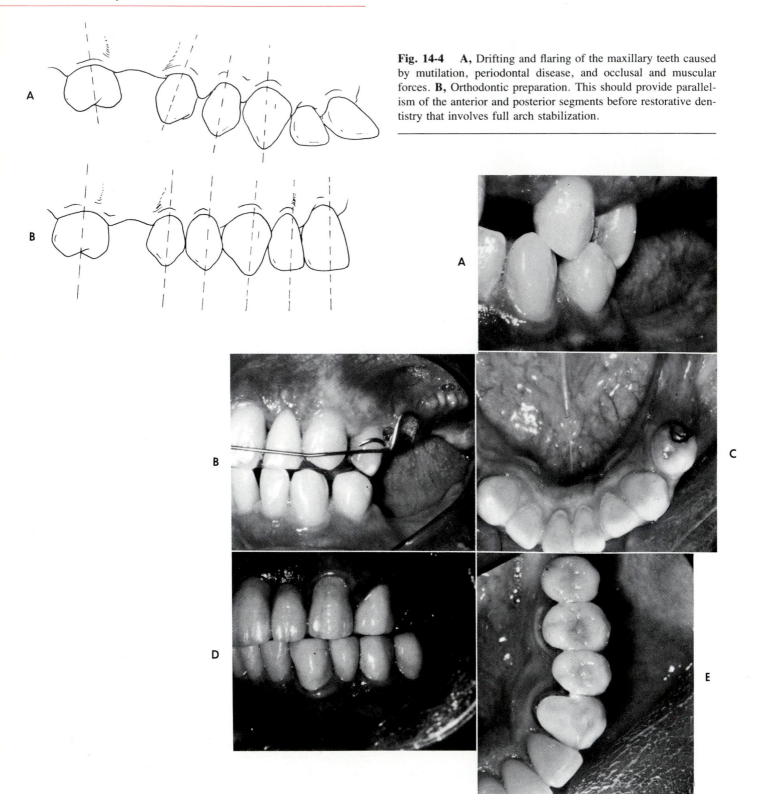

Fig. 14-4   **A,** Drifting and flaring of the maxillary teeth caused by mutilation, periodontal disease, and occlusal and muscular forces. **B,** Orthodontic preparation. This should provide parallelism of the anterior and posterior segments before restorative dentistry that involves full arch stabilization.

Fig. 14-5   **A,** First premolars; the only teeth present in the left maxillary and mandibular quadrants of a 56-year-old black man. **B,** A combination of fixed and removable appliances was used to move the mandibular first premolar one pontic space distally in the left quadrant. **C,** Preoperative. Note the lower left first premolar adjacent to the canine. **D,** Final restoration. Distal movement of the first premolar abutment created a pontic space between the canine and the distal premolar abutment. **E,** Better distribution of abutments allowed for this lower left four-unit restoration, preventing the need for a distal extension partial denture or implants.

esis of periodontal disease,[82] interproximal cleaning, or placement of restorative materials.[74]

Acceptable occlusal plane and potential for incisal guidance at satisfactory vertical dimension. To establish the acceptable occlusal plane for a mutilated dentition exhibiting bite collapse, the Hawley bite plane (Fig. 14-8) is usually inserted with the platform of the anterior plane adjusted at a right angle to the long axis of the lower incisors.[8] This allows for the location of centric relation at an acceptable vertical relationship.

Even with extended platforms in Class II patterns, patients can usually speak well. However, if the vertical dimension is excessive, they will whistle involuntarily and complain of muscle fatigue in the morning or the acrylic will develop etched lines or wear streaks. When properly adjusted at the correct vertical height, there will be simultaneous bilateral neuromuscular activity. Be sure that no contact occurs between the posterior teeth during excursive movements and no interferences between anterior teeth while on the bite plane. Such interferences will prevent the patient from dem-

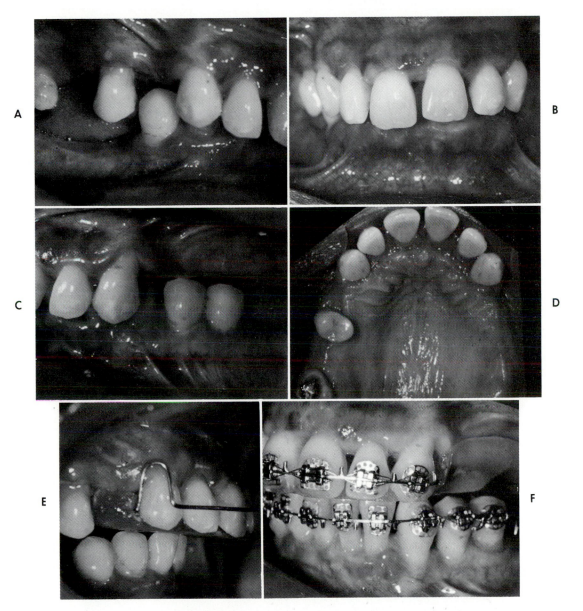

Fig. 14-6   **A,** No natural tooth stops in a 45-year-old black woman. The initial tooth contact in centric relation was between the mandibular first premolar and the maxillary second premolar. **B,** Anteriorly, the mandible fits within the maxillary arch. **C,** No tooth contact on the left side. **D,** Soft tissue indentations indicate the location of lower incisor contact with the palate. **E,** Severe maxillary protrusion. A Hawley bite plane was used to locate centric relation at the acceptable vertical. **F,** After maxillary and mandibular alignment a splint was placed before maxillary segmental osteotomy. The osteotomy positioned the maxillary canines axially to contact the lower dentition bilaterally.   *Continued.*

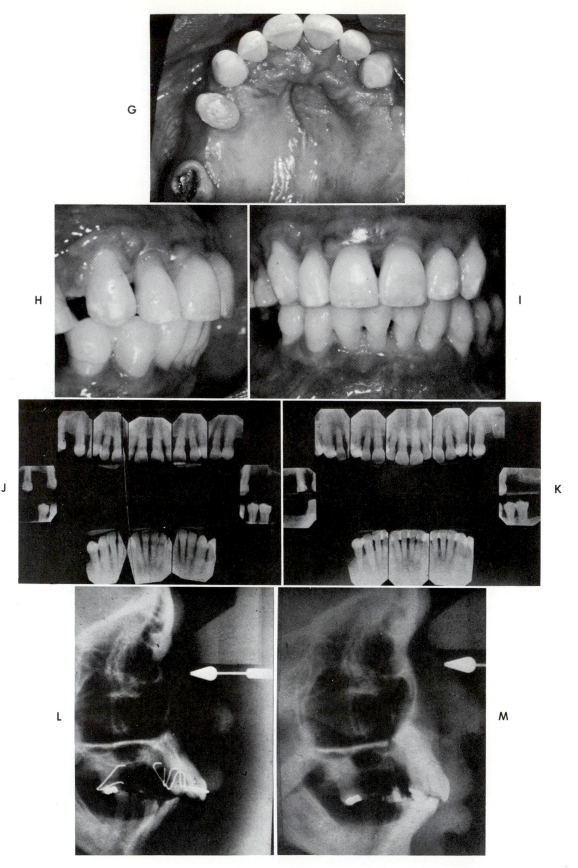

Fig. 14-6, cont'd **G,** After surgery, occlusal platforms placed on the maxillary canines support the vertical dimension. **H,** Three-year post-treatment. **I,** Lower anteriors bonded with composite resin as a form of retention. **J,** Pretreatment. **K,** Three-year post-treatment. **L,** Pretreatment cephalogram. Acceptable vertical dimension. **M,** One-year post-treatment.

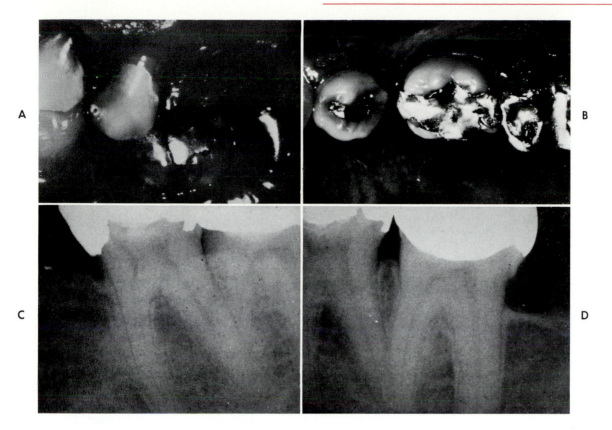

Fig. 14-7   A, Note the collapse of the lower left first and second molars into the second premolar space. **B,** Occlusolingual view. **C,** Inadequate embrasure and root proximity. **D,** Distal view. Poor root position that should be corrected before restorative dentistry.

onstrating simultaneous bilateral neuromuscular activity and correct location of centric relation.

The curve of Spee should be mild to flat bilaterally. This is difficult to achieve if supraerupted molars are present. However, the most extruded posterior segment will be the ruling factor in determining the potential for an orthodontic solution at an acceptable vertical. Adult molars with amalgam restorations and with normal pulpal recession, adult molars often can be occlusally reduced 2 to 4 mm and still allow for placement of restorations without the need for devitalization. With the aid of heavy musculature, molars may be intruded 1 to 2 mm in treatment. The unilateral orthodontic treatment of an accentuated occlusal plane should be avoided; one side cannot be left extruded.

Adequate occlusal landmark relationships. As previously described for adult patients, the transverse dimension is the most difficult to correct and maintain orthodontically, the sagittal next, and the vertical least. However, when teeth are to be restored, they must be positioned to achieve acceptable buccolingual landmarks. Posterior crossbites involving severe transverse skeletal dysplasias that are not to undergo surgery should be positioned so that the maxillary buccal cusps contact the lower central fossae with the crossover for incisal guidance in the premolar area or the canine positions (Fig. 14-9).

Better lip competency and support. Many adults have long upper lips that preclude significant maxillary retraction. In cases requiring anterior restorations, retraction should be done to achieve lip competency while maintaining lip support. The restoration then can be shaped to provide incisal guidance on the canines or by 1 or 2 mm palatal extension of the incisors. Incisors extended more than 1 or 2 mm palatally will cause constant palatal soft tissue irritation. In some of Class II, division 1 cases (when orthognathic surgery is rejected) the lower incisors can be advanced into a more procumbent position than the usual orthodontic norm to establish incisal guidance. With the aid of bilateral posterior restorations, the incisors will be stabilized when in relatively flared positions (IMPA 105° to 120°[2]). In some Class III patients as well, the maxillary incisors can be kept in stable relation (even though more flared than normal) with posterior restorations. Adults usually are anxious about changes of the upper lip. Inadequate support may create a change of anteroposterior and vertical position of the upper lip and increase wrinkling. This often makes the face seem prematurely aged and is a major esthetic concern of adults, especially women.

Improved crown/root ratio. In adult patients who have lost bone on individual teeth, the length of the clinical crown can be reduced with the high speed handpiece; and as the

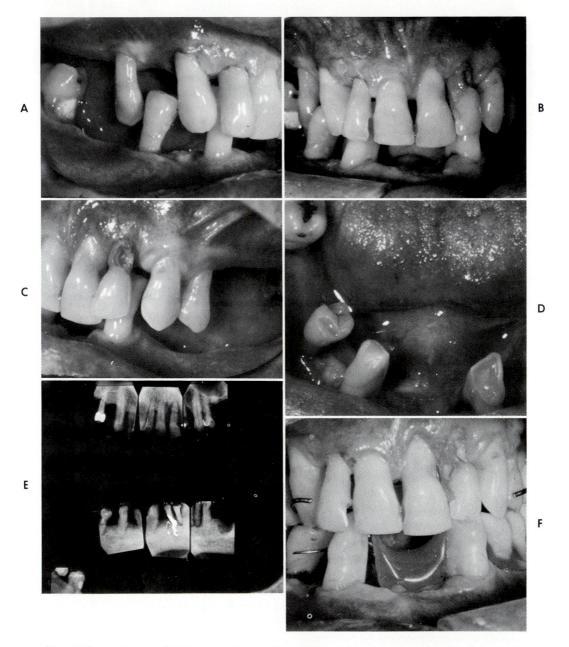

Fig. 14-8 **A** through **C,** No occlusal stops bilaterally in a 61-year-old patient. The lower right premolar had only soft tissue attachment. **D,** Lower canines tipped lingually and mobile. **E,** Preoperative. **F,** Upper and lower removable appliances placed to support the vertical height and move each lower canine labially over its basal support.

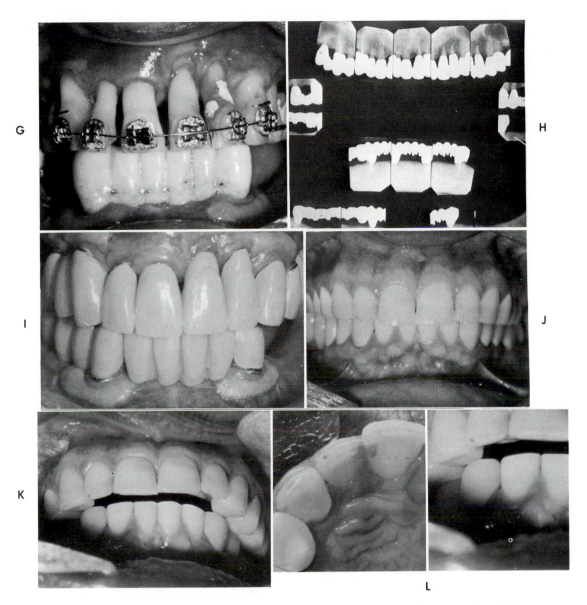

Fig. 14-8, cont'd   **G,** Once the lower canines were axially positioned, the restorative dentist (Dan Casullo, Philadelphia) placed a provisional restoration. A platform was then added to the upper appliance (to determine the satisfactory vertical) and the maxillary incisors were aligned. **H,** Seven-year postoperative. **I,** Final restoration. **J,** Severe Class II in another patient. Orthognathic surgery was refused. The long upper lip precluded maxillary retraction. Note the mild curve of Spee. **K,** Posterior segments aligned. Composite restorative material providing incisal guidance. **L,** Note the canine buildup, allowing for Bennett movement. (*I* through *L* courtesy Dan Casullo.)

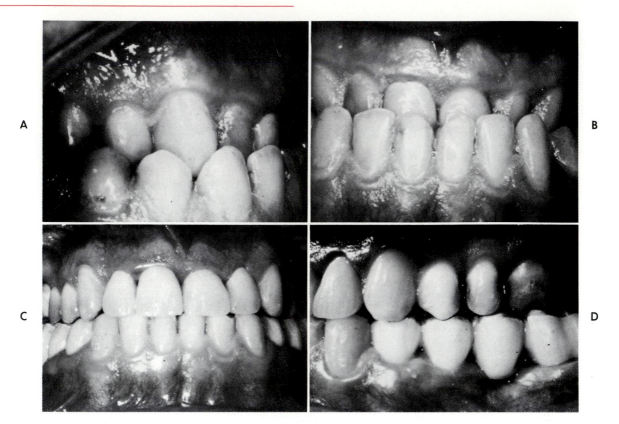

Fig. 14-9 **A** and **B,** Class III with severe transverse skeletal discrepancy. Required lower posterior reconstruction. **C,** The anterior segment could be positioned normally to provide incisal guidance. The posterior occlusion was left in crossbite because of the maxillary transverse deficiency. **D,** Note the occlusal scheme. Allows the crossbite to occur in the premolar area.

tooth is erupted orthodontically (the same amount of bone will remain on the clinical root), the ratio of crown-to-root will be improved.[40,41,42]

Improvement or correction of mucogingival and osseous defects. Proper repositioning of prominent teeth in the arch will improve gingival topography (Fig. 14-10, *A* and *B*). In adolescents the brackets are placed to level marginal ridges and cusp tips. In adults the goal should be to level the crestal bone between adjacent cementoenamel junctions (Fig. 14-10, *C* to *H*). It has been demonstrated that the need for osseous and mucogingival surgery may be diminished by favorable changes of the osseous and soft tissue topography during tooth movement. Therefore, attachments should be placed on individual teeth to allow the leveling of the attachment apparatus. This will create more physiologic osseous architecture with the potential to correct certain osseous defects.[93] During leveling stages any teeth that have erupted above the occlusal plane should be grossly reduced occlusally. Also continuous adjustment should be done to prevent the patient from contacting individual posterior teeth prematurely and causing occlusal trauma.

Better self-maintenance of periodontal health. The location of the gingival margin is determined by axial inclination and alignment of the tooth. Clinically it appears that

there is improved self-maintenance of periodontal health with proper tooth position.[67,69,70] This can be seen in adult patients during correction of bite collapse and accelerated mesial drift (Fig. 14-11).

Patients who need weekly periodontal maintenance during initial leveling phases of therapy may require less frequent scaling and root planing as periodontal status improves. Poor tooth position and improper tooth preparation before irreversible restorative dentistry are local causative factors that may be contributory to periodontal disease. For better periodontal health on an individual pattern basis, teeth should be placed properly over their basal bone support. In the nonsurgical management of skeletal Class III and Class II malocclusions, there is a delicate balance between periodontally desirable tooth positions and achievement of other nonsurgical treatment objectives.

Esthetic and functional improvement. As stated previously, a plan should provide acceptable dentofacial esthetics and allow for improved muscle function, normal speech, and masticatory improvements. This is possible when a therapeutic occlusion is provided that enables the anterior teeth to function as disarticulators and the posterior teeth to support the vertical dimension.[8]

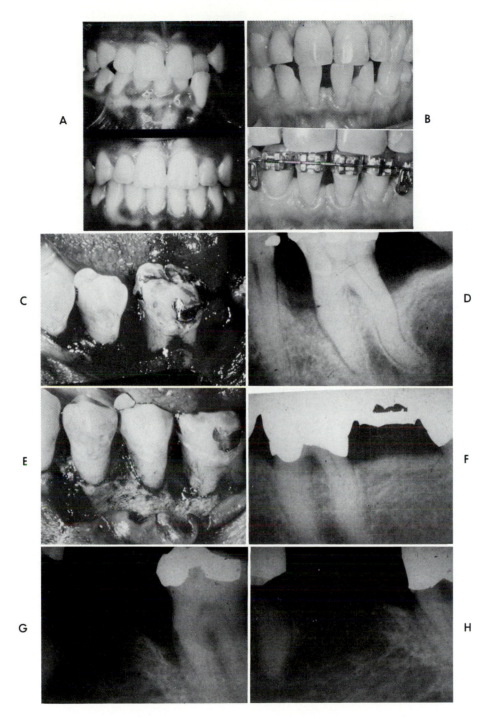

Fig. 14-10 **A,** Before correction of an incisor crossbite. Note the normal gingival position on the labially displaced lower left lateral incisor in a 14-year-old patient. After lower incisor alignment the gingival margins were confluent. **B,** Narrow zone of attached gingiva in a 61-year-old patient. As the lower incisors were retracted and allowed to erupt, more gingiva was created incisogingivally. **C,** Gingival tissue reflected for root surface preparation. Note the large osseous defect in the lower left molar before tooth movement in a 38-year-old patient. **D,** First molar before control of inflammation, occlusal rest, and tooth movement. **E,** New bone formation 3 months after tooth movement and stabilization. **F,** Ten-year postoperative. No further periodontal destruction, without any periodontal maintenance. **G,** Preoperative. Before eruption of the second molar in a 58-year-old patient. Note the evidence of an osseous defect on the mesial. **H,** Postorthodontic stabilization. Improved osseous topography after tooth movement. (*C* to *E* courtesy Clark Kvistad, Seattle, and Morton Amsterdam, Philadelphia.)

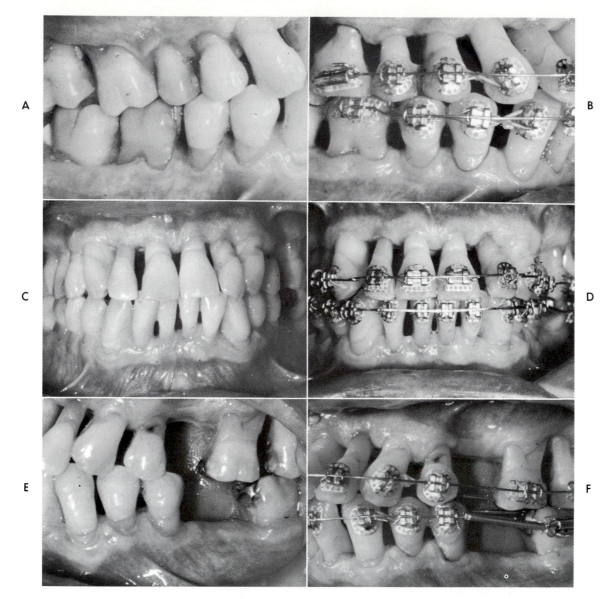

Fig. 14-11 **A, C,** and **E,** Gingival form after control of inflammation and occlusal therapy with a bite plane in a 58-year-old man. In patients with posterior bite collapse, the posterior teeth are disarticulated with a Hawley bite plane appliance during scaling and root planing. **B, D,** and **F,** Axial positioning of the teeth. Note the changes in gingival form. (The topography has improved as the bite collapse was corrected and the teeth were properly positioned.) In addition, it is easier to control gingival inflammation once better tooth position has been established.

Attainment of traditional orthodontic treatment objectives. The traditional goals would be the objectives for patients who have normal to mild skeletal dysplasias and complete dentitions. However, these goals are not realistic for mutilated dentitions with uncorrected severe skeletal dysplasias. To attempt to achieve ideal tooth positions, such as usually possible with Class I skeletal relations, and to seek Andrews' *Six keys to normal occlusion* in these patient types would usually constitute undersirable overtreatment. This is not to say that the orthodontic therapy provided is any less precise; rather, it suggests a need to customize the

orthodontic treatment for the individual patient so that the achievement of any one goal (perhaps esthetic) does not undermine a less obvious but important functional need.

Problem-oriented synthesis of the dental needs of each case will help determine specific treatment objectives that must be established before the orthodontic treatment plan can be determined. To begin treatment without knowing specific goals or else with unrealistic goals, can lead to treatment failure. Treatment efficiency and proper timing are essential in dealing with adult patients. Unlike the typical adolescent, an adult may exhibit rapid (within 2 to 3 months) periodontal breakdown and bone loss. Therefore adult therapy requires the establishment of individualized treatment goals and efficient mechanotherapy, so completion *(get in and get out)* occurs as expeditiously as possible.

Adult Diagnostic Considerations

Diagnostic Process Using a Problem Oriented Approach

The adult patient presents more numerous and more demanding problems and therefore requires a collection of more specialized data pertinent to the patient's dental and orthodontic problem and a highly skilled mechanism to interpret it. We use the problem-oriented medical record (POMR) of Weed,[99] which takes the following into account:

1. The tremendous growth in medical knowledge
2. The resulting increase in specialization
3. The fragmentation of knowledge that has followed this increase
4. The consequential impossibility of relying on memory for adequate patient care

The needs that prompted development of the POMR have also impacted on dentistry, particularly on adult orthodontics. Profitt and Ackerman have modified the problem oriented medical record and discuss it in Chapter 1. The format and mechanisms used for interpreting problems into orthodontic dental records are important steps in improving the practitioner's understanding of the adult patient and in providing treatment measures that can optimize the overall treatment result. The problem-oriented dental records significantly aid in making the appropriate diagnosis because they require that the patient's problems be listed and that a plan be developed to manage each problem.[68,70] This is a

significant improvement over the *morphologically oriented* diagnostic method that dates from the introduction of Angle's original classification of malocclusion (Fig. 14-12).

Diagnostic Steps

1. Accurate collection of data
2. Analyze data base
3. Develop problem list
4. Prepare tentative treatment plan with consideration of available options
5. Interact with those who are involved; discuss plans and options (may include other providers); clarify sequence; acquire patient acceptance
6. Final treatment plan

PERIODONTAL DIAGNOSIS

The orthodontist must make an accurate assessment of the patient's potential for bone loss or gingival recession during orthodontic tooth movement. A common problem occurs when the orthodontist assumes that the general dentist will provide skilled inflammation control for a patient with incipient periodontal disease. After months of tooth movement and occasional clenching or grinding instigated by movement interferences, the radiograph may exhibit significant bone loss (Fig. 14-13, *A* and *B*). Consequently, regaining control of periodontal inflammation is harder than maintaining it from the beginning. The orthodontist needs to monitor every adult case closely and collaborate with the periodontal specialist to properly treat adult patients.

Periodontal disease continues to be an outlandishly large percentage of dental malpractice claims. The basis for

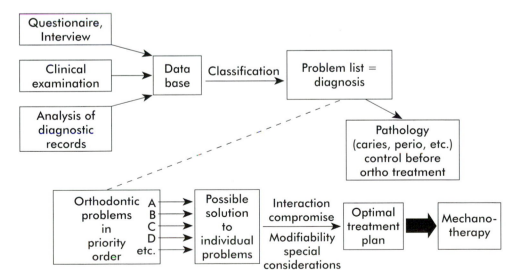

Fig. 14-12 Demonstrates the disciplined diagnostic process that precedes the actual treatment. This approach assures the processing of important information before irreversible changes take place as a result of therapy. The problem-oriented mechanism is important for adult treatment. (From Proffit WR, White RP: *Surgical-orthodontic treatment*, St Louis, 1991, Mosby.)

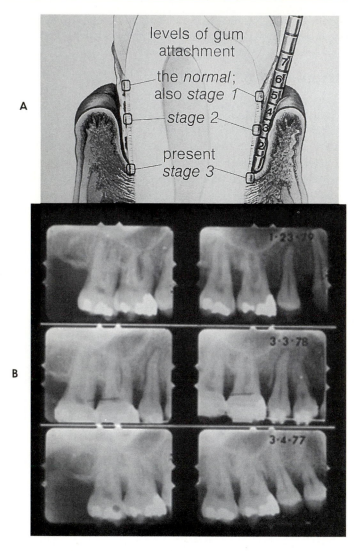

Fig. 14-13 **A,** Schematic illustrations demonstrate the changing levels of gingival attachments as the periodontal disease progresses. **B,** Radiograph showing bone loss at mesial and distal of tooth #3 during orthodontic movement. Inflammation and occlusal control are required during orthodontic movement to prevent an accelerated advance of periodontal disease.

the litigation . . . appears to originate from a number of sources:
- *Poor case selection*
- *Poor office procedure in insisting that prospective patients be periodontally stable*
- *Patient reluctance or refusal of periodontal checkups*
- *Dentist's acquiescence in the patient's neglectful behavior*
- *Ill-defined protocol between orthodontist and general dentist (or periodontist)*[1]

Therefore, appropriate management of several factors is needed to prevent negative periodontal sequelae during orthodontic treatment:

1. Awareness and vigilance of the orthodontist and the staff must be heightened
2. Awareness and vigilance of the patient must be frequently reinforced
3. Awareness of *risk factors* related to periodontal breakdown must be reviewed

General factors:
- Family history of premature tooth loss (indication of immune system deficiency in resistance to chronic bacterial infection associated with periodontal disease)
- General health status and evidence of chronic diseases (i.e., diabetes)
- Nutritional status
- Current stress factors
- *Life stage* of women[24]

Local factors:
- Tooth alignment (i.e., marginal ridge, CEJ relationship)
- Plaque indices
- Occlusal loading
- Crown to root ratio
- Grinding, clenching habits
- Restorative status

DIAGNOSIS OF TEMPOROMANDIBULAR JOINT DYSFUNCTION
Temporomandibular Disorders

Since the signs and symptoms of temporomandibular disorders (TMD) often increase in frequency and severity during adult treatment; it is imperative that orthodontists be familiar with diagnostic and treatment parameters of temporomandibular disorder. A recent study (Howard 1990) showed that the majority of 3,428 TMD patients were between the ages of 15 and 45 (mean age 32.9 years). However, it is important to note that "Craniomandibular disorders are self-limiting, or they fluctuate over time as suggested by declining incidence with age."[38] Unfortunately, knowledge regarding the natural history or course of TMD is limited.[75,83]

In a prevalence study Schiffman et al. (1990) found in the group that they treated that TMD problems were divided into several types:

• Muscle disorders	23%
• Joint disorders	19%
• Muscle-joint combinations	27%
• Normal	31%

It is important to note that prevalence data frequently overstate the clinical significance of the problem, since many patients have mild signs that may be transitory and are better left untreated.

The orthodontist treating adults would be wise to have a separate TMD questionnaire to supplement other health history information as part of the initial evaluation process. The goals of such a questionnaire would be to answer the following questions:

INTERNATIONAL HEADACHE SOCIETY'S CLASSIFICATION AND DIAGNOSTIC CRITERIA FOR HEADACHE DISORDERS, CRANIAL NEURALGIAS, AND FACIAL PAIN*

1. Migraine
2. Tension-type headache
3. Cluster headache and chronic paroxysmal hemierania
4. Miscellaneous headaches, unassociated with structural lesion
5. Headache associated with head trauma
6. Headache associated with vascular disorders
7. Headache associated with nonvascular intracranial disorders
8. Headache associated with substances or their withdrawal
9. Headache associated with noncephalic infection
10. Headache associated with metabolic disorder
11. Headache or facial pain associated with disorder of cranium, neck, eyes, ears, nose, sinuses, teeth, mouth, or other facial or cranial structures
12. Cranial neuralgias, nerve trunk pain, and deafferentation pain
13. Headache not classifiable

*From Cephalgia, vol 8, suppl 7, Oslo, Norway, 1988 Norwegian University Press, Publications Expediting.

 RECOMMENDED DIAGNOSTIC CLASSIFICATION FOR CATEGORY 11 (HEADACHE/FACIAL PAIN ASSOCIATED WITH THE FOLLOWING STRUCTURES)

11.1 Cranial bones including mandible
11.2 Neck
11.3 Eyes
11.4 Ears
11.5 Nose and sinuses
11.6 Teeth and related oral structures
11.7 Temporomandibular joint disorders
11.8 Masticatory muscle disorders

From McNeill C, editor: *Craniomandibular disorders: guidelines for evaluation, diagnosis, and management*, Chicago, 1990, Quintessence.
**Comment:* Most disorders of the skull and mandible (e.g., congenital abnormalities, aplasia, hypoplasia, osteolysis, hyperplasia, neoplasia, and fracture) are not accompanied by facial pain. Important exceptions are osteomyelitis, pain associated with altered function, multiple myeloma, and Paget's disease.

1. What type of TMD does the patient have? Muscle, joint, combination, psychosomatic?
2. Where is most of the problem located?
3. Is there pain? What is the degree of pain? What is the frequency of pain? Is the pain chronic or acute? "Chronic pain syndromes are defined as persistent pain that lasts more than 6 months with significant associated behavioral and psychosocial factors."[65]
4. Has there been previous treatment for this problem? What treatment? How long? How effective? Any medication?
5. What is the patient's understanding of his or her condition? Does he or she need a program designed to educate?
6. Is there an occlusal factor that may be exacerbating the problem? Are there occlusal habits that are known or are apparent?

Differential diagnosis may not be established until there are more assessments, records, and imaging. However, the orthodontist must have a clear perspective of diagnostic possibilities. To do this the authors have referenced the American Academy of CMD Consensus Report and will present their diagnostic criteria classified according to the International Headache Society's Classification and Diagnostic Criteria for Headache Disorders, Cranial Neuralgias, and Facial Pain. The following Tables 14-1 through 14-3

TABLE 14-1

Disorders of Cranial Bones Including Mandible

Disorder	Description
Agenesis	Condylar aplasia is a failure in development of the cranial bones or mandible.
Hypoplasia	Incomplete development or underdevelopment of cranial bones or mandibular condyle that is congenital or acquired.
Condylolysis	Mandibular condylolysis is related to a lytic event. The condyle becomes progressively smaller and may disappear.
Hyperplasia	Overdevelopment of the cranial bones or mandible that is congenital or acquired.
Neoplasia	A neoplasm is a new, abnormal, uncontrolled growth of the cranial bones or mandible. Benign tumors are most commonly found in the TMJ (e.g., osteoma, chondroma, and chondromatosis). Malignant tumors (e.g., osteosarcomas, chondrosarcomas) are exceedingly rare.

From McNeill C, editor: *Craniomandibular disorders: guidelines for evaluation, diagnosis, and management*, Chicago, 1990, Quintessence.

TABLE 14-2

Temporomandibular Joint Disorders

Disorder	Description
Deviation in form	Irregularities of intra-capsular soft and hard articular tissues
Disc displacement with reduction	Alteration, usually abrupt, of the disc-condyle structural relationship during mandibular translation; usually characterized by reciprocal clicking
Disc displacement without reduction	Altered disc-condyle structural relationship that is maintained during translation; can be acute or chronic
TMJ hypermobility	Excessive disc and/or condylar translation usually well beyond the eminence
Dislocation	A condition in which the condyle is positioned anterior to the articular eminence and/or disc and is unable to return to a closed position
Synovitis	An inflammation in the synovial lining of the TMJ
Capsulitis	Inflammation of the joint capsule; usually includes an inflammation of the synovium
Osteoarthrosis	Osteoarthrosis is a degenerative noninflammatory condition of the joint, characterized by structural changes of the joint surfaces
Osteoarthritis	Osteoarthritis is a degenerative condition accompanied by secondary inflammation (synovitis of the TMJ)
Polyarthritides	Arthritis caused by a generalized systemic polyarthritis condition
Ankylosis	Ankylosis is restricted mandibular movement with deviation to the affected side on opening
Fibrous ankylosis	Fibrous ankylosis is produced by adhesions within the TMJ
Bony ankylosis	The union of the bones of the TMJ by proliferation of bone cells, resulting in complete immobility of that joint

Adapted from McNeill C, editor: *Craniomandibular disorders: guidelines for evaluation, diagnosis, and management*, Chicago, 1990, Quintessence.

TABLE 14-3

Masticatory Muscle Disorders

Disorder	Description
Myofacial pain	Myofacial pain is a regional aching pain associated with localized tenderness in firm bands of muscle and tendons.
Myositis	Myositis is a painful generalized inflammation usually of the entire muscle; may occur in tendinous attachments of muscle as well.
Tendomyositis Tendonitis	Inflamed tendons
Spasm	Muscle spasm is a sudden, involuntary contraction of a muscle.
Reflex splinting	Reflex rigidity of a muscle occurring as means of avoiding pain caused by movement of the parts (i.e., muscle guarding).
Muscle contracture	Muscle contracture is chronic resistance of a muscle to passive stretch, as a result of fibrosis.
Hypertrophy	Muscle hypertrophy is a generalized abnormal enlargement of muscle tissue.
Neoplasm	Craniofacial muscle neoplasia is a new, abnormal, and uncontrolled growth of muscle tissue (e.g., myxoma, myxosarcoma, rhabdomyosarcoma).

Adapted from McNeill C, editor: *Craniomandibular disorders: guidelines for evaluation, diagnosis, and management*, Chicago, 1990, Quintessence.

are summarized from Chapter 3 to classify temporomandibular disorders.

Treatment Planning

Differences Between Adolescent and Adult Orthodontic Patients

As orthodontists become more aware of the need to integrate adult patients into their practices and since adolescents have been the customary recipients of orthodontic care in the past, it is of value to compare the two age groups particularly in the area of treatment planning. It is hoped that through an understanding of the similarities and differences between adolescent and adult patients, less stereo-

typed and more customized treatment can be rendered for each patient problem.

Several authors have stated what they consider to be the major differences between adolescent and adult patients. Levitt[53] offered that in adult patients "there is no growth, only tooth movement." Barrer,[10] who has had clinical experience with both adult and adolescent patients, stated that the adult, unlike the child, "is a relentless patient, who will not cover our deficiencies in skills or our errors in the use of mechanical procedures by helpful settling in post-treatment." Finally, Ackerman[2] had identified an important treatment difference, "In a child, one occasionally calls on another specialist. [On the other hand] it is a rare adult whom one treats orthodontically without finding it necessary to collaborate with another specialist."

The authors have a combined 40 years of clinical experience studying and treating adult orthodontic patient problems, which has made them aware of the many ways in which adult patients differ from the traditional adolescent patient. In this portion of the chapter we will describe and classify these differences, ranging from the initial examination of the patient to the final retention procedures. The five major categories in which adult patients exhibit significant differences from their adolescent counterparts follow:

1. Clarification and individualization of treatment objectives—this requires specific study of the problem and the indicated therapeutic refinements.
2. The diagnostic process—a problem-oriented approach to diagnosis is an absolute necessity.
3. Treatment plan selection—a more systematic and detailed analysis is required for adults than for adolescents.
4. Acceptance of recommended therapy—the patient's thorough understanding of and agreement with the recommended treatment are necessary.
5. Identifying adult case types—using an adult classification system is helpful in maintaining the orthodontist's and the staff's attention on the individual patient's needs.

To understand applicable factors better in each of these categories, we shall note specific variables and show how the two patient groups differ (Tables 14-4 through 14-12).

Adult Patient Management

Methods to Enhance the Success Rate

Adult patients present an ongoing challenge before, during, and after the prescribed treatment. To meet this challenge and to improve the quality of care for each patient, there are several steps in the areas of behavioral and clinical management that orthodontists treating adults should integrate into their professional activities.

Adult behavioral management

1. Advanced continuing education courses

   Since a large percentage of adult patients (1) have conditions that require multidisciplinary therapy, and (2) require treatment in areas of emerging knowledge, it is helpful to seek continuing education that provides an opportunity to update the orthodontic clinician's knowledge and skills in the specialty areas of periodontics, orthognathic surgery, TMD management, and restorative dentistry. In addition, there often are opportunities to enroll with other specialty providers in multidisciplinary courses that augment each provider's ability to play an efficient role in the delivery of care.

2. Refined consultation techniques

   Methods of consultation or case presentation vary from orthodontist to orthodontist. When reviewing records with the adult, particularly patients who require dual or multiple providers (60% to 70%), it is valuable to employ a consultation format designed to inform and educate. For patients with tooth size discrepancies, borderline or atypical extraction problems, restorative uncertainties, or some unique surgical situation, using a diagnostic setup on mounted models is usually informative and sometimes quite revealing to both the orthodontist and the patient.

   For cephalometric analysis of the patient with a skeletal disharmony, the Broadbent-Bolton transparencies or the Jacobson templates are helpful. They have proved to be graphic tools enabling the orthodontist to translate cephalometric data into a visually understandable reference for the patient who is considering orthodontics and orthognathic surgery.

   Also, the Unitek Troyer patient education series chart enables orthodontic-orthognathic patients to consider anticipated changes resulting from combined therapy in a more informed way. The skeletal disharmony patient, particularly one with a borderline skeletal-dental problem, requires a clearer explanation regarding therapeutic alternatives than do many other patients.

   Educating and informing the patient about the presence and significance of moderate or advanced periodontal disease can be a delicate process if the referring dentist has not discussed this with the patient.

   Frequently the orthodontist's hygienist may have made the patient aware of the existence of this problem at the initial examination. The orthodontist will then be in a better position to refer the patient to a periodontist for needed therapy. A recent publication (*Quintessence*) provides excellent schematics that help to educate patients.

   Other innovative consultation devices (i.e., a *before and after* photographic album, a *before and after* photographic bulletin board, and videotaped interviews with similarly treated adults) can greatly enhance the patient's knowledge and confidence. Grateful patients, who have successfully undergone complex treatment, will often provide a reassuring person-to-person consultation with a prospective patient regarding their own experiences with a proposed treatment modality. This is a frequently used educational procedure for patients who are considering orthognathic surgery. A patient who has already received the projected care is uniquely qualified to fill any knowledge voids, especially in areas of family care and inconvenience, work interference, rate of recovery, pain and discomfort. Finally, adult patients who are about to undergo multidisciplinary therapy seem to appreciate dual or multispecialist consultation so that all questions and information exchanges can be addressed on one occasion, thereby increasing patient trust regarding a shared level of agreement, permitting unanimous approval and understanding of upcoming treatment. Dual or multispecialist consultations also aid in organizing the timing and the sequencing of steps needed to complete the planned therapy.

3. Appliance modifications for adult treatment to reduce concern about appearance[28,31,54]

   Numerous appliances are available to provide forces for tooth movement within a biologically sound range. Two basic appliances, removable and fixed, are widely used. Within the categories are a multitude of choices, and it is logical that each orthodontist will employ the one that is both comfortable for the patient and reliable in accomplishing the desired treatment goals.

Text continued on p. 782

TABLE 14-4

Factors in Selection of a Treatment Plan: Comparison Between Adolescents and Adults, Existing Oral Pathosis (Fig. 14-14, *A* through *F*)

Factors	Comparisons	
Dental caries	**Adolescents**	More likely to have simple limited carious lesions, but more susceptible to caries
	Adults	More likely to have recurrent decay, restorative failures, root decay, and pulpal pathosis
Periodontal disease	**Adolescents**	More resistant to bone loss, but highly susceptible to gingival inflammation
	Adults	Higher susceptibility to periodontal bone loss
Faulty restorations	**Adolescents**	Few significant restorative problems
	Adults	Frequent restorative problems with economic and treatment planning implications
TMJ adaptability	**Adolescents**	Small percentage with symptoms because of high degree of TMJ adaptability; infrequent symptoms
	Adults	Frequent appearance of symptoms with dysfunction
Occlusal awareness	**Adolescents**	Infrequent cause of problem
	Adults	Heightened; may lead to accelerated enamel wear with adverse change in supporting tissues

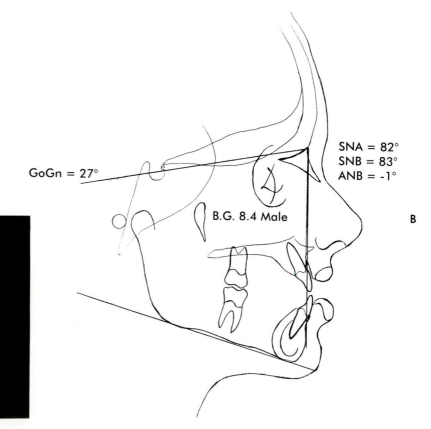

Fig. 14-14   A, Child (8:4) with Class III malocclusion. Cephalogram in retruded relationship. **B,** Tracing of cephalogram in retruded relationship.

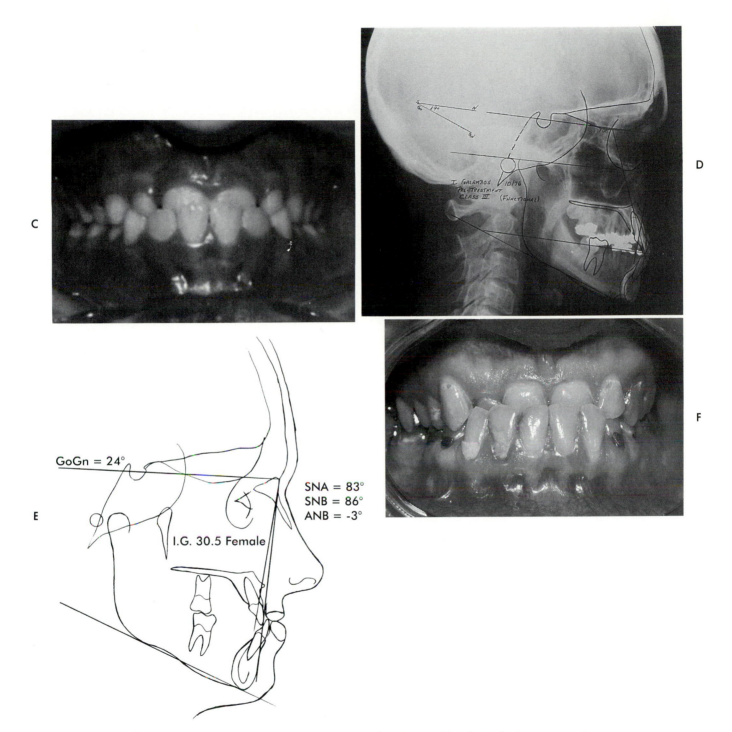

GoGn = 24°

SNA = 83°
SNB = 86°
ANB = -3°

I.G. 30.5 Female

Fig. 14-14, cont'd   C, Intra-oral photograph of an 8-year-old patient who has a convenience bite. **D,** Cephalometric radiograph of the mother of the boy shown in *A,* and *C.* The cephalometric comparison with her son illustrates the difference in the amount of dental treatments and the degree to which the Class III skeletal problem has developed. **E,** Tracing of cephalogram showing skeletal Class III with −3° ANB difference. **F,** Intra-oral photograph showing anterior crossbite and, in comparison to *C,* illustrates the difference in restorative problems that may impact treatment planning, prognosis, and cost of treatment.

TABLE 14-5

Factors in Selection of a Treatment Plan: Comparison Between Adolescents and Adults,
Skeletal Relationships (Fig. 14-15, *A* and *B*)

Factors	Comparisons	
Growth factors	**Adolescents**	Because of growth, an orthopedic treatment option is available; stable correction of skeletal discrepancies is possible; sequence of difficulty of orthodontic correction (most to least) is vertical, anteroposterior, transverse
	Adults	No growth with minimal skeletal adaptability; therefore, surgical procedures are frequently necessary for moderate to severe skeletal disharmonies; stable correction in skeletal transverse problems requires surgically assisted RPE; mandibular deficiency problems require sagittal split osteotomy and mandibular advancement; mandibular excess problems require mandibular set-back, and vertical maxillary excess with or without open bite requires LeFort osteotomy. Combination problems may require combination surgery depending on severity (see Fig. 14-15 for range of treatment capacities.)
Dentofacial esthetics	**Adolescents**	Reasonable concern; frequently matched to severity of condition
	Adults	Concern occasionally disproportionate to degree of existing problem

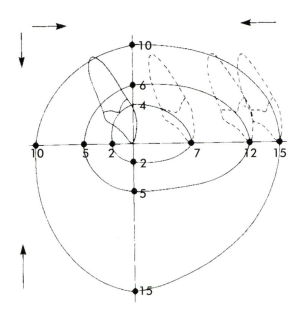

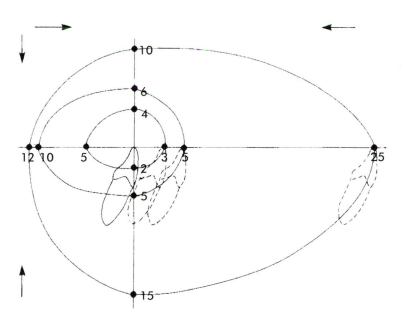

Fig. 14-15 "Envelope of discrepancy" (From Chapter 1, Proffit) Range of correction in sagittal (*AP*) and vertical planes of space. Envelope of discrepancy for transverse plane of space (from Vanarsdall), is shown in Fig. 14-43, *A* and *B*.

TABLE 14-6

Factors in Selection of a Treatment Plan: Comparison Between Adolescents and Adults,
Biologic Considerations (Fig. 14-16, *A* and *B*)

Factors	Comparisons	
Neuromuscular maturity	**Adolescents**	Significant potential for adaptability of stomatognathic system allowing a variety of biomechanical choices (i.e., Class II elastics, etc.)
	Adults	Mechanical options are limited because of lack of neuromuscular adaptability; also tendency toward iatrogenic transitional occlusal trauma, coinciding with orthodontic occlusal changes
Growth	**Adolescents**	Frequently a significant factor in selection of treatment plan; usually a positive factor in resolution of many adolescent malocclusions; however, overly optimistic assessment of potential growth changes in the adolescent may lead to disappointment and compromises in treatment result
	Adults	No growth present; therefore potential for significant skeletal alterations without orthognathic procedures is minimized (Behrents); dental camouflage option available for mild to moderate skeletal disharmonies (Compare 14-16, *A* with 14-16, *B*.)
Periodontal susceptibility	**Adolescent**	More resistant to bone loss as result of periodontal disease, but highly susceptible to gingival inflammation
	Adults	Higher degree of susceptibility to bone loss as result of periodontal disease; may be particularly evident during orthodontic therapy in which major occlusal changes are occurring; need for modification of mechano therapy
Rate of tooth movement[76]	**Adolescents**	Predictable and rapid, particularly during eruptive stages when permanent root development is not yet completed
	Adults	Initially somewhat slower, but more rapid and predictable once initial movement has begun

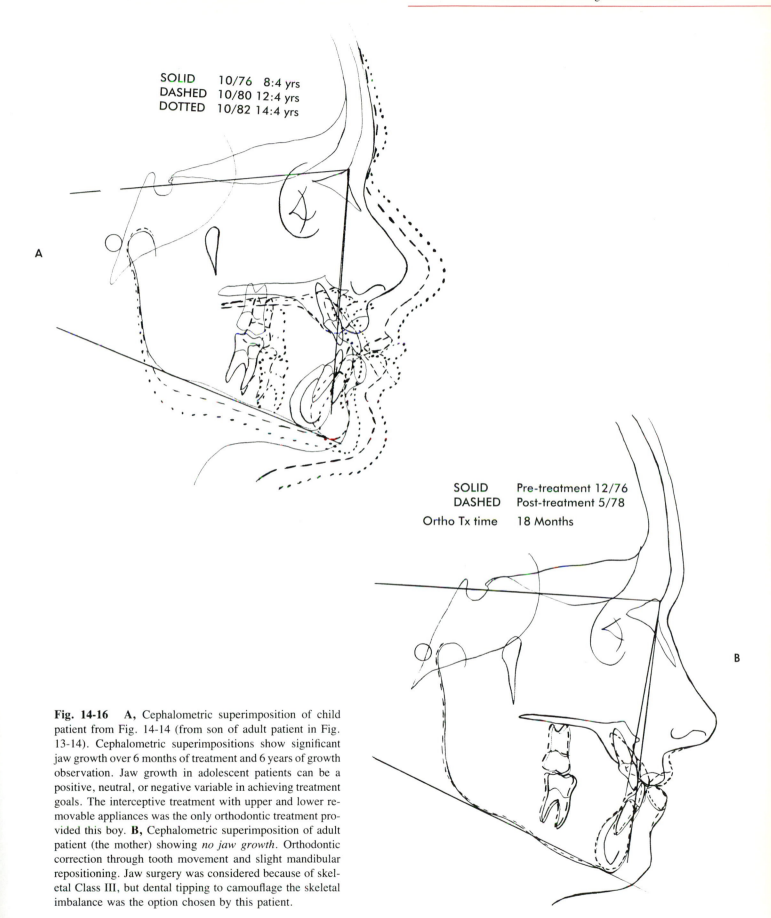

SOLID   10/76 8:4 yrs
DASHED 10/80 12:4 yrs
DOTTED 10/82 14:4 yrs

A

SOLID   Pre-treatment 12/76
DASHED   Post-treatment 5/78

Ortho Tx time   18 Months

B

Fig. 14-16 **A,** Cephalometric superimposition of child patient from Fig. 14-14 (from son of adult patient in Fig. 13-14). Cephalometric superimpositions show significant jaw growth over 6 months of treatment and 6 years of growth observation. Jaw growth in adolescent patients can be a positive, neutral, or negative variable in achieving treatment goals. The interceptive treatment with upper and lower removable appliances was the only orthodontic treatment provided this boy. **B,** Cephalometric superimposition of adult patient (the mother) showing *no jaw growth*. Orthodontic correction through tooth movement and slight mandibular repositioning. Jaw surgery was considered because of skeletal Class III, but dental tipping to camouflage the skeletal imbalance was the option chosen by this patient.

TABLE 14-7

Factors in Selection of a Treatment Plan: Comparison Between Adolescents and Adults, Therapeutic Approaches Available (Fig. 14-17)

Factors	Comparisons	
Tooth movement	**Adolescents**	Most require some tooth moving forces
	Adults	Most require some moving forces
Orthopedics	**Adolescents**	About half require orthopedics
	Adults	Effective only in a small percentage
Orhtognathic surgery	**Adolescents**	Major skeletal alterations needed in 1% to 5%
	Adults	Alterations needed in 10% to 20%
Restorative dentistry	**Adolescents**	Smaller percentage require it; when teeth are congenitally missing, frequently orthodontic therapy is useful in space closure or space redistribution, thus avoiding the need for restorative dentistry
	Adults	Frequently required for space re-opening where teeth have been lost and for abutment preparation and stabilization of occlusal relationship; integrated restorative plan can greatly reduce duration of fixed appliance treatment
Combination treatment	**Adolescents**	Uncommon
	Adults	Required in 80% of orthodontic restorative treatments

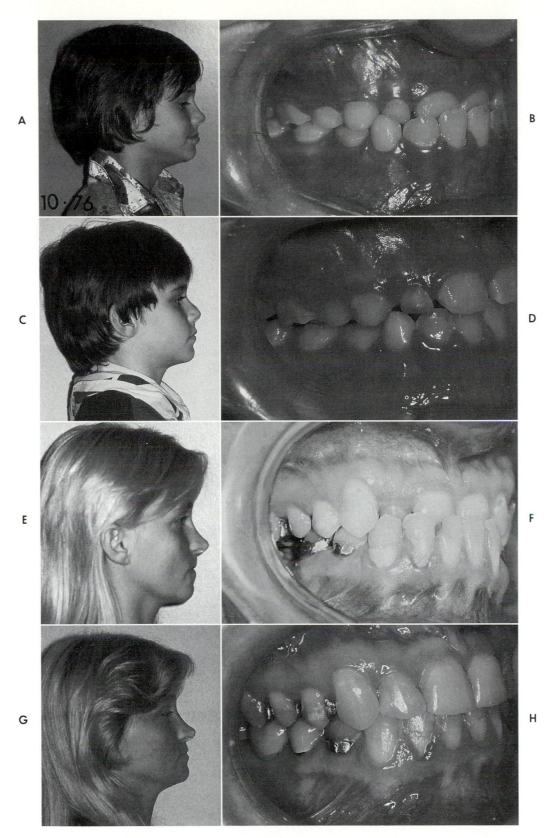

Fig. 14-17 **A** through **H,** A comparison of the mother and son from Fig. 14-14. It is evident that therapeutic approaches and treatment needs of these patients differ greatly. **A** through **B,** Shows the 8-year-old before removable appliance treatment. **C** through **D** Shows the profile and occlusal change 4 months after the appliances were placed. On the other hand, the mother (Fig. 14-17, **E** through **H**) required extensive corrective treatment, which lasted 18 months. Jaw surgery was a consideration, but because of a 1.5 mm functional shift, the dental movement of the upper and lower incisors was effective in camouflaging the skeletal imbalance.

TABLE 14-8

Factors in Selection of a Treatment Plan: Comparison Between Adolescents and Adults, Extraction versus Nonextraction Therapy (Fig. 14-18)

Factors	Comparisons	
Extraction controversy	**Adolescents**	A treatment plan of four-premolar extraction is used frequently to resolve crowding symmetrically, as well as protrusions, and seems justified in the immature face; space gaining techniques are also available
	Adults	Four-premolar extractions less frequent to resolve crowding; upper premolar extractions are a common alternative; asymmetric extraction and stripping of overbulked restorations.
Strategic extraction		Irreversible damage to periodontal tissue (Fig. 14-18) or to adjacent teeth (Fig. 14-19) may force orthodontists into unusual treatment plans for adults; careful analysis may lead to strategic extraction to solve alignment problems, as well as to eliminate existing damaged teeth

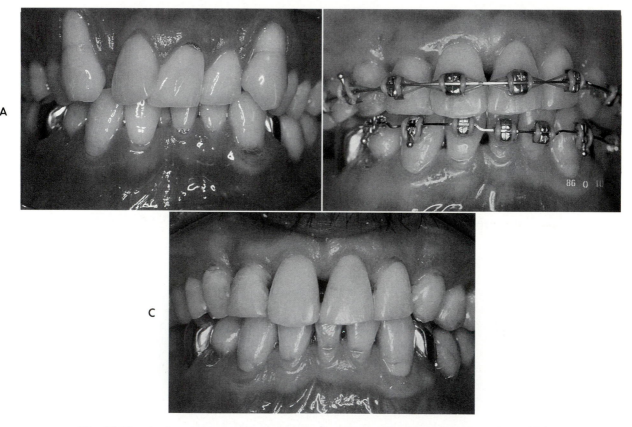

Fig. 14-18   **A,** Anterior intra-oral photograph of a 32-year-old adult male with tooth sensitivity to hot and cold. Large composites in labiogingival surface of ectopic #6 and #11. Significant lower crowding. **B,** Orthodontic treatment in progress. *Strategic extraction* of #6, #11, and #25 was recommended as part of the orthodontic treatment plan. **C,** Finished result with healthy teeth #5 and #12 replacing damaged canines. This is an unusual extraction treatment. Had this patient been seen as an adolescent, the more conventional extraction of first premolars may have been recommended before canine damage occurred.

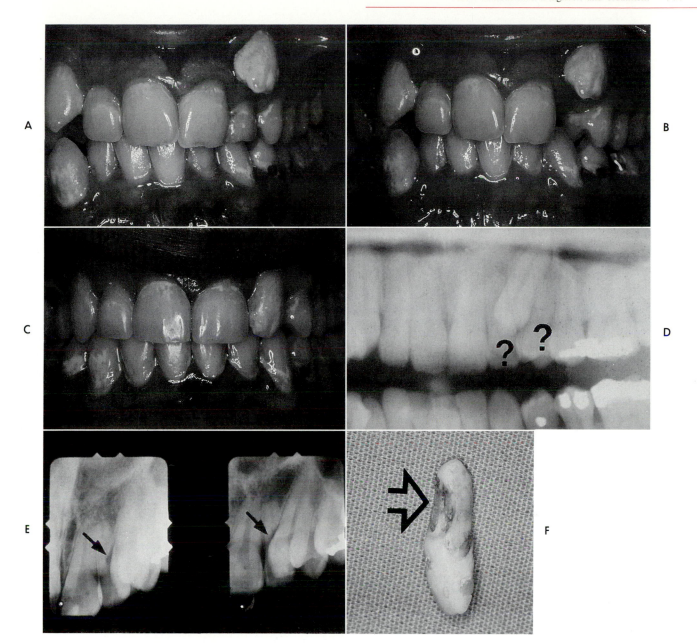

Fig. 14-19   A, Anterior intra-oral photograph of an adult male (21) who presents with severe crowding of the upper arch (12 mm arch deficiency) and moderate crowding of the lower arch (7 mm arch deficiency). **B,** Anterior intraoral after *strategic extraction* of #10 and conventional extraction of #5, #20, and #29. **C,** Anterior intra-oral photograph, post-treatment, demonstrating #11 replacing #10 and #12 replacing #11. Excellent function and acceptable dental esthetics were achieved. **D,** Panorex showing the extraction dilemma that presented itself in this adult case. **E,** Periapical of the area shows apparent radiolucency of lateral incisor caused by ectopic position of #11. **F,** Extracted lateral with *arrow* showing labial surface of lateral root resorbed into pulp canal. *Strategic extraction* elminated a major dental liability in this case.

TABLE 14-9

Factors in Selection of a Treatment Plan: Comparison Between Adolescents and Adults,
Anchorage Requirements

Factors	Comparisons	
Anchorage potential	**Adolescents**	More frequent incorporation of headgear to maximize anchorage and the retraction of anterior teeth
Headgear cooperation molar distalization	**Adults**	Greater anchorage potential because completely erupted first and second molars, as well as accentuated mesial drift particularly in mandibular arch; fewer adult cases will be categorized as maximum anchorage problems; implants in conjunction with restorative dentistry[86]; several molar distalization techniques are being developed as options to avoid headgear wear with adults (Fig. 14-20)

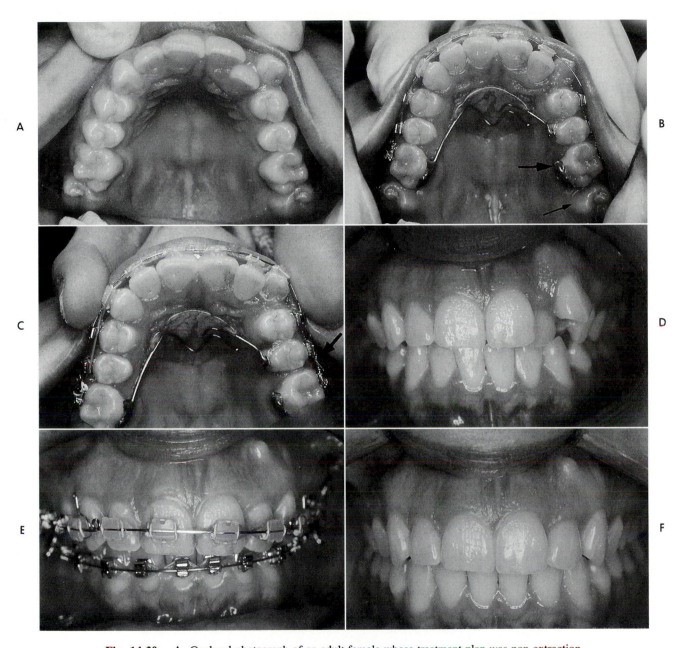

Fig. 14-20 **A,** Occlusal photograph of an adult female whose treatment plan was non-extraction for severe unilateral (upper left) crowding. **B,** Upper occlusal view, with appliances. Bonded transpalatal Nance holding arch with #3, #13, and #14 bonded for anchorage. Small arrow showing distalized second molar. Larger arrow shows release of Nance wire at #14 to allow distal movement. **C,** Arrow to distalizing spring which is moving the first molar distally. Class II elastics are also worn to sliding hook at #12. **D,** Frontal intra-oral view of pretreatment malocclusion. **E,** Frontal intra-oral view after 16 months of treatment. **F,** Frontal intra-oral view after 22 months of treatment and now in retention.

TABLE 14-10

Factors in Selection of a Treatment Plan: Comparison Between Adolescents and Adults, Missing Teeth (Dental Mutilation) (Fig. 14-21)

Factors	Comparisons	
Missing teeth	**Adolescents**	Early treatment control during eruption stages facilitates space closure without prostheses (i.e., congenitally missing maxillary laterals or missing second premolars)
	Adults	Frequent problems involving anterior and posterior teeth require restorative commitment for treatment planning and temporary tooth replacement during fixed appliance therapy; supra-eruption is a problem in posterior bite collapse; occlusal plane management is critical; implants as a restorative option have become a reliable alternative[45,52]

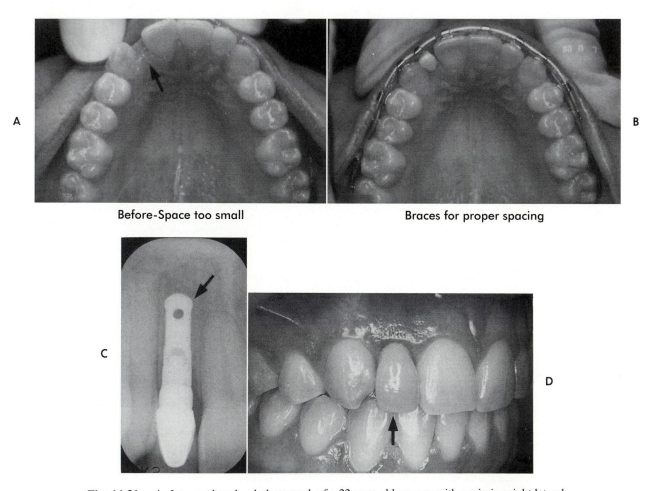

A   Before-Space too small

B   Braces for proper spacing

C

D

Fig. 14-21 **A,** Intra-oral occlusal photograph of a 22-year-old woman with a missing right lateral incisor; 3 mm space is too small for tooth replacement. **B,** Orthodontic appliances open space. Space opening and lateral incisor replacement was the treatment plan chosen to create optimum symmetry and esthetics, as well as and to maintain posterior occlusal balance with *canine rise* in lateral excursions. **C,** Radiograph with arrow showing osseointegrated mini-implant in place. **D,** Intra-oral side view with arrow to crown on the implant. Good esthetics and good occlusal function have been achieved.

TABLE 14-11

Factors in Selection of a Treatment Plan: Comparison Between Adolescents and Adults, Restorative Dentistry (Existing, Planned, and/or Needed) (Fig. 14-22)

Factors	Comparisons	
Restorative dentistry	**Adolescents**	Infrequent problem
	Adults	Appliance placement and orthodontic movement of existing bridgework possible but difficult; for total correction of occlusal relationship, existing bridges and anterior crowns frequently require replacement; important consideration in comprehensive treatment is to give the patient the best result; temporary (provisional) restoration should be avoided before orthodontics, but if it is absolutely necessary, it must follow original axial inclinations of tooth so bracket position and ultimate tooth changes will be accurate

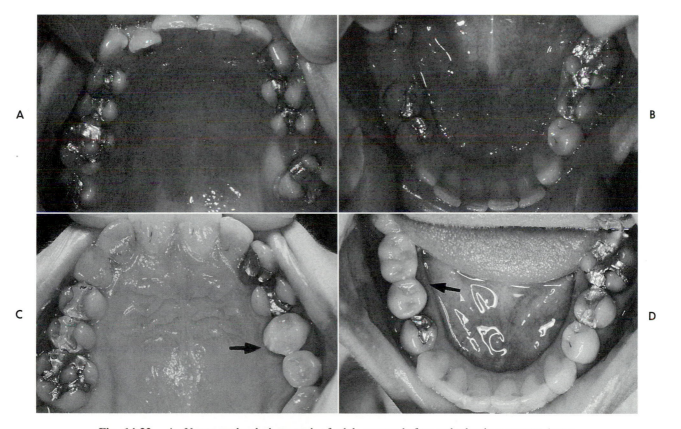

Fig. 14-22   A, Upper occlusal photograph of adult woman before orthodontic treatment (same patient as in Fig. 14-14). **B,** Lower occlusal photograph of adult woman before orthodontic treatment. **C,** Upper occlusal photograph after tooth movement and during restorative treatment; three units of bridgework *(arrow)* and several replaced amalgams have been completed. **D,** Lower occlusal photograph after tooth movement and restorative treatment; three units of bridgework, right posterior *(arrow).*

Continued.

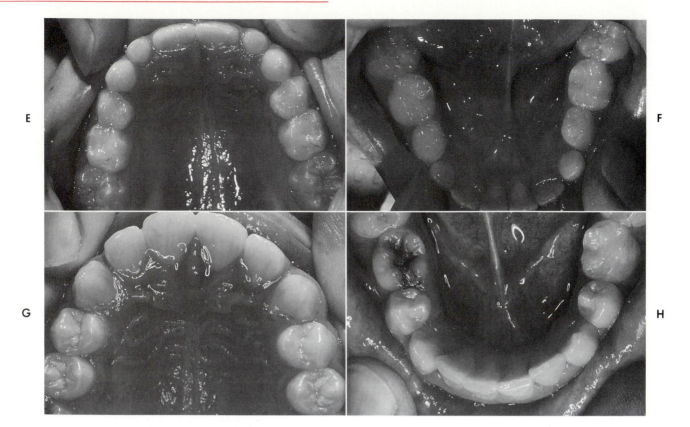

Fig. 14-22, cont'd   **E** through **F,** Upper and lower occlusal of an 8-year-old son of the patient (Fig. 14-14). Note lack of restorative needs in this patient. **G** through **H,** Upper and lower occlusal of same boy as in **E** and **F** at age 12; minor restorative problems. Comparing mother and son in *A* through *H* clearly illustrates the additional treatment planning and cost considerations that adult treatment may present, compared to the child or adolescent patient. The orthodontic and restorative treatment cost (over 2 years) was 600% higher for the adult than the child patient of the same family.

Adult clinical management
1. Periodontal considerations (See Chapter 13.)

Periodontal preparation of adults before orthodontic therapy. Successful adult orthodontic treatment for many patients will depend on the periodontal preparation before treatment and the maintenance of periodontal health throughout all phases of mechanotherapy. Gingival inflammation must be eliminated by acceptable oral hygiene measures and removal of accretions on the teeth (usually by scaling and root planing). The occlusion also must be controlled during periods of stress and severe bruxism throughout orthodontic treatment, so that occlusal trauma[56,95] and excessive tooth mobility will be prevented.[94] The Hawley bite plane is used for disarticulation as necessary throughout treatment (Fig. 14-23).

Gingival tissue. The orthodontist should make a clinical distinction between thin, delicate gingival tissue and normal or thickened tissue that is in the labiolingual plane.[14,27] The thin friable tissue is more prone to undergo recession during orthodontics than normal or thick tissue.

In addition, if there is a minimal zone of attached gingiva, particularly on abutment teeth, it is prudent to place free gingival grafts to help control inflammation before orthodontic treatment begins. It is important to note that the orthodontist *controls the timing* of the referral for grafting procedures. The prognosis for successful gingival grafts and prevention of bone loss is better if these are done before any recession has taken place.

Osseous surgery. As a rule, orthodontics should logically precede definitive osseous surgery. The optimal approach is as follows: (1) complete the orthodontic therapy; (2) establish a stable occlusion; and (3) wait a minimum of 6 months before requesting the periodontist to intervene for definitive periodontal procedures.

2. Inflammation control

Several visits with a periodontist or hygienist will not suffice to prepare a periodontally compromised adult properly for orthodontic correction. Meticulous root surface preparation and curettage are required. In patients with significant bone loss, furcation involvement, and

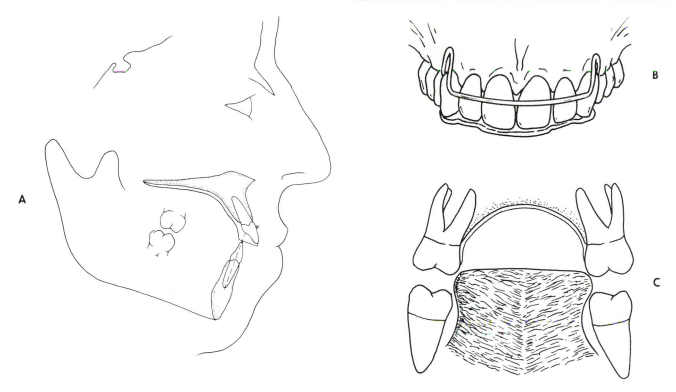

Fig. 14-23   A, Proper placement of the maxillary Hawley bite plane. Right angle to the lower incisors. **B,** The labial bow adds stability to the appliance, and the platform should allow for smooth guidance in excursive movements. **C,** Except in extreme anterior deep bite cases (usually Class II, division 2), the posterior teeth will be only minimally discluded. With normal neuro-musculature, the tongue will not be placed between the posterior teeth.

severe pocket depths, it may be necessary for the periodontist to do open-flap procedures[7] for removal of diseased gingival tissue and to accomplish proper root surface preparation before orthodontic therapy. Better visualization and access may allow deeper pocket areas and tortuous root configurations to be root planed properly. Before open-flap debridement, in cases in which there is advanced periodontal disease, control of adverse occlusal factors using the Hawley bite plane is essential.

Gingival bleeding provides the most reliable index for determining the presence of clinically significant gingivitis,[32] and before placement of appliances there should be no significant gingival bleeding on gentle probing.

Healthy tissue will not bleed when a thin Michigan probe is gently inserted into the sulcus. To keep the patient free of inflammation during treatment, root planing and curettage should be scheduled as frequently as necessary to prevent significant bleeding. Also, to assess disease activity, the tendency to bleed should be evaluated at each appointment. If this inflammation control is not rigidly adhered to, irreversible bone loss (Fig. 14-24) will inevitably result in the periodontally susceptible patient.

3. Removable appliances

Within the removable appliance group there are appliances designed for both diagnostic purposes and for tooth movement.

The diagnostic appliances are generally bite planes and splints. The acrylic splints are acrylic and wire bite planes with several features that are helpful, depending on the patient's problem. Some of the ways in which these appliances prove useful follow:
- For neuromuscular deprogramming
- As therapeutic adjuncts to reduce joint inflammation and pain
- As intermediaries during corrective orthodontic therapy to avoid transitory occlusal trauma or treatment induced TMJ symptoms

Removable appliances thus serve the patient as a *crutch* during specific treatment stages. Some patients whose problems cannot be therapeutically resolved without surgery, instead will choose to wear a bite plane splint permanently to help maintain a symptom-free joint. Although tooth movement appliances are in a separate group, there are occasions when one appliance can be diagnostic initially and then therapeutic once the di-

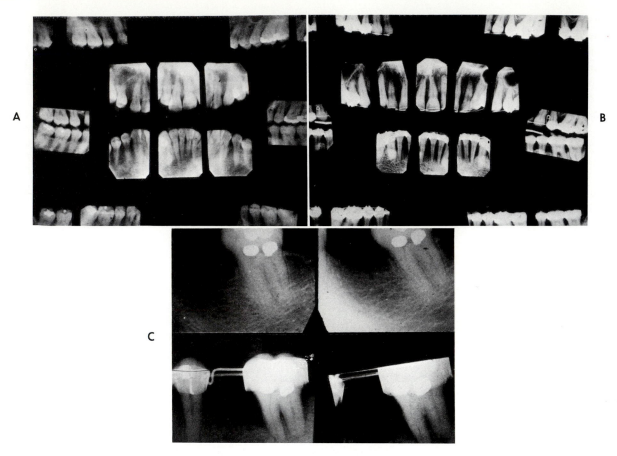

Fig. 14-24 **A,** Preoperative. **B,** After several months with appliances. Note the severe bone loss. **C,** Normal bone support round the molars *(top radiographs* before appliance placement. The radiolucency after appliance insertion was caused by the patient's parafunctional habits and inadequate inflammation control.

agnostic phase has been completed.

We use the following appliances for adults:

- *The sagittal appliance* for distalizing buccal segments or individual teeth, thereby reducing he need for extraoral anchorage (headgear). This type of appliance with a spring-loaded jackscrew is particularly useful for patients who have had maxillary mesial buccal segment drift and thus require distal movement to create or to regain space. Frequently, a bite plane is employed with this appliance to open the bite and allow more rapid distal tooth movement without occlusal or intercuspal interference.

- *The slow palatal expander (Schwarz plate)* for mild to moderate dental transverse discrepancy cases. This appliance has the potential for addition of an anterior or posterior bite plane to minimize the resistance of occlusal or intercuspal interference during the occlusal correction. Also bite planes on a palatal expander can deprogram an existing mandibular functional shift. However, skeletal transverse problems in adults resist treatment with this type of appliance and usually require surgical intervention for a stable correction.

- *The Phase I appliance* is used for reducing the length of time the patient must wear fixed appliances, for testing patient acceptance of the treatment plan, and to initiate tipping movements that may be more efficiently handled by a removable appliance. Orthodontists using Stage I removable appliances appreciate the rapid tooth movement initiated by such appliances. In addition, the use of this type of appliance frequently provides early insight regarding the patient's degree of motivation that would otherwise be unattainable without a much longer treatment commitment.

- *Bite plane therapy* is used in periodontally susceptible or already compromised bite collapse cases (and for diagnostic aspects in the treatment of TMD patients) and for disarticulation to find the centric relationship at the acceptable vertical dimension. It is during this phase of treatment that an evaluation can be made of the patient's response to the removal of adverse local factors and thus help the clinician determine not only the prognosis but also the best therapy for the patient.

Preorthodontic inflammation management and occlusal control can be done by the general dentist or the periodontist, but the orthodontist should monitor this phase and evaluate patient response over time before initiating the orthodontic phase of treatment. In addition, obviously, all caries control should have been completed, overhanging margins corrected, over-bulked contacts reduced, irregular marginal ridges reshaped, and endodontic procedures completed.

4. Fixed appliances

   Accurate predictable inter-arch and intra-arch tooth positioning in most adults requires the use of fixed orthodontic appliances. With continued advancement in bracket design featuring prescribed torque and other angulations, the orthodontist now has the capability of more precise tooth movement with shorter periods of therapy. Advancements in bonding techniques, new compositions and types of fixed appliances have become available, thereby adding to the orthodontist's armamentarium of prescribable options. Pretorqued, preangulated, stainless steel labially affixed appliances are described elsewhere in this text and are generally regarded as the most predictable appliances for accomplishing desired tooth movements in all three planes of space. However, plastic brackets, porcelain brackets, mini-brackets, such as the Hanson Speed appliance, and lingual or *invisible* appliances have additional appeal to adult patients because of their more cosmetic appearance.

   Although plastic and porcelain brackets have cosmetic advantages, they also present significant mechanical disadvantages for certain types of tooth positioning problems. From an analysis of the patient's records, the orthodontist must determine whether the problem is treatable (i.e., treatment goals achievable) within the limitations imposed by the use of *cosmetic appliance* choices. The initial choice can be altered during treatment, but it is wise nonetheless to provide for an alternative treatment plan (and appliance if needed) that will accomplish the treatment goals efficiently and predictably, especially when treating adults.

5. Occlusal control

   Occlusal control during the leveling phase of treatment in advanced cases can be accomplished with the aid of the Hawley bite plane and posterior sectional arches (see Fig. 14-10). To prevent excessive forces from bruxism and clenching, it may also be necessary to insert bite planes during stressful periods throughout the course of orthodontic care. Fortunately, once the posterior segments have been axially positioned and the transverse correction made, it is more difficult for the patient to traumatize posterior segments by parafunctional habits.

6. Treatment of the periodontally involved adult[94]

   Periodontally involved/compromised patients who have experienced shifting migration, extrusion, flaring, or lost teeth can benefit from orthodontics designed to correct local causative factors, predisposing malpositions, and certain bony and periodontal pockets.[96] Clin-ical evidence in periodontics shows overwhelmingly that changing local environmental factors can improve periodontal health and reduce the frequency of long-term periodontal maintenance. Orthodontics is one of the most dramatic means available to modify local factors and site specificity of the disease process.

Patients who have already been affected by periodontal disease and have lost significant tooth support are at risk for recurrent episodes of active disease; this group especially is susceptible because of their past history. In the United States 80% of adults have experienced some degree of periodontitis, and 95% of the elderly have moderate to severe periodontal disease.[72] Movement of teeth for periodontally susceptible or previously comprised patients in the presence of inflammation can result in increased loss of attachment and/or irreversible crestal bone loss. Fortunately, research and clinical studies have shown that dentitions with a history of periodontitis or teeth with reduced attachment height can be moved without significant loss of attachment.[91] Identification of susceptible sites or areas and control of the inflammatory lesion is critical to successful therapy. All patients, however, will have some degree of inflammation, and it is critical to ensure that periodontitis remains stable or quiescent throughout orthodontic treatment.

Periodontal Preparation and Occlusal Management During Active Therapy (See Chapter 13)

Before beginning tooth movement, inflammation should be reduced by root planing and curettage. As previously pointed out, it may be necessary to perform open-flap curettage for direct vision. All members of the inter-disciplinary dental team must accept responsibility for adequate oral physiotherapy and mechanical maintenance of gingival health in deep pocket areas. This is achieved by root planing, tooth polishing, and curettage throughout tooth movement on a basis as frequent as necessary to keep the periodontium free of significant inflammation. Bleeding upon gentle instrumentation or probing is the most reliable clinical indication of significant inflammation. If, during curettage, blood pools in the gingival margin surrounding a tooth, too much inflammation will be present to do tooth movement for a periodontally susceptible patient. The frequency of visits during tooth movement will be determined not by orthodontic adjustments but by the necessity to control soft tissue inflammation during appliance therapy. This could be on a biweekly basis in the 60- to 70-year-old patient. A periodontally susceptible patient should never be placed on a 2- to 3-month recall program for removal of subgingival microbiota as has been suggested in the literature.[15] The frequency of removal of subgingival microorganisms must be titrated for the particular patient to prevent crestal bone loss. Studies that have reported on repopulation of the gingival bacteria do not apply to orthodontic patients.

Control of Occlusal Parafunction and Modification of Periodontal Susceptibility

In addition to frequently controlling soft tissue inflammation, it is necessary to prevent excessive tooth mobility during treatment. An investigation done with Squirrel monkeys concluded that increasing tooth mobility superimposed upon reduced but healthy periodontal tissues is without effect upon the level of connective tissue attachment.[77] This level in inflammatory control may be unrealistic for clinical patients who are periodontally susceptible: who have systemic factors (e.g., pregnancy), reduced oral hygiene, and will be subjected to significant tooth mobility.

Significance of Tooth Mobility

Many experimental studies have demonstrated that traumatic lesions in the presence of a healthy periodontium do not initiate loss of attachment or periodontitis. Investigations using the beagle dog[56] and those in monkeys[80] have improved our understanding of the relationship between inflammation and occlusal trauma.

Studies in the beagle dog by Svanberg have shown that trauma from occlusion that had created increased tooth mobility can also cause increased vascularity, increased vascular permeability, and increased osteoclastic activity during a traumatic phase lasting approximately 60 days.[89] Once a stable, permanent hypermobility was established, vascularity and osteoclastic activity returned to normal. These findings led Svanberg to suggest that only through measurements taken at intervals can one determine the existence of progressively increasing mobility that may be diagnosed as trauma from occlusion. Jiggling occlusal forces have been found to aggravate active periodontitis, accelerate loss of connective tissue attachment, and possibly diminish gain in re-attachment after periodontal treatment.[23,55] A recent study to evaluate the association between trauma from occlusion and severity of periodontitis concluded that teeth with increased mobility have greater pocket depths and less bone support than teeth without these findings.[78] A University of Pennsylvania study designed to evaluate initial alignment and leveling of teeth and also to determine the effect of probing depths on healthy teeth,[95] indicated that test teeth in this study did not show significant change (i.e., increase in the plaque or sulcular bleeding indices between the initial appointment and the appointment at which maximal tooth mobility was recorded) to ensure that any increase in probing depth could not be caused by increased periodontal inflammation. Eleven patients served as their own controls. The test teeth that became mobile, demonstrated an increase in probing depth by an average of 1.09 ± 0.53 mm between the initial appointment and the appointment at which the maximal tooth mobility value was recorded. Therefore, it was concluded that during orthodontic alignment and leveling, teeth with significant increase in mobility will also have an increase in probing depth and that severely rotated teeth will have a greater increase in mobility. The findings of this preliminary study would indicate that increased tooth mobility has a detrimental effect on the periodontium and that increased probing depth would indicate an increased periodontal risk such as an increase in the patient's susceptibility to periodontal disease. Therefore, subgingival microbiota should be removed during periods of increased mobility, and appropriate steps taken to prevent further tooth mobility in patients who have already demonstrated periodontal susceptibility.

Parafunctional habits can not only increase tooth mobility and traumatize the attachment but can also slow tooth movement. Therefore, the orthodontist must control occlusal forces during orthodontic treatment, especially at the initial stage of leveling and alignment of posterior segments.

Control of Occlusion

There are three critical ways to control occlusal forces during appliance therapy: *disarticulation* or *disclusion* of the teeth moved, *selective grinding* with the high speed drill, and *modification of mechanotherapy* for the periodontally susceptible or compromised individual.

Disarticulation. The Hawley bite plane (see Fig. 14-23) is used for disarticulation (and for diagnosis of TMD patients), to establish centric relation at the acceptable vertical dimension and as necessary throughout orthodontic treatment to prevent excessive tooth mobility. During the leveling stages the bite plane is used (in conjunction with posterior sectional arch wires) to allow teeth to move free of occlusal forces. The appliance is worn at all times, except while eating or sleeping (Fig. 14-25, *H*). A significant biomechanical advantage of disarticulation (or disclusion) in the adult is that it allows the mesially inclined tooth crowns to tip distally to an upright position with only slight mesial movement of their root apices, thereby creating space in the mandible distal to the canines for alignment of crowded lower anterior teeth. If the posterior teeth are not disarticulated, occlusal forces may cause the buccal segment roots to move mesially so that no space is gained distal to the canines during uprighting. Note also that uprighting of posterior teeth, free of occlusal forces, requires much less time and reduces the hazard of mesial root movement.

Selective grinding. The typical adult malocclusion is characterized by posterior teeth that have moved and tipped mesially (accentuated mesial drift) and bite collapse. There is less wear on the mesial marginal ridges than on the distal marginal ridges of mesially inclined posterior teeth. Once these teeth start to upright, the mesial marginal ridges need to be reshaped so that the occlusal table will be perpendicular to the long axis of the tooth. Many teeth need to be extruded to correct osseous defects and to level the crestal bone but must not be allowed to remain in premature contact once eruption has occurred.

Therefore, at each appointment, the bite plane is removed and selective grinding is done as necessary to ensure simultaneous bilateral contact with the posterior teeth when

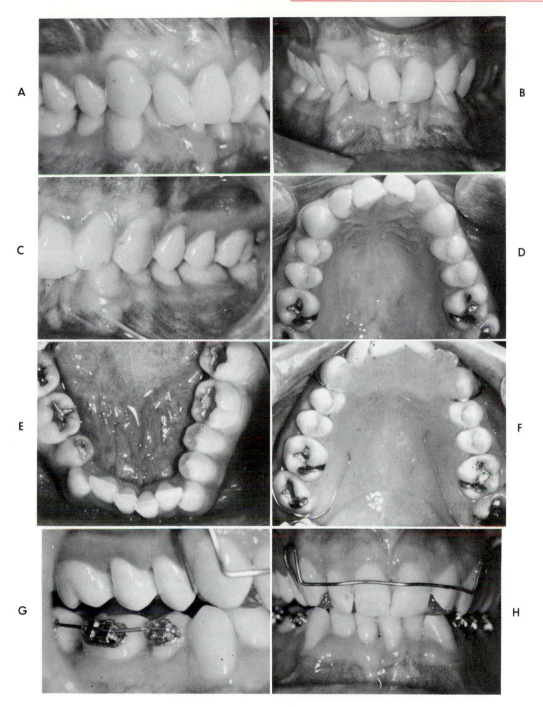

Fig. 14-25   Sequence used in periodontally susceptible adults. **A** through **E,** Preoperative. Mild Class II skeletal pattern in a 33-year-old man with strong musculature who has experienced some periodontal bone loss. **F,** The Hawley bite plane acts as a diagnostic aid to determine centric relation, control the occlusion during leveling of the posterior segments, and expedite tooth movement. **G** and **H,** Lower posterior segments bonded. The bite plane is worn full time (except during eating) to prevent adverse occlusal forces during leveling and alignment of these segments.

Continued.

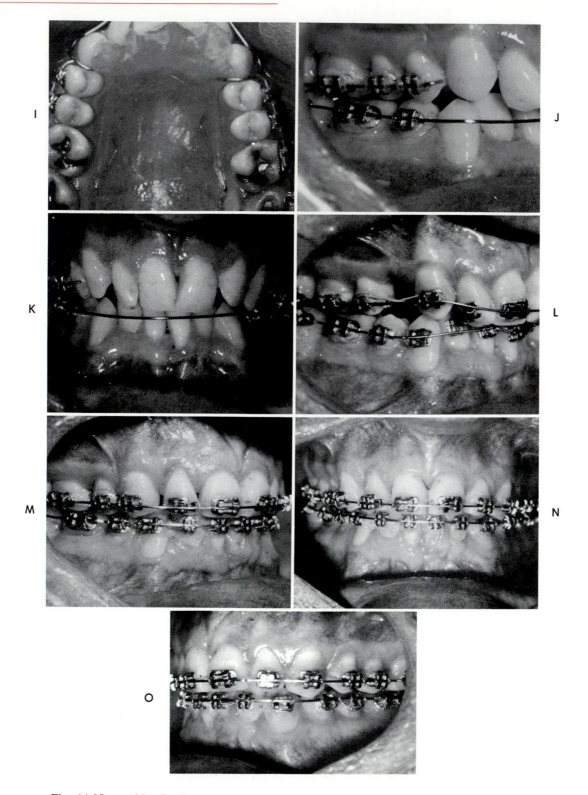

Fig. 14-25, cont'd   **I,** Clasps removed in the maxillary arch. Note that upon insertion of the maxillary sectional arches the acrylic has been cut away 4 to 5 mm from the palatal aspects of the posterior teeth. **J,** Extraction of the maxillary first premolar delayed until the bite has opened. **K,** The lower anterior teeth, which contact the bite plane, are bypassed by the full lower arch. A full archwire is frequently needed for buccolingual control. **L,** Once the posteriors are aligned, the premolars are extracted and upper and lower anterior teeth are bonded. The bite plane is discarded, and working mechanics (space closure) is started. **M** through **O,** Beginning of the finishing and detailing stage.   *Continued.*

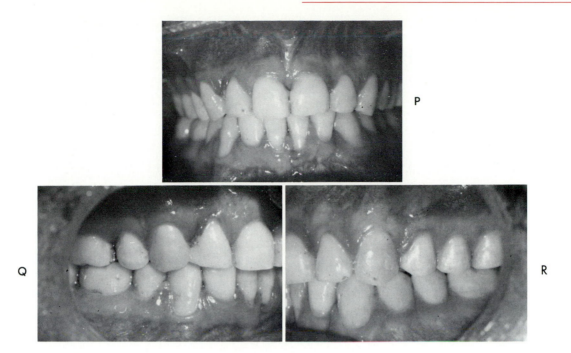

Fig. 14-25, cont'd   **P** through **R,** Post-treatment.

in centric relation. Once a malocclusion involving mesially inclined posterior teeth has been uprighted, the posterior segments will not be stable unless selective grinding is used to reshape the occlusal surfaces along with any required operative and restorative dentistry to ensure simultaneous bilateral contact along the long axis when in centric relation. The objectives of selective grinding then are to allow leveling of the attachment to crestal bone and leveling of the marginal ridges to achieve simultaneous bilateral occlusion.

Modification of mechanotherapy. With traditional multibonded techniques in nonperiodontally involved patients, both arches are usually bonded and full-continuous arch wires are placed. In the adult patient (for reasons stated previously), we delay appliance placement on both the maxillary and mandibular anterior segments. This approach is well accepted by adults who invariably prefer no brackets on the anterior teeth during the initial 9 to 12 months that it takes for posterior segments to be axially aligned and for the transverse correction to be made (Fig. 14-25, *J* and *K*). The objective is to first set-up the posterior occlusion before placing appliances on the anterior segments—these are moved last. Once posterior teeth are aligned and axially positioned, the bite plane is removed and the upper and lower anterior teeth are bonded. Space closure is begun and anterior alignment is completed. In Class II cases in which upper premolars may need to be extracted, the extractions can be delayed and then maxillary canines can be immediately retracted into the extraction site, minimizing the time for maxillary space closure. It is more difficult to traumatize

posterior segments by parafunctional habits once the teeth have been axially positioned. However, if significant bruxism and clenching during stressful periods cause increased mobility, an immediate impression should be taken for a bite plane. The patient should be given a bite plane for disarticulation and referred for inflammatory control (scaling and root planing) as well. Once mobility patterns have been reduced, mechanotherapy can be continued.

THE CONCEPT OF TREATMENT SEQUENCING

An important advantage of categorizing patients into *provider* groups is in the area of patient education, particularly as it relates to sequence of treatment. After the diagnostic process takes place, it is necessary for the various practitioners involved to be precise in outlining the steps of treatment and the rationale for these steps to their patients. Patients under dual provider and multiple provider care must also be educated to the *plateaus of treatment progress* and how these relate to their well-being.[71] These plateaus include the following:
1. Active disease
2. Disease arrested
3. Disease controlled
4. Contributing structural malrelationships corrected
5. Periodontal defects corrected
6. Restorative and reconstructive dentistry completed
7. Optimal oral health maintained

Failure to adequately educate patients in this area will result in high rates of noncompliance.

Text continued on p. 814.

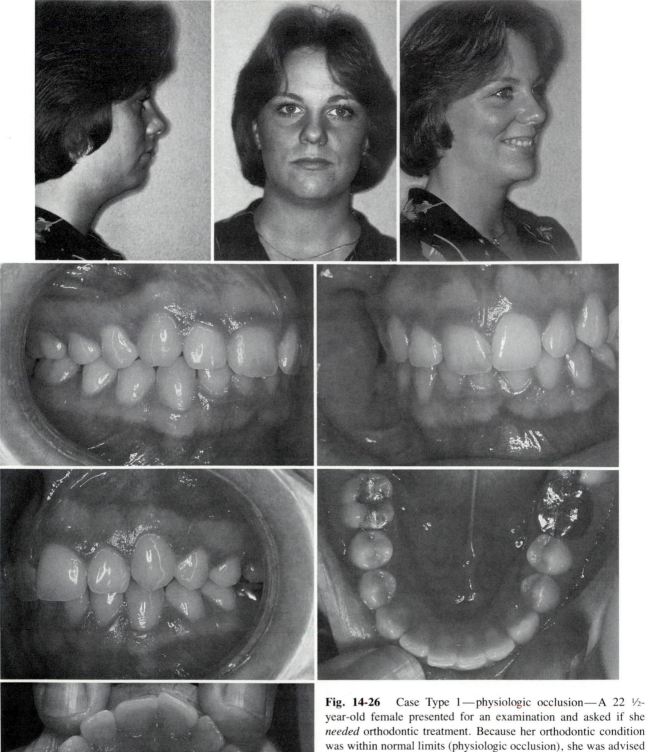

Fig. 14-26 Case Type 1—physiologic occlusion—A 22 ½-year-old female presented for an examination and asked if she *needed* orthodontic treatment. Because her orthodontic condition was within normal limits (physiologic occlusion), she was advised that no treatment was needed at this time and that she could be placed on observation. Data indicates that 69 adult patients of the 1370 examined (approximately 5%) are in the Case Type *physiologic occlusion: no treatment; physiologic occlusion: observation.*

TABLE 14-12

Adult Orthodontic Patient Types (Classified according to most significant treatment needs)

Case type	Characteristics of major problem areas	Associated systems are healthy and in balance	Treatment provider and treatment responsibilities of designated provider
Physiologic occlusion (exhibits no signs of existing pathosis) (Fig. 14-26)	Mild dental malalignment; normal occlusion or malocclusion that is esthetically acceptable with healthy associated systems	Occlusal stability No decay and lack of occlusal wear Psychological balance Periodontal health TMJ asymptomatic No speech impairment No occlusal awareness No functional disorders	Orthodontist Consultation and patient education (i.e., *present condition requires no orthodontic treatment*). Relieve concern of referring dentist that condition probably *won't get worse* Make patient aware of existing health levels Document present condition with radiographs, color slides, and/or study models Recall or re-evaluate Restorative dentist Periodic monitoring of oral health needs
Psychological disorientation (Fig. 14-27, A through E)	Concern about minor dental condition far exceeding *real* significance of the problem	Dentition aligned Skeletal balance TMJ asymptomatic Periodontal health	Restorative dentist Inform patient Orthodontist Make patient aware of dental health status Psychologist/psychiatrist Psychological counseling as needed
Adjunctive orthodontics (Fig. 14-28, A through H)	Mild or moderate dental-skeletal malrelationship with periodontal and/or restorative needs	Periodontal resistance All other systems within normal limits (WNL)	Periodontist, restorative DDS, or hygienist Caries and inflammatory control Restorative dentist Patient acceptance of restorative or prosthetic commitment Orthodontist Limited orthodontic treatment objectives Stabilization and retention (usually sectional appliances) Restorative DDS/periodontist Restorative therapy and periodontal therapy as needed
Corrective orthodontics (Fig. 14-29, A through P)	Mild to moderate dental-skeletal disharmony Unsatisfactory dentofacial esthetics	Psychologic balance Skeletally WNL orthodontically periodontal resistance TMJ asymptomatic No tooth replacement required	Restorative DDS or hygienist Caries and inflammatory control Orthodontist Comprehensive orthodontic therapy (extraction/non-extraction) Restorative DDS or hygienist Scaling and curettage at 3 to 6 month intervals Orthodontist Retention Restorative DDS Periodic monitoring of oral health needs

Continued.

TABLE 14-12

Adult Orthodontic Patient Types (Classified according to most significant treatment needs)—cont'd

Case type	Characteristics of major problem areas	Associated systems are healthy and in balance	Treatment provider and treatment responsibilities of designated provider

Orthognathic surgery (Fig. 14-30, A through M)	Dental-skeletal and/or neuromuscular disharmonies of moderate to severe degree	Other systems may be affected secondary to existing major problem areas
		
		Periodontal resistance
			Restorative DDS or Hygienist
			  Caries and inflammatory control
			Orthodontist
			  Presurgical intra-arch orthodontic preparation
			  Re-evaluate records
			Oral surgeon
			  Orthognathic surgery to correct skeletal-dental disharmony
			Orthodontist
			  Postsurgical orthodontic therapy
			  Retention records
			Oral surgeon or plastic surgeon
			  Adjunctive surgical procedures (genioplasty, rhinoplasty, facelift, etc.)

Periodontally susceptible (Fig. 14-31, A through H)	Dental-skeletal malrelationship with moderate to advanced bone loss
	Primary and/or secondary occlusal trauma may be present
		Emotional balance
		TMJ asymptomatic
		Other systems may be affected as secondary consequence of existing major problem area
			Restorative DDS or hygienist
			  Caries and inflammatory control
			Periodontist or hygienist
			  Maintenance of root surface preparation
			Periodontist
			  Subgingival removal of microbiota
			  Gingival grafting procedures
			Orthodontist
			  Comprehensive orthodontic therapy
			  Selective grinding
			  Retention
			Periodontist
			  Periodontal re-evaluation and definitive periodontal procedures
			Restorative DDS
			  Restorative dentistry as required

Temporomandibular joint dysfunction (Fig. 14-32, A through L)	Dental-skeletal malrelationship with joint dysfunction
	TMJ symptoms
		Periodontal resistance
		Other systems may be affected secondary to existing major problem areas
			Restorative DDS or orthodontist
			  Diagnostic appliance to achieve relief of symptoms and to determine degree of skeletal disharmony and need for further diagnosis
			Psychotherapist
			  Counseling as needed
			Orthodontist
			  Occlusal therapy
			  Comprehensive orthodontics
			  Selective grinding

Enamel wear beyond that expected for chronologic age (Fig. 14-33, *A* through *I*)	Heavy musculature (mandibular deficiency)
	Dental-skeletal deep-bite
	Periodontal resistance
	Other systems WNL
		Oral surgeon
		  Orthognathic surgery
		Restorative DDS
		  Restorative dentistry
		Restorative DDS
		  Caries or inflammatory control
		  Occlusal control
		Orthodontist or oral surgeon
		  Comprehensive orthodontics (orthognathic surgery may be a necessary adjunct)
		Periodontist
		  Periodontal surgery
		  Crown lengthening
		Restorative DDS
		  Restorative dentistry as needed

Dental mutilations (Fig. 14-34, *A* through *L*)	Premature loss of teeth or congenitally missing teeth
	May involve bite collapse and loss of vertical height
	Periodontal resistance
	Associated systems WNL but may be affected as secondary consequence of major problem area
		Restorative DDS
		  Caries and inflammatory control
		  Occlusal control with modified treatment goals
		Orthodontist
		  Comprehensive orthodontic treatment with modified goals
		Periodontist
		  Adjunctive periodontal treatment before restorative dentistry
		Restorative DDS
		  Tooth replacement through restorative dentistry

ADULT CASE TYPE
Psychologic Disorientation

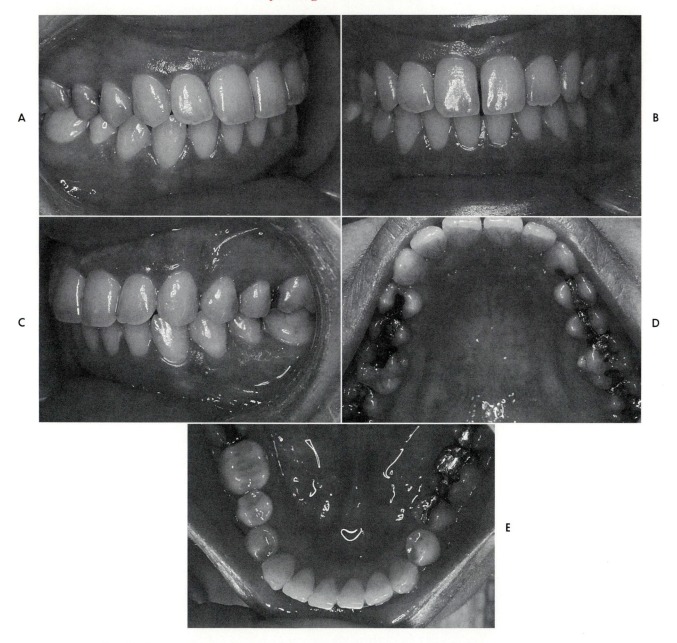

Fig. 14-27 Psychologic disorientation—The above clinical photographs illustrate a 37-year-old female who is extremely self conscious about the space between her incisors. She has had the space for a long time but now believes that it interferes with the attractiveness of her smile, as well as her overall attractiveness. Her concerns are disproportionate to the degree of the dental problem. Consideration of the underlying cause of her self-esteem deficiency may need to be addressed before dental therapies begin.

ADULT CASE TYPE
Adjunctive Orthodontics

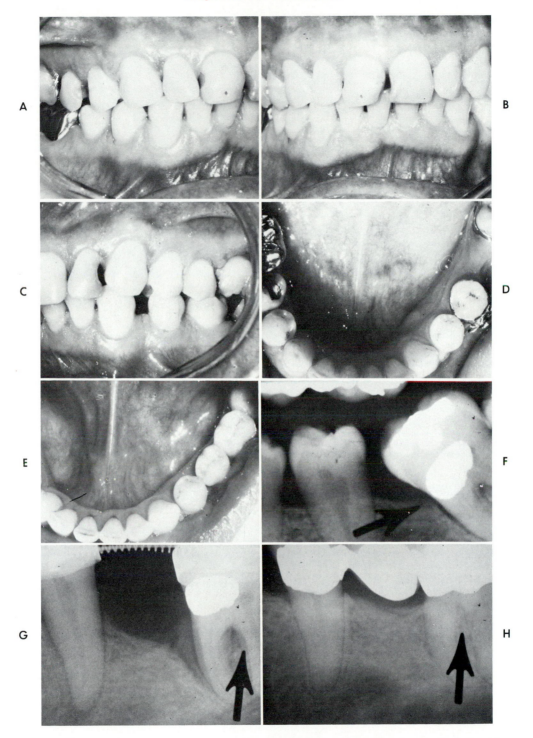

Fig. 14-28   Adult-type adjunctive orthodontics. **A** to **C,** Pretreatment. Class I occlusal relationship with unilateral absence of the lower left first molar. Also arch collapse accompanied by dental shifting. **D,** Stabilization. Sectional arch in place after removal of the fixed orthodontic appliances used during the active stage. This patient had appliances from the right canine to the left second molar. **E,** Posttreatment. Abutment teeth uprighted and restorations in place. **F,** Pretreatment. Note the vertical defect on the mesial root surface of the tipped second molar. **G,** Five months after initiation of mechanotherapy. Osteoid fills the area of the previous vertical defect on the mesial. **H,** Eighteen months after bridge insertion. Maturation of bone in the mesial defect and interradicular area.

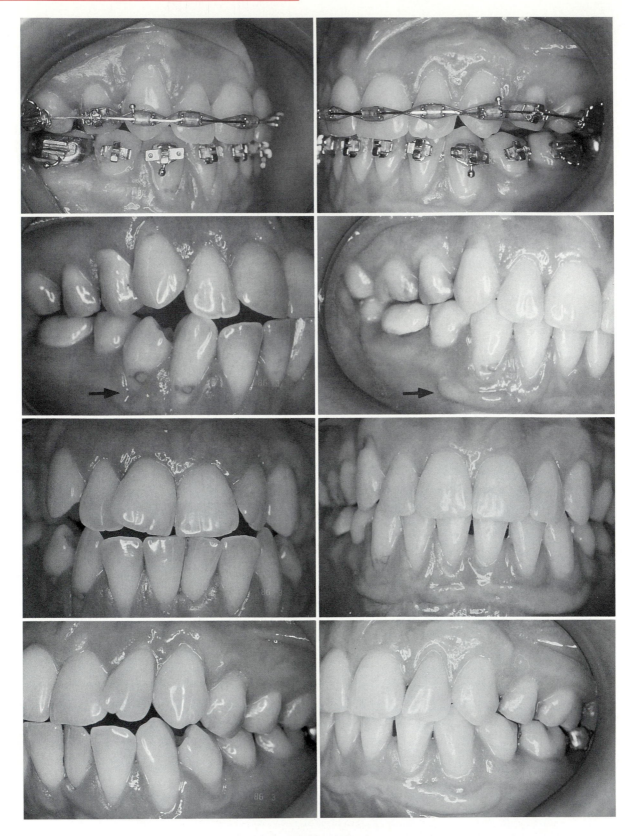

Fig. 14-29 Section VII; case type 4; corrective orthodontics. This patient was a 38-year-old female who wanted to improve her bite, and her smile esthetics. She was concerned about being unable to close her lips. Because of the crowding, maxillary and mandibular dental protrusion, and gingival recession, the treatment plan called for the extraction of four first premolars and full braces. Gingival grafting was done in the early stages of tooth movement.

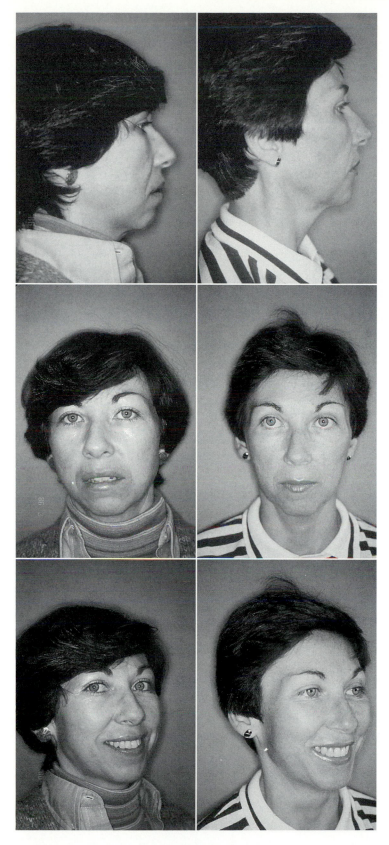

Fig. 14-29, cont'd   Data from the adult treatment-need study indicate 25.5% of adults examined will require conventional orthodontic treatment only (solo provider mode). No other specialists were involved in major treatment planning steps. Note: This patient required gingival grafts as part of her therapy, but she needed no ongoing periodontal management.   *Continued.*

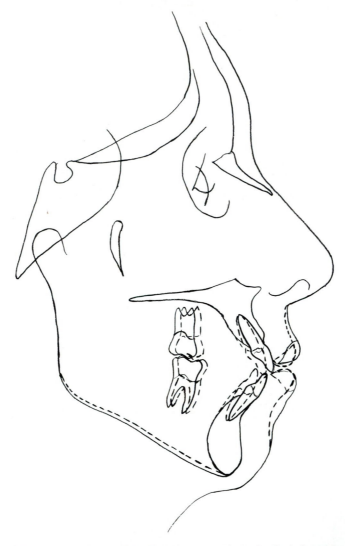

Fig. 14-29, cont'd Pretreatment (solid). Post-treatment (dashed). Cephalometric super-imposition showing favorable lip response to the orthodontic retraction of the upper and lower incisors.

ADULT CASE TYPE
Othognathic Surgery

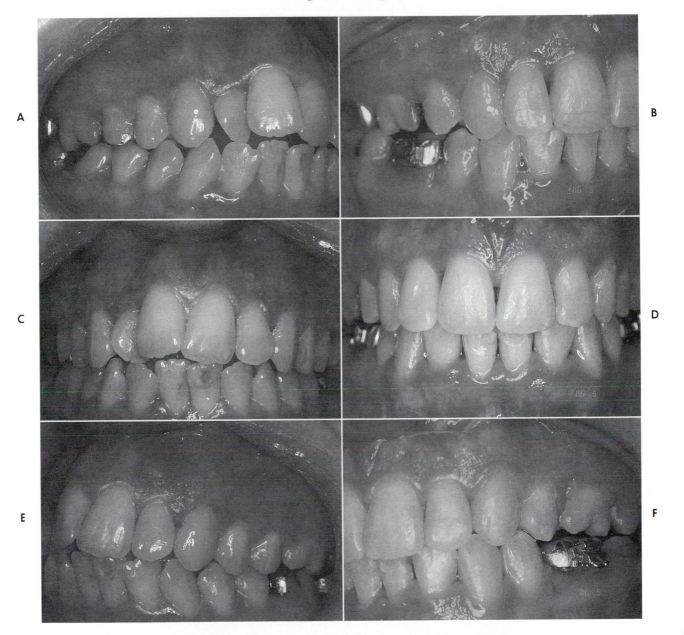

Fig. 14-30 A-M   Section VII; type 5; orthognathic surgery—This 27-year-old woman presented for evaluation with the following chief concerns: overbite; self-conscious about appearance of teeth; and awareness of a clenching habit. Her mouth was heavily restored; #29 had deep decay and was in need of root canal therapy.

This patient was presented with the treatment plan alternatives of extraction and braces, which would give partial correction, or extraction, braces and jaw surgery for full correction. Since she sought a long-term correction and better facial balance, the orthodontic-surgical plan was accepted: orthodontic treatment: full braces with the extraction of four second premolars; orthognathic surgery: LeFort osteotomy with maxillary impaction 5 mm at the first molars, 2 mm at the incisors. Genioplasty with 2.5 mm vertical reduction and 5 mm advancement. **A,C,E,** Pretreatment intra-oral condition. **B,D,F,** Post-treatment intra-oral correction.

Continued.

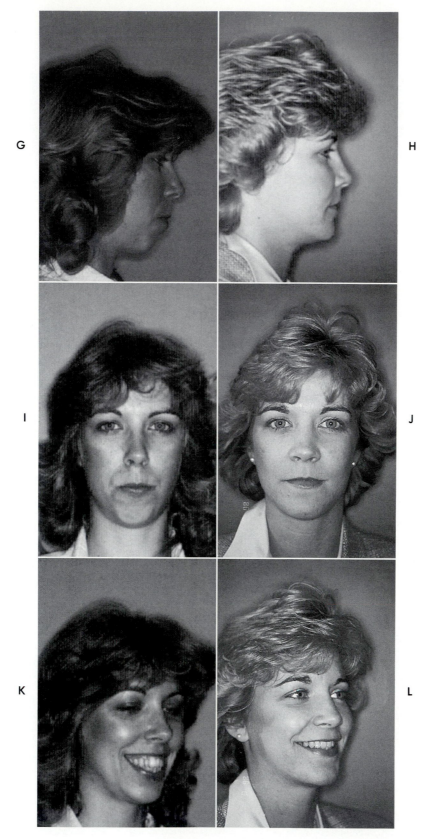

Fig. 14-30, cont'd   **G,H,I,** Pretreatment facial photographs. **J,K,L,** Post-treatment facial relationships.

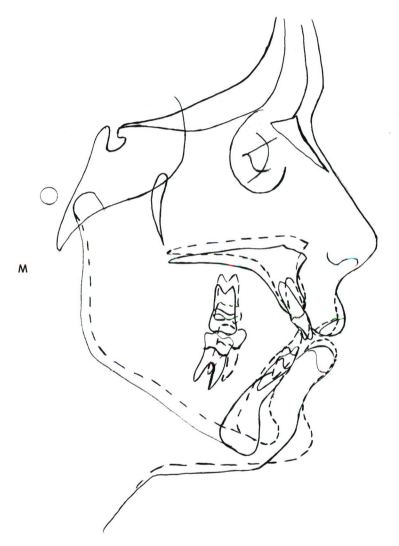

Fig. 14-30, cont'd   M, Cephalometric superimposition. Pretreatment *(solid line)*; post-treatment *(dashed line)*. Data from assessment of treatment needs for adult patients indicate that 15.2% of adults will require an orthodontic surgical component to optimally resolve their condition.

ADULT CASE TYPE
Periodontal Disease

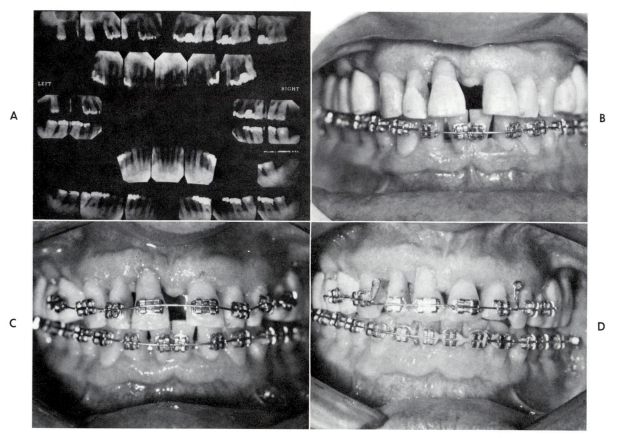

Fig. 14-31 Advanced generalized bone loss in a 48-year-old man. **A,** Pretreatment. **B,** All posterior tooth movement accomplished with disarticulated posterior arches (as in Fig. 14-25). Posterior provisionals then placed bilaterally in the maxillary arch for tooth replacement and stability, and the lower anterior segment bonded. **C,** Maxillary anterior teeth bonded at the same time as the lowers. Brackets bonded to the maxillary posterior provisionals. **D,** Final movement. Retraction of the maxillary anteriors to achieve lip competency and incisal guidance.

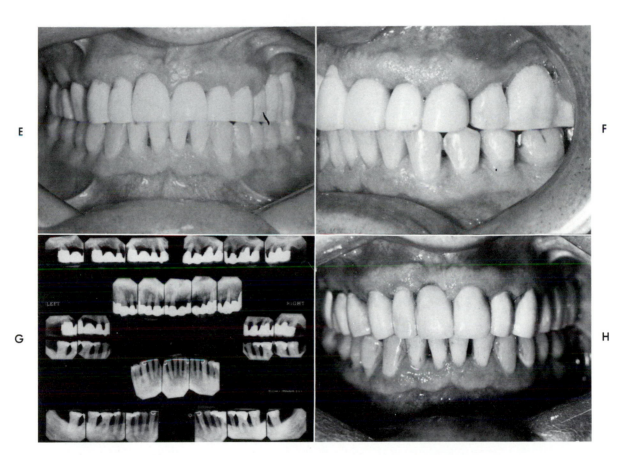

Fig. 14-31, cont'd　**E,** One year after tooth movement and maxillary provisional restoration. **F,** Lower anteriors retained with a bonded 3 to 3. When a precise posterior occlusal scheme is employed, there is no tendency for the accentuated mesial drift to return. **G,** Six years post-treatment. **H,** Final maxillary restoration.

ADULT CASE TYPE
Temporal Mandibular Joint Dysfunction

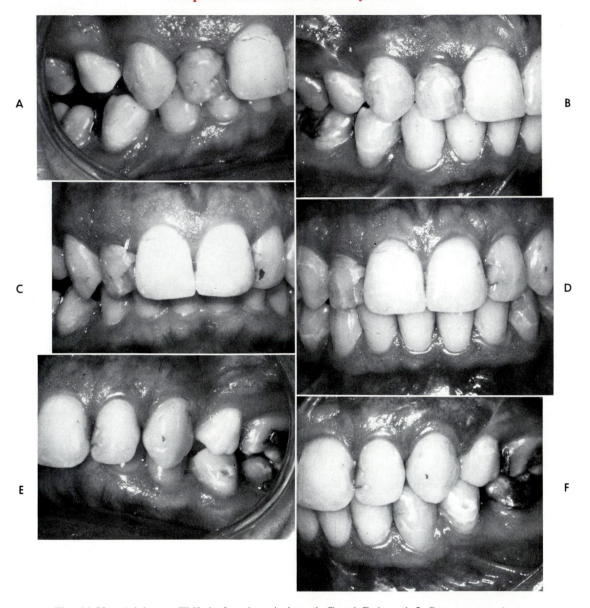

Fig. 14-32   Adult-type TMJ dysfunction. **A** through **C** and **G** through **I,** Pretreatment. A previously treated (four premolar extraction) orthodontic condition. The patient's chief concerns were severe episodes of headache and muscle pain. After symptomatic relief with splint therapy (2½ months), retreatment was done using fixed orthodontic appliances (straight wire edgewise). In conjunction with the orthodontic therapy, orthognathic surgery was included to correct the skeletal imbalances.

G   H   I

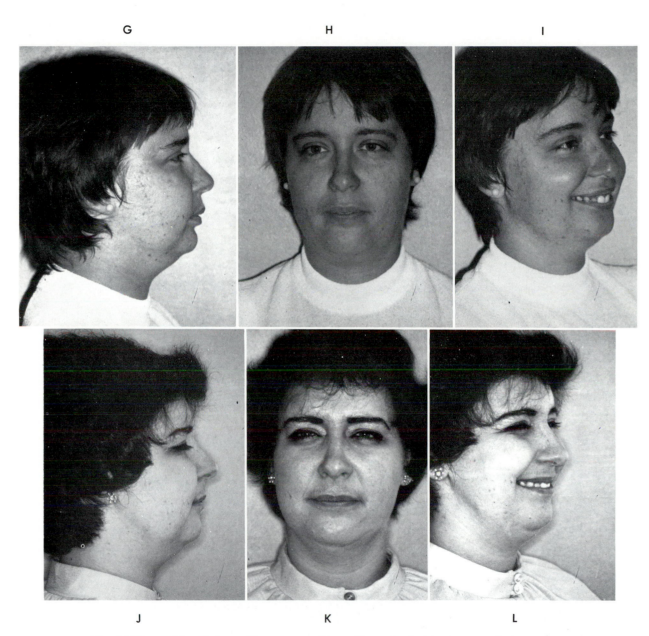

J   K   L

Fig. 14-32, cont'd   Orthognathic treatment: (1) maxillary subapical (canine to canine) osteotomy for intrusion and 3 mm setback; and (2) mandibular sagittal split osteotomy and advancement. **D** through **F** and **J** through **L,** Eighteen months after treatment. Occlusal correction and skeletal harmony. The temporomandibular joint problems have not recurred, and the patient is scheduled for posterior crowns on molars with large failing amalgam restorations. Splint therapy, 2½ months; presurgical orthodontics, 20 months; postsurgical orthodontics, 8 months.

ADULT CASE TYPE
Enamel Wear

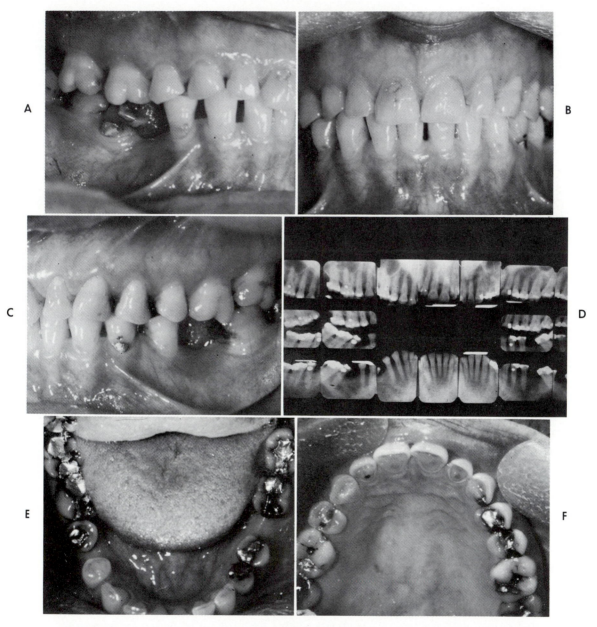

Fig. 14-33 Adult-type enamel wear. **A through C,** Class I with loss of posterior support in a 57-year-old patient, primarily because of caries. **D,** Pretreatment. Good bone support, with no evidence of active periodontal disease. **E,** Extensive amalgam restorations and anterior tooth wear in the lower arch. **F,** The maxillary incisors are in danger of fracturing because of retrograde wear on the palatal aspect.

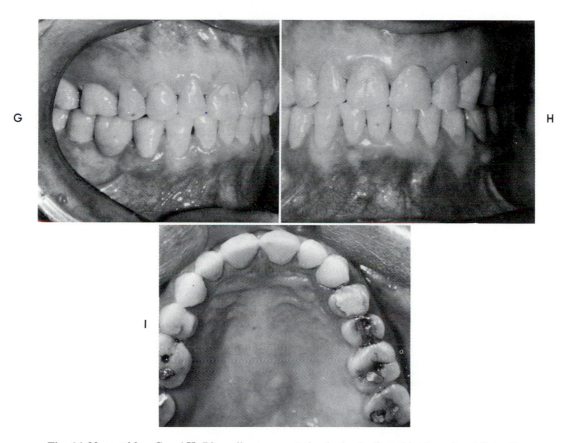

Fig. 14-33, cont'd   G and **H,** Bite collapse corrected orthodontically and bridges place bilaterally in the lower arch. **I,** Three years posttreatment. Composite restoration material used to build up the severely worn anterior teeth.

ADULT CASE TYPE
Dental Mutilation

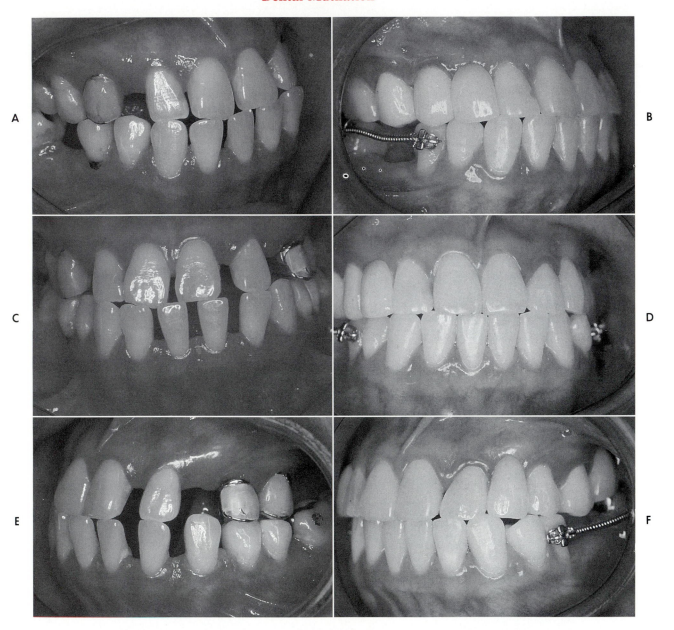

Fig. 14-34 A-L   Section VII: case type 9; dental mutilation. There are similarities between this type and the adjunctive (Case type 3) in that both case types have patients with missing teeth. Case type 9, however, has teeth missing for longer duration. The clinical example illustrates a 38-year-old woman with six missing teeth (#6, #11, #14, #15, #19, #30). The teeth have been missing for over 20 years, and there has been considerable drifting, with subsequent bite changes. The cephalometric tracing shows a −4° ANB difference with a high angle (42° GoGn SN). There is also an obvious tongue thrust or tongue posture problem. The treatment consisted of full braces to redistribute spaces, upright #18 and #31 as abutments, and to leave the skeletal relationship alone. The restorative phase is not yet complete because of the patient's financial problems. Stability remains good 6 years after treatment completion.   *Continued.*

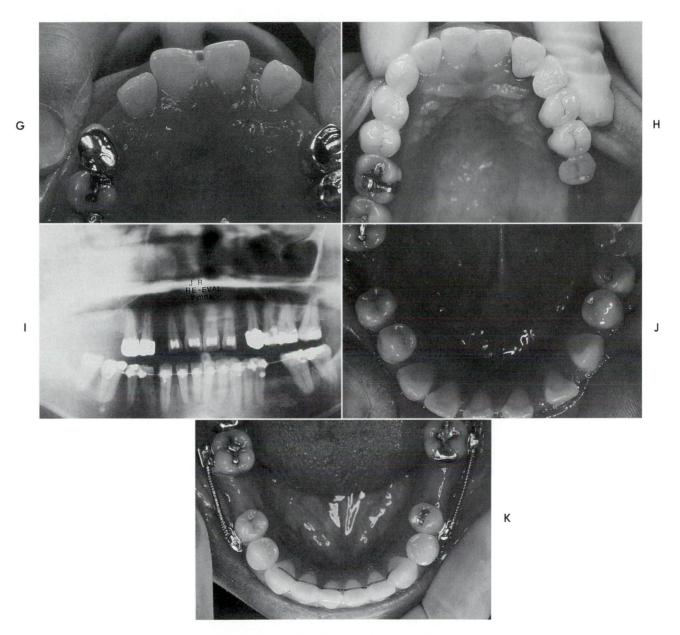

Fig. 14-34, cont'd   For legend see opposite page.

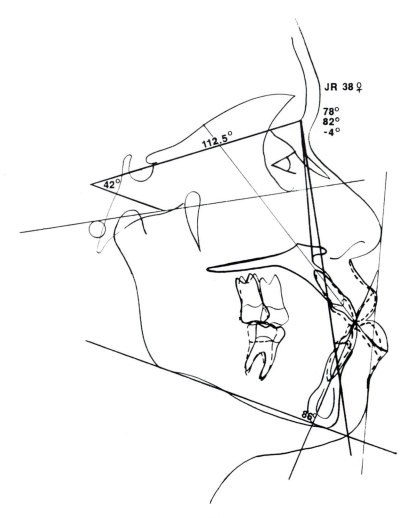

Fig. 14-34, cont'd   For legend see p. 808.

ADULT CASE TYPE
Combination Therapy

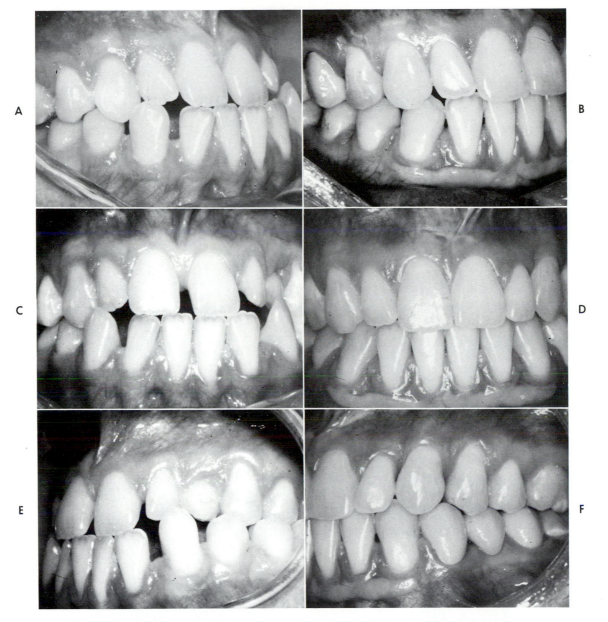

Fig. 14-35 Adult-type combination therapy (periodontal soft tissue grafting, orthodontics, orthognathic surgery, and restorative dentistry). **A, C, E, G, I,** and **M** through **O,** Pretreatment. This patient required combination therapy involving four dental specialists. She had a skeletal Class III malocclusion with facial asymmetry to the left. Her left maxillary canine was impacted and ankylosed; tooth 3 was missing, and gingival stripping had occurred in the lower anterior segment. Surgery; mandibular setback; rotation to the right. **B, D, F, H, J** through **L,** and **P** through **R,** Eighteen months after appliance removal. Mild overcorrection of the mandibular position. Gingival grafting *(arrows)* preceded the orthodontic tooth movement because of the thin gingival tissue and the need to decompensate the lower anterior teeth before orthognathic surgery. Redistribution of the mandibular anterior space and incisor decompensation resulted in the need for a bridge in the lower left quadrant. Presurgical treatment time, 18 months; postsurgical treatment time, 8 months.

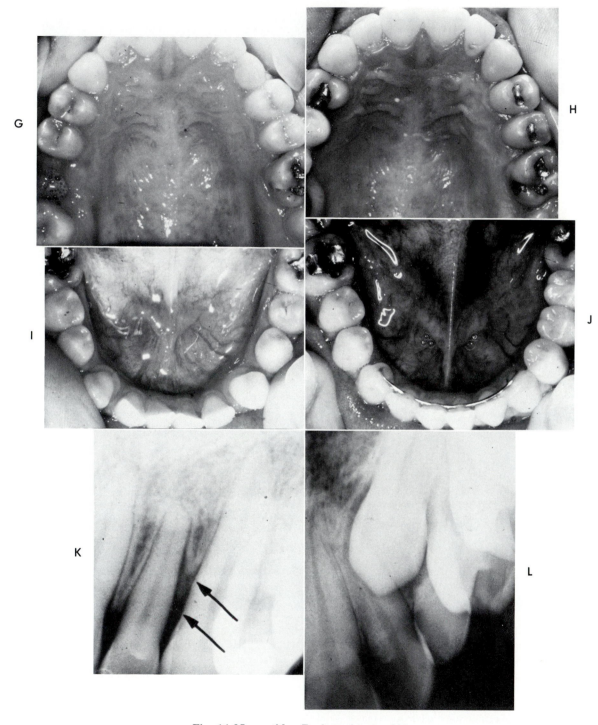

Fig. 14-35, cont'd For legend see p. 811.

M   N   O

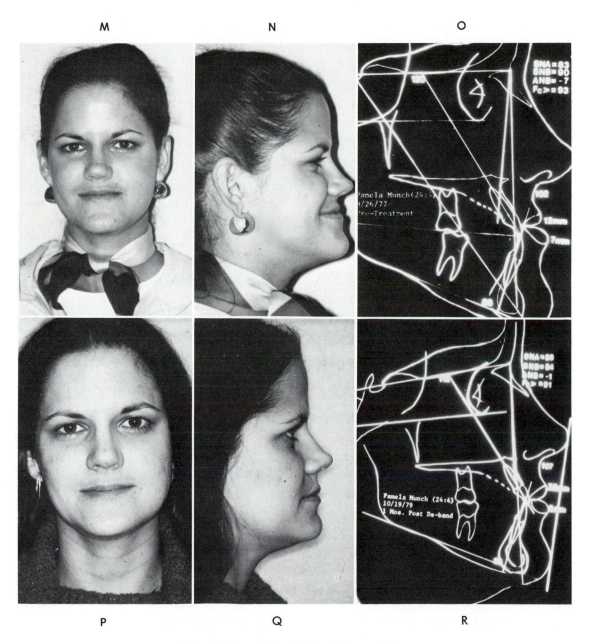

P   Q   R

Fig. 14-35, cont'd   For legend see p. 811.

Periodontal Considerations

One of the most frequently overlooked aspects of orthodontic treatment for adults is the patient's level of periodontal health before the placement of fixed orthodontic appliances. Frequently, the orthodontist is responsible for determining the level of periodontal health so that thorough measures can be undertaken to stop the advancement of the periodontal destruction during tooth movement.

For the orthodontist the periodontal health of adult patients may be classified in one of three categories: incipient periodontal disease, moderate periodontal disease, or advanced periodontal disease as illustrated in the table below:

Each level of periodontal disease requires different therapy with consistent monitoring throughout fixed mechanotherapy to ensure that the disease is arrested and inflammation is controlled. Careful compliance with these steps

TABLE 14-13
Classification of Periodontal Health of Adult Patients

Level of periodontal disease	Therapy prescribed	Provider
Incipient periodontal disease	1. Scaling and curettage 2. Patient education for home care 3. 2 to 6 month maintenance intervals while in fixed appliances	General dentist
Moderate periodontal disease	1. Oral physiotherapy 2. Scaling 3. Definitive osseous surgery 6 to 8 weeks before orthodontics	Periodontist
	4. Orthodontic tooth movement	Orthodontist
	5. 4 to 16 week maintenance intervals during orthodontics	
	6. Periodontal re-evaluation 12 weeks after appliances are removed	Periodontist
Advanced periodontal disease	1. Oral physiotherapy 2. Scaling 3. Periodontal curettage (open flap clean-out)	Periodontist
	4. Orthodontics	Orthodontist
	5. Periodontal reevaluation	Periodontist
	6. Temporization (if needed)	General dentist
	7. Definitive osseous surgery	Periodontist
	8. Final restorative dentistry	General dentist

will help assure that there is no loss of the supporting alveolar bone during orthodontic treatment.

Though various types of procedures have been recommended to control periodontal disease, it should be remembered that conservative approaches are effective in the treatment of cooperative patients with periodontal disease and no orthodontic appliances should be applied to patients who are undergoing periodontal treatment. Adult orthodontic patients generally have 12 to 30 months of fixed appliance therapy, and these appliances interfere with *convenient* oral physiotherapy with the additional potential negative effects of iatrogenic transitional occlusal traumatism induced during certain stages of orthodontic tooth movement.

Management of Dentofacial Deformities

Patients with skeletal imbalances who plan to undergo orthognathic procedures require our utmost attention and care. Although they have the potential to receive the greatest benefits from the combined therapy, they also are exposed to the greatest risk. Each step in this outline (see box on p. 815) is essential for consistent success and quality outcomes. Note: Step 16 in the Sequence, post-treatment (6 to 12 months) records, is often skipped. However, it is critical for refinement and improvement of future team efforts. This step can become an important *in-house* approach to the TEAM's continuing education protocol.

Dual and multiple provider patients need treatment sequencing information, as illustrated in Fig. 14-36, so that standardized communication of the treatment plan is available to the patient and to all providers.

The key elements are as follows:
- Orthodontic diagnosis
- List of dental problems
- Sequence of treatment to manage problems
- Rating of severity
- Rating of prognosis with treatment (Include a discussion of limiting factors.)
- Addressing patient concerns

Retention and Stability Following Active Appliance Therapy

Retention is another critical and challenging aspect of comprehensive orthodontic treatment for adult patients. Proper diagnosis of causative factors (orthodontic, periodontal, psychologic) is essential to achieving treatment objectives best suited for each patient. Also the patient's compliance with the complete regimen of therapy, especially restorative dentistry and orthognathic surgery, provides the underlying framework for orthodontic therapy that offers stability. The principles of retention are clearly discussed in Chapter 16, and those principles are applicable to patients with complete natural dentitions regardless of age. There are, however, special considerations regarding adult retention that should be mentioned.

TREATMENT SEQUENCE FOR PATIENTS WITH MAJOR DENTO-FACIAL SKELETAL IMBALANCES

1. Multiple provider team selection
   - Orthodontist
   - Periodontist
   - Restorative dentist
   - Oral surgeon
   - Psychologist
2. Goal clarification for team members
   - Function
   - Reliable methods
   - Esthetics
   - Stability
   - Health
3. Clinical awareness of dentofacial deformity
   - Self, DDS, friend
4. General assessment of patient
   - A good candidate?
5. Evaluation of preliminary records by the dental team
   - Splint therapy for diagnosis of TMJ dysfunction if needed
6. Completion of diagnostic records
   - May include lifestyle assessment by clinical psychologist
   - May require more sophisticated TMJ studies
7. Multidisciplinary review of dentofacial problem based on patient records
8. Explanation to patient of available treatment options
   - Recommend optimal treatment plan
9. Consultation with patient and spouse by dental providers
   - Risk/benefit ratio
   - Fees and insurance coverage
   - Treatment time
   - Other concerns
10. Patient acceptance of treatment plan

11. Comprehensive orthodontic treatment (usually 8 to 10 months before surgery)
    - Orthodontic movement to decompensate tooth positions
    - Coordinate arches in anticipation of surgical repositioning
    - Align teeth and correct rotations
12. Presurgical reevaluation records
    - Complete records
    - Prediction tracing (detailed movements planned)
    - Model surgery
    - Determination of specific fixation needs
    - Patient/spouse review
    - Reevaluation by psychologist
13. Orthognathic surgery
    - Choose simplest procedure(s) to achieve goals and to satisfy needs of the patient
14. Postsurgical period
    - Early: 2 to 3 weeks fixation
    - Late: 3 to 8 weeks fixation
    - Reevaluation of surgical procedure
    - Meeting between patient and psychologist for update and support
15. Evaluation of surgery stability
    - Orthodontic finishing, occlusal adjustments, and retention procedures
    - Optional continuation of contact with psychologist
16. Post-treatment records
    - One-year post-treatment
    - Reevaluation with dental team, especially oral surgeon and psychologist
17. Treatment experience (used in management of future cases)
    - Positive reinforcement
    - Problem-solving
    - Reevaluation of degree of success in achieving goals
    - Treatment evaluations by patient and all providers

Evaluation Before Debonding or Debanding

1. Root parallelism—this must be verified by panoramic or periapical radiographs before appliance removal.
2. Coincidence of centric relation and habitual occlusion—this should be evaluated clinically and may require deprogramming appliances.
3. Incisal guidance—this should be evaluated clinically and in some cases with mounted study models.
4. Joint symptoms—these are assessed clinically and appropriate therapy is provided.
5. Excursive movements—these are examined clinically and augmented in some cases with mounted study models.
6. Patient input—patients should be encouraged to discuss

the existing dentofacial esthetics before appliance removal. Many patients will point out concerns that may be correctable with minor modifications in mechanotherapy.

7. Reaffirmation of restorative commitment—this is to be reviewed with the patient and discussed with the restorative dentist and periodontist. The timing of the restorative procedures and the coordination of restorative treatment with the orthodontic retention schedule are important.
8. Periodontal considerations re-evaluated—this is done clinically with radiographs; check mobility and fremitus, perform probing, and make soft tissue assessment.
9. Re-evaluation of anterior and posterior tooth size dis-

TREATMENT CONFERENCE REPORT

Re: Barbara S. (40:2)   Date: 10-84

I. Classification and Diagnostic Description of Malocclusion

1. Class III mandibular excess with maxillary posterior vertical excess and open bite

II. List of Dental Problems: (mild / moderate / severe)

1. Periodontitis (moderate)
2. Restorative—several old restorations failing (moderate)
3. TMJ—disc displacement with reduction; frequent headaches (moderate)
4. Class III mandibular excess (moderate)
5. Anterior openbite—chewing difficult (moderate)
6. Posterior crossbite (moderate)
7. Lower incisor crowding (moderate)

III. Treatment Sequence Recommended at This Time

1. Periodontal—inflammation control; deep scaling and periodontal preparation for tooth movement
2. TMJ—lower splint to evaluate headache symptoms and mandibular position
3. Temporary crowns—#8, #9 for better periodontal environment
4. Oral surgery consult for orthognathic treatment plan and TMJ evaluation (also insurance approval)
5. Orthodontic treatment to prepare for jaw surgery
6. Extraction of #24 to allow for alignment of lower incisors
7. Re-evaluation records with mounted models to decide on lower jaw surgery only or upper or lower jaw surgery for anterior stability of openbite correction
8. Jaw surgery
9. Finish orthodontics
10. Periodontal evaluation and osseous surgery if needed
11. Complete needed restorative dentistry

Reference Charting							
Deciduous				Permanent			
A B C D E|F G H I J				1 2 3 4 5	6 7 8|9 10 11	12 13 14 15 16
T S R Q P|O N M L K				32 31 30 29 28	27 26 25|24 23 22	21 20 19 18 17

IV. Overall Problem Severity (0-10 scale; ideal to severe)

Due to perio, TMJ, restorative and orthognathic—severity equals 8

V. Limiting Factors in Achieving "Text Book Ideal" Result   Prognosis: (0-10; ideal to severe) 2

1. TMJ problem may persist, as displaced disc is not being corrected; improved occlusion should reduce muscle spasms
2. Perio condition needs constant management by periodontist and home care by patient
3. Restorative treatment needs are significant, and treatment by general dentist will follow bite correction

VI. Patient Concerns and Current Plan of Action

1. Patient wants to improve bite; she had previous orthodontic disappointment (4 years of braces as a teenager by nonspecialist)
2. Patient wants to improve appearance of teeth
3. She is encouraged that something can be done

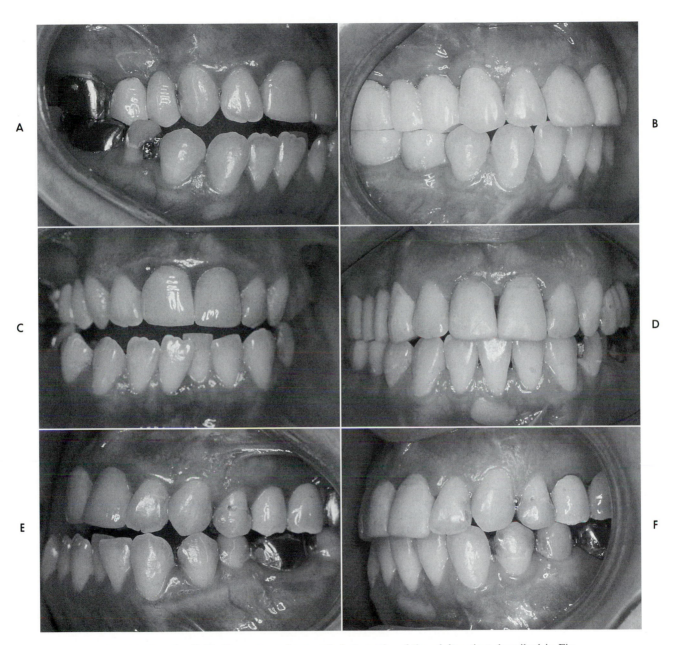

Fig. 14-37   **A, C, E,** Pretreatment intra-oral photographs of the adult patient described in Fig. 14-36 (Treatment Conference Report). **B, D, F,** Post-treatment intra-oral photographs. The patient has received periodontal therapy, orthodontics as well as jaw surgery, and is in provisional restorations at this time.   *Continued.*

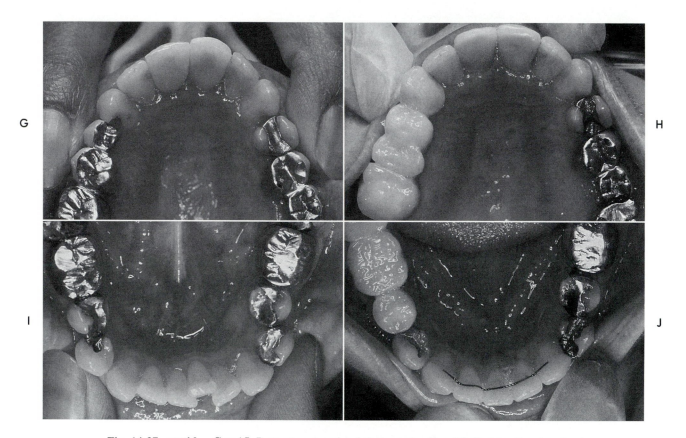

Fig. 14-37, cont'd   **G** and **I,** Pretreatment occlusal photographs. **H** and **J,** Post-treatment occlusal photographs showing improved arch form with a lower incisor extraction. There was a tooth size discrepancy which allowed this procedure to be effective.

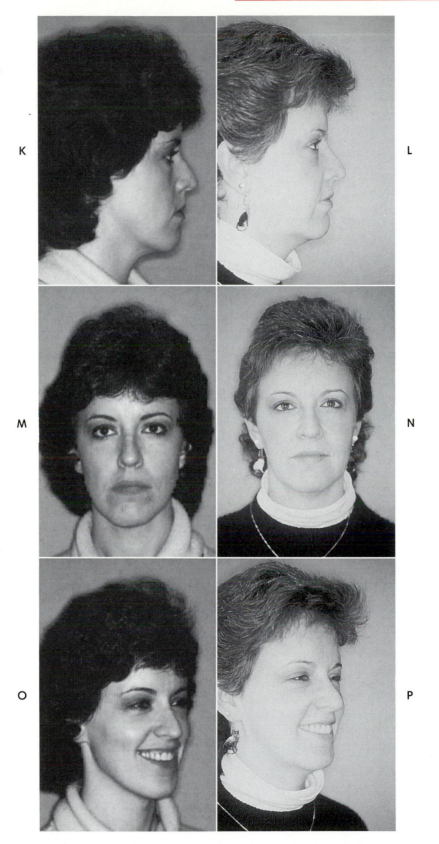

Fig. 14-37, cont'd   K, M, O, Pre-treatment facial photographs. **L, N P,** Post-treatment facial photographs showing minor facial change with the LeFort surgery and mandibular auto-rotation and surgical set-back.   *Continued.*

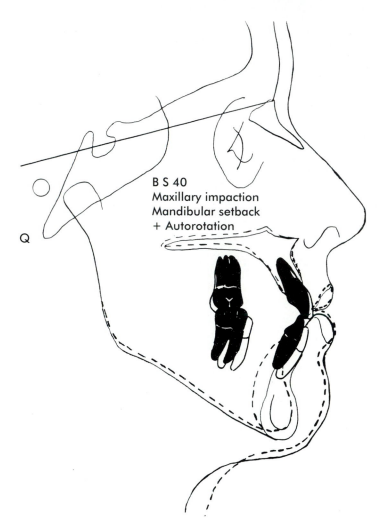

Fig. 14-37, cont'd   **Q,** Cephalometric superimposition showing 3 mm impaction at the first molars and 0 mm impaction at the incisors. There was mandibular auto-rotation and a mandibular set-back of approximately 6 mm at *B* point.

crepancies—this should be done to inform the patient and the general dentist of additional measures that may be necessary to resolve tooth size discrepancies. Plans should be made to correct these discrepancies without adversely altering the posterior occlusal relationships or incisal guidance (i.e., acid etch *add on* technique).

10. Anticipated retention problems—plans and provisions should be made and entered on the patient's chart if retention problems are anticipated so problem-solving steps can be easily recalled in the future as necessary.

11. Reassess original malocclusion—this is helpful to determine the specific anatomic retention needs of the case (i.e., skeletal or dental deepbite, openbite, overcorrections).

Abnormal Musculature

When the patient has abnormal lip, tongue, or cheek muscle activities, it is incumbent on the orthodontist to prepare the patient for long-term use of fixed retainers and tongue cribs at night.

Periodontal Surgical Retention Procedures

Procedure	Indications	Time
Fiberotomy[3,21] (Fig. 14-38)	Any significantly rotated teeth, especially maxillary and mandibular anterior teeth (e.g., maxillary lateral incisors in Class II, division 2, type problems)	Just before debanding after mild (5° to 10°) overcorrection Before fixed appliance removal

Procedure	Indications	Time
Gingivectomy or gingivoplasty (Fig. 14-39)	To enhance alignment and overbite correction where significant vertical changes have been made orthodontically	Before fixed appliance removal

Procedure	Indications	Time
Labiolingual tissue reflections with interproximal sutures (Fig. 14-40)	To maintain incisors and canines previously labially or lingually displaced	After root positioning and just before fixed appliance removal

Coordination of debonding or debanding with other treatment providers

1. Post-treatment radiographs
2. Periodontal re-evaluation and treatment
3. Restorative treatment and retention considerations—these require that stabilizing sectional appliances be removed by the restorative dentist before placement of restorations. Also maxillary and mandibular Hawley retainers may be needed with tooth replacements when the restorative procedure includes anterior tooth replacement.
4. Duration of the retention period—this will vary according to the case type, overall restorative treatment plan, orthodontic result, and various causative factors (which

---

RETAINER DESCRIPTION

Type	Indications
Noninterfering acrylic and wire (Hawley retainer)	To retain most maxillary arches
Hawley with tongue cribs	To aid in management of residual neuromuscular problems, especially postural tongue habits; worn at night, with regular Hawley during daytime
Tooth positioner	Orthognathic patients, especially those having undergone double jaw procedures and significant vertical muscular changes to help refine residual discrepancies; not indicated for periodontally involved patients on long-term basis
Fixed (bonded) retainer	Lower anterior segments; also to maintain maxillary anterior segments not treated with surgical intervention (e.g., hypertonic mentalis muscle, long term)

Restorative Dentistry	Indications
Limited techniques Composite add-on reshaping	To fill in space beneath contact area in patients with bell-shaped incisors who previously had overlapped teeth; some lower incisor extractions may also require this reshaping for esthetics and proper incisal positioning
Amalgam (Class II), inlay or onlay	To correct posterior tooth size discrepancies and reestablish interproximal contact relationships in bite collapse, after debanding, and before selective grinding
Comprehensive restorative procedures (crown and bridge)	Mutilated dentitions that require immediate posterior provisional restorations for stabilization to be followed by permanent restorative dentistry
	Bonded anterior tooth replacement should be considered in conjunction with maxillary Hawley retainer for optimal esthetics; if labial bow from Hawley crosses occlusal area, the provisional restoration should be grooved to allow proper wire accommodation and positioning without occlusal interference
	During alterations of provisional restoration, contact area of anterior teeth can be bonded as retention measure if there are frequent changes in retainer needs

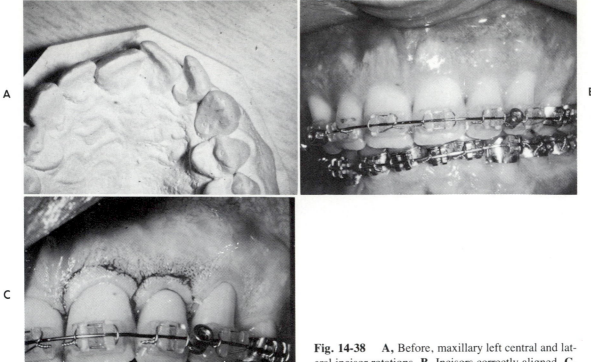

Fig. 14-38 **A,** Before, maxillary left central and lateral incisor rotations. **B,** Incisors correctly aligned. **C,** Before appliance removal; a circumferential fiberotomy to enhance posttreatment stability.

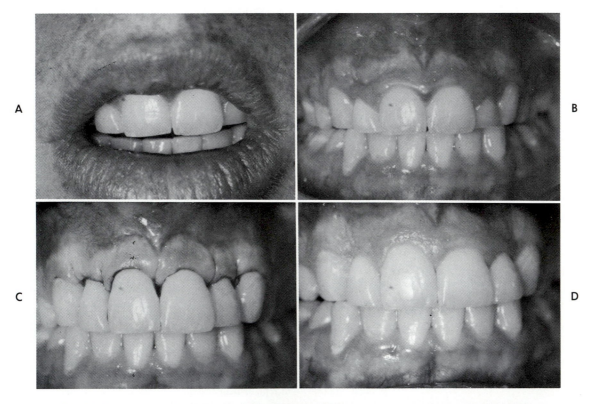

Fig. 14-39 **A,** Note the short upper lip and exposed gingiva in a post-treatment mouth breather. **B,** Erythematous gingiva covers 50% of the anatomic crowns of this 14-year-old boy's maxillary anterior segment. **C,** To enhance post-treatment stability and improve esthetics and gingival health, an internal beveled gingivectomy was performed. Note the interproximal absorbable sutures. **D,** One year postretention. Maintenance of tooth position and periodontal health.

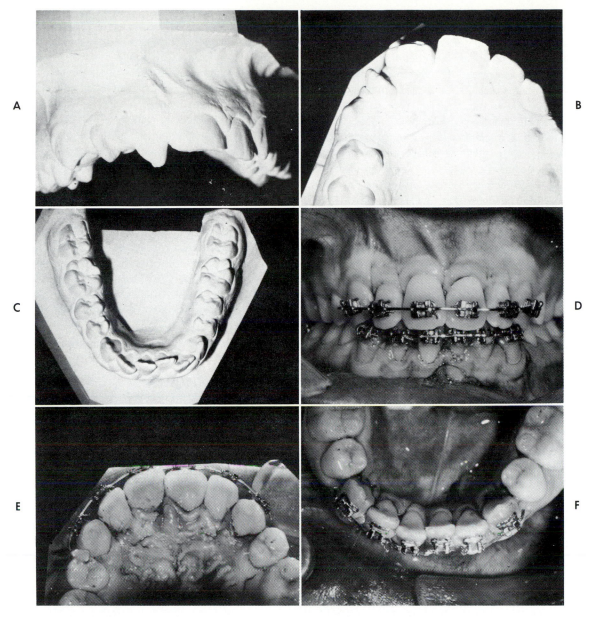

Fig. 14-40 **A** through **C,** Before incisor rotations and labiolingual positioning. **D,** Retreatment after maxillary and mandibular incisor relapse. Labial and lingual reflections were performed and interproximal absorbable sutures were placed to adapt the gingival tissue. **E** and **F,** Note the overcorrections in both segments, as advocated by Swain.

again must be customized to the individual patient). Generally, the retention period for adults is longer. The weaning period from the removable retainers also takes place over a longer time. To enhance the overall stability of treatment, selective grinding for centric and anterior disclusion during excursive movements is essential. If there is significant (1 or 2 mm) CR to CO discrepancy, occlusal adjustment is required. A Hawley appliance with a bite plane will help eliminate muscle dysfunction and facilitate selective grinding to a stable centric relation position.

Adult Stability

Whether a case may have been treated by extraction or nonextraction, retention is necessary for stabilization. Each individual malocclusion requires special planning for post-treatment stabilization during the retention phase of treatment. Many changes will occur in patients after completion of orthodontic therapy, but it is well documented today that growth in small amounts occurs in the adult patient.[20,25,84] Behrents[11] documented facial growth in the adult years. He showed that rotation of the mandible continued forward in males and backward in females; further eruption of teeth occurred, as well as dentitional compensations. There were changes in the soft tissue profile (in particular in the nose and chin) that must be understood to treat adults in the best fashion. Israel documented that the craniofacial skeleton increases in size into adult years.[43,44] Susanne documented facial growth continuing into the fourth through to the sixth decade.[89] Data has shown there can be from 12% to 15% of dentofacial growth that can occur in adults.[11] The occlusion has been identified as another significant factor in post-treatment change. With interarch relationships changing during growth the teeth will contact occlusally in different ways, and there will be compensating changes in the teeth resulting in occlusal changes. The occlusal contacts and excursive movements must be evaluated at all retention visits, and if significant change has occurred, selective grinding may be required. Williamson and Roth have indicated the importance of treating to centric relation and the instability that can be introduced when a therapeutic occlusion is created orthodontically and a discrepancy between maximum intercuspation and centric relation exists.[87,101]

Treating a Class I relationship for adolescents or teenage patients in which the skeletal bases are normal, is usually satisfactory and often quite stable. Unfortunately these are not the clinical circumstances presented by most adult patients. Frequently, they have skeletal Class II problems, more appropriately treated with extraction in the upper arch only; the outcome is finished with a Class II molar relationship that usually requires occlusal adjustment by selective grinding that may or not be done. A tooth size discrepancy is created by removing maxillary first premolars only, and this approach has been shown by Servoss to be less stable than extraction in both arches. Also, the effects of the periodontium in creating instability in post-treated orthodontic cases is well documented.[85] Picton and Moss have shown that the effects of transseptal fibers upon the teeth with a constant and mesial migration of the dentition throughout life could cause incisor irregularities and crowding. Hixon and Horowitz in their 1969 text stated that "the significant point is that orthodontic therapy may temporarily alter the course of continuous physiological changes and possibly for a time can even reverse them. However, following mechanotherapy and a period of retention restraint, the developmental maturation process resumes." In addition, there has been the apical base school throughout the history

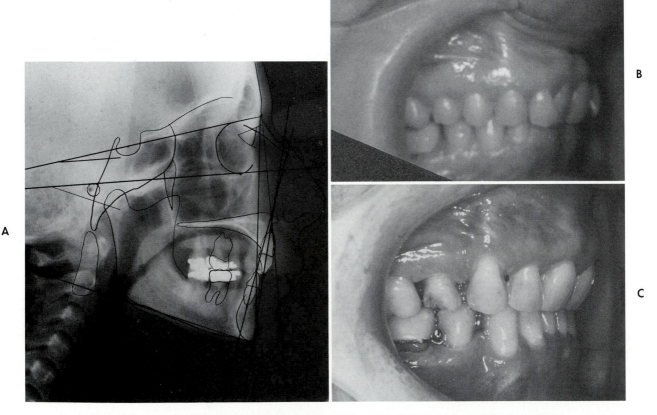

Fig. 14-41 **A,** This cooperative patient demanded that appliances be removed because of poor esthetics, extremely mobile teeth, and periodontal problems. Observe on the post-treatment Cephalometric film an upper incisor to NA at 14° with an IMPA of 87°. **B,** Preoperative right lateral intra-oral view. **C,** Post-orthodontic right lateral view showing gingival recession and compensated position of maxillary incisors.

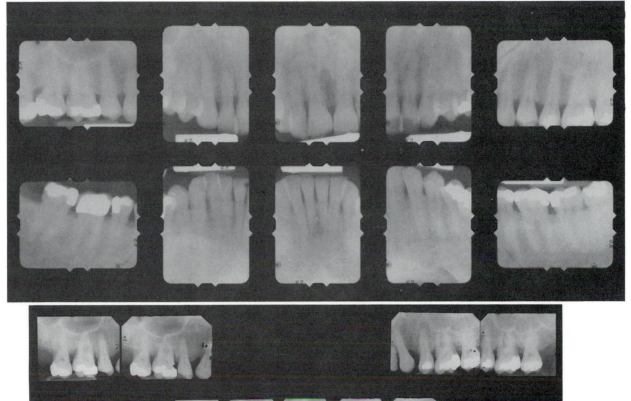

D

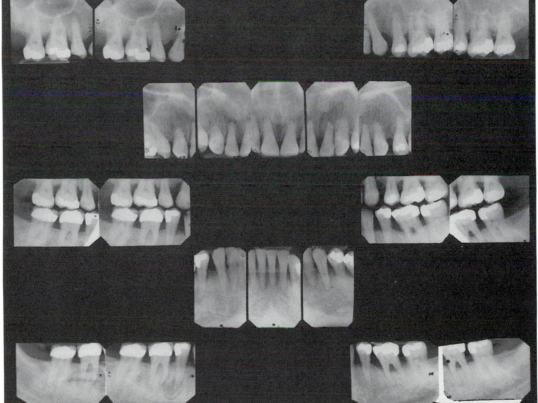

E

Fig. 14-41, cont'd   D, Pretreatment periapical radiographs exhibiting normal root length and minimal attachment loss. **E,** Post-treatment radiographs after 3 years in appliances, showing loss of attachment, widened PDL spaces, root resorption, and lack of arch integrity.

of orthodontics (discussed in Chapter 16). Holdaway cautioned that good facial harmony could be achieved as long as the apical base did not exceed a range permitting compensating dental adjustments.[36] Apical base discrepancies are tremendously limiting factors in adult treatment.

Observe a Class II adult female patient who received extraction of upper and lower first premolars because of sagittal skeletal discrepancy of 8° ANB and a rather normal vertical pattern (an FMA of 22°); note that more dental compensation was placed in the upper incisors than the lower incisors (Fig. 14-41, A and C). Also observe the unesthetic dentofacial change. In addition, the patient experienced significant loss of attachment, root resorption (over a two or three-year period of time), and generalized spacing as the result of an inability to close extraction spaces in this severe sagittal discrepancy. Fig. 14-41, B through E, demonstrates that there are skeletal limitations of orthodontic treatment, particularly in adult patients. The sagittal limitations without camouflaging the skeletal discrepancy, with a normal vertical relationship would be approximately a Class II ANB of 7° or 8° (this would exclude bimaxillary protrusion) and in the Class III skeletal problems, an ANB of −3° usually would require restorative procedures or orthognathic surgery to achieve compensated anterior tooth stability. With patterns that involve vertical open bite, excessive face height, and associated muscle problems, it is common with the use of vertical elastics to encounter more root blunting or root resorption. Clinicians are well aware of the problems of Class II elastics in high angle cases tending to tip the occlusion plane, moving the lower dentition forward, and creating periodontal problems resulting in discrepancies in centric relation and habitual occlusion.

The familiar long face problem exhibits excessive eruption of maxillary teeth, maxillary transverse constriction, excessive overjet, anterior open bite and associated mouth breathing. This patient, with a long face and a gingival smile, who elected to go through orthodontic treatment first, could only have been improved to look as he does on the right through the use of the Le Fort I osteotomy technique (Fig. 14-42, A and B).

Common pitfalls in adult treatment leading to instability are as follows:
1. Tendency to extract premolars in borderline cases, and extracting in the lower arch as well, when the mandibular dentition is more distally placed
2. With vertical excess problems of lip incompetency, extracting upper premolars only
3. Attempting to close excessive extraction spaces when the problem should be treatment planned for alignment of the teeth, and using prosthetic replacements to replace teeth rather than attempting space closure

A significant report was made by Casko and Shepherd in the Angle Orthodontist in 1984 in which they evaluated 79 untreated adults with ideal Class I dental occlusions, and none of the patients subjectively were thought to have poor or unacceptable profiles. They discovered that the cephalometric values for the skeletal discrepancies in this group were far beyond mean figures often used as treatment goals. Proffit and Ackerman illustrate the envelope of discrepancy in the sagittal and vertical dimensions in Chapter 1. As well, cases must be evaluated in the transverse dimension for transverse skeletal discrepancy and this can best be done at the present time with the use of the (P/A) radiograph. A significant skeletal discrepancy in a transverse dimension diagnosed by only looking at the dentition and by attempting

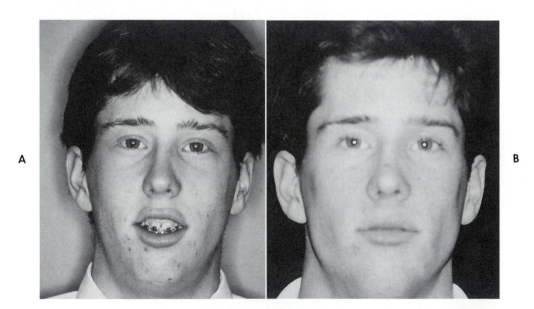

A

B

Fig. 14-42 **A,** Long face patient, who initially refused surgery, and after 1½ years of orthodontics requested to be reevaluated for a maxillary impaction. **B,** Postorthognathic surgery. Observe excellent lip competency.

to use arch wires to laterally expand the teeth on a constricted maxillary apical base frequently creates buccal gingival recession as one of the possible side effects of camouflaging patients wtih transverse dysplasias. Clinicians must develop an envelope of discrepancy concept for the transverse dimension, as well as in the sagittal and vertical dimension (Fig. 14-43, *A* and *B*). With transverse skeletal problems for the adult, treatment options are to leave the patient in crossbite, use restorative dentistry to change the contour of the posterior teeth to achieve a more normal dental buccolingual landmark relationship through restorative dentistry, or correct the skeletal pattern by surgically assisted palatal expansion correcting the skeletal problem surgically. If we camouflage the transverse skeletal deficiency by only moving the teeth it may cause periodontal problems, mainly buccal gingival recession, and instability of the occlusal

scheme. The effective surgical procedure to use was reported in August, 1976.[48]

In the transverse dimension the clinician may elect to camouflage the skeletal discrepancy by tipping the teeth, creating occlusal instability and periodontal problems, or should the surgical procedure be used, the expansion appliance should have acrylic that covers the palate. With an effective surgical procedure, tissue borne appliances do not create excessive pressure on the palatal mucosa and will not create vascular ischemia by pressure against the palatal tissue. Tooth borne appliances alone, however, tend to allow for more dental tipping than is seen with appliances that have acrylic on the palate. Therefore, *Hyrax-type* appliances are not recommended. This case illustrates significant dental tipping that occurred as a result of using that appliance (Fig. 14-44). The more effective appliance is the Haas-type ap-

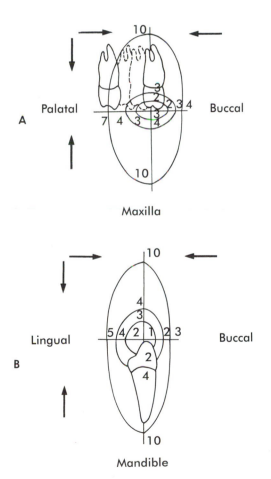

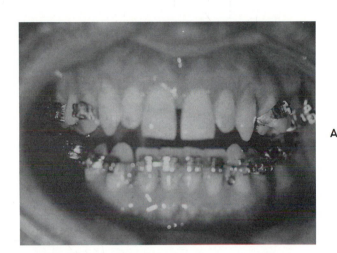

A

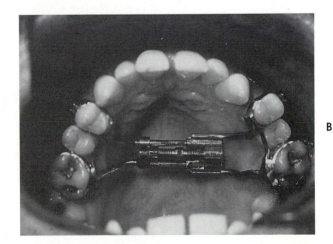

B

Fig. 14-43 **A,** "Transverse "envelope of discrepancy" for the maxilla. **B,** Transverse envelope for the mandible. Inner circle indicates movement possible with orthodontic's alone and the outer red circle indicates the potential with the aid of orthognathic surgery on the left side of the mandible.

Fig. 14-44 **A,** From the anterior view, note obvious tipping of buccal segments with the appliance being used in conjunction with orthognathic surgery to widen the palate. **B,** Occlusal view of Hyrax-type expander and tipped posterior segments.

Pre   Post

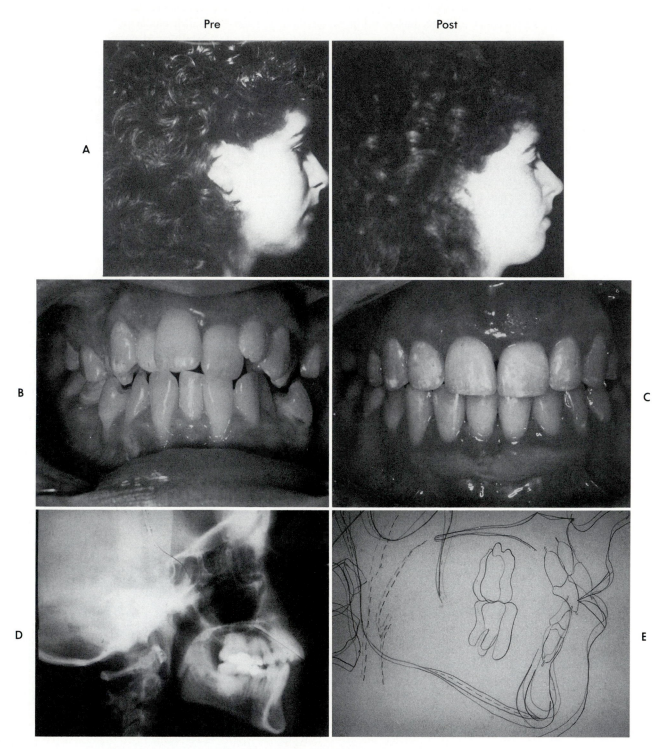

Fig. 14-45 **A,** Pre- and post-treatment facial profile photographs indicate little change with removal of four premolars. **B,** Pretreatment alignment. **C,** Post-treatment alignment. **D,** Pretreatment cephalometric film shows the anterior open bite and overjet. **E,** Cephalometric superimposition illustrates upper incisor retraction to obtain incisal guidance. **F,** Note spaces mesial and distal to the lower right molar when patient demanded that appliances be removed. **G,** The large mandibular molar provisional was placed at the time appliances are removed.

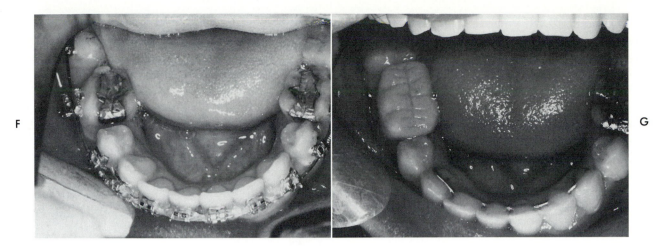

Fig. 14-45, cont'd   For legend see opposite page.

pliance. The surgical procedure involves raising the mucoperiosteal tissue in the buccal vestibule bilaterally in the maxilla and a horizontal osteotomy is made through the lateral wall of the maxilla 4 to 5 mm, superior to the posterior teeth. In addition, to facilitate the separation of the maxilla, an osteotome is used between the central incisors to separate the palate. Usually the procedure is a day surgery and does not require that the patient stay overnight in the hospital.

For the Class II orthodontic patient, extraction is necessary with skeletal deformities, vertical growth patterns, and bimaxillary protrusions, and in the maxillary arch only. Therefore, for the Class II patient, Fig. 14-45 shows an example of limitations that exist in adult treatment. The pre- and post-treatment photographs (Fig. 14-45, A) demonstrate little change in the patient's profile, but her dental alignment is much better (Fig. 14-45, B and C). The upper teeth have been bilaterally retracted several millimeters to couple the upper incisors and the lower arch (Fig. 14-45, D and E). Once the patient *demanded* that all appliances be removed before complete space closure, a retainer was bonded to the lower, canine to canine. The lower right molar had a large amalgam filling and was crowned so that mesiodistal contact (arch integrity) was maintained through the second molar (Fig. 14-45, F and G). An operative restoration was placed on the patient's left side and *immediate* removable retainers were inserted. An impression was taken of the upper arch with instructions for the laboratory to carve off all the brackets, and at the time the case was debonded the retainer was placed *immediately* because of the muscle problem (tongue thrust). The patient was given two retainers for the maxillary arch. One was worn during the day (a regular removable retainer) for an indefinite period of time, until it could be left out during the day. The termination of the daytime wear was indicated when the patient felt no pressure on the teeth at the insertion of the night crib appliance. The day appliance

may be required for up to a year, but the night crib is used indefinitely. The crib appliance at night prevents the tongue from being placed between the anterior teeth that would allow for eruption of molars and a return of the open bite. The tongue appliance that is given to all patients with a forward resting tongue posture problem is illustrated in Fig. 14-46, A and B.

Patients who exhibit a tongue placement habit can also be recognized by their forward tongue placement during speech. Retention requires special consideration for post-treatment stability, as indicated in Fig. 14-46. The forward resting tongue posture problem is significant, particularly for the adult patient who has maintained the habit of placing his or her tongue between the anterior segment beyond the adolescent years. An article was reported in the *Angle Orthodontist* in 1989 by Denison, Kokich, and Shapiro titled "Stability of Maxillary Surgery in Openbite vs Non-openbite Malocclusion." The sample was divided into three groups and based upon the degree of pretreatment overbite, open bite subsample; results show clearly that the three subsamples tested responded differently during the post-treatment interval. Forty-two and nine tenths percent of the subsample with pretreatment open bite showed a significant increase in facial height, significant eruption of maxillary molars, and significant decrease in overbite; 26.6% of the open bite sample and 16.7% of the overlap subsamples showed a significant increase in facial height, significant eruption of posterior teeth, and no change in overbite. The incisal contact sample had no significant post-treatment changes. Possible reasons for post-treatment instability and one of the factors that was not taken into consideration in retention with this study population was the forward placement of the tongue crib that was to be worn at night only. Open bite that recurred in 42.9% of subjects with pretreatment of open bite could have been reduced with the use of a tongue crib retainer at night. As stated earlier, patients commonly place

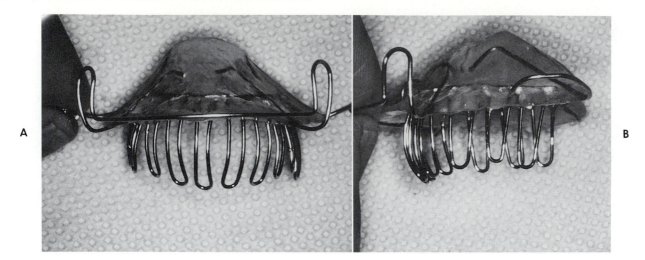

Fig. 14-46 **A,** Anterior view of the tongue crib that is used as a retainer indefinitely. **B,** The appliance has a labial bow with ring clasps, and the crib extends back to the second molar area and to the lingual mucogingival junction of the mandible when the patient is in maximum intercuspation.

their tongue between the anterior segments, allowing the vertical eruption at the molars that will result in recurrence of the dental open bite.

For skeletal Class II patients it may be necessary to advance the lower incisors (compensation is placed in the mandibular dentition not in the maxillary incisors) and place tooth material bilaterally in the posterior segments of the mandible, as seen in Fig. 14-47, where two restorations were placed in the mandible. In Class III cases we may compensate the maxillary incisors for the Class III skeletal pattern by adding tooth material in the maxillary posterior segments bilaterally to maintain a more procumbent maxillary incisors, without allowing the upper incisors to be placed into permanent trauma or fremitus because of the Class III skeletal pattern. Fig. 14-48 exhibits a Class III case in which the maxillary centrals are moved to the midline; two bridges were placed in the maxillary posterior segments, allowing the anterior teeth to be stable without putting permanent trauma on the upper anterior teeth. To remove the appliance and merely insert an upper and lower removable retainer would not insure stability. Placing two retainers without reshaping old restorations that have been carved up in the preorthodontic occlusion will not achieve stability. When there are tooth size discrepancies or when teeth are taken out, it may be necesssary to reshape remaining teeth with bonding material. It is much easier to establish intimate occlusion and stability for a patient that does not have old fillings and restorations. Patients with old crowns that were carved to a previous malocclusion or large restorations and amalgams that need to be reshaped also require occlusal adjustment by selective grinding to create a definitive occlusion that coordinates maximum intercuspation and central relation.

Adaptations that occur with aging have been well described by Behrents. The adult orthodontic patient will need

to have indefinite retention in the mandibular anteriors. The Sillman collection at University of Pennsylvania features long-term records of Class I individuals (who received minimal or no treatment) that had well-aligned incisors at age 13 but had crowding at 22 years of age, together with normal dentitional compensations of aging. Prerestorative space or pontic areas that are created in treatment require indefinite retention, and the forward tongue position, particularly in adults, requires a crib to be worn at night for an indefinite time.

There are three important situations that demand indefinite retention. Patients with generalized spacing in which the arches are large and the tooth structure is not sufficient to close all the space. When there is lip competency, the objective should be to transfer the space to the posterior segments and add tooth material in the posterior areas to achieve arch integrity. With adult patients the objective is to keep the restorative dentistry in the posterior segments and have natural tooth material in the anterior; but with the tooth size discrepancies in the anterior area, it may be necessary to correct the tooth material problem where the tooth size exists. If the discrepancy is in the anterior teeth, we have to do bonding and reshaping on the anterior group; if the discrepancy is in the posterior teeth, we should correct the problem in the posterior area. Commonly, with generalized spacing problems (arch size larger than tooth size) the objective is not to allow the anterior teeth to retract, which is difficult to accomplish with the heavy musculature cases. The tongue accommodates by forward placement, and, therefore, the anterior teeth are maintained in their labiolingual position, where they are stable; the incisor spaces are closed by moving incisors mesially to the midline and advancing the canine and premolar teeth mesially, shifting the space to the posterior segments.

Again, it is recommended that the orthodontist refer to

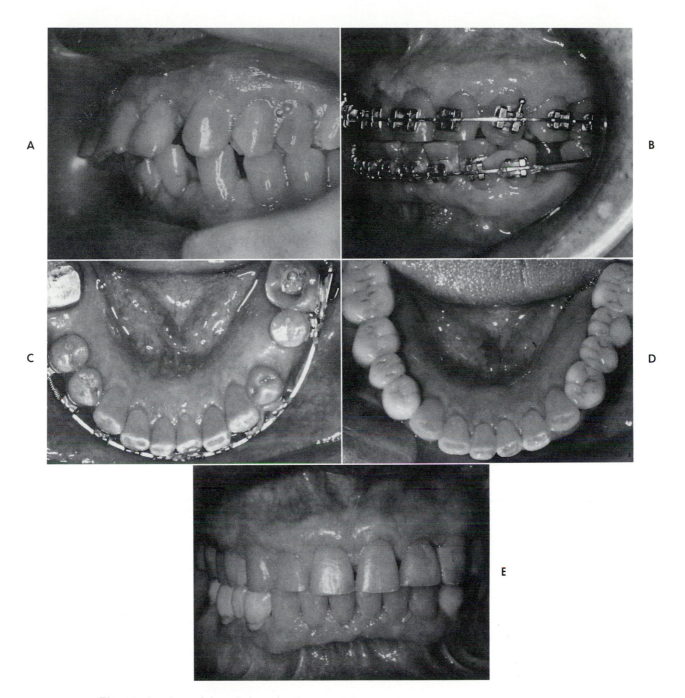

Fig. 14-47 **A,** Left lateral view of a 59-year-old Class II adult. **B,** Lower incisors, canines, and first premolars were advanced to obtain a Class I dental relationship and incisal guidance. **C,** Mandibular arch after pontic space was created in lower left quadrant between the premolars and before pontic space had been created between the mandibular right premolars. **D,** Postrestorative occlusal view with the bridges having been placed bilaterally, which allows the more procumbent incisors to remain stable. **E,** The compensated mandibular incisors remain stable 7 years post-treatment.

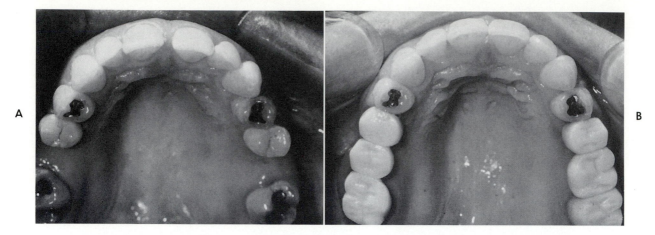

Fig. 14-48 **A,** Occlusal view of the maxillary arch in a Class III patient who is missing posterior teeth bilaterally. If a Class III patient has an ANB greater than $-3°$, space can be created bilaterally in the maxillary posterior areas and bonding material can be added mesiodistally to achieve arch integrity and to maintain more procumbent maxillary incisor stability, without occlusal trauma. **B,** The incisors are advanced and centered on the midline, and restorations have been placed bilaterally in posterior areas.

the basic concepts of retention outlined in Chapter 16. Those concepts and research findings can guide clinicians in further integrating a retention approach that is optimal for each patient.

REFERENCES

1. AAO Risk Management Teleconference, 1988.
2. Ackerman JL: The challenge of adult orthodontics, *J Clin Orthod* 12:43, 1978.
3. Ahrens DG, Shapira Y, Kuftinec M: An approach to rotational relapse, *Am J Orthod* 80:83, 1981.
4. Aimamo J: Relationship between malalignment of teeth and periodontal disease, *Scand J Dent Res* 80:104, 1972.
5. Alpern MC, Nuvelle DG, Wharton MC: TMJ diagnosis and treatment in multidisc environments and follow-up study, *Angle Orthod* 58(2):101-126, 1988.
6. American Association of Orthodontists: Study of the availability of orthodontic services, *Am J Orthod* 68:326, 1975.
7. Ammons WF, Smith DH: Flap curettage: rationale, technique, and expectations, *Dent Clin North Am* 20:215, 1976.
8. Amsterdam M: Periodontal prosthesis: twenty-five years in retrospect, *Alpha Omegan*, December, 1974.
9. Amsterdam M, Abrams L: *Periodontal prosthesis in periodontal therapy.* In Goldman HM, Cohen DW, editors: *Periodontal therapy,* ed 6, St Louis, 1980, Mosby.
10. Barrer HG: The adult orthodontic patient, *Am J Orthod* 72:619, 1977.
11. Behrents RG: *A treatise on the continuum of growth in the aging craniofacial skeleton,* Ann Arbor, 1984, The University of Michigan.
12. Bell WH, Proffit WR, White RP: *Surgical correction of dentofacial deformities,* Philadelphia, 1980, WB Saunders.
13. Berns JM: *What is periodontal disease?* Chicago, 1982, Quintessence.
14. Blazi S, Vanarsdall RL: Correlation of visual assessment and instrumental recording of the thickness of attached gingiva, Unpublished research, University of Pennsylvania, 1983.
15. Boyd RL, Leggott PJ et al: Periodontal implications of orthodontic treatment in adults to reduced or normal periodontal tissues versus

adolescents, *Am J Orthod Dentofac Orthop* 96(3):191-198, 1989.
16. Brandt S: The future of orthodontics, *J Clin Orthod* 10:668, 1976.
17. Brown IS: Effects of orthodontic therapy on periodontal pockets. I. Clinical findings, *J Periodontol* 44:742, 1973.
18. Case C: *Dental orthopedia and correction of cleft palate,* Chicago, 1921, CS Case.
19. Dibbets JMH, Van der Weele LT: Prevalence of joint noises as related to age and growth; *J Craniomand Disord Facial Oral Pain* 6:3, 157-168, 1992.
20. Dubin DS, Sandusky C: Changes in tooth contact following treatment, *Am J Orthod Dentofac Orthop* 90:375-382, 1986.
21. Edwards JG: A surgical procedure to eliminate rotational relapse, *Am J Orthod* 57:35, 1970.
22. Epker BN, Fish LC: *Dentofacial deformities,* 2 vols, St Louis, 1986, Mosby.
23. Ericsson I, Lindhe J: Effect of longstanding jiggling on experimental periodontitis in the beagle dog, *J Clin Periodont* 9:497-503, 1982.
24. Folkers SA, Weine FS, Weissman DP: Periodontal disease in the life stages of women, *Compend Cont Educ Dent* 13(10):852-860, 1992.
25. Gazit E, Lieberman MA: Occlusal contacts following orthodontic treatment, *Angle Orthod* 55:316-320, 1985.
26. Geiger A, Hirschfeld L: *Minor tooth movement in general practice,* ed 3, St Louis, 1974, Mosby.
27. Goaslind GD et al: Thickness of facial gingiva, *J Periodontol* 48:768, 1977.
28. Goldstein MC, Bruno MH, Yurfest P: Esthetic orthodontic appliances for adult, *DCNA* 33(2):183-193, 1989.
29. Gorman JC: Treatment with lingual appliances: the alternative for adult patients; *Int J Adult Orthod Orthognath Surg* 3:131-149, 1987.
30. Gottlieb EL, Nelson AH, Vogels DS III: 1990 JCO study of orthodontic diagnosis and treatment procedures, Part I. Results and trends, *J Clin Orthod* 45-156, 1990.
31. Grant DA, Stern IB, Everett FG: *Periodontics: in tradition of Orban and Gottlieb,* ed 5, St Louis, 1979, Mosby.
32. Greenstein G, Canton J, Polson AM: Histologic characteristics associated with bleeding after probing and visual signs of inflammation, *J Periodontol* 52:420, 1981.
33. Griffiths CS, Abby M: Effects of malalignment of teeth in the anterior segments on plaque accumulation, *J Clin Periodontol* 8:481, 1981.

34. Hampf G, Adberg V, Sanders B: Experience from a facial pain unit, *J Craniomand Disord Fac Oral Pain* 4:267-277, 1990.

35. Harris EF, Baker WC: Loss of root length and crestal bone height before and during treatment in adolescent and adult orthodontic patients, *Am J Orthod Dentofac Orthop* 98(5):463-469, 1990.

36. Holdaway RA: Changes in relationship of points A and B during orthodontic treatment, *Am J Orthod* 42:176-193, 1956.

37. Holmes TH, Rahe RH: Social readjustment rating scale, *J Psychosom Res* 11:213, 1967.

38. Howard JA: *Temporomandibular joint disorders, facial pain and dental problems of performing artists.* In Sataloff R, Brandfonbrenner A, Leberman R, editors: *Textbook of performing arts medicine*, New York, 1990, Raven Press.

39. Huser MC, Baehni PC, Lang R: Effort of orthodontic bands on microbiologic and clinical parameters, *Am J Orthod Dentofac Orthop* 97:3, 213-218, 1990.

40. Ingber JS: Forced eruption. I. A method of treating isolated one and two wall infrabony osseous defects—rationale and case report, *J Periodontol* 45:199, 1974.

41. Ingber JS: Forced eruption II. A method of treating nonrestorable teeth-periodontal and restorative considerations, *J Peridontol* 47:203, 1976.

42. Ingber JS: Forced eruption: alteration of soft tissue cosmetic deformities, *IJ Periodont Res* 9:6, 416-425, 1989.

43. Israel H: Recent knowledge concerning craniofacial aging, *Angle Orthod* 43:176-184, 1973.

44. Israel H: Evidence for continued apposition of adult mandibular bone from skeletized materials, *J Prosthet Dent* 41:101-104, 1978.

45. Ive JC: Orthodontic treatment enhances the use of endosseous implants to replace missing teeth, *Angle Orthod* 60(2):153-157, 1990.

46. Jeffcoat MK, Reddy MS: Progression of probing attachment loss in adult periodontitis, *J Periodontol* 62(3):185-189, 1991.

47. Kampe T, Hannery H, Stom W: Five year follow-up of adolescents with intact and restored dentitions: a comparative anamnestic and clinical study, *J Cranio Disorder Fac Oral Pain* 5(2):121-129, 1991.

48. Kennedy J, Bell W et al: Osteotomy as an adjunct to rapid maxillary expansion, *Am J Orthod* 70:123-137, 1976.

49. Kingsley NW: A treatise on oral deformities as a branch of mechanical surgery, New York, 1880, D Appleton.

50. Kraut RA, Hammer HS, Wheeler JJ: Use of endosteal implants as orthodontic anchorage, *Compend Cont Educ Dent* 9(10):796-797, 800-801, 1988.

51. Kvam E: Traumatic ulcers and pain in adults during orthodontic treatment, *Community Dent Oral Epidemiol* 17(3):154-157, 1989.

52. LaSuta EP: Orthodontic considerations in prosthetic and restorative dentistry, *DCNA* 32(3):1447-1456, 1988.

53. Levitt HL: Adult orthodontics, *J Clin Orthod* 5:1130, 1971.

54. Levitt HL: Modification of appliance design for the adult mutilated dentition, *J Adult Orthod Orthognoth Surg* 1:9-21, 1988.

55. Linde J: Textbook of clinical periodontology, ed 2, Copenhagen, 1989, Munksgaard, p. 245.

56. Linde J, Svanberg G: Influence of trauma from occlusion on progression of experimental periodontitis in the beagle dog, *J Clin Periodontol* 1:3, 1974.

57. Lindegaard B et al: Need and demand for orthodontic treatment, *Tandlaegbadet* 75:1198, 1971.

58. Lischer BE: *Principles and methods of orthodontia*, Philadelphia, 1912, Lea & Febiger.

59. Lundstrom A: Malocclusion of the teeth regarded as a problem in connection with the apical base, *Int J Orthod Oral Surg* 11:591, 1925.

60. Lytle JD: The clinicians index of occlusal disease: definition, recognition, and management, *Int J Periodont Rest Dent* 10(2):103-122, 1990.

61. MacDowell JN: *MacDowell Orthodontia*, Chicago, 1901, Blakely.

62. Machen DE: Legal aspects of orthodontic practice: risk management concepts, *Periodont Dis Orthod Prac* 95(5):445-447, 1989.

63. Machen DE: Developing protocols for adult patients, *Am J Orthod Dentofac Orthop* 98(5):476-477, 1990.

64. Marks MH: *Tooth movement in periodontal therapy.* In Goldman HM, Cohen DW, editors: *Periodontal therapy*, ed 6, St Louis, 1980, Mosby.

65. McNeill C, editor: *Cranio-mandibular disorders: guidelines for evaluation, diagnosis, and management*, Chicago, 1990, Quintessence.

66. Melsen B: Adult orthodontics: factors differentiating the selection of biomechanics in growing and adult individuals, *Int J Adult Orthod Orthod Surg* 3(3):167-177, 1988.

67. Miller TE: Orthodontic therapy for the restorative patient, Part I. The biomechanical aspects, *J Prosthet Dent* 61(3):268-276, 1989.

68. Miller G, Vanarsdall R: *Initial preparation for periodontal therapy.* In Goldman HM, Cohen DW, editors: *Periodontal therapy*, ed 6, St Louis, 1980, Mosby.

69. Morgan DH, Hall WP, Vamvas SJ: *Disease of the temporomandibular apparatus: a multidisciplinary approach*, St Louis, 1977, Mosby.

70. Musich DR: *Problem oriented record.* In Graber TM, Swain BF, editors: *Current orthodontic concepts and techniques*, ed 2, Philadelphia, 1975, WB Saunders.

71. Musich DR: Assessment and description of the treatment needs of adult patients evaluated for orthodontic therapy. Part I, II, III. *Int J Adult Orthod Orthognath Surg* 1:55-67, 101-117, 251-274, 1986.

72. National Institute of Dental Research: *Oral health of United States adults, the national survey or oral health in U.S. employed adults and seniors: 1985-86*, No DHHS (NIH) 87-2868, Bethesda, Md, 1987, National Institute of Dental Research.

73. Neiderud A, Ericsson I, Lindhe J: Probing pocket depth of mobile/nonmobile teeth, *J Clin Periodontol* 19:754-759, 1992.

74. Nevins M: Interproximal periodontal disease: the embrasure as an etiologic factor, *Int J Periodontol Rest Dent* 6:9, 1982.

75. Nickerson JW, Boering G: Natural course of osteoarthrosis as it relates to internal derangement of the temporomandibular joint, *Oral Maxillofac Surg Clin North Am* 1:27-45, 1989.

76. Norton LA: The effect of aging cellular mechanism on tooth movement, *DCNA* 32(3):437-446, 1958.

77. Perrier M, Polson A: The effect of progressive and increasing tooth hypermobility on reduced but healthy periodontal supporting tissues, *J Periodont* 53:152, 1982.

78. Philstrom BL et al: Association between signs of trauma from occlusion and periodontitis, *J Periodontol* 57:1-6, 1986.

79. Polson AM, Heijl LC: Occlusion and periodontal disease, *Dent Clin North Am* 24:783, 1980.

80. Polson AM, Meiner SW, Zander HA: Trauma and progression of marginal periodontitis in squirrel monkeys. Part III. Adaptation of interproximal alveolar bone to repetitive injury, *J Periodont Res* 12:279-289, 1976.

81. Proffitt WR, White RP: Surgical-orthodontics treatment, St Louis, 1991, Mosby.

82. Ramfjord SP, Ash MM: Periodontology and periodontics, Philadelphia, 1979, WB Saunders.

83. Rasmussen OC: Clinical findings during the course of temporomandibular arthropathy, *Scand J Dent Res* 89:285-288, 1981.

84. Razdolsky Y, Sadowsky C, BeGole EA: Occlusal contacts following orthodontic treatment: a follow-up study, *Angle Orthod* 59:181-185, 1989.

85. Reitan K: Experiments of rotation of teeth and their subsequent retention, *Trans Eur Orthod Soc* 34:124-140, 1958.

86. Roberts WE, Marshall KJ: Rigid endosseous implant utilized as anchorage to protract molars and close an atrophic extraction site, *Angle Orthod* 60(2):135-163, 1992.

87. Roth RH: Functional occlusion for the orthodontist, *J Clin Orthod* 15:1-4, 1981.

88. Schiffman E, Fricton JR: *Epidemiology of TMJ and craniofacial pain.* In Fricton JR, Kroening RJ, Hathaway KM, editors: *TMJ and craniofacial pain: diagnosis and management*, St Louis, 1988, Ishiyaku Euro America, pp. 1-10.

89. Susanne C: *Aging, continuous changes of adulthood.* In Johnston FE, Roche AF, Susanne C, editors: *Human physical growth and maturation,* New York, 1978, Plenum Press, pp. 111-124.

90. Svanberg G: *Effect of trauma from occlusion on the peridontium.* In McNamara JA Jr, editor: *Malocclusion and the periodontium,* Monograph Number 15: Craniofacial Growth Series, Ann Arbor, 1983, University of Michigan, pp. 101-125.

91. Thilander B: Orthodontic treatment in dentitions with reduced periodontal support, *Revue Belge de Medecine Dentaire* 37:119-125, 1982.

92. Vanarsdall RL: *Uprighting the inclined mandibular molar in preparation for restorative treatment.* Continuing dental education series, vol 1, No. 2, Philadelphia, 1977, University of Pennsylvania Press.

93. Vanarsdall RL: Orthodontics, provisional restorations and appliances, *Dental Clin North Am* 33(3):479-496, 1989.

94. Vanarsdall RL: *Tooth movement as an adjunct to periodontal therapy.* In Genco R, Goldmann H, Cohen DW, editors: *Contemporary periodontics,* St Louis, 1990, Mosby.

95. Vanarsdall RL: *Treatment of the periodontally involved adult.* In Hösl E, Baldauf A, editors: *Mechanical and biological basics in orthodontic therapy,* Heidelberg, 1991, Hüthig.

96. Vanarsdall R, Lemay J, Lindhe J: The effect of tooth mobility on probing depths, *Compend Cont Educ Dent* (suppl 12) pp. S433-S437, 1988.

97. Viazis AD, DeLong R et al: Enamel surface abrasion from ceramic orthodontic brackets: a special case report. *Am J Orthod Dentofac Orthop* 96(6):514-518, 1989.

98. Waddell G, Birscher M et al: Symptoms and Syns: physical disease or illness behavior, *Tx Med J* 289:739-741, 1984.

99. Weed LL: *Medical records, medical education, and patient care: the problem oriented record as a basic tool,* Cleveland, 1969, Case Western Reserve Press.

100. Williamson EH: JCO interviews: Dr. Eugene Williamson on occlusion and TMJ dysfunction. I. *J Clin Orthod* 14-333, 1981.

101. Williamson EH: *Occlusal concepts in orthodontic diagnosis and treatment.* In Johnston LE, editor: *New vistas in orthodontics,* Philadelphia, 1985, Lea & Febiger, pp. 122-147.

102. Zachrisson BU, Brobakken BL: Clinical comparison of direct versus indirect bonding with different bracket types and adhesives, *Am J Orthod* 74:62, 1978.

Orthodontics and Orthognathic Surgery: Principles of Combined Treatment

DAVID R. MUSICH

And so it came to pass that a heavenly angel in white, bearing his forms and charts, appeared before him and said, "Fear not, for I will lead you to a small room, where He shall appear before you shortly." And the angel placed him in a contoured vinyl manger and draped him in swaddling drool cloth, where upon a brilliant light appeared unto him and shown brightly in his face for what seemed like hours. And it came to pass that from this blinding light He came forth, and placing His hands about this trembling man's face, He said unto him, "Woe is thee, ye of little chin and mutant jaw. I have seen witness to your tablets of plaster and x-rays, and I say unto you: Lay down before me and go forth before Thine knife; for even the jaw bone of an ass shall wear better than yours. For it has been born upon you as stomatognathic dysfunction secondary to skeletal dysplasia of the maxilla and mandible." And so this Man looked upon the charts and tablets and x-rays and saw that it was bad, and so it was that on the 28th day he would go before the knife.

And in celebration of this solemn event he declared a final feast with friends, that all might chew in his honor with hearty food and drink, and with much laughter and joy. And it was good. And so he sent forth notice throughout the city that all who bear witness herein should come forth on the 18th day of February and partake of this: The Last Supper

Jim Eaton—Orthognathic patient

(Dinner invitation, 1 week before his jaw surgery)

Proposals regarding the general goals of an orthodontic treatment procedure have been presented throughout the development of our specialty:

Case (1921)[10]:
Correct malocclusions to normal *function esthetic* relationship, and *beautifying facial* outlines

Ackerman/Proffit (1970)[1]:
To establish optimal proximal and occlusal contact of the teeth within the framework of acceptable facial esthetics, normal function, and reasonable stability

Lindquist (1985)[33]:
The improvement of facial esthetics; alignment of teeth evenly; good occlusal relationships, both static and functional; psychologic benefits; the maintenance of healthy supporting structures; and the prodution of a stable dentition

Roth (1992)[56]:
I would divide my goals into five categories: facial esthetics, dental esthetics, functional occlusion, periodontal health, and stability.

Although there is an apparent consistency in treatment goals among orthodontic leaders, many differences exist over the specific meanings of terms such as *stability, facial balance, esthetics,* and even *function*. For example, does the term *stability* always mean *without continual retention?* Is long term mechanical retention to create stability ac-

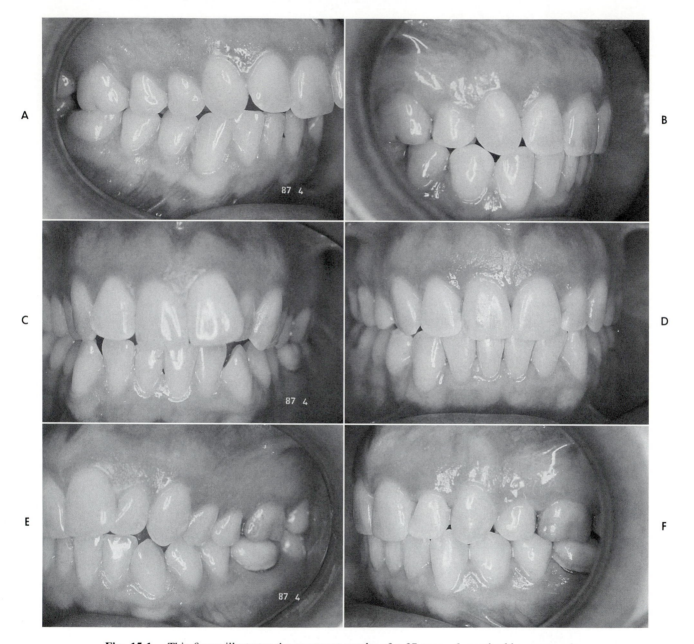

Fig. 15-1 This figure illustrates the treatment results of a 37-year-, 6-month-old woman, who sought treatment to correct her crowding and her overjet. Teeth numbers 5 and 12 were extracted, and upper and lower braces were worn for 30 months. **A** and **B,** Right, pretreatment and post-treatment. **C** and **D,** Center, pre- and post-treatment. **E** and **F,** Left, pre- and post-treatment. **G** and **H,** Profile, pre- and post-treatment. **I** and **J,** Frontal, pre- and post-treatment. **K,** Cephalometric superimposition of pretreatment *(solid lines)* and post-treatment *(dashed lines)* changes. The patient's response to the question, "Are you happy with the outcome?" "Yes. The smile is more attractive. I am definitely more happy with the way my teeth look." A surgical option to do a LeFort impaction of the maxilla was discussed.

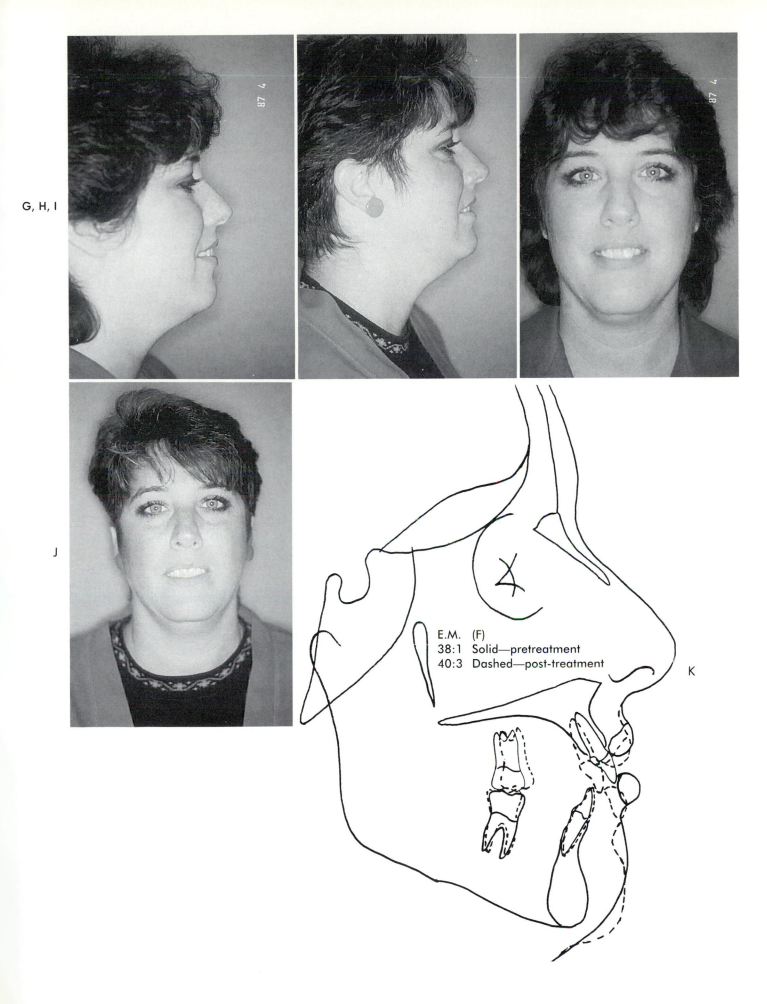

G, H, I

J

E.M. (F)
38:1 Solid—pretreatment
40:3 Dashed—post-treatment

K

ceptable as suggested by Dahl and Zachrisson[11]? Who is the judge of esthetics—the orthodontist, the surgeon, the spouse, the parent, or the patient? Each of these important people may judge differently the esthetics of the profile, the smile, the tooth angulation, and the chin (see Chapter 10).

In addition to the problems of having uniform definitions for the terms that are used to describe the specialty's accepted treatment objectives, situations frequently arise when a clinician must *prioritize* the treatment objectives. A patient, for example, may have a moderate chewing problem and incipient myofacial imbalance caused by a mild skeletal open bite (high angle mandibular deficiency) (Fig. 15-1). The ideal treatment plan is orthodontics and jaw surgery to achieve stability, function, and facial balance; a secondary plan may be the extraction of upper first premolars to close the bite. The functional goal is prioritized, but the stability (extraction space rebound), vertical excess, facial balance (naso-labial angle change) are compromised (deprioritized). Therefore, developing a way to understand the treatment goals that the prospective patient seeks and also having an effective way of communicating the treatment goals that the orthodontist can achieve, are essential prerequisites for achieving successful results. This is especially true when treating patients with *skeletal jaw malrelationships*.

The process that most clearly allows clarification of goals is well described by Proffit (Fig. 15-2). A problem list is carefully developed by the orthodontist and reviewed with the patient, thereby providing an opportunity to discuss alternative treatment options that are available to achieve desirable outcomes. The patient and the orthodontist then must come to an agreement on the plan that both believe will provide the best possible outcome with the least exposure to risk. Frequently, the plan of action cannot be finalized until other members of the *provider team* have each had input into the treatment plan and sequence.

The treatment planning approach that includes significant patient input requires more of the practitioner's time and, at a humanistic level, more emphasis on educating the patient and less emphasis on arbitrary directives. From a risk-management perspective, the steps in the problem-oriented approach of Proffit, if well-documented, will provide an excellent record to assist the clinician in the event that the patient subsequently initiates legal action for any reason, as noted by Machen.

In evaluating this case, several factors appear to have been deemed important by the jury in determining that the practitioner fulfilled his obligations to the patient. First, the practitioner performed a complete evaluation and suggested a course of treatment designed to correct the patient's problem. Second, an alternative plan was made available that was clearly identified as a compromise. Third, the potential risks and complications asso-

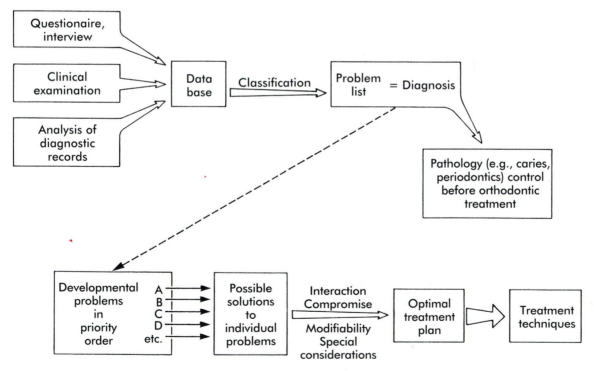

Fig. 15-2   Proffit has effectively modified the concept of *problem-oriented diagnosis,* which was developed by our medical colleagues in the 60s. This problem-oriented process is important in surgical orthodontic planning to organize the data and to help prioritize the goals of the treatment plan. (From Proffit WR, White RP: *Surgical-orthodontic treatment,* St Louis, 1990, Mosby.)

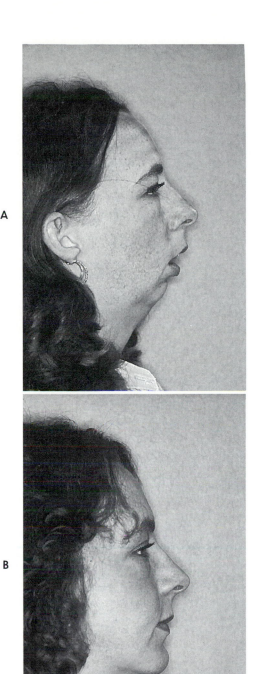

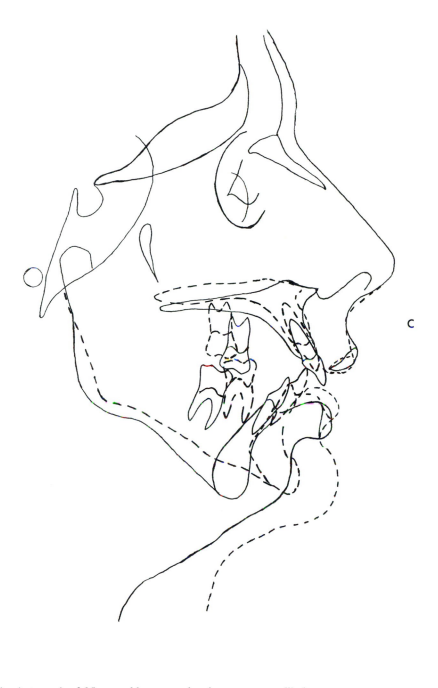

Fig. 15-3 **A,** Presurgical profile photograph of 25-year-old woman showing severe mandibular deficiency and chin deficiency. **B,** Postsurgical profile photograph 3 months after completion of orthodontics and 10 months after jaw surgery. She reported that it took longer than 1 year to recognize her own reflection in a mirror. **C,** Superimposition of a lateral cephalometric tracing. This patient had:

- Maxillary LeFort Impaction—6 mm at 1st molars and 6 mm at incisors
- Mandibular autorotation and advancement—10 mm advancement at *B* point
- Advancement genioplasty—13 mm advancement at *Pg* (*Pg* change is due to mandibular advancement, autorotation, and advancement genioplasty.)

ciated with the alternative treatment were presented to, discussed with, and acknowledged by the patient. And, finally, a paper trail existed confirming each of the above-mentioned steps.[35]

Following the steps in Fig. 15-2 may seem time consuming, but they will prove to be invaluable because technologic capabilities that are now available to change the form and function of the stomatognathic system are profound and require judicious care in their use (Fig. 15-3).

NEED VERSUS DEMAND

In an early publication describing the use of the *problem oriented* approach to medical situations, Weed[65] stated that the only limitations to treatment are:

1. Hazard
2. Cost
3. Pain

Inasmuch as the orthodontic-orthognathic treatment of skeletal dysplasias remains as *elective procedures* in most

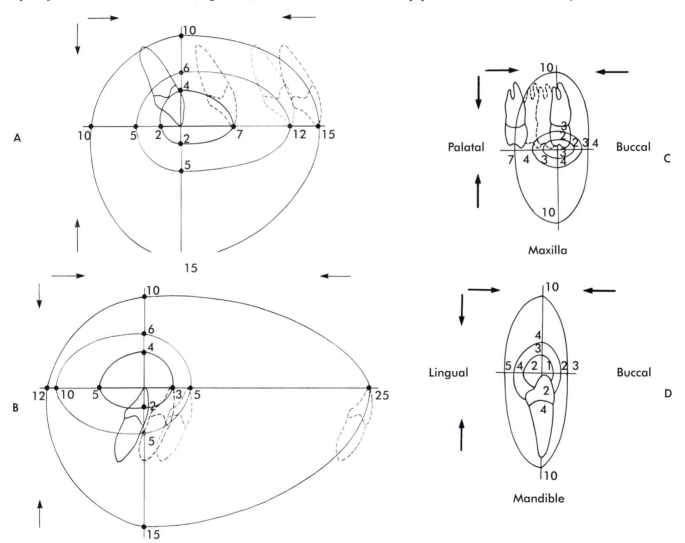

Fig. 15-4 A, Envelope of discrepancy for maxillary alterations. **B,** Envelope of discrepancy for mandibular alterations. **C** and **D,** The transverse envelope of discrepancy is another valuable guide in planning treatment for patients who require an increase or a decrease in the lateral dimensions of their jaws. (From Vanarsdall RL, Mershon Lecture, 1991.) The envelope of discrepancy shows the amount of change in all three planes of space that could be produced by orthodontic tooth movement alone *(inner circle* of each diagram); orthodontic tooth movement combined with growth modification in a growing child *(middle circle)*; and orthognathic surgery *(outer circle)*. Note that the possibilities of each treatment are not symmetric with regard to the planes of space. For example, greater tooth movement is possible anteroposteriorly than vertically, growth modification is more effective in mandibular deficiency than in mandibular excess, and surgery to move the lower jaw back has greater potential than surgery to advance it. (From Proffit WR, White RP: *Surgical-orthodontic treatment,* St Louis, 1990, Mosby.)

cases, further discussion is warranted regarding the need/
demand considerations. Proffit has helped to clarify this
discussion with the following statement:

> *The indication for surgical-orthodontic treatment is that
> a skeletal or dento-alveolar deformity is so severe that
> the magnitude of the problem lies outside the envelope
> of possible correction by orthodontics alone.*[8]

To further aid orthodontists in their treatment planning
decisions, Proffit and Ackerman created an envelope of
discrepancy (Fig. 15-4) for the sagittal plane.[49] Proffit also
helped to identify, through data extrapolation, the approximate number of the major types of malocclusions that could
benefit from orthognathic surgery.

If it is assumed that individuals were counted twice because of overlap in the long face category (some long face
patients have Class II malocclusions and some have Class
III), the total number of persons in the United States who
could benefit from combined orthodontic-orthognathic procedures is, therefore, estimated to be 1.2 million (Tables
15-1 through 15-3). Although this estimate seems to be quite
high, as the *hazards* of orthognathic techniques decrease,
the probability is that more and more of this group will seek
combined therapy.

In the author's 1986 paper assessing the treatment needs
of 1370 consecutively examined adult patients, optimal
treatment plans were presented to each patient.[40-42] In this
group of adults who were evaluated in a private practice
setting, 25.5% were determined to be solo provider patients
(orthodontic treatment only, no surgical treatment), 45.2%
were dual provider patients (two dental specialists to properly manage their treatment needs), and 24.3% of the patients required multiple provider care (Fig. 15-5). Jaw surgery was recommended to 15.4% of the patients in conjunction with orthodontics. Not all patients chose to have
surgery as part of their treatment plan.

TECHNOLOGICAL ADVANCES

Advances in several areas have *decreased the surgical
risk* to patients undergoing orthognathic surgery. A brief
discussion of advances in the following areas will be presented in this section:

- Anesthetic technique
- Edema control
- Infection control
- Surgical procedures
- Fixation techniques

Modified hypotensive anesthetic technique as described
by Anderson[2] has given the surgeon the capability to perform
complicated orthognathic surgical procedures in highly vascular areas, with minimal blood loss. The following hypotensive technique is used at the University of North
Carolina[20]:

1. Induction by sodium thiopental
2. Muscle relaxation via vecuronium

TABLE 15-1
Estimated Prevalence of Mandibular Deficiency Severe
Enough to Indicate Surgery

	%*	No.†
Prevalence of skeletal Class II malocclusion	10.0	22,500,000
At appropriate age for surgical treatment	65.0	14,625,000
Severe enough to warrant surgery	5.0	731,250
Mandibular advancement	70.0	510,000
Maxillary setback	10.0	67,500
Both	20.0	145,000
New patients added to population yearly‡	0.5	21,250

* At 225,000,000 US population.
† At 4,250,000 live births per year.

TABLE 15-2
Estimated Prevalence of Class III Problems Severe
Enough to Indicate Surgery

	%*	No.†
Prevalence of skeletal Class III malocclusion	0.6	1,350,000
At appropriate age for surgical treatment	65.0	877,500
Severe enough to warrant surgery	33.0	290,000
Mandibular setback	45.0	130,000
Maxillary advancement	35.0	101,000
Both	20.0	58,000
New patients added to population yearly‡	0.2	8,500

* At 225,000,000 US population.
† At 4,250,000 live births per year.

TABLE 15-3
Estimated Prevalence of Long Face Problems Severe
Enough to Indicate Surgery

	%*	No.†
Prevalence of severe anterior open bite	0.6	1,350,000
At appropriate age for surgical treatment	65.0	877,500
Severe enough to warrant surgery	25.0	220,000
(Superior repositioning of maxilla)		
New patients added to population yearly‡	0.2	6,375

* At 225,000,000 US population.
† At 4,250,000 live births per year.

3. Manual ventilation with oxygen and isoflurane until
   paralysis
4. Endotracheal tube placed
5. Local anesthetic to area of incision
6. Fifty percent nitrous oxide added to anesthetic gas
7. Isoflurane delivery adjusted to achieve systolic pressure of 100 to 110 torr
8. Isoflurane increased 20 minutes before osteotomy and
   arterial pressure in 85 to 90 torr range; other intra-
   venous IV drugs may be used; mean arterial pressure
   not allowed to fall below 60 torr

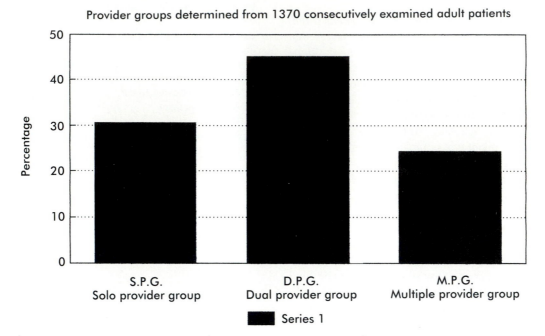

Fig. 15-5 A summary diagram showing the percentage of adults in each of the provider groups. The provider groups were defined as follows: *Solo provider*—a group of patients who have dental problems that require one primary dental provider. *Dual provider*—a group of patients who have dental problems that require two providers (i.e., orthodontics and jaw surgery; orthodontics and periodontics, etc.). *Multiple provider*—a group of patients who have dental problems that require the interaction of three or more primary dental providers (i.e. orthodontics, orthognathics, and restorative treatment). (From Musich DR: 1986.[40, 41])

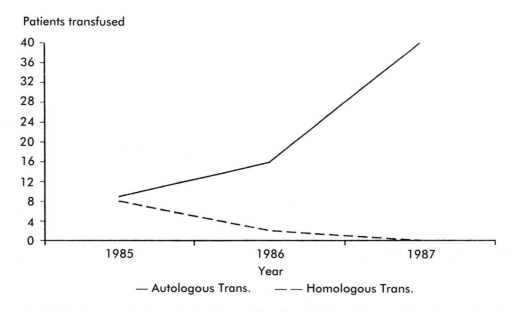

Fig. 15-6 Preoperative deposit of autologous blood has eliminated the use of homologous blood transfusion for orthognathic surgery. (Modified by Dr. Myron Tucker. From Hegtvedt AK, Collins ML, White RP: *Int J Adult Orthod Orthognath Surg* 2:185, 1987.)

9. Fluids replaced by Ringers lactate, and homologous blood not transfused unless patient beomes hemodynamically unstable

The recent concern for orthognathic patients regarding transfusion with *tainted* blood has been resolved with the use of predeposited autologous blood. Tucker's modification of Hegtvedt's data[20] shows the significant decrease in the need for transfusion during orthognathic procedures in the graph in Fig. 15-6.

Control of Edema

Postoperative swelling related to orthognathic procedures requires special attention. Excessive swelling can lead to limited mandibular function, swallowing difficulties, pain and airway obstruction. Measures to control edema include:

1. Minimizing surgical trauma
2. Decreasing operating time
3. Careful hemostasis
4. Pharmacologic control of inflammation process

The pharmacologic control is achieved primarily through the use of corticosteroids. Although corticosteroids can produce toxic effects to leukocyte function, short-term use has minimal negative effects. Studies by Shaberg and co-workers[59] have quantified the degree of reduction in post-surgical facial swelling through the use of computerized tomography (CT). Their findings indicate a 61% reduction in edema during the first 24 hours after a LeFort I osteotomy and a 38% reduction at 24 hours after transoral vertical ramus osteotomy. The patients were medicated with methylprednisolone.

In addition, reduction in edema for orthognathic patients has been accomplished through nonpharmacologic approaches.

1. Immediate 30° head elevation after surgery
2. Early ambulation of the patient, thereby using gravity to decrease edema
3. Pressure dressings to decrease dead space, enhance hemostasis, and control edema

Infection Control

Infection occurs infrequently after orthognathic procedures, and when it does occur, the "infection is usually local and responds well to I & D and systemic antibiotics, usually just penicillin."[20] Prophylactic antibiotics are still used, with

---

ROUTINE POSTOPERATIVE ORDERS FOR ORTHOGNATHIC SURGERY AT THE UNIVERSITY OF NORTH CAROLINA

1. Operation: LeFort I osteotomy, BSSO, genioplasty
2. Condition: stable, *jaws not wired*
3. Vitals q15min. until stable, then q1h × 4, then q4hr
4. Allergies: none
5. Activity: Out of bed with assistance this PM
6. Diet: Clear liquids as tolerated
7. IV D5 1/2NS at _____ cc/hour (according to fluid calculations)
8. K⁺ Penicillin G 1 million units IV q4hr, next dose at _____ (or other appropriate antibiotic)
9. Solumedrol 125 mg IV q4hr, next dose at _____ (or other appropriate IV corticosteroid preparation)
10. Morphine sulfate 2 mg IV × 4 maximum in recovery room only
11. Demerol 50 mg/Phenergan 12.5 mg IM q4hr prn moderate to severe pain (or other appropriate IV or IM pain medication)
12. Tylenol with codeine elixir 15-30 cc PO q4hr prn mild to moderate pain (or other appropriate PO pain medication)
13. Compazine 10 mg IM q4hr prn severe nausea and vomiting (or other IV, IM, or PR antiemetic)
14. Otrivin 0.1% nasal spray—2 squirts each nostril prn congestion
15. Hydrocortisone ointment to lips at all times (or other appropriate lubricant)
16. Humidified 40% oxygen via face bucket
17. Record intake and output
18. Elevate head of bed 30 degrees
19. Light oral suction at bedside
20. Ice chips ad lib PO; otherwise NPO until positive bowel sounds
21. Ice packs to face × 12 hours
22. Dietary consultation in AM
23. Coughing and deep breathing q2hr while awake
24. NG tube to light intermittent suction (if maxillary surgery)
25. Foley catheter to straight drain (or D/C Foley in recovery room if satisfied with urine output)
26. Neuro checks q2hr (if cranial bone harvested)
27. Physical therapy consultation in AM (if iliac bone harvested)
28. Labs: urinalysis in AM (CBC and electrolytes ordered if unusually concerned about amount of blood loss or renal function; otherwise ordered on second postoperative day after maxillary surgery)
29. Wire cutters at head of bed (if wire maxillomandibular fixation used)
30. Please contact Dr. _____ at pager # _____ if there are any problems or questions, or if:

BP: 180 < systolic < 100	Severe nausea and vomiting
100 < diastolic < 50	No void by 8 hr postoperatively

Pulse: >100 or <50
Temperature >101.5

*From Hegtvedt AA: *Oral and maxillofacial Surgery Clinics of North America*, vol 2, No. 4, 1990, p. 864.

Problem	Surgical procedure
Mandibular deficiency	Sagittal split osteotomy with advancement

A

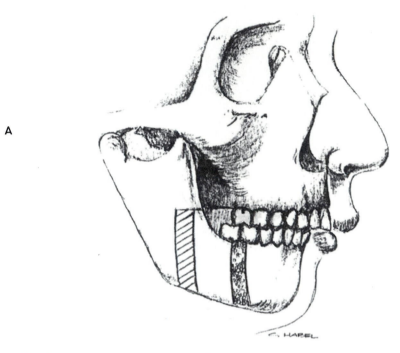

Problem	Surgical procedure
Mandibular excess	Sagittal split osteotomy with set-back (shown) or subcondylar vertical osteotomy (not shown)

B

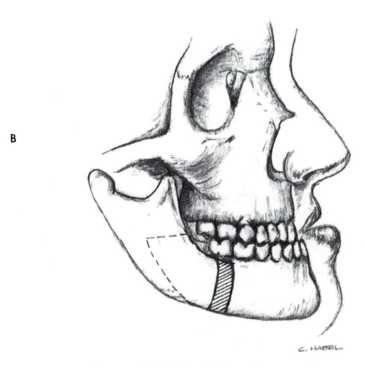

Fig. 15-7 For legend see opposite page.

1 ml unit of penicillin given intravenously just before surgery and continuing every 4 hours for 12 hours after surgery. An alternative to penicillin G is cefazolin (Kefzol).

The box on p. 845 shows routine postoperative orders for orthognathic surgery at the University of North Carolina. A review of this table may give the orthodontist a better appreciation for the overall postoperative management that the orthognathic patient requires.

SURGICAL PROCEDURES

Oral and maxillofacial surgeons have studied the effects of a wide range of surgical techniques during the past 20 years.

- Safety of the techniques
- Reduced morbidity—neurologic and vascular
- Minimal external scarring
- Stability of procedures
- Enhanced rate of healing
- Reduced surgical time under anesthesia

A schematic illustration of some of the most common surgical procedures that are currently performed to correct skeletal malocclusions is shown in Fig. 15-7.

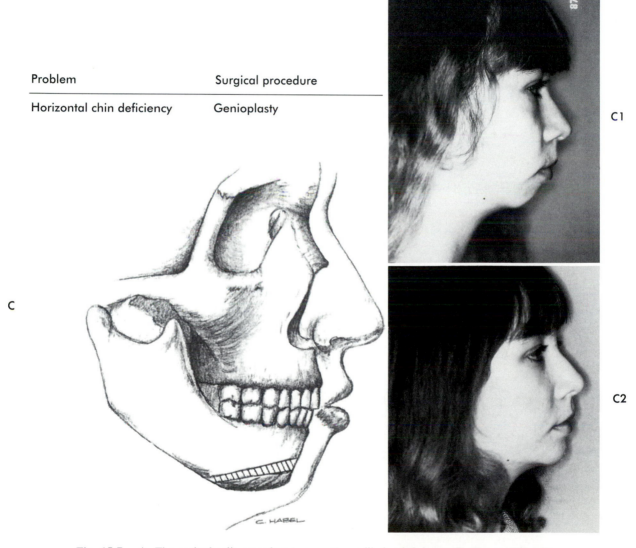

Problem	Surgical procedure
Horizontal chin deficiency	Genioplasty

Fig. 15-7   A, The sagittal split procedure to correct mandibular deficiency. **B,** The sagittal split procedure to correct mandibular excess. **C,** The genioplasty procedure can be used to reduce the chin vertically and horizontally or to reduce the chin vertically and lengthen it horizontally. The genioplasty has other combinations of surgical movements to enhance the muscle balance and the esthetics of the lower facial one third. **C1,** Pregenioplasty. **C2,** Postgenioplasty.   *Continued.*

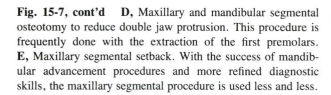

Problem	Surgical procedure
Double jaw protrusion	Segmental set-back of anterior maxilla and anterior mandible

Fig. 15-7, cont'd   D, Maxillary and mandibular segmental osteotomy to reduce double jaw protrusion. This procedure is frequently done with the extraction of the first premolars. **E,** Maxillary segmental setback. With the success of mandibular advancement procedures and more refined diagnostic skills, the maxillary segmental procedure is used less and less.

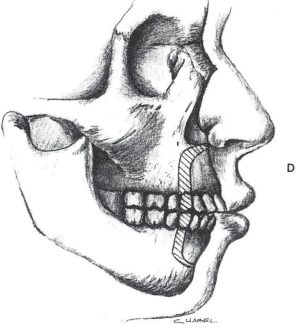

D

Problem	Surgical procedure
Maxillary protrusion	Maxillary anterior set-back

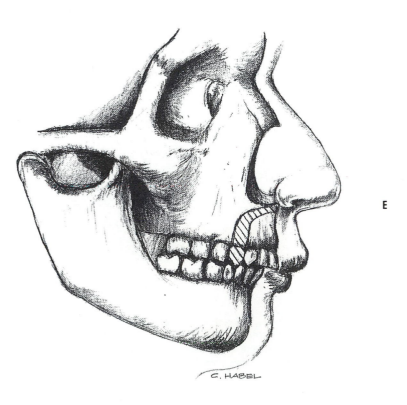

E

Problem	Surgical procedure
Excess vertical growth of maxilla	LeFort osteotomy with maxillary impaction

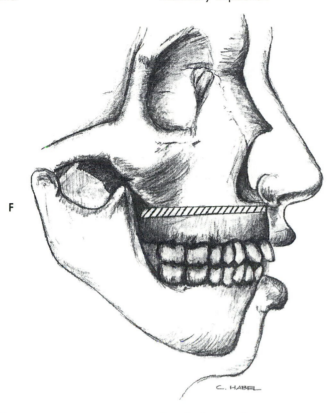

F

Fig. 15-7, cont'd   F, The LeFort osteotomy has a number of modifications, has proven to be safe, and has a high degree of stability. Excess vertical maxillary growth is one problem that is readily solved with a LeFort procedure. **G,** The LeFort procedure to advance the maxilla in a maxillary deficiency problem.

Continued.

Problem	Surgical procedure
Maxillary horizontal deficiency	LeFort osteotomy with maxillary advancement

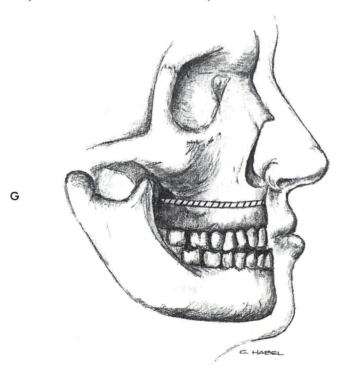

G

Problem	Surgical procedure
#1 Class III with maxillary deficiency and mandibular excess or,	LeFort osteotomy of maxilla to advance and/or impact and sagittal split osteotomy of mandible to set-back
#2 Also, Class III maxillary vertical excess and mandibular horizontal excess	

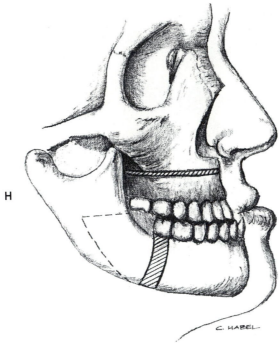

Problem	Surgical procedure
Mandibular deficiency Type III (high mandibular plane angle)	LeFort osteotomy for maxillary impaction Sagittal split osteotomy for mandibular advancement

Fig. 15-7, cont'd   H, Surgery combining the LeFort procedure with the mandibular sagittal split to resolve a maxillary deficiency/mandibular excess problem. **I,** The LeFort procedure with the sagittal split mandibular advancement procedure for a mandibular deficiency with open bite.

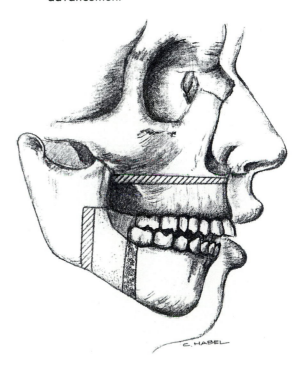

Problem	Surgical procedure
Asymmetric facial growth	Differential LeFort of the maxilla; sagittal split with rotation of the mandible. Genioplasty (optional)

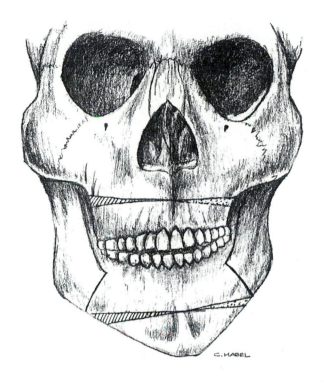

J1

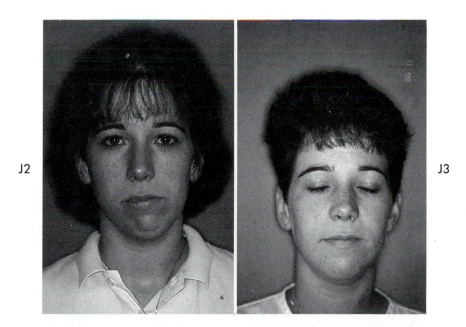

J2   J3

Fig. 15-7, cont'd   J1, Frontal view of a differential LeFort of the maxilla and sagittal split rotation of the mandible and a differential genioplasty to resolve a facial asymmetry problem. **J2,** Presurgical frontal photograph of patient showing moderate degree of facial asymmetry. **J3,** Postsurgical frontal photograph showing surgical correction using osteotomies described in *Fig. 15-7, J1.   Continued.*

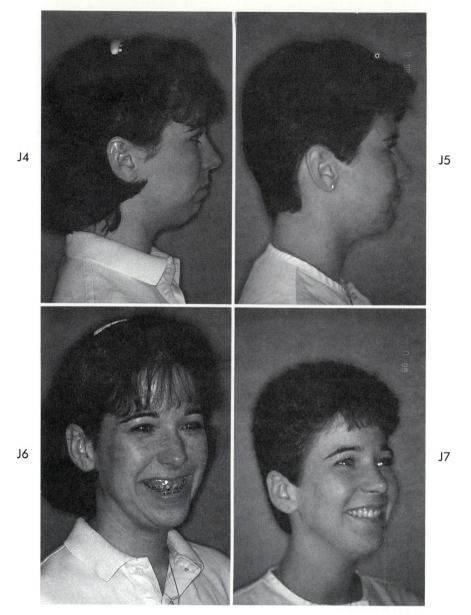

Fig. 15-7, cont'd   J4, Presurgical profile photograph of patient with mandibular deficiency and asymmetry. **J5,** Postsurgical profile photograph. **J6,** Presurgical smiling photograph showing vertical maxillary excess. **J7,** Postsurgical smile photograph demonstrating improved smile esthetics.

FIXATION

Immobilization of bone fracture sites is a necessity for proper healing of the bone. Acceptance of the new technological advances in orthognathic surgery by patients and the orthodontic community has been greatly influenced by the recent changes in fixation techniques.

For many years interdental fixation with arch bars was the method of choice for fixation of orthognathic surgery patients. As presurgical orthodontic treatment became state of the art in the late 1960s, interdental fixation, with modified orthodontic appliances, and *surgical arch wires,* with soldered hooks, replaced arch bars.

Limitations imposed by periodontally compromised teeth, short rooted teeth, mutilated dentitions, and double jaw procedures led to a requirement for more stable forms of fixation using the skeletal bases. The fixation period lasted for 6 to 10 weeks, with numerous reports of postsurgical depression.[30,62]

Patients described their fixation period of convalescence as one in which their interactions with the outside world, spouse, children, friends, and business associates, changed dramatically. Weight loss of 5 to 25 pounds was reported, as loss of appetite, temporomandibular joint (TMJ) pain, and facial muscle pain became frequent concerns.

Lack of jaw mobilization, particularly in patients with

existing degenerative joint disease, may exacerbate TMJ pathology under certain postsurgical conditions.[46]

In 1980, the introduction of rigid fixation technique into the oral surgery literature helped eliminate one of the major hurdles for many patients considering jaw surgery. The obvious advantage is that early jaw mobilization allowed the following:

1. Normal ability to communicate
2. More normal diet
3. Less time off from work
4. Less sense of being *handicapped* or feeling *stigmatized*
5. Better oral hygiene during healing

Certain controversial aspects of rigid fixation are currently being assessed at major teaching centers. Concerns regarding *condyle torque*, TMJ overload, and reduced postsurgical adaptation of skeletal structures have led some clinicians to hypothesize that certain rigid fixation tehniques are a causative factor in postsurgical condyle resorption.

Transoral lag screw techniques, which tend to distalize the condyles, may compress and hold diskal tissue in pathologic position. These changes may be sufficient to start progressive condyle resorption. Rigid fixation sagittal split osteotomies may be contra-indicated in this group of patients because the condyles may be loaded by the soft tissue stretch produced by the mandibular advancement, with no skeletal suspension to help counter that stretch.[4]

Some surgeons continue their orthognathic surgery using previously successful skeletal fixation. Until more long-term data is reported, clarifying possible latent negative effects of the rigid fixation technique for mandibular surgery, there will continue to be less than 100% use of this technique. Examples of several fixation modalities can be seen in the postsurgical cephalograms shown in Figs. 15-8 through 15-11. The patient's choice is obviously in favor of rigid fixation methods for all types of jaw surgery, as long as stability and safety are not sacrificed.

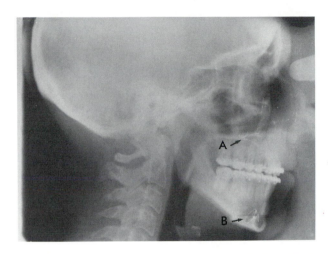

Fig. 15-8   Lateral cephalogram of a patient *(MP, 21Y 8M, F)* 2 weeks after a LeFort osteotomy and A-P vertical reduction genioplasty. The patient is in intermaxillary dental fixation (IMF) with maxillo-mandibular elastics to immobilize the lower jaw. *Arrow A* shows the surgical wires that helped to stabilize the maxilla. *Arrow B* indicates stabilizing wire to chin.

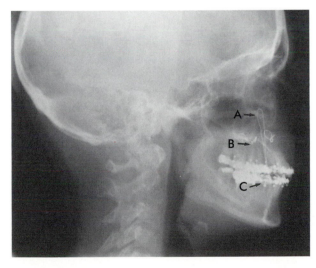

Fig. 15-9   Lateral cephalogram of a patient *(GA, 26Y 4M, F)* 2 weeks after a differential LeFort osteotomy to close a 6 mm openbite. *Arrow A*—orbital skeletal suspension wire; *arrow B*—surgical wire to stabilize LeFort surgery; *arrow C*—intra-maxillary ligation wires. This patient had skeletal fixation and IMF to assure proper healing of the LeFort procedure.

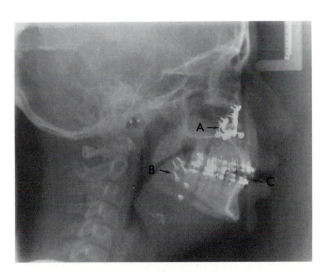

Fig. 15-10   Lateral cephalogram of a patient *(KC, 27Y 11M, F)* 2 weeks after a LeFort and a mandibular advancement and autorotations. *Arrow A*—rigid fixation plates to maxilla to stabilize LeFort osteotomy; *arrow B*—rigid fixation screws to mandible to stabilize the sagittal split osteotomy for mandibular advancement; *arrow C*—apparent post-surgical openbite caused by radiolucent surgical splint.

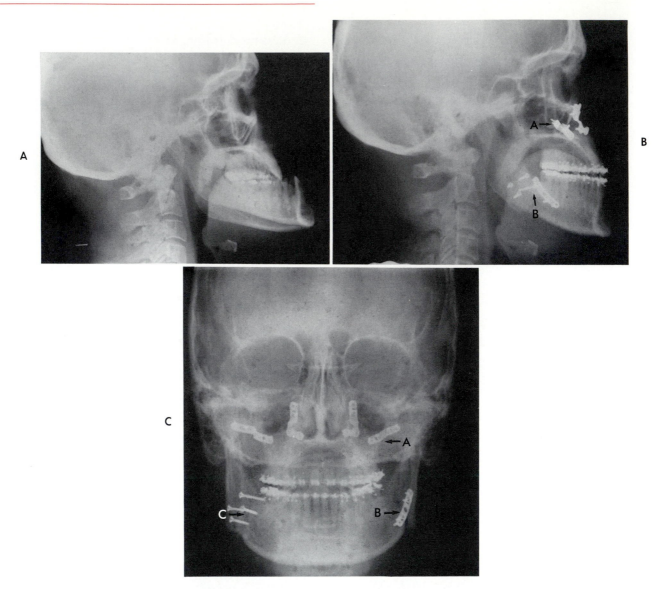

Fig. 15-11   A, Pretreatment lateral cephalogram of a patient *(LC, 33Y 10M),* with a severe maxillary deficiency and severe mandibular excess. **B,** Postsurgical lateral cephalogram showing advancement of maxilla and mandibular set-back. *Arrow A*—rigid fixation plates stabilizing the maxillary LeFort advancement; *arrow B*—rigid fixation screws and plate stabilizing sagittal split mandibular set-back. **C,** Postsurgical frontal cephalogram. *Arrow A*—maxillary fixation plates; *arrow B*—mandibular fixation screws; *arrow C*—mandibular fixation plate. This patient delayed surgery for 9 years to avoid 8 weeks of intermaxillary fixation and the *downtime* from work. Five days after his double jaw surgery he returned to work. His case was stabilized with rigid fixation devices only.

The rate of return of chewing capacity, range of motion and functional comfort are greatly affected by the type of surgery, the type of fixation, and the postoperative management. Studies have shown that there is an accelerated functional improvement if physical therapy is added to the postsurgical regimen.[63] Fig. 15-12 illustrates the basic flow chart for jaw rehabilitation that is used by the University of North Carolina's surgical team.[53]

DIFFERENTIAL DIAGNOSIS AS APPLIED TO SKELETAL MALOCCLUSIONS

For the majority of patients who seek orthodontic procedures, there is a significant *elective component* to this health care decision. Although it is necessary to carefully examine the patient for pathology and medical problems that may be present, the orthodontist generally focuses most of his other attention on diagnostic considerations of the struc-

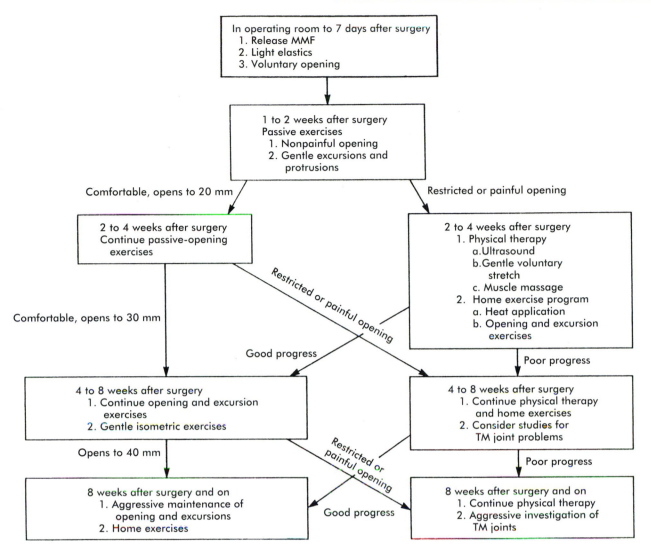

Fig. 15-12 Flow chart for jaw rehabilitation.

tural imbalances (Table 15-4). This process has been termed a *search for truth* by Proffit.[53] Whether the structural diagnostic process is a search for truth, a search for understanding, or simply the definition of a problem, it is a process that requires skill and experience. Fundamental to the diagnostic process is the *standardization* of high-quality records, *consistency* of record *analysis* and *clarity* of thought.

A variety of *tools* to help orthodontists make accurate differential diagnoses of malocclusions, especially skeletal disharmonies, have been discussed frequently in the orthodontic literature. The diagnostic aids most frequently employed by orthodontists have been ascertained through a national poll of practicing orthodontists (Table 15-5).

Some of the most popular cephalometric analyses rely on angular and linear measurements to describe dental and skeletal facial relationships. Frequently cephalometric analyses have been used as the cornerstone of the differential diagnostic process of skeletal imbalances. Many of the popular

analyses in use are limited by the lack of correlation with angular or linear measurements to soft tissue contours. In the 1990 JCO study[18] the three most routinely used cephalometric analyses were Steiner (43%), Ricketts (27%), and Downs (25%). In 1978, Burstone[9] and others developed a cephalometric appraisal system specifically designed to assess and plan for orthognathic surgery. The system was called the Cephalogram for Orthognathic Surgery (COGS).

The COGS analysis can be useful in diagnosing the nature of a facial dysplasia and abnormalities in position of teeth. If one is aware of the limitations of a two-dimensional cephalometric analysis, it can serve as a first step in diagnosis and detailed planning of treatment for the orthognathic surgical patient.

Cephalometric analyses using a template method (Jacobson[23]) and the Moorrees mesh[39] have the capacity to graphically qualify (demonstrate which jaw is not in bal-

TABLE 15-4

Medical Problems Significant for Surgical-Orthodontic Treatment

Condition	Significance	Comments
Diabetes mellitus	Susceptible to periodontal breakdown during orthodontic treatment; decreased resistance to infection; poor wound healing	Maintenance of excellent control necessary
Hyperthyroidism	Increased metabolic rate, tendency to osteoporosis	Infection may create crisis; psychologic instability possible
Adrenal insufficiency	Decreased stress tolerance, delayed healing	Knowledge of steroid dosage important
Pregnancy	Major hormonal changes, increased susceptibility to periodontal breakdown	Defer surgical treatment; limited orthodontic treatment acceptable but careful periodontal monitoring required
Rheumatic heart disease, other heart disease	Susceptible to endocarditis	Antibiotic coverage required for invasive procedures; in orthodontics, for banding but not for bonding or routine adjustments
Bleeding disorders (e.g., hemophilia, von Willebrand's disease, thrombocytopenia)	Susceptible to bleeding	Replace missing clotting factors before surgery; in orthodontics, bonded attachments instead of bands, avoid aspirin and related drugs for pain control
Sickle cell anemia	Susceptible to sickle cell crisis, bone loss	Not good candidates for general anesthesia, therefore usually not considered for orthognathic surgery
Allergy-immune problems	Excessive reaction to drugs, other antigens	Rarely, nickel content in stainless steel orthodontic appliances causes problem
Rheumatoid arthritis	Episodic involvement of multiple joints, possible destruction of TM joint	Manipulation of TM joint tends to exacerbate problem; avoid functional appliances, Class II elastics, and mandibular advancement
Osteoarthritis	Progressive involvement of multiple joints, possibly including TM joint, with increasing age	Orthodontics or orthognathic surgery has little effect for better or worse on involved TM joints
Behavioral disorders	Depends on degree of control; patients often on potent medications	Drug effects may slow orthodontic tooth movement; bizarre reactions to surgery possible

In all instances, surgical-orthodontic treatment would be undertaken only after these and related conditions are under medical control.[53]

ance) and quantify (demonstrate the degree to which each jaw, both dental and skeletal component, contribute to the imbalance).

> *The Broadbent Bolton template proved to be a simple, quick, and reliable* tool *to employ in consultation with the treating oral surgeon and with patients to demonstrate the direction and approximate amount of surgery to correct the skeletal disharmony.*[42]

Proffit has discussed the use of the template analysis in his surgical text; he pointed out that the template may appear to be somewhat less scientific than a table of cephalometric measurements with standard deviations, but the "template is a visual analogue of a table and is just as valid."[53]

Proffit further states:

What the template does is place the emphasis on the

analysis itself, that is deciding what the distortions are, rather than on an intermediate measurement step that too often becomes an end in itself rather than just a means to an end.

The author has found that the *template approach* to cephalometric analysis allows an assessment of skeletal landmarks compared to age-matched norms. The use of nasal superimposition fully integrates the nose into cephalometric assessment and allows the clinician to assess soft tissue compensation for skeletal imbalance. I have found that approach excellent for diagnosis and planning treatment for skeletal dysplasias.

In addition, a concise approach to differential diagnosis was presented by Epker and Wolford et al.[16] in a classic article discussing mandibular deficiency syndrome. In this two part paper the clinical, cephalometric features of man-

TABLE 15-5

Most Frequently Used Orthodontic Records

	Panorex	Lat ceph	PA ceph	Diag set-up	Trim model	Mounted models	Photos
Pretreatment	92%	98%	13%	8%	82%	19%	88%
Progress	49%	29%	1%	1%	13%	5%	19%
Posttreatment	78%	69%	3%	1%	51%	9%	15%

From Gottlieb EL, Nelson AH, Vogel DS: 1990 JCO study of orthodontic diagnosis and treatment procedures, *J Clin Orthod* 25(3):145-156, 1991.

dibular, horizontal deficiencies were defined further by adding (1) the vertical component—Type I (low mandibular plane angle—vertical deficiency); (2) Type II (normal mandibular plane angle); and (3) Type III (high mandibular plane angle—vertical excess). Epker and co-workers went on to correlate the type of mandibular deficiency with the preferred surgical treatment. The description of Angle Class II problems, such as mandibular deficiencies, when appropriate, is an important step in differential diagnosis. Further categorization of the horizontal mandibular deficiencies into Types I, II, and III vertical categories, with specific surgical solutions, provides a clear visualization for both mandibular deficiencies and mandibular excess problems.

This author has chosen to use the Epker/Wolford approach to diagnostic descriptions, integrated with the diagnostic steps of quantification and the rating of severity, to illustrate diagnostic and treatment differences of the basic types of mandibular deficiency problems and mandibular excess problems (Figs. 15-13 through 15-17). The Bolton template was employed to show the skeletal deviations from the *template ideal*. The process of differential diagnosis of the structural problem, then, includes the following steps:

1. Classification: (The use of Angle's traditional system of classification is still important and also aids in codification for insurance purposes.)
2. Qualification: Determine problem location. (Is it upper jaw only, lower jaw only? Is the problem all skeletal or part skeletal and part dental?) Can the vertical aspect of the problem be included as was suggested by Wolford et al.?
3. Quantification: (Determine how much each jaw contributes to the problem—percent or mm.)
4. Rate severity: A 0 to 10 scale encompasses a rating of severity of anteroposterior, transverse, and vertical problems in addition to tooth alignment, dental pathology, TMJ status, psychosocial factors, and degree of motivation. Although each of the problems could be rated individually, the concept of using one number to rate the whole constellation of problems helps the patient understand, in a relative way, the severity of their current condition. A "O" rating means ideal or no problems, where as a rating of "10" indicates a severe dentoskeletal imbalance with possible pathologic sequelae. This number can also be used to project the prognosis of treatment outcome with the various treatment options under consideration.

TREATMENT PLANNING AND TREATMENT OPTIONS

With the safety of jaw surgery improving because of technique modifications and with the anesthetic risks being reduced, orthognathic surgical procedures create a range of treatment options that can be both exciting and confusing to the orthodontist and to his or her patients. It can be exciting when a patient with a double jaw treatment problem accepts the optimal treatment plan and when the result achieved matches both the patient's and the doctor's expectations (Fig. 15-18). Confusion in treatment planning can occur, however, when there is an orthodontic problem that is both skeletal and dental in nature, with both jaws contributing to the malrelationship (Fig. 15-19).

Upper-lower jaw; skeletal-dental. The following three steps should be taken:

1. Treatment options must be discussed
2. Anticipated outcomes analyzed
3. *Trade-offs* considered (Proffit's *interaction-compromise*)

The basic concepts of treatment planning for patients with skeletal imbalances are discussed by Proffit in Chapter 1 and also in his textbook.[53] The orthodontist must consider certain key elements to provide consistent treatment planning.

The orthodontist treatment planning for patients with malocclusions plays a *pivotal* role in guiding the patient to a treatment plan that will satisfy the patient's needs for both short-term concerns and long-term function and stability. Although the aforementioned three steps seem simple, there are several specific treatment planning modalities in which orthodontists must strive to gain expertise in order to achieve maximum effectiveness. In each of these modalities, the orthodontist should be able to answer the following questions:

1. Clarification and individualization of treatment goals
   Pertinent questions:
   • Is it imperative that every patient be assigned a treatment plan exemplifying a *textbook ideal* result?
   • When will a *practical* result *suffice?*
   • Whose concept of facial esthetics and balance takes precedence?
   • Is it acceptable to achieve *stability* with mechanical approaches: lifetime bonded retainers and/or lifetime removable retainers?

Text continued on p. 867.

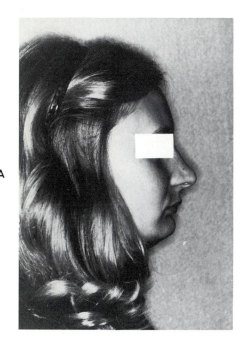

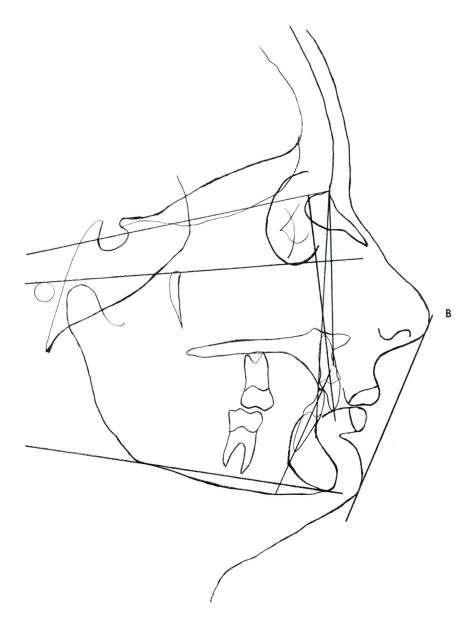

Fig. 15-13
Patient (BB, 27Y 2M, F)

Classification:	Class II, division 2, deepbite, telescoping crossbite.
Qualification:	Mandibular anteroposterior deficiency and vertical deficiency
Quantification:	One hundred percent mandibular skeletal deficiency: mandibular vertical deficiency, severe; moderate horizontal excess in chin area camouflages the skeletal deficiency of mandible
Severity:	8/10
Prognosis:	1.0/10 with orthodontics and jaw surgery

A, Pretreatment profile photograph showing classic appearance of mandibular deficiency Type I. Frequently, these patients are conventionally classified Angle, Class II, division 2 problems and have excess horizontal chin development, requiring A-P reduction after the mandible is advanced.
B, Lateral cephalometric tracing with conventional orthodontic angular criteria shown.

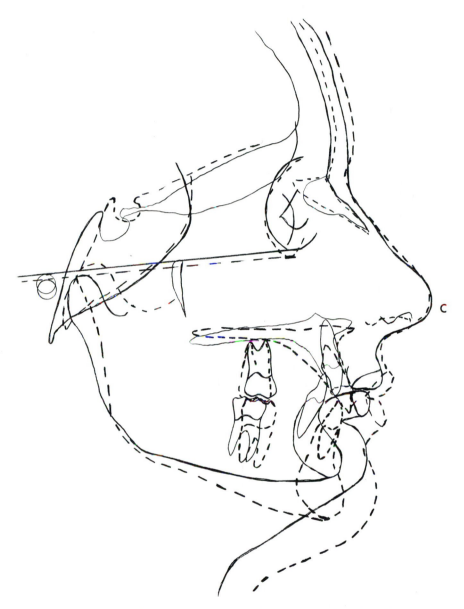

Fig. 15-13, cont'd   C, Lateral cephalometric tracing with Bolton template *(dotted line)* positioned
for nasal superimposition and FH reference plane parallel.

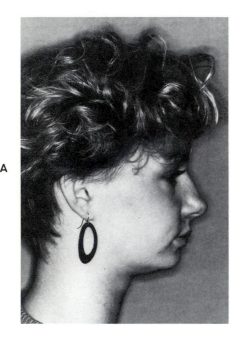

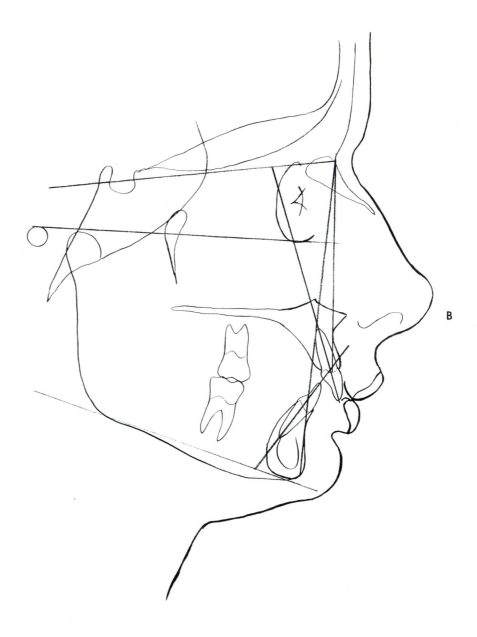

A   B

Fig. 15-14
Patient (JT, 17Y 11M, F)

Classification: Class II, division 1
Qualification: Mandibular deficiency (Type II)
Quantification: 100% mandibular deficiency with normal maxillary skeletal and dental position
                  as seen through template analysis (14C)
Severity: $^{7}/_{10}$
Prognosis: $^{0.5}/_{10}$ with jaw surgery

A, Pretreatment facial profile of patient with mandibular deficiency Type II (medium mandibular
plane angle). **B,** Cephalometric tracing with conventional measures shows SNA at 84.5 and SNB
at 78. Because of the SNA measurement, some might think in terms of a combination Class II—
part maxillary protrusion/part mandibular retrusion. See template assessment, *C.*

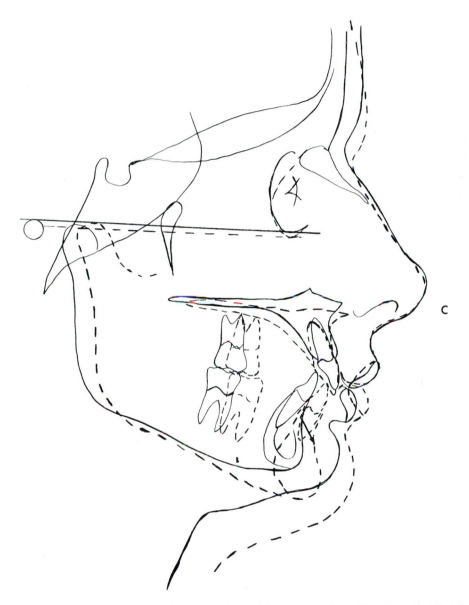

Fig. 15-14, cont'd   C, Bolton template comparison with nasal superimposition shows that facial
imbalance is present because of a 5 mm to 6 mm horizontal and vertical deficiency in point B's
position *(arrow)*. (See Applied Principles section for completed case.)

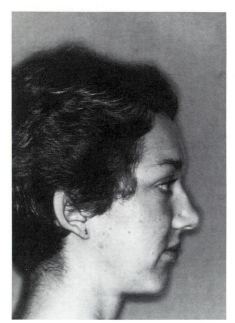

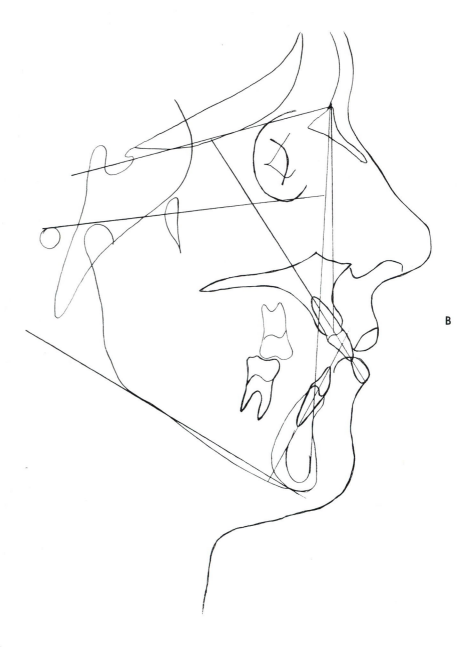

Fig. 15-15
Patient (LG, 26Y 4M, F)

Classification: Class II, division 1
Qualification: Mandibular deficiency (Type III) with openbite
Quantification: Maxillary posterior vertical excess in 100% mandibular deficiency
Severity: $^8/_{10}$ (patient also has TMJ pain, disc displacement with reduction)
Prognosis: TMJ (re-evaluate) occlusal function $^{1.9}/_{10}$

A, Pretreatment facial profile of a patient with mandibular deficiency Type III high mandibular plane angle. Note classic characteristics of clockwise opening of slope of body of mandible, mild lip incompetence, retrognathic appearance with long lower ⅓. **B,** Cephalometric tracing with conventional measurements with SNA at 77 suggesting an underdeveloped maxilla and retruded mandible.

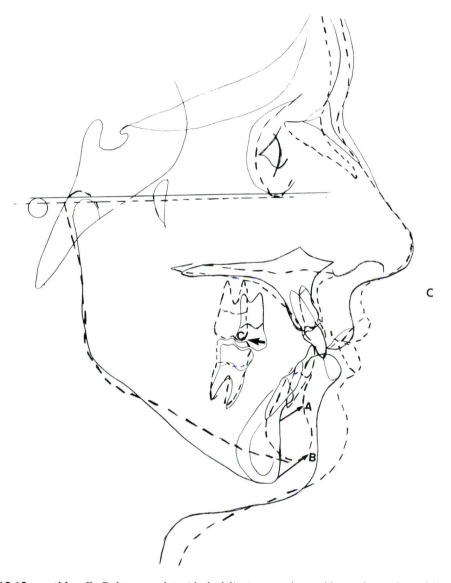

Fig. 15-15, cont'd C, Bolton template *(dashed line)* comparison with nasal superimposition clearly shows the facial imbalance. *Arrow A* shows B point to B point comparison; *arrow B* shows Pogonion to Pogonion comparison; *arrow C* shows patient's first molar to be vertically excessive. Bolton template suggests differential LeFort to affect the molars but not the incisors, mandibular autorotation and mandibular advancement. (See full pre- and post-treatment records in Applied Principles section of this chapter.)

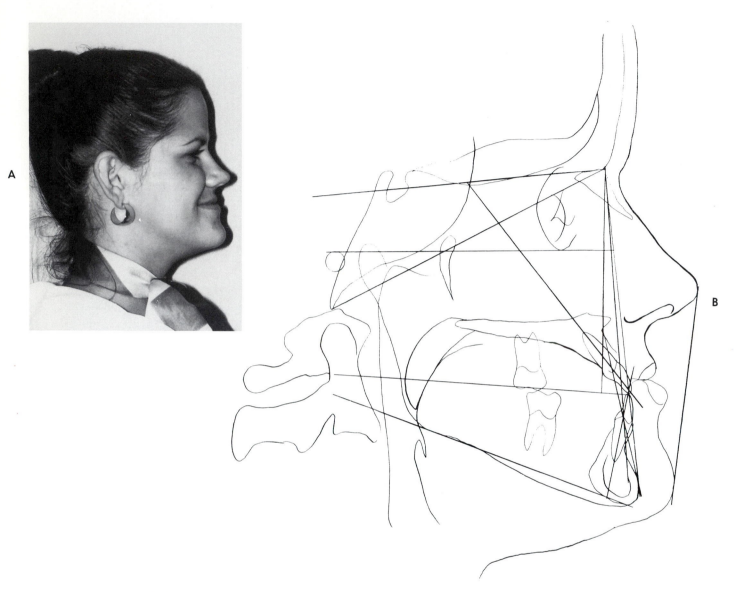

Fig. 15-16
Patient (PM, 24Y 3M, F)

Classification:	Class III mandibular excess (Type I i.e., low mandibular plane angle)
Qualification:	Mandibular skeletal excess with significant maxillary dentoalveolar compensation and relative protrusion
Quantification:	100% mandibular excess
Severity:	8.5/10 severe skeletal problem; impaction of No. 11, dental spacing and mucogingival deficiency
Prognosis:	2/10 prognosis estimated at 2 because of impacted canine and other dental problems that require management; patient has a good attitude to handle complicating factors in treatment

A, Pretreatment facial profile of the patient described above. Mandibular excess is evident.
B, Pretreatment cephalometric tracing with conventional measurements. SNA = 84; SNB = 89. (Mandibular plane angle makes this a Type I category.)

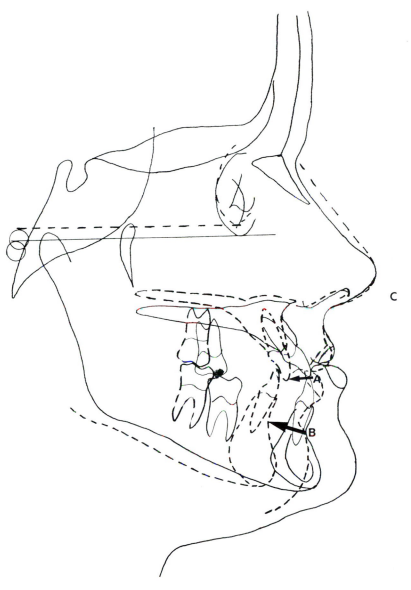

Fig. 15-16, cont'd   C, Bolton template assessment *(dashed line)* clearly demonstrates the areas
of dental and facial imbalance. *Arrow A* illustrates the compensation of the upper incisors; *arrow
B* shows the degree of mandibular excess. Note that, although the upper incisors are *flared* several
millimeters, the soft-tissue lip is only slightly forward of the template.

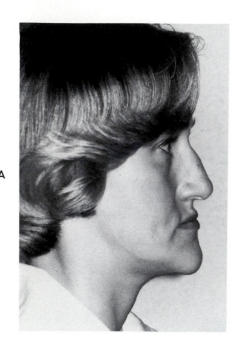

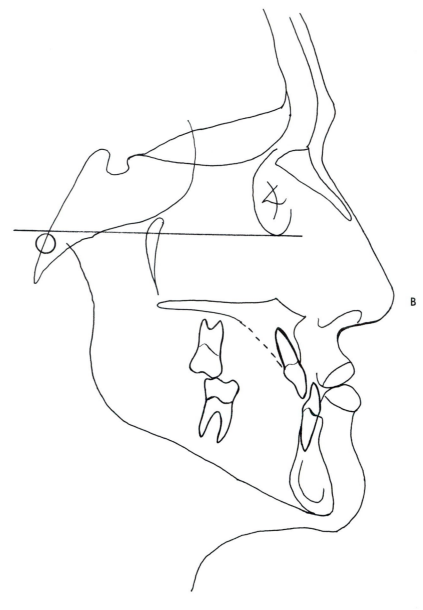

Fig. 15-17
Patient (EF, 30Y 8M, F)

Classification: Class III skeletal
Qualification: Mandibular excess (Type II i.e., moderate mandibular plane angle)
Quantification: 100% mandibular excess (see Fig. 15-16, C)
Severity: 7/10 caused by skeletal severity and long-standing dental compensation of the lower incisors
Prognosis: 3/10 prognosis good with full orthodontics and jaw surgery (chin excess and nasal form may require cosmetic procedure for ideal outcome)

A, Pretreatment facial profile of the patient described above with significant degree of mandibular excess. **B,** Pretreatment cephalometric tracing with conventional measurements. SNA = 81; SNB = 87.

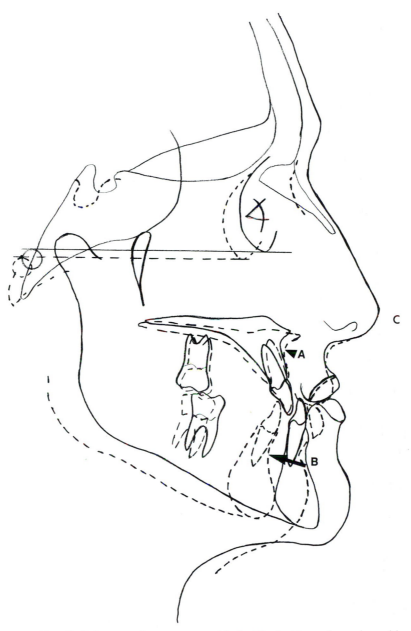

Fig. 15-17, cont'd   C, Bolton template assessment *(dashed line)* with nasal superimposition and
parallel FH clearly demonstrates the facial imbalance. *Arrow A* shows that the *A* point of the
standard and the patient's *A* point are close in their position; *arrow B* shows the difference between
the *B* point of the patient's and the Bolton standard.

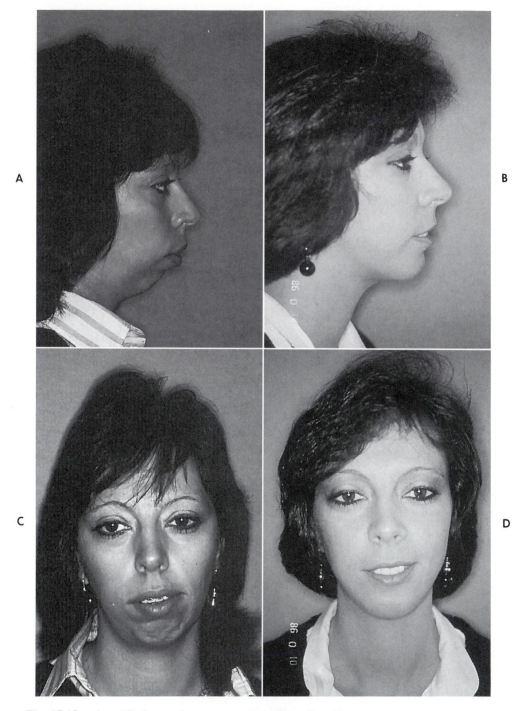

Fig. 15-18   **A** and **B,** Pre- and post-treatment profiles. **C** and **D,** Pre- and post-treatment frontal views. Results match patient's and doctor's expectations. Two-jaw surgery was done. (See Fig. 15-7, J.)

2. Differential diagnosis
   Pertinent questions:
   - At what point does a nonsurgical problem become a surgical problem?
   - Is the surgical-nonsurgical decision made by the patient, the orthodontist, the surgeon, or the insurance company?
   - What is a *borderline* surgical case? Are there many cases that fall into this category?
3. Extractions
   Pertinent questions:
   - Will extraction of teeth be effective for orthodontically camouflaging the malocclusion?
   - Is extraction of premolars needed to decompensate a condition before surgery?
   - Is extraction of premolars being planned for alignment purposes *only?*
   - Should molar or bicuspid extraction be planned to maximize autorotation?
   - What happens when several of the above extraction considerations are applicable to one patient?
4. *Acceptable compromises* of Steiner[61] (Fig. 15-20)
   Pertinent questions:
   - Can patients with a 5° or greater (ANB) difference have an acceptable result without surgery? Under what conditions?
   - Should the concept of *acceptable compromise* be redefined with the understanding of new surgical capabilities?
5. Visualized treatment objectives
   Pertinent questions:
   - Can cephalometric predictions be routinely achieved?
   - Do patients have an overly optimistic perception of the outcome?
   - Will computerized video predictions be an integral part of the VTOs in the future?[58]
   - Is computerized imaging a treatment planning tool, a marketing tool, or both?
6. Patient expectations[6,5,28]
   Pertinent questions
   - Are a patient's presurgical expectations a predictor of their postsurgical satisfaction?
   - What percent of surgical-orthodontic patients eventually indicate that they are satisfied with the treatment outcome?
   - Are immediate postsurgical patients prone to be less satisfied than expected, and if so, why?

Therapeutic Diagnosis

Because of the range of treatment plan options, the concept of therapeutic diagnosis is even more viable today than it was when it was initially introduced.

Ackerman and Proffit[1] discuss this:

Therapeutic diagnosis is not a substitute for established procedures; nor should it become a cover for fuzzy think-
ing in diagnosis. Where uncertainty exists despite a careful diagnostic evaluation, however, there is danger in formulating a rigid treatment plan. Systematic evaluation of the initial response to orthodontic treatment can help a great deal in making the difficult diagnostic and treatment planning decisions, especially as concerns the basic question of extraction or non-extraction. Borderline cases in which the treatment response should be considered before one decides to extract, are more common than many diagnostic systems indicate. It is strength, not weakness, to recognize true uncertainty.

The process calls for using therapeutic aids as indicated in Table 15-6.

Borderline Case Concept

Borderline surgical-non-surgical cases frequently require initial therapy, followed by re-evaluation records to allow thorough review of treatment compromises if the surgical approach is not undertaken. A case may be a definite surgical case but *borderline* in terms of the number of osteotomies. Consideration regarding what is *practical* and safe versus the achievement of a hypothetic ideal is important.

In essence, borderline surgical cases have moderate skeletal malrelationships that affect both jaws equally, Class II maxillary protrusion and mandibular deficiency. In such cases, dental camouflage can be considered appropriate rather than surgical correction. Another borderline case example would arise when a surgical plan has been selected and a decision must be made between double jaw surgery or surgery on just one jaw, leaving a mild asymmetry or a mild degree of vertical excess. Sometimes the added risks of a double jaw procedure, in relation to the minor gains anticipated, allow a single osteotomy to be the procedure of choice.

Generally, wisdom gained through experience and communication with the oral surgeons and the patient will assist the orthodontic planning, using the concept of borderline considerations. In this group of patients the orthodontist needs to exercise the discipline that is intrinsic in the Ackerman-Proffit *problem-oriented* approach to treatment planning. The significant step in borderline cases is the analysis of *interaction and compromises* (see Fig. 15-2).

Treatment Timing

The orthodontist is the key person in deciding the appropriate time to initiate treatment plans that are:
1. Orthodontic only
2. Orthopedic and orthodontic (growth modification)
3. Orthodontic and surgical

General concepts that are accepted for specific treatment problems will be reviewed in this section. The principles presented require individual application to the patient whose treatment is being planned.

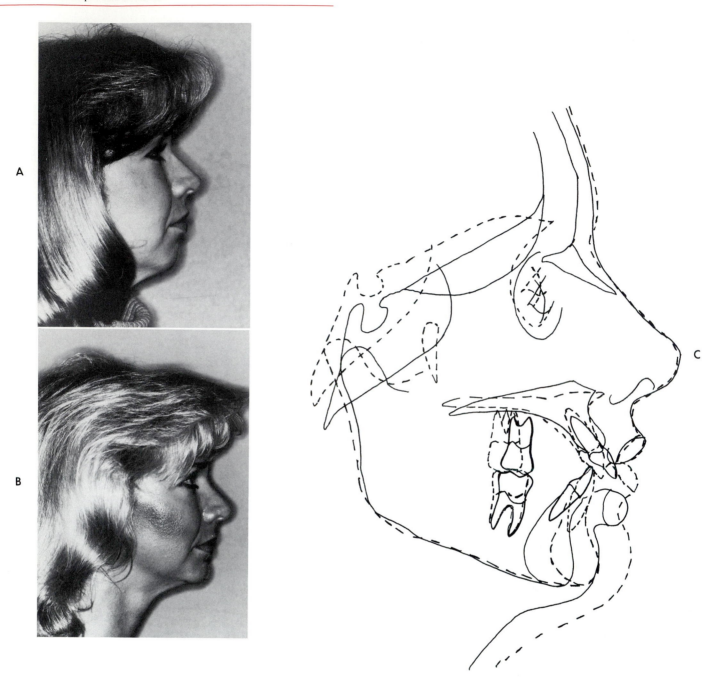

Fig. 15-19 (SL, 39Y 4M, F) **A,** Pretreatment profile of patient with Class II, division 1, malocclusion. **B,** Post-treatment profile photograph that shows the profile changes after numbers 5, 12, and 21 were extracted. (Number 27 was previously removed.) Orthodontic appliances were worn 20 months, and an advancement genioplasty was done. This procedure had less morbidity than a mandibular advancement. **C,** Cephalometric tracing using Bolton template with superimposition method discussed previously. The tracing compared to Bolton standard shows a maxillary protrusion and a mandibular skeletal deficiency with lower incisors compensated forward. Because of the moderate maxillary, mandibular, and chin imbalances, the patient could be treated in many different ways.

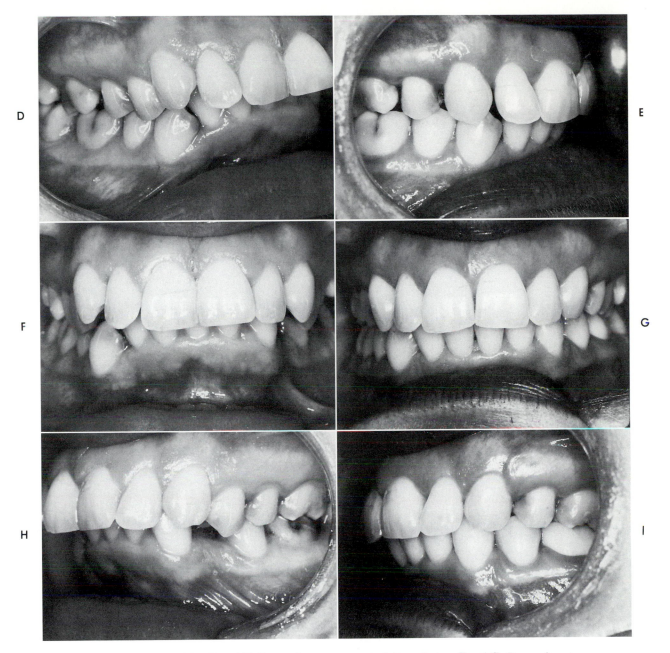

Fig. 15-19, cont'd   D and **E,** Pre- and post-treatment, right occlusion. **F** and **G,** Pre- and post-treatment, center occlusion. **H** and **I,** Pre- and post-treatment, left occlusion. (See discussion on p. 855.)

Acceptable compromises of Steiner
Steiner diagram

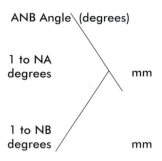

Relocation of upper and lower incisors (compromises) for Class II skeletal patterns

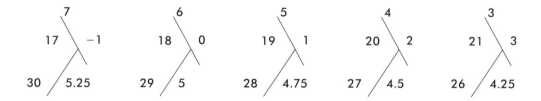

Location of upper and lower incisors for Class I skeletal patterns

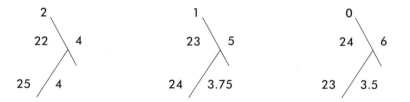

Relocation of upper and lower incisors (compromises) for Class III skeletal patterns

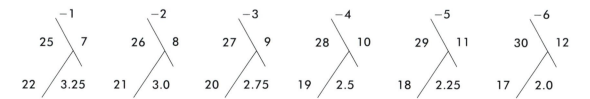

Fig. 15-20 This figure illustrates a modification of Steiner's acceptable compromises and demonstrates the orthodontic solution to skeletal Class II and Class III problems through incisor relocation. The concepts of *acceptable compromises* that were valid in 1950 and 1960 need reevaluation with more recent surgical technology that can minimize compromise. This is especially true in skeletal Class II cases with ANB differences greater than 5° and Class III cases with ANB differences greater than −2°.

TABLE 15-6

Therapeutic Aids

Appliance	Used to assess	Duration
Bite splint Superior repositioning splint (SRS)	Neuromuscular habits and to deprogram muscles of mastication	1 to 6 months re-evaluate new cephalogram and mounted study models
High pull headgear orthopedic effect limited to growing patient	1. Degree of patient co-operation 2. Orthopedic response of Class II with vertical maxillary growth	6 to 12 months (possibility of continuation)
DeLaire face mask	1. Orthopedic response in Class III with mild to moderate maxillary deficiency 2. Maxillary horizontal growth acceleration	6 to 12 months (possibility of continuation)
Chin cup	1. Orthopedic response in Class III with mild mandibular excess 2. Restrain or redirect mandibular growth, primarily in early years 3. Reprogramming of jaw muscles with psuedo skeletal class III problems	6 to 24 months
Fixed appliances to level and align	Combination maxillary protrusion and mandibular deficiency (Class II, division 2 type) Evaluate: Upper lip contour and option between upper premolar extraction and mandibular advancement	6 months

From: Kiyak HA, Bell R: *Psychosocial considerations in surgery and orthodontics*. In Proffit WR, White RP, editors: *Surgical orthodontic treatment*, St. Louis, 1990, Mosby.[27]

Maxillary Deficiency

Deficiency of the maxilla with anteroposterior and transverse components is best managed in the mixed dentition stage. The orthopedic effect is predictable and the early treatment staging enhances the environment for future harmonious growth.

It is not too late to plan treatment for many patients with maxillary deficiency in the early permanent dentition stage, but the stability of the results may be somewhat less than if the patient were treated earlier.[37] (See Chapter 9.)

Mandibular Excess

Patients who have a family history of moderate to severe mandibular excess and demonstrate the growth pattern coincident with mandibular growth imbalance are best treated when growth is complete, as verified by wrist films or headplate superimposition (Fig. 15-21).

It is important to note that some patients have mild mandibular excess, mild maxillary deficiency and a functional forward shift of the mandible (Fig. 15-22). The combination of these factors creates the clinical appearance of a severe Class III mandibular excess pattern. Accurate recording of mandibular position, early orthopedics, and some compensatory camouflage (compensate upper incisor labially and compensate lower incisor lingually) may allow satisfactory nonsurgical management. It is exactly this type of patient who benefits from *therapeutic diagnosis* and periodic re-evaluation of growth. Care must be taken to not *over-treat*

these patients orthodontically through camouflage if the mandibular excess growth continues.

Mandibular Deficiency

The degree of the deficiency (mild, moderate, severe) and the type of the deficiency (Type I [low angle], Type II [medium angle], Type III [high angle] will be factors in deciding the treatment timing. Based on a study of 12 patients, ages 8 to 16 years, Wolford et al.[71] have concluded that:

The surgical-orthodontic correction of mandibular deficiency in actively growing children by mandibular advancement using a modified sagittal osteotomy has proven to be an acceptable procedure.

Most orthodontists will attempt conservative (nonsurgical) measures on this particular age group to limit maxillary horizontal growth and enhance mandibular growth. In female patients the mandibular growth rate slows earlier than it does in males. For severe cases of pure mandibular deficiency or for mandibular deficiency with asymmetry, surgery can be recommended in conjunction with orthodontic treatment in the 14- to 16-year age range for females.

For males, there is evidence of protracted mandibular growth until age 21 to 23. Although a mandibular deficiency will not self correct, the maxillo-mandibular growth differential can be used with directional force orthopedics to significantly improve many low and medium mandibular plane

Text continued on p. 876.

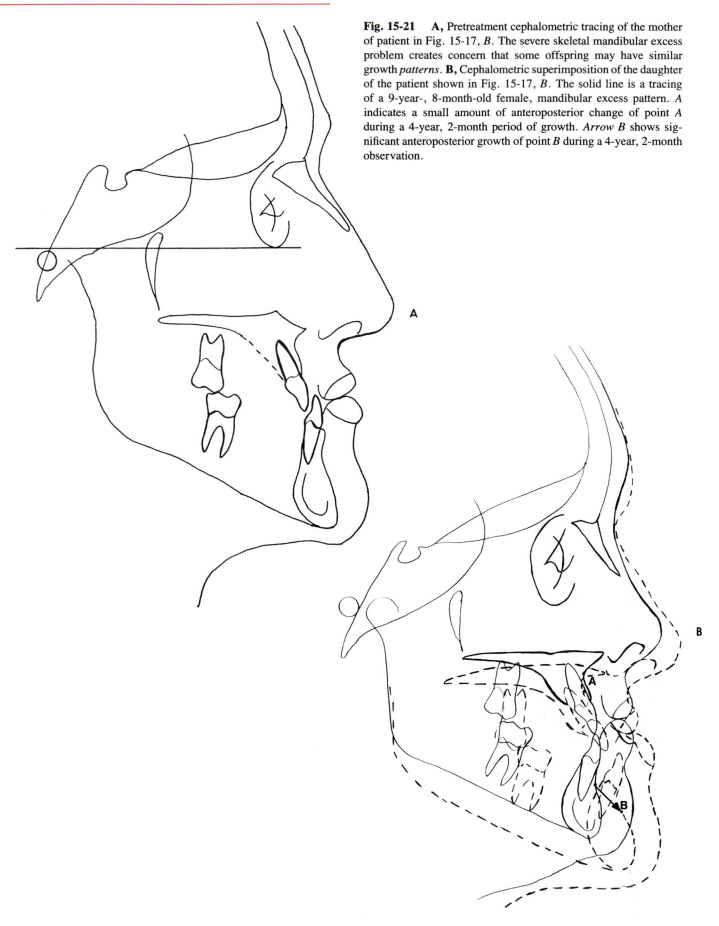

Fig. 15-21 **A,** Pretreatment cephalometric tracing of the mother of patient in Fig. 15-17, *B*. The severe skeletal mandibular excess problem creates concern that some offspring may have similar growth *patterns*. **B,** Cephalometric superimposition of the daughter of the patient shown in Fig. 15-17, *B*. The solid line is a tracing of a 9-year-, 8-month-old female, mandibular excess pattern. *A* indicates a small amount of anteroposterior change of point *A* during a 4-year, 2-month period of growth. *Arrow B* shows significant anteroposterior growth of point *B* during a 4-year, 2-month observation.

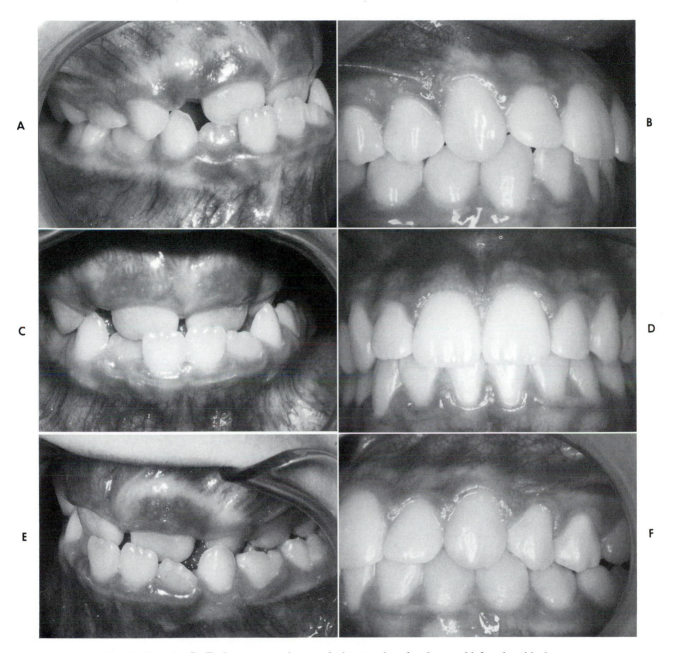

Fig. 15-22   A, C, E, Pretreatment intra-oral photographs of a 6-year-old female with the appearance of a significant Class III problem. There is a functional shift of the mandible to the left and forward, which makes the problem look worse than it is. **B, D, F,** Post-treatment views.

Continued.

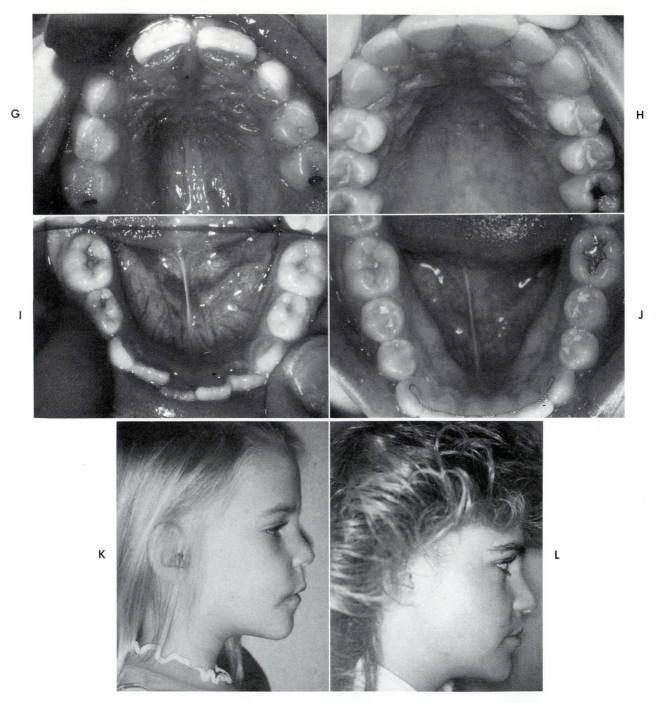

Fig. 15-22, cont'd   G, I, K, Pretreatment. **H, J, L,** Three year post-treatment intra-oral photographic series. Treatment consisted of three phases: Phase 1 (6 years to 6 months)—removable appliance to correct anterior crossbite; Phase 2 (7 years, 6 months to 8 years)—rapid palatal expander and partial upper anterior braces; Phase III (11 years, 6 months to 13 years)—full braces and periodic Class III elastics. **K,** Pretreatment facial profile at 6 years, 0 months. **L,** Three years postretention facial photograph (16 years, 1 month).

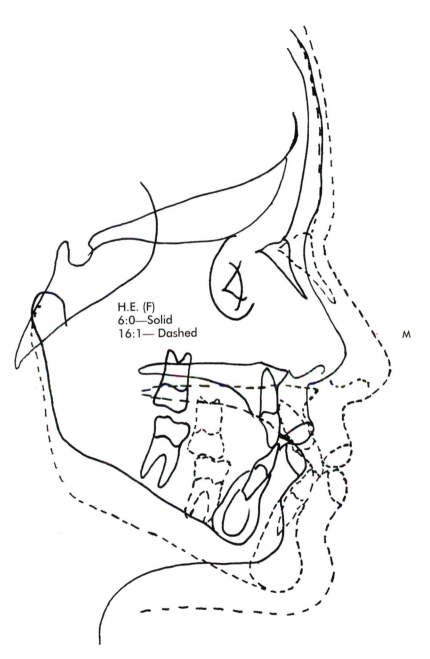

H.E. (F)
6:0—Solid
16:1— Dashed

M

Fig. 15-22, cont'd   M, Cephalometric superimposition (solid 1978; dashed 1988) which illustrates ten years maxillary and mandibular growth and treatment with some upper and lower incisor compensation for the mild lower jaw growth excess.

angles (Class II mandibular deficiency Type I, Type II) to the point that surgery would not be necessary.

In patients who have moderate and severe mandibular deficiency Type III, both males and females will usually require orthodontics and surgery to achieve facial balance, stability, and good function. The timing of surgical intervention in these cases is ultimately dependent on (1) growth factors; (2) emotional maturity; (3) self-image considerations; (4) college plans and related treatment logistics; (5) insurance factors; and (6) the patient's and family's perception of relative need.

Facial Asymmetry

One of the most challenging treatment planning decisions in which orthodontists are involved is the management of facial asymmetry cases. Key questions must be addressed early in the analysis of the case:

1. Is the developing asymmetry a result of trauma?[51] A careful history must be taken. An excellent discussion of acute care of condylar fracture can be found in Proffit's text.[53]
2. Is the asymmetry affecting maxilla and mandible? Is it getting worse with time? Panoramic x-rays and serial PA cephalograms, as well as a submental vertex radiograph, are necessary to aid in this assessment.[18,57]
3. Is functional appliance therapy effective in these asymmetry cases? Some authors have shown good improvement with a functional appliance approach.[38] Severe cases of hemifacial microsomia, however, may require orthopedics to prepare for staged surgery to correct the growth imbalance.
4. What is appropriate timing for surgical intervention? An early consultation with a surgeon who is familiar with the range of considerations present in asymmetry cases is desirable. Periodic functional and emotional assessment is also desirable in preparing the patient for the corrective steps. Orthopedic measures can be taken, but orthodontists need to avoid patient *burn-out* and disappointment, if surgery will still be needed, especially in cases of moderate and severe asymmetry.

In patients who have condylar hypertrophy, a scintigraphy analysis (isotope uptake) can help in determining the appropriate timing based on *hot spot* analysis. Waiting until the hypertrophy *burns itself out* is the most judicious way to proceed in condylar hypertrophy cases. A review of this problem is presented by Obwegeser and Makek.[48]

SEQUENCE OF TREATMENT FOR THE ORTHOGNATHIC PATIENT

Although many believe that the sequence of treatment starts with the patient interview-examination, the most important steps take place long before the surgeon or orthodontist meet the patient with skeletal jaw imbalances. The feedback loop sequence described in the box on p. 877 schematically demonstrates 17 significant steps that, if fol-

lowed, will provide an excellent opportunity for patient and doctors to achieve the treatment success desired.

Sequence

In the sequence of treatment for patients with major dentofacial imbalances (box on p. 877), steps 1, 2, and 17 are most frequently underemphasized. Because of this deficiency in private office policies, the author will review these steps to emphasize the reasons, for their importance:

Step 1: multiple provider team selection

The dentist will refer skeletal malocclusion patients to the orthodontist if there is confidence that the patient will receive appropriate state-of-the-art care.

The orthodontist has to select surgeons who are experienced and well trained in the spectrum of orthognathic procedures. A periodontist, a psychologist, and a physical therapist are also key *team members*.

Step 2: goal clarification

The *provider team* should share similar concepts of treatment goals. Occlusal goals, esthetic goals, and stability of outcomes can mean different things to different providers. Periodic group meetings oriented to individual case analysis offers an opportunity for team members to discuss their concept of the treatment goals that apply to the individual patient.

Steps 3-16: these steps are commonly performed by provider groups and are self-explanatory.

By following the general concepts stated in each step, the orthodontist will automatically spend time with the patient and will be able to address most of the patient's presurgical and postsurgical concerns. Communicating the sequence of treatment to the patient and the general dentist can be done through the use of the treatment conference report shown in Fig. 15-23.

Orthodontists and their staffs need to constantly be reminded, through appropriate chart designation, of those patients who have orthognathic treatment plans. These patients frequently have increased anxiety and extra questions that need to be addressed to maintain their confidence and trust. At the presurgical consultation (step 12) it is important to listen to the patient and to determine his or her physical, dental, and emotional readiness for surgery.

Kiyak and co-workers[27-30] have done numerous studies assessing patient's responses to current ortho-surgical treatment modalities. A thorough review of their work is necessary to help orthodontists and their staffs appreciate the range of feelings that orthognathic patients report before and after the surgical procedure. Table 15-7 describes the psychologic considerations during the various treatment steps for a patient who is having jaw surgery.

SEQUENCE OF TREATMENT FOR PATIENTS WITH SIGNIFICANT DENTOFACIAL IMBALANCES

1. Multiple provider team selection
   - Orthodontist
   - Periodontist
   - Restorative dentist
   - Oral surgeon
   - Psychologist
2. Goal clarification for team members
   - Function
   - Reliable methods
   - Esthetics
   - Stability
   - Health
3. Clinical awareness of dentofacial deformity
   - Self, D.D.S., friend
4. General assessment of patient
   - A good candidate?
   - Periodontal status
5. Evaluation of preliminaty records by the dental team
   - Splint therapy for diagnosis of TMJ dysfunction, if needed
6. Completion of diagnostic records
   - May include lifestyle assessment by clinical psychologist
   - May require more sophisticated TMJ studies
7. Multidisciplinary review of dentofacial problem based on patient records
8. Explanation to patient of available treatment options
   - Recommended optimal treatment plan
9. Consultation with patient and spouse by dental team providers
   - Risk-benefit ratio
   - Fees and insurance coverage
   - Treatment time
   - Other concerns
10. Patient acceptance of treatment plan

11. Comprehensive orthodontic treatment (usually 8 to 18 months before surgery)
    - Orthodontic movement to decompensate tooth positions
    - Coordinate arches in anticipation of surgical repositioning
    - Align teeth and correct rotations
12. Presurgical reevaluation records
    - Complete records
    - Prediction tracing (detailed movements planned)
    - Model surgery
    - Determination of specific fixation needs
    - Patient-spouse review
    - Reevaluation by psychologist
13. Orthognathic surgery
    - Choose simplest procedure(s) to achieve professional goals and to satisfy needs of the patient
14. Postsurgical period
    - Early: 2 to 3 weeks fixation
    - Late: 3 to 8 weeks fixation
    - Reevaluation of surgical procedure
    - Meeting between patient and psychologist for update and support
15. Evaluation of surgery stability
    - Orthodontic finishing, occlusal adjustments, and retention procedures
    - Optional continuation of contact with psychologist
16. Post-treatment records
    - One-year post-treatment
    - Reevaluation with dental team, especially oral surgeon and psychologist
17. Treatment experience (used in management of future cases)
    - Positive reinforcement
    - Problem-solving
    - Reevaluation of degree of success in achieving goals
    - Treatment evaluations by patient and all providers

Step 17: treatment experience

This step is seldom incorporated in the sequence routine policy of private orthodontic and surgical practices. To gain the most from this step, all team members would review postsurgical records and discuss the positives and negatives of the overall treatment plan, sequence of treatment and provider interaction. Each completed case would provide an opportunity for the providers to consider *feedback* from each other and the patient. This step would be the most powerful, continuing education program in which a practitioner could participate. Having each orthognathic patient complete a post-treatment questionnaire also would provide additional feedback and would be an integral part of practice maturation.

APPLIED CONCEPTS FOR SPECIFIC CASE TYPES

Certain concepts that have been discussed in this chapter will now be integrated and applied to case types previously introduced in the differential diagnosis section. A summary of the concepts that are presented in this chapter and that are fundamental to consistent excellence in the management of skeletal disharmonies are as follows:

- *Treatment goals* that are defined and agreed upon in principle by the providers.
- *Technique advancements* that are used to enhance the safety of all orthognathic procedures.
- *Current capacity to alter* dentofacial structures is significant. Because the potential degree of change is so great,

Treatment Conference Report

Re: _____   Date: _____

I. *Classification and diagnostic description of malocclusion:*

_____

II. *List of Dental Problems:* (mild / moderate / severe)   *Dental treatments available:*

_____   _____

_____   _____

_____   _____

_____   _____

_____   _____

_____   _____

III. *Treatment sequence recommended at this time:*

1. _____

2. _____

3. _____

4. _____

5. _____

6. _____

7. _____

8. _____

9. _____

10. _____

Reference charting		
Deciduous		**Permanent**
A B C D E F G H I J		1 2 3 4 5 6 7 8 | 9 10 11 12 13 14 15 16
T S R Q P O N M L K		32 31 30 29 28 27 26 25 | 24 23 22 21 20 19 18 17

IV. *Overall problem severity:* (0-10 scale) _____

V. *Limiting factors in achieving "text book ideal" result:*   Prognosis: (0-10) _____

1. _____

2. _____

3. _____

4. _____

VI. *Patient concerns and current plan of action:*

1. _____

2. _____

3. _____

Fig. 15-23   Treatment conference report—sample of reporting mechanism to send to general dentist and to give to patient or parent.

TABLE 15-7

Psychosocial Considerations in Clinical Interaction

Treatment stage	Steps in psychologic management
A. Initial assessment	1. Explore motives for treatment and expectations from treatment in detail. Why treatment? Why now instead of last or next year? 2. Consider using an auxiliary with a warm personality to do at least part of the interview. Patients often are intimidated by the doctor and may not reveal their true concerns. 3. Be careful not to create unrealistic expectations—it is better not to discuss the specifics of treatment procedures before the diagnostic workup has been completed, but a broad outline including the possibility of surgery should be presented.
B. Orthodontic consultation	1. The spouse, a family member, or a close friend should attend if at all possible—but be careful about invasion of patient's privacy. 2. Begin with a discussion of the patient's problems; be sure doctor and patient agree as to what is most important; then describe how the problems might be solved, beginning with the most important problem and presenting the alternatives. 3. Encourage—indeed, insist on—an early appointment with the surgeon if surgical treatment may be needed.
C. Surgical consultation	1. Review patient's records with same general approach as the orthodontist, emphasizing the problems and their possible solutions. 2. Discuss the functional and esthetic benefits of surgery, in that order. It is better to tell patients they will have functional benefits and esthetic changes than the reverse. Functional changes nearly always are appreciated; esthetic changes may not be. 3. Provide more detail about the surgical experience, to the extent the patient has questions, but keep the discussion relatively general. Many details can wait until just before surgery. 4. Consider using patient education materials at this stage, such as booklets, video cassettes, and videodisc. 5. Offer now to help with insurance preauthorization.
D. Presurgical treatment	1. Evaluate the patient's personality characteristics and psychologic stability in more detail. Focus on: neuroticism, degree of external locus of control, introversion in males, mood states (particularly depression and current major life events), and tendency for patient to be a *vigilant coper.*
E. Immediate presurgery	1. Review the planned surgery in detail, but take the patient's psychologic profile into account. Patients who expect the worst are more likely to experience it. 2. Discuss with family members and close friends the importance of their psychologic and emotional support postsurgically. Be sure the *significant other* is prepared for changes in the patient's facial appearance so that they do not express shock or dismay.
F. Immediate postsurgery	1. Expect a period of mood swings and negative emotions, which usually peak at about 2 weeks. Reassure the patient, family, and friends that these emotions are normal and will soon disappear. 2. A visit from the orthodontist and, perhaps, flowers or a *care package* of easy-to-eat foods keep the patient from feeling forgotten.
G. Postsurgical orthodontics	1. Negative emotions and mood swings are more likely to be seen by the orthodontist in patients who return for finishing orthodontics more quickly and in older patients. Reassurance and psychologic support may be needed. 2. Remember that a decrease in satisfaction and facial body image occurs if active treatment takes more than 6 months postsurgically. If treatment has not been completed by this time, progress should be reviewed with the patient and an anticipated completion date discussed.

From: Kiyak HA, Bell R: *Psychosocial considerations in surgery and orthodontics.* In Proffit WR, White RP, editors: *Surgical orthodontic treatment,* St. Louis, 1990, Mosby.[27]

the responsibility of the surgeon and orthodontist planning treatment is also great. Psychosocial and emotional balance may be at risk.

- *The differential diagnosis process* generates a problem list and treatment planning options. The so-called *textbook ideal* result should be considered and discussed with all patients; however, not all patients have the resources or the desire for *state-of-the-art treatment.*
- *Treatment planning* will, therefore, create alternative options. The *good, better, best* approach to patient education will yield understanding and trust.

- *Borderline cases* (i.e., Class II with moderate lower jaw deficiency) can benefit from therapeutic diagnosis with initial leveling and alignment. Then assess facial balance with the mandible postured forward.
- *Standardized sequencing* through the 17 steps presented in the box on p. 877 will assure a well-educated patient and a well-prepared treatment team.

An important part of orthognathic treatment planning involves a surgical prediction. The hard tissue changes are relatively easy to predict; however, soft tissue changes are less predictable. In Table 15-8 from Jensen, Sinclair, and

TABLE 15-8

Current Concepts of Facial Growth

Treatment	Soft-tissue change	Notes
Anteroposterior movement of incisors: maxillary or mandibular, forward or back, surgical or orthodontic	60% to 70% of incisor movement	1, 2
Vertical movement of incisors	Minimal unless jaw rotates	3, 4, 5
Mandibular advancement	Soft tissue: chin 1:1 with bone, lower lip 60% to 70% with incisor	6
Maxillary advancement	Nose: slight elevation of tip	7, 8
	Base of upper lip: 20% of point A	
	Upper lip: 60% of incisor protraction, shortens 1 to 2 mm	
Mandibular setback	Chin: 1:1	5
	Lip: 60%	
Maxillary setback	Nose: no effect	3
	Base of upper lip: 20% of point A	
	Upper lip: 60% of incisor	
	Advancement lower lip: variable, may move back	
Mandibular setback plus maxillary advancement	Changes similar to a combination of the two procedures separately	
Maxillary superior repositioning	Nose: usually no effect	7
	Upper lip: shortens 1 to 2 mm	
	Lower lip: rotates 1:1 with mandible	
Mandibular advancement plus maxillary superior repositioning	Chin: 1:1	9
	Lower lip: 70% of incisor	
	Upper lip: shortens 1 to 2 mm	
	80% of any incisor advancement	
	Nose: slight elevation of tip	
Mandibular inferior border repositioning	Soft tissue forward: 60% to 70% bone	
	Chin: Up—1:1 with bone	
	Back—50% bone	
	Laterally—60% bone	
	Down—?	

1. Little difference occurred with surgery or orthodontics.
2. If both upper and lower incisors are retracted (bimaxillary protrusion), lip movement stops when lips come into contact.
3. Lip shortens 1 to 2 mm with vestibular incision (more if surgical technique is poor).
4. Lip rotates with mandible 1:1.
5. If face height increases, lip may uncurl and lengthen.
6. If lip uncurls, it will go forward less.
7. Nose change is usually temporary.
8. Less soft-tissue change occurs after cleft-lip repair.
9. Data from Jensen AC, Sinclair PM, Wolford IM: Soft tissue changes associated with double jaw surgery, *Am J Orthod Dentofac Orthop* 101(3)266-275, 1992.

Wolford's work, a variety of general guidelines are used to predict soft tissue changes in the lateral cephalometric view. However, the most difficult soft tissue predictions with current surgical treatments are predictions of changes in the frontal view. Current video technology may help the surgeon and the patient visualize the facial changes that are part of the treatment plan under consideration.[58] The patients in Figs. 15-24 and 15-25 illustrate the outcome of treatment that uses the concepts described in this chapter. The patient in Fig. 15-24 is a classic skeletal Class II, mandibular deficiency, Type II. (See template assessment in Fig. 15-14, *C.*

The patient in Fig. 15-25 represents a classic, skeletal Class II, mandibular deficiency, Type III (see template assessment Fig. 15-15,*C.*

The treatment outcomes of two types of Class III, skeletal mandibular excess are shown in Fig. 15-26 and 15-27. The

patient in Fig. 15-26 represents a classic patient whose skeletal problem can be described as Class III, mandibular excess, Type II. (Refer to template superimposition in Fig. 15-17,*C.*) Complete surgical correction of the mandibular excess was dependent on lower incisor decompensation from pretreatment incisor to mandibular plane angle of 77° to presurgical angulation of 89°.

The patient in Fig. 15-27 demonstrates a classic example of mandibular excess, Type III (high mandibular plane with openbite). Generally, patients with high mandibular plane angles and open bites require a maxillary LeFort procedure with impaction, as well as a mandibular procedure. Both a maxillary and mandibular procedure were performed on this patient. The patient in Fig. 15-28 illustrates a well-treated patient who was not fully satisfied with her treatment (see legend for Fig. 15-28, *L*).

Text continued on p. 894.

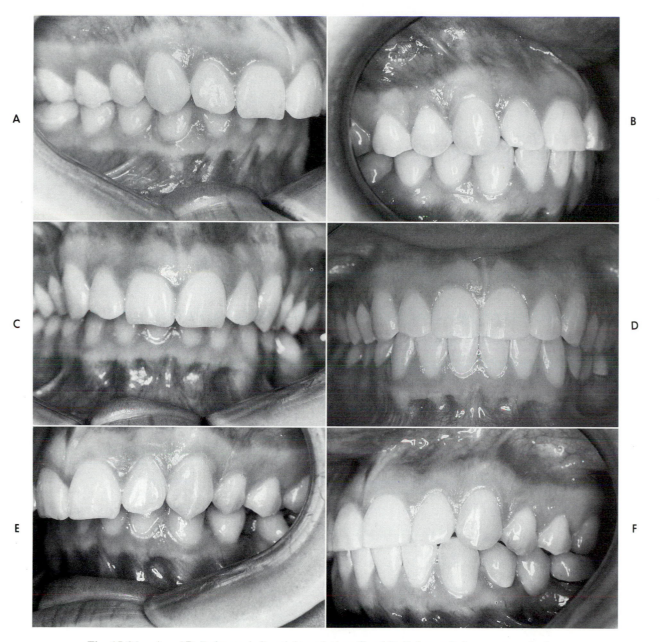

Fig. 15-24 **A** and **B,** Before and after, right occlusion. **C** and **D,** Before and after, center occlusion.
E and **F,** Before and after, left occlusion. *Continued.*

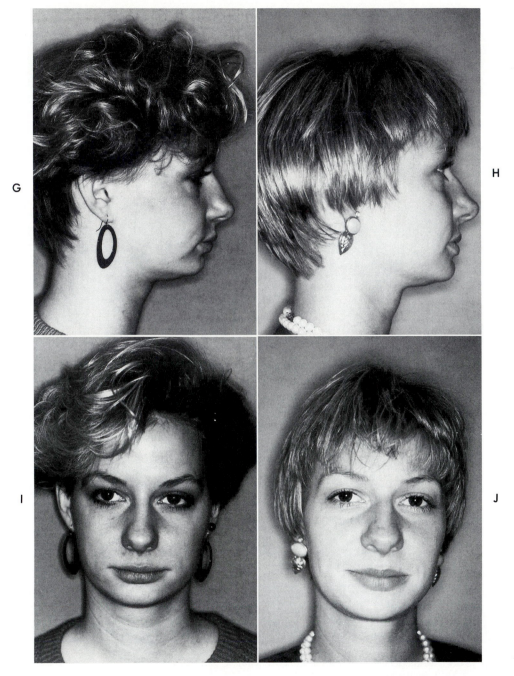

Fig. 15-24, cont'd   **G** and **H,** Before and after, profile views. **I** and **J,** Before and after, full face.

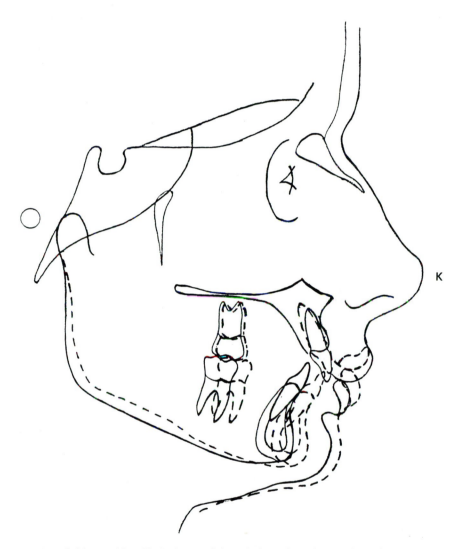

Fig. 15-24, cont'd   K, Before *(solid)* and after *(dashed)* superimpositions.

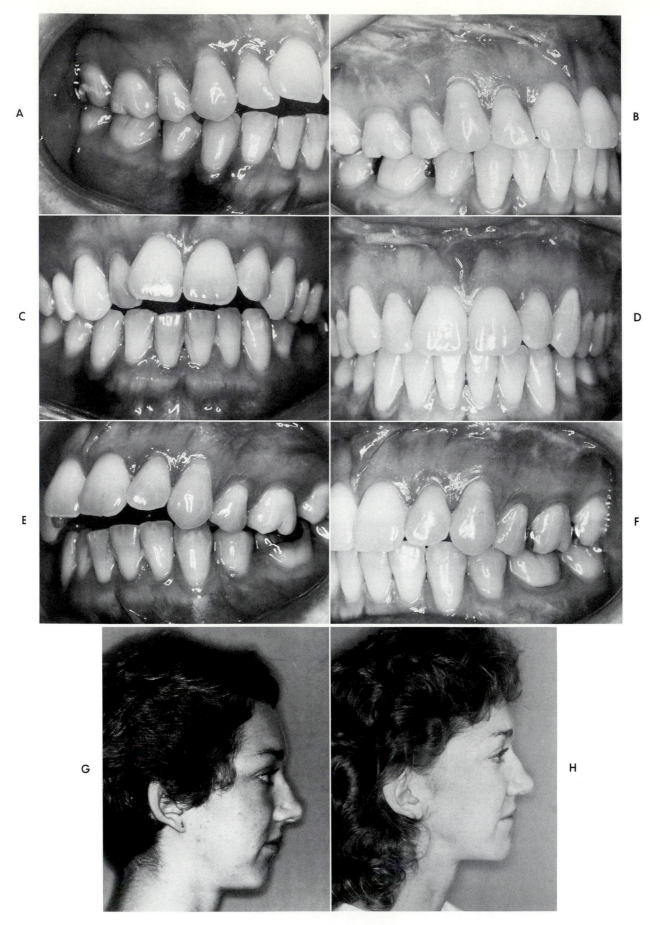

Fig. 15-25 For legend see opposite page.

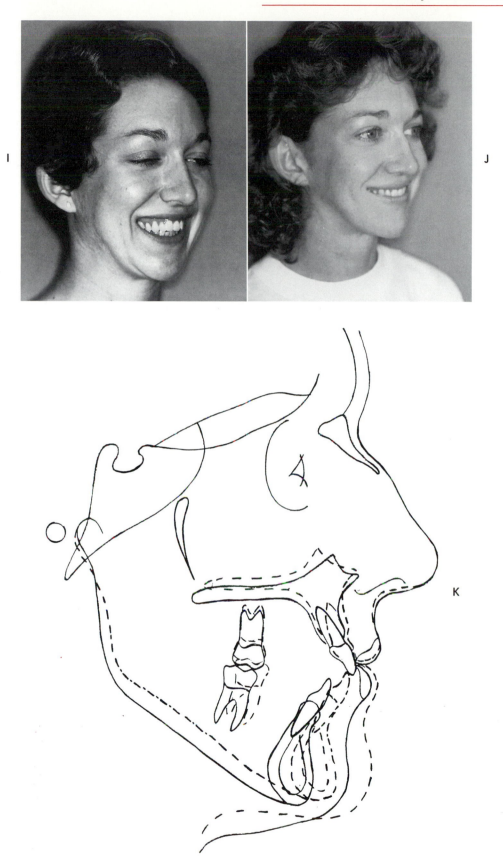

Fig. 15-25   **A** and **B,** Before after, right occlusion. **C** and **D,** Before and after, center occlusion. **E** and **F,** Before and after, left occlusion. **G** and **H,** Before and after, profile views. **I** and **J,** Before and after, smiling views. **K,** Before and after superimpositions.

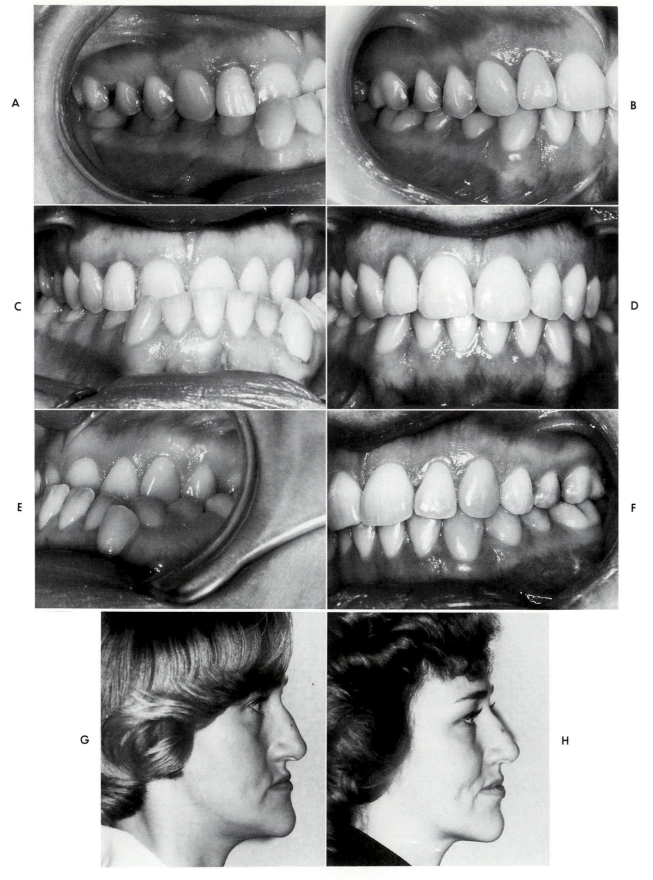

Fig. 15-26 For legend see opposite page.

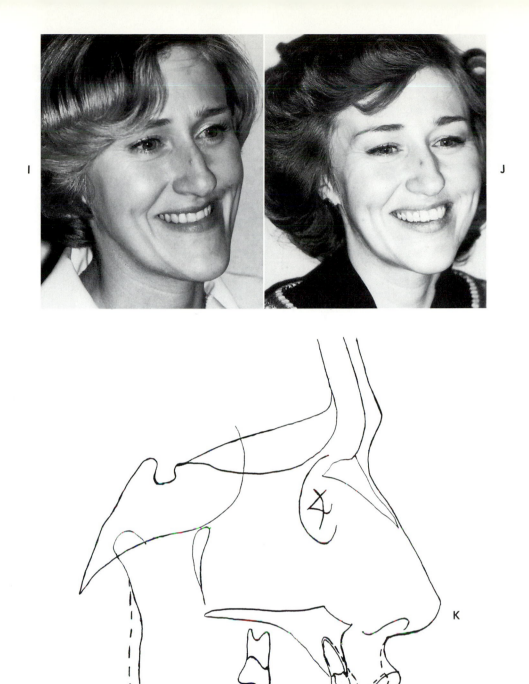

Fig. 15-26   **A** and **B,** Before and after, right occlusion. **C** and **D,** Before and after, center occlusion. **E** and **F,** Before and after, left occlusion. **G** and **H,** Before and after, profile view. **I** and **J,** Before and after, smiling views. **K,** Before and after cephalometric superimpositions.

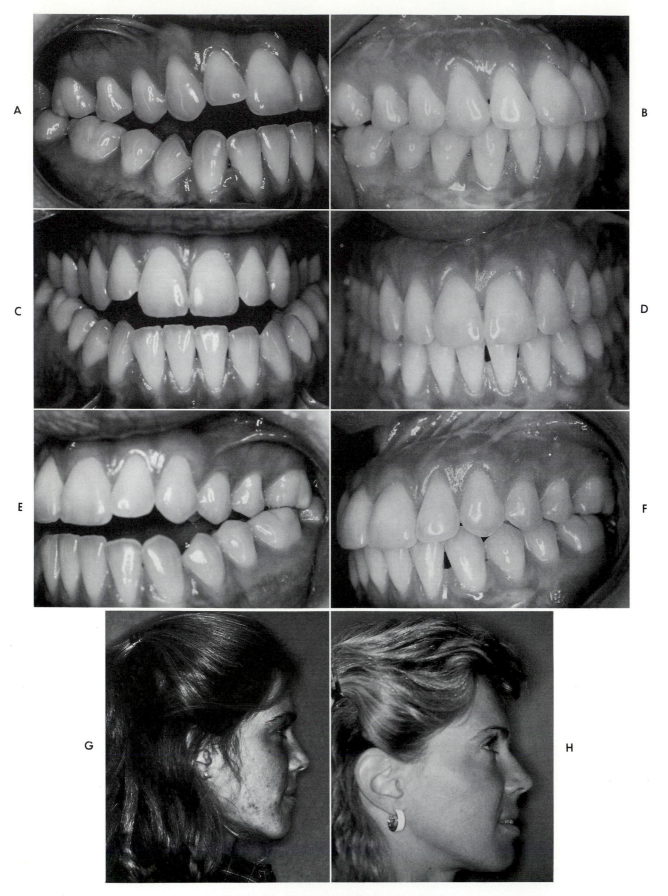

Fig. 15-27 For legend see opposite page.

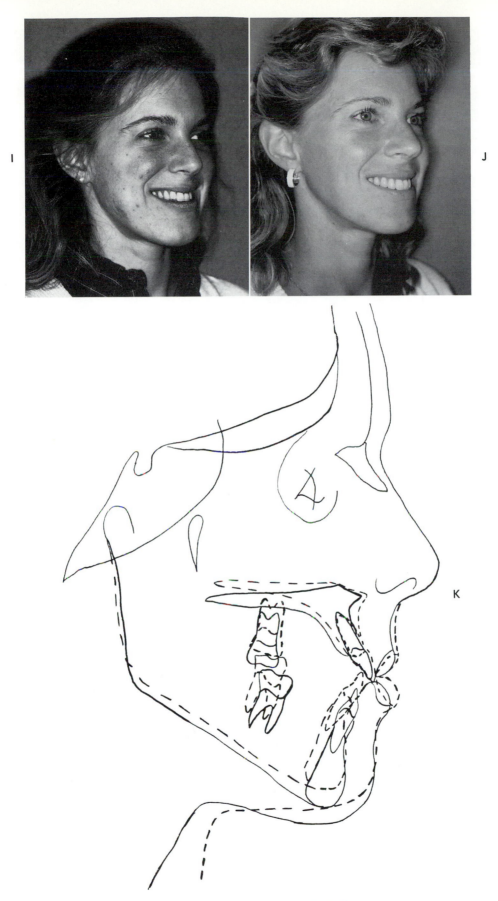

Fig. 15-27 **A** and **B,** Before and after, right occlusion. **C** and **D,** Before and after, center occlusion. **E** and **F,** Before and after, left occlusion. **G** and **H,** Before and after, profile views. **I** and **J,** Before and after, smiling views. **K,** Before and after superimpositions.

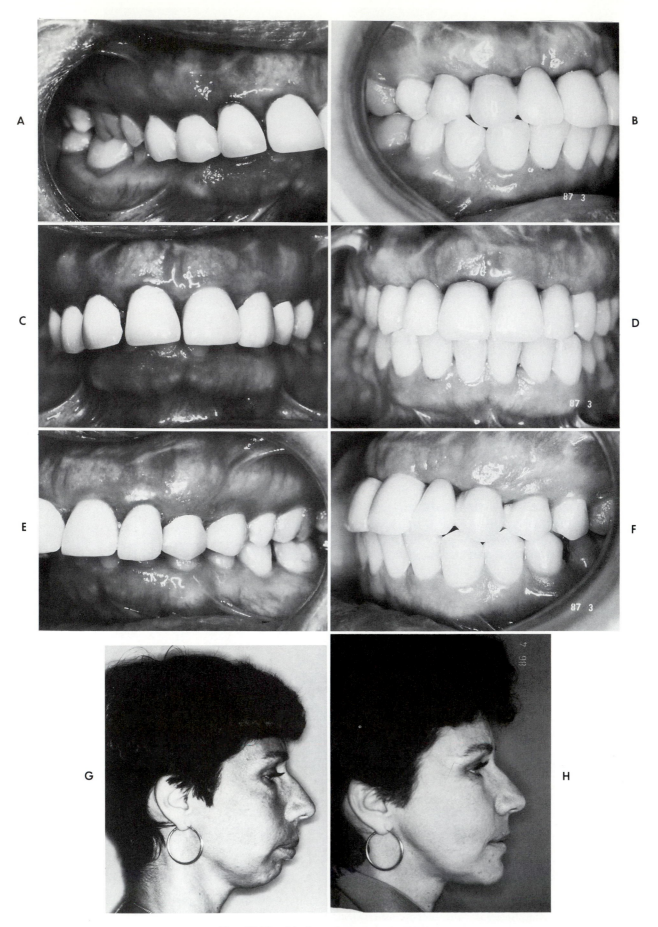

Fig. 15-28 For legend see opposite page.

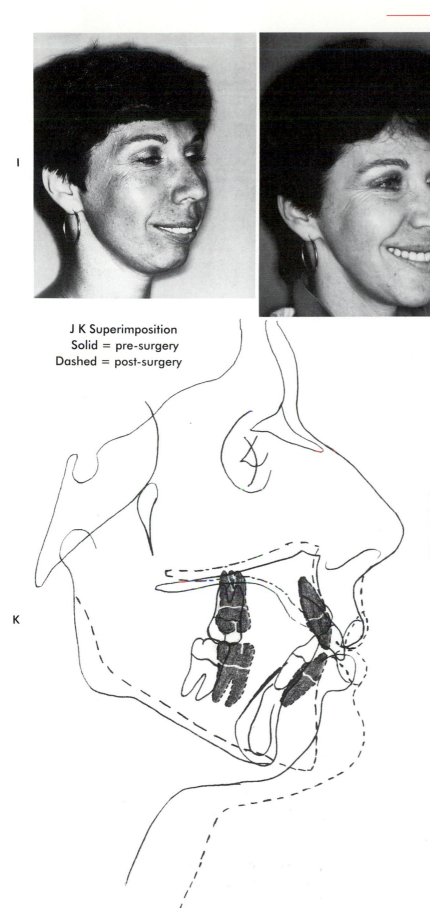

J K Superimposition
Solid = pre-surgery
Dashed = post-surgery

Fig. 15-28   **A, C, E,** Pretreatment intra-oral photographs. **B, D, F,** Post-treatment photographs. **G,** Pretreatment, profile. **H,** Post-treatment profile. **I,** Pretreatment ¾ view, smiling. **J,** Post-treatment, ¾ view, smiling. **K,** Cephalometric superimposition; *solid line* shows pretreatment and *dashed line* indicates post-treatment.

- LeFort osteotomy with impaction 5.0 mm and *A* point move distally 2.0 mm
- Mandibular auto-rotation and advancement; *B* point came forward 13.0 mm
- Vertical reduction and advancement genioplasty; *Pg* came forward 16.0 mm   *Continued.*

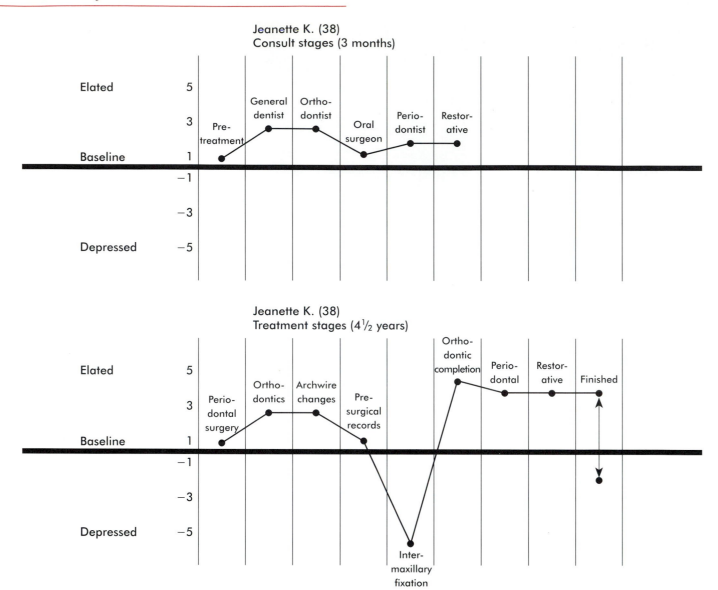

Fig. 15-28, cont'd **L,** Graph showing patient's attitude changes during a program of *state-of-the-art* comprehensive dentistry. Her post-treatment *negative* feelings were related to residual TMJ discomfort and also feeling that she wasn't fully informed about some of the *downsides* of the multidisciplinary treatment that she experienced.

STABILITY

Of the treatment goals discussed in this chapter's introduction, orthodontists and surgeons are alike in their ongoing quest to recommend and to provide procedures that give lasting stability to their patients. Lindquist,[33] in a previous edition of this text, stated:

The idea is that all the objectives must be brought into proper balance. At the center of the spokes is stability (Fig. 15-29). If the treatment is not stable, production of the other objectives will not last.

The stability of orthognathic procedures has been one of the most studied aspects of the techniques in use. In a review article assessing the stability of the sagittal split osteotomy for mandibular advancement by McDonald,[36] the author cited 34 references that reported on the stability of one type of surgery for one type of jaw correction.

Stability is a key goal of both orthodontic treatment and orthognathic treatment—the lack of stability is considered a complication, particularly as it relates to the surgical aspect of the correction. In order to discuss the general concept of stability, it is important to consider several factors necessary to achieve stability:

Orthodontic considerations

1. Proper differential diagnosis
2. Growth factors and timing of the referral
3. TMJ stability when planning the treatment
   CR-CO discrepancies
   Asymmetric growers

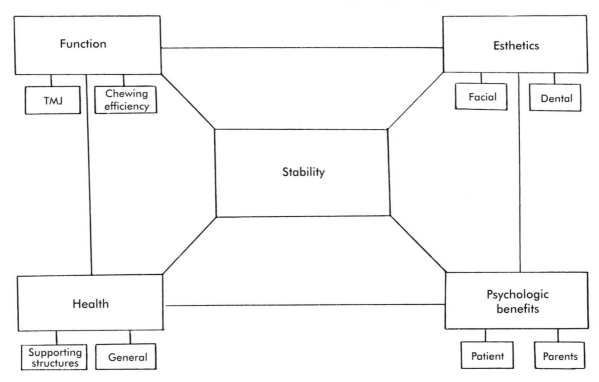

Fig. 15-29 Lindquist's chart of orthodontic treatment objectives showing that stability of the result is *central* to the balance of the overall objectives.

4. Dental stability
   Crown to root ratio is important (periodontal health must be maintained)
   Also, temporary crowns can be a source of instability during intra-dental fixation
5. Presurgical orthodontic preparation that reduces dental compensations

Surgical considerations

1. Treatment plan
   Surgery on which jaw
   Single or double jaw procedures, especially for openbite
2. Design of osteotomy
   Maintain blood supply and accomplish objectives
3. Type of fixation
   Dental, skeletal, rigid, semi-rigid, or combination
4. Muscles of mastication and blood supply
   In sagittal split of mandible it is advisable not to strip pterygomasseteric attachment to avoid ischemia and delayed healing
5. Suprahyoid muscle pull
   Cervical brace or myotomy
6. Type of mandibular rotation
   Downward and backward clockwise movement is more stable than upward, forward movement
7. The stability decreases as the magnitude of surgical correction increases, especially in:
   Maxillary vertical deficiencies
   Mandibular horizontal deficiencies

8. Stable condylar position applies to presurgical assessment, surgical control of proximal segment, and patient's post-surgical adaptation to new neuro-muscular and functional environment; also, Arnett[4] has described the condition of idiopathic female condyle resorption that may be responsible for late condyle changes (*cheerleaders'* syndrome, AVN or condylolysis)
   These findings led us to hypothesize that a small portion of the female population is prone to condylar resorption secondary to increased joint load that is tolerated well by the general female population.[4] (Fig. 15-30).
9. Neuromuscular adaptation—the surgical procedures that change the skeletal structures, also change long-standing neuromuscular patterns of the stomatognathic system; achieving a balance or an equilibrium of the skeletal structures, dental structures, and muscles is the ultimate biologic challenge for the orthognathic team. Although the procedures provided today are based scientifically on a variety of working hypotheses, the relapse problems that still occur are reminders that some of the treatment provided may have components of empiricism

Planning treatment for orthognathic cases has the potential of aiding the stability of the treatment outcome through:

1. *Proper differential diagnosis of those patients who would most benefit from combined therapy.* The classic example is the Class III grower. The orthodontist must determine through differential diagnostic studies and growth forecasting that this patient has a mandibular excess case.

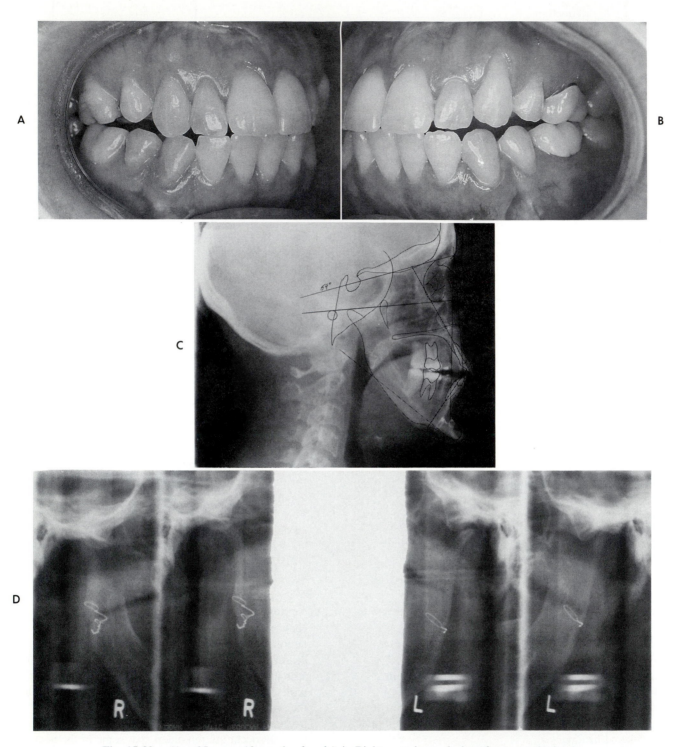

Fig. 15-30   (Age 35 years, 10 months; female) **A,** Right posterior occlusion after two orthodontic treatments and two separate orthognathic procedures. **B,** Lateral posterior occlusion after two orthodontic treatments and two separate orthognathic procedures. **C,** Lateral cephalogram after the two separate orthodontic and surgical treatments. Note lack of incisal contact. Patient states that the "open bite is progressively getting worse." **D,** Right condyle showing degenerative changes. Left condyle showing degenerative changes similar to those described by Arnett.[4]

In borderline situations, an early phase of treatment can test, through therapeutic diagnosis, the skeletal modifiability, as well as test for the presence of functional shifts. In other cases surgery is clearly needed. However, the orthodontist may still resolve the maxillary transverse deficiency and the anterior alignment during Phase I, while anticipating the second phase of braces at ages 16 to 20, and surgery when facial growth is complete. The orthodontist plays a major role in guiding these cases to completion. Too long a period in Phase I treatment may *over compensate* the teeth and interfere with corrective surgical therapy later.

This is also true of moderate to severe mandibular deficiency, Type III (downward and backward growth) patterns. Early introduction of the concept of combined therapy (orthodontics and surgery) *conditions* parents to the necessity of surgical correction and begins the psychologic preparation of the patient. (Care must be taken that the terminology used does not frighten nor stigmatize the young patients. This author recommends having preliminary surgical consultations *with the parents only* for patients under the age of 16).

2. *Growth factors and the timing of the referral.* Post-treatment growth is a factor that is known by orthodontists to be a destabilizing factor of orthodontic treatment results. In a study by this author, 19 out of 50 (38%) adult patients who required retreatment, did so because of growth changes that moderately or severely altered the original orthodontic correction.

If the differential growth is minimal, the occlusal change can be handled by 4 to 8 months of orthodontic retreatment. On the other hand, if growth undermines an orthodontic correction, the retreatment via surgery is not easily accepted by the patient.

To avoid growth induced complications, the following guidelines should be considered:

a. For moderate and severe Class III mandibular excess patients, surgery should be delayed until standardized cephalograms demonstrate completion of mandibular growth. In males, this could be as late as 22 to 24 years of age.

b. For asymmetry patients with unilateral hypertrophy, surgery should be delayed until bone scans demonstrate cessation of growth activity of the hypertrophic condyle.

c. For mandibular deficiency patients, it has been reported that surgery can be successfully done before growth is complete.[60,71] In males there is some risk of the mandible growing past the Class I correction, but the risk is apparently small as the normal rebound tendency of the mandibular advancement may be offset by a late differential growth spurt of the mandible. In Snow's study, the postsurgical mandibular growth appeared to be mainly in the vertical plane.[60]

d. For patients with excessive vertical growth (Class I, II), the maxillary LeFort procedure can be safely done before growth is complete. The effect of this procedure on the future growth of the nasal cartilage is not fully understood. There is, however, risk that premature double jaw surgery for mandibular deficiency type III patients will be vitiated if the mandible persists in a downward and backward growth mode and reopens the bite.[45]

e. For the maxillary transverse deficiency patients, orthopedic expansion is effective for females up to 14 years of age and for males up to 18 years of age. Successful orthopedic expansions have been reported in both groups at older ages, especially with surgical assistance. Predictability of nonsurgical orthopedic success decreases as the age of the patient increases.

f. Psychosocial needs may supercede growth factors when the patient has a severe growth imbalance. Self-esteem considerations during adolescence require concern, and two-stage sequential surgery may be desirable for those patients whose psychic and social development are affected by their jaw growth imbalance (Fig. 15-31).

g. Timing of the referral to the maxillofacial surgeon and the initial patient education process are important responsibilities of the orthodontist. The orthodontist should try to determine the patient's level of awareness regarding the growth imbalance. If a patient is totally unaware that his or her condition may require surgical adjuncts, the education process may take longer and require more than one consultation with the orthodontist to create sufficient understanding to pursue the consultation with the surgeon.

This author has used consultation aids, such as the template method of cephalometric analysis, before and after photographs of other cases (Fig. 15-32), the Troyer patient education series, and the Ortho Ed information tapes to help patients understand the concepts relevant to their problems.

3. *TMJ Stability.* The orthodontic literature emphasizes the importance of planning treatment based on a reproducible condyle-fossa relationship.[69]

This concept is all the more true when diagnosing and planning orthognathic patients (Fig. 15-33). The orthodontist's skill at diagnosing and documenting functional shift problems in the occlusion is quite important. Without such skill, a mandibular functional shift may make a case look better than it is, causing a treatment plan to fail because of *under-treatment;* or, at the other extreme, a case (e.g., psuedo Class III) that looks worse than it is due to functional forward shift, causing treatment plan failure by *over-treatment:* insisting on surgery when the case can be managed with conventional treatment only.

The time to diagnose mandibular shifts is *before initiating* treatment; it is accomplished through the use of superior repositioning deprogramming splints, leaf gauge

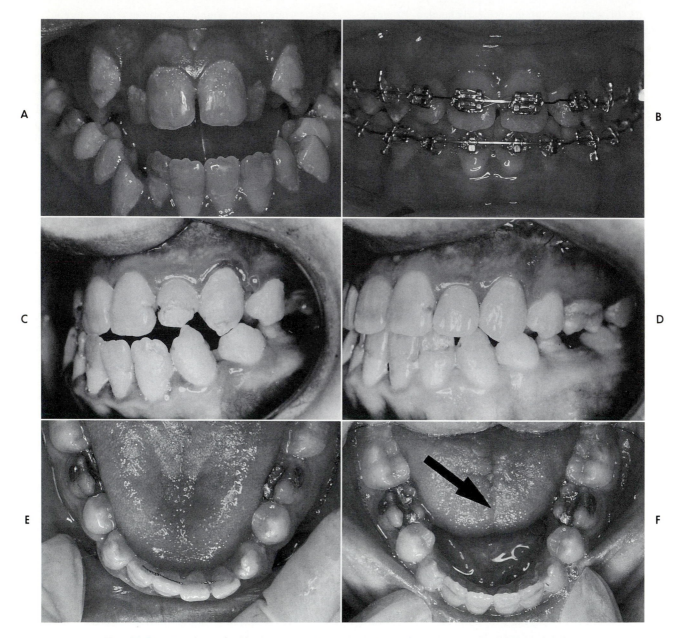

Fig. 15-31 Because of self-esteem and chewing problems, this patient requested surgery before growth was complete, being aware of the possibility of Phase II surgery after growth. **A,** (Age 15 years, 4 months)—pretreatment frontal occlusion photograph showing severe openbite. **B,** (Age 16 years, 7 months)—after 4 bicuspid extractions, orthodontic preparation, maxillary LeFort impaction and mandibular set-back. **C,** (Age 19 years, 1 month)—left occlusion photograph 30 months after jaw surgery, showing Class III and anterior open bite relapse. The relapse was predicted, and Phase II surgery was planned. **D,** (Age 23 years, 0 months)—left occlusion photograph after Phase II orthodontics and *partial glossectomy*. No osteotomies were performed in Phase II. **E,** (Age 19 years, 1 month)—lower occlusal photograph. Note large tongue and displaced left incisors. **F,** Lower occlusal view after partial glossectomy *(arrow)*.

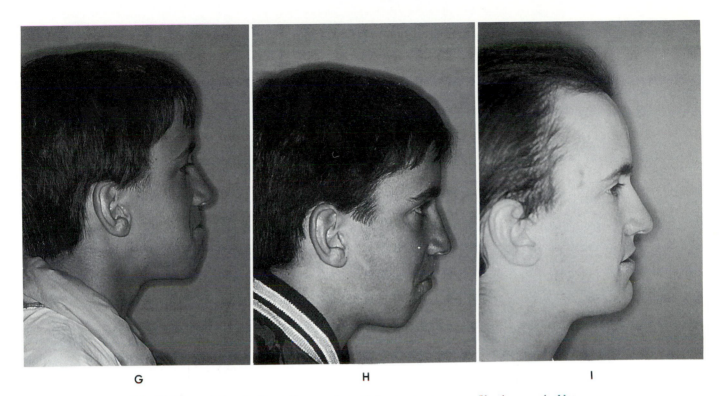

G   H   I

Fig. 15-31, cont'd   **G,** (Age 15 years, 4 months)—pre-treatment profile photograph. Note mandibular excess III (clockwise rotating). **H,** (Age 16 years, 7 months)—post-surgical profile photograph showing significant change in mandibular excess appearance. **I,** (Age 23 years, 0 months)—post-treatment profile appearance showing good facial balance.

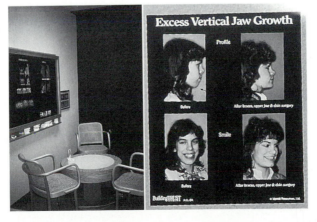

Fig. 15-32   **A,** Consultation room with photograph display board to illustrate *before* and *after* possibilities to prospective surgical patients. **B,** Consultation photograph of treated vertical excess problem to illustrate *before* and *after* possibilities to prospective surgical patients.

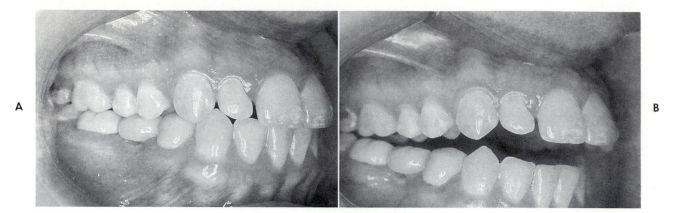

Fig. 15-33 **A,** Pretreatment right posterior occlusion of patient with myofacial pain and joint noises. Two surgeons who examined her said that she did not need jaw surgery. **B,** Right posterior occlusion of the same patient 1 month after anterior repositioning splint therapy. Significant muscle deprogramming occurred with splint therapy. Full records taken at this time indicted that maxillary LeFort and mandibular surgery were needed.

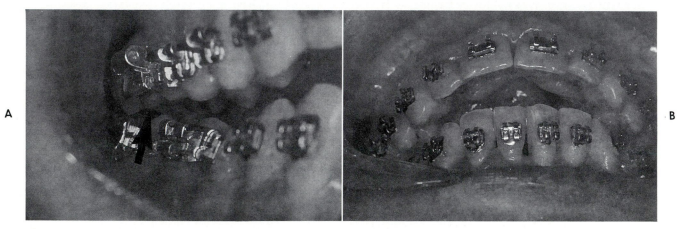

Fig. 15-34 *Postsurgical* (mandibular set-back from a vertical subcondylar osteotomy) *photographs* showing posterior prematurity *(arrow)* and poor postsurgical occlusal result. Inadequate presurgical leveling and inadequate fixation caused this problem. The patient had several excessively mobile periodontally involved teeth that were used for *interdental fixation*. There was no skeletal fixation to completely stabilize the mandibular position during healing.

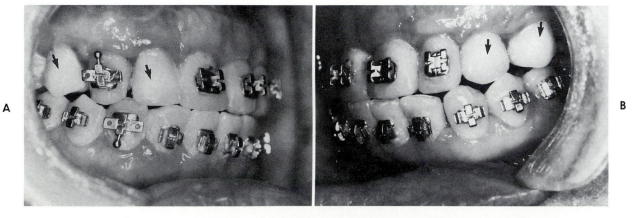

Fig. 15-35 **A and B,** Postsurgical and immediate postfixation right and left posterior occlusion, showing the loss of four brackets from plastic temporary crowns *(arrows)*. Also, note the surgical over correction of a severe skeletal mandibular deficiency problem.

condyle seating, or careful mandible manipulation. If such discrepancies are not detected before appliance placement but show up during treatment, the clinician has an obligation to document and inform the patient of the diagnostic data arising during treatment and to advise the patient of any recommended change in the plan. It is then the patient's decision to pursue the surgical plan or to reject it.

Undetected functional shifts in maxillary vertical excess and mandibular deficiency cases can lead to a treatment plan that calls for LeFort impaction only. In the operating room, when the patient is under general anesthetic, if the surgeon discovers a hidden mandibular deficiency, at that point he or she has to decide to perform a surgery containing a built-in compromise and relapse potential or to do double jaw surgery for which there is no treatment plan, no patient consent, and no insurance pre-approval. Such a situation has the potential to create medico-legal problems.

Other TMJ stability concerns will be addressed in the next section of this chapter: complications.

4. *Dental unit stability.* One aspect of dental instability is due to unfavorable crown-to-root ratio, secondary to bone loss from periodontal disease, or due to short roots—genetic or acquired. The orthodontist should be able to detect tooth mobility problems and advise the surgeon of the need for fixation that is skeletal rather than inter-dental (Fig. 15-34). Another form of dental instability features temporary crowns cemented as part of a perio-restorative program. Not only do brackets break from these crowns easily, but also the crowns dislodge from the teeth easily (Fig. 15-35).

Therefore, inter-dental fixation in a patient with temporary crowns is not advisable.

5. *Presurgical orthodontic preparation.* Arch leveling should be inclusive of second molars. In mandibular excess cases the upper second molar is frequently supraerupted (Fig. 15-36), and in mandibular deficiency cases the lower second molar may be supraerupted. These distal teeth, if not leveled vertically, can interfere with proper occlusal seating at the time of surgery, creating condylar distraction and instability.

If the surgical treatment plan calls for segmental intrusion, the arch may require segmental leveling to satisfy the stability and esthetic requirements of the case. Continuous archwires may cause instability through unwanted incisor extrusion (in an open bite case), causing less skeletal correction of the open bite and relapse that would be dental in origin.

There are nine key responsibilities of the surgeon to maximize the stability of the orthognathic outcome. These were presented earlier in this section of the chapter and require periodic review with the surgeon as treatments are planned.

Proffit et al.[50] and Quejada et al.[54] have presented excellent papers regarding the stability of the LeFort superior repositioning procedures. The inferior repositioning procedure is less stable, and a good review of this procedure is provided by Wessberg and Epker.[66]

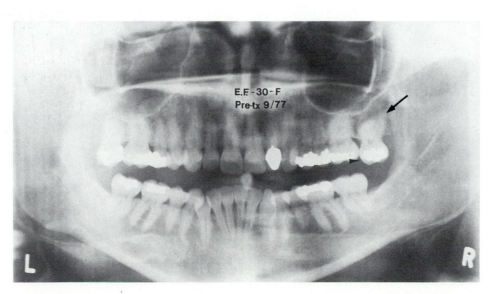

Fig. 15-36 Pretreatment panorex of several mandibular excess problems (patient previously shown in Fig. 15-17). Note the supraerupted right second molar *(arrow)*.

The sagittal split advancement of the mandible has proven to be an excellent procedure, and in most cases, it, too, is quite stable. Will[68] has reviewed the factors that affect mandibular stability.

COMPLICATIONS

The risks that orthodontic patients are exposed to during routine orthodontic therapy are minimal by comparison with the complications that may occur during orthognathic procedures. Not only must practicing orthodontists understand all of the differential diagnostic considerations of the patient who has skeletal imbalances, but they should also have a high level of awareness of the *risk factors* associated with the orthognathic procedures recommended. As the range of corrective surgeries has increased, so have the reported negative sequelae.

In the previous section of this chapter, the undesirable risk factors of instability were discussed and referenced. This section will focus on a variety of other complications that have been associated with orthognathic procedures.

The complications related to orthognathics can be divided into the following categories:

Physical well-being
Stomatognathic function
Emotional well-being
Oral health sequela

1. *Physical well-being*
   - Excessive blood loss[13,14,32]
   - Neurologic injury—anesthesia, paresthesia
     a. Hypoesthesia—decreased sensation[64]
     b. Hyperpathia—increased sensation
     c. Dysesthesia—altered sensation that is painful
   - Allergic reaction to anesthetic, antibiotic, or anti-inflammatory drugs[20]
   - Postoperative infections
     a. Surgical site
     b. Skeletal fixation wires
     c. Rigid fixation plates

Current modalities for infection prevention techniques are discussed by Hegtvedt.[20] In addition, orthodontists can aid the surgeon in reducing potential iatrogenic incidence of nidi of infection by using soldered or slide-on surgical hooks, well-secured brackets, and stainless ligatures (*not alastics* because their force decays rapidly, and they are not radiopaque; if alastic ligatures inadvertently fall into the surgical site, they are difficult to locate and remove). Fig. 15-37 shows the postsurgical migration of a molar bracket that broke off the left first molar during surgery. Fortunately, there was no subsequent infection.

- Bone fractures (Fig. 15-38):
  Reports exist in the literature of unfavorable surgical splits of the mandible, including buccal plate fracture associated with impacted third molar teeth that were extracted at the time of the mandibular osteotomy. When sagittal split procedures are planned for mandibular deficiency or mandibular excess, the third molars should be removed 6 to 12 months before the osteotomy. Where unfavorable splits occur, the stability of the procedure is jeopardized and an increased incidence of neuropathies may be noted. It would seem that the incidence of unfavorable splits is technique and operator

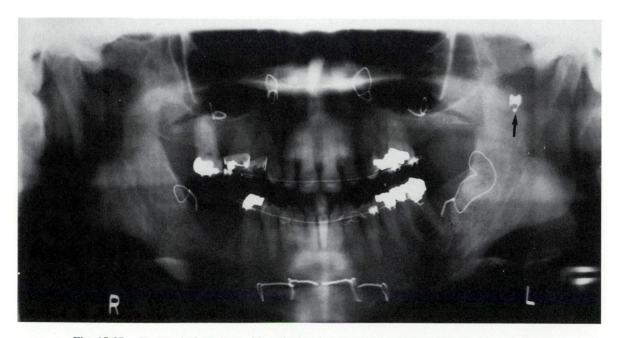

Fig. 15-37 Postsurgical panorex with molar bracket *(arrow)* that broke off during surgery. It has migrated to the coronoid notch.

dependent, and extra care to avoid this undesirable side effect is most important.

• Delayed healing and nonhealing:
This group of complications occurs most often when the surgical and postsurgical plans do not go smoothly. Intra-operative complications, such as those previously discussed, and including unfavorable splits in the sagittal split or unfavorable downfracture in the LeFort osteotomy, can result in incomplete bone healing.[74] Also, an inaccurate preoperative medical assessment (see Table 15-6) or postoperative surgical traumatic occlusion can result in poor bone healing and fibrous unions.

• Retrieval of rigid fixation devices:
A serious disadvantage of mini-plates and screws used in rigid fixation is the need for their removal because of *potential risk of stress-protection-induced osteopenia*.[7,8] Also there is concern regarding inflammatory reactions from corrosion of these metal devices.[17,70]

Current research efforts are being undertaken to as-

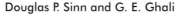

Douglas P. Sinn and G. E. Ghali

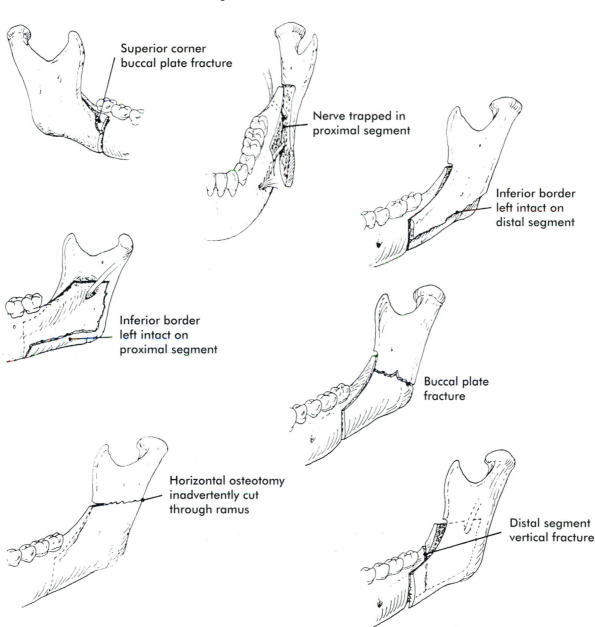

Fig. 15-38 Common types of unfavorable splits. (From O'Ryan FS: *Complications of orthognathic surgery: mandibular surgery.* In *Selected readings in oral and maxillofacial surgery,* vol 1, no 1, 1989.)

sess the effectiveness of biodegradable (resorbable) plates and screws.[7,8,34]

Orthopedic repair materials of resorbable poly (L-Lactide) (PLLA), polyglycolide (PGA), and polydioxanon (PDA) are being strength tested as a maxillofacial surgery fixation device. Future improvement in the rate of resorption and reliability of these materials may provide a modality for fixation that is biologically absorbed with time.

• Secondary surgery:

A percentage of orthognathic patients has to return to the operating room for secondary surgery because of dissatisfaction with the surgical outcome—some return before release from the hospital following their first surgery; others return months or years after their initial surgical procedure (Fig. 15-39). The most common reasons include:

a. Early relapse—condyle distraction[73]
b. Posthealing relapse
c. Unfavorable split
d. Patient dissatisfaction with the esthetic result. (In the early years of the LeFort procedure, many patients had their maxilla impacted beyond an esthetic smile line.)

Overimpaction of the maxilla may occur for several reasons:

1. Removal of an excessive amount of bone from the lateral walls
2. Thin, concave maxillary bone that may collapse on loading
3. The use of overly tight suspension wires that tend to pull the maxilla superiorly
4. Excessive masticatory function that overides the stability of the bony interfaces
5. Lack of bony contact
6. Poor treatment planning

Correction of overimpaction cannot be achieved short of surgically repositioning the maxilla inferiorly and returning the dento-alveolar portion to its original position. This would necessitate interpositional bone grafting, rigid internal fixation and also might entail concomitant mandibular surgery.[67]

• Sinus complications:

Several authors studying postsurgical patients have found that a higher percentage than expected report sinus problems after LeFort procedures.[12,30] Other authors indicate that postsurgical sinus disease is no greater than that seen in the general population.[47] Post-

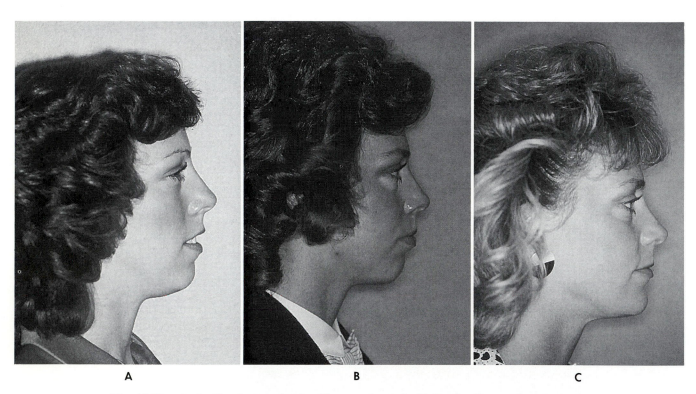

| A | B | C |

Fig. 15-39 A, Profile photograph of a 21-year-, 1-month-old female who sought orthodontic treatment to correct three impacted canines and a *gummy smile.* **B,** Profile photograph (age 23 years, 8 months) 6 months after full braces and jaw surgery. Vertical maxillary excess, vertical chin excess were not changed in accordance with the presurgical plan and patient returned 5 years after the first treatment to have more surgical correction of the vertical excess, vertical chin excess, and lip incompetence. **C,** Profile photograph (29 years, 1 month) following an additional 4.5 mm of maxillary impaction in addition to a vertical reduction, advancement genioplasty.

surgically, the maxillary sinus function may have been altered to interfere with proper drainage, causing sinus-type headaches, or sinuses may congest more frequently, causing interference with nasal breathing. Although this complication may seem relatively minor, it can have an adverse effect on the quality of life activities of the patients *having to deal with chronic sinus flare-ups* on a day-to-day basis.

2. *Stomatognathic function*
   - Decreased efficiency and discomfort during chewing: Two common causes of postsurgical occlusal inefficiency are:
     a. Posterior open bites caused by overseated condyles during mandibular surgery
     b. Excessive superior positioning of the posterior maxilla, especially when there are inadequate posterior vetical stops in the area of the osteotomy
   - TMJ dysfunction, discomfort, and pain:
   Orthognathic surgery in some cases is justified because it has the potential to reduce TMD symptoms. Karabouta and Martis[25] reported that TMD symptoms declined from 40% to 11% of the sample. However, 4% of previously asymptomatic patients developed TMD symptoms postoperatively. In another study Kerstens et al.[26] found a 66% reduction in TMD symptoms; they also found 11.5% of preoperative asymptomatic patients experienced symptoms postoperatively. Many of these patients who developed symptoms postoperatively may have had latent TMD problems that were *stirred up* by the altered joint loading that followed jaw surgery. Management requires a team effort and appropriate care, depending on the nature of the problem.
   - Limitation in range of motion:
   A program of physical therapy is prescribed for most orthognathic patients shortly after the release of fixation. If there is mandibular hypomobility following jaw surgery, it should be noted that it could have an intra-capsular or an extra-capsular cause.

Intra-capsular problems are characterized by a sharp pain localized in the temporomandibular joints. Extra-capsular problems are characterized by less intense dull pain that is generalized and diffused and may or may not be aggravated by mandibular movements; often the pain is alleviated by biting.[15]

A prospective study of 55 orthognathic patients by Aragon et al.[3] found that the maximal incisal opening (MIO) decreased in most of these patients postsurgically. The percent of MIO decrease was dependent on the surgery performed.

Procedure	Percent MIO Reduction
Sagittal split osteotomy (SSO)	29% (mean)
Vertical subcondylar osteotomy (VSO)	10% (mean)
LeFort I (LFI)	2% (mean)
LeFort I and SSO (LFI/SSO)	28% (mean)
LeFort I and VSO (LFI/VSO)	9% (mean)

3. *Emotional well-being*
   Since orthognathic procedures can significantly alter facial appearance, it is not surprising that there are numerous articles[6,24,28-30] investigating the postsurgical emotional response of the patients. It should be noted here that, in the author's experience, negative emotional responses seldom occur with single jaw mandibular advancement or mandibular set-back procedures, since these procedures mainly affect the patient's profile, and, therefore, the changes are not readily observed by the patient. Changes that occur with single jaw LeFort or LeFort with mandibular advancement or mandibular set-back cause the frontal facial appearance alterations immediately and the patient has to adapt to the new look.
   - Self-esteem changes caused by unexpected facial changes:
   In Jacobson's study[24] the majority of patients (80%) said that orthodontic-orthognathic treatment positively influenced their lives, 4% said that treatment had a negative influence on social activities. Kiyak et al.[29] found in their 55-patient study, that at the 9-month postoperative interval there was a significant decline in the patients' self-esteem from an early postsurgical period. The orthodontist and staff who follow these patients postsurgically need to be aware of the potential for emotional *highs* and *lows* during the postsurgical period. Having a psychologist available, who is aware of the needs of orthognathic patients and who is able to intercept significant patient emotional problems is imperative.
   - Unprepared for changes in intra-personal relationships:
   As the surgical technology has improved to allow more stable, functional results, so, too, has the capacity to alter a person's appearance and his or her identity. The preponderance of orthognathic patients are females between 20 and 40 years. Many of these surgical candidates are married, with husbands and young children. When this person returns home from the hospital after a LeFort osteotomy and genioplasty, she is swollen, black-blue (bruised), and may be in fixation with limited speech and eating capacities.

   If the husband and children, as well as other immediate family members in the support group, are not fully prepared for her to return looking *so differently,* there will be significant stress and disruption of normal family functions. As patient #13 of Kiyak's 1982 study stated, "I would not recommend this surgery to anyone without counseling."

   Postsurgical patients have many good ideas regarding ways to enhance the recovery process. Patient #05 of Kiyak's 1982 paper stated:

Much more time is needed to prepare the patient with facts and information. I was unprepared for the bleeding and earaches, leaving the hospital so soon—less than 24 hours after surgery. I lost more weight than expected and really suffered psychologically and felt little support dur-

ing the fixation period. Maybe the patients could be invited to form a mutual support group.

- *Depression:*
Postsurgical depression is a phenomenon that receives little attention in the orthognathic literature and has only recently been discussed as a legitimate complication of jaw surgery.[62] Generally, dentists are not properly trained to medically handle depression, even

Adapted from Holmes TH, Rahe RH: Social readjustment rating scale; *J Psychosom Res* 11:213, 1967.

TABLE 15-9
Social Readjustment Rating Scale

Life event	Mean value
Death of spouse	100
Divorce	73
Marital separation from mate	65
Detention in jail or other institution	63
Death of close family member	63
Major personal injury or illness	53
Marriage	50
Being fired at work	47
Marital reconciliation with mate	45
Retirement from work	45
Major change in health or behavior of family member	44
Pregnancy	40
Sexual difficulties	39
Gaining new family member: through birth; adoption; oldster moving in	39
Major business readjustment: merger; reorganization; bankruptcy	39
Major change in financial state: *worse off* or *better off* than usual	38
Death of a close friend	37
Changing to different line of work	36
Major change in number of arguments with spouse: either more or less than usual regarding childrearing; personal habits	35
Taking on mortgage greater than $70,000: purchasing home; business	31
Foreclosure on mortgage or loan	30
Major change in responsibilities at work: promotion; demotion; lateral transfer	29
Son or daughter leaving home: marriage; attending college	29
In-law troubles	29
Outstanding personal achievement	28

Familiarity with the social readjustment rating scale of Holmes and Rahe (above) and good communication with the patient will aid the patient during stressful periods. This scale can be used by adding the stress points that occur during certain life experiences. For example, if 200 stress points accrue within a 3 to 6 month period, the odds are good (3 to 1) that this person will be overtaken by illness. A score of 300 or more means that there is approximately an 80% chance of responding to the stress physically and even suffering a nervous breakdown.

if it is likely to be a transitory state of mind for the orthognathic patient. On the other hand, as the orthodontic member of the health care team, it is our duty to recognize the symptoms of depression, discuss it with the patient and family, refer, and interact with the psychologist to aid in the patient's recovery.

In addition, the orthodontist should try to be aware of other stressful events in the patient's life that may add to his or her anxiety level during the 2 to 3 years that we follow these patients. The chart of Holmes and Rahe[22] in Table 15-9 that assigns a numerical score to events that may occur in a lifetime will aid the orthodontist and his or her staff to assess stress factors that may be affecting orthognathic and TMJ patients.

Although the current literature does discuss the postsurgical sequelae of depression,[23,24,26-30] the author's personal experience is that patients with rigid fixation show rapid psychological rebound and fewer signs of depression than the patients of 5 to 10 years ago who were in intermaxillary fixation for 6 to 10 weeks.

4. *Oral Health Sequelae*
- Bone loss:
  a. Periodontal disease exacerbation
     Although this complication is not reported frequently, the exacerbation of existing periodontitis is a potentially serious problem. Doyle[12] reported that 14% of his consecutively evaluated orthognathic patients have bone loss following orthodontic-orthognathic procedures. Patients with mild, moderate, or advanced periodontal disease require strict supervision and management by a specialist before the orthognathic procedure. Patients with moderate or advanced periodontal disease are at a high risk for further periodontal breakdown after orthognathic surgery because of ensuing dietary changes, oral hygiene interferences (depending on mode of fixation), and transitory occlusal trauma.
  b. Gingival deficiency with recession:
     Doyle[12] also reported that of his sample of 50, only 4 required gingival grafts following jaw surgery; he did indicate that 10 other patients were being monitored for inadequately attached gingiva. It was not clear if the gingival problem existed before the osteotomy or if the osteotomy site caused the tissue deficiency—as can happen in the area of the lower incisors following genioplasty.
- Pulpal changes:
  The osteotomies that are done often approximate root apices—particularly LeFort I procedures and segmentals. Occasionally, following an osteotomy the affected tooth will start to change color, lose its vitality, and require a root canal. The likelihood of vitality loss is minimal, but it does occur. Careful preparation by the orthodontist and surgical planning by the surgeon should eliminate this annoying complication.

- Tooth Loss

Tooth loss is an infrequent sequela, but it does warrant a brief discussion. Tooth loss occurs as in Fig. 15-40 because of inadequate apical root space (4.0 mm is the desired amount of separation between apices). Proper preparation of the area to be segmented will reduce the probability of tooth loss sequelae.

Summary of Complications

Although this discussion of complications associated with orthognathic surgical procedures is far from complete, it should give the orthodontist an awareness of some of the more frequent postsurgical sequelae that he or she will have to manage with the oral surgeon for the overall well-being of the patients. It is recommended that orthodontists who are referring patients for orthognathic surgery, review the informed consent policy of the surgeon's office so that the orthodontist and staff can help patients understand any unclear aspects of this information.

Contemporary surgical practices in the United States will generally review potential negative sequelae with the patient before surgery.

Chapter Summary

This chapter began with a discussion of treatment goals and the technologic advances that have helped the orthodontic-surgical team enhance the lives of many of their patients with facial skeletal disharmonies. The end of the chapter intentionally concluded with a discussion of complications. The addition of new surgical technology has broadened the scope of the orthodontist's treatment capacity and at the same time has expanded his or her responsibilities.

In John Naisbitt's book *Megatrends*, there is an excellent thought that applies to the field of surgical-orthodontics:

Technology is always on the verge of liberating us from personal discipline. Only it never does and it never will.[44]

As the orthodontic specialty and the surgical specialty continue to study factors that reduce risk and enhance success, it is both the surgeon's and the orthodontist's responsibility to integrate these new findings into the care of their patients.

ACKNOWLEDGEMENT

The author wishes to extend his appreciation to the patients and surgeons whose efforts made this chapter possible. Special thanks to Elizabeth Barrett for her many hours of assistance. Her expertise greatly enhanced this work.

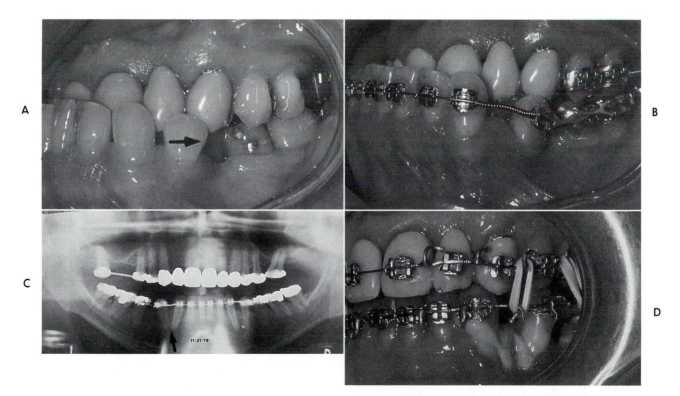

Fig. 15-40 **A,** Photograph of lateral posterior occlusion of adult male with severe CEJ problem. Segmental surgery was planned to intrude the lower incisors before mandibular set-back surgery. **B,** Left first premolar tipped distally to make room for osteotomy. **C,** Panorex shows inadequate space at the apical area for a safe segmental procedure. Surgery proceeded, however. **D,** Postsurgical infection at area of number 21 and number 22 required extraction of number 21 and necessitated bridgework, for which there was no plan.

REFERENCES

1. Ackerman JG, Proffit WR: Treatment response as an aid in diagnosis and treatment planning, *Am J Orthod* 57:5, 490-496, 1970.
2. Anderson JA: Deliberate hypotensive anesthesia for orthognathic surgery: controlled pharmacologic manipulation of cardiovascular physiology, *Int J Adult Orthod Orthognath Surg* 1:133, 1986.
3. Aragon SB, Van Sickels JE et al: The effects of orthognathic surgery on mandibular range of motion, *J Oral Maxillofac Surg* 43:938-943, 1985.
4. Arnett GW, Tamborello JA: Progressive Class II development: female idiopathic condyle resorption, *Oral Maxillofac Surg Clin North Am* 2:699-716, 1990.
5. Athanasiou AE, Melsen B, Ericksen J: Concerns, motivation, and experience of orthognathic surgery patients: a retrospective study of 152 patients, *Int J Adult Orthod Orthognath Surg* 4:47-55, 1989.
6. Auerbach SM, Meredith J et al: Psychological factors in adjustment to orthognathic surgery, *J Oral Maxillofac Surg* 42:435-440, 1984.
7. Bos RRM, Rozema FR, Boering G et al: Bone plates and screws of bioabsorbable poly (L-lactide): an animal pilot study, *J Oral Maxillofac Surg* 27:467-476, 1989.
8. Bos RRM, Rozema FR, Boering G et al: Bioresorbable osteosynthesis in maxillofacial surgery—present and future, *Oral Maxillofac Clin North Am* 2(4):745-750, 1990.
9. Burstone CJ, Randall JB et al: Cephalometrics for orthognathic surgery, *J Oral Surg* 36:269-277, 1978.
10. Case C: *Dental orthopedia and correction of cleft palate*, Chicago, 1921, CS Case.
11. Dahl EH, Zachrisson BU: Long-term experience with direct-bonded lingual retainers, *J Clin Orthod* 25(10):619-630, 1991.
12. Doyle MG: Stability and complications in 50 consecutively treated surgical-orthodontic patients: a retrospective longitudinal analysis from private practice, *Int J Adult Orthognath Surg* 1:23-36, 1986.
13. Epker BN: Vascular considerations in orthognathic surgery: I mandibular osteotomies, *Oral Surg Oral Med Oral Pathol* 57(4):467-472, 1984.
14. Epker BN: Vascular considerations in orthognathic surgery: II maxillary osteotomies, *Oral Surg Oral Med Oral Pathol* 57:473-478, 1984.
15. Epker BN, LaBlanc JP: Orthognathic surgery: management of postoperative complications, *Oral Maxillofac Surg Clin North Am* 2(4):109-133, 1990.
16. Epker BN, Wolford LM, Fish LC: Mandibular deficiency syndrome II: surgical considerations for mandibular advancement, *Oral Surg* 45:349-363, 1978.
17. French HG, Cook SD, Haddad RJ: Correlations of tissue reaction to corrosion in osteosynthetic devices, *J Biomed Mater Res* 18:817-828, 1984.
18. Gottlieb EL, Nelson AH, Vogel DS: 1990 JCO study of orthodontic diagnosis and treatment procedures, *J Clin Orthod* 25(3):145-156, 1991.
19. Grayson B, Cutting C, Bookstein FL et al: The three-dimensional cephalogram: theory technique and clinical application, *Am J Orthod Dentofac Orthop* 94:327-337, 1988.
20. Hegtvedt AK: *Intra-operative and post-operative patient care.* In West RA, editor: *Oral and maxillofacial clinics of North America*, Philadelphia, 1990, WB Saunders.
21. Hegtvedt AK, Collins ML, White RP: Minimizing the risk of transfusion in orthognathic surgery: use of pre-deposited blood, *Int J Adult Orthod Orthognath Surg* 2:185, 1987.
22. Holmes TH, Rahe RH: Social adjustment rating scale, *J Psychosom Res* 11:213, 1967.
23. Jacobson A: The proportionate template, *Am J Orthod* 75:156-172, 1979.
24. Jacobson A: Psychologic aspects of dentofacial esthetics and orthognathic surgery, *Angle Orthod* 54:18-35, 1984.
25. Karabouta I, Martis C: The TMJ dysfunction syndrome before and after sagittal split osteotomy of the ramus, *J Maxillofac Surg* 13:185-188, 1985.
26. Kerstens HC, Tuinzing DB, VanderKwast WA: Temporomandibular

joint symptoms in orthognathic surgery, *J Craniomaxillofac Surg* 17:215, 1989.
27. Kiyak HA, Hohl T, Sherrick P et al: Sex differences in motives for and outcomes of orthognathic surgery, *J Oral Surg* 39:757-764, 1981.
28. Kiyak HA, McNeill RW, West RA: Predicting psychologic responses to orthognathic surgery, *J Oral Maxillofac Surg* 40:150-155, 1982.
29. Kiyak HA, McNeill RW, West RA: The emotional impact of orthognathic surgery and conventional orthodontics, *Am J Orthod* 88:224-234, 1985.
30. Kiyak HA, West RA, Hohl T et al: The psychologic impact of orthognathic surgery: a 9 month follow-up, *Am J Orthod* 81:404-412, 1982.
31. Lanigan DT: Hemorrhage associated with orthognathic surgery, *Oral Maxillofac Surg Clin North Am* 2:4, 887-899, 1990.
32. Lanigan DT, Hey JH, West RA: Major vascular complications of orthognathic surgery: hemorrhage associated with LeFort osteotomies, *J Oral Maxillofac Surg* 48:561-573, 1990.
33. Lindquist JD: *The edgewise appliance.* In Graber TM, Swain BF, editors: *Orthodontics: current principles and techniques*, St Louis, 1985, Mosby.
34. Leenslag JW, Pennings AJ: Synthesis and morphology of high molecular weight poly (L-Lactide) VI: plates and screws for internal fixation, *Biomaterials* 8:70-73, 1987.
35. Machen DE: Legal aspects of orthodontic practice, *Am J Orthod Dentofac Orthoped*, 1991.
36. McDonald WR: Stability of mandibular lengthening: a comparison of moderate and large advancements, *Oral Maxillofac Surg Clin North Am* 2(4):729-735, 1990.
37. McNamara JA: An orthopedic approach to the treatment of Class III malocclusion in young patients, *JCO* 21(9):598-608, 1986.
38. Melsen B, Bjerregaard J, Bundgaard M: The effect of treatment with functional appliance on a pathologic growth pattern of the condyle, *Am J Orthod* 90:503-512, 1986.
39. Moorrees CFA, Lebrets L: The mesh diagram in cephalometrics, *Angle Orthod* 32:214-231, 1962.
40. Musich DR: Assessment and description of the treatment needs of adult patients evaluated for orthodontic therapy: characteristics of the dual provider group, *Int J Adult Orthod Orthognath Surg* 1(2):101-117, 1986.
41. Musich DR: Assessment and description of the treatment needs of adult patients evaluated for orthodontic therapy: characteristics of the solo provider group, *Int J Adult Orthod Orthognath Surg* 1(1):55-67, 1986.
42. Musich DR: "Evaluation of the Broadbent/Bolton templates as a treatment planning tool for patients with skeletal jaw disharmonies." Unpublished paper presented to Eastern Component, Boston, 1988, Angle Society.
43. Musich DR, Crossetti HC: Assessment and description of the treatment needs of adult patients evaluated for orthodontic therapy: characteristics of the multiple provider group, *Int J Adult Orthod Orthognath Surg* 1(4):251-274, 1986.
44. Naisbitt J: *Megatrends*, New York, 1982, Warner Books.
45. Nanda SK, Rowe TK: Circumpubertal growth spurt related to vertical dysplasia, *Angle Orthod* 59:113, 1989.
46. Nitzan DW, Dobvich MF: Temporomandibular joint fibrous ankylosis following orthognathic surgery: report of eight cases, *Int J Adult Orthod Orthognath Surg* 4:7, 1989.
47. Nustad RA, Fonseca RJ, Zeitler D: Evaluation of maxillary sinus disease in maxillary orthognathic patients, *Int J Adult Orthod Orthognath Surg* 1:195-202, 1986.
48. Obwegeser HL, Malek MS: Hemimandibular hypertrophy hemimandibular elongation, *J Maxillofac Surg* 14:183-208, 1986.
49. Proffit WR, Ackerman JL: *Diagnosis and treatment planning.* In Graber TM, Swain BF, editors: *Orthodontics: Current concepts and techniques*, St Louis, 1985, Mosby.
50. Proffit WR, Phillips C, Turvey TA: Stability following superior repositioning of maxilla by LeFort I osteotomy, *Am J Orthod Dentofac Orthop* 92:151, 1987.

51. Proffit WR, Vig KWL, Turvey TA: Fractures of the mandibular condyle: frequently an unsuspected cause of facial asymmetry, *Am J Orthod* 78:1-24, 1980.

52. Proffit WR, White RP: Who needs surgical orthodontic treatment? *Int J Adult Orthod Orthognath Surg* 5(2):81-89, 1990.

53. Proffit WR, White RP: *Surgical orthodontic treatment,* St Louis, 1990, Mosby.

54. Quejada JG, Bell WH, Kawamura H et al: Skeletal stability after inferior maxillary repositioning, *Int J Adult Orthod Orthognath Surg* 2:67, 1987.

55. Ricketts RM: JCO roundtable: diagnosis and treatment planning, 26(9):586, 1992.

56. Roth R: JCO roundtable: diagnosis and treatment planning, *J Clin Orthod* 26(9):585-586, 1992.

57. Rune B, Sarnes KV et al: Roentgen stereometry in the study of craniofacial anomalies—the state of the art in Sweden, *Br J Orthod* 13:151-157, 1986.

58. Sarver DM, Johnson KW: Video imaging: techniques for superimposition of cephalometric radiography and profile images, *Int J Adult Orthod Orthognath Surg* 5(4):241-248, 1990.

59. Shaberg SJ, Stuller CB, Edwards SM: Effects of methyprednisolone on swelling after orthognathic surgery, *J Oral Maxillofac Surg* 42:797, 1984.

60. Snow MD, Turvey TT et al: Surgical mandibular advancement in adolescents: post-surgical growth related to stability, *Int J Adult Orthod Orthognath Surg* 6:3, 143-150, 1991.

61. Steiner CC: Cephalometrics for you and me, *Am J Orthod* 39:729, 1953.

62. Stewart TD, Sexton J: Depression: a possible complication of orthognathic surgery, *J Oral Maxillofac Surg* 44:94, 1986.

63. Storum KA, Bell WH: The effect of physical rehabilitation on mandibular function after ramus osteotomies, *J Oral Maxillofac Surg* 44:94, 1986.

64. Walter WM, Gregg JM: Analysis of post-surgical neurologic alterations in the trigeminal nerve, *J Oral Surg* 37:410, 1979.

65. Weed LL: *Medical records, medical education, and patient care: the problem oriented record as a basic tool,* Cleveland, 1969, Case Western Reserve Presentation.

66. Wessberg GA, Epker BN: Surgical inferior repositioning of the maxilla: treatment considerations and comprehensive management, *Oral Surg* 52:349, 1981.

67. West RA: Vertical maxillary dysplasia: diagnosis, treatment planning, and treatment response—a reappraisal, *Oral Maxillofac Surg Clin North Am* 2(4):775-794, 1990.

68. Will LA, West RS: Factors affecting stability of the sagittal split osteotomy for mandibular advancement, *J Oral Maxillofac Surg* 47:813, 1989.

69. Williamson EH: *Orthodontic implications in diagnosis, prevention, and treatment of TMJ dysfunction.* In Graber TM, Swain BF, editors: *Orthodontics: current principles and techniques,* St Louis, 1985, Mosby.

70. Winter GD: Tissue reactions to metallic wear and corrosion products in human patients, *J Biomed Mater Res* 8:11-26, 1974.

71. Wolford LM, Schendel SA, Epker BN: Surgical orthodontic correction of mandibular deficiency in growing children (long-term result), *J Maxillofac Surg* 7:61-72, 1979.

72. Wolford LM, Walker G, Schendel S et al: Mandibular deficiency syndrome, Part I, clinical delineation and therapeutic significance, *Oral Surg Oral Med Oral Pathol* 45(3):329-348, 1978.

73. Worms FW, Speidel TM et al: Post-treatment stability and esthetics of orthognathic surgery, *Angle Orthod* 50(4):251-273, 1980.

74. Van Sickels JE, Tucker MR: Management of delayed union and nonunion of maxillary osteotomies, *J Oral Maxillofac Surg* 48:1039-1044, 1990.

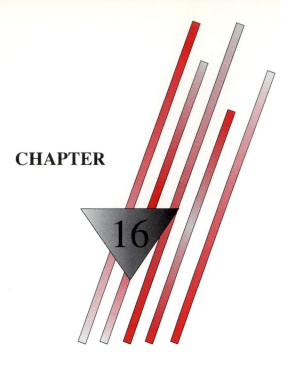

Retention and Relapse

DONALD R. JOONDEPH
RICHARD A. RIEDEL

A working definition of retention in relation to orthodontics might be stated as follows: *the holding of teeth in ideal esthetic and functional positions*.

The requirements for retention are often decided at the time of diagnosis and treatment planning. The correct diagnosis and logical treatment plan and its timing must be directed toward ideal esthetics, ideal function, and the permanent maintenance of these ideals. A satisfactory balance of utility, beauty, and stability often simplifies (and may even avoid) retention by mechanical appliances. On the other hand, incorrect diagnosis or treatment complicates the requirements for retention. Gross expansion of the dental arches, severe changes in arch form, incomplete correction of anteroposterior malrelationships, and uncorrected rotations may require retentive measures, but there is little point in attempting to classify them.

Orthodontists have long been aware of the fact that teeth that have been moved in or through bone by mechanical appliances have a tendency to return to their former positions. It is the purpose of retention to counteract this tendency.

The type of retentive measures and the duration of their use *allegedly* are determined by how many teeth have been moved and how far,[27] the occlusion and age of the patient,[28] the cause of a particular malocclusion, the rapidity of correction,[6] the length of cusps and health of tissues involved, relationships of the inclined planes,[33,34] size of the arches or arch harmony, muscular pressure, approximal contact, cell metabolism, and atmospheric pressure.[128]

Some authors have suggested that rotations be corrected by overrotation in the opposite direction,[103] that elastics be worn continuously,[26] that retention depend on a fixed type of appliance, that retention depend upon modification of structure and function of tissues,[75] that slight movement is more difficult to retain than extensive movement,[48] that oc-

cipital retention is most desirable for certain cases,[93] that we should correlate treatment with development, that function is the most important factor in retention, that appliances should be removable[30] and not depend on teeth for retention,[96] that overcorrection of all malpositions should be attempted, that retention is dependent on bone change—which is in turn related to endocrine dysfunction—that functional adaptation of occlusion occurs with growth, that retention is a problem of the apical base or apical base limitation,[81] that mandibular incisors should be maintained upright over basal bone,[47,135] that there may be discrepancies in tooth sizes that cause problems in retention,[21] that early treatment is more desirable than treatment at a later age,[85] that intercanine and intermolar widths should be maintained as in the original malocclusion,[130] that it is desirable to attempt functional treatment (i.e., to achieve muscle balance), that it is desirable to use mild forces, and that there are limitations to moving teeth imposed on the orthodontist by the arch itself.[138]

HISTORY OF RETENTION

For many years clinicians did not agree about the need for retention. Hellman[53] said in summary, "We are in almost complete ignorance of the specific factors causing relapses and failures." Different philosophies or schools of thought have developed, and our present-day concepts generally combine several of these theories.

The occlusion school. Kingsley[64] stated, "The occlusion of the teeth is the most potent factor in determining the stability in a new position." Many early writers* considered that proper occlusion was of prime importance in retention.

---

*References 9, 28, 33, 34, 48, 52, 61, 75, 84, 88, 94, 98, 101, 110, 120, 132.

The apical base school. In the middle 1920s a second school of thought formed around the writings of Axel Lundström,[81] who suggested that the apical base was one of the most important factors in the correction of malocclusion and maintenance of a correct occlusion. McCauley[86] suggested that intercanine width and intermolar width should be maintained as originally presented to minimize retention problems. Strang[129] further enforced and substantiated this theory. Nance[92] noted that "arch length may be permanently increased only to a limited extent."

The mandibular incisor school. Grieve[47] and Tweed[135,136] suggested that the mandibular incisors must be kept upright and over basal bone.

The musculature school. Rogers[109] introduced a consideration of the necessity of establishing proper functional muscle balance, which has been corroborated by others. Orthodontists have come to realize that retention is not a separate item apart from orthodontic treatment but that it is part of treatment itself and must be included in treatment planning. Hellman[53] aptly phrased it:

Retention is not a separate problem in orthodontia but is a continuation of what we are doing during treatment. It is not a definite stage of treatment requiring a new technique; therefore, there is no need for a separate machinery to carry it through. Retention is but a letting off of what we have been doing during treatment. The changes that we do make in our machinery are to ease up on the strains and stresses and to wean the tissues away from the effects of all our tinkering so that any change that is made should be a reduction in appliance. This can be done by changing either the type of the appliance or the amount of time wearing it. A complete result must be accomplished before retention is applied.

Stability has become a prime objective in orthodontic treatment, for without it either ideal function or ideal esthetics, or both, may be lost.[46] Retention depends on what is accomplished during treatment. Care must be exercised to establish a proper occlusion within the bounds of normal muscle balance and with careful regard to the apical base or bases available and the relationships of these bases to one another.

BASIC THEOREMS

Theorem I. *Teeth that have been moved tend to return to their former positions.*[24,46,89] There is little agreement as to the reason for this tendency; suggested influences include musculature,[143] apical base,[81,91,106] transseptal fibers,[104] and bone morphology. Whatever the reason, many clinicians agree that teeth should be held in their corrected positions for some time after changes are made in their positions. Only a few orthodontists have suggested that retention is routinely unnecessary.[38,88]

Theorem 2. *Elimination of the cause of malocclusion will prevent recurrence.*[80] Until more is known about the causative factors that are related to particular types of malocclusion, little can be done about their elimination. When obvious habits, such as thumb or finger sucking or lip biting are causes of malocclusion, little difficulty is presented in diagnosis. It is important, however, in regard to retention, that the causative factors for a given malocclusion be prevented from recurring. One of the most insidious habits that operate against satisfactory retention is tongue posture, which results in anterior and sometimes lateral open bites. The mere fact that the patient has been directed along a course of tongue therapy and has been able to meet all the exercise requirements of the therapist on command does not guarantee correction.[122,131]

In fact, several authors have suggested that open bite malocclusion may be secondary to mouth breathing resulting from nasopharynx obstruction. This could be due to anatomic blockage, allergic disease,[24] or adenoid hyperplasia[72]; or it could be habitual, which would necessitate a compensatory low anterior tongue posture to be able to breathe. Dentofacial changes associated with this functional alteration appear to become more severe with age[24] and are a challenge to diagnose accurately and to treat successfully and retain. This retention problem has been discussed by Lopez-Gavito et al.,[78] who conducted a long-term evaluation of patients with initial anterior open bites. They found that despite attempts to control posterior maxillary vertical changes during appliance therapy and retention, 35% of the patients who presented with an initial open bite had an open bite of 3 mm or more 10 years after retention.

Theorem 3. *Malocclusion should be overcorrected as a safety factor.* It is common practice on the part of many orthodontists to overcorrect Class II malocclusions into an edge-to-edge incisor relationship. One must be aware, however, that these overcorrections may be the result of overcoming muscular balance rather than absolute tooth movement. The unrestricted use of Class II elastics sometimes produces a mesial displacement of the mandible, which is almost impossible to detect until elastics have been discontinued long enough to allow normal mandibular posture. Quessenberry's study[102] (using full-time intermaxillary coil springs) suggests that the most retruded mandibular position can be determined and reduplicated after release of these mechanics. Class II forces tend to have the greatest effect on tooth position rather than jaw position.

The same phenomenon may be seen in the use of Class III elastic forces. The use of elastics must be likened to the use of traction forces in orthopedic surgery, in which muscular forces are overcome by constant pull. However, absolute overcorrection is possible and has been demonstrated in many instances. Overcorrection of deep overbite is an accepted procedure in many practices.

Certainly, satisfactory maintenance of overbite correction is dependent on establishment of satisfactory correction during treatment.

One of the most irritating types of relapse is the tendency for a previously rotated tooth to attempt to rotate toward its former position. Overrotation has not often been carried out, and there is *no evidence to indicate that it is successful in preventing return to the former position.* It is often possible to prevent anterior teeth from erupting in a rotated position by providing space for them to erupt unimpeded, either by orthodontic appliances or by the early extraction of deciduous teeth. The principle is that if a tooth has never been rotated it would certainly have less tendency to rotate at some later time.

Recently, hope for increased stability of corrected rotations after surgical intervention has been elaborated by Allen,[3] Boese,[20] Brain,[23] and Edwards.[37]

Theorem 4. *Proper occlusion is a potent factor in holding teeth in their corrected positions.*[44] From the standpoint of reducing the potential of irritations to the periodontium, an excellent functional occlusion is certainly to be desired. Orthodontists often blame overfunction or pounding of the mandibular canines by the maxillary canines for relapse in the mandibular anterior area.[99] The everyday evidence presented by the tremendous wear that many teeth undergo would indicate that they do not move in response to repeated grinding and tapping until bone has been so thoroughly destroyed that it does not prevent their migration or until fibrous tissue builds up to such a degree that it actually moves the teeth and function of these teeth is not possible. Certainly we have all observed instances of mandibular anterior irregularity or collapse, in which canines either have not yet erupted or are not actually in occlusion. Studies evaluating stability of the mandibular arch[78] show no difference in long-term response between patients with anterior tooth contact when compared to individuals with anterior open bite malocclusions devoid of canine contact in centric positions and functional excursions. It is evident that orthodontists often consider the denture from a static viewpoint (i.e., with the teeth in occlusion as seen on study casts). It is doubtful that proper intercuspation or interlocking is *the* most potent factor in retention.

Theorem 5. *Bone and adjacent tissues must be allowed time to reorganize around newly positioned teeth.* Some type of either fixed or rigid appliance or an appliance only inhibitory in nature, and not dependent on the teeth, should be used. Histologic evidence shows that bone and tissue around teeth that have been moved are altered and considerable time elapses before complete reorganization occurs. Some authors have said that retainers should be fixed, such as the *G wire,*[27] the band and spur type of attachment,[25] and bands soldered together. Other authors believe that retainers should be only inhibitory in nature and have no positive fixation to allow for the natural functioning of teeth; it has been suggested that the mandibular lingual arch admirably suits this description.[105,142] Oppenheim[96] argued that appliances should be only inhibitory and that repair of tissues around the teeth occurs much more rapidly if no fixed retaining appliance is used.

All these suggestions are based on the presumption that mature bone will assure greater stability for the teeth. Present-day orthodontic concepts, however, regard bone as being a plastic substance and consider tooth position to result from

an equilibrium of the muscular forces surrounding the teeth.[57] The placement of retentive appliances, then, is an admission of inadequate orthodontic correction or of a predetermined decision to place teeth in relatively unstable positions for esthetic reasons. Whether stability increases with prolonged retention is one of the most interesting points of discussion in regard to retention planning and is the phase of treatment that is most difficult to quantify. Documentation and control of such variables as cooperation, length of retention time, growth, and appliance design make this type of investigation difficult to interpret.

Theorem 6. *If the lower incisors are placed upright over basal bone, they are more likely to remain in good alignment.* Therefore attention should be directed to the proper angulation and placement of the mandibular incisor segment.* It is obvious that the difficulty of evaluating this contention revolves around proof of the fact that incisors have been placed upright over basal bone. We have been able to define upright: perpendicular to the mandibular plane, 5° or some other specified angulation to the occlusal plane or Frankfort horizontal plane, etc. However, no one can specify where basal bone begins or ends, and there seems to be no satisfactory method of measuring it.[58,59,79,106]

It has sometimes been assumed that teeth that are upright are also over basal bone. However, there are cases in which the roots of mandibular incisors have been moved labially to a considerable degree in the process of uprighting these teeth. It is significant that many malocclusions present with mandibular incisors upright and *over basal bone,* and yet these teeth are both crowded and rotated. Teeth that supposedly have the attributes of stability can actually be in a state of malocclusion (Fig. 16-1).

From a purely mechanical standpoint there is a certain amount of virtue in inclining the mandibular incisors slightly to the lingual. Those who have set mandibular anterior teeth during fabrication of a diagnostic setup have noted that if the teeth are aligned with a labial inclination, attempts to push them lingually must result in expansion in the canine area or in collapse of the teeth. On the other hand, if the anterior teeth are inclined lingually, further pressure to the lingual does not cause collapse, and tipping to the labial only creates spacing. If the clinician must make any errors in positioning of mandibular incisor teeth, it is probably well to err in the direction of a lingual rather than a labial inclination.

If the patient is growing, the mandibular anterior segment may exhibit a physiologic migration in relation to the mandibular body in a distal direction that is apart from orthodontic treatment.[14,16-18] It can be readily seen that if the mandibular anterior section is moved lingually during orthodontic treatment, this movement may be in harmony with the normal expected migration of these teeth; hence, retentive care may be minimized.[115] However, we believe that mandibular arch form plays a more important role in stable

---

*References 47, 54, 74, 126, 139, 135, 136.

mandibular tooth alignment than does the relative antero-posterior relationship of mandibular denture to base. (This subject will be discussed further later.)

Theorem 7. *Corrections carried out during periods of growth are less likely to relapse*. Therefore orthodontic treatment should be instituted at the earliest possible age. There seems to be little direct evidence to substantiate this statement, but it is plausible. If orthodontists are in any way able to influence growth and development of the maxilla or mandible, then *certainly* it is logical to presume that this growth can be influenced only while the patient is growing.[65,85,90,145] In 1924 Matthew Federspiel[40] said, "I am free to confess that we find it almost impossible to treat a true type of distoocclusion without extraction after the developmental period and keep it in position." When treatment depends on a retardation or change of direction of growth (as implied in headgear or functional appliance therapy), then treatment must be instituted early during periods of active growth.

Early diagnosis and treatment planning appear to afford several advantages in long-term stability. Institution of early treatment can prevent progressive, irreversible tissue or bony changes,[95] maximize the use of growth and development with concomitant tooth eruption, allow interception of the malocclusion before excessive dental and morphologic compensations (which may become more difficult to treat and retain than the primary malocclusion symptom), and allow correction of skeletal malrelationships while sutures are morphologically immature and more amenable to alteration.

Much has been said about changes in muscle balance established by changing the positions of teeth, which in turn will promote rather than retard normal growth. Whether malrelations in muscle balance have as much influence on growth and development as has been supposed is difficult to say. It might be mentioned that changes in muscle balance in a normal direction would allow for more normal development of the dentition; in relation to retention, normal muscle balance should allow for normal arch alignment.

Theorem 8. *The further teeth have been moved, the less likelihood there is of relapse*. Thus, when it has been necessary to move teeth a great distance, the patient will probably need less retentive attention—or perhaps it is desirable to move teeth further during the process of orthodontic treatment.

It is possible that positioning far from the original environment will produce equilibrium states permitting more satisfactory occlusions, but the wisdom of this rule has not yet been put to the test. Little real evidence supports the statement that the further teeth have been moved, the less relapse tendency they will have. In fact, the opposite may be true. It may be more desirable through guidance of eruption and early interception of skeletal dysplasias to *minimize* the need for future extensive tooth movement, with the resultant impact on the functional environment and such local factors as supracrestal fibers.

Theorem 9. *Arch form, particularly in the mandibular arch, cannot be permanently altered by appliance therapy*. Therefore treatment should be directed toward maintaining the arch form presented by the malocclusion as much as possible.[129] The evidence brought to our attention by Hayes Nance[92] and others, that attempts to alter mandibular arch form in the human dentition generally meet with failure, has been accepted realistically by some orthodontists. In 1944 Dallas McCauley[86] made the following statement: "Since these two mandibular dimensions, molar width and cuspid width, are of such an uncompromising nature, one might establish them as fixed quantities and build the arches around them." Strang[129] said essentially the same thing in 1946: "I am firmly convinced that the axiom of the mandibular canine width may be stated as follows: The width as measured across from one canine to the other in the mandibular denture is an accurate index to the muscular balance inherent to the individual and dictates the limits of the denture expansion in this area of treatment."

Reports of Cases

A number of investigations of orthodontically corrected malocclusions several years after retention have been made by various authors.[89,125] In almost every instance mandibular intercanine width tended to return to or maintain the original dimension after all of the retaining appliances had been removed for several years. One of the few reports of postretention cases, which seems to conflict with the theorem of the relative stability of the intercanine width, is that of Walters,[140,141] who told of maintaining slight increases in mandibular intercanine width after all retention had been removed for what he termed *an adequate period*. Arnold[7] later pointed out that at least 5 years must elapse before an apparent maintenance of increased intercanine width can be accepted. In one of his patients the intercanine width was increased by 4.2 mm during treatment. After a year without retention there was a contraction of 1 mm, so that the gain in intercanine width was still 3.2 mm. However, after a 5-year postretention period, there was an effective intercanine width gain of only 0.7 mm (Fig. 16-2).

During the same year, Amott[4] conducted an examination of patients out of retention whose malocclusion had been treated without the extraction of any permanent teeth. The results of this investigation also indicated that with the exclusion of *an* exceptional case, in which 5.5 mm of intercanine width increase was maintained for 7 years (Fig. 16-3), the postretentive intercanine widths were similar to or the same as pretreatment intercanine dimensions. Riedel[108] reported previously on several groups of patients who were at least 5 years out of retention and whose mandibular intercanine widths had returned to their original dimensions. Similar and stronger evidence has been found in cases 10 years out of retention.[43,146]

It has frequently been suggested that if the mandibular canines are moved into a more posterior position in relation to the mandibular basal arch increased intercanine width can

Text continued on p. 917.

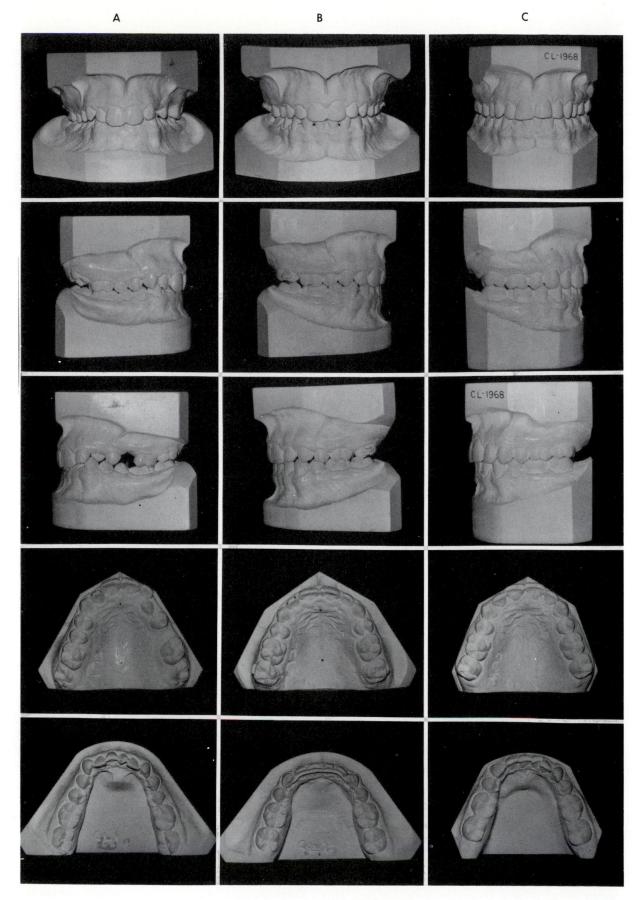

A   B   C

Fig. 16-1 For legend see opposite page.

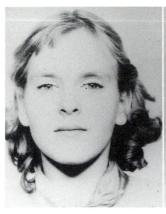 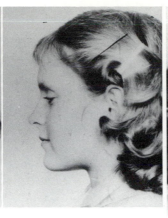 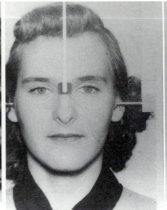 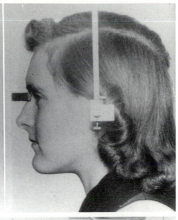

D

E

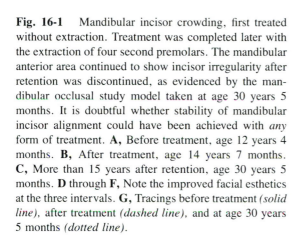

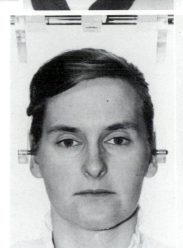 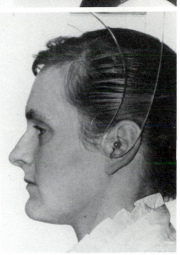

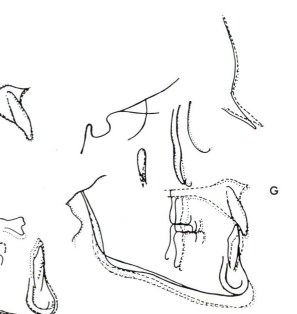

F

Fig. 16-1 Mandibular incisor crowding, first treated without extraction. Treatment was completed later with the extraction of four second premolars. The mandibular anterior area continued to show incisor irregularity after retention was discontinued, as evidenced by the mandibular occlusal study model taken at age 30 years 5 months. It is doubtful whether stability of mandibular incisor alignment could have been achieved with *any* form of treatment. **A,** Before treatment, age 12 years 4 months. **B,** After treatment, age 14 years 7 months. **C,** More than 15 years after retention, age 30 years 5 months. **D** through **F,** Note the improved facial esthetics at the three intervals. **G,** Tracings before treatment *(solid line),* after treatment *(dashed line),* and at age 30 years 5 months *(dotted line).*

G

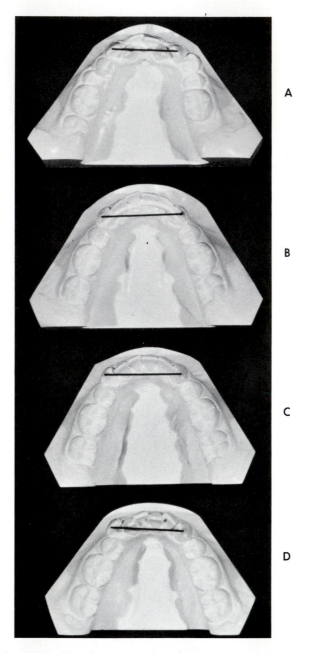

Fig. 16-2 **A,** Malocclusion. **B,** After completion of treatment. **C,** One year postretention. **D,** Five years postretention. Intercanine widths: before treatment, 24.2 mm; after treatment, 28.4 mm; 1 year postretention, 27.4 mm; 5 years postretention, 24.9 mm. Note that after 1 year without retention there had been a contraction of only 1 mm yet after 5 years the total intercanine gain was but 0.7 mm. This illustrates the distorted conclusion, based on a 1-year postretention period rather than 5 years, that would be drawn regarding the amount of posttreatment adjustment in this case. (From Arnold M: Thesis, University of Washington, 1962.)

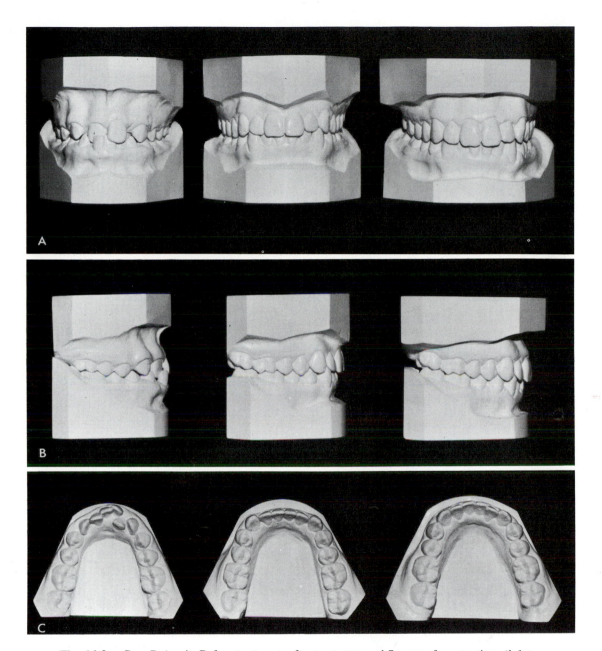

Fig. 16-3 Case R.A., **A,** Before treatment, after treatment, and 7 years after retention, *(left to right).* **B** and **C,** Before treatment, after treatment, and postretention (7 mm of expansion held). (From Amott RD: Thesis, Northwestern University, 1962.)

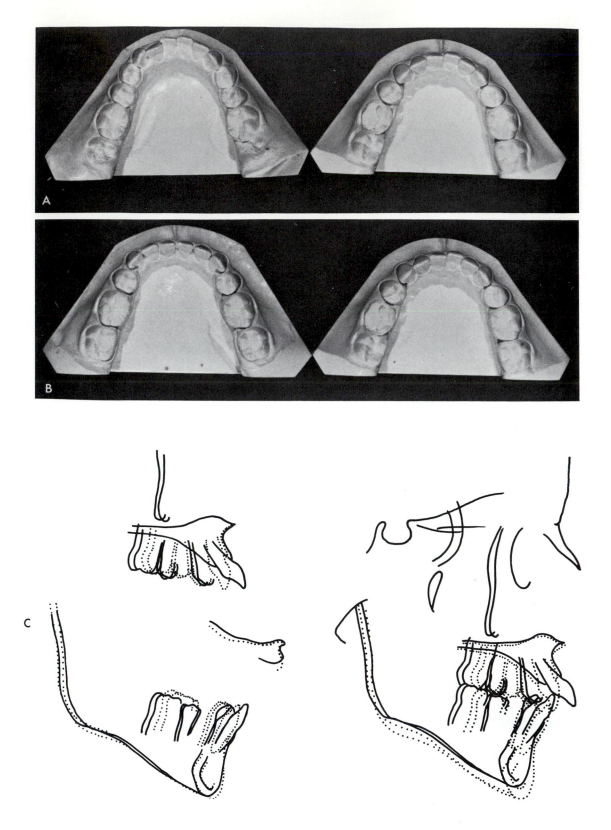

Fig. 16-4   **A,** Pretreatment *(left)*. Three weeks after the lower retainer was lost *(right)*. Intercanine width has decreased to within 0.5 mm of the original dimension. **B,** At the time lower retainer was placed *(left)*. (Canines expanded 4 mm at the end of treatment.) Three weeks later *(right)*. (Canines contracted almost to original width.) **C,** Definite distal movement of the mandibular canines between pretreatment and post-treatment models.

be expected to hold. This expectation may be presumed to be completely logical, but all of the evidence collected to date seems to indicate that distal mandibular canine movement, whether by tipping or bodily repositioning, has little to do with increasing intercanine width and correlates poorly with degree of incisal crowding (Fig. 16-4). The following are some of Arnold's[7] conclusions:

1. The intercanine width in patients who had no retaining devices for a period of 5 years or more shows a remarkable tendency to return to or to approach that of the original malocclusion.

2. No significant effect on resultant intercanine width is demonstrated following premolar extraction therapy.

3. The original intercanine width, when it is intelligently and judiciously employed, can serve as a valuable clinical guide to orthodontic diagnosis and treatment (Fig. 16-5).

Further evidence is provided by Dona,[35] Little et al.,[77] Shapiro,[117] and Welch.[144]

Little et al.[77] examined patients treated with first premolar

extraction and routine edgewise mechanics at least 10 years out of retention and stated that long-term alignment was variable and unpredictable. They found that no descriptive characteristics (e.g., Angle Class, length of retention, age at initiation of treatment, or sex) and no measured variables (initial or end-of-active-treatment alignment, overbite, overjet, arch width, or arch length) were of value in predicting long-term stability. Arch width and length typically were decreased after retention, whereas crowding was increased. This occurred despite treatment maintenance of initial intercanine width or treatment expansion or constriction. Their conclusion was that success at maintaining satisfactory mandibular anterior alignment is less than 30%, with nearly 20% of the cases likely to show crowding many years after removal of retainers.

Using this same sample, Shields et al.[119] evaluated the relationship of cephalometric changes to mandibular incisor alignment and found that combinations of pretreatment and post-treatment cephalometric parameters (e.g., incisor position and facial growth) were poor predictors of long-term

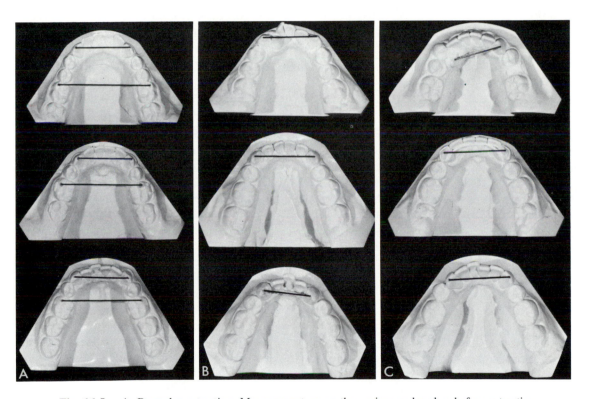

Fig. 16-5 **A,** Premolar extraction. Measurement across the canines and molars before extraction *(top),* after extraction *(middle),* and after retention *(bottom).* Note the incisor irregularity after retention, despite maintenance of the pretreatment intercanine width and extraction of the premolars. **B,** Postretention variability. Intercanine widths were 26.7 mm before treatment *(top),* 29.3 mm after treatment *(middle),* and 23 mm after retention *(bottom).* The patient lost an incisor in an accident, but the remaining incisors are crowded despite premolar and incisor extraction and reduced intercanine width. **C,** Postretention variability with an effective increase in intercanine width. The measurement was 23.8 mm before treatment *(top),* 29.5 mm after treatment *(middle),* and 27.4 mm 5 years after retention *(bottom).* Note that the left canine was lingually impacted, leading to an effective intercanine gain of 3.6 mm. Measurement from 3̄| to |4 (before treatment) is almost the same as from |3 to |3 after retention.

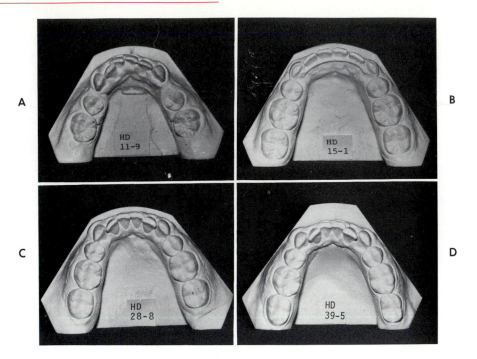

Fig. 16-6 Case H.D. **A,** Before treatment (11 yr, 9 mo). **B,** After treatment (15 yr, 1 mo). **C,** Ten years postretention (28 yr, 8 mo). **D,** Twenty-five years after retention (age 39 yr, 5 mo). Note the increase in mandibular incisor crowding between the 10 and 20 year postretention records.

mandibular incisor stability. Additionally, postretention changes in cephalometric parameters failed to explain postretention crowding.

The exact number of years out of retention provides no certainty relative to the stability of arch alignment. Witness case *H.D.* (Fig. 16-6) before treatment, after treatment, 10 years postretention, and 20 years postretention. Further crowding took place between 10 and 20 years out of retention. This is only one of many cases that exhibit postretention changes of various degrees.

Two of Shapiro's conclusions[117] are important additions to our knowledge of postretention changes: (1) Class II, division 2, malocclusions demonstrated a significantly greater ability to maintain intercanine width expansion as compared to Class I and Class II, division 1, treated malocclusions; (2) arch length reduction in Class II, division 2, was significantly less than in Class I and Class II, division 1, during treatment and from pretreatment to 10 years postretention.

GENERAL CONSIDERATIONS
Extraction of Incisors

The extraction of *two* mandibular incisors may satisfy the requirements of maintaining arch form without expansion of intercanine width. A question that arises in the orthodontist's mind when considering mandibular incisor extraction is the possibility that the overbite may be deepened.

Note that we mention the extraction of two mandibular incisors, not one, and this is the key point in mandibular incisor extraction. Extraction of one mandibular incisor usually does create problems of deep overbite, at least when a normal tooth size relationship is present before the extraction. If maxillary canines are related in their normal positions to mandibular canines, then maxillary incisors must naturally fall into either a greater overbite or overjet. However, when *two* mandibular incisors are removed, the mandibular teeth are so rearranged that the mandibular canines become lateral incisors. If the central incisors are removed, the mandibular lateral incisors become central incisors. Note also that the mandibular first premolars assume the place of the mandibular canines and the maxillary canines must occlude along the distal inclined planes of the mandibular first premolars. When two mandibular incisors have been removed, the usual relationship of the anterior teeth is end to end; the mandibular arch in its anterior area is usually slightly larger than it would have been with four incisors present instead of two incisors and two canines. It is usually necessary to trim the mesiodistal widths of the mandibular centrals or laterals (whichever remain), the canines, and the first premolars to create a harmonious tooth size relationship between these teeth and the maxillary six anterior teeth (Figs. 16-7 and 16-8).

When a patient has one mandibular incisor already removed, a most logical consideration is to remove another mandibular incisor and two maxillary units, probably the

A   B   C   D

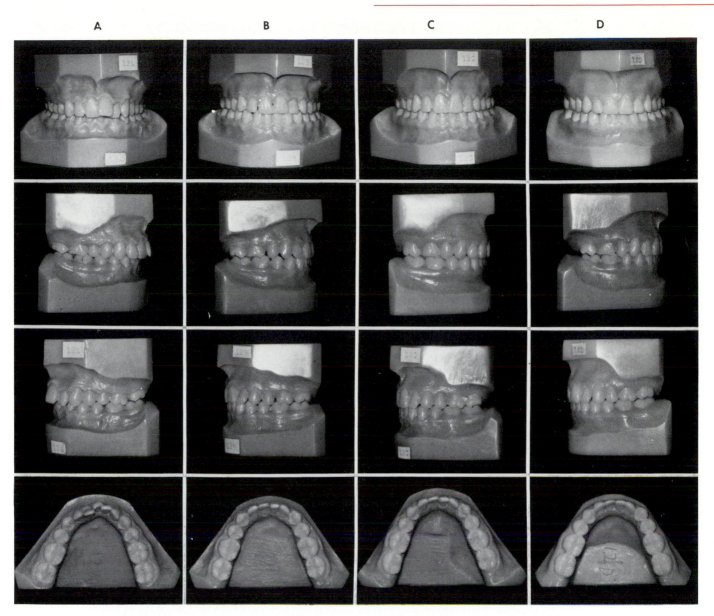

Fig. 16-7   Stability achieved after lower incisor extractions for a Class I malocclusion. **A,** Before treatment. **B,** After treatment. **C,** Approximately 8 years after retention. **D,** At age 30 years 7 months. A mandibular central incisor had been previously extracted. The remaining mandibular central incisor was removed with the maxillary second premolars.

first premolars. There are some instances in which the maxillary laterals are either missing or deformed; and if the maxillary laterals are removed, spaces can be closed with canine against central, using the first premolar as a maxillary canine to occlude with the new mandibular arch (Fig. 16-9).

To clarify the point concerning maintenance of mandibular arch form and intercanine width, we can examine an attempt to realign the mandibular anterior segment in a case in which there was considerable crowding and minimal intercanine width. When mandibular first premolars are ex-

tracted, the simple realignment of mandibular anterior teeth and canines in normal arch form results in a greatly increased intercanine width, which in all likelihood cannot be maintained. On the other hand, if mandibular intercanine width is maintained as presented, the arch form cannot be anything but pointed or V-shaped (Fig. 16-9). A satisfactory solution involves the extraction of two mandibular central incisors. The consequent intercanine width is little changed, whereas mandibular arch form has been maintained in a form similar to the original.

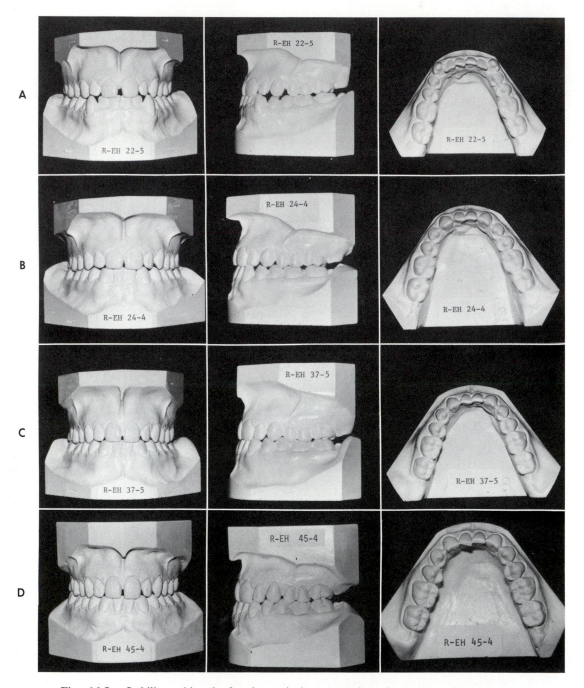

Fig. 16-8 Stability achieved after lower incisor extractions for a Class III malocclusion. **A,** Before treatment (22 yr, 5 mo). **B,** After treatment (24 yr, 4 mo). **C,** Six years postretention (37 yr, 5 mo). **D,** Fourteen years postretention (45 yr, 4 mo).

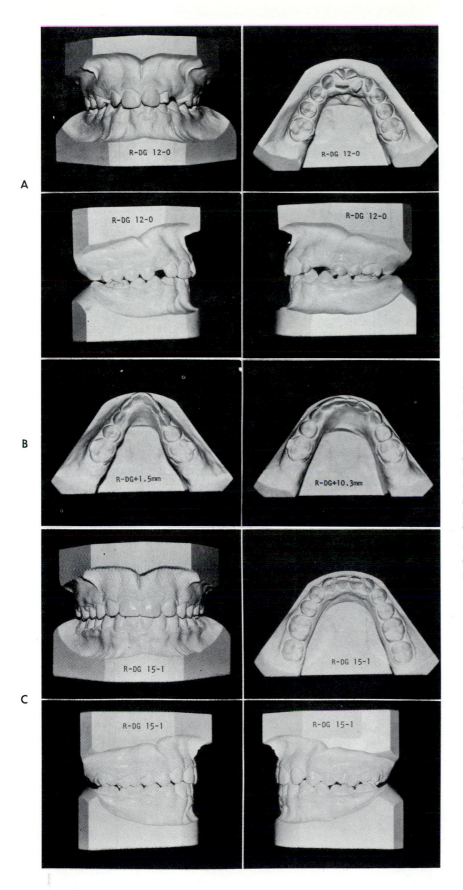

Fig. 16-9 **A,** Age 12 years. Considerable crowding with inflammation of the gingival tissue labial to the central incisors. **B,** Mandibular arch diagnostic setup showing first premolar extraction, where the intercanine width is maintained as in the original *(left),* and a similar setup with an attempt to maintain normal arch form. The intercanine width was expanded 10.3 mm and would almost certainly have relapsed after retention was discontinued. **C,** After treatment, age 15 years 1 month. The mandibular central and maxillary lateral incisors were removed. The maxillary left lateral was congenitally missing, and the right lateral was malformed.   *Continued.*

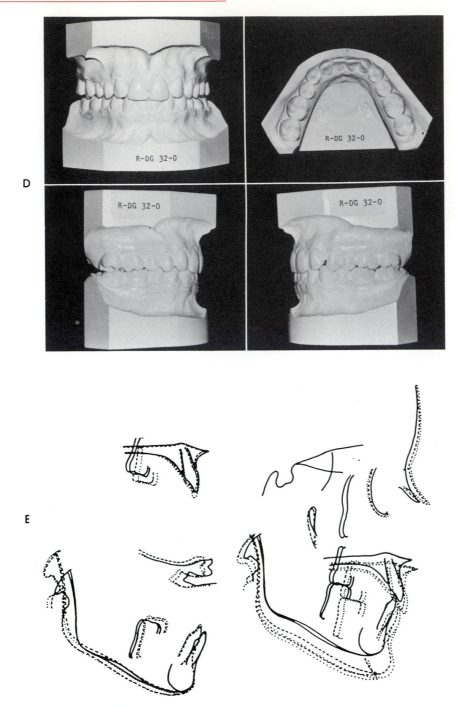

Fig. 16-9, cont'd   D, Fifteen years after retention, age 32 years. Note the satisfactory mandibular incisor alignment. **E,** Changes in the maxilla and mandible *(left)* and changes in over-all growth *(right).* Note the considerable modification in contour at *B* point.

Contraindications

This is not to suggest that all problems of mandibular anterior crowding can be solved with the extraction of mandibular anterior teeth. The following are two drawbacks to such treatment:

1. In instances of minimal crowding, spaces tend to open between the canines and centrals or the canines and laterals (whichever are maintained). Spacing in this

area can be irritating to the patient; food impaction is embarrassing and esthetics is unpleasant. In all mandibular two-incisor extraction cases examined 10 or more years after retention, none of the patients maintained spaces in the mandibular arch. Some slight irregularities have been seen (particularly rotations of either incisors or canines), but the problem of spacing is only a temporary one.

A   B   C

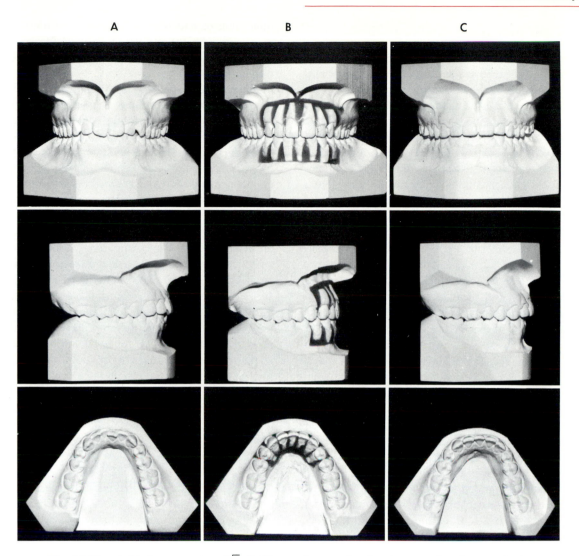

Fig. 16-10   A, Before extraction of ⌐1. **B,** Diagnostic setup showing the extraction, interproximal marking, and trimming of the maxillary anterior teeth. **C,** After extraction.

2. Generally, the most protruded mandibular incisors are removed, and then immediately, the mandibular denture becomes more posterior relative to the mandibular base. It is difficult if not impossible to move the whole mandibular denture forward to assume its previous relation with pogonion, and facial esthetics may suffer as a result of this recessive positioning of the mandibular denture.

A third possible problem includes the anatomic differences in shape of the mandibular canines as compared to the normal mandibular lateral incisors; occasionally, the color of these teeth differs as well. Some of these drawbacks are compensated for by the fact that the mandibular anterior segment is less visible than the maxillary, being covered by the lower lip during normal functional activities.

One of the indications for mandibular incisor extraction is the type of problem that is frequently seen when mandibular anterior teeth are considerably crowded and/or protruded (i.e., recession of the gingival tissues on the facial aspect of the most protruded incisor teeth). Because of reduced bone height, these tissues rarely recover position enough to provide a normal clinical crown; and extraction of these teeth, rather than the mandibular first premolars, should be considered whenever periodontal problems involving the lower anteriors are seen.

All these considerations, of course, presume that the patient has a malocclusion that *requires* extraction. Mandibular incisor extraction should be confined to particularly crowded mandibular anterior segments.

Instances occur in which the extraction of one mandibular incisor will allow a satisfactory occlusal relationship. Patients occasionally have tooth size discrepancies of such a type that the removal of one mandibular incisor allows for a normal tooth size relationship with the maxillary anterior teeth (Fig. 16-10). Slight mandibular crowding concomitant with good facial esthetics may also preclude extraction of the premolars.

TOOTH SIZE DISCREPANCY

Tooth size discrepancy is an often overlooked problem in retention. Ballard[10] reported that 90% of the casts of 500 patients he examined had tooth size discrepancies.

When maxillary anterior teeth are too large in relation to mandibular anterior teeth, the maxillary teeth must be placed in one of the several following positions: (1) deeper overbite; (2) greater overjet; (3) combinations of greater overbite and overjet; (4) crowded anterior segment; or (5) out of proper occlusion buccal segment (the maxillary teeth fitting into a more or less distal relation with the mandibular because the posterior teeth generally do not remain stabilized in an end-to-end occlusion).

If the mandibular anterior teeth are too large, compensations can include (1) an end-to-end incisor relationship; (2) spacing in the maxillary anterior segment; (3) crowding in the mandibular incisor area; or (4) improper occlusion distal to and including the maxillary lateral, with the maxillary posterior teeth in mesial relation to the mandibular posterior teeth. It is possible to estimate and determine these discrepancies by making a trial setup or by using a mathematical formula that can determine the degree of the area in which a tooth size discrepancy exists.[22]

Proximal reduction of tooth size. It is logical to have measurements of all orthodontic casts before consultation appointments. Tooth size ratios can be established and the degree and location of abnormality noted.

When anterior tooth size discrepancies exceed 2.5 mm in patients whose teeth are otherwise normally formed (excluding pegged or undersize maxillary lateral incisors), a trial setup is usually indicated. If the teeth cannot be occluded in a normal relationship in a trial setup without proximal reduction, then the clinician must resort to stripping these teeth in the mouth. If a banded appliance is used, proximal reduction should be initiated before its fitting and cementation. With the advent of bonded appliances, interproximal stripping can be accomplished with more ideal control and ease during the finishing stages of therapy.

Between 2 and 4 mm of enamel can be removed from the maxillary or mandibular six anterior teeth, and it is sometimes desirable to include the maxillary or mandibular first premolars as well. When tooth size discrepancies exceed this dimension, it is logical to consider some other type of approach to treatment, such as extraction of a single incisor (usually done in the case of an excess in the mandibular anterior section). If excess exists in the maxillary anterior section, the greatest amount of enamel can be removed from the distal surfaces of the maxillary centrals, maxillary laterals, and maxillary canines. Occasionally, the maxillary first premolars can be trimmed at the mesial surface. Enamel thicknesses can be determined from good periapical radiographs, and the enamel cap should not be trimmed so far that dentin is exposed in the proximal area. It is also unwise to remove so much enamel from the contact area that crown width becomes narrower than the cervical dimension or narrower than the root or roots of the teeth themselves, for it will then be unlikely that the spaces between the teeth can be closed and maintained in a normal contact relationship.

The procedure involved in stripping anterior teeth usually includes the use of lightning strips to break open contact areas, a limited use of lightning or diamond disks to reduce the greater bulk of enamel, and the completion of final trimming with lightning strips and coarse and fine sandpaper strips so that the original contour of the tooth crown can be maintained and the tooth enamel kept smooth. If stripping is done by completing the reduction of one proximal surface at a time, it is easier to visualize or measure the amount of tooth enamel removed. If both surfaces in a proximal area are reduced at the same time, using double-sided abrasion strips, it will be difficult to determine from which of these surfaces the greater amount of enamel has been removed. If the clinician proceeds from right to left, removing 0.25 mm on all surfaces from the distal of one canine to the mesial of the other, then the procedure can be reversed and another 0.25 mm can be removed starting from the distal of the left canine and moving to the mesial of the right. A total of 0.5 mm gained in each interproximal space reduces the tooth size discrepancy by approximately 2.5 mm. Proximal tooth reduction should be done on a diagnostic setup and the amounts and locations transferred clinically to the dentition.

Axial Inclination

Another consideration that is little discussed in the orthodontic literature is the axial inclination of the maxillary and mandibular incisor teeth. In many instances, orthodontists are brought to the realization that the further they have retracted mandibular incisors, the further must the maxillary incisors be retracted. Tipping maxillary and mandibular incisors into a too upright relation usually results in deep anterior overbite. Periodontists suggest that there are potentially damaging functional implications to this type of occlusion.[124] (Bolton[22] found that in excellent occlusions the angles of the *labial* surfaces of the maxillary and mandibular central incisors to their occlusal plane totaled approximately 177°. In other words, the labial surfaces of these teeth in profile formed almost a straight line.)

It is interesting to note that the technique of measuring the axial inclinations of maxillary to mandibular anterior teeth is not really a satisfactory one from a functional standpoint. Drawing a line from incisal edge through root tip may be a convenient technique for cephalometric tracing, but it certainly does not take into account variations in crown-root relationships which may be present. From an esthetic viewpoint it would be more desirable to measure the relationship of the labial surfaces of the crowns of the anterior teeth, and from a functional standpoint perhaps the angulation of the lingual surfaces of the maxillary anterior teeth and their relation to the labial surfaces of the mandibular incisors might be just as important (Fig. 16-11).

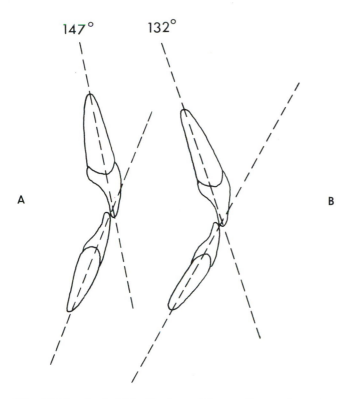

Fig. 16-11 **A,** Axial inclinations of the maxillary and mandibular central incisors form an angle of 147°. Labial surfaces of the crowns in profile meet at almost 180°. **B,** The axial inclinations of the maxillary and mandibular incisors form an angle of 132°, yet the crown surfaces are almost exactly in the same relative functional position as in **A.**

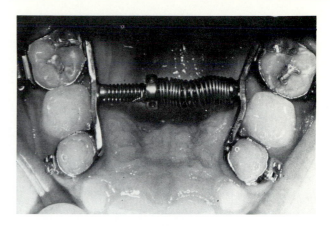

Fig. 16-12 Mini-expander with a 2-pound compressed coil and a ligature wire tied adjacent to the turnscrew to maintain its position. The patient is seen once every 3 to 4 weeks.

Transverse Discrepancies

Numerous authors[67,68,133,134] have documented the tendency for relapse associated with rapid palatal expansion techniques. Typically the clinician must significantly overcorrect in the transverse dimension, anticipating that a more normal relationship will occur during the relapse stages. Additionally, the expansion appliance must be maintained passively or a removable appliance placed to aid in transverse retention.

Storey[127] has documented experimentally that rapid expansion results in a predominantly destructive process in which the sutural connective tissue becomes disrupted and edematous with enlarged blood vessels or hemorrhaging. This is followed by eventual *filling in* of immature bone as a healing response. The growing of bone of sufficient maturity requires a slow steady rate of formation with lateral separation of bones on the order of 0.5 to 1.0 mm per week. Results of Storey's experiments show that slow separation with continued physiologic growth of bony serrations within the suture provides the best form of retention with the least potential for relapse.

Castro,[29] Cotton,[32] and Hicks[55] have further evaluated experimentally and clinically the stability of palatal expansion

with light continuous forces and have concluded that this technique is more stable than rapid expansion.

Anatomically, the limitation of palatal expansion is not fusion of the midpalatal suture but rather changes in the morphology of the suture caused by maturation. As the patient ages, further intercuspation and interdigitation of bony serrations take place until the suture becomes mechanically difficult to expand at older ages. These changes in sutural morphology may occur as early as 13 to 14 years of age. We believe that early expansion with light forces, done before these maturation changes, will allow maximum skeletal separation, with normal physiologic bone deposition enhancing the long-term stability in this plane of space.

Clinically we use a modified *mini-expander* in which either a two-pound or a four-pound coil is substituted. Coils are fabricated to deliver the desired force on full compression (Fig. 16-12). It has been our experience that excellent clinical results are achieved using a 2-pound force when the patient is in the mixed dentition and a 4-pound force when the patient is in the permanent dentition. The clinical results achieved with this type of expansion procedure are illustrated in Figs. 16-13 and 16-14.

Relationship of Third Molars

Although some authors[15,73,114,118] have attributed the presence of third molars to long-term mandibular dental stability, other investigators* have published data suggesting that third molars play very little if any role in long-term mandibular arch changes.

Ades et al.[1] compared four groups of patients who were a minimum of 10 years out of retention and had the following bilateral mandibular third molar status: third molars erupted into good alignment and function, third molar agenesis, third molar impaction, and third molar extraction at least 10 years

---

*References 1, 63, 107, 116.

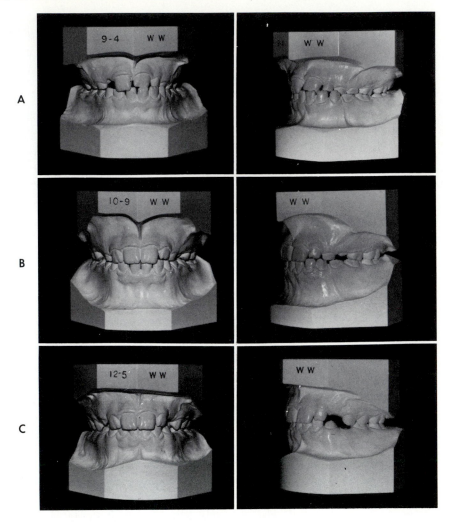

Fig. 16-13 **A,** Age 9 years, 4 months. Bilateral maxillary constriction and resultant mandibular functional shift to the left. **B,** After 8 weeks of expansion with a 2-pound force. Excellent axial control of the maxillary buccal segments. **C,** Two years after expansion with no retention. Excellent stability.

before the postretention records. They found no differences in mandibular incisor crowding, arch length, intercanine width, and eruption pattern of mandibular incisors and molars between the groups. In the majority of cases some degree of mandibular incisor crowding took place after retention but was not significantly different between third molar groups. This suggests that the recommendation for mandibular third molar removal with the objective of alleviating or preventing mandibular incisor irregularity may not be justified (Fig. 16-15).

Growth Factors

Growth is an aid in the correction of many types of orthodontic problems, but it also may cause relapse in treated orthodontic patients. Orthodontists take advantage of growth when treating patients in the transitional dentition period with headgear anchorage[76] or functional appliances. Cephalometric records indicate that cervical traction influences the normal downward and forward growth of the maxillary alveolar process, and it is possible that the growth of the maxilla itself may be retarded or redirected.[41,123,145] The normal forward movement of the maxillary molars seems to be restrained while the mandible continues in its course of growth, and a normal tooth relationship may eventually be reached.[42,50,69] (Other, more complicated, changes occur, but it is not possible to examine them in this chapter.)

We find essentially the same thing occurring in treatment of Class II cases—that is, the maxillary buccal segments are not so much moved distally en masse (although the maxillary buccal segment crowns may be tipped distally and a certain amount of distal bodily movement may occur), but correction takes place as a result of mandibular growth or forward translation of the mandibular teeth.[5,90]

It may be undesirable to leave maxillary buccal segments tipped distally, particularly if there will be no further man-

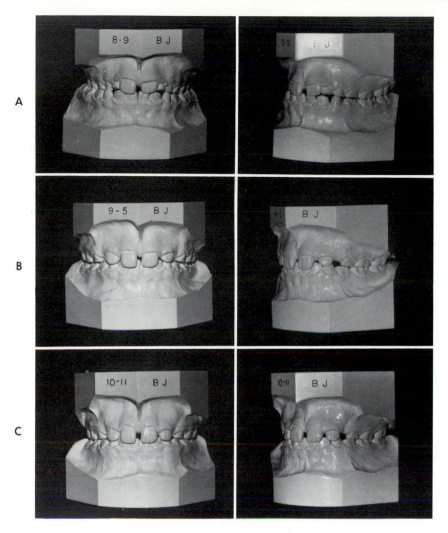

Fig. 16-14 **A,** Age 8 years, 9 months. Bilateral maxillary constriction has resulted in a bilateral maxillary lingual crossbite. **B,** After 10 weeks of expansion with a 2-pound force. Note the excellent axial control and the absence of bite opening. **C,** Eighteen months after expansion with no retention. Excellent stability.

dibular growth. In most instances these distally tipped teeth upright themselves again, with the crowns moving in a mesial direction. If, however, sufficient mandibular forward growth occurs, the occlusion may continue to remain satisfactory.

The forward translation of the mandibular denture on its base after use of Class II elastics or functional appliances is generally regarded as being undesirable, for apparently the mandibular posterior teeth do not migrate distally again. Mandibular anterior teeth, in their attempt to upright to their former positions, frequently break contact and crowd to the lingual.

Regulating Mandibular Growth

Although it is now accepted that retardation or redirection of maxillary growth can be achieved by the orthodontist,

some evidence suggests that mandibular growth can be similarly altered.

Many orthodontists have attempted to restrain mandibular growth by the use of a chin cup or backward force against the mandible, usually at the area of the chin. Cephalometric superimpositions of young children (4 to 7 years of age) suggest that full-time distal force to the mandible can reduce anterior growth increments (Fig. 16-16). It must be kept in mind however that short-term changes may not reflect long-term alteration of growth. Evidence suggests that in spite of early positive changes, that by complete maturation there is no statistically significant difference in mandibular growth increment between patients treated with chin cup therapy and untreated controls.

Injury to the condyles, which are the growth centers, through disease or trauma, may also effect partial or complete retardation of mandibular growth; but this is unpredictable and almost impossible to control, except for the possibility of causing complete cessation of growth (as in removal of the condyles themselves). Exceptions might include the use of the Milwaukee brace, with which investigators[2,36,51] have shown significant alteration in mandibular growth.

In the other direction it has been suggested that vigorous Class II mechanics against the mandibular arch will cause forward mandibular repositioning through what has become known as the Tweed response.[56] Many clinicians favor the idea that the free and uninhibited use of Class II pull against the mandibular arch will cause greater than average forward mandibular growth. However, proof for this thinking has not been adequate. A comparison of patients treated by Dr. Tweed with those treated at the University of Washington[66] produced the following conclusions.

Changes in the forward positioning of the chin were unpredictable and varied greatly in each group. There was no conclusive evidence to indicate that Tweed was able to produce a greater forward positioning of the chin through his treatment technique. The girls treated by Tweed showed the same mean net change for the forward positioning of the chin as did those treated at the University of Washington. There was a greater retraction of the maxillary apical base, and the retraction of the mandibular apical base was less than that of the maxillary apical base—these changes showing a trend for greater retraction in the patients treated by Tweed. The greatest significant difference between the two groups involved linear and angular reductions in the protrusion of the lower incisors.

A study of the soft tissue outlines of Class II, division 1, malocclusions treated by Tweed and at the University of Washington[11] also showed significantly greater retraction of the soft tissues of the upper lip in the Tweed cases.

The rationale for using functional appliances has been discussed in earlier chapters in this book; however, it is clear that for these appliances to be successful, they must be used at the younger ages, when facial growth and concomitant dental eruption potential are at their maximum (see Chapters 7 and 8).

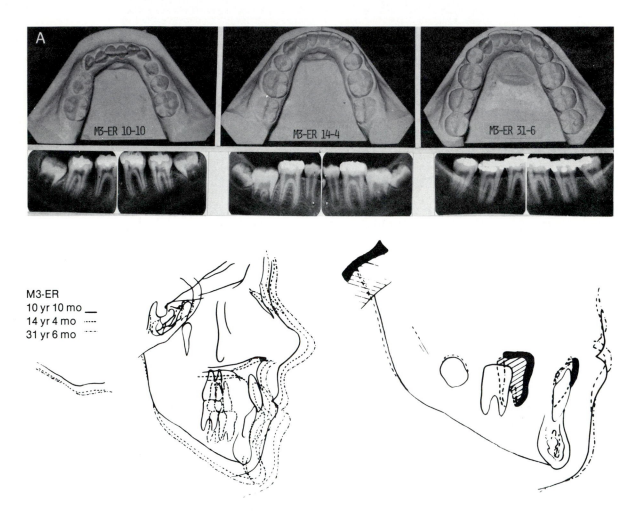

Fig. 16-15   Study models and periapical radiographs (pretreatment, post-treatment, and postretention) plus overall and mandibular superimpositions of patients with the following: **A,** bilaterally erupted third molars *(M3-ER)*. **B,** Bilateral third molar agenesis *(M3-AG)*. **C,** Bilaterally impacted third molars *(M3-IM)*.

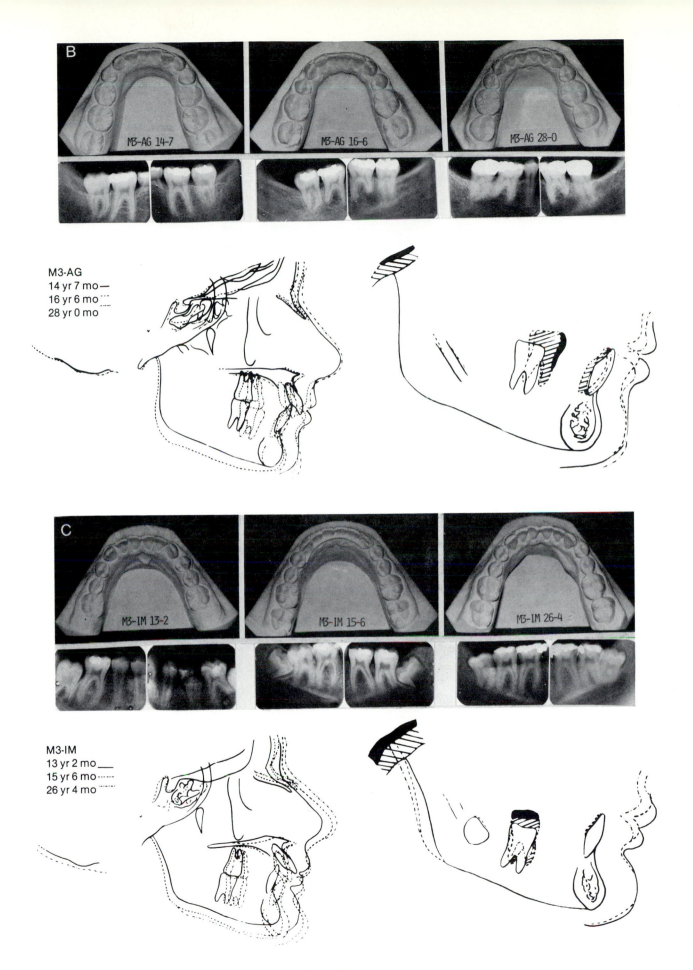

B

MB-AG 14-7 MB-AG 16-6 MB-AG 28-0

M3-AG
14 yr 7 mo—
16 yr 6 mo····
28 yr 0 mo

C

MB-IM 13-2 MB-IM 15-6 MB-IM 26-4

M3-IM
13 yr 2 mo___
15 yr 6 mo····
26 yr 4 mo

Fig. 16-15, cont'd

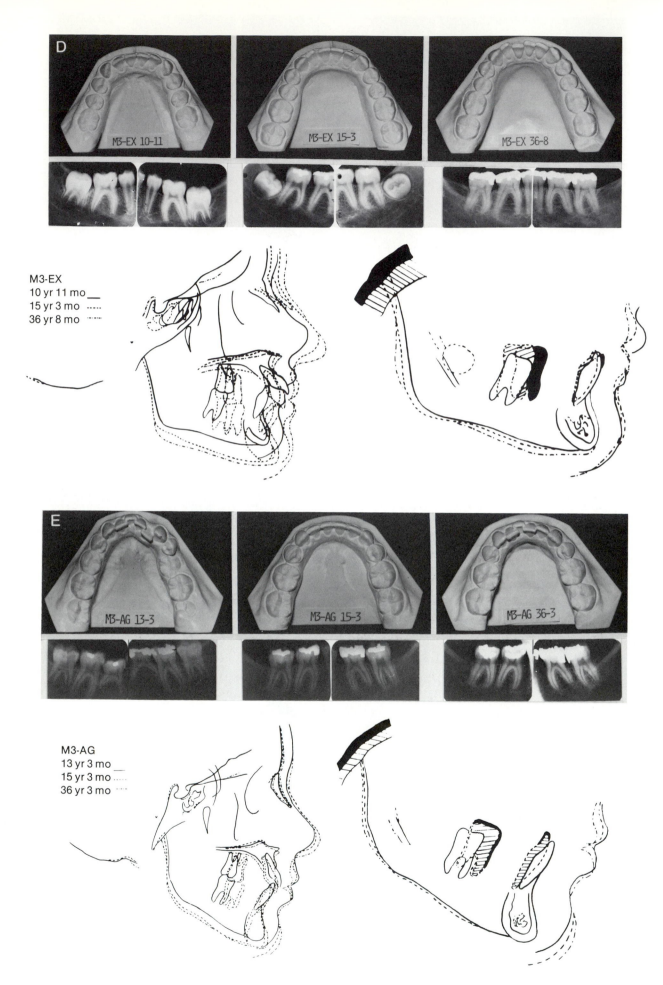

Fig. 16-15, cont'd

Sex Differences

In any discussion of growth the clinician also must be aware that the sex of the patient must be considered when planning treatment and retention. Statistics derived by Baird,[8] Baum,[12,14] and Petraitis[100] from measurements in patients with excellent occlusion indicate that there is a marked difference between the maturation of skeletal and dental patterns of males and females. An analysis of the skeletal and dental patterns of girls aged 11 to 13 establishes that they are not significantly different from those of women. On the basis of this and other investigations it may be concluded that, on the average, the female skeletal and dental pattern matures by the thirteenth year.[19] In boys the skeletal and dental patterns mature somewhat after the fifteenth year on the average. This knowledge is significant in the treatment of skeletal Class II malocclusions, particularly in girls. Certainly the clinician must start treatment before the maturation of the skeletal pattern, independent of dental maturation, if growth is to be influenced at all.

Further Implications of Growth

The implications of continued mandibular growth in the case of a true Class III malocclusion are so well known that few orthodontists attempt to complete orthodontic treatment or surgery until the child has ceased to grow. However, there are other growth peculiarities that are of interest to the orthodontist. The amount and direction of mandibular growth may be of great importance in the correction and retention of corrected malocclusions.

In the patient shown in Fig. 16-17, correction of a Class II malocclusion was accomplished by means of headgear therapy, extraction of premolars, and full banding with Class II elastic traction until normal occlusion was achieved. After treatment was completed, however, the patient's mandible continued to grow in a backward and downward direction, tending to cause a recurrence of the Class II relationship. Maxillary posterior retraction was continued during retention in an attempt to maintain a normal occlusion.

In another instance, in what was apparently a Class I malocclusion corrected with the extraction of four first premolars and complete orthodontic treatment (Fig. 16-18), continued mandibular growth after treatment produced a more or less unilateral type of Class III relationship.

Maturation changes can and do occur, particularly in boys, in relation to the apical bases and alveolar processes. In some, a so-called *swing* of the facial structures occurs out from beneath the cranium in late adolescence.[121] This may have the effect of reducing the angle of convexity, reducing the differences in apical base relationships, and

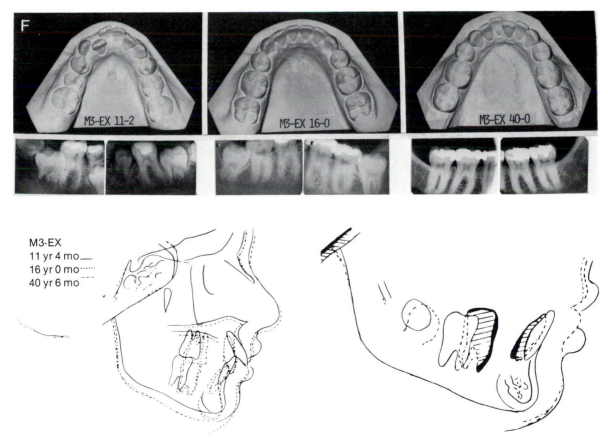

M3-EX
11 yr 4 mo
16 yr 0 mo
40 yr 6 mo

Fig. 16-15, cont'd   D, Bilaterally extracted third molars *(M3-EX).* **E,** Bilateral third molar agenesis *(M3-AG)* (note the amount of crowding). **F,** Bilaterally extracted third molars *(M3-EX).* (treatment completed at least 10 years before final records).

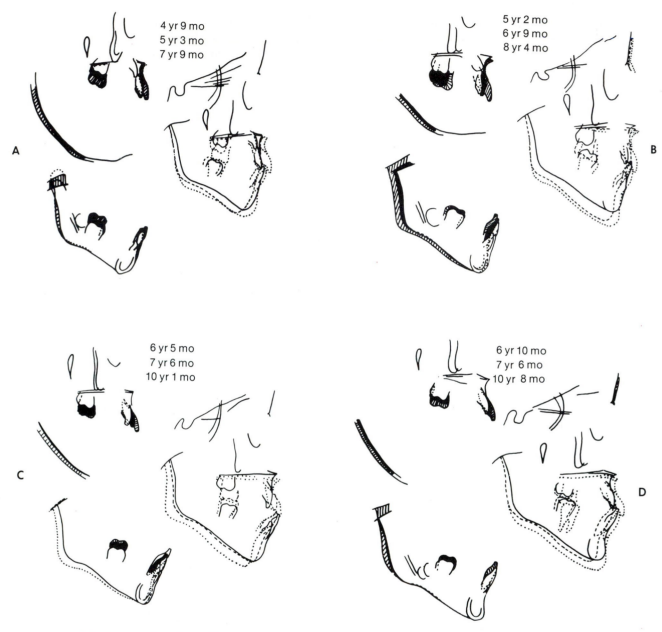

Fig. 16-16 Overall maxillary and mandibular superimpositions of patients who have undergone chin cup therapy for the following age periods: **A,** from 4.9 to 5.3 (no therapy from 5.3 to 7.9); **B,** 5.2 to 6.9 (no therapy from 6.9 to 8.4); **C,** 6.5 to 10.1 (whole time) (note the lack of change at articulare and the mandibular growth pattern); **D,** 6.10 to 7.6 (discontinued from 7.6 to 10.8).

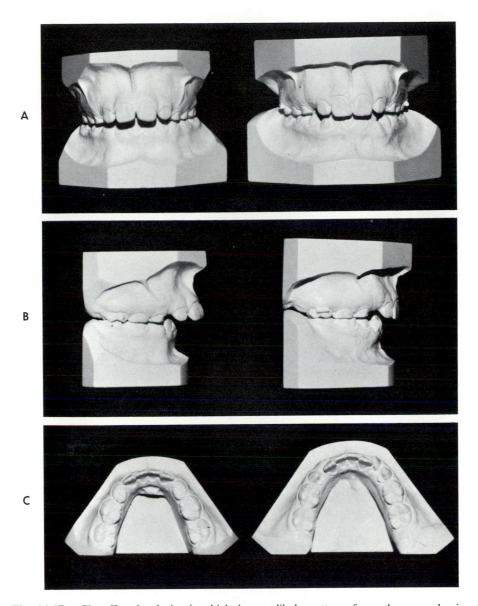

Fig. 16-17   Class II malocclusion in which the mandibular pattern of growth was predominantly downward and backward during headgear use in the mixed dentition and full treatment. There was some forward recovery of the mandible during retention while the maxillary headgear was still being worn. **A** and **B,** Before treatment *(left)* and after headgear to 6|6 only *(right).* **C,** Lower arch. Note the alignment resulting from extraction of the deciduous canines *(left)* and the mandibular premolars *(right).*   *Continued.*

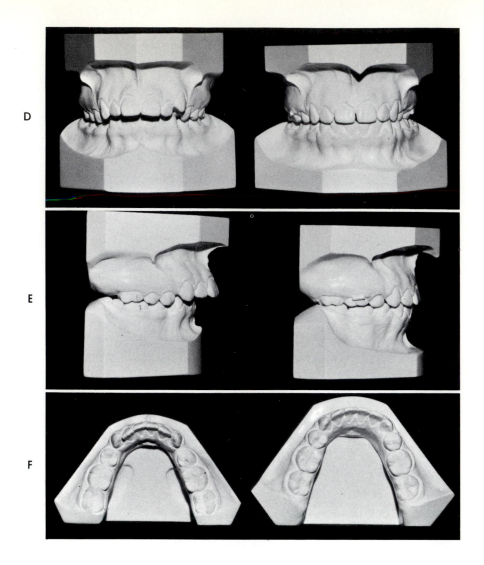

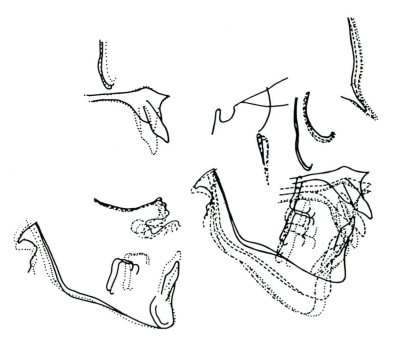

G

Fig. 16-17, cont'd **D** to **F,** At the time of maxillary premolar extraction *(left)* and the final head films *(right).* **G,** The head film tracing shows three periods of growth: during mixed dentition headgear, during full treatment, and during retention. Superimposed on the original tracing.

A   B   C   D

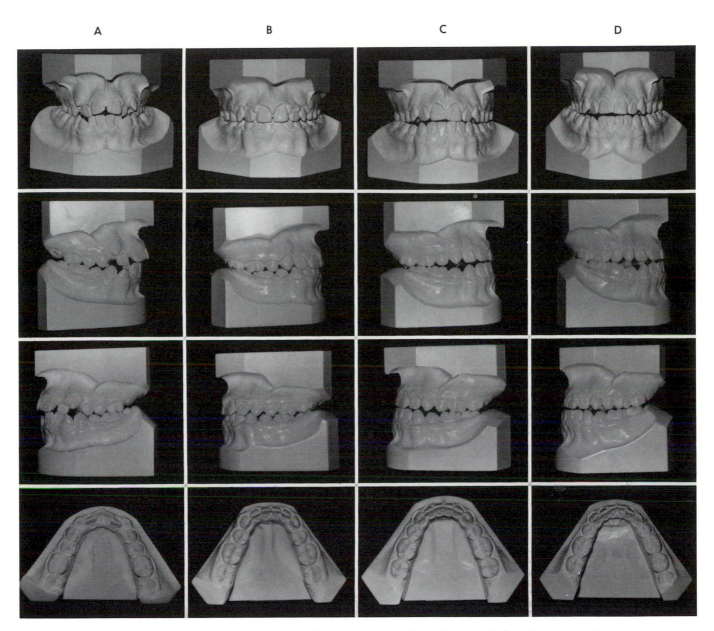

Fig. 16-18   Class I occlusion, **A,** before treatment (age 11 yr, 5 mo) and, **B,** at band removal (age 13 yr, 1 mo). **C,** Postretention relapse into a Class III (age 15 yr, 4 mo). **D,** Further relapse at 17 years of age. Note the stability of anterior alignment, probably because of reduced intercanine width during treatment.   *Continued.*

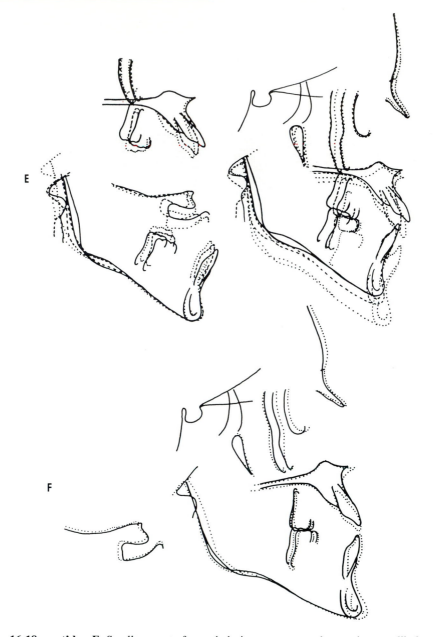

Fig. 16-18, cont'd **E,** Small amount of growth during treatment and excessive mandibular growth after retention. Note that the continued lingual migration of the mandibular incisors after treatment is almost proportionate to the retraction achieved during treatment. **F,** Final tracing from **E** followed by a tracing 1½ years later after tongue posture therapy. There has been an apparent change to a more anterior growth pattern for the mandible and an increase in the open bite. Orthodontic treatment (and possibly surgery) may be instituted when further growth changes cease.

increasing the compensatory angulation of maxillary and mandibular incisors to one another. A restriction of the mandibular denture may be produced in the process, resulting in uprighting of the mandibular incisors. The buccal segments may tend toward a Class III relationship. Usually the occlusal plane flattens, the mandibular plane decreases in relation to the Frankfort horizontal, and often the overbite is reduced. It has been demonstrated[13,39,115] that during growth the permanent dentition has a natural tendency to become more recessive in relation to the body of the mandible and that, particularly in boys, the mandibular denture can be expected grow to erupt distally relative to pogonion.

Continued posterior traction may be desirable on the maxillary arch in corrected Class II malocclusions, especially in patients whose mandibular growth is primarily downward or downward and backward. In boys particularly, continued retention in the maxillary and mandibular incisor areas may be desirable until growth changes have been completed.

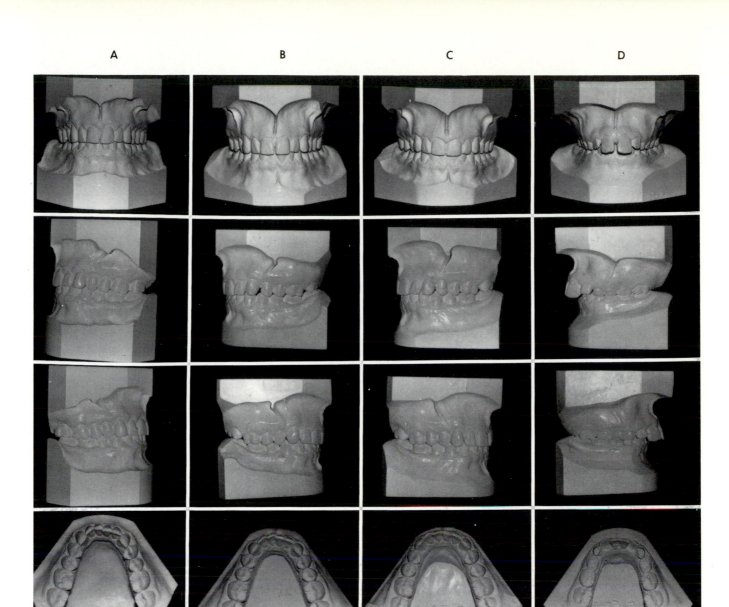

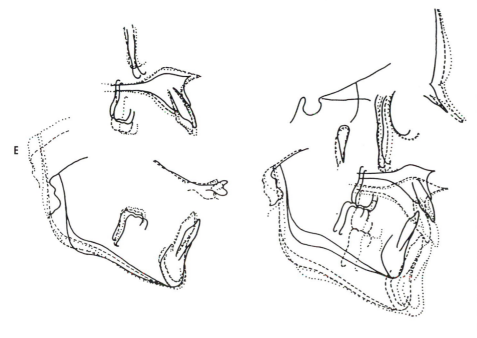

Fig. 16-19 Class II malocclusion treated with Kloehn headgear, maxillary incisor bands, mandibular lingual arch, and maxillary Hawley plate. **A,** Before treatment (age 9 yr) and, **B,** after appliance removal (age 15 yr, 3 mo). **C,** Four years after treatment (age 19 yr, 2 mo), and, **D,** 19 years after retention (age 39 yr, 4 mo). Postretention mandibular incisor instability was possibly due to continued mandibular forward growth. **E,** Growth changes from the malocclusion until retention was stopped. Postretention changes *(dotted line)* may have contributed to the mandibular incisor collapse and maxillary incisor spacing. Note the continued lingual migration of the mandibular incisors during treatment, almost as if Class III traction had been applied, typical of the direction in which these teeth move during prolonged headgear therapy to the maxillary arch. Note also the amount of postretention horizontal mandibular growth with no appliance therapy.

Some orthodontists make it routine practice to retain the mandibular anterior segment in boys until total skeletal growth is completed (Fig. 16-19).

Functional appliances may play an important role during the retention period to assist in maintaining correction of skeletal components. These types of removable appliances can be worn during sleep to prevent changes in maxillomandibular position that may take place through continued unharmonious growth. They are also effective in encouraging differential eruption and tooth movement in compensation for skeletal changes resulting from growth and/or relapse.

Recovery from Tooth Movements

With the possible exception of those who have an open bite malocclusion,[111] patients who have a Frankfort mandibular plane angle within the normal range can generally be expected to show a reduction in the angle with continued growth. If during orthodontic treatment the angle has increased, it may be expected to return to its former dimension or less. If there will be no further growth, the return of the original mandibular plane angle will probably not occur. If, on the other hand, further growth is forthcoming and maxillary and mandibular teeth are retained in a position of minimum overbite, the consequent increase in posterior facial height and leveling of the mandibular plane may occur without an increase in overbite.

Increases in the angulation of the occlusal plane to the sella-nasion plane or the Frankfort horizontal plane during orthodontic treatment are probably also undesirable, since the general tendency is for a decrease in the angle between the occlusal plane and the Frankfort horizontal. Some treatment techniques attempt first to tip the occlusal plane downward in the back and upward in the front to prepare for the later tipping up in back and down in front that will occur with Class II mechanics. If no further growth is forthcoming after the occlusal plane has been tipped to increase its angulation to the Frankfort plane, then the subsequent recovery change of the occlusal plane angle may mean the production of an end-to-end relationship in the buccal segments or a deepened anterior overbite.[90] If, however, the mandibular posterior teeth have been previously tipped in a distal direction, they may recover by tipping mesially, maintaining a Class I relationship with the maxillary posterior teeth, provided the maxillary posteriors do not tip forward an equal or greater distance.

Apical base. Changes may also occur in the apical base relationships. For instance, what is recorded as an angle of convexity of 12° in a boy of 8 may some day be an angle of convexity of only 3°, perhaps less. Hence, when attempting to relate incisors in both inclination and bodily position by means of a standard such as the A-N-B angle or angle of convexity, the clinician must be aware of the implications of future growth changes in these relationships and of the results that may be produced by orthodontic

treatment. It must be recognized that the normal mandibular denture is sometimes carried upward and backward away from pogonion and that bony additions may occur at the pogonion itself; thus the relationship of the mandibular incisor teeth to pogonion at age 9 to 12 is certainly not a permanent position for these teeth[31,76] (Fig. 16-19, D).

It has been suggested that the careless orthodontist can easily lose or *burn* mandibular and maxillary anchorage in extraction cases and not allow for sufficient retraction of the incisor teeth. Although it is true that instances have been recorded in which the injudicious application of mechanics has allowed space closure primarily by mesial movement of the posterior teeth, there are a number of instances in which, with minimal crowding, the orthodontist has found it difficult if not impossible to prevent retraction of the mandibular and, consequently, the maxillary anterior teeth. When we have attempted to maintain mandibular incisor teeth in their original anteroposterior positions and extraction was a part of treatment therapy, we have been all too often discouraged to see the mandibular anterior teeth move lingually despite all attempts to maintain them in their original position (Fig. 16-20).

Experimental results. Experiments have been conducted to attempt to define the effects of tooth movement procedures.

Holdaway[56] suggested that during treatment the permanent maxillary first molar is frequently tipped distally, with the apex as a pivotal point, and that it recovers by tipping mesially, with the apex again as a pivotal point.

Wallman[139] examined 37 patients treated by Tweed with lateral head films before treatment, after treatment, and 1½ to 4 years after appliances were discontinued. He found a variety of changes in the recovery of moved maxillary molars. They tipped mesially after treatment, moved bodily mesially at the same time, moved only bodily mesially, continued to tip distally, continued to move bodily distally, and, in short, showed a range of movement that covered most of the possible movements that anyone could expect. Wallman *did* find that the maxillary molars were the least variable of all the teeth in their recovery attempts and that 83% of all the changes in the recovered maxillary molars fell into two categories. In 19 instances the crown moved forward and the root moved back. In 11 instances, the crown moved forward and the root moved forward, usually the crown more than the root. In only 3 instances did the crown tip forward with the apex of the root as a pivotal point.

In most instances there was little bodily distal movement of the maxillary permanent molars during or after treatment.[5]

Holdaway[56] further suggested that, in relation to the mandibular posterior teeth, once the crown was tipped distally and the roots were tipped mesially during orthodontic treatment, the tooth tended to recover, with a pivotal point in the area of the gingival margin; that is, the crown tipped mesially and the roots distally. Wallman[139] concluded that

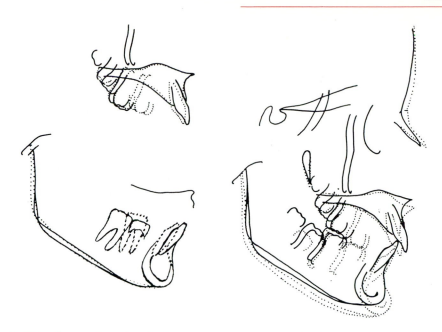

Fig. 16-20   Treated Class II malocclusion in which the mandibular deciduous second molars were removed (permanent second premolars were absent) and an attempt was made to move the mandibular molars forward without retracting the incisors. A mandibular chin cup was used with elastics pulling from the chin cup spurs back to the mandibular molars to aid their forward movement. Despite these efforts, the incisors were bodily retracted to a considerable degree and the chin became relatively more prominent.

there was no typical recovery of the mandibular first permanent molar. In 10 instances the crown did move anteriorly and the root posteriorly, although not necessarily in equal amounts. In 7 cases the crown and the root moved posteriorly, usually the root more than the crown. In 4 instances the crown and root moved anteriorly, usually the crown more than the root. In 4 instances also the crown alone moved anteriorly. These movements accounted for only 25 of the 37 cases. No hard and fast rules could be laid down about the recovery of mandibular permanent molars from the effects of orthodontic treatment.

One common characteristic was found concerning the maxillary and mandibular incisors and their recovery from orthodontic treatment. If these teeth had been depressed during treatment, typically they tended to erupt again after treatment was discontinued. In 89% of the cases, the maxillary incisors moved forward after treatment. In 12 instances, the crown and root moved anteriorly, with the crown moving more than the root; in 6 instances the root moved more than the crown (both root and crown moving anteriorly); in 6 instances there was an equal anterior movement of the root and crown, and in 5 instances the crown alone tipped anteriorly. The mandibular incisor was less regular in its recovery pattern—sometimes tipping labially, sometimes lingually, sometimes moving bodily in either direction, or sometimes combining bodily movement and crown tipping movements labially or lingually.

Recently Van Dyke[137] made similar observations on post-treatment changes in incisor and molar positions of a group of 64 cases treated by the Utah Tweed group.

Rapidity of treatment. A further implication that may be derived from growth studies is that rapid orthodontic treatment may not necessarily be the most desirable. There may be instances when slower orthodontic treatment takes advantage of growth (if it is at all possible to restrain maxillary growth and/or enhance mandibular growth).

Duration of retention. Orthodontists have not yet decided how long to use retention appliances.[104] Does prolonged retention provide for greater stability later? Will the use of retainers for 5 or 10 years provide for an adult dentition that shows less relapse than retention for a year, or 6 months, or not at all? Is prolonged mechanical restraint desirable? To date, no satisfactory comparison has been made of patients with similar malocclusions similarly treated but having *greatly* different retention times. This question has been almost totally disregarded or at least remains unanswered to the present date. There is difficulty, of course, in maintaining continuous retention. Another difficulty is to determine exactly how long (months or years) and how much (hours each day) removable retainers have been used post-treatment.

Musculature. Not much attention has been given in this chapter to musculature. Although there has been a great deal learned about the functioning of the oral and facial muscles, little of this information has been translated into useful clinical procedures.

An exception is the use of certain mechanical devices[45,107] that make use of the labial musculature to modify tooth position or to control tongue position. However, there is still not much knowledge about whether orthodontic techniques can direct, control, or retrain muscles or patterns of muscular behavior.

Electromyography will no doubt provide further information of value, but its place in relation to retention is still nebulous.[62] Whereas tongue thrusting and deviate swallowing have been frequently described, there has been no definitive exploration of the effects of tongue and speech therapy on orthodontic results. The techniques of the therapy have been elaborated, but their long-term results are still unknown.[80,122,131]

Equilibration. There was a time when occlusal equilibration soon after completion of orthodontic therapy was expected to provide stability of the corrected malocclusion. More recently periodontists have emphasized the desirability of the so-called canine-protected occlusion, in contrast to Schuyler's principles of occlusion.

We have adopted a conservative approach in the attempt to achieve stability with equilibration after orthodontic treatment that includes removal of obvious interferences in centric relation and elimination of cross-tooth and cross-arch deflective interferences. We do not find it desirable to at-tempt to achieve perfect functional balance soon after the completion of orthodontic treatment. It is our impression that there are factors other than functional overloads which contribute to the changes that occur after treatment, and it is certainly disconcerting to have a denture that was completely equilibrated after treatment undergo post-treatment changes that completely distort the hard-won relationships.

Restorations can be recontoured, cusps and incisal edges adjusted, and teeth esthetically recontoured where either excessive function or lack of function has produced undesirable arrangements. Periodic observation of post-treatment changes and equilibration and adjustment of certain teeth are, no doubt, desirable and functionally useful; but whether these procedures operate effectively against postretention relapses is debatable. The frequent occurrence of post-treatment open bite casts doubt on the efficacy of early post-treatment equilibration.

CLINICAL APPLICATIONS

Retention planning is divided into three categories, depending on the type of treatment instituted: (1) no retention; (2) limited retention, in terms of both time and appliance wearing; (3) permanent or semipermanent retention.

1. No retention required

A   B

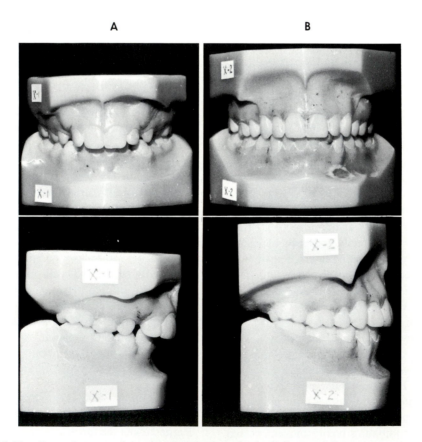

Fig. 16-21 Extraction was the only procedure used. **A,** Before and **B,** several years after. (Courtesy Matt Lasher.)

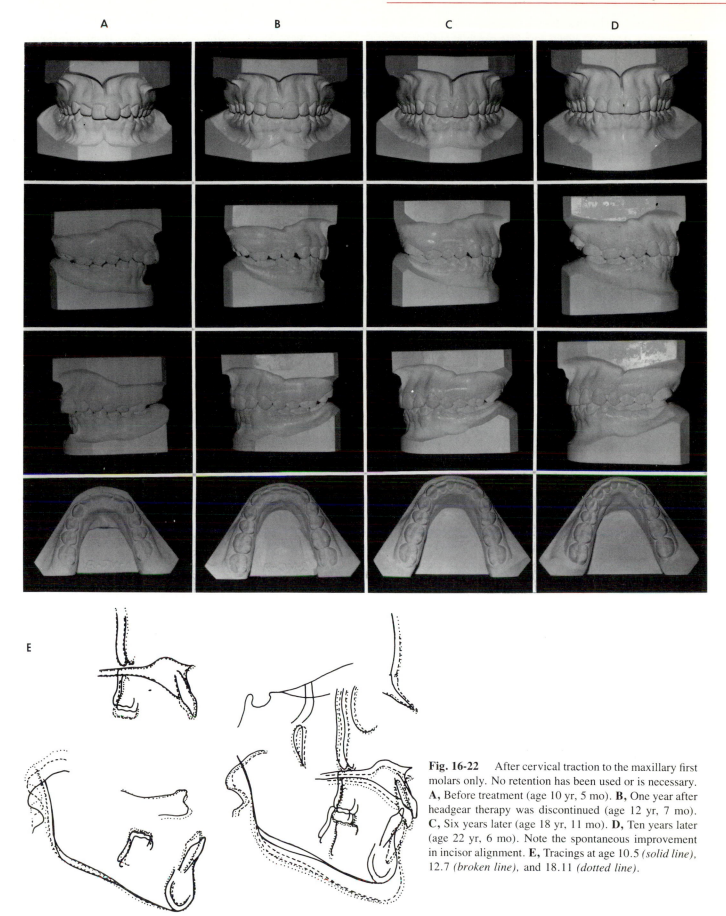

Fig. 16-22   After cervical traction to the maxillary first molars only. No retention has been used or is necessary. **A,** Before treatment (age 10 yr, 5 mo). **B,** One year after headgear therapy was discontinued (age 12 yr, 7 mo). **C,** Six years later (age 18 yr, 11 mo). **D,** Ten years later (age 22 yr, 6 mo). Note the spontaneous improvement in incisor alignment. **E,** Tracings at age 10.5 *(solid line)*, 12.7 *(broken line)*, and 18.11 *(dotted line)*.

a. Corrected crossbites
   (1) Anterior: when adequate overbite has been established
   (2) Posterior: when axial inclinations of posterior teeth remain reasonable after corrective procedures have been completed (It may be suggested in regard to posterior crossbites that overcorrection is a desirable procedure.)

b. Dentitions that have been treated by serial extraction (The percentage of complete satisfaction here is probably low and is dependent on the degree of perfection desired by the orthodontist. When it is possible to extract mandibular second premolars or when they are absent, the resultant occlusions will often be more satisfactory than those in first premolar extraction cases.[87])
   (1) High canine extraction cases (Fig. 16-21)
   (2) Cases calling for extraction of one or more teeth (e.g., subdivision types of malocclusion, or when the posterior teeth are in Class II relationship and the anterior teeth in a normal occlusion)

c. Corrections that have been achieved by retardation of maxillary growth, whether dental or skeletal (once the patient has passed through the growth period) (Fig. 16-22)

d. Dentitions in which the maxillary and mandibular teeth have been separated to allow for eruption of teeth previously blocked out (Typical examples are *partially impacted mandibular* second premolars and maxillary canines.)

2. Limited retention*

a. Class I nonextraction cases characterized by protrusion and spacing of maxillary incisors (These require retention until normal lip and tongue function has been achieved.)

b. Class I or Class II extraction cases (These probably require that the teeth be held in contact, particularly in the maxillary arch, until lip and tongue function can achieve a satisfactory balance, as in the nonextraction group. It is especially true in extraction cases that the maxillary incisors can be retracted so far as to be unrestrained by lip pressure and to impinge on the space occupied by the tongue before treatment. It is generally desirable to use a maxillary Hawley type of retainer until normal functional adaptation has occurred; and it is sometimes also desirable to use either a maxillary Kloehn headgear, whose force is directed to the permanent first molars, or a labiobuccal type of appliance, with cervical or occipital resistance applied at night.[70,97] The time of application of this type of

retention can be reduced as the patient adapts to new tooth positions, proceeding from full-time wearing of appliances to nighttime wear only—perhaps every other night, once or twice a week, and finally discontinuing all retention as tooth positions remain stable. It is particularly true in the corrected Class II malocclusion that continued mandibular growth will reduce the need for retention more rapidly; conversely, corrections of adult dentitions probably require longer retentive procedures. It is probably undesirable to predetermine a time schedule for removing retentive appliances in these cases, and the time of retention is dependent directly on the patient's reactions during retention. Lip exercises and tongue-training lessons may be advantageous in this group of corrected cases.)

c. Corrected deep overbites (In either Class I or Class II malocclusions, these usually require retention in a vertical plane.[83,112,121])
   (1) Anterior teeth depressed to achieve overbite correction (Then a bite plate on a maxillary retainer is desirable. To be effective in retaining overbite correction, the bite plate should be worn continuously for perhaps the first 4 to 6 months, including while the patient is eating. It is in deep overbite cases that overcorrection is usually desirable and equilibration and adjustment to functional occlusion are necessary. Often the incisal edges of the anterior teeth are unworn and require spot grinding and adjusting.)
   (2) Overbite correction achieved as a result of bite opening (If the mandible has been *forced* away from the maxilla, vertical dimensions should be held until growth [i.e., mandibular ramal height] can catch up.)
      (a) A measure of bite opening can be assessed in the degree of change between the mandibular plane and a cranial base plane, such as the Frankfort or sella-nasion. Positive changes of the mandibular plane angle suggest continued retention until growth recoveries can occur or until it is determined that continued growth is either of the same type or not occurring at all.*
   (3) Severe occlusal plane tipping (This may also require extended retention protocols and possibly additional maxillary restraint as well. Examination of cephalometric films taken at approximately 6-month intervals will reveal

---

*Most typical orthodontic cases probably fall into this category. Many corrections require time to allow muscular adaptation and sometimes to maintain the correction until growth has been completed.

---

*This would suggest that it is desirable to correct deep overbites before the completion of facial growth. The work of Matthews[85] in this field suggests that beneficial results may be achieved by beginning overbite correction as early as the deciduous dentition.

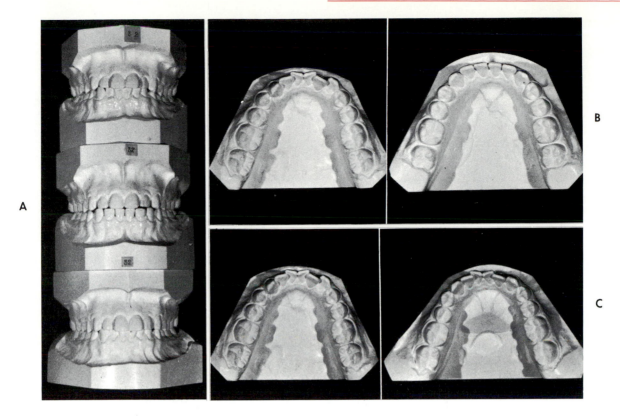

Fig. 16-23   Peculiar tendency for recurrence of rotations after a 2-year retention period. **A,** Before treatment, after treatment, and 6½ years after retention *(top to bottom).* **B,** Before *(left)* and after treatment *(right).* **C,** Note the relapse to the original rotations and intercanine widths, before *(left)* and after treatment *(right).*

whether adaptive growth changes have taken place.)

d. Early correction of rotated teeth[103,104] to their normal positions
   (1) Perhaps before root formation has been completed (Fig. 16-23)
   (2) In the mandibular incisor area (Here a removable type of appliance having a labial bow is probably best. In this area, the occlusal splint type retainer or cast lower partial, as suggested by Lande, may be useful [Fig. 16-24]. More recently gingivectomy procedures have offered hope for increased stability of corrected rotations. Early correction of rotations or severing of transseptal fibers may prove to be more satisfactory.*
   (3) Transseptal fiber surgery (This offers the best possibility of achieving post-treatment stability of rotated teeth. The gold-plated nickel-silver or G wire, as originally advocated by Angle, can be affixed to the lingual of gold or stainless steel bands and carried either from canine to canine or premolar to premolar while being contoured to contact the lingual surfaces of the mandibular anterior teeth. Refer to the canine-to-canine retainer technique illustrated by Paul Lewis.[71])

e. Cases involving ectopic eruption of teeth or the presence of supernumerary teeth (These require varying retention times, usually prolonged, and occasionally a fixed or permanent retentive device such as joined lingual pinlays in maxillary central incisors or the soldering together of inlays on neighboring teeth [Fig. 16-25].)
   (1) Supernumerary teeth (One frequently encounters these in the maxillary area; and on their removal, the maxillary incisors often erupt slowly and incompletely. When the latter have been brought to a normal level through orthodontic therapy, it is probably desirable to leave the appliance in a passive state for several months before retaining this area, for these teeth seemingly have a tendency to intrude themselves when released.)
   (2) Excessive spacing between maxillary incisors

---

*References 3, 20, 23, 37, 96.

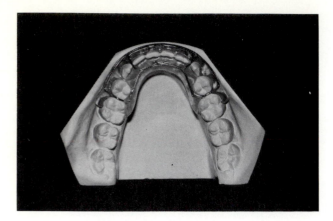

Fig. 16-24 Mandibular splint retainer. Wire position can be altered to avoid passing through an extraction site or coming in contact with the maxillary dentition.

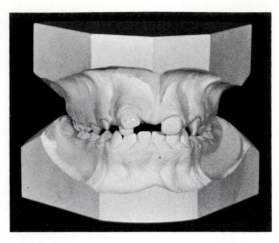

Fig. 16-25 Wide space between maxillary central incisors after the removal of supernumerary teeth. Prolonged or fixed retention may be necessary to maintain space closure.

(Prolonged retention after space closure is required where supernumerary teeth have been present.)
   f. Class II, division 2, types of corrected malocclusion (Corrected division 2 malocclusion generally requires extended retention to allow for the adaptation of musculature. These cases may have some increase in mandibular intercanine width, which is maintained out of retention. Refer to Shapiro.[117])

3. **Permanent or semipermanent retention**
   a. Cases in which expansion has been the choice of treatment, particularly in the mandibular arch (These may require either permanent or semipermanent retention to maintain normal contact alignment. In many instances patients have esthetically desirable dentofacial relationships, and extraction of permanent teeth would create esthetically undesirable results. The orthodontist may be faced with a choice between stability and esthetics, and it is often the patient's esthetic requirements that win out. Occasionally, mild mandibular crowding can be relieved by interproximal stripping whereas other cases will require that the patient wear a retainer indefinitely if normal contact is to be maintained.)
   b. Cases of considerable or generalized spacing (These may require permanent retention after space closure has been completed. It is sometimes possible and desirable to accumulate excess space in the posterior segments and to place bridges to fill the excess thus created.)
   c. Instances of severe rotation (particularly in adults) or severe labiolingual malposition (These sometimes require permanent retention, as provided by the placement of a bridge, the placement of soldered lingual pinlays on incisors, or the fusing together of anterior jacket crowns.)

   d. Spacing between maxillary central incisors in otherwise normal occlusions (This sometimes requires permanent retention, particularly in adult dentitions.)

RETENTION APPLIANCES

The Hawley retainer[52] is one of the most frequently used retentive devices available to the clinical orthodontist. The palatal or lingual portion is usually constructed of acrylic and may completely cover the palatal mucosa or may be constructed in a horseshoe shape contacting the lingual surfaces of the teeth and some of the palatal mucosa. A labial bow of round stainless steel 0.020 to 0.036 inch wire usually is constructed to contact the labial surfaces of four or six maxillary anterior teeth. If it is constructed to cross incisally to the contact area between the canine and the lateral incisor, occlusal or bite interference in the area of the mandibular canine may be minimized. If such construction is resorted to, then it is desirable to include a restraint on the labial of the canines to prevent their extrusion or labial drift (Fig. 16-26).

The clinician may wish to alter the type and position of retention clasps to avoid traumatic occlusal interferences and to assist in eruption guidance or minor tooth movements (Fig. 16-27). Additionally, the labial bow and retention clasps should not pass through extraction sites if possible because they may aggravate the tendency for space to reopen, especially in adult patients.

Circumferential maxillary retainers provide excellent retention with the added benefit of eliminating potential occlusal interferences (Fig. 16-28). *Keeper* wires may be placed between the lateral incisors and canines to enhance the stability of the labial wire. Labial bow tension can also be efficiently adjusted through incorporation of recurved loops. Palatal acrylic should be extended distally to retain second molar position. This is particularly important in pa-

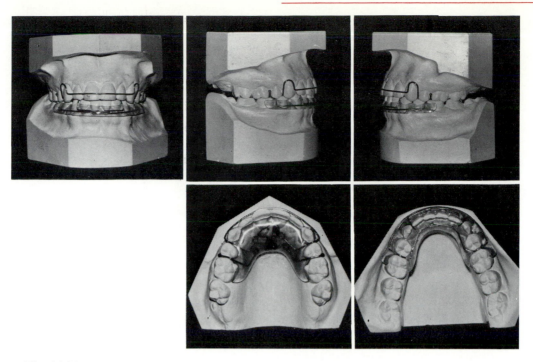

Fig. 16-26   Typical Hawley and splint retainers. Note that the models should be articulated in occlusion to ensure that the patient is not prematurely contacting on retainer wires or acrylic.

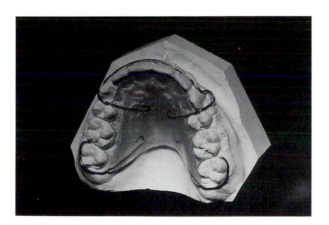

Fig. 16-27   Maxillary Hawley retainer with *C* clasps to guide second molar eruption.

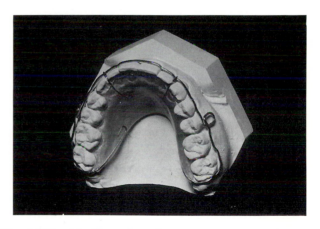

Fig. 16-28   Maxillary circumferential retainer. Palatal acrylic can be reduced to minimize the impact on speech and swallowing patterns.

tients that have undergone changes in transverse dimension during active treatment, such as surgical or sutural maxillary expansion.

Pontics should be included in retainer design to enhance esthetics and to retain the edentulous area(s) during the transition from fixed appliances to prosthetic replacement (Fig. 16-29). Following placement of implants, the retainer should be relieved in the gingival area to allow maintenance of dental esthetics while avoiding tissue impingement during the osseointegration stage. The retainer may be adjusted after completion of the prosthetic phase by simply recontouring the palatal acrylic to fit the final restoration.

The size of a retainer may also be altered to accommodate special needs. A mandibular spring retainer for instance may include only the six anterior teeth to eliminate the difficulty of seating such an appliance over buccal segment undercuts (Fig. 16-30), which are fairly common in adult patients with long clinical crown heights or undercuts created by lingual crown torque (Fig. 16-30).

Fixed retention appliances may also be used to more

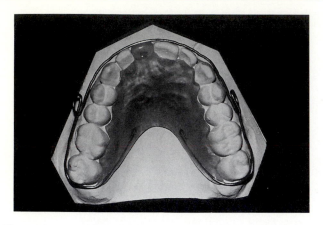

Fig. 16-29   Maxillary circumferential retainer with pontic to replace missing right central incisor.

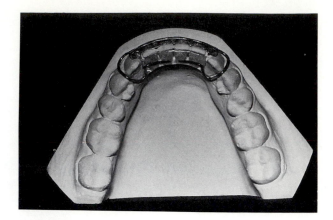

Fig. 16-30   Mandibular spring retainer modified to maintain only anterior tooth position.

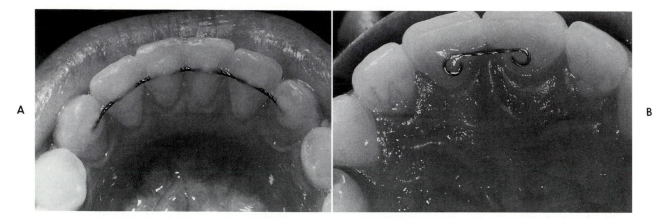

Fig. 16-31   **A,** Mandibular bonded retainer. A braided wire is bonded to each tooth while allowing physiologic tooth movement. **B,** A bonded retainer may be used to prevent relapse of a maxillary diastema. The retainer must be positioned and contoured to prevent premature mandibular incisor contact.

rigidly retain potential areas of relapse to reduce the dependency upon patient compliance (Fig. 16-31). The development of bonding materials has facilitated the fabrication of segmental retainers that splint two or more teeth together to maintain intra-arch tooth position. The wires used for such retainers should be flexible enough to allow physiologic tooth movement. Removable retainers may be fabricated to fit over bonded retainers to minimize potential relapse in the other planes of space and to maintain inter-arch relationships. Eventually, however, fixed retainers should be removed and consideration given to fabricating removable retainers to be used on an as-needed basis to minimize long-term relapse and maturation changes.

The Positioner in Retention Planning

The positioner appears to be particularly beneficial in re-establishing normal tissue tone and firmness where gingival hyperplasia has occurred during treatment. The advantages of the positioner are that it is clean, is unlikely to be broken, tends to stimulate tissue tone, and works constantly toward maintenance or improvement of tooth position. Its disadvantages are its limited time of wear (since the patient can neither eat nor talk with the positioner in place) and the possibility that it may keep teeth loose by producing intermittent forces contrary to natural muscle balance. The positioner is probably contraindicated in patients who have a tendency for nasal airway obstruction.

It has been said that the positioner creates deep overbites. However, we believe that it tends rather *not to prevent* the recurrence of a deep overbite because of the limited time it is generally used. If a positioner is to be used on what has been a deep overbite malocclusion, then it is expedient to construct a maxillary retainer with a bite plane to be used when the patient is unable to wear the positioner. It also

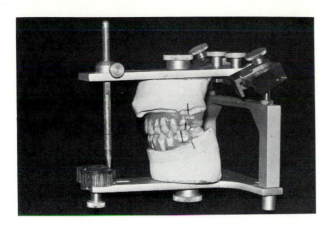

Fig. 16-32 Diagnostic setup completed on an adjustable articulator after a facebow transfer. Fabrication of the positioner on this type of instrument will allow the patient to bite into the positioner without altering condylar position.

may be desirable to construct and place a positioner that fits over a fixed appliance (e.g., a mandibular lingual wire).

Positioner setups and fabrication should be done on an adjustable articulator after a facebow transfer (Fig. 16-32). This will allow the patient to function into the positioner without altering condylar position.

DURATION OF RETENTION

As may be noted from the literature, various authors suggest anything from no retention whatsoever[38] to permanent retention.[77] We advise them that some form of mandibular retention will probably be maintained until evidence of completion of growth is forthcoming, and consideration should be given to the use of retainers on an as-needed basis indefinitely to ensure maintenance of tooth relationships.) Retainers of various kinds are shown to the patients before orthodontic treatment, and they are thus prepared for the retentive phase that will follow active treatment.

RECOVERY AFTER RELAPSE

If, despite the observance of utmost care in treatment and retention, relapse occurs, the following suggestions may be useful:

1. Retreatment may take the form of rebanding or rebonding most if not all teeth. Admittedly, this is an extreme measure, but an interested and cooperative patient may deserve that kind of consideration. It is sometimes expedient to consider the removal of certain teeth, particularly where the relapse occurs in the form of crowding. In other instances permanent retention may be the preferable procedure. In any case an attempt should be made to discover and eliminate the factors that appear contributory to the relapse.

2. The mandibular lingual arch serves admirably to realign teeth in instances of mandibular collapse or crowding. Light pressure against the mandibular anterior teeth may be used to realign them.

3. Springs and clasps can be added to a maxillary Hawley retainer to assist in repositioning and controlling labiolingual deviations.

4. Spring retainers using both facial and lingual acrylic for added leverage and labial bows for increased flexibility may be used for minor realignment. Teeth are sectioned and aligned on the retainer model and the active retainer is fabricated to the realigned relationship (Fig. 16-33). The same retainer(s) may be used after alignment to maintain the correction achieved.

5. The maxillary labiobuccal retainer, Kloehn-type headgear, or functional appliances may be used against the maxillary arch to provide recorrection in instances of relapse toward a Class II relationship.

6. Habit training in the form of tongue and lip therapy may be beneficial when abnormal habit patterns have caused orthodontic relapses. Removable appliances are also helpful as tongue restraints.

7. Equilibration and trimming may be all that is necessary to achieve esthetic and functional satisfaction for the patient and the orthodontist. (Interproximal stripping or

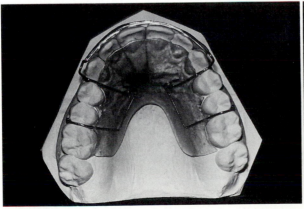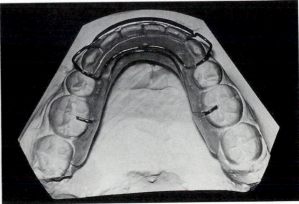

Fig. 16-33 Maxillary and mandibular spring retainers. Incisors have been realigned in the working model.

reduction in crown width sometimes reduces the tendency for further relapse.)

8. In certain cases it may be desirable to suggest that the patient accept minimal relapses rather than continue with prolonged treatment or retention.

In summary it can be said that retention is not a separate problem or phase of orthodontics but is and will continue to be a problem to be considered in diagnosis and treatment planning. As Oppenheim[96] so aptly phrased it, "Retention is the most difficult problem in orthodontia; in fact, it is *the* problem."

REFERENCES

1. Ades A, Joondeph D et al: A long-term study of the relationship of third molars to mandibular dental arch changes, *Am J Orthod Dentofac Orthop* 97:323-335, 1990.
2. Alexander RG: The effects on tooth position and maxillofacial vertical growth during treatment of scoliosis with the Milwaukee brace, *Am J Orthod* 52:161, 1966.
3. Allen RL: "A study of the regression phenomenon of orthodontically rotated teeth in the human patient with and without surgical removal of the supra-alveolar fiber apparatus." Thesis, University of Washington, 1969.
4. Amott RD: "A serial study of dental arch measurements on orthodontic subjects." Thesis, Northwestern University, 1962.
5. Andreasen G, Naessig C: Experimental findings on mesial relapse of maxillary first molars, *Angle Orthod* 38:51, 1968.
6. Angle EH: Malocclusion of the teeth, ed 7, Philadelphia, 1907, SS White Dental Manufacturing Co.
7. Arnold M: "A study of the changes of the mandibular intercanine and intermolar width during orthodontic treatment and following a five or more years post-retention period." Thesis, University of Washington, 1962.
8. Baird FP: "A cephalometric evaluation of the skeletal and dental patterns of 7- to 9-year-old children with excellent occlusions." Thesis, University of Washington, 1952.
9. Baker HA: Discussion of Dr. Pullen's paper, *Dent Items Interest* 29:389, 1907.
10. Ballard ML: Asymmetry in tooth size: a factor in the etiology, diagnosis and treatment of malocclusion, *Angle Orthod* 14:67, 1944.
11. Bash VP: "A method of defining the soft-tissue profile." Thesis, University of Washington, 1958.
12. Baum AT: A cephalometric evaluation of the normal skeletal and dental pattern of children with excellent occlusion, *Angle Orthod* 21:96, 1951.
13. Baum AT: Age and sex differences in the dento-facial changes following orthodontic treatment and the significance in treatment planning, *Am J Orthod* 47:355, 1961.
14. Baum AT: Orthodontic treatment and the maturing face, *Angle Orthod* 36:121, 1966.
15. Bergstrom K, Jensen R: Responsibility of the third molar for secondary crowding, *Dent Abstr* 6:544, 1961.
16. Björk A: Facial growth in man studied with the aid of metallic implants, *Acta Odontol Scand* 13:9, 1955.
17. Björk A: Variations in the growth pattern of the human mandible: longitudinal radiographic study by the implant method, *J Dent Res* 42:400, 1963.
18. Björk A: A sutural growth of the upper face: studied by the implant methods, *Eur Orthod Soc Trans* p. 1, 1964.
19. Björk A, Helm S: Prediction of the age of maximum pubertal growth in body height, *Angle Orthod* 37:134, 1967.
20. Boese LR: "Increased stability of orthodontically rotated teeth following gingivectomy." Thesis, University of Washington, 1968.
21. Bolton W: The clinical application of a tooth size analysis, *Angle Orthod* 28:113, 1958.
22. Bolton WA: Disharmony in tooth size and its relation to the analysis and treatment of malocclusion, *Angle Orthod* 28:113, 1958.
23. Brain WE: The effect of surgical transsection of free gingival fibers on the regression of orthodontically rotated teeth in the dog, *Am J Orthod* 55:50, 1969.
24. Bresolin D, Shapiro PA, Shapiro GG et al: Mouth breathing in allergic children: its relationship to dentofacial development, *Am J Orthod* 83:334, 1983.
25. Brodie AG: The fourth dimension in orthodontia, *Angle Orthod* 24:15, 1954.
26. Canning E: *Orthodontia: a textbook and treatise on malocclusion*, Denver, 1919, Dental Specialty, pp. 135-145.
27. Case C: Principles of retention in orthodontia, *Int J Orthod Oral Surg* 6:3, 1920.
28. Case C: *Retention of dental orthopedia*. In *Dental orthopedia and correction of cleft palate*, Chicago, 1921, CS Case Company.
29. Castro CM: "Slow maxillary expansion: a clinical study of the skeletal and dental response during and following the application of low magnitude force." Master's thesis, University of Washington, 1979.
30. Chapman H: Orthodontics: retention, *Int J Orthod Oral Surg Radiogr* 12:781, 1926.
31. Cole HJ: Certain results of extraction in the treatment of malocclusion, *Angle Orthod* 18:103, 1948.
32. Cotton LA: Slow maxillary expansion: skeletal versus dental response to low magnitude force in *Macaca mulatta*, *Am J Orthod* 73:1, 1978.
33. Dewey M: Some principles of retention, *Am Dent J* 8:254, 1909.
34. Dewey M: *Practical orthodontia*, St Louis, 1920, Mosby, pp. 300-308.
35. Dona AA: "An analysis of dental casts of patients made before and after orthodontic treatment." Thesis, University of Washington, 1952.
36. Eastham RM: An evaluation of stabilizing appliances for Milwaukee brace patients, *Am J Orthod* 60:445, 1971.
37. Edwards JG: A study of the periodontium during orthodontic rotation of teeth, *Am J Orthod* 54:931, 1968.
38. Englert G: Further determination and implementation of a clinical ideology, *Angle Orthod* 30:14, 1960.
39. Enlow DH, Hunter WS: A differential analysis of sutural and remodeling growth in the human face, *Am J Orthod* 52:823, 1966.
40. Federspiel M: On gnathostatic diagnosis in orthodontics, *Int J Orthod* 10:783, 1924.
41. Frederick DL: "Dentofacial changes produced by extraoral highpull traction to the maxilla of the *Macaca mulatta*: a histologic and serial cephalometric study." Thesis, University of Washington, 1969.
42. Funk AC: Mandibular response to headgear therapy and its clinical significance, *Am J Orthod* 53:182, 1967.
43. Gallerano R: "Mandibular anterior crowding, a postretention study." Thesis, University of Washington, 1976.
44. Goldstein A: The clinical testing of orthodontic results, *Am J Orthod* 51:723, 1965.
45. Graber TM: Muscles, malformation, and malocclusion, *Am J Orthod* 49:418, 1963.
46. Graber TM: Postmortems in post-treatment adjustment, *Am J Orthod* 52:331, 1966.
47. Grieve GW: The stability of a treated denture. *Am J Orthod Oral Surg* 30:171, 1944.
48. Guilford SH: *Orthodontia*, Philadelphia, 1893, Spangler & Davis, pp. 61-63.
49. Hambleton RS: The soft-tissue covering of the skeletal face as related to orthodontic problems, *Am J Orthod* 50:405, 1964.
50. Harris J: A cephalometric analysis of mandibular growth rate, *Am J Orthod* 48:161, 1962.
51. Hassig FH: "A cephalometric and histologic study in *Macaca mulatta* of the changes in the craniofacial complex during and following modified Milwaukee brace therapy." Thesis, University of Washington, 1969.
52. Hawley CA: A removable retainer, *Dent Cosmos* 61:449, 1919.

53. Hellman M: *Fundamental principles and expedient compromises in orthodontic procedures.* In *Transactions of the American association of orthodontists,* St Louis, 1945, Mosby, p. 46.

54. Hernandez JL: Mandibular bicanine width relative to overbite, *Am J Orthod* 36:455, 1969.

55. Hicks EP: Slow maxillary expansion: a clinical study of the skeletal versus dental response to low-magnitude force, *Am J Orthod* 73:121, 1978.

56. Holdaway RA: Changes in relationship of points A and B, *Am J Orthod* 42:176, 1956.

57. Horowitz SL, Hixon EH: Physiologic recovery following orthodontic treatment, *Am J Orthod* 55:1, 1969.

58. Howes AE: Case analysis and treatment planning based upon the relationship of tooth material to its supporting bone, *Am J Orthod Oral Surg* 33:499, 1947.

59. Howes AE: Model analysis for treatment planning: a portion of a symposium on case analysis and treatment planning, *Am J Orthod* 38:183, 1952.

60. Huggins DG, Birch RH: A cephalometric investigation of upper incisors following their retraction, *Am J Orthod* 50:852, 1964.

61. Jackson VH: *Orthodontia and orthopedia of the face,* Philadelphia, 1904, JB Lippincott.

62. Jacobs RM, Brodie AG: The analysis of perioral muscular accommodation in young subjects with malocclusion, *Angle Orthod* 36:325, 1966.

63. Kaplan R: Mandibular third molars and postretention crowding, *Am J Orthod* 66:411, 1974.

64. Kingsley N: *Treatise on oral deformities,* New York, 1880, Appleton.

65. Kloehn SJ: At what age should treatment be started? *Am J Orthod* 41:262, 1955.

66. Knell JD: "A cephalometric evaluation of the dento-facial changes with specific reference to the mandible occurring during treatment of Class II, division I, malocclusion." Thesis, University of Washington, 1957.

67. Krebs A: Expansion of the midpalatal suture studied by means of metallic implants, *Eur Orthod Soc Trans* 34:163, 1958.

68. Krebs A: Midpalatal suture expansion studied by the implant method over a seven year period, *Eur Orthod Soc Trans* 40:131, 1964.

69. Lagerstrom LO, Brodie AG: A quantitative method for measuring changes in the maxilla due to growth and orthodontic procedures, *Angle Orthod* 37:241, 1967.

70. Lewis PD: The labiobuccal retainer, *Angle Orthod* 29:1, 1959.

71. Lewis PD: Arch width, canine position, and mandibular retention, *Am J Orthod* 63:481, 1973.

72. Linder-Aronson S: Adenoids: their effect on mode of breathing and nasal airflow and their relationship to characteristics of the facial skeleton and the dentition, *Acta Otolaryngol* (suppl. 265), p. 1, 1970.

73. Lindquist B, Thilander B: Extraction of third molars in cases of anticipated crowding in the lower jaw, *Am J Orthod* 81:130, 1982.

74. Lindquist JT: The lower incisor: its influence on treatment and esthetics, *Am J Orthod* 44:112, 1958.

75. Lischer BE: *Orthodontics,* Philadelphia, 1912, Lea & Febiger, pp. 184-185.

76. Litowitz R: A study of the movements of certain teeth during and following orthodontic treatment, *Angle Orthod* 18:113, 1948.

77. Little RM, Wallen TR, Riedel RA: Stability and relapse of mandibular anterior alignment: first premolar extraction cases treated by traditional edgewise orthodontics, *Am J Orthod* 80:349, 1981.

78. Lopez-Gavito G, Wallen T, Little RM, Joondeph Dr: Anterior openbite malocclusion: A longitudinal ten-year post-retention evaluation of orthodontically treated patients, *Am J Orthod* 87:175-186, 1985.

79. Lude JC: Technique for the determination of the size of the mandibular apical base: its application to growth studies, *Angle Orthod* 37:272, 1967.

80. Ludwig MK: An analysis of anterior open-bite relationship changes during and following orthodontic treatment, *Angle Orthod* 36:204, 1966.

81. Lundström A: Malocclusions of the teeth regarded as a problem in connection with the apical base, *Int J Orthod Oral Surg* 11:591, 1925.

82. Lundström A: Changes in crowding and spacing of the teeth with age, *Dent Pract* 19:218, 1969.

83. Magill JM: Changes in the anterior overbite relationship following orthodontic treatment in extraction cases, *Am J Orthod* 46:755, 1960.

84. Markus MB: A review and consideration of the problem of retention, *Am J Orthod Oral Surg* 24:203, 1938.

85. Matthews R: Clinical management and supportive rationale in early orthodontic therapy, *Angle Orthod* 31:35, 1961.

86. McCauley DR: The cuspid and its function in retention, *Am J Orthod* 30:196, 1944.

87. McNeill RW, Joondeph DR: Congenitally absent maxillary lateral incisors: treatment planning considerations, *Angle Orthod* 43:24, 1973.

88. Mershon JV: *The removable lingual arch appliance.* In *The first international orthodontic congress,* St Louis, 1927, Mosby, p. 279.

89. Mills JRE: A long-term assessment of the mechanical retroclination of the lower incisors, *Angle Orthod* 37:165, 1967.

90. Moore AW: Orthodontic treatment factors in Class II malocclusion, *Am J Orthod* 45:323, 1959.

91. Moorrees CFA, Chadha JM: Available space for the incisors during dental development, *Angle Orthod* 35:12, 1965.

92. Nance H: Limitations of orthodontic treatment in the permanent dentition, *Am J Orthod* 33:253, 1947.

93. Nelson B: What does extraoral anchorage accomplish? *Am J Orthod* 38:422, 1952.

94. Northcroft G: The problem of retention with a view to permanence of result and minimum of danger, *Br Dent J* 36:898, 1915.

95. Ochsenbein C, Maynard JG: The problem of attached gingiva in children, *J Dent Child* 41:1, 1974.

96. Oppenheim A: The crisis in orthodontia. I. Tissue changes during retention. Skogsborg's septotomy, *Int J Orthod Dent Child* 20:640, 1934.

97. Oppenheim A: Biologic orthodontic therapy and reality, *Angle Orthod* 5:159; 6:69, 153, 1936.

98. Ottolengui R: Discussion of Dr. Pullen's paper. *Dent Items Interest* 29:388, 1907.

99. Parker WS: The significance of clinical evidence, *Angle Orthod* 35:61, 1965.

100. Petraitis BJ: "A cephalometric study of excellent occlusion and Class I malocclusion of children and adults." Thesis, University of Washington, 1951.

101. Pullen HH: Some considerations in retention, *Dent Items Interest* 29:287, 1907.

102. Quessenberry JL: Serial cephalometric analysis of the mandible and dental arches following Class II intermaxillary forces. Thesis, University of Washington, 1969.

103. Reitan K: Tissue rearrangement during retention of orthodontically rotated teeth, *Angle Orthod* 29:105, 1959.

104. Reitan K: Clinical and histologic observations on tooth movement during and after orthodontic treatment, *Am J Orthod* 53:721, 1967.

105. Reitan K: Principles of retention and avoidance of post-treatment relapse, *Am J Orthod* 55:776, 1969.

106. Richardson ER, Brodie AG: Longitudinal study of maxillary width, *Angle Orthod* 34:1, 1964.

107. Richardson M: Late third molar genesis: its significance in orthodontic treatment, *Angle Orthod* 50:121, 1980.

108. Riedel RA: A review of the retention problem, *Angle Orthod* 30:179, 1960.

109. Rogers AP: Making facial muscles our allies in treatment of retention, *Dent Cosmos,* July 1922.

110. Salzmann JA: *Principles of orthodontics,* Philadelphia, 1943, JB Lippincott.

111. Schudy FF: Vertical growth versus anteroposterior growth as related to function and treatment, *Angle Orthod* 34:75, 1964.

112. Schudy FF: The control of vertical overbite in clinical orthodontics, *Angle Orthod* 38:19, 1968.

113. Schwartz H: The case against biomechanics, *Angle Orthod* 37:52, 1967.

114. Schwarze CW: *The influence of third molar germectomy: a comparative long-term study.* In *Transactions of the third international orthodontic congress,* St Louis, 1975, Mosby, p. 551.

115. Shafer A: Behavior of the axes on human incisor teeth during growth. *Angle Orthod* 19:254, 1949.

116. Shanley LS: The influence of mandibular third molars on mandibular anterior teeth, *Am J Orthod* 48:786, 1962 (abstract).

117. Shapiro PA: Mandibular arch form and dimension, *Am J Orthod* 66:58, 1974.

118. Sheneman JR: "Third molar teeth and their effect upon the lower anterior teeth: a survey of forty-nine orthodontic cases five years after band removal." Thesis, St. Louis University, 1968.

119. Shields T, Little R, Chapko M: Stability and relapse of mandibular anterior alignment: a cephalometric appraisal of first premolar extraction cases treated by traditional edgewise orthodontics, *Am J Orthod* 87:27-38, 1985.

120. Simon P: *Fundamental principles of a systematic diagnosis of dental anomalies,* Boston, 1926, Stratford Press.

121. Simons ME, Joondeph DR: Change in overbite: a ten year post-retention study, *Am J Orthod* 64:349, 1973.

122. Speidel TM, Isaacson RJ: Tongue thrust therapy and anterior dental open bite, *Am J Orthod* 62:287, 1972.

123. Sproule W: "Dentofacial changes produced by extraoral cervical traction to the maxilla of the *Macaca mulatta:* a histologic and serial cephalometric study." Thesis, University of Washington, 1968.

124. Stallard H: Survival of the periodontium during and after orthodontic treatment, *Am J Orthod* 50:584, 1964.

125. Steadman HR: A philosophy and practice of orthodontic retention, *Angle Orthod* 37:175, 1967.

126. Stoner MM, Lindquist JT, Vorhies JM et al: A cephalometric evaluation of fifty-seven consecutive cases treated by Dr. Charles H. Tweed, *Angle Orthod* 26:68, 1956.

127. Storey E: Tissue response to the movement of bones, *Am J Orthod* 64:229, 1973.

128. Strang RHW: *Textbook of orthodontia,* Philadelphia, 1933, Lea & Febiger, p. 582.

129. Strang RHW: Factors of influence in producing a stable result in treatment of malocclusions, *Am J Orthod* 32:313, 1946.

130. Strang RHW, Thompson WM: *Textbook of orthodontia,* ed 5, Philadelphia, 1958, Lea & Febiger, pp. 1, 764.

131. Subtelny JD, Sakuda M: Open bite: diagnosis and treatment, *Am J Orthod* 32:27, 1946.

132. Talbot ES: *The irregularities of the teeth,* Philadelphia, 1903, SS White Dental Manufacturing.

133. Thörne NAH: Experiences on widening the median maxillary suture, *Eur Orthod Soc Trans* 32:279, 1956.

134. Thörne NAH: Expansion of the maxilla: spreading the midpalatal suture; measuring the widening of the apical base and the nasal cavity on serial roentgenograms, *Am J Orthod* 46:626, 1960 (Abstract).

135. Tweed CH: Indications for extraction of teeth in orthodontic procedure, *Am J Orthod Oral Surg* 30:405, 1944.

136. Tweed CH: Why I extract teeth in the treatment of certain types of malocclusion, *Alpha Omegan* 1952.

137. Van Dyke TR: "A serial cephalometric study of the mandibular denture and soft tissue changes in patients five or more years out of retention." Thesis, University of Washington, 1973.

138. Waldron R: Reviewing the problem of retention, *Am J Orthod Oral Surg* 28:770, 1942.

139. Wallman RH: "A cephalometric roentgenographic investigation of changes occurring in certain teeth as a result of orthodontic therapy." Thesis, University of Washington, 1958.

140. Walters DC: Changes in the form and dimensions of dental arches resulting from orthodontic treatment, *Angle Orthod* 23:3, 1953.

141. Walters DC: Comparative changes in mandibular canine and first molar widths, *Angle Orthod* 32:232, 1962.

142. Webster RL: Retention, *Am J Orthod* 34:897, 1948.

143. Weinstein S: Minimal forces in tooth movement, *Am J Orthod* 53:881, 1967.

144. Welch KN: "A study of treatment and post-retention dimensional changes in mandibular dental arches." Thesis, University of Washington, 1965.

145. Weislander L: The effect of orthodontic treatment on the concurrent development of the craniofacial complex, *Am J Orthod* 49:15, 1963.

146. Witzel D: Long-term stability of the mandibular arch following differential management of arch length deficiencies. Thesis, University of Washington, 1978.

INDEX